EQUINE
ANESTHESIA

Second Edition

Monitoring and Emergency Therapy

EQUINE ANESTHESIA

Second Edition

Monitoring and Emergency Therapy

William W. Muir, DVM, MSc, PhD, DACVA, DACVECC
Regional Director, American Academy of Pain Management
Veterinary Clinical Pharmacology Consulting Services
Columbus, Ohio

John A.E. Hubbell, DVM, MS, DACVA
Professor of Anesthesia
Department of Veterinary Clinical Science
College of Veterinary Medicine
The Ohio State University
Columbus, Ohio

with 539 illustrations

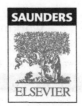

SAUNDERS

ELSEVIER

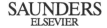

11830 Westline Industrial Drive
St. Louis, Missouri 63146

EQUINE ANESTHESIA: MONITORING AND EMERGENCY THERAPY,   ISBN: 978-1-4160-2326-5
SECOND EDITION

Notice

Knowledge and best practice in this field are constantly changing. As new research and experience broaden
our knowledge, changes in practice, treatment and drug therapy may become necessary or appropriate.
Readers are advised to check the most current information provided (i) on procedures featured or (ii) by the
manufacturer of each product to be administered, to verify the recommended dose or formula, the method
and duration of administration, and contraindications. It is the responsibility of the practitioner, relying on
their own experience and knowledge of the patient, to make diagnoses, to determine dosages and the best
treatment for each individual patient, and to take all appropriate safety precautions. To the fullest extent of
the law, neither the Publisher nor the Authors assumes any liability for any injury and/or damage to persons
or property arising out of or related to any use of the material contained in this book.

The Publisher

Library of Congress Cataloging-in-Publication Data

Equine anesthesia : monitoring and emergency therapy / [edited by]
William W. Muir, John A. E. Hubbell.—2nd ed.
    p. ; cm.
    Includes bibliographical references and index.
    ISBN 978-1-4160-2326-5 (hardcover : alk. paper)
1. Horses—Surgery. 2. Veterinary anesthesia. I. Muir, William,
1946- II. Hubbell, John A. E.
    [DNLM: 1. Anesthesia—veterinary. 2. Horses—surgery. SF 951
M9455e 2009]
    SF951.E54 2009
    636.1'089796—dc22

2008042056

Vice President and Publisher: Linda Duncan
Senior Acquisitions Editor: Anthony Winkel
Developmental Editor: Maureen Slaten
Publishing Services Manager: Patricia Joiner-Myers
Senior Project Manager: Joy Moore
Design Direction: Mark Oberkrom

Printed in the United States of America

Last digit is the print number: 9 8 7 6 5 4 3 2

Contributors

Richard M. Bednarski, DVM, MS, DACVA
Associate Professor
Department of Veterinary Clinical Sciences
College of Veterinary Medicine
The Ohio State University
Columbus, Ohio
Tracheal and Nasal Intubation
Anesthetic Equipment

Lori A. Bidwell, DVM, DACVA
Head of Anesthesia
Rood & Riddle Equine Hospital
Lexington, Kentucky
Anesthetic Risk and Euthanasia

John D. Bonagura, DVM, MS, DACVIM
(Cardiology, Internal Medicine)
Professor and Head of Clinical Cardiology Services
Member, Davis Heart & Lung Research Institute
Department of Veterinary Clinical Sciences
College of Veterinary Medicine
The Ohio State University
Columbus, Ohio
The Cardiovascular System

Joanne Hardy, DVM, MSc, PhD, DACVS, DACVECC
Clinical Associate Professor of Surgery
Department of Large Animal Clinical Sciences
College of Veterinary Medicine & Biomedical Sciences
Texas A&M University
College Station, Texas
Venous and Arterial Catheterization and Fluid Therapy

John A.E. Hubbell, DVM, MS, DACVA
Professor of Anesthesia
Department of Veterinary Clinical Science
College of Veterinary Medicine
The Ohio State University
Columbus, Ohio
History of Equine Anesthesia
Monitoring Anesthesia
Local Anesthetic Drugs and Techniques
Peripheral Muscle Relaxants
Considerations for Induction, Maintenance, and Recovery
Anesthetic-Associated Complications
Cardiopulmonary Resuscitation
Anesthetic Protocols and Techniques for Specific Procedures
Anesthetic Risk and Euthanasia

Carolyn L. Kerr, DVM, DVSc, PhD, DACVA
Associate Professor of Anesthesiology
Department of Clinical Studies
Ontario Veterinary College
University of Guelph
Guelph, Ontario, Canada
Oxygen Supplementation and Ventilatory Support

Phillip Lerche, BVSc, DAVCA
Assistant Professor – Clinical
Department of Veterinary Clinical Sciences
The Ohio State University
Columbus, Ohio
Perioperative Pain Management

Nora S. Matthews, DVM, DACVA
Professor and Co-Chief of Surgical Sciences
Department of Small Animal Clinical Sciences
College of Veterinary Medicine & Biomedical Sciences
Texas A&M University
College Station, Texas
Anesthesia and Analgesia for Donkeys and Mules

Wayne N. McDonell, DVM, MSc, PhD, DACVA
Professor Emeritus, Anesthesiology
Department of Clinical Studies
Ontario Veterinary College
University of Guelph
Guelph, Ontario, Canada
Oxygen Supplementation and Ventilatory Support

William W. Muir, DVM, MSc, PhD, DACVA,
DACVECC
Regional Director, American Academy
    of Pain Management
Veterinary Clinical Pharmacology Consulting Services
Columbus, Ohio
History of Equine Anesthesia
The Cardiovascular System
Physical Restraint
Monitoring Anesthesia
Principles of Drug Disposition and Drug Interaction
    in Horses
Anxiolytics, Nonopioid Sedative-Analgesics, and Opioid
    Analgesics
Local Anesthetic Drugs and Techniques
Intravenous Anesthetic Drugs
Intravenous Anesthetic and Analgesic Adjuncts to
    Inhalation Anesthesia
Peripheral Muscle Relaxants
Perioperative Pain Management
Considerations for Induction, Maintenance, and Recovery
Anesthetic-Associated Complications
Cardiopulmonary Resuscitation
Anesthetic Protocols and Techniques for Specific
    Procedures
Anesthetic Risk and Euthanasia

James T. Robertson, DVM, DACVS
Equine Surgical Consultant
Woodland Run Equine Veterinary Facility
Grove City, Ohio
Physical Restraint
Preoperative Evaluation: General Considerations

N. Edward Robinson, BVetMed, MRCVS, PhD
Honorary Diplomate, ACVIM
Matilda R. Wilson Professor
Department of Large Animal Clinical Sciences
College of Veterinary Medicine
Michigan State University
East Lansing, Michigan
The Respiratory System

Richard A. Sams, PhD
Professor and Program Director
Florida Racing Laboratory
College of Veterinary Medicine
University of Florida
Gainesville, Florida
*Principles of Drug Disposition and
    Drug Interaction in Horses*

Colin C. Schwarzwald, Dr.med.vet., PhD, DACVIM
Assistant Professor
Section of Internal Medicine
Equine Department
Vetsuisse Faculty of the University of Zurich
Zurich, Switzerland
The Cardiovascular System

Claire Scicluna, DVM
Clinique Vétérinaire du Plessis
Chamant, France
Preoperative Evaluation: General Considerations

Roman T. Skarda, DVM, PhD, DACVA (Deceased)
Professor
Department of Veterinary Clinical Sciences
College of Veterinary Medicine
The Ohio State University
Columbus, Ohio
Local Anesthetic Drugs and Techniques

Eugene P. Steffey, VMD, PhD, DACVA
Professor Emeritus
Department of Surgical and Radiological Sciences;
Pharmacologist
K.L. Maddy Equine Analytical Chemistry Laboratory
California Animal Health and Food Safety Laboratory
University of California, Davis
Davis, California
Inhalation Anesthetics and Gases

Ann E. Wagner, DVM, MS, DACVA, DACVP
Professor, Anesthesia
Department of Clinical Sciences
College of Veterinary Medicine & Biomedical Sciences
Colorado State University
Fort Collins, Colorado
Stress Associated with Anesthesia and Surgery

Kazuto Yamashita, DVM, PhD
Professor
Department of Small Animal Clinical Sciences
School of Veterinary Medicine
Rakuno Gakuen University
Ebetsu, Hokkaido, Japan
*Intravenous Anesthetic and Analgesic Adjuncts to Inhalation
    Anesthesia*

Dedication

This edition is dedicated to our friend, the late Dr. Roman T. Skarda. Romi Skarda was a colleague and friend for over 30 years. A Diplomate of the American College of Veterinary Anesthesiologists, Romi was recognized as the world's expert on local and regional anesthesia of animals, especially horses. His contributions to the scientific liter-ature, book chapters, and teaching materials contributed immeasurably to the advancement of equine medicine and surgery. A consummate entertainer, magician, and always the life of any party, Romi will be remembered as the most compassionate, gentlest, and strongest man either one of us has known.

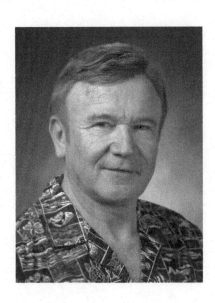

Contents

EQUINE

Second Edition

ANESTHESIA

Monitoring and Emergency Therapy

Acknowledgments

We would like to extend our sincerest thanks to the past and current veterinary technicians, interns, residents, and faculty members of the Equine Medicine and Surgery Section of the Department of Veterinary Clinical Sciences at The Ohio State University. Special recognition to:

Anesthesia Technical Support and Advice
Amanda English
Carl O'Brien
Renee Calvin
Deana Vonschantz (New England Equine, Dover, NH)

Review, Critique, Editing
Dr. Anja Waselau
Dr. Martin Waselau
Dr. Ashley Wiese
Dr. Yukie Ueyama

Dr. Tokiko Kushiro
Dr. Deborah Grosenbaugh
Dr. Lindsay Culp
Dr. Juliana Figueiredo
Dr. Turi Aarnes

Graphics, Illustrations, and Photographs
Marc Hardman
Jerry Harvey
Tim Vojt

Library and Editorial Assistance and Typing
Barbara Lang
Dr. Jay Harrington
Susan Kelley
Robin Bennett

The first edition of this book, published in 1991, was written "to provide the specialist interested in equine surgery and anesthesia, the veterinary surgeon, technical support staff, and veterinary students with a thorough and in-depth discussion of equine anesthesiology." The preface to that edition noted that the evolution of the practice of equine anesthesia had been slow but that the incidence of postoperative myopathy had dropped dramatically because of the adoption of improved monitoring techniques and methods for cardiopulmonary support, including the use of vasopressors and mechanical ventilation. Much has been learned from the writings and research of those interested in equine anesthesia (see Chapter 1; "Those who don't know history are destined to repeat it." *Edmund Burke*) and the 17 years that have passed since the first publication of this text. Most of the original contributors have agreed to rewrite, update, and expand their original contributions to further define the art and science of equine anesthesia. New chapters on pain management; anesthetic adjuncts; and techniques for induction, maintenance, and recovery from anesthesia focus on areas of increased concern and a need for improvement. They provide a relatively succinct presentation of what is known and offer suggestions for future direction. A new chapter on anesthesia of donkeys and mules broadens the text to include other members of the genus *Equus* encountered by the equine veterinarian.

Anesthetic risk in horses is greater than that in dogs, cats, or humans. Mortality data suggest that the risk of death from anesthesia in otherwise normal horses ranges from 0.1% to 1%. Factors known to contribute to this risk include youth or old age; longer durations of anesthesia; stress; and emergency procedures, particularly colic. Anesthetic risk is greater at night than during the day, but even the simplest anesthetic procedure in horses carries an increased risk of complications. At least one third of the deaths associated with equine anesthesia have been attributed to cardiac arrest. It is important to note that approximately 25% of all horses that die do so from injuries occurring during recovery from anesthesia. Surely we can do better. The cardiopulmonary effects of all current anesthetic drugs have been determined, and dependable monitoring techniques have evolved and been investigated in horses. In our experience there are few complications that are "new"; and most complications, if discovered promptly, can be averted. Another one third of anesthetic-associated deaths in horses are attributed to fractures or myopathy in the postoperative period. The goal of recovery from anesthesia should be the calm, coordinated resumption of a standing posture on the first attempt within a time frame that does not exacerbate the consequences of recumbency. Multiple methods have been proposed to attain this goal, but none has emerged as universally acceptable.

Clearly the horse is unique among the commonly anesthetized domestic species, and some level of stress accompanies every anesthesia. Procedures designed to reduce pain and stress and improve the horse's quality of life throughout the anesthetic experience require greater focus. Toward this end the education of all involved in the practice of equine anesthesia cannot be overemphasized. Furthermore, the employment of educated, trained, experienced, and ultimately certified personnel should be a prerequisite to the practice of equine anesthesia. The first edition of this text was dedicated to two pioneers in equine surgery and anesthesia: Drs. Albert Gabel and Robert Copelan. They epitomize the foundation upon which the science and art of equine practice was built: Dr. Gabel's passion and inquisitiveness and Dr. Copelan's persistence (still practicing at 82 years of age) and emphasis on perfection. In addition, we recognize Dr. Peter Rossdale whose dedicated service as chief editor of the *Equine Veterinary Journal* has become synonymous with a persistence for excellence in equine veterinary science. The future for equine anesthesia is clear and will be enhanced by the attributes of passion, perseverance, persistence, and pursuit of excellence and realized by the efforts of dedicated, vigilant equine anesthetists.

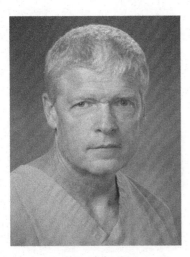

William W. Muir

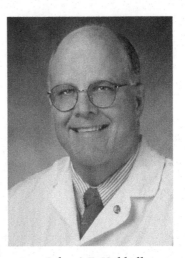

John A.E. Hubbell

History of Equine Anesthesia

William W. Muir
John A.E. Hubbell

In comparison with the ancients, we stand like dwarfs on the shoulders of giants.

BERNARD OF CHARTRES

Those who don't know history are destined to repeat it.

EDMUND BURKE

Reports that say that something hasn't happened are always interesting to me, because as we know, there are known knowns; there are things we know we know. We also know there are known unknowns; that is to say we know there are some things we do not know. But there are also unknown unknowns — the ones we don't know we don't know. And if one looks throughout the history of our country and other free countries, it is the latter category that tend be the difficult ones.

DONALD H. RUMSFELD
(FEB. 12, 2002, DEPARTMENT OF DEFENSE NEWS BRIEFING)

DEFINING ANESTHESIA IN EQUINE PRACTICE: AN EMERGING SCIENCE

Equine anesthesia is a species-specific art and science (Table 1-1). The word *anesthesia* was first defined in Bailey's English Dictionary in 1751 as "*a defect in sensation.*" Historically the word *anesthesia* has held special significance because it is associated with the public demonstration of surgical anesthesia in humans by William Morton in America in October 1846.[1,2] This single dramatic and widely publicized event in the wake of earlier unpublicized successes (Crawford Long used ether to remove a tumor from the neck of a patient on March 30, 1842) established the idea that drugs could and should be administered to render patients free from surgical pain. Bigelow[1] states, "*No single announcement ever created so great and general excitement in so short a time. Surgeons, sufferers, scientific men, everybody, united in simultaneous demonstration of heartfelt mutual congratulation (pp 175-212).*" Most important, Morton's demonstration heralded a true paradigm shift, as defined by T.S. Kuhn,[3] in that it represented an unprecedented crystallization of thought of sufficient magnitude to attract an enduring group of adherents while being open-ended enough to serve as a new direction and model for future research. This crystallization of thought was made possible by the efforts of a dedicated scientific community, including Sir Humphrey Davy, Michael Faraday, Henry Hill Hickman, Crawford Long, Horace Wells, J.Y. Simpson, J. Priestley, John Snow (1813-1856; heralded as the first anesthesiologist), and others.[3] However, like a typical character in George Orwell's *1984*, Morton (as many other practitioners of anesthesia) was "*the victim of history rewritten by the powers that be*," dying almost destitute because of attempts to patent his new invention. This paradigm shift (crystallization of thought) fostered the secularization of pain, and a moral transformation that neither humans nor animals should be subjected to or allowed to suffer pain.

The word *anesthesia* became synonymous with unconsciousness that provided insensibility to pain, a viewpoint that persisted for the next 50 years. As the clinical use of neuromuscular blocking drugs, opioids, barbiturates, and diethyl ether became more commonplace, the term was redefined in 1957 by Woodbridge to include four specific components: sensory blockade (analgesia); motor blockade (muscle relaxation); loss of consciousness or mental blockade (unconsciousness); and blockade of undesirable reflexes of the respiratory, cardiovascular, and gastrointestinal systems.[4] Woodbridge believed a single drug or a combination of drugs could be used to achieve the different components of anesthesia, a concept that led to the development of drug combinations to produce a state of "balanced anesthesia." Various prominent anesthesiologists have proposed alternative definitions. Prys-Roberts (1987)[5] suggested that anesthesia should be considered "*drug-induced unconsciousness...the patient neither perceives nor recalls noxious stimulation*"; Pinsker (1986)[6] proposed "*paralysis, unconsciousness, and the attenuation of the stress response*"; and Eger (1993)[7] "*discussed reversible oblivion and immobility.*" Interestingly, a recent edition (27th) of *Stedman's Medical Dictionary* (2005) provides the following definition—"*1. Loss of a sensation resulting from pharmacological depression of nerve function or from neurological dysfunction. 2. Broad term for anesthesiology as a clinical specialty*"— that is not as descriptive as Woodbridge's, although multiple qualifiers have been added (e.g., local, regional, general, surgical, dissociative (Figure 1-1).

Given recent advances in our current understanding of the pharmacodynamics (drug concentration-effect) of anesthetic drugs in horses and the differing anesthetic requirements for surgery (e.g., orthopedic; abdominal), any definition of anesthesia should include any and all effects that protect the patient from the trauma of surgery or produce desirable supplements to anesthesia, including treatments that provide analgesia long after the administration of anesthetic drugs.[8] This viewpoint continues to gain acceptance, as evidenced by detailed manuscripts in the *Equine Veterinary Journal*, the *American Journal of Veterinary Research*, and the *Journal of Veterinary Anesthesia and Analgesia* describing the anxioltic, hypnotic, analgesic, and muscle relaxant effects of α_2-adrenoceptor agonists/dissociative anesthetic/centrally acting muscle relaxant drug combinations (e.g., detomidine/ketamine/guaifenesin) for total intravenous anesthesia (TIVA); the use of inhalant anesthetics (e.g., isoflurane, sevoflurane, desflurane) in combination with various intraoperative anesthetic adjuncts

Table 1–1. Historical events important in equine anesthesia

Time period	Historical event
Before 1500s (Herbalism)	Plant extracts produced: atropine, opium, cannabis
1500-1700 (Emerging)	Anesthesia defined as "a defect in sensation" Ether (1540) Needles (intravenous access)
1800s (Developing)	Anesthesia comes of age: William Morton (1846) demonstrates ether anesthesia in America: "Gentlemen, this is no humbug." Key drug developments: • Peripheral muscle relaxants: curare (1814) • Inhalant anesthetics: carbon dioxide (1824), nitrous oxide (N_2O, 1844), chloroform (1845), ether (Mayhew, 1847) • Intravenous: chloral hydrate (Humbert, 1875) • Local anesthetic: cocaine (1885) • Equipment: face masks, orotracheal tubes, inhalant anesthetic apparatus • Anesthetic record keeping

1900-1950 (Achieving)	Key drug developments:
	• Chloral hydrate (combinations with magnesium sulfate, pentobarbital)
	• Barbiturates (pentobarbital, thiopental)
	• Local anesthetic drugs and techniques developed (procaine)
	• Peripheral muscle relaxants (succinyl choline)
	• Compulsory Anesthetic Use Act in the UK (1919)
	Key texts:
	• E. Stanton Muir, *Materia Medica and Pharmacy* (1904)
	  ▪ Atropine, cannabis, humulus, herbane, chloral, cocaine, codeine, morphine, narcotina, heroin, ethyl alcohol, chloroform, ether
	• L.A. Merillat, *Principles of Veterinary Surgery* (1906)
	  ▪ First American surgeon to devote dedicated attention to anesthesia
	• Sir Frederick Hobday, *Anesthesia and Narcosis of Animals and Birds* (1915)
	  ▪ First English text on veterinary anesthesia: introduces concepts of preanesthetic medication; pain relief; and local, regional, and spinal anesthesia
	• J.G. Wright, *Veterinary Anaesthesia* (1942; ed 2, 1947)
	  ▪ Cannabis, chloral hydrate, pentobarbital, thiopental, chloroform, ether, morphine, bulbocapnine
	• E.R. Frank, *Veterinary Surgery Notes* (1947)
	  ▪ Chloral hydrate and magnesium sulfate, pentobarbital, procaine

1950-2000 (Extending)	Art becomes a science
	Controlled studies conducted on horses
	Key drug developments:
	• Central muscle relaxants (e.g., guaifenesin, diazepam)
	• Peripheral muscle relaxants (e.g., atracurium)
	• Phenothiazines (e.g., promazine, acepromazine)
	• α_2-Agonists (e.g., xylazine, detomidine, medetomidine, romifidine)
	• Dissociative anesthetics (e.g., ketamine, tiletamine)
	• Hypnotics (e.g., propofol)
	• Inhalants (e.g., cyclopropane, methoxyflurane, halothane, isoflurane, enflurane, sevoflurane, desflurane)
	Species-specific anesthetic equipment and ventilators
	Monitoring techniques and equipment
	Key texts:
	• J.G. Wright, *Veterinary Anaesthesia*, (ed 3, 1952; ed 4, 1957)
	• J.G. Wright, L.W. Hall, *Veterinary Anaesthesia and Analgesia*, ed 5 (1961)
	  ▪ Subsequent editions by L.W. Hall and K.W. Clarke
	• L.R. Soma, *Textbook of Veterinary Anaesthesia* (1971)
	  ▪ Chapter 23, written by L.W. Hall, describes anesthesia in horses
	• W.V. Lumb, E. Wynn Jones, *Veterinary Anaesthesia* (1973)
	• C.E. Short, *Principles and Practice of Veterinary Anesthesia* (1987)
	  ▪ Chapter 13, Part 1: "Special considerations of equine anesthesia"
	  ▪ Chapter 13, Part 8: "Anesthetic considerations in the conditioned animal"
	• W.W. Muir, J.A.E. Hubbell, *Equine Anesthesia: Monitoring and Emergency Therapy* (1991)
	  ▪ First text on anesthesia completely devoted to the horse

(Continued)

Table 1–1. **Historical events important in equine anesthesia—Cont'd**

Time period	Historical event
1950-2000 Extending (Cont'd)	Detailed anesthetic records
	Species-specific designed anesthetic equipment and ventilators
	Monitoring techniques and equipment
	"Point of care" blood chemistry (e.g., pH, PO_2, PCO_2) equipment
	Anesthesia universally taught as part of veterinary school curriculum
	American (1975) and European (1993) colleges established
	Information transfer (computer networks and assisted learning)
2000-present	Refinement in equine anesthetic equipment
	Development of computerized ventilators and respiratory monitoring equipment
	Holothane discontinued in the United States; replaced by isoflurane and sevoflurane
	Deflurane investigated for clinical use in horses
	Advanced monitoring techniques, including telemetry and minimally invasive methods for the determination of cardiac output, used at veterinary teaching hospitals
	Key texts:
	• T. Doherty, A. Valverde, eds, *Manual of Equine Anesthesia and Analgesia* (2006)
	• P.M. Taylor, K.W. Clarke, *Handbook of Equine Anesthesia*, ed 2 (2007)

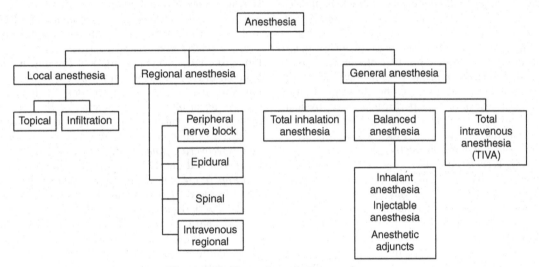

Figure 1–1. Types of anesthetic procedures.

(e.g., ketamine, lidocaine, medetomidine, morphine); and the administration and infusion of analgesic drugs before, during, and after the anesthetic event. The "ideal" anesthetic state (e.g., sedation, analgesia, muscle relaxation, loss of consciousness) in horses is best achieved by administering multiple drugs in combination or sequence to produce the desired effects on consciousness and pain. The advantages of this "multimodal" approach include, but are not limited to, an increase in the potential for additive or synergistic beneficial anesthetic effects, an increase in the scope of anesthetic activity (e.g., analgesia and muscle relaxation), and the potential to reduce side effects or an adverse event. The disadvantages include the potential for adverse drug interactions, resulting in a greater potential for side effects (e.g., bradycardia, ileus, ataxia), adverse events (e.g., hypotension, respiratory depression), and prolonged recovery from anesthesia. It is mandatory that the equine anesthetist become knowledgeable and proficient in administrating a select group of drugs that provide the aforementioned anesthetic qualities if the "best" outcome is to be achieved (Figure 1-2).

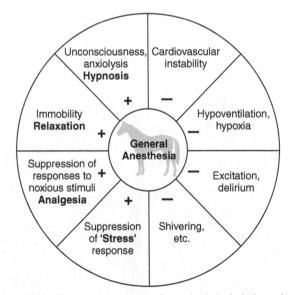

Figure 1–2. The key components of anesthesia include loss of consciousness (hypnosis), analgesia, muscle relaxation, and suppression of stress. Drugs that produce anxiolysis and reduce stress are frequently administered as preanesthetic medication.

THE EVOLUTION OF EQUINE ANESTHESIA

The practice of anesthesia evolved from an art to a science during the 1800s.[9] H.H. Hickman administered carbon dioxide to animals in 1824 to render them unconscious.[10–13] However, before 1850 (and for a long time thereafter), the practice of equine anesthesia remained an art overly dependent on herbal remedies (Atropa mandragora, opium, henbane, hemlock) and physical restraint ("a heavy hand").[12,13] The practical advantages of anesthesia and its potential benefits for equine surgery were advocated by G.H. Dadd 1 year after Morton's demonstration (1847) and recorded in his book *Modern Horse Doctor* (1854).[12,13] It is apparent from these writings that the medical care of horses was, for the most part, left to untrained individuals. Books such as Edward Mayhew's *The Illustrated Horse Doctor*, published in 1880,[14] were written to "*render the gentleman who had consulted it independent of his groom's dictation;…enable any person who had read it capable of talking to a veterinary surgeon without displaying either total ignorance or pitiable prejudice; and which, in cases of emergency, might direct the uninitiated in the primary measures necessary to arrest the progress of the disease; and…might even instruct the novice in such a manner as would afford a reasonable prospect of success.*" Such texts covered all of the known maladies of the day, including simple ophthalmia, staggers, gutta serena, nasal gleet, and scald mouth. Most surgeries were performed with physical restraint of the horse rather than anesthesia (Figure 1-3). Directions for casting the horse included statements such as: "*Let it be hobbled and never, during the operation, hear any sound but soothing accents. Animals do not understand words, creatures may not be able to literally interpret; but they comprehend all that the manner conveys.*" Mayhew may have been the first individual to use diethyl ether in horses, although similar experiments in animals, including horses, were reported in France, Germany, Russia, and the United States. Mayhew's experiences (1847) caused him to comment with skepticism, "*The results of these trials are not calculated to inspire any very sanguine hopes. We cannot tell whether the cries emitted are evidence of pain or not but they are suggestive of agony to the listener, and, without testimony to the contrary, must be regarded as indicative of suffering…. There has yet been no experiment that I know of made to ascertain the action of the vapor on the horse; but I cannot anticipate that it will be found of service to that animal…. We should be cautious lest we become cruel under the mistaken endeavour to be kind.*" Others of this era were more optimistic than Mayhew. Percivall, a graduate physician and veterinarian, stated in that same year, "*We must confess we augur more favourably of the inferences deducible from them [Mayhew's experiments] than he would seem to. To us it appears questionable whether the cries emitted by the animals during experiments are to be regarded as evidence of pain.*"[12,13]

Within 1 year of Morton's demonstration, "ether mania" had reached its peak, only to subside primarily because of Simpson's (1847) demonstration of the advantages of chloroform compared to ether: "*1st. A much less quantity will produce the same effect. 2nd. A more rapid, complete and generally more persistent action, with less preliminary excitement and tendency to exhilaration and talking. 3rd. The inhalation is far more agreeable and pleasant than that of ether. 4th. As a smaller quantity is used, the application is less expensive, which becomes an important consideration if brought into general use. 5th. The perfume is not unpleasant, but the reverse, and more evanescent. 6th. No particular instrumental inhaler is necessary.*"[1] However, skepticism, pragmatism, and reluctance to change were the order of the day, with comments from equine surgeons warning (Box 1-1), "*It is, in my opinion, very doubtful whether chloroform will ever become an efficient agent in veterinary practice on the horse, as I believe these two bad-conditioned animals [neurotomy surgeries in two horses] suffered more in being reduced to a state of insensibility, and in recovering from the state, than they did from the operation performed*"; and "*We very often delude ourselves in regard to the operation of medicines, which seldom effect what we suppose them to do. For this reason it is proper that we should be sceptical with regard to new remedies, which hardly ever maintain the character bestowed upon them by their first employers.*" An editorial in the *Veterinarian* in 1848 suggested, "*abandoning the use of this potent chemical [chloroform] agent as an anesthetic, at least for practical purposes, [instead] let us turn our attention to it as an internal remedy*"; and other writings suggested that ether and chloroform be reserved for internal use (as vermicides) and that during the 1850s "*Horses continued to be bled and purged with vehemence, and operated on without benefit of anesthesia.*" However, these

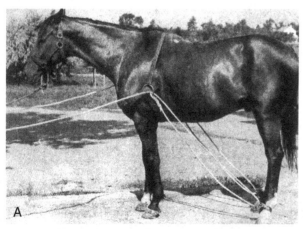

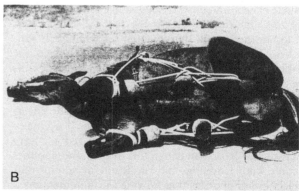

Figure 1–3. A and **B,** The use of hobbles, casting harnesses, and ropes were an essential part of equine "anesthesia" until inhalants and dissociative anesthetics were introduced.

viewpoints gradually did change; and, as R. Jennings in *The Horse and His Diseases* (1860) states: "*In severe operations, humanity dictates the use of some anesthetic agent to render the animal insensible to pain. Chloroform is the most powerful of this class, and may be administered with perfect safety, provided a moderate quantity of atmospheric air is inhaled during its administration. Euphoric ether acts very feebly upon the horse, and cannot therefore be successfully used.*" J.N. Nave commented in his text *Veterinary Practice, or Explanatory Horse Doctor* (1873): "*Chloroform may be administered to the horse for the same purpose as it is given to man.... I would not recommend its use in any but the more important operations*"; and A. Leotard in his *Manual of Operative Veterinary Surgery* (1892) states that for large animals, "*Chloroform used singly has proved itself to be the most effective and safest of all.*"

L.A. Merillat was one of the first veterinary surgeons in the United States to emphasize anesthesia, albeit cautiously, in his *Principles of Veterinary Surgery* (1906) stating: "*Anesthesia in veterinary surgery today is a means of restraint and not an expedient to relieve pain. So long as an operation can be performed by forcible restraint...the thought of anesthesia does not enter into the proposition.*"[13] However, Merillat devoted over 30 pages of his text to anesthesia and anesthetics and suggests "*that the practitioner of the near future will take advantage of the expedient that made the rapid advancement of human surgery possible.*"[13] Merillat listed fatalities from chloroform in horses to be 1/800 (0.125%), a percentage far less than the 1% (1/100) reported in more recent reports for equine perioperative fatalities, albeit the surgical procedures performed were of relatively short duration and heavily dependent on the use of physical restraint (hobbles).[15]

Sir Frederick Hobday published the first English textbook totally devoted to veterinary anesthesia in 1915.[16] Commenting on chloroform, Hobday stated, "*For the horse and dog, chloroform is by far the best general anesthetic both in regard to its utility and cheapness and, also, its safety.*" He went on to say, "*It must of course, like all toxic drugs, be used with discretion and in a skillful and proper manner by a careful anesthetist.*" Hobday recognized that on occasion, especially when complex surgery was contemplated, the veterinary

surgeon would do well to seek the assistance of another, saying, "*it is of no avail to have done any operation, however clever, if the patient succumbs to the anesthetic*" and "*there must always be a certain amount of risk taken by everybody when the anesthetist is an amateur.*" Further, Hobday recognized that economic barriers existed in the provision of safe anesthesia and encouraged the development of "safer" techniques when he said, "*The sentimental public, too, must not forget that for several reasons the services of a qualified veterinary surgeon to act as anesthetist only, whilst his colleague operates (as in human practice), is not always possible. So that if a safe agent can be used which renders the operation to all intents and purposes practically painless and at the same time guarantees the safe return of the patient, the use of such an agent is preferable to one that gives an element of risk.*" Induction to anesthesia and particularly recovery were identified as particular points of stress and he recommended that, "*care must be taken not to remove the hobbles or other restraint before the animal can get up properly or stand steadily, as otherwise there may be an accident to itself or the assistants from blundering about.*" Always the progressive, Hobday concluded, "*The progress of anesthetics in veterinary surgery has not been as rapid as it ought to have been.*"

Years later, Hall[10] commented on Hobday's zeal for using chloroform during the Sir Frederick Hobday memorial address (1982), stating, "*There is no reason to disbelieve his statement that he personally administered chloroform to thousands of horses without mishap.*" Hall goes on to point out that Hobday "*blamed the method of administration rather than the agent itself for any fatality,*" an opinion that has always been and remains a critical issue in the practice of equine anesthesia. Hobday also pointed out that it was "*safer to chloroform a horse than a dog or cat, one indisputable reason being that the larger animal was perforce hobbled and secured in such a position that its lungs could expand and the chest was not pressed upon by human hands.*" An additional factor was the use of lower amounts of anesthetic because of the use of physical restraint. One of the many significant contributions of Hobday's text was the introduction of the concept of preanesthetic medication to: (1) suppress excitement, (2) reduce the anesthetic requirement (providing safer anesthesia); (3) decrease the total anesthesia time; and (4) shorten and improve recovery from anesthesia.

J.G. Wright (1940) credited Hobday as "*the great pioneer of anesthesia for animal surgery in this country [England]*" and with being the first to use cocaine as a local anesthetic in horses. Wright actively taught both the use and safety of diethyl ether and chloroform in horses as detailed in the first four editions of his book *Veterinary Anesthesia* (first published in 1942).[17] The slow development and universal application of veterinary anesthetic techniques had many causes, however, including a general lack of knowledge and experience, differing opinions and expectations, and a lack of emphasis at most veterinary teaching institutions before 1950.

Despite slow development (1850 to 1950), equine anesthesia emerged from herbalism and physical restraint to a science capable of rendering patients insensible to pain. Smithcors (1957)[12] commented on the tardy pace by stating, "*The reasons for veterinarians later (1850 to 1950) being reluctant to make any considerable use of general anesthetics are not immediately apparent.... Although much progress in anesthesiology had been made in human medicine, veteri-*

nary clinical teachers took few steps to include this adjunct to surgery in school practice.... It is likely that more than a few simply thought of anesthesia as an unnecessary refinement to a practice where a heavy hand was accounted a major asset." These statements remind us of the aphorism, "the easiest pain to bear is someone else's," and of the Roman writer Celsius who encouraged "pitilessness" as an essential character of surgeons. This attitude prevailed in human medicine until 1846, when William Morton demonstrated the surgical benefit of diethyl ether, but lingered in equine surgical practice perhaps until the 1950s.[18,19] Smithcors[12] ends his essay by stating, "Whether it be accounted in the name of humanity to the animal, or for the safety and ease of the surgeon, the relatively recent development (1940s and 1950s) of high calibre techniques of anesthesiology must be considered a major advance in veterinary medicine."

RECENT DEVELOPMENTS (1950 TO TODAY)

Throughout the 1940s and 1950s, Wright's teachings at the Beaumont Hospital of the Royal Veterinary College and his texts served as a resource on anesthetic drugs, principles, and techniques for those interested in animal, especially equine, anesthesia.[20,21] He stated (*Veterinary Anesthesia and Analgesia*, ed 4, 1957), "Of the inhalation anesthetics, chloroform is the most potent used in the horse, although... whether or not prenarcosis with chloral hydrate or Cannabis indica is induced will depend chiefly on the size of the animal and the magnitude and duration of the operation to be performed." By the 1950s Cannibus indica was no longer administered to horses because it produced "hyperesthetic activity and the animal (horse) behaved in a maniacal fashion, kicking wildly." In 1961 Wright and Hall[22] summarized earlier experiences with chloroform in horses by stating, "Over the years chloroform has acquired the reputation of being the most dangerous of all the anesthetic agents. However, it seems more than likely that many workers have overestimated the danger associated with the use of chloroform in horses." Commenting on the inhalation of chloroform they state, "This can be applied only to the recumbent animal and the horse must be cast either with ropes or by inducing anesthesia in the standing animal with thiopentone sodium. The dose of thiopentone used for this purpose should not exceed 1 g for 200 lb body weight.... After a period of two to three minutes a second dose of half the initial dose of chloroform is given." Regarding diethyl ether they comment, "There is general agreement that, using the ordinary methods of administration described for chloroform, it is an impossibility to obtain concentrations of ether sufficient to provoke anesthesia in the horse." They also note, "because of its potency, halothane (used in horses by Hall in 1957) is a most useful inhalation anesthetic for the horse. It is about twice as potent as chloroform and may be regarded as a much less dangerous anesthetic agent. Halothane and chloroform both reduce cardiac output and blood pressure but an overdose of halothane causes respiratory failure long before it produces circulatory failure whereas an overdose of chloroform results in almost simultaneous respiratory and circulatory arrest." They go on to point out that "it is usual to restrain the animal with hobbles for about 30 minutes after the administration of the anesthetic is discontinued."

Succinylcholine was introduced to equine anesthesia in 1955 in North America through the publication of articles in the *Journal of the American Veterinary Medical Association* and the *Cornell Veterinarian*.[23,24] A depolarizing, neuromuscular blocking drug with no anesthetic or analgesic qualities, succinylcholine produced recumbency within 30 to 60 seconds of intravenous injection with durations of action of 2 to 8 minutes. Apnea was usually present for a period of 1.5 to 2.5 minutes, and recovery occurred with "a complete lack of excitement." A later article published in 1966 noted the "psychological effects" of succinylcholine administration.[25] The series of case reports touted succinylcholine as an aid to "taming" and noted that, after an administration of succinylcholine to a 4-year-old Quarter Horse stallion, "all the fight had left him and he stood with a crushed and dejected attitude."[25] Despite its lack of anesthetic or analgesic properties and its potential to cause aortic rupture because of systemic hypertension, the use of succinylcholine continued in the horse for approximately 25 years because its administration allowed short surgical procedures (e.g., castration) to be performed and its induction and recovery characteristics were as good as or better than other available techniques. The description and adoption of xylazine and ketamine for short-term anesthesia years later removed any justification for the use of succinylcholine as a sole agent in the horse.[26] During the 1960s and early 1970s, Dr. Hall and others such as E.P. Steffey investigated the cardiopulmonary effects of halothane and other inhalants, paving the way for the expansion of their use in equine anesthesia.[11] The late 1960s introduced the use of guaifenesin (then glyceryl guaiacolate) to the practice of equine anesthesia.[27] Guaifenesin, a centrally acting skeletal muscle relaxant, produced some sedation and minimum-to-no analgesia. Guaifenesin had to be given in larger volumes but found popularity because its use allowed for a reduction in the dose of the hypnotic drugs thiopental or thiamylal.[28] This reduction in dose produced an anesthetized state with reduced cardiopulmonary depression and was associated with improved induction and recovery from anesthesia.

The first α_2-adrenoceptor agonist, xylazine, was introduced into general equine practice in the early 1970s and was followed shortly thereafter by the adoption of xylazine and ketamine for short-term anesthesia.[26,29] Xylazine produced sedation, muscle relaxation, and analgesia, the quality of which was more predictable than seen after phenothiazine administration.[29] The discussion from an early paper indicated, "xylazine may, in time, prove to be an almost invaluable sedative for horses...." The use of xylazine and ketamine was the first of many α_2-agonist dissociative anesthetic drug combinations that continue to evolve to this day. Xylazine and ketamine were easily administered with two intravenous injections, produced 10 to 15 minutes of good-quality anesthesia with reasonable maintenance of cardiopulmonary function, and were associated with rapid recovery. The horse stood squarely within an hour of the beginning of the procedure.[26] The adoption of xylazine and ketamine and subsequently an α_2-adrenoceptor agonist followed by the administration of ketamine-diazepam for short-term intravenous anesthesia or induction to inhalant anesthesia is probably one of the most significant events in equine anesthesia in the last 50 years.

What was largely an art before the 1970s became a powerfully effective science in the years that followed. Hall devoted over 20 pages (318 to 343) to equine anesthesia in Soma's *Textbook of Veterinary Anesthesia*.[30] Hall commented that both chloroform and ether "*still have a place in equine practice,*" although he emphasized halothane as "*the principal inhalant anesthetic to be used in horses.*" Methoxyflurane, although very popular in dogs and cats at this time, "*would seem to be only of academic interest (in horses) to the practical anesthetist. Induction of anesthesia is very slow, changes in the depth of anesthesia can only be achieved very gradually and recovery is slow.*" He went on to state, "*Choral hydrate, the best basal narcotic for horses, has been used in veterinary practice for many years.*" Guaifenesin, a centrally acting muscle relaxant introduced in Germany in the 1950s and administered to horses by M. Whethues, R. Fritsch, K.A. Funk, and U. Schatzman since the 1960s, was given only cursory mention. Hall finished the chapter by stating, "*It is probable that in veterinary anesthesia generally, too little attention is paid to the relief of pain in the postanaesthetic and postoperative periods, and the use of analgesics in this period warrants further study.*"

Improved monitoring techniques identified hypotension and ventilation abnormalities as significant factors in the development of anesthetic complications in the 1980s. Rhabdomyolysis had been a frequent significant complication of equine anesthesia. Numerous anesthetic protocols and padding strategies were devised in an attempt to prevent "tying-up." In 1987 Dr. Jackie Grandy and her coworkers[31] showed a direct link between arterial hypotension and postanesthetic myopathy. Grandy demonstrated that hypotensive horses (mean arterial blood pressure 55 to 65 mm Hg for 3.5 hours) were predisposed to postanesthetic myopathy. All of the horses were normal on recovery when mean arterial blood pressure was maintained above 70 mm Hg. This work and subsequent studies established the importance of monitoring and maintaining arterial blood pressure in anesthetized horses.

Arterial blood gas monitoring came to prominence in the 1980s and led to a number of investigations of ventilation-perfusion abnormalities, hypoventilation, and hypoxia in anesthetized horses.[32] The realization that the arterial partial pressure of oxygen in anesthetized horses frequently falls below 100 mm Hg spurred numerous studies investigating the causes of hypoxia and potential therapies.[33,34] No consensus has evolved as to the best ventilatory strategy or the immediacy of need to treat. The realization that some horses hypoventilate (arterial partial pressure of carbon dioxide in excess of 60 to 70 mm Hg) leads to somewhat divergent viewpoints regarding the acid-base benefits of maintaining normocarbia versus the circulatory benefits of relatively mild hypercarbia. The debate continues with the proventilator group currently holding forth.

In 1991 the first text devoted specifically to the horse was published,[35] with more than 500 pages devoted to issues associated with the administration and consequences of anesthetic drug administration to horses. The goal of the text was to detail the evolution and use of equine anesthesia protocols and deemphasize the need for a heavy hand for equine restraint. Since that time two additional texts devoted to equine anesthesia and analgesia have been published.[36,37] These texts were written as handbooks to be used at the horse's side and are a testimony to the increased interest in and dedication toward improving the practice of equine anesthesia. Today computerization; global networking; and new and faster methods for recording, storing, and transferring information continue to influence how equine anesthesia is performed. Numerous scientific contributions describing the effects of inhalant anesthetics, the stress response, and TIVA in horses and many others describing the pharmacodynamics and toxicity of inhalant and intravenous anesthetic drugs, the use of anesthetic adjuncts, and new and improved monitoring techniques provide ample reading on subjects directly pertaining to both the basic and applied science of equine anesthesia (Figure 1-4).

One highly significant, but less recognized, advance has been the development of a critical mass of educated and trained individuals skilled in the art and science of equine anesthesia. A thorough review of several sources, including the proceedings of the American Association of Equine Practitioners (AAEP; established in 1954), the British Equine Veterinary Association (BEVA; established in 1961), veterinary surgery and anesthesia texts, and numerous manuscripts, revealed that the essential ingredient missing from the practice of equine anesthesia before 1970 was not a lack of appreciation by earlier practitioners of its importance or use, but a relative absence of knowledgeable and dedicated equine anesthetists. The science of veterinary anesthesia has achieved formal and universal recognition as an independent field of study as evidenced by the formation of the American College of Veterinary Anesthesia in 1975 and the European College of Veterinary Anesthesia in 1993. Both organizations were founded on the principles of the dissemination of knowledge, the advancement of science, and the development and maintenance of minimum standards of care. The development of veterinary anesthesia teaching (continuing education) and training programs for both professional and technical practitioners of anesthesia has been a major focus of these groups. Academia has fostered and supported the development of training programs to better serve the profession and the public and has developed focused research areas that provide a resource for continuing education.

Private specialty equine practices have begun to advance the science of equine anesthesia by employing individuals

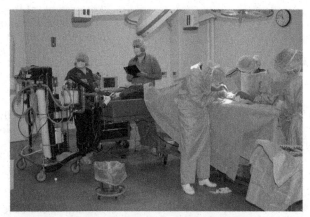

Figure 1–4. Modern equine surgical anesthesia facilities provide highly skilled, dedicated anesthesia personnel and equipment to ensure the best possible outcome.

with keen interest and advanced training. There is a growing realization that a dedicated surgeon cannot devote her or his full attention and concentration to the surgery while providing the best anesthesia possible. Entry-level anesthetists will need innate or acquired "horse sense" and an appreciation of the effects of anesthetic drugs and how best to monitor their patients' well-being. Practitioners of equine anesthesia should become educated and develop an applied understanding of equine physiology (neurology, respiratory, cardiovascular, endocrine, acid-base, and fluid and electrolyte balance), pharmacology (pharmacokinetics, pharmacodynamics, toxicology, drug interactions), chemistry/physics (vapor pressures, solubility coefficients, dissociation constants, pressure, flow, resistance, anesthetic circuits), electronics (computers, monitors [electrocardiogram, electroencephalogram]) and principles of emergency medicine and therapy (cardiopulmonary resuscitation and shock). The self-imposed education and vigilance provided by veterinary anesthetists has significantly impacted the consequences (morbidity) and safety (mortality) of anesthesia in horses while significantly improving patient well-being and lengthening the duration that equine surgery can be safely performed.

The horse stands alone as being one of the most challenging of the common species that are anesthetized. The significance of this challenge is dramatized by a twofold to threefold greater morbidity and a tenfold greater mortality reported for horses (approximately 1%) compared to that for dogs and cats (approximately 0.1%) and 100-fold greater death rate compared to that reported for humans.[38-40] Interestingly, this percentage (1%) has not changed from values originally reported by Lumb and Jones in the first (1973) edition of their text *Veterinary Anesthesia*.[41] Death rates

Table 1–2. Importance of general categories for producing anesthetic-associated morbidity and mortality in horses

Category	Estimated percent
Species	20-25
Drugs	<5
Equipment and facilities	<5
Surgery	<15
Human error	55-60

associated with equine surgery/anesthesia are even more dramatic, reaching values in excess of 10% when obstetric/colic patients are considered.[39] One is led to ponder the cause for such high death rates in horses, particularly since recent (1998) figures from veterinary teaching hospitals and private equine specialty practices suggest a much lower number in noncolic/obstetric patients (Table 1-2).[42-43] These reports would suggest that focusing on anesthesia and attaining advanced training could reduce anesthetic mortality. We believe that Robert Smith was right when he said, *"There are no safe anesthetic drugs, there are no safe anesthetic techniques; there are only safe anesthetists."* We cannot change the temperament or the anatomy and physiology of the horse. We can educate and develop skilled individuals to perform anesthesia to reduce the human error component of anesthetic mortality. This issue, (i.e., error) is relevant to a discussion of the current and future state of the art because error is intrinsic to all human endeavors (Table 1-3).[44] Human error is the most common cause for adverse events, including mortality associated with equine anesthesia. Human error can be categorized based

Table 1–3. Common reasons why anesthetic problems occur

Problem	Reason for occurrence
Human error	Failure to obtain an adequate history or physical examination
	Lack of familiarity with the anesthetic machine or drugs being used
	Incorrect drug administration (incorrect drug, dosage, route or concentration)
	Failure to devote sufficient time or attention to the patient
	Failure to recognize and respond to signs of patient stress or distress
Equipment failure	Carbon dioxide absorber exhaustion
	Empty oxygen tank
	Misassembly of the anesthetic machine or breathing circuit
	Endotracheal tube obstruction or problems
	Vaporizer problems
	One-way valve or "pop-off" valve problems
Adverse effects of anesthetic drugs	There are no safe anesthetic drugs
	Reducing adverse effects is maximized by:
	Evaluation of the patient and any potential risk factors
	Familiarity with the effects, side effects, and contraindications of different drugs
	Individualizing the selection of the anesthetic protocol, often including multiple drugs to achieve balanced anesthesia
Patient-related factors	Aged or young
	Colic
	Trauma
	Fracture
	Pregnancy
	Systemic diseases (cardiovascular, respiratory, hepatic, or renal disease)
	Breed predispositions (hyperkalemic periodic paralysis, myelomalacia)
	General poor condition

on lack of knowledge, lack of experience, lack of instruction, lack of supervision, complacency, task saturation, and personnel fatigue (Box 1-2). Errors in drug selection and dose and route of administration (e.g., intracarotid injections) in conjunction with inadequate monitoring and a general lack of familiarity with resuscitation procedures all contribute significantly to human error–associated anesthetic complications.[44] One study estimated that the main factors responsible for the high anesthetic mortality rate in horses were the horses' physical status and the knowledge, skill, and experience of the person performing anesthesia.[42] The issue is not whether human error occurs but how it can be minimized. In many instances it is not the first error but rather the second (failure to recognize the error) that results in complications. Human error will always remain a primary cause of accidents; but knowledge, an understanding of causality, competence, and a constructively critical team approach can reduce its occurrence. *Obstacles are those frightful things you see when you take your eyes off the goal.* HENRY FORD

THE FUTURE

Many practical issues (e.g., long-term analgesia, hypoxemia, hypotension, recovery quality, drug-related hangover), and new horizons (e.g., immune system modulation, cytokine pathophysiology) require continued investigation. New ideas, drugs, techniques, and equipment continue to evolve. Equine anesthesia, unlike human anesthesia, will continue to require the administration of drugs or techniques that permit control of consciousness with loss of sensation (analgesia) or loss of consciousness and analgesic adjuncts to perform even minor surgical procedures.[45] Although insurrections may occur, the next major advance in anesthesia depends on as yet unrecognized advances in technology and molecular pharmacology. The most immediate issue impacting the practice of equine anesthesia is the immediacy and availability of information (e.g., CABDirect, PubMed, BiosisPreviews on line), the globalization of information transfer, and computer network-based education. The role of anesthetists in equine surgery will become unquestioned and mandatory. Continued research will be required to provide the qualitative and quantitative data necessary to remove dogma and evaluate new approaches.

There is much left to accomplish. The ideal anesthetic drug or combination of drugs has yet to be developed. Monitoring techniques, practices, and equipment remain poorly developed or adapted for use in horses and are difficult to use during recovery. The maintenance and recovery phases of anesthesia remain major issues in horses as evidenced by the comparatively high mortality rates and the incidence of accidents leading to euthanasia (i.e., fractures). Methods for improving pulmonary gas exchange, limiting ventilation perfusion inequalities, and ensuring adequate tissue perfusion need to be developed. These ongoing challenges, combined with an ever-increasing emphasis on prevention and treatment of pain, continue to receive special attention in shaping anesthetic protocols.

This is an exciting time; we hope the next generation of equine anesthetists is ready for the challenges that await them. Horses are a vital part of a grand industry and play an essential role in the lives of many people. In closing, we offer an excerpt from a poem entitled, *The Horse*, written by Ella Wheeler Wilcox and published in *Poetry's Plea For Animals* in 1927:

The world as we see it now
Is only half man-made;
As the horse recedes with a parting bow
We know the part he has played.
For the wonderful brain of man,
However mighty its force,
Had never achieved its lordly plan
Without the aid of the horse.

REFERENCES

1. Bigelow HJ: A history of the discovery of modern anaesthesia. In Clarke EH et al, editors: *A century of American medicine 1776-1876*, Brinklow, 1876, Old Hickory Bookshop, pp 175-212.
2. Calverley RK, Scheller M: Anaesthesia as a specialty: past, present and future. In Barash PG, Cullen BF, Stoelting EK, editors: *Clinical anaesthesia*, ed 2, Philadelphia, 1992, Lippincott, pp 3-33.
3. Kuhn TS: *The structure of scientific revolutions*, ed 3, Chicago, 1996, The University of Chicago Press, pp 43-51.
4. Woodbridge PD: Changing concepts concerning depth of anaesthesia, *Anaesthesiology* 18:536-550, 1957.
5. Prys-Roberts C: Anaesthesia: a practical or impractical construct? (editorial), *Br J Anaesth* 59:1341-1345, 1987.
6. Pinsker MC: Anaesthesia: a pragmatic construct, *Anesth Analg* 65:819-820, 1986.
7. Eger EI: What is general anaesthetic action? (editorial), *Anesth Analg* 77:408, 1993.
8. Kissin I: A concept for assessing interactions of general anaesthetics, *Anesth Analg* 85:204-210, 1997.
9. Caton D: The secularization of pain, *Anaesthesiology* 62:493-501, 1985.
10. Hall LW: Equine anaesthesia: discovery and rediscovery, *Equine Vet J* 15:190-195, 1983.
11. Weaver BMQ: The history of veterinary anaesthesia, *Vet Hist* 5:43-57, 1988.
12. Smithcors JF: The early use of anaesthesia in veterinary practice, *Br Vet J* 113:284-291, 1957.
13. Smithcors JF: History of veterinary anaesthesia. In Soma LR, editor: *Textbook of veterinary anaesthesia*, Baltimore, 1971, Williams & Wilkins, pp 1-23.
14. Mayhew E: *The illustrated horse doctor*, Philadelphia, 1880, Lippincott.
15. Johnston GM: The risks of the game: the confidential enquiry into perioperative equine fatalities, *Br Vet J* 151:347-350, 1995.
16. Hobday F: *Anaesthesia and narcosis of animals and birds*, London, 1915, Baillière Tindall & Cox.
17. Wright JG: *Veterinary anaesthesia*, London, 1942, Baillière Tindall & Cox, pp 1-6, 85-106, 120-129.

18. James W: The varieties of religious experience. In *A study in human nature*, New York, 1982, Penguin Books, pp 297-298.
19. Holzman RS: The legacy of Atropos, the fate who cut the thread of life, *Anaesthesiology* 89:241-249, 1998.
20. Wright JG: *Veterinary anaesthesia*, ed 2, London, 1948, Baillière Tindall & Cox, pp 85-107, 119-128.
21. Wright JG: *Veterinary anaesthesia*, ed 3, London, 1952, Baillière Tindall & Cox, pp. 160-188.
22. Wright JG, Hall LW: Inhalation anaesthesia in horses. In *Veterinary anaesthesia and analgesia*, ed 5, London, 1961, Williams & Wilkins, pp 262-281.
23. Belling TH, Booth NH: Studies on the pharmacology of succinylcholine chloride in the horse, *J Am Vet Med Assoc* 126:37-42, 1955.
24. Stowe CM: The curariform effect of succinylcholine in the equine and bovine species: a preliminary report, *Cornell Vet* 45:193-197, 1955.
25. Miller RM: Psychological effects of succinylcholine chloride immobilization on the horse, *Vet Med Small Anim Clin* 61: 941-943, 1966.
26. Muir WW, Skarda RT, Milne DW: Evaluation of xylazine and ketamine hydrochloride for restraint in horses, *Am J Vet Res* 38:195-201, 1977.
27. Gertsen KE, Tillotson PJ: Clinical use of glyceryl guaiacolate in the horse, *Vet Med Small Anim Clin* 63:1062-1066, 1968.
28. Jackson LL, Lundvall RL: Effect of glyceryl guaiacolate-thiamylal sodium solution on respiratory function and various hematologic factors of the horse, *J Am Vet Med Assoc* 161: 164-168, 1972.
29. Clarke KW, Hall LW: Xylazine—a new sedative for horses and cattle, *Vet Rec* 85:512-517, 1969.
30. Soma LR: Equine Anesthesia. In Soma LR, editor: *Textbook of veterinary anesthesia*, Baltimore, 1971, Williams & Wilkins, pp. 318-343.
31. Grandy JL et al: Arterial hypotension and the development of postanesthetic myopathy in halothane-anesthetized horses, *Am J Vet Res* 48:192-197, 1987.
32. Nyman G, Hedenstierna G: Ventilation-perfusion relationships in the anaesthetized horse, *Equine Vet J* 21:274-281, 1989.
33. Moens Y: Arterial-alveolar carbon dioxide tension difference and alveolar dead space in halothane-anesthetized horses, *Equine Vet J* 21:282-284, 1989.
34. Wilson DV, Soma LR: Cardiopulmonary effects of positive end-expiratory pressure in anesthetized, mechanically ventilated ponies, *Am J Vet Res* 51:729-734, 1990.
35. Muir WW, Hubbell JAE, editors: *Equine anesthesia: monitoring and emergency therapy*, St. Louis, 1991, Mosby.
36. Doherty T, Valverde A, editors: *Manual of equine anesthesia and analgesia*, Oxford, 2006, Blackwell Publishing.
37. Taylor PM, Clarke KW: *Handbook of equine anaesthesia*, ed 2, Edinburgh, 2007, Saunders Elsevier.
38. Johnston GM, Steffey E: Confidential enquiry into perioperative equine fatalities (CEPEF), *Vet Surg* 24:518-519, 1995.
39. Mee AM, Cripps PJ, Jones RS: A retrospective study of mortality associated with general anaesthesia in horses: emergency procedures, *Vet Rec* 142:307-309, 1998.
40. Johnston GM et al: Confidential enquiry of perioperative equine fatalities (CEPEF-1): preliminary results, *Equine Vet J* 27:193-200, 1995.
41. Lumb WV, Jones EW: *Veterinary anaesthesia*, Philadelphia, 1973, Lea & Febiger, pp 629-631.
42. Jones RS: Comparative mortality in anaesthesia, *Br J Anaesth* 87:813-815, 2001.
43. Bidwell LA, Bramlage LR, Rood WA: Equine perioperative fatalities associated with general anaesthesia at a private practice—a retrospective case series, *Vet Anaesth Analg* 34:23-30, 2007.
44. Arnstein F: Catalogue of human error (review), *Br J Anaesth* 79:645-656, 1997.
45. Roy JE, Prichap LS: The anesthetic cascade: a theory of how anesthesia suppresses consciousness, *Anesthesiology* 102:447-471, 2005.

The Respiratory System

N. Edward Robinson

1. The horse's unique anatomy, size, and weight make it particularly vulnerable to anesthetic-related disturbances in pulmonary function and gas (PO_2; PCO_2) exchange.
2. Anesthetized horses are particularly susceptible to compression atelectasis when placed in recumbent, particularly dorsal (supine), positions.
3. All anesthetic drugs (e.g., inhalant anesthetics) depress respiratory drive, inspiratory and expiratory muscle function, ventilation (rate, volume), and the horse's response to hypercarbia and hypoxia.
4. Most anesthetics, but particularly inhalant anesthetics, markedly attenuate or abolish hypoxic pulmonary vasoconstriction (HPV) and alter the distribution of pulmonary blood flow.
5. All anesthetic drugs, but particularly inhalant anesthetics, depress laryngeal function and surfactant production and decrease mucus clearance.
6. The primary causes for hypoxemia in horses are hypoventilation, ventilation-perfusion ($\dot{V}A/\dot{Q}$) mismatching, right-to-left shunting of blood flow ($\dot{Q}$), and diffusion impairment.
7. Varying degrees of upper airway obstruction (nasal edema) should be expected following longer surgical procedures, particularly if the horse is supine or in a head-down position during surgery.
8. Respiratory embarrassment from anesthesia often extends into the recovery period, requiring vigilant monitoring and oxygen supplementation.

The function of the respiratory system is impaired in part from the effects of the preoperative and anesthetic drugs and in part as a result of recumbency and positioning when a healthy horse is anesthetized. Additional complications arise as a result of preexisting disease and the interactions of drugs with the disease processes when a sick horse is anesthetized. Knowledge of anatomy and respiratory physiology is crucial to the maintenance of respiratory function for delivery of oxygen and elimination of carbon dioxide. Respiratory function in horses is always altered by anesthetic drugs and, when combined with the effects of body position (supine; head down), can be responsible for significant derangement of arterial blood gas values (PaO_2; $PaCO_2$) and oxygen delivery (see Appendix A).

VENTILATION OF THE LUNG

Minute, Dead-Space, and Alveolar Ventilation

Ventilation is the movement of gas in and out of the alveoli. The volume of each breath, tidal volume (VT), and respiratory frequency (f) determine the volume of air breathed per minute, which is known as minute ventilation (Vmin). Respiratory frequency, VT, and Vmin average approximately 15 per minute, 5 L (10 ml/kg), and 75 L/min (150 ml/kg/min), respectively, in the resting horse of approximately 480 kg body weight.[1] The changes in Vmin necessitated by metabolism can be accommodated by changes in either VT or f.

Air flows into the alveoli through the conducting airways (i.e., nares, nasal cavity, pharynx, larynx, trachea, bronchi, and bronchioles). Conducting airways are also called the anatomic dead space because no gas exchange occurs within them (Figure 2-1). A portion of each VT, and therefore of alveolar ventilation (VA), ventilates the anatomic dead space (VD), and a portion of VA participates in gas exchange. VA is regulated by control mechanisms to match the oxygen uptake and carbon dioxide elimination necessitated by metabolism.

Dead space ventilation also occurs in poorly perfused alveoli where gas exchange cannot occur optimally (see Ventilation Perfusion Matching Under Anesthesia later in the chapter). Physiological dead space describes the sum of the anatomic and alveolar dead space. The ratio of physiological dead space ventilation to Vmin (also known as the dead space/tidal volume ratio, VD/VT) approximates 60% in the standing unsedated horse.[2]

Because the volume of the anatomic dead space is relatively constant, changes in VT and respiratory frequency can alter VD/VT. Small VTs ventilate primarily the anatomic dead space; thus VD/VT is high. Conversely, an increased VD as occurs during exercise provides a greater fraction of ventilation to the alveoli so that VD/VT becomes low.[2] Equipment used for anesthesia should not increase the dead space. Excessively long endotracheal tubes or overly large face masks should be avoided because they increase mechanical dead space.

Muscles of Respiration

Ventilation requires energy to stretch the lungs and thorax and to overcome the frictional resistance to breathing. Respiratory muscles provide the energy necessary for inhalation, but during exhalation the elastic force stored in the stretched lung and thorax provides much of the energy. Therefore in most animals at rest inhalation is an active process, whereas exhalation is passive. Horses are an exception to this general rule; they have an active phase of exhalation even at rest.[3] If the horse is breathing spontaneously during anesthesia, the muscles provide the driving force; but if the horse's ventilation is being controlled, the ventilator provides the driving force to move the lungs and thorax.

The diaphragm is the primary inspiratory muscle. During contraction the dome of the diaphragm is pulled caudally

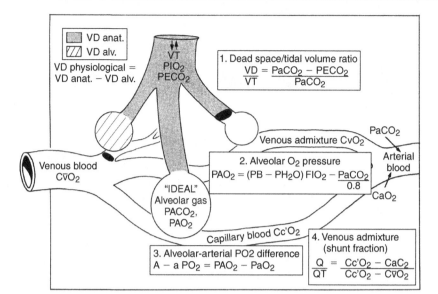

Figure 2–1. Diagrammatic representation of the lung illustrating anatomic, alveolar, and physiological dead space and important relationships.

and thereby enlarges the thoracic cavity. The tendinous center pushes against the abdominal contents, elevating intraabdominal pressure, which displaces the caudal ribs outward. As with any muscle, the efficacy of diaphragmatic contraction depends on the resting length of the muscle fibers. When a horse is recumbent, the diaphragm is displaced forward by the abdominal contents during anesthesia so that its fibers may be stretched beyond their optimal length and diaphragmatic function may be less than optimal.[4]

The external intercostal muscles are also active during inhalation, moving the ribs forward and outward. However, the relative contributions of diaphragmatic and costal movement to ventilation in the conscious and anesthetized horse are undefined. Other inspiratory muscles include those connecting the sternum and head such as the sternohyoid and sternocephalic muscles. These muscles contract during strenuous breathing and move the sternum rostrally.

The subatmospheric pressure generated within the thorax during inhalation enlarges the lungs and causes airflow though the airways. The resulting subatmospheric pressure within the airways tends to collapse the external nares, pharynx, and larynx. Contraction of adductor muscles attached to these structures is essential to prevent their collapse. α_2-Agonists (xylazine; detomidine) relax the upper airway muscles and make the upper airway prone to collapse during inhalation, which tends to obstruct airflow.

The abdominal muscles and internal intercostals are the expiratory muscles. Contraction of abdominal muscles increases abdominal pressure, which forces the relaxed diaphragm forward and reduces the size of the thorax. Contraction of the internal intercostals also decreases the size of the thorax by moving the ribs caudally and downward.

Mechanics of Ventilation

The respiratory muscles generate work to stretch the chest wall and lung and overcome frictional resistance to airflow. At the end of a tidal exhalation, a volume of air known as functional residual capacity (FRC; approximately 45 ml/kg) remains in the lung. The pressure in the pleural cavity (Ppl)

at FRC is approximately 5 cm H_2O subatmospheric (–5 cm H_2O). During inhalation Ppl decreases (more negative) by 5 to 10 cm H_2O as the thorax enlarges and the respiratory muscles work to stretch the elastic lung and thorax and generate airflow through the airways. The change in Ppl during each breath is determined by the change in lung volume (ΔV), lung compliance (C), airflow rate (V), respiratory resistance (R), acceleration (a), and inertia of the respiratory system (I):

$$\Delta Ppl = \Delta V/(C) + RV + I$$

The resting horse breathes slowly, flow rates are low, acceleration is minimal, and the primary work of the respiratory muscles is to overcome the elasticity of the lung. Flow rates increase, and more energy is used to generate flow against the frictional resistance of the airways when respiratory rate increases. Increases in frequency usually increase flow rate and also acceleration and therefore inertial forces. Otherwise inertial forces are usually negligible. Respiratory disease can change both elasticity and resistance and increase the work of breathing. As a consequence, it is necessary to use higher airway pressures when ventilating a horse with lung disease.

Pulmonary Elasticity

The lung is an elastic structure because of its content of elastin and also because the fluid lining the alveoli generates surface tension forces. When the thorax is opened and pleural pressure becomes atmospheric, the lung collapses to its minimal volume as a result of its inherent elasticity. Some air remains trapped within the alveoli at the minimal volume behind closed peripheral airways. Documentation of the elasticity of the lung requires generation of a pressure-volume curve by inflating the lung and concurrent measurement of the difference between the airway pressure and the pressure surrounding the lung (i.e., pleural pressure in the intact animal). This pressure difference required for inflation of the lung is known as transpulmonary pressure (PL).

A high pressure is required to exceed the critical opening pressure of the bronchioles when the lung is inflated with air from the gas-free state (Figure 2-2). This high critical opening pressure may be required during anesthesia to

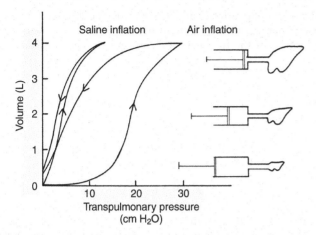

Figure 2–2. Diagrammatic representation of pressure-volume curves generated by inflating a degassed lung with air and saline. Note the hysteresis in the air pressure-volume curve and the lack of hysteresis in the saline pressure-volume curve. Inflation of the lung with saline requires less pressure than inflation of the lung with air because of the absence of surface tension forces in the saline-inflated lung.

reinflate areas of atelectasis. Once the bronchioles open, the lung inflates more easily until its elastic limits are reached at a PL of approximately 30 cm of H_2O. The volume of air in the lung at this point is the total lung capacity (TLC). The lung does not deflate along the same pressure-volume curve; less pressure is required to maintain a given volume than during inflation. This difference in lung elastic properties between inflation and deflation is known as pressure-volume hysteresis. The lung is gas free only in the fetus and for a few seconds after birth until the first breath is taken. Usually the lung inflates from FRC, about 40% to 45% of TLC. It then exhibits little hysteresis, in part because the bronchioles are already open and their critical opening pressure does not need to be exceeded. However, under anesthesia FRC decreases, and airways may close, resulting in more pressure-volume hysteresis than in the conscious animal.

Connective tissues such as elastin and collagen contribute to the elasticity of the lung, but surface tension forces that arise in the fluid film overlying the alveolar epithelium are also responsible. Collapse of alveoli under the effect of surface tension is impeded by the presence of pulmonary surfactant, which reduces surface tension on the alveolar lining fluid. Pulmonary surfactant is a mixture of lipids and proteins, the most common lipid component being dipalmitoyl phosphatidylcholine. It is produced in type II alveolar cells, and its hydrophilic and hydrophobic portions cause it to seek the surface of the alveolar lining. The alveolar surface area shrinks as lung volume decreases, and surfactant molecules become concentrated, reducing surface tension and promoting alveolar stability. The proteins in surfactant facilitate its recruitment to the alveolar surface and also have antibacterial properties.

The conscious animal reactivates surfactant by sighing and expanding the alveolar surface several times per hour. Horses will not sigh under anesthesia or if the cranial abdomen of the thorax is painful. As a consequence, airways may close, and alveoli may collapse. Regular deep breaths can be substituted for sighs to help prevent alveolar collapse.

Interactions on the Lung and Chest Wall

The lung and thorax interact mechanically because the visceral and parietal pleura are maintained in close apposition by a thin layer of pleural fluid. The pressure-volume curves of the lung and thorax and total respiratory system are illustrated in Figure 2-3. At slightly below 50% TLC, the respiratory system is at equilibrium, and the inward elastic recoil of the lung is balanced by the outward recoil of the chest wall. This equilibrium position is FRC in most mammals; but in the horse, which always exhales actively, FRC is slightly below the equilibrium volume. The lung has little elastic recoil below FRC, but the thorax resists deformation so that residual volume—the volume of air in the lung at the end of a maximum exhalation—is determined by the limits to which the rib cage can be compressed. Above FRC, lung and chest wall elastic recoil both increase. The lung approaches its elastic limits at TLC, but the chest wall is still compliant.

The slope of the lung pressure-volume curve is known as lung compliance (C). Compliance obviously varies with the state of lung inflation because the pressure-volume curve is nonlinear. Compliance is usually measured over the VT range. It is the compliance of the combined lungs and thoracic wall that determines the pressures needed to provide adequate ventilation. In normal horses, lung compliance averages 1 to 2 L/cm of H_2O. If lung compliance decreases below this value (e.g., because of pulmonary edema or lung fibrosis), more pressure is needed to maintain ventilation. Dynamic lung compliance (Cdyn) is compliance measured during tidal breathing. Cdyn is also decreased by lung fibrosis and diffuse obstruction of the peripheral airways. For example, it is not unusual for Cdyn to be as low as 0.25 L/cm of H_2O in horses with heaves.

Frictional Resistance to Breathing

The frictional resistance between air molecules and the walls of the air passages opposes the flow of air through the tubes of the upper airway and tracheobronchial tree during ventilation. The nasal cavity, pharynx, and larynx provide more than 50% of this resistance (Figure 2-4).[5]

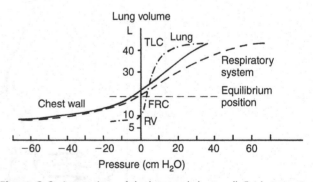

Figure 2–3. Interactions of the lung and chest wall. Expiratory pressure-volume curves are shown for the lung, the chest wall, and the total respiratory system. At the equilibrium position, the elastic recoil of the lung and chest wall are equal and opposite, so that there is zero recoil by the total respiratory system. In the horse functional residual capacity *(FRC)* is just below the equilibrium position. At residual volume *(RV)* the lung has little elastic recoil, but the chest wall greatly resists further compression. At total lung capacity *(TLC)* the lung pressure-volume curve is almost horizontal, indicating that the lung is reaching its elastic limits, but the chest wall is still compliant.

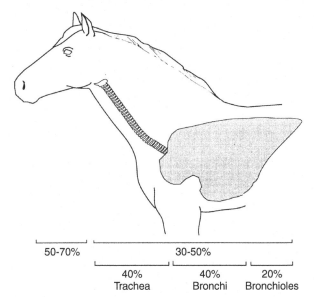

50-70%	30-50%		
	40% Trachea	40% Bronchi	20% Bronchioles

Figure 2–4. Approximate partitioning of the resistance to airflow in the horse.

In the anesthetized horse the resistance of the endotracheal tube generally replaces the upper airway resistance (see Chapter 14). Therefore it is important to use the largest diameter tube compatible with the horses's airway size.

The tracheobronchial tree in horses has more than 40 branches lined by a secretory, ciliated epithelium. The large airways, trachea, and bronchi are supported by cartilage. The bronchi ramify in the lung in association with the pulmonary arteries and larger veins; the three structures are contained in the bronchovascular bundle. The smaller branches of the tracheobronchial tree are the bronchioles, which lack cartilage and a connective tissue sheath. Alveoli surround the intrapulmonary airways, and the alveolar septa attach to the outer layers of the bronchovascular bundle and the walls of the bronchioles. The alveolar septa are always under tension, which provides radial traction around the airways and maintains their patency. This interdependence between alveolar septa and bronchi/bronchioles means that the bronchi/bronchioles dilate as the lung inflates and narrow during exhalation (Figure 2-5). The reduction in lung volume in dependent lung regions in the anesthetized recumbent horse can lead to excessive airway narrowing and even closure of some of the bronchioles.

The branching pattern of the tracheobronchial tree and the diameter of the different branches have important effects on the function of the airways. For example, the cross-sectional area of the tracheobronchial tree increases only a little between the trachea and the first four generations of bronchi but increases dramatically toward the periphery of the lung. Consequently the velocity of airflow diminishes progressively from the trachea toward the bronchioles. The high-velocity turbulent airflow in the trachea and bronchi produces the lung sounds heard through a stethoscope in a normal animal. Laminar low-velocity flow in the bronchioles produces no sound. A consequence of the airway branching pattern is that airways greater than 2 to 5 mm in diameter contribute more of the tracheobronchial resistance than the bronchioles (see Figure 2-4).

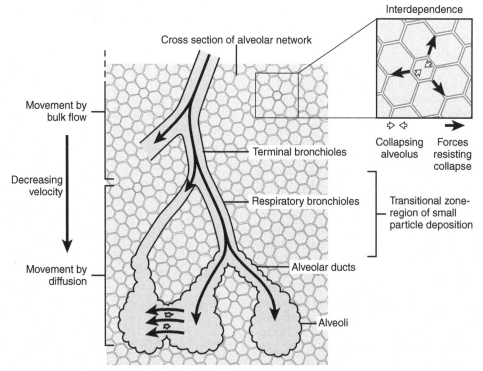

Figure 2–5. Normal flow of gas from the respiratory bronchioles to the alveoli. Obstruction of a small airway leading to a group of alveoli can be compensated for by the movement of gas between adjacent alveoli via the pores of Kohn, thereby preventing collapse of alveoli downstream from the obstruction. The alveoli are connected to each other via shared walls and to airways via collagen and elastin. These connections allow forces to be shared among alveoli and provide the basis for structural interdependence, making it difficult for a single alveolus to collapse. (Modified from Schwartzstein RM, Parker MJ: *Respiratory physiology: a clinical approach,* Philadelphia, 2006, Lippincott Williams & Wilkins, p 22.)

Airway resistance is usually less than 1.2 cm H_2O/L/sec in normal horses, but in diseases such as heaves, resistance can increase to as much as 4 cm H_2O/L/sec. Resistance is determined by the radius and length of the airways. Airway length changes very little during normal breathing or during disease, but radius can be altered by several passive and active forces. As noted previously, airways dilate as the lung inflates because they are mechanically linked to the alveolar septa in which tension increases as lung volume increases. There is smooth muscle in the walls of the airways from the trachea to the alveolar ducts. Smooth muscle actively regulates airway diameter in response to neural regulation, circulating catecholamines, and release of inflammatory mediators.

Stimulation of the vagus nerve parasympathetic innervation narrows all airways, but especially the bronchi (Table 2-1).[6,7] Activation of submucosal tracheobronchial irritant receptors by irritant materials such as dust causes reflex bronchoconstriction, the afferent arm of which is by way of the parasympathetic system.

Tracheal smooth muscle receives sympathetic nerves, but there is little or no sympathetic nerve supply to the intrapulmonary airway smooth muscle of horses.[8] For this reason, most of the relaxation of tracheobronchial smooth muscle occurs following activation of α_2-adrenoceptors (α_2-agonists; xylazine, detomidine, romifidine) by circulating epinephrine released from the adrenal medulla rather than from local release of norepinephrine from sympathetic nerve endings in the airways. Another bronchodilator system, the nonadrenergic noncholinergic inhibitory nervous system, is present in the trachea and large bronchi.[8] The nerve fibers are in the vagus, and the neurotransmitter is nitric oxide/vasoactive intestinal peptide. The factors that activate this system are presently unknown.

Airway smooth muscle also contracts in response to many of the inflammatory mediators, particularly histamine and the leukotrienes. Airway inflammation leads to the phenomenon known as airway hyperresponsiveness. When animals have hyperresponsive airways, their smooth muscle contracts in response to small doses of irritants or mediators that would cause no effect in a healthy animal. Horses with a history of heaves or with inflammatory airway disease may have hyperresponsive airways that bronchoconstrict and are difficult to ventilate.[9,10]

Anesthetic Effects on the Airway Smooth Muscle

Volatile anesthetics such as halothane, isoflurane, sevoflurane, and desflurane relax airway smooth muscle and therefore cause bronchodilation.[11,12] The inhibitory effects of halothane, isoflurane, and desflurane are similar in the trachea; but in the more peripheral airways halothane is the most potent inhibitor, desflurane is the least, and isoflurane has intermediate effects.[13,14] The mechanisms of relaxation involve (1) inhibition of inward calcium currents through voltage-dependent calcium channels, (2) inhibition of IP3-induced calcium release from the sarcoplasmic reticulum, and (3) decreased sensitivity of contractile mechanisms to calcium.[12] Intravenous anesthetics thiopental, ketamine, and propofol also inhibit airway smooth muscle tone by reducing calcium influx into smooth muscle. Benzodiazepines have similar effects. However, the inhibitory effects of intravenous agents are less than that of inhaled anesthetics.[15] Xylazine and acepromazine have been reported to cause

bronchodilation in ponies.[16,17] Barbiturates, opioids, many muscle relaxants, drug vehicles, and cardiovascular drugs have the potential to release histamine from airway mast cells and therefore may cause bronchospasm.

Dynamic Airway Compression

Dynamic airway compression occurs when the pressure surrounding the airway exceeds the pressure within the airway lumen. Dynamic compression occurs during inhalation in the external nares, pharynx, and larynx because pressure within the airways is subatmospheric and the airways are surrounded by atmospheric pressure. Contraction of the abductor muscles of the nares, pharynx, and larynx during inhalation is necessary to prevent collapse of these regions. Anesthesia reduces the tone in the abductor muscles and inhibits that contraction during inhalation. This can lead to a respiratory collapse of the upper airway in the nonintubated heavily sedated or anesthetized horse.

Dynamic collapse of the intrathoracic airways occurs during forced exhalation when intrapleural pressure exceeds pressures within the intrathoracic airway lumen. Dynamic collapse of the intrathoracic airways occurs during the forced expiratory effort exhibited by horses with obstructive lung disease. Cough is a forced exhalation during which dynamic collapse narrows the larger airways. During cough the high air velocity through the narrowed portion of the airway facilitates removal of foreign material.

Distribution of Ventilation

Intrapleural pressure is more subatmospheric in the uppermost part of the thorax than in the lowermost parts in the standing horse (Figure 2-6).[18] Consequently the lung is more distended and therefore less compliant dorsally than ventrally. Air preferentially enters the more compliant dependent regions, resulting in a vertical gradient of ventilation in the standing horse (see Figure 2-6).[19] However, the relative distention of different regions of lung is only one of the factors affecting ventilation distribution. The distribution of air within the lung also depends on local lung compliance and airway resistance, which is altered in horses (Figure 2-7). Region A represents a healthy piece of lung with normal compliance and a normal airway; region B has a disease such as interstitial pneumonia in which compliance is decreased but the airways are normal; and region C has a normal compliance but a narrowed airway. When the same decrease in pleural pressure is applied to each region, regions A and C fill to the same volume because they have similar compliance, but C fills more slowly than A because of its obstructed airway. Like region A, region B fills rapidly but, because of its reduced compliance, achieves a lesser volume than regions A and C. An increase in respiratory rate can cause even greater abnormalities in ventilation distribution. Because region C takes a long time to fill, it has inadequate time to fill when breathing rate increases.

The distribution of ventilation is very uneven in the recumbent animal, especially in the supine and laterally recumbent positions, because of reductions in lung volume and changes in the pleural pressure gradient. The decrease in lung volume may be so great, and pleural pressure may become so positive that the peripheral airways close in the dependent regions of lung. The lung volume at which airway closure occurs is known as closing volume (Figure 2-8).

Table 2–1.   Autonomic regulation of the respiratory system

Effector response	Anatomic pathway	Neurotransmitter	Receptor	Intracellular coupling	Action	Notes
Bronchodilation	Sympathetic	Norepinephrine	β_2-adrenoceptor	$G\alpha_e$: adenylyl cyclase-↑cAMP	Relaxes airway smooth muscle	Sympathetic nerves on the supply airway smooth muscle in the trachea and large bronchi. Norepinephrine is only a weak agonist for the β_2-adrenoceptor.
	Sympathetic	Norepinephrine	α_2-adrenoceptor		Inhibits release of acetylcholine from postganglionic neurons supplying airway smooth muscle	
	Sympathetic: adrenal medulla	Epinephrine	β_2-adrenoceptor	$G\alpha_e$: adenylyl cyclase:↑cAMP	Relaxes airway smooth muscle	Epinephrine is a potent agonist for the β_2-adrenoceptor.
	Parasympathetic	Acetylcholine	M_2 muscarinic	$G\alpha_i$: adenylyl cyclase-↓cAMP in postganglionic parasympathetic neuron	Inhibits release of acetylcholine from postganglionic neurons supplying airway smooth muscle	In many inflammatory conditions of the airways, the prejunctional M_2 muscarinic receptor becomes dysfunctional.
	iNANC	NO		Guanylyl cyclase inside airway smooth muscle	Relaxes airway smooth muscle	iNANC nerves form the primary neural bronchodilator mechanism in most of the horse's tracheobronchial tree.

Function	Autonomic system	Neurotransmitter	Receptor	Signal transduction	Effect	Comments
Bronchoconstriction	Parasympathetic	Acetylcholine	M_3 muscarinic	$G\alpha_q$; PLC - IP_3 & DAG-↑Ca^{+2}	Contracts airway smooth muscle	The primary autonomic system causing smooth muscle contraction.
	eNANC	Excitatory neuropeptides such as substance P.	NK_1	$G\alpha_q$; PLC - IP_3 & DAG-↑Ca^{+2}		Increased activity of this system may facilitate smooth muscle contraction in some inflammatory airway diseases.
Mucus secretion and mucociliary clearance	Sympathetic	Norepinephrine	β_2-adrenoceptor	$G\alpha_e$; adenylyl cyclase-↑cAMP	Increases mucus secretion and mucociliary clearance	
	Sympathetic: adrenal medulla	Epinephrine	β_2-adrenoceptor	$G\alpha_e$; adenylyl cyclase-↑cAMP	Increases mucus secretion and mucociliary clearance	
	Parasympathetic	Acetylcholine	M_3 muscarinic	$G\alpha_q$; PLC - IP_3 & DAG-↑Ca^{+2}	Increases mucus secretion and mucociliary clearance	
	iNANC	NO		Activates guanylyl cyclase-↑cGMP	Relaxes airway smooth muscle	iNANC nerves form the primary neural bronchodilator mechanism in most of the horse's tracheobronchial tree.
	eNANC	Excitatory neuropeptides such as substance P	NK_1	$G\alpha_q$;- PLC - IP_3 & DAG-↑Ca^{+2}	Increases mucus secretion	
Pulmonary circulation	Sympathetic	Norepinephrine	α_1-adrenoceptor	$G\alpha_q$;- PLC - IP_3 & DAG-↑Ca^{+2}	Contract pulmonary vascular smooth muscle	Decreases compliance of pulmonary circulation but does not increase vascular resistance.
	Parasympathetic	Acetylcholine	M_3 muscarinic	Unclear	Relaxes pulmonary vascular smooth muscle	Probably endothelium dependent via release of nitric oxide.

cAMP, Cyclic adenosine monophosphate; *cGMP*, cyclic guanosine monophosphate; *DAG*, diacylglycerol; $G\alpha_e$, G protein α_e; $G\alpha_z$, G protein α_z; $G\alpha_q$, G protein α_q; IP_x, inositol-1,4,5 triphosphate; M_z acetylcholine M_2 receptor; *NANC*, nonadrenergic noncholinergic (*i*, inducible; *e*, endothelial); *PLC*, phospholipase C.

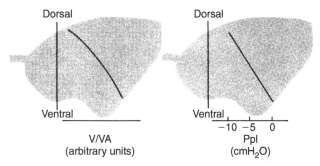

Figure 2–6. Vertical gradient of pleural pressure *(right)* and the distribution of ventilation *(left)* as a function of the height of the lung in the horse. Pleural pressure increases from the dorsal toward the ventral part of the lung, and ventilation per unit lung volume *(V/VA)* also increases down the lung. (Modified from Amis TC, Pascoe JR, Hornof W: Topographic distribution of pulmonary ventilation and perfusion in the horse, *Am J Vet Res* 45:1597-1601, 1984 [Fig 2, Pg 1598].)

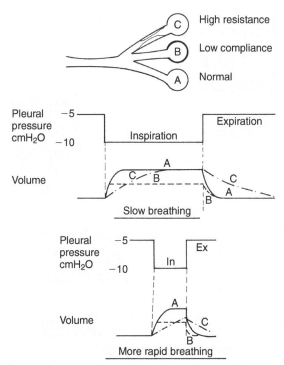

Figure 2–7. Effects of mechanical properties of the lung on the distribution of ventilation. See text for explanation.

Collateral Ventilation and Interdependence

Collateral ventilation and interdependence tend to restore homogeneity to ventilation distribution (see Figure 2-5). The collateral movement of air between adjacent regions of lung, most probably through anastomosing respiratory bronchioles, occurs only to a small degree in horses.[20] This is because adjacent lung lobules are separated by almost complete interlobular connective tissue septa. Interdependence is the mechanical interaction between adjacent regions of lung and between the lung and chest wall. If one region of lung is ventilating asynchronously with adjacent regions, the pull of adjacent lung tissue tends to make the asynchronous region ventilate more synchronously with the remainder of the lung.

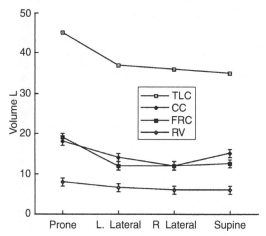

Figure 2–8. Effect of posture on lung volumes in the anesthetized horse. *TLC,* total lung capacity; *RV,* residual volume; *CC,* closing capacity. All lung volumes are decreased by recumbency, but CC exceeds FRC only in the supine animal. (From Sorenson PR, Robinson NE: Postural effects on lung volumes and asynchronous ventilation in anesthetized horses, *J Appl Physiol* 48:97, 1980.)

Postural and Anesthetic Effects on Lung Volumes and Ventilation Distribution

Anesthetized horses develop a large alveolar-arterial oxygen difference as a result of postural effects on the distribution of blood flow and especially ventilation.[21,22] Ventilation of the down lung is impeded mechanically during recumbency, and functional residual capacity is reduced. The causes of these changes have received considerable investigation.

Functional Residual Capacity

Functional residual capacity decreases when the horse is anesthetized and becomes recumbent (see Figure 2-8).[23,24] The decrease in FRC is in part a result of recumbency but is also caused by the anesthetic drug effects because anesthetic agents such as isoflurane decrease FRC more than intravenous agents do.[23] The transmural pressure acting on different parts of the diaphragm is one of the causes of the decrease in FRC under anesthesia.[25] Because the abdominal contents are fluid, pressure within the abdomen increases from its dorsal to its ventral part. By contrast there is no pressure gradient from the most dorsal to the most ventral alveoli because they are air filled. Thus transdiaphragmatic pressure increases from the dorsal to the ventral parts of the diaphragm. The position of the horse's diaphragm is different in different postures (Figure 2-9).[24] In standing horses the transdiaphragmatic pressure increases from the spine to the sternum so that the diaphragm slopes deeply forward and down, with the apex of the diaphragm at the base of the heart. A large part of the lung is dorsal to the diaphragm. When the horse assumes lateral recumbency, the transdiaphragmatic pressure gradient causes the diaphragm to encroach on the thorax adjacent to the dependent lung. Thus, radiographically, the dependent lung is smaller and more dense than the upper lung in the laterally recumbent horse. In dorsal recumbency the diaphragm overlies much of the lung, and the pressure gradient causes the diaphragm adjacent to both lungs to encroach on the thorax. Radiographically both lungs are reduced in size and increased in density. There may be other causes of the

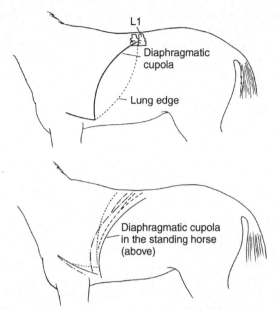

Figure 2–9. Composite line drawing illustrating *(top)* general diaphragmatic outline of a standing horse and *(bottom)* changes in the diaphragmatic outline with anesthesia and positional changes. *Bottom:* Conscious standing *(-)*, anesthetized sternal recumbency *(--)*, anesthetized dorsal recumbency *(.....)*, and anesthetized left lateral recumbency *(.-.-.)*. (From McDonell WN, Hall LW, Jeffcott LB: Radiographic evidence of impaired pulmonary function in laterally recumbent anesthetized horses, *Equine Vet J* 11:28, 1979.)

reduction in FRC, such as a reduction in the tone of the muscles of the thorax and limitation of the motion of the thorax by contact with the surgery table.

Effect of Positive-Pressure Ventilation

Attempts to improve gas exchange by use of positive end-expiratory pressure (PEEP) in spontaneously ventilating horses have been relatively unsuccessful.[26-28] PEEP applied to the whole lung increases FRC but may not exceed the opening pressure of closed airways in the lower lung (see Chapter 17). TLC (defined during positive-pressure inflation of the lung) and FRC are reduced proportionally in the anesthetized horse, suggesting that inflation pressures as great as 45 cm H_2O are insufficient to recruit closed airways in some parts of the lung, presumably the dependent regions.[29] Radiographic evidence also suggests that the latter is true. The upper lung increases in size during positive-pressure ventilation, but the lower lung does not.[4,24] However, selective application of PEEP to the dependent parts of the caudal lobes of dorsally recumbent horses improves gas exchange, probably because PEEP increases regional FRC.[30] When PEEP is applied to the whole lung along with positive-pressure ventilation, FRC increases progressively at PEEP of 10, 20, and 30 cm of H_2O. However, greater than 20 cm of H_2O PEEP is necessary to improve gas exchange.[31] Airway pressures greater than 30 cm of H_2O are necessary to reduce shunt fraction during high-frequency positive-pressure ventilation,[32] and inflation pressures of up to 55 cm of H_2O in combination with PEEP of 20 cm of H_2O improves gas exchange in anesthetized ponies.[33] These findings all suggest that high pressures are necessary to reopen closed airways in the lung of the anesthetized horse.

Ventilation Distribution

The reduction in FRC in the recumbent anesthetized horse presumably leads to airway closure in dependent regions, which is responsible in part for uneven distribution of ventilation, leading to ventilation perfusion inequalities and hypoxemia. The slope of phase III of the single-breath nitrogen washout curve is steeper in the laterally recumbent and supine horse than in the prone anesthetized horse.[29] This indicates that ventilation distribution is less uniform when the horse is not prone. The effect of posture on the relationship between FRC and the onset of airway closure is less clear. Although the onset of phase IV of the single-breath nitrogen washout curve (taken to be the onset of airway closure) occurs at higher lung volumes in lateral recumbency than in the prone posture, only in the supine posture does closing capacity exceed FRC (see Figure 2-8).[29] Scanning techniques show a progressive decrease in the ventilation-perfusion ratio from the top down in each lung of laterally recumbent horses, suggesting a reduction of ventilation in dependent regions.[34]

BLOOD FLOW

The lung receives blood flow from two circulations. The pulmonary circulation receives a total output of the right ventricle, perfuses the alveolar capillaries, and participates in gas exchange. The bronchial circulation, a branch of the systemic circulation, provides nutrient blood flow to airways and other structures within the lung.

Pulmonary Circulation

The main pulmonary arteries accompanying the bronchi are elastic, but the smaller arteries adjacent to the bronchioles and alveolar ducts are muscular. The terminal branches of the pulmonary arteries—the pulmonary arterioles—consist of endothelium and an elastic lamina and lead into the pulmonary capillaries, which form an extensive branching network of vessels within the alveolar septum. Not all capillaries are perfused in the resting animal, so that vessels can be recruited when pulmonary blood flow increases (e.g., during exercise). Pulmonary veins with thin walls conduct blood from capillaries to the left atrium and also form a reservoir of blood for the left ventricle.

Vascular Pressures and Resistance

Even though the pulmonary circulation receives the total output of the right ventricle, pulmonary arterial systolic, diastolic, and mean pressures average only 42, 18, and 26 mm Hg, respectively, in the horse at sea level.[35,36] This observation shows that the pulmonary circulation has a low vascular resistance compared with the systemic circulation (see Chapter 3). Pulmonary wedge pressure (mean 8 mm Hg) is only slightly greater than left atrial pressure, showing that the pulmonary veins provide very little resistance to blood flow. Pulmonary vascular resistance (PVR) is calculated as

$$PVR = (PPA - PLA)/\dot{Q}$$

where PPA is mean pulmonary arterial pressure, PLA is left atrial pressure, and $\dot{Q}$ is cardiac output.

Approximately half of vascular resistance in the pulmonary circulation is precapillary, and capillaries themselves provide a considerable portion of resistance to blood flow.

Unlike the systemic circulation, arterioles do not provide a large resistance, and consequently pulmonary capillary blood flow is pulsatile.

Passive Changes in Vascular Resistance

Passive changes in vascular resistance result from changes in lung and vascular volumes and transpulmonary, intravascular, and interstitial pressures. The changes in pulmonary vascular resistance during lung inflation reflect the opposing effects on capillaries and large vessels. At residual volume, pulmonary vascular resistance is high because arteries and veins are narrowed. As the lung inflates to FRC, resistance decreases, primarily because of dilation of arteries and veins. Further inflation above FRC increases vascular resistance, primarily because the cross-section of alveolar capillaries changes from circular to elliptical.

Pulmonary vascular resistance is low in the resting horse, and it decreases even further when pulmonary blood flow or arterial pressure increases, as occurs during exercise. Increasing either pulmonary arterial or left atrial pressure or increasing vascular volume decreases pulmonary vascular resistance by distending already perfused vessels and recruiting previously unperfused vessels.

Vasomotor Regulation

Although pulmonary arteries have both sympathetic and parasympathetic innervation, the function of this autonomic supply is unclear. The pulmonary vasculature is subjected to a variety of vasodilator and vasoconstrictor chemical mediators released from nerves and inflammatory cells. Some mediators such as catecholamines, bradykinin, and prostaglandins are metabolized by the vascular endothelium; thus the effects may be modified by endothelial damage. Prostaglandins maintain a tonic vasodilator effect on the pulmonary circulation. Nitric oxide is a pulmonary vasodilator that is released from the pulmonary endothelium during exercise[37,38] or under the influence of some endothelial-dependent vasodilators such as acetylcholine.[39] Administration of nitric oxide or its precursor nitroglycerin reduces pulmonary vascular resistance in resting horses[40] and foals[41] and therefore could provide temporary relief of pulmonary hypertension.

Alveolar hypoxia is a potent constrictor of small pulmonary arteries; this phenomenon is known as hypoxic pulmonary vasoconstriction (HPV). This response redistributes pulmonary blood flow toward better-ventilated regions of lung. The vasoconstrictor response to hypoxia is most vigorous in cattle and pigs, less vigorous in horses, and trivial in sheep and dogs. The response is more vigorous in neonates and older animals. There are also regional differences in the magnitude of hypoxic vasoconstriction that redistributes pulmonary blood flow to the dorsal caudal regions of the lung under hypoxic conditions.[42] Constriction of the pulmonary arteries in response to hypoxia involves oxidant and redox signaling that leads to a rise in intracellular calcium concentration within pulmonary arterial smooth muscle. Endothelial cell signals also seem to be important during sustained hypoxia.[43,44]

The ability of local alveolar hypoxia to cause a local reduction in blood flow has been clearly demonstrated.[45] Local blood flow is greatly reduced by a combination of vessel closure as the lung collapses and vasoconstriction in response to local hypoxia under conditions of atelectasis when there is no ventilation to a collapsed region of lung. The amount of flow redistribution away from the hypoxic region of lung is a complex function of the volume of the hypoxic region, pulmonary vascular pressures, and the degree of hypoxia.[45] Anesthetic agents tend to inhibit HPV and flow redistribution (see Pulmonary Blood Flow and its Distribution Under Anesthesia later in the chapter).

Distribution of Pulmonary Blood Flow

Until quite recently gravity was thought to be of major importance in the determination of the distribution of pulmonary blood flow; and elegant models that incorporated pulmonary arterial and venous pressures and alveolar pressure were used to explain the distribution of blood flow within the lung. Equine anesthesiologists were the first to question the role of gravity by demonstrating that the caudal part of the caudal lobe of the horse lung receives the greatest blood flow, regardless of the posture of the horse (Figures 2-10, A and B and 2-11, A and B).[46] Other groups[47-49] then showed that in standing quadrupeds, the dorsal caudal region of the lung receives the highest blood flow and this distribution becomes more accentuated during exercise, even in horses.[50] Regional distribution of blood flow is fractal;[51] the fractal dimension is determined by the branching pattern of the pulmonary circulation and the relative resistances of various vascular pathways. However, there are also regional differences in mechanisms controlling blood vessel diameter that play a part in the distribution.[39,42] However, gravity is not unimportant. In a laterally recumbent anesthetized horse, pulmonary hypotension could mean that the uppermost part of the upper lung is less well perfused than the more dependent parts of the lung. It is also worth noting that many anesthetic agents relax pulmonary vascular smooth muscle and this in itself may cause changes in resistance that alter the distribution of flow.

Bronchial Circulation

The bronchial circulation, which provides nutrient flow to airways, large vessels, and visceral pleura, receives approximately 2% of the output of the left ventricle.[52,53] Bronchial arteries follow the tracheobronchial tree to the terminal bronchioles, forming a plexus in the peribronchial connective tissue and under the epithelium along the length of the airways. Bronchial vessels anastomose with the pulmonary circulation at the level of the terminal bronchiole. Most anastomoses occur at the capillary or venular level. The bronchial blood flow to the large extrapulmonary airways drains into the azygos vein; intrapulmonary bronchial blood flow enters the pulmonary circulation at both the prepulmonary and postpulmonary capillary level.

Inflow pressure to the bronchial circulation is systemic arterial pressure, but outflow pressure varies, depending on whether venous drainage is by way of the azygos vein or pulmonary circulation. The bronchial artery blood flow is low in quietly standing horses and averages only 1% to 2% of pulmonary artery flow. Bronchial artery flow is reduced (about threefold) to a greater degree than pulmonary artery flow during halothane anesthesia and therefore is not responsible for an alveolar-arterial gradient during dorsal recumbency.[54] Changes in pressure in both the systemic and pulmonary vascular bed affect the magnitude of bronchial blood flow. Increasing systemic pressure increases flow,

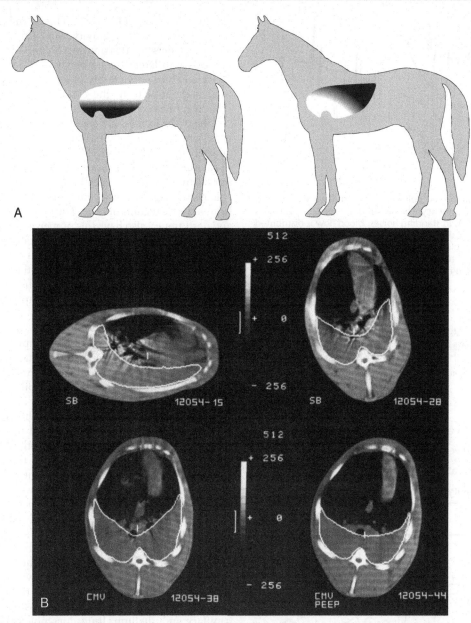

Figure 2–10. A, Distribution of blood flow in the lung of the horse at rest if gravity dependent *(left)* and in conscious horses *(right)*. **B,** Transverse computed tomography scans of a pony during anesthesia in left lateral recumbency *(upper left)*, dorsal recumbency *(upper right)*, mechanical ventilation *(lower left)*, and mechanical ventilation with PEEP of 10 cm H₂O *(lower right)*. Note the appearance of large dense areas encircled by a white line in dependent lung regions. Note also the heart as a white area in the middle of the thorax. (**A** From Marlin DJ, Vincent TL: Pulmonary blood flow. In McGorum BC et al, editors: *Equine respiratory medicine and surgery,* Edinburgh, 2007, Saunders Elsevier, p 37. **B** From Nyman G et al: Atelectasis causes gas exchange impairment in the anaesthetized horse, *Equine Vet J* 22:320, 1990.)

but increasing pulmonary vascular pressures (downstream pressure) reduces and may even reverse flow.

Pulmonary Blood Flow and Its Distribution Under Anesthesia

Anesthesia results in changes in posture, lung volumes, cardiac output, and vascular pressures and resistance, all of which can alter blood flow distribution that contributes to the mismatching of ventilation and blood flow (Box 2-1). Changes in cardiac output alter not only the distribution of blood flow and gas exchange in the lung but also the delivery of oxygen to the tissues. For this reason, there have been

many studies of the effects of anesthetic agents on cardiac function (see Chapters 3, 10, 12, and 15).

Positive-pressure ventilation and PEEP tend to decrease cardiac output (see Chapter 17). These procedures decrease venous return to the right atrium by increasing intrathoracic pressure. Positive-pressure ventilation also increases alveolar pressure, which compresses pulmonary capillaries and increases pulmonary vascular resistance (see Chapter 17 Figure 2-12). Sometimes high airway pressures coupled with PEEP are necessary to improve oxygen exchange under anesthesia. A recent paper suggested that this can be done in ponies with only slight detriments to cardiovascular function.[33]

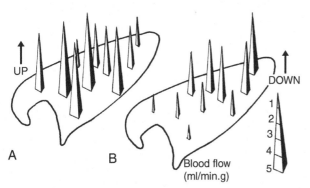

Figure 2-11. Distribution of pulmonary blood flow in standing horses and in dorsal recumbency. The height of the pyramid indicates the magnitude of flow. **A**, In standing horses, blood flow is distributed preferentially to the cranial and ventral portions of the lung. **B**, In dorsally recumbent horses, blood flow is distributed preferentially to the caudal dorsal portions of the lung. (From Dobson A et al: Changes in blood flow distribution in equine lungs induced by anesthesia, *Q J Exp Physiol* 70:288, 1985.)

Box 2-1	Factors Affecting Blood Flow Distribution in the Horse's Lung

- Cardiac output
- Posture
- Lung volume
- Vascular pressures and resistance
- Positive-pressure ventilation
- Positive end-expiratory pressure (PEEP)
- Hypoxic pulmonary vasoconstriction (HPV)

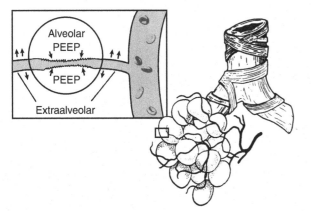

Figure 2-12. Schematic showing the effects of PEEP on ventilation and capillary blood flow in the anesthetized horse.

Before the distribution of blood flow was measured in the lungs of anesthetized horses, their poor oxygen exchange was hypothesized to be a result of the preferential distribution of blood flow to the poorly ventilated dependent lung. However, actual measurements of blood flow distribution using microspheres demonstrated that this is not the case. In dorsally (supine) recumbent horses, blood flow is distributed preferentially to the most dependent lung region, the diaphragmatic lobe adjacent to the spine and the diaphragm

(Figures 2-10, *B* and 2-11).[46] This is the distribution that might be expected if gravity were the dominating force. However, the same distribution of blood flow persists when horses are in lateral recumbency and even in the standing conscious horse. Therefore blood flow seems to be distributed preferentially to the caudal most part of the caudal lobe, regardless of the animals' posture.[46,47]

One of the factors that could affect blood flow distribution is HPV, which normally redistributes flow to the better-oxygenated alveoli (see Box 2-1). Halothane, enflurane, and isoflurane depress HPV in a concentration-dependent manner[55,56] so that animals that are anesthetized with these agents are less able than unanesthetized animals to divert blood flow away from hypoxic regions of lung. The newer agents sevoflurane[57] and desflurane[58] also have this propensity, but the effect is not as clinically important.[59-61] Nitrous oxide, barbiturates, and propofol[62,63] have less depressant effects on hypoxic constriction than the halogenated agents. For the latter reason PaO_2 is better maintained under propofol than with halogenated agents when one lung needs to be collapsed during surgery.

Pulmonary Fluid Exchange

The lung continuously produces lymph as a result of the net fluid movement from the pulmonary microvasculature into the pulmonary interstitium. Normally the lymphatics remove fluid from the arterioles, capillaries, and veins at the same rate as it is produced in the alveoli and therefore remain dry.[64] This is even the case in the exercising horse in which 5 or more liters per minute of fluid are transferred from the pulmonary circulation into the lung.[65] When the capacity of lymphatics is overloaded, fluid accumulates in the pulmonary interstitium and eventually leaks into the alveoli, resulting in pulmonary edema.

Fluid filtration normally occurs between the capillary and the interstitial tissue on the "thick" side of the alveolar septum where a layer of interstitium is interposed between the endothelium and the epithelial basement membrane. On the "thin" side of the septum, the capillary endothelium shares a basement membrane with the alveolar epithelium, and there is no interstitial tissue (Figure 2-13). Because the alveolar epithelium is less permeable than the capillary endothelium, fluid does not leak into the alveoli unless the epithelium is damaged or there is considerable fluid accumulation in the interstitium.

Forces described in the Starling equation govern the movement of fluid across the endothelium:

$$Qf = Kfc[(Pmv - Pif) - \alpha(\pi mv - \pi if)]$$

where Qf is the amount of fluid flowing per minute, Kfc is the capillary filtration coefficient, Pmv is microvascular hydrostatic pressure, Pif is interstitial fluid hydrostatic pressure, πmv and πif are microvascular and interstitial colloid osmotic (oncotic) pressures, respectively; and α is the colloid reflection coefficient (see Figure 2-13).

The net filtration force favors fluid movement from the capillaries to the interstitium of the lung (see Figure 2-13). The fluid flux between the capillaries in the interstitium varies with changes in vascular permeability and hydrostatic and oncotic pressures. Left heart failure or the excessive administration of intravenous fluids raises capillary hydrostatic pressure, which increases fluid filtration across pulmonary capillaries and may cause pulmonary edema. Pulmonary

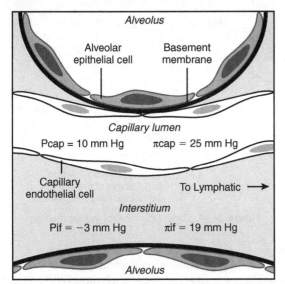

Figure 2–13. Forces determining fluid filtration across the alveolar capillary. *Pcap,* Capillary hydrostatic pressure; *Pif,* interstitial fluid hydrostatic pressure; *πcap,* capillary oncotic pressure; *πif,* interstitial fluid oncotic pressure. Note the shared basement membrane between the epithelium and endothelium on one side of the capillary and the wider interstitial space on the other side of the capillary. Note also the tighter junctions between alveolar epithelial cells and between capillary endothelial cells.

edema can result from a decrease in plasma oncotic pressure (hypoproteinemia), which can be caused by starvation or overly vigorous administration of intravenous fluids. Increased vascular permeability occurs after severe hypoxia and in many inflammatory lung diseases such as pneumonia because of the effects of neutrophil products, probably oxygen radicals, on the endothelium. Protein-rich fluid leaks into the interstitium, elevating interstitial fluid oncotic pressure and causing osmotic attraction of water from the vasculature.

Fluid filtered from capillaries moves through the interstitium toward the perivascular and peribronchial tissues where lymphatics are located. Lymphatic vasomotion, valves, and the pumping action of the lungs during breathing aid fluid transport along lymphatics. Lymphatics can accommodate large increases in fluid flux, and compliant peribronchial and perivascular spaces also provide intrapulmonary sinks for fluid accumulation. Fluid does not accumulate in the lung unless there is a large increase in the amount of fluid

being filtered from the capillaries. Alveolar flooding occurs after the peribronchial capacity is exceeded; fluid probably enters the airspaces across the alveolar epithelial cells or at the level of the bronchioles. The foaming of clinical pulmonary edema results from the mixing of air, edema fluid, and surfactant within the airways.

Changes in vascular permeability in the lung and pleura can be a complicating factor in anesthesia. Sepsis and endotoxin both increase fluid flux from the pulmonary vasculature. An increase in pulmonary vascular pressure caused, for example, by intravenous fluid administration, could cause pulmonary edema in a horse exposed to gram-negative bacterial endotoxin. In addition, pulmonary edema associated with airway obstruction could result in negative-pressure pulmonary edema (NPPE). Inspiratory efforts against a closed glottis can cause a precipitous decrease in mean intrathoracic pressure and an increased transmural pressure gradient for all intrathoracic vascular structures. The large transmural pressure gradient at the level of the capillary increases permeability and alters Starling forces; both changes promote the movement of fluid from capillaries to the interstitial space. When the transmural pressure gradient is large enough, stress failure of the capillary occurs, resulting in hemorrhagic pulmonary edema.[66] Recent evidence suggests that anesthetics such as propofol and isoflurane may provide some protection for the lung against oxidant stress that accompanies endotoxemia and other injuries.[67,68]

GAS EXCHANGE

Alveolar Gas Composition

Air contains 21% oxygen both at sea level and on the top of Mount Everest. Despite the similarity of oxygen percentage, climbers become hypoxic on Mount Everest because it is not the fraction of oxygen that is important for gas exchange; rather, it is the partial pressure (also called tension) and, more important, the partial pressure difference between the two parts of the body that results in gas transfer (Table 2-2).

The oxygen tension of a dry gas mixture is determined by barometric pressure (PB) and the fraction of oxygen (FiO_2) in the gas mixture:

$$PO_2 = PB \times FiO_2$$

Table 2–2.	Effect of altitude on oxygen partial pressure			
Altitude (feet)	Altitude (meters)	Barometric pressure (mm Hg)	PiO_2 ($FiO_2 = 0.21$)	PAO_2 ($FiO_2 = 0.21$)
Sea level	—	760	159.6	109.6
500	153	733	156.7	106.7
1000	305	746.3	153.9	103.9
2000	610	706.6	148.4	98.4
3000	915	681.2	143.1	93.1
4000	1220	656.3	137.8	87.8
5000	1526	632.5	132.8	82.8
10,000	3050	522.7	109.8	59.8

FiO_2, Fraction of inspired oxygen; PiO_2, partial pressure of inspired oxygen, PAO_2, alveolar partial pressure of oxygen.
The calculated PAO_2 assumes a $PaCO_2$ of 40 mm Hg. However, as animals ascend to altitude, they hyperventilate in response to the hypoxia; therefore $PaCO_2$ decreases with increasing altitude. This tends to raise the PAO_2.

Atmospheric FiO_2 is 0.2; thus PiO_2 in dry air at sea level is 160 mm Hg:

$$PiO_2 = 760 \times 0.21 = 160 \, mm \, Hg$$

In cities at high altitude such as Denver (5280 ft), PB is 633 mm Hg; thus PO_2 is also low (133 mm Hg).

During inhalation air is warmed to body temperature and humidified. The concentration of other gases is reduced by the presence of water vapor molecules; therefore PO_2 decreases slightly as inhaled air enters the body. The PO_2 of humidified gas is calculated as:

$$PO_2 = (PB - PH_2O) \times FiO$$

where PH_2O is the partial pressure of water vapor at the body temperature (50 mm Hg at the horses's normal temperature of 38° C) and FiO_2 is the fraction of oxygen in inspired air. Therefore the PO_2 of warmed, completely humidified gas in the conducting airways is:

$$PO_2 (760-50) \times 0.21 = 149 \, mm \, Hg$$

The average alveolar oxygen tension (PAO_2) can be calculated from the alveolar gas equation:

$$PAO_2 = (PB - PH_2O) \times FiO_2 - PACO_2/R$$

This equation shows that alveolar oxygen tension is determined by the inspired oxygen tension and the exchange of oxygen for carbon dioxide. The respiratory exchange ratio (R): CO_2 production/O_2 consumption. Assuming R = 0.8, $FiO_2 = 0.21$, $PACO_2 = 40$ mm Hg, $PH_2O = 50$ mm Hg, and PB = 760 mm Hg, PAO_2 averages 99 mm Hg at sea level.

The more clinically useful form of the alveolar gas equation substitutes arterial carbon dioxide partial pressure ($PaCO_2$) for $PACO_2$ as follows:

$$PAO_2 = (PB - PH_2O) \times FiO_2 - PaCO_2/R$$

The amount of carbon dioxide in inspired air is negligible. Exchange of oxygen and carbon dioxide occurs continually within the alveoli. The alveolar partial pressure of carbon dioxide ($PACO_2$) is determined by CO_2 production ($\dot{V}CO_2$) in relation to alveolar ventilation (VA):

$$PACO_2 = K \times \dot{V}CO_2/VA$$

For clinical purposes, this equation can also be written:

$$PaCO_2 = K \times \dot{V}CO_2/VA$$

This equation shows that, if $\dot{V}CO_2$ increases, VA must also increase if $PACO_2$ and therefore $PaCO_2$ remain constant. If VA does not increase sufficiently, $PACO_2$ and $PaCO_2$ increase. Similarly, if $\dot{V}CO_2$ remains constant and VA decreases, $PACO_2$ and $PaCO_2$ increase. The alveolar gas equation shows that, whenever $PACO_2$ increases, PAO_2 decreases and vice versa.

The inverse relationship between $PACO_2$ and VA is made use of when capnography is used to monitor ventilation during anesthesia. A capnograph continually measures the percentage or partial pressure of CO_2 in the expired air (see Chapter 8). When it is attached to the endotracheal tube of the anesthetized horse, the end-tidal PCO_2 provides a reasonable estimate of $PACO_2$ and $PaCO_2$ for routine monitoring of ventilation. However, in critical cases it is advisable to monitor blood gas tensions directly because ventilation/perfusion inequalities can result in a difference between end-tidal and arterial PCO_2 ($ETCO_2$-$PaCO_2$ gap).[69]

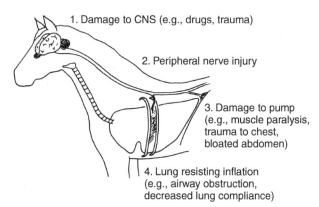

1. Damage to CNS (e.g., drugs, trauma)

2. Peripheral nerve injury

3. Damage to pump (e.g., muscle paralysis, trauma to chest, bloated abdomen)

4. Lung resisting inflation (e.g., airway obstruction, decreased lung compliance)

Figure 2–14. Causes of alveolar hypoventilation.

Alveolar hypoventilation, a decrease in alveolar ventilation in relation to CO_2 production, elevates $PACO_2$ ($PaCO_2$) and decreases PAO_2. Alveolar hypoventilation is observed when tranquilizers, sedatives, anesthetic drugs, or injury depresses the central nervous system; when there is severe airway obstruction; or when there is damage to the thorax and respiratory muscles (Figure 2-14). Use of inhalation anesthetics is routinely associated with alveolar hypoventilation in horses, and for this reason positive pressure ventilation should always be available.[70]

The $PACO_2$ (and $PaCO_2$) decrease during alveolar hyperventilation because ventilation is greater than needed to eliminate CO_2 being produced by the body. Hyperventilation occurs when the drive to ventilate is increased by stimuli such as hypoxia, increased production of hydrogen ions, or an increase in body temperature. Animals kept at high altitude routinely hyperventilate to increase the delivery of oxygen to their lungs. For this reason it is usual for $PaCO_2$ to be less than the normal of 40 to 45 mm Hg in areas such as the Rocky Mountain States. Overly vigorous use of the ventilator also can cause hypoventilation in the anesthetized horse.

Diffusion

Mixing of gases in the terminal airspaces and exchange of oxygen and carbon dioxide between the alveolus and pulmonary capillary blood and between systemic capillaries and tissues occurs by diffusion. The physical properties of the gas, the surface area available for diffusion (A), the thickness of the air-blood area (x), and the driving pressure gradient of the gas between the alveolus and the capillary blood (PAgas – Pcapgas) determine the rate of gas movements between the alveolus and the blood:

$$VO_2 = [D \times A \times (PAgas - Pcapgas)]/x$$

The alveolar surface area available for diffusion is that part of the surface that is occupied by perfused pulmonary capillaries. When pulmonary vascular pressures increase (e.g., during exercise), the surface area available for diffusion increases because previously unperfused capillaries are recruited. When pulmonary arterial pressure decreases (e.g., during hypovolemic shock), loss of perfused capillaries decreases the available surface area for gas exchange.

The barrier separating air and blood, which is less than 1 μm thick in the lung, includes a layer of liquid and surfactant lining the alveolar surface, an epithelial layer (usually from type I epithelial cells), a basement membrane and variable thickness interstitium, and a layer of endothelium. For oxygen to be brought into contact with the erythrocyte and hemoglobin, it must also diffuse through the plasma.

The driving pressure for gas diffusion ($PAO_2 - PcapO_2$) varies during inhalation and exhalation and also along the length of the capillary. Cyclic fluctuations in PAO_2 occur as fresh air is delivered to the lung. Blood enters the lung with a low PO_2, which then rises progressively as blood flows along the alveolar capillaries. Alveolar oxygen tension (PAO_2) averages 100 mm Hg, and in the resting animal mixed venous blood entering the lung has an oxygen tension (PvO_2) of approximately 40 mm Hg. The driving pressure gradient of 60 mm Hg causes rapid diffusion of oxygen into the capillary, where it combines with hemoglobin. Hemoglobin provides a sink for oxygen and helps maintain a gradient for oxygen diffusion. Normally equilibration between alveoli and capillary oxygen tensions occurs within 0.25 seconds, approximately one third of the time the blood is in the capillary.

The PAO_2 and therefore the driving pressure for oxygen transfer are increased when horses breathe oxygen-enriched gas mixtures. For example, when a horse breathes 100% oxygen, PAO_2 is over 600 mm Hg, and the driving pressure for oxygen diffusion is more than 500 mm Hg ($PaO_2 \approx FiO_2 \times 5$). Carbon dioxide is 20 times more diffusible than oxygen because of its greater solubility. For this reason, transfer of carbon dioxide is accomplished with a lesser driving pressure gradient ($PACO_2 = 40$ mm Hg, $PvCO_2 = 46$ mm Hg), and failure of diffusion equilibrium for carbon dioxide is rare.

Matching of the Ventilation and Blood Flow

Gas exchange is accomplished by the close approximation of air and blood in the peripheral airspaces of the lung. The matching of ventilation to blood flow ($\dot{V}/\dot{Q}$ matching) is the most important determinant of gas exchange. Examination of the distribution of $\dot{V}/\dot{Q}$ ratios in the standing horse by use of the multiple inert gas technique has confirmed that, despite its size, the horse, like other mammals, has a narrow distribution of $\dot{V}/\dot{Q}$ ratios (i.e., ventilation and blood flow are well matched) (Table 2-3 and Figure 2-15).[71,72]

Anesthesia and disease cause abnormalities in the distribution of both ventilation and blood flow. This causes $\dot{V}/\dot{Q}$ inequalities and therefore impairs gas exchange (see Fig. 2-15; Figure 2-16). The ideal gas exchange unit in the lung receives ventilation and blood flow with a $\dot{V}/\dot{Q}$ ratio of 0.8. Other regions of the lung receive a reduced amount of ventilation but continue to receive blood flow.

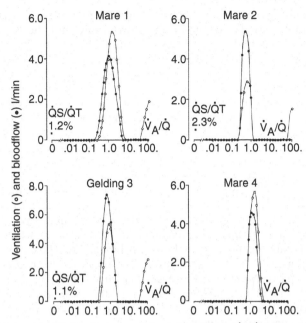

Figure 2–15. Ventilation-perfusion distribution ($\dot{V}A/\dot{Q}$). Horse 4 shows good matching of ventilation and perfusion with unimodal distributions and a narrow base. Horses 1, 2, and 3 show bimodal $\dot{V}A/\dot{Q}$ distributions with an additional mode within high $\dot{V}A/\dot{Q}$ regions. Moreover, minor shunts ($\dot{Q}S/\dot{Q}T$) are seen in horses 1, 2, and 3. (From Hedenstierna G et al: Ventilation-perfusion relationships in the standing horse: an inert gas elimination study, *Equine Vet J* 19:517, 1987.)

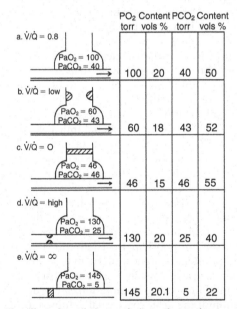

Figure 2–16. The effect of ventilation-perfusion ratios on the composition of pulmonary capillary blood. **A,** Normal alveolus with a $\dot{V}/\dot{Q}$ ratio of 0.8. The composition of mixed venous and capillary blood is shown. **B,** Low $\dot{V}/\dot{Q}$ ratio caused by an incomplete airway obstruction. This results in low oxygen content and increased carbon dioxide content. **C,** Right-to-left shunt ($\dot{V}/\dot{Q} = 0$) caused by a complete airway obstruction. The capillary blood leaving the alveolus has the same composition as mixed venous blood. **D,** High $\dot{V}/\dot{Q}$ ratio unit caused by incomplete obstruction of the pulmonary artery. Pulmonary artery CO_2 content is decreased, but oxygen content is not increased because of the shape of the oxyhemoglobin dissociation curve. **E,** Alveolar dead space ($\dot{V}/\dot{Q}$ = infinity) caused by complete obstruction of a blood vessel. The capillary blood adjacent to the alveolus has the same composition as the alveolar gas but does not participate in overall gas exchange because there is no net blood flow past this alveolus.

Table 2–3.	Ventilation-perfusion ($\dot{V}/\dot{Q}$) relationships and associated blood gas abnormalities[92]	
$\dot{V}/\dot{Q}$ Ratio	**Term**	**Consequences**
1	$\dot{V}/\dot{Q}$ Match	Normal PaO_2
>1	Dead space ventilation	↓PaO_2, ↑$PaCO_2$
<1	Venous admixture	↓PaO_2 Normal or ↓$PaCO_2$

Modified from Marino PL: *The ICU Book*, ed 3, Philadelphia, 2007, Lippincott Williams & Wilkins, p 368.

Such regions are said to have low $\dot{V}/\dot{Q}$. The oxygen content of blood leaving such regions is low, and the CO_2 content is high. The extreme form of low $\dot{V}/\dot{Q}$ ratio is a right-to-left shunt, which has a $\dot{V}/\dot{Q}$ ratio of zero. Normal horses have an intrapulmonary shunt fraction of less than 1%,[71] but the venous outflow of the bronchial and coronary veins into the oxygenated blood leaving the lungs may result in a total shunt fraction of 5%. Right-to-left shunts can occur within the lung (e.g., through areas of atelectasis or through complex cardiac defects such as tetralogy of Fallot). When blood passes through a right-to-left shunt, it does not participate in gas exchange, and the blood leaving such a region of lung has the same composition as mixed venous blood. When this blood mixes with oxygenated blood coming from the normal parts of the lung, it causes hypoxemia, the magnitude of which depends on the size of the shunt blood flow (Box 2-2). Right-to-left shunts slow the rate of increase of the arterial partial pressure of inhalant anesthetics but speed the delivery of injectable anesthetics to the systemic circulation, thereby slowing and speeding the production of anesthesia respectively.

Right-to-left shunts are relatively unusual in unanesthetized animals, but less extreme low $\dot{V}/\dot{Q}$ regions of lung are very common. These arise when regional ventilation is decreased by bronchial or bronchiolar obstruction with mucus or bronchospasm, by stiffening of the lung parenchyma as a consequence of fibrosis, or when there is alveolar flooding with edema or exudates. In the anesthetized horse low $\dot{V}/\dot{Q}$ regions can occur because portions of the dependent lung may not be ventilating well but continue to receive blood flow.[73] The amount of shunting increases because of resorption atelectasis when such anesthetized animals breathe oxygen rather than air.[74]

Ventilation is high in relation to blood flow in high $\dot{V}/\dot{Q}$ regions of lung. This occurs when pulmonary blood flow to part of the lung is reduced (e.g., by pulmonary hypotension). The blood leaving such a unit has a higher PO_2 and a lower PCO_2 and blood from an ideal $\dot{V}/\dot{Q}$ unit. The CO_2 content of this blood is low, but because of the shape of the oxyhemoglobin dissociation curve, the oxygen content of the blood is increased only trivially. The extreme form of high $\dot{V}/\dot{Q}$ is dead space, which has a $\dot{V}/\dot{Q}$ ratio of infinity. Anatomic dead space is the volume of the conducting airways, and alveolar dead space describes the air ventilating unperfused or poorly perfused alveoli. The latter can occur when pulmonary arterial pressure is so low that capillaries are unperfused or when vessels are obstructed by thrombi. The amount of wasted ventilation can be determined by calculation of the dead space/tidal volume ratio (VD/VT) (the Bohr equation):

$$VD/VT = (PaCO_2 - PECO_2)/PaCO_2$$

where $PECO_2$ equals the partial pressure of CO_2 in mixed expired gas. Blood in the pulmonary veins is composed of venous blood from thousands of individual gas exchange units with a whole variety of $\dot{V}/\dot{Q}$ ratios. The PO_2 and PCO_2 of this blood is not a simple flow-weighted average of the constituent tensions. The total gas content must be considered because oxygen and CO_2 are transported in chemical combination and in solution. An elevation of PO_2 in blood from high $\dot{V}/\dot{Q}$ regions does not compensate for the depressed

PO_2 and oxygen content from the low $\dot{V}/\dot{Q}$ regions because of the shape of the oxyhemoglobin dissociation curve. For this reason $\dot{V}/\dot{Q}$ inequalities usually cause hypoxemia (low PaO_2). Because the CO_2 dissociation curve is almost linear over the physiological range and because mixed venous and ideal alveolar PCO_2 differ only by approximately 6 mm Hg, $\dot{V}/\dot{Q}$ inequalities generally do not elevate $PaCO_2$.

Increasing overall $\dot{V}/\dot{Q}$ inequality depresses PaO_2 and increases the alveolar dead space, venous admixture, and the alveolar-arterial oxygen difference [(PA-aO_2)]. Normally the PA-aO_2 is less than 20 mm Hg. This difference occurs because there is a degree of $\dot{V}/\dot{Q}$ inequality even in normal lungs and because venous blood draining the bronchial and coronary circulations mixes with the oxygenated blood draining from the alveoli.

Box 2–2   Determining the Magnitude of $\dot{V}/\dot{Q}$ Inequality and Shunting

Distribution of ventilation and perfusion can be evaluated by use of scanning techniques. Ventilation distribution is evaluated after horses have inhaled radiolabeled gases (krypton) and perfusion scans after intravenous injection of neutron activated microspheres (e.g., gold). Even if ventilation and perfusion scans are conducted almost simultaneously, it is difficult to use them to determine $\dot{V}/\dot{Q}$ matching in the various regions of the lung.

For the latter purpose the multiple inert gas technique was developed. A number of gases of varying solubility are dissolved in saline and infused intravenously. As blood passes through the lung, these gases come out of solution to differing degrees, depending on the $\dot{V}/\dot{Q}$ ratio of a region of lung. If the blood gas partition coefficient of each inert gas is known, by collecting the expired air, a model of the lung $\dot{V}/\dot{Q}$ distribution can be derived to explain the elimination and retention of these gases. This technique has provided a lot of valuable information that helps in understanding $\dot{V}/\dot{Q}$ distributions in a variety of conditions, including the anesthetized horse. However, unfortunately the technique is too cumbersome to be used routinely in clinical situations.

The magnitude of right-to-left shunting can be determined by allowing animals to breathe 100% oxygen for 15 minutes. This causes the blood leaving ventilated alveoli to be saturated with oxygen. The shunt fraction can then be calculated as:

$$Qs/Qt = (Cc'O_2 - CaO_2)/(Cc'O_2 - CvO_2)$$

where C = oxygen content in arterial (a), mixed venous (v), and pulmonary capillary (c') blood. $Cc'O_2$ is calculated from PAO_2 assuming 100% saturation of hemoglobin (see Figure 2-18). The magnitude of the A-aDO_2 when an animal is breathing pure oxygen is an indication of the amount of blood passing through shunts.

In the normal lung end-tidal and arterial PCO_2 are almost identical. As the magnitude of $\dot{V}/\dot{Q}$ mismatching increases, especially the regions of high $\dot{V}/\dot{Q}$ that constitute the alveolar dead space, end-tidal PCO_2 becomes less than $PaCO_2$, and an arterial to end-tidal PCO_2 ($P_{a-ET}CO_2$) gradient develops. Measurement of this gradient has been used to evaluate $\dot{V}/\dot{Q}$ matching in anesthetized horses.[77]

Ventilation Perfusion Matching Under Anesthesia

There is an almost immediate large increase in the alveolar-arterial oxygen difference when a horse is anesthetized, which is reflected in a decrease in PaO$_2$, particularly when the horse is positioned on its back (Table 2-4 and Figure 2-17).[22,27] Subsequently PA-aO$_2$ increases only slightly over time.[22] The PA-aO$_2$ is greater in dorsal than lateral recumbency and is quite small when the horse is in the prone posture.[75-77] Gas exchange immediately improves when horses are turned from dorsal recumbency to the prone position, suggesting that atelectasis is not the major cause of the large PA-aO$_2$.[75] However, minimal improvement in gas exchange occurs after horses have been in dorsal recumbency for more than 2 hours and then are turned to lateral recumbency. Inhalant anesthesia is an essential component of impaired gas exchange because recumbency alone does not cause hypoxemia.[77]

Measurements of the distribution of $\dot{V}/\dot{Q}$ ratios in the anesthetized horse lung by means of the multiple inert gas technique show that the fraction of cardiac output passing through right-to-left shunts is much greater in anesthetized than in awake horses and also is greater in dorsal than in lateral recumbency.[73] Interestingly, anesthesia does not produce a large increase in blood flow to low $\dot{V}/\dot{Q}$ regions except for right-to-left shunts (see Figure 2-15). These findings suggest that gas exchange impairment during anesthesia results from blood flow to regions of lung that are not ventilated rather than blood flow to regions served by intermittently closed airways. Right-to-left shunts can be reduced by selective mechanical ventilation of the dependent lung regions.[30] This tends to confirm that the persistent airway closure is the cause of shunting.

Anesthesia also is associated with an increase in the amount of physiological dead space, especially when horses are in dorsal recumbency. The increase in physiological dead space is less when ventilation is controlled compared to spontaneous breathing.[78]

Use of dissociative anesthetics in combination with α$_2$-agonists has become a popular method of anesthesia for short-duration procedures in the field. The gas exchange problems associated with these anesthetic techniques are less than with inhalant anesthetics;[79,80] and for this reason dissociative anesthesia is very suitable for use in the field. Although some $\dot{V}/\dot{Q}$ abnormalities are associated with these procedures, hypoventilation does not occur, right-to-left vascular shunts do not develop, there is no diffusion limitation, and delivery of oxygen to the tissues is maintained quite well. When anesthetized horses breathe air, slight hypoxemia may develop. Although administering 100% oxygen increases PaO$_2$ as expected, this results in an increase in right-to-left shunting, most likely because the presence of pure oxygen in the dependent alveoli leads to absorption atelectasis. For the latter reason and because tissue oxygenation is maintained with air breathing, it may not be necessary to supplement recumbent horses with oxygen when dissociative anesthetic methods are used in the field.

Blood Gas Tensions

Arterial oxygen (PaO$_2$) and carbon dioxide (PaCO$_2$) tensions are the end result of the individual processes involved in gas exchange and therefore are affected by the composition of inspired air, alveolar ventilation, alveolar-capillary diffusion, and ventilation-perfusion matching. Blood gas tensions are measured in arterial samples that are obtained anaerobically and kept on ice until measurements can be made with an accurately calibrated blood gas machine. Blood gas tensions increase with increasing temperature; thus for accurate work, especially calculations of gas exchange, the blood gas values should be corrected to body temperature rather than reported at the temperature of the blood gas machine.[94] For routine monitoring temperature correction is not necessary (Table 2-5).

Conscious horses usually breathe air containing 20.9% oxygen (FiO$_2$ = 0.209), but under anesthesia FiO$_2$ is often increased, resulting in an increase in PiO$_2$. The daily fluctuations in barometric pressure caused by atmospheric

Table 2–4.	Sources of hypoxemia[93]	
Source	A-a PO$_2$	PvO$_2$
Hypoventilation	Normal	Normal
$\dot{V}/\dot{Q}$ mismatch	Increased	Normal
DO$_2$/VO$_2$ imbalance	Increased	Decreased

A-a PO$_2$, alveolar-arterial oxygen difference; *DO$_2$*, oxygen delivery; *PvO$_2$*, venous oxygen tension; *VO$_2$*, oxygen uptake. Modified from Marino PL: *The ICU Book*, ed 3, Philadelphia, 2007, Lippincott Williams & Wilkins, p 375.

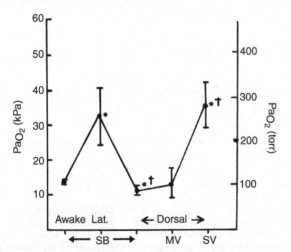

Figure 2–17. Arterial oxygen tension (mean ± SEM) in the awake standing horse (FiO$_2$ = 0.21) and during anesthesia in the lateral and dorsal recumbent positions (FiO$_2$ >0.92). *SB*, Spontaneous breathing; *MV*, general mechanical ventilation; *SV*, selective mechanical ventilation with PEEP 20 cm H$_2$O; *, significantly different from the awake value; †, significantly different from the previous value. (From Nyman G et al: Selective mechanical ventilation of dependent lung regions in the anesthetized horse in dorsal recumbency, *Br J Anesth* 59:1031, 1987.)

Table 2–5.	Effect of temperature on PO$_2$, PCO$_2$, and pH		
Temperature (°C)	PO$_2$	PCO$_2$	pH
39	91	44	7.37
37	80	40	7.40
30	51	30	7.50

conditions cause only trivial changes in PiO_2, but the decrease in barometric pressure that occurs at higher altitudes results in a major decrease in PiO_2 (see Table 2-2). Altitude-induced changes in PiO_2 must always be considered when evaluating blood gas tensions.

Examining $PaCO_2$ assesses adequacy of alveolar ventilation. The $PaCO_2$ is elevated above the normal value of around 40 mm Hg when animals hypoventilate and is decreased during hyperventilation. Hypoventilation also decreases PAO_2 and PaO_2; hyperventilation increases these tensions. Horses anesthetized with inhalant or injectable anesthetic drugs tend to hypoventilate because of the depressant effects of anesthetic drugs on respiratory control centers and muscle respiration, including the diaphragm. Changes in alveolar ventilation affect PaO_2 but, in the absence of changes in $\dot{V}/\dot{Q}$ distribution, do not change the $PA\text{-}aO_2$.

Diffusion abnormalities, $\dot{V}/\dot{Q}$ mismatching, and right-to-left shunts impair the transfer of oxygen from the alveolus to arterial blood, increase the $PA\text{-}aO_2$, and reduce PaO_2. $PaCO_2$ is rarely elevated by these problems because the hypoxemia stimulates ventilation, keeping $PaCO_2$ normal or even below normal.

Increasing FiO_2 elevates PaO_2 in horses with normal lungs. As $\dot{V}/\dot{Q}$ mismatching becomes more extreme (especially in the presence of right-to-left shunts), increasing FiO_2 increases PaO_2 only modestly. Concurrently the $PA\text{-}aO_2$ widens.

Many anesthetic drugs decrease cardiac output. When this occurs, the PO_2 of mixed venous blood decreases because of reduced delivery of oxygen to the tissues in the face of continuing oxygen demand. This decrease in mixed venous oxygen tension reduces PaO_2 and increases the $PA\text{-}aO_2$ (even if the degree of $\dot{V}/\dot{Q}$ inequality or the shunt fraction remains unchanged). This occurs because the mixed venous blood with low oxygen content is passing through shunts and low $\dot{V}/\dot{Q}$ regions and being mixed with the oxygenated blood leaving the remainder of the lung.

Gas Transport

When blood in the pulmonary capillaries flows past the alveoli, oxygen diffuses from the alveolus into the blood until the partial pressures equilibrate (i.e., there is no further driving pressure difference). Some of the oxygen dissolves in the plasma; but, because oxygen is poorly soluble, most combines with hemoglobin. Even though the amount of oxygen dissolved in plasma is small, it increases directly as partial pressure increases. Approximately 0.3 ml of oxygen dissolves in each deciliter of blood at the normal PAO_2 of 100 mm Hg. When a horse breathes pure oxygen, PaO_2 about 600 mm Hg, 1.8 ml of oxygen dissolves in each deciliter of plasma.

Hemoglobin

Mammalian hemoglobin consists of four-unit molecules, each containing one heme and its associated protein. Heme is a protoporphyrin consisting of four pyrroles with a ferrous iron at the center. The ferrous iron combines reversibly with oxygen in proportion to PO_2. The hemoglobin molecule is spheroidal; an amino acid side chain is attached to each heme. The amino acid composition of the side chains and their conformation greatly affects the affinity of hemoglobin for oxygen and defines the different types of

mammalian hemoglobin. Adult hemoglobin contains two α- and two β-amino acid chains. Each hemoglobin molecule can reversibly bind up to four molecules of oxygen. The reversible combination of oxygen with hemoglobin is shown in the oxyhemoglobin dissociation curve (Figure 2-18).

The oxygen content of blood (i.e., the oxygen combined with hemoglobin) is determined by PO_2 (Box 2-3; see Figure 2-18). The oxyhemoglobin dissociation curve is virtually flat above a PO_2 of approximately 70 mm Hg. Further increases in PO_2 add little oxygen to hemoglobin, and the hemoglobin is said to be saturated with oxygen. When saturated, 1 g of hemoglobin can hold 1.36 to 1.39 ml of oxygen. Therefore blood from a resting horse with 15 g of hemoglobin per deciliter has an oxygen capacity of 21 ml of oxygen per deciliter of blood (volumes percent).

The oxyhemoglobin dissociation curve has a steep slope below PO_2 of 60 mm Hg. This is the range of tissue PO_2 at which oxygen is unloaded from the blood. Tissue PO_2 varies, depending on the blood flow/metabolism ratio, but "average" tissue PO_2 is 40 mm Hg (the same as mixed venous PO_2). Blood exposed to a PO_2 equaling 14 mm Hg loses 25% of its oxygen to the tissues. More oxygen is unloaded from the blood in rapidly metabolizing tissues where tissue PO_2 is low. The oxygen that remains in combination with hemoglobin forms a reserve that can be drawn on in emergencies.

The oxyhemoglobin dissociation curve can also be displayed with percent saturation of hemoglobin as a function of PO_2. Percent saturation is the ratio of oxygen content to oxygen capacity (the amount of oxygen combined with hemoglobin when saturated), and hemoglobin is over 95% saturated with oxygen when it leaves the lungs in horses at sea level. Mixed venous blood is 75% saturated with oxygen

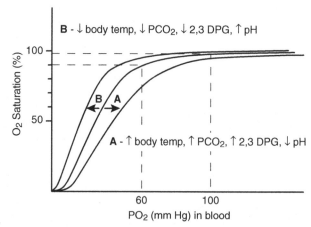

Figure 2-18. Oxygen-hemoglobin dissociation curve. The oxygen saturation (the percentage of hemoglobin in the oxyhemoglobin state) is plotted as a function of PO_2. Note the sigmoid shape of the curve. Above a partial pressure of about 60 mm Hg, the curve is relatively flat, with oxygen saturations above 90%. Below a PO_2 of 60 mm Hg, the oxygen saturation decreases rapidly (i.e., the oxygen comes off the hemoglobin). The PO_2 of 100 mm Hg shown on the graph corresponds to a normal alveolar PO_2 (at sea level) and translates to an oxygen saturation of nearly 100%. Factors that shift the curve to the right include increased body temperature, increased PCO_2, increased 2,3 DPG, and decreased pH. Factors that shift the curve to the left include decreased body temperature, decreased PCO_2, decreased 2,3 DPG, and increased pH. (From Schwartzstein RM, Parker MJ: *Respiratory physiology: a clinical approach,* Philadelphia, 2006, Lippincott Williams & Wilkins, p 109.)

when PO_2 is 40 mm Hg. Pulse oximeters allow easy evaluation of the percent saturation of hemoglobin in vivo.

The relationship between PO_2 and oxyhemoglobin saturation is not fixed but varies with blood temperature, pH, and the intracellular concentration of certain organic phosphates (see Figure 2-18). An increase in tissue metabolism produces heat, which elevates blood temperature and shifts the oxyhemoglobin dissociation curve to the right (increases P_{50}) (i.e., the PO_2 at which hemoglobin is 50% saturated). Such a shift facilitates dissociation of oxygen from hemoglobin and releases oxygen to the tissues. Conversely, excessive cooling of the blood, as occurs in hypothermia, shifts the dissociation curve to the left; thus the tissue PO_2 must be lower to release oxygen from hemoglobin.

The shift in the oxyhemoglobin dissociation curve that results from a change in PCO_2 (known as the Bohr effect) is caused in part by combination of CO_2 with hemoglobin, but mostly by the production of hydrogen ions, which decreases pH (Box 2-4). A change in pH alters the structure of hemoglobin and the accessibility of oxygen to the binding sites on heme (Figure 2-19). An increase in PCO_2 or a decrease in

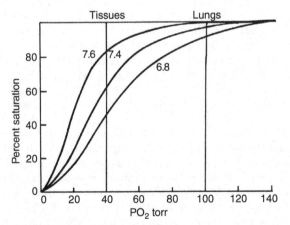

Figure 2–19. Effect of a change in blood pH on a mammalian oxyhemoglobin dissociation curve. A decrease in blood pH shifts the dissociation curve to the right, thereby decreasing the affinity of hemoglobin for oxygen. An increase in pH increases the affinity of hemoglobin for oxygen.

pH shifts the oxyhemoglobin dissociation curve to the right and facilitates the unloading of oxygen. These are the conditions that occur in metabolically active tissues that have increased need for the oxygen.

Organic phosphates, especially diphosphoglycerate (DPG) and adenosine triphosphate (ATP), also regulate the combination of oxygen with hemoglobin. The oxyhemoglobin dissociation curve is shifted to the right when concentrations of DPG are high, as occurs under anaerobic conditions, and the unloading of oxygen is facilitated. The DPG concentrations decrease when blood is stored; this can limit the ability of transfused blood to release oxygen to the tissues. Storing equine blood in citrate-phosphate-dextrose with supplemental adenine (CPDA-1) maintains acceptable concentrations of DPG.[81]

Carbon Dioxide Transport

Carbon dioxide is transported in the blood in solution in plasma and in two chemical combinations (see Box 2-4; Figure 2-20). Carbon dioxide is produced in the tissues and diffuses down a concentration gradient into the blood. When the blood leaves the tissues, PCO_2 has risen from 40 to approximately 46 mm Hg; exact values depend on the blood flow/metabolism ratio.

Approximately 5% of the carbon dioxide in the blood is transported in solution. The majority of CO_2 diffuses into the red cell where it undergoes one of two chemical reactions. Some combines with water and forms carbonic acid, which then dissociates into bicarbonate and hydrogen ion:

$$H_2O + CO_2 \rightleftharpoons H_2CO_3 \rightleftharpoons H^+ + HCO_3^-$$

This reaction also occurs in plasma, but in the red cell the presence of carbonic anhydrase accelerates the hydration of carbon dioxide several hundredfold. The reversible reaction is kept moving to the right because H⁺ is buffered by hemoglobin and the HCO_3^- diffuses out of the erythrocyte into the plasma.

The addition of CO_2 to venous blood is facilitated by the deoxygenation of hemoglobin occurring concurrently in the tissue capillaries. The deoxyhemoglobin is a better buffer than oxyhemoglobin and combines readily with H⁺, which facilitates the formation of HCO_3^- from CO_2. This effect of CO_2 on oxygen transport is known as the Haldane effect (Box 2-4).

Carbamino compounds, the second chemical combination in which CO_2 is transported in the blood, are formed by coupling of CO_2 to the amino groups of proteins, particularly hemoglobin. Although carbamino compounds account for only 15% to 20% of the total CO_2 content of the blood, they are responsible for 20% to 30% of the CO_2 exchange occurring between the tissues and the lungs.

All of the reactions depicted in Figure 2-20 are reversed when blood reaches the lungs. Exposure of arterial blood to the lower PCO_2 of the alveolus causes diffusion of CO_2 from the plasma and the erythrocyte, thus causing the reactions shown in Figure 2-20 to move to the left. Simultaneously the oxygenation of hemoglobin releases hydrogen ions. These combine with bicarbonate, forming carbonic acid, which dissociates to release carbon dioxide.

The blood content of CO_2 as a function of PCO_2 is depicted in the carbon dioxide equilibrium curve (Figure 2-21). Two curves are shown: one for oxygenated blood and one for

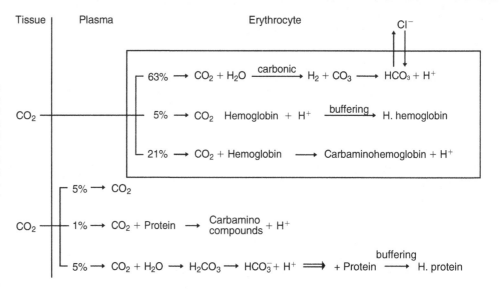

Figure 2–20. Reactions involved in the loading of carbon dioxide into the blood. From the tissues carbon dioxide diffuses into the plasma and erythrocyte and undergoes a variety of reactions that result in the production of bicarbonate and hydrogen ion. Hydrogen ion is then buffered by proteins in the plasma and by hemoglobin. In the lung, all the reactions shown in this illustration are reversed.

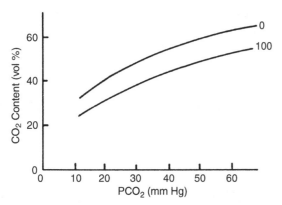

Figure 2–21. Carbon dioxide dissociation curve. Carbon dioxide content of blood is shown as a function of carbon dioxide tension (PCO_2). Two curves are shown: one for fully oxygenated blood (100% saturation) and one for deoxygenated blood (0% saturation). Deoxygenated blood has a higher carbon dioxide content than oxygenated blood at a given PCO_2 because deoxyhemoglobin is a better buffer than oxyhemoglobin.

deoxygenated blood. The curves are almost linear and have no plateau in the physiological range: CO_2 can be added to the blood as long as the buffering capacity for hydrogen ions is available. The greater CO_2 content of deoxygenated blood resulting from the greater buffering capacity of deoxyhemoglobin is clearly visible.

The transports of oxygen and CO_2 in the blood have mutual interactions through the Bohr and Haldane effects. In the lungs addition of oxygen to the blood makes hemoglobin a poor buffer, which aids in unloading CO_2 (Haldane effect). In the tissue capillaries the high concentration of CO_2 reduces the affinity of hemoglobin for oxygen and thereby assists in the unloading of oxygen (Bohr effect).

CONTROL OF BREATHING

Respiratory control mechanisms monitor the chemical composition of the blood, the effort exerted by the respiratory muscles on the lungs, and the presence of foreign materials in the respiratory tract. This information is integrated with other nonrespiratory activities such as thermoregulation, vocalization, and parturition to produce a pattern of breathing that maintains gas exchange.

A feedback control diagram for the respiratory system is shown in Figure 2-22. The central controller regulates the activity of the respiratory muscles, which by contracting give rise to alveolar ventilation. Changes in alveolar ventilation affect blood gas tensions and pH, which are monitored by chemoreceptors; signals are returned to the central controller, and necessary adjustments are made in ventilation. Mechanoreceptors in the lungs monitor the degree of stretch of the lungs and changes in the airways and vasculature. Stretch receptors in the respiratory muscles monitor the effort of breathing.

Central Control of Respiration

Respiratory rhythm originates in the medulla and is modified by higher brain centers and inputs from peripheral receptor.[82] Within the medulla two groups of neurons fire in association with respiration. The dorsal respiratory group (DRG) is located in the ventral lateral portion of the nucleus tractus solitarius, and the ventral respiratory group (VRG) is located in the nucleus ambiguus and nucleus retroambiguus. The DRG neurons fire primarily during inhalation, and the VRG neurons fire during both inhalation and exhalation. The DRG axons project by way of bulb or spinal pathways to innervate true spinal motor neurons (primarily those supplying the diaphragm), and the VRG. Axons from the VRG project to spinal motoneurons of both expiratory and accessory inspiratory muscles. Anesthetic drugs produce dose-dependent depression of all aspects of central nervous system control of breathing. Barbiturates, propofol, and newer inhalant anesthetics (isoflurane, sevoflurane) are particularly potent respiratory depressants (see Chapters 12 and 15).

The exact neural networks responsible for rhythmic breathing are not well understood, but several models have

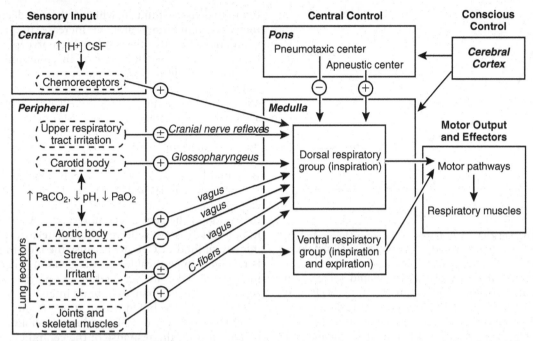

Figure 2–22. Relationship between sensory input, central control, and motor output in regulation of ventilation. Information from various sensors is fed to the control centers, the output of which goes to the respiratory muscles. By changing ventilation, the respiratory muscles reduce perturbations of the sensors (negative feedback).

been proposed.[82] Rhythmic respiration appears to result from rhythmic inhibition of inspiratory activity. The strength of inspiratory activity is increased when chemoreceptors are activated by hypoxia, hypercapnia, or acidosis. Termination of inspiration can be a result of inputs from pulmonary stretch receptors or from a central pontine off-switch.

Pulmonary and Airway Receptors

Three types of receptors with vagal afferents have been identified within the lung: slowly adapting stretch receptors and irritant receptors, both of which have myelinated afferents, and C-fibers with unmyelinated axons. Slowly adapting stretch receptors are associated with smooth muscle in the trachea and main bronchi but to a lesser degree in the intrapulmonary airways. They are stimulated when intrathoracic airways are stretched during lung inflation and are thought to be responsible for the inhibitory effect of lung inflation on breathing.

Rapidly adapting stretch or irritant receptors are unmyelinated nerve endings ramifying between epithelial cells in the larynx, trachea, large bronchi, and intrapulmonary airways. They are activated by mechanical deformation of the airways during lung inflation, bronchoconstriction, and mechanical irritation of the airway surface by an endotracheal tube. Irritant gases, dusts, histamine release, and a variety of other stimuli can also cause these receptors to respond. Stimulation of rapidly adapting irritant receptors leads to cough, bronchoconstriction, mucus secretion, and hyperpnea (i.e., protective responses to clear irritant materials from the respiratory system). Activation of receptors in the nasal cavity elicit sniffing and snorting; whereas stimulation of laryngeal and pharyngeal receptors may cause cough, apnea, or bronchoconstriction. Cooling activates receptors within the pharynx. Increasing airflow causes evaporation

from the mucosal surface and cooling of the latter receptors. For this reason these receptors are involved in adjustments of respiratory effort to maintain appropriate airflow.

Chemoreceptors

Chemoreceptors monitor oxygen, CO_2, and hydrogen ion concentration [H^+] at several sites in the body. Both CO_2 and hydrogen ion apparently are more important than oxygen in the minute-by-minute regulation of breathing. Small changes in $PaCO_2$ and [H^+] produce major changes in ventilation, whereas small changes in PaO_2 within the physiological range have little effect on breathing.

Chemoreceptors are located at several sites in the body. Peripheral chemoreceptors provide the respiratory response to hypoxia. Hypercapnia and changes in blood [H^+] are detected by both the peripheral and the central chemoreceptors.

Peripheral Chemoreceptors

The carotid bodies are located close to the bifurcation of the internal and external carotid arteries, and the aortic bodies surround the aortic arch. The carotid bodies are small structures with very high blood flow per kilogram. The aortic bodies are supplied by the vagus nerve, and a branch of the glossopharyngeal nerve supplies the carotid body. Axons within these nerves are primarily afferent except for a few efferents to blood vessels.

Firing rates in the carotid body afferents increase when the carotid bodies are perfused with blood that is hypoxic, hypercapnic, or acidotic. There is an almost linear increase in ventilation as PCO_2 increases and pH decreases. The response to decreasing PO_2 is nonlinear. Modest increases in firing rate and ventilation occur as PO_2 decreases from unphysiologically high levels of 500 mm Hg down to 70 mm Hg.

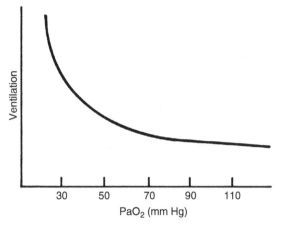

Figure 2–23. Effect of PaO_2 on ventilation in a conscious horse. As PaO_2 decreases, ventilation increases, particularly below $PaO_2 = 60$ mm Hg.

Further decreases in PO_2 cause a more rapid increase in ventilation, particularly below 60 mm Hg (i.e., the PO_2 at which hemoglobin begins to desaturate; Figure 2-23). PO_2 may be more important than oxygen content as a stimulus to the carotid bodies because neither modest anemia nor carbon monoxide poisoning increase ventilation. Carotid bodies contribute to ventilatory drive in the resting equine. Hypoventilation and failure to acclimate to high altitude follow carotid body denervation in ponies.[83,84]

Central Chemoreceptors

Increases in the concentration of CO_2 in inspired air are accompanied by increases in Vmin in horses.[85] The ventilatory response to CO_2 is mediated by way of a medullary chemoreceptor. Chemosensitive areas have been localized to the ventral lateral surface of the medulla, lateral to the pyramids, and medial to the roots of the seventh through the tenth and twelfth cranial nerves. The central chemoreceptor apparently responds to changes in the pH of the

interstitial tissue fluid in which it lies. A decrease in pH increases ventilation, and an increase in pH decreases ventilation. Because the central chemoreceptor is bathed by brain interstitial fluid that is in communication with cerebrospinal fluid (CSF), changes in ventilation can be induced by changes in the composition of arterial blood and by changes in the [H⁺] of CSF. All anesthetics and many sedatives (acepromazine, α_2-agonists) depress the ventilatory response to CO_2, shifting the Vmin – CO_2 relationship down to the right (Figure 2-24).

The central chemoreceptor is separated from the blood by the blood-brain barrier, which is freely permeable to CO_2 but less permeable to H⁺ and HCO_3^-. An increase in blood PCO_2 causes a rapid increase in the PCO_2 and a decrease in pH in the region of the central chemoreceptor. An acute increase in blood [H⁺] is not reflected immediately by a decrease in interstitial fluid or CSF pH because the blood-brain barrier is relatively impermeable to hydrogen ion. Therefore acute increases in [H⁺] are detected by the peripheral chemoreceptors. However, changes in brain interstitial fluid pH may follow those in the blood within 10 to 40 minutes.

The composition of CSF and brain interstitial fluid has a major effect on the response of the central chemoreceptor. The buffering capacity of the CSF is reduced if the $[HCO_3^-]$ of the CSF decreases, as occurs in metabolic acidosis. An increasing PCO_2 then causes a greater decrease in CSF pH than would occur in the presence of normal buffering capacity so that the ventilatory response to CO_2 is more vigorous than normal. Conversely, in metabolic alkalosis the CSF $[HCO_3^-]$ increases, and the response to CO_2 is depressed.

Effects of Drugs on Ventilation and Control of Breathing

Premedicant and anesthetic drugs are used to restrain horses and alleviate pain, but a side effect is respiratory depression (Table 2-6). The effects of these drugs on VT, respiratory rate, and Vmin have been reviewed extensively

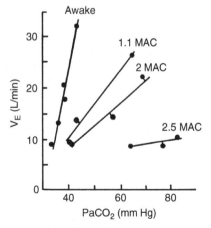

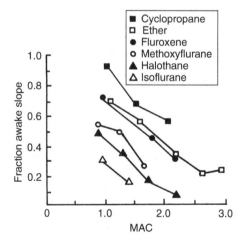

Figure 2–24. Effect of inhalation anesthetics on respiratory control. *Left,* Effect of increasing alveolar concentrations of halothane on the ventilatory response to carbon dioxide. As halothane concentration increases, the rise in minute ventilation (Vmin), caused by an increase in $PaCO_2$, is decreased. *Right,* Effect of increasing concentration of different anesthetic agents on the slope of the CO_2 response curve. All anesthetic agents depress the response to CO_2, but the depression is greatest with the newer inhalation agents. (*Left* from Munson ES et al: The effects of halothane, fluroxene, and cyclopropane on ventilation: a comparative study in man, *Anesthesiology* 27:718, 1966. *Right* from Hornbein TF, Severinghaus JW: Regulation of breathing: drug effects. In Hornbein TF, editor: *Lung biology in health and disease: regulation of breathing,* vol 17, part II, New York, 1978, Marcel Dekker, p 1260.)

Table 2–6. Effects of drugs used for chemical restraint and anesthesia on respiratory variables in horses*

	f	Vt	Vmin	PaCO$_2$	Respiratory center	Response to hypoxia
Inhalation	↑→↓	↓	↓	↑	↓ Sensitivity	↓
N$_2$O	—	↓		—↑	Minimum effect	—
Injectables						
Barbiturates	↓	↓	↓	↑	↓ Sensitivity	↓
Cyclohexamines	↓	↓	↓	↑	↓ Sensitivity	↓
Guaifenesin	—↓	—↓	—↓	—↑	No change	↓
Opioids						
Conscious	↓	↑	—	—		
Unconscious	↓	↓	↓	↑	↑ Threshold	↓
Opioid agonist/antagonist	—	—	—	—	↑ Threshold	—
Sedatives/tranquilizers						
Phenothiazines	—	↑	≈	—	↓ Sensitivity	↓
α$_2$Agonists	↓	↑↓	—↓	—↑	↓ Sensitivity ↑ Threshold	

↑, Increase; ↓, decreased; — minimum change; f, respiratory rate; PaCO$_2$, arterial partial pressure of carbon dioxide; Vt, tidal volume; Vmin, minute ventilation.
*Assumes minimal effective dosages have been used.

(see Figure 2-24).[86,87] Although Vmin is most easily measured to quantify the effects of a drug, it reflects not only the effect of the drug on respiratory control but also its effects on the metabolic rate and lung and respiratory muscle function. To determine drug effects on respiratory control, investigators measure the effect on the response to carbon dioxide, hypoxia, or an external resistive load.

Injectable and Inhalation Anesthetics

All injectable and inhalation anesthetics depress respiration and increase PaCO$_2$. Carbon dioxide retention is caused by the progressive decrease in VT and respiratory rate that occurs with increasing anesthetic depth. In general, VT and respiratory frequency decrease as the dose of anesthetic drug increases. Thiopental and propofol almost always produce a transient period of apnea when administered as an intravenous bolus for induction to anesthesia. Ventilatory depression is most profound in horses with compromised respiratory function so that the rise in PaCO$_2$ during anesthesia is greater in the horse with chronic lung disease than in the normal horse. Lower dosages of dissociative anesthetics (ketamine, tiletamine) are less depressant than thiopental, propofol, or guaifenesin and much less depressant than inhalant anesthetics (see Chapters 12 and 15). Halothane, sevoflurane, isoflurane, and desflurane depress ventilation and cause a dose-dependent increase in PaCO$_2$ in horses.[70,77,88,89] Prolonged isoflurane anesthesia at constant MAC causes progressive CO$_2$ retention without a concomitant rise in Vmin, suggesting a progressive loss of the response to CO$_2$.[89]

Inhalation anesthetics depress the increase in Vmin that normally occurs in response to inhalation of carbon dioxide (see Figure 2-24). Older anesthetics such as cyclopropane and ether produce relatively less respiratory depression than the newer drugs such as isoflurane. Although 1 MAC of nitrous oxide depresses the response to CO$_2$ profoundly, nitrous oxide spares the response to CO$_2$ when administered with inhalant anesthetics.

The ventilatory response to hypoxia is also depressed and may even be eliminated by very low concentrations of inhalation anesthetics. The effect may be direct on the carotid bodies, because the response to doxapram, a respiratory stimulant acting on the carotid bodies, is also lost.[90] Therefore hypoxemia does not illicit an increase in ventilation in the anesthetized horses.

Opioids

Most opioids can depress Vmin in a dose-dependent manner in horses that are anesthetized. Opioid effects on breathing may be exerted through opiate receptors located in close proximity to the medullary respiratory centers. Respiratory depression is caused by a reduction in VT or respiratory frequency or both. The ventilatory response to CO$_2$ is shifted to the right, and the slope of the response curve may be decreased. The ventilatory response to hypoxia may also be reduced. The respiratory depressant effects of clinical doses of opioids administered to horses are negligible compared to the effects of inhalant anesthetics. Endogenous opiates do not appear to play a major role in the control of breathing because the opiate antagonist naloxone has no effect on breathing in normal animals. However, naloxone or naltrexone, opioid antagonists, will reverse opioid-induced respiratory depression.

Sedatives and Tranquilizers

Like inhalation anesthetics and opioids, sedatives and tranquilizers also depress the respiratory system. Vmin is decreased, but the response to carbon dioxide is only minimally depressed by sedating doses of drug. However, anesthetic doses of barbiturates elevate PaCO$_2$ and significantly depress the response to CO$_2$. Acepromazine decreases respiratory frequency in horses but increases VT so that minute ventilation is unchanged. Acepromazine also slightly depresses the response to both carbon dioxide and hypoxia.[85]

The α_2-adrenergic receptor agonists xylazine and detomidine are widely used as sedatives for horses. Detomidine at doses up to $160\,\mu g/kg$ has no effect on respiratory rate in normal horses but may reduce the rate in horses with chronic airway disease.[91] Xylazine consistently reduces respiratory rate but does not cause hypoxemia.[91,92]

Muscle Relaxants

By virtue of their effects on muscles of respiration, muscle relaxants such as guaifenesin and diazepam can depress ventilation. Peripheral neuromuscular blocking drugs cause respiratory paralysis (see Chapter 19).

References

1. Willoughby RA, McDonnell WN: Pulmonary function testing in horses, *Vet Clin North Am Large Anim Pract* 1:171-191, 1979.
2. Pelletier N, Leith DE: Ventilation and carbon dioxide exchange in exercising horses: effect of inspired oxygen fraction, *J Appl Physiol* 78:654-662, 1995.
3. Koterba AM et al: Breathing strategy of the adult horse (Equus caballus) at rest, *J Appl Physiol* 64:337-346, 1988.
4. Benson GJ et al: Radiographic characterization of diaphragmatic excursion in halothane-anesthetized ponies: spontaneous and controlled ventilation systems, *Am J Vet Res* 43:617-621, 1982.
5. Art T, Serteyn D, Lekeux P: Effect of exercise on the partitioning of equine respiratory resistance, *Equine Vet J* 20:268-273, 1988.
6. Broadstone RV et al: In vitro response of airway smooth muscle from horses with recurrent airway obstruction, *Pulm Pharmacol* 4:191-202, 1991.
7. Mason DE, Muir WW, Olson LE: Response of equine airway smooth muscle to acetylcholine and electrical stimulation in vitro, *Am J Vet Res* 50:1499-1504, 1989.
8. Yu M et al: Inhibitory nerve distribution and mediation of NANC relaxation by nitric oxide in horse airways, *J Appl Physiol* 76:339-344, 1994.
9. Derksen FJ et al: Airway reactivity in ponies with recurrent airway obstruction (heaves), *J Appl Physiol* 58:598-604, 1985.
10. Hoffman AM, Mazan MR, Ellenberg S: Association between bronchoalveolar lavage cytologic features and airway reactivity in horses with a history of exercise intolerance, *Am J Vet Res* 59:176-181, 1998.
11. Hirshman CA, Bergman NA: Factors influencing intrapulmonary airway caliber during anesthesia, *Br J Anaesth* 65:30-42, 1990.
12. Yamakage M, Namiki A: Cellular mechanisms of airway smooth muscle relaxant effects of anesthetic agents, *J Anesth* 17:251-258, 2003.
13. Mazzeo AJ et al: Differential effects of desflurane and halothane on peripheral airway smooth muscle, *Br J Anaesth* 76:841-846, 1996.
14. Mazzeo AJ et al: Topographical differences in the direct effects of isoflurane on airway smooth muscle, *Anesth Analg* 78:948-954, 1994.
15. Cheng EY et al: Direct relaxant effects of intravenous anesthetics on airway smooth muscle, *Anesth Analg* 83:162-168, 1996.
16. Broadstone RV et al: Effects of xylazine on airway function in ponies with recurrent airway obstruction, *Am J Vet Res* 53:1813-1817, 1992.
17. Watney GC et al: Effects of xylazine and acepromazine on bronchomotor tone of anaesthetised ponies, *Equine Vet J* 20:185-188, 1988.
18. Derksen FJ, Robinson NE: Esophageal and intrapleural pressures in the healthy conscious pony, *Am J Vet Res* 41:1756-1761, 1980.
19. Amis TC, Pascoe JR, Hornof W: Topographic distribution of pulmonary ventilation and perfusion in the horse, *Am J Vet Res* 45:1597-1601, 1984.
20. Robinson NE, Sorenson PR: Collateral flow resistance and time constants in dog and horse lungs, *J Appl Physiol* 44:63-68, 1978.
21. Gillespie JR, Tyler WS, Hall LW: Cardiopulmonary dysfunction in anesthetized, laterally recumbent horses, *Am J Vet Res* 30:61-72, 1969.
22. Hall LW, Gillespie JR, Tyler WS: Alveolar-arterial oxygen tension differences in anaesthetized horses, *Br J Anaesth* 40:560-568, 1968.
23. McDonell WN, Hall LW: Functional residual capacity in conscious and anesthetized horses, *Br J Anaesth* 46:802-803, 1974.
24. McDonell WN, Hall LW, Jeffcott LB: Radiographic evidence of impaired pulmonary function in laterally recumbent anaesthetised horses, *Equine Vet J* 11:24-32, 1979.
25. Benson GJ et al: Radiographic characterization of diaphragmatic excursion in halothane-anesthetized ponies: spontaneous and controlled ventilation systems, *Am J Vet Res* 43:617-621, 1982.
26. Beadle RE, Robinson NE, Sorenson PR: Cardiopulmonary effects of positive end-expiratory pressure in anesthetized horses, *Am J Vet Res* 36:1435-1438, 1975.
27. Hall LW, Trim CM: Positive end-expiratory pressure in anaesthetized spontaneously breathing horses, *Br J Anaesth* 47:819-824, 1975.
28. Swanson CR, Muir WW: Hemodynamic and respiratory responses in halothane-anesthetized horses exposed to positive end-expiratory pressure alone and with dobutamine, *Am J Vet Res* 49:539-542, 1988.
29. Sorenson PR, Robinson NE: Postural effects on lung volumes and asynchronous ventilation in anesthetized horses, *J Appl Physiol* 48:97-103, 1980.
30. Nyman G et al: Selective mechanical ventilation of dependent lung regions in the anaesthetized horse in dorsal recumbency, *Br J Anaesth* 59:1027-1034, 1987.
31. Wilson DV, Soma LR: Cardiopulmonary effects of positive end-expiratory pressure in anesthetized, mechanically ventilated ponies, *Am J Vet Res* 51:734-739, 1990.
32. Wilson DV, Suslak L, Soma LR: Effects of frequency and airway pressure on gas exchange during interrupted high-frequency, positive-pressure ventilation in ponies, *Am J Vet Res* 49:1263-1269, 1988.
33. Wettstein D et al: Effects of an alveolar recruitment maneuver on cardiovascular and respiratory parameters during total intravenous anesthesia in ponies, *Am J Vet Res* 67:152-159, 2006.
34. Hornof WJ et al: Effects of lateral recumbency on regional lung function in anesthetized horses, *Am J Vet Res* 47:277-282, 1986.
35. Erickson BK, Erickson HH, Coffman JR: Pulmonary artery, aortic, and oesophageal pressure changes during high-intensity treadmill exercise in the horse: a possible relation to exercise-induced pulmonary haemorrhage, *Equine Vet J* (suppl) 9:47-52, 1990.
36. Milne DW, Muir WW, Skarda RT: Pulmonary arterial wedge pressures: blood gas tensions and pH in the resting horse, *Am J Vet Res* 36:1431-1434, 1975.
37. Mills PC et al: Nitric oxide and exercise in the horse, *J Physiol* 495:863-874, 1996.
38. Mills PC, Marlin DJ, Scott CM: Pulmonary artery pressure during exercise in the horse after inhibition of nitric oxide synthase, *Br Vet J* 152:119-122, 1996.

39. Pelletier N et al: Regional differences in endothelial function in horse lungs: possible role in blood flow distribution? *J Appl Physiol* 85:537-542, 1998.

40. Manohar M: Effects of glyceryl trinitrate (nitroglycerin) on pulmonary vascular pressures in standing thoroughbred horses, *Equine Vet J* 27:275-280, 1995.

41. Lester GD, DeMarco VG, Norman WM: Effect of inhaled nitric oxide on experimentally induced pulmonary hypertension in neonatal foals, *Am J Vet Res* 60:1207-1212, 1999.

42. Starr IR et al: Regional hypoxic pulmonary vasoconstriction in prone pigs, *J Appl Physiol* 99:363-370, 2005.

43. Aaronson PI et al: Hypoxic pulmonary vasoconstriction: mechanisms and controversies, *J Physiol* 570:53-58, 2006.

44. Wolin MS, Ahmad M, Gupte SA: Oxidant and redox signaling in vascular oxygen sensing mechanisms: basic concepts, current controversies, and potential importance of cytosolic NADPH, *Am J Physiol* 289:L159-L173, 2005.

45. Marshall BE et al: Hypoxic pulmonary vasoconstriction in dogs: effects of lung segment size and oxygen tension, *J Appl Physiol* 51:1543-1551, 1981.

46. Dobson A, Gleed RD, Meyer RE, et al: Changes in blood flow distribution in equine lungs induced by anaesthesia, *Q J Exp Physiol* 70:283-297, 1985.

47. Hlastala MP et al: Pulmonary blood flow distribution in standing horses is not dominated by gravity, *J Appl Physiol* 81:1051-1061, 1996.

48. Walther SM et al: Pulmonary blood flow distribution in sheep: effects of anesthesia, mechanical ventilation, and change in posture, *Anesthesiology* 87:335-342, 1997.

49. Walther SM et al: Pulmonary blood flow distribution has a hilar-to-peripheral gradient in awake, prone sheep, *J Appl Physiol* 82:678-685, 1997.

50. Bernard SL et al: Minimal redistribution of pulmonary blood flow with exercise in racehorses, *J Appl Physiol* 81:1062-1070, 1996.

51. Glenny RW, Robertson HT: Fractal properties of pulmonary blood flow: characterization of spatial heterogeneity, *J Appl Physiol* 69:532-545, 1990.

52. Baile EM: The anatomy and physiology of the bronchial circulation, *J Aerosol Med* 9:1-6, 1996.

53. Deffebach ME et al: The bronchial circulation. Small, but a vital attribute of the lung, *Am Rev Respir Dis* 135:463-481, 1987.

54. Gleed RD, Dobson A, Hackett RP: Pulmonary shunting by the bronchial artery in the anaesthetized horse, *Q J Exp Physiol* 75:115-118, 1990.

55. Johnson DH, Hurst TS, Mayers I: Effects of halothane on hypoxic pulmonary vasoconstriction in canine atelectasis, *Anesth Analg* 72:440-448, 1991.

56. Slinger P, Scott WA: Arterial oxygenation during one-lung ventilation: a comparison of enflurane and isoflurane, *Anesthesiology* 82:940-946, 1995.

57. Ishibe Y et al: Effect of sevoflurane on hypoxic pulmonary vasoconstriction in the perfused rabbit lung, *Anesthesiology* 79:1348-1353, 1993.

58. Loer SA, Scheeren TW, Tarnow J: Desflurane inhibits hypoxic pulmonary vasoconstriction in isolated rabbit lungs, *Anesthesiology* 83:552-556, 1995.

59. Kerbaul F et al: Effects of sevoflurane on hypoxic pulmonary vasoconstriction in anaesthetized piglets, *Br J Anaesth* 85:440-445, 2000.

60. Kerbaul F et al: Sub-MAC concentrations of desflurane do not inhibit hypoxic pulmonary vasoconstriction in anesthetized piglets, *Can J Anaesth* 48:760-767, 2001.

61. Lesitsky MA, Davis S, Murray PA: Preservation of hypoxic pulmonary vasoconstriction during sevoflurane and desflurane anesthesia compared to the conscious state in chronically instrumented dogs, *Anesthesiology* 89:1501-1508, 1998.

62. Abe K et al: The effects of propofol, isoflurane, and sevoflurane on oxygenation and shunt fraction during one-lung ventilation, *Anesth Analg* 87:1164-1169, 1998.

63. Karzai W, Haberstroh J, Priebe HJ: Effects of desflurane and propofol on arterial oxygenation during one-lung ventilation in the pig, *Acta Anaesthesiol Scand* 42:648-652, 1998.

64. Taylor AE et al: Fluid balance. In Crystal RG et al, editors: *The lung: scientific foundations*, Philadelphia, 1997, Lippincott-Raven, pp 1549-1566.

65. Vengust M et al: Transvascular fluid flux from the pulmonary vasculature at rest and during exercise in horses, *J Physiol* 570:397-405, 2006.

66. Tute AS et al: Negative pressure pulmonary edema as a post-anesthetic complication associated with upper airway obstruction in a horse, *Vet Surg* 25:519-523, 1996.

67. Balyasnikova IV et al: Propofol attenuates lung endothelial injury induced by ischemia-reperfusion and oxidative stress, *Anesth Analg* 100:929-936, 2005.

68. Reutershan J et al: Protective effects of isoflurane pretreatment in endotoxin-induced lung injury, *Anesthesiology* 104:511-517, 2006.

69. Koenig J, McDonell W, Valverde A: Accuracy of pulse oximetry and capnography in healthy and compromised horses during spontaneous and controlled ventilation, *Can J Vet Res* 67:169-174, 2003.

70. Steffey EP et al: Effects of desflurane and mode of ventilation on cardiovascular and respiratory functions and clinicopathologic variables in horses, *Am J Vet Res* 66:669-677, 2005.

71. Hedenstierna G et al: Ventilation-perfusion relationships in the standing horse: an inert gas elimination study, *Equine Vet J* 19:514-519, 1987.

72. Wagner PD et al: Mechanism of exercise-induced hypoxemia in horses, *J Appl Physiol* 66:1227-1233, 1989.

73. Nyman G, Hedenstierna G: Ventilation-perfusion relationships in the anaesthetised horse, *Equine Vet J* 21:274-281, 1989.

74. Marntell S, Nyman G, Hedenstierna G: High inspired oxygen concentrations increase intrapulmonary shunt in anaesthetized horses, *Vet Anaesth Analg* 32:338-347, 2005.

75. Gleed RD, Dobson A: Improvement in arterial oxygen tension with change in posture in anaesthetised horses, *Res Vet Sci* 44:255-259, 1988.

76. Mitchell B, Littlejohn A: The effect of anaesthesia and posture on the exchange of respiratory gases and on the heart rate, *Equine Vet J* 6:177-178, 1974.

77. Steffey EP et al: Body position and mode of ventilation influences arterial pH, oxygen, and carbon dioxide tensions in halothane-anesthetized horses, *Am J Vet Res* 38:379-382, 1977.

78. Neto FJ et al: The effect of changing the mode of ventilation on the arterial-to-end-tidal CO_2 difference and physiological dead space in laterally and dorsally recumbent horses during halothane anesthesia, *Vet Surg* 29:200-205, 2000.

79. Kerr CL, McDonell WN, Young SS: Cardiopulmonary effects of romifidine/ketamine or xylazine/ketamine when used for short-duration anesthesia in the horse, *Can J Vet Res* 68:274-282, 2004.

80. Marntell S et al: Effects of acepromazine on pulmonary gas exchange and circulation during sedation and dissociative anaesthesia in horses, *Vet Anaesth Analg* 32:83-93, 2005.

81. Mudge MC, Macdonald MH, Owens SD: Comparison of 4 blood storage methods in a protocol for equine pre-operative autologous donation, *Vet Surg* 33:475-486, 2004.

82. Richerson GB, Boron WF: Control of ventilation. In Boron WF, Boulpaep EL, editors: *Medical physiology: a cellular and molecular approach*, Philadelphia, 2003, Saunders, pp 712-734.

83. Bisgard GE et al: Hypoventilation in ponies after carotid body denervation, *J Appl Physiol* 40:184-190, 1976.

84. Bisgard GE, Orr JA, Will JA: Hypoxic pulmonary hypertension in the pony, *Am J Vet Res* 36:49-52, 1975.

85. Muir WW, Hamlin RL: Effects of acetylpromazine on ventilatory variables in the horse, *Am J Vet Res* 36:1439-1442, 1975.

86. Hornbein TF: Anesthetics and ventilatory control. In Covino BG et al, editors: *Effects of anesthesia*, Bethesda, 1985, American Physiological Society, pp. 75-90.

87. Pavlin EG, Hornbein TF: Anesthesia and control of ventilation. In Fishman AP, editor: *Handbook of physiology*, section 3: the respiratory system, Bethesda, 1986, American PhysiologicalSociety.

88. Fisher EW: Observations on the disturbance of respiration of cattle, horses, sheep, and dogs caused by halothane anesthesia and the changes taking place in plasma pH and plasma CO2 content, *Am J Vet Res* 22:279-286, 1961.

89. Steffey EP et al: Cardiopulmonary function during 5 hours of constant-dose isoflurane in laterally recumbent, spontaneously breathing horses, *J Vet Pharmacol Ther* 10:290-297, 1987.

90. Knill RL, Manninen PH, Clement JL: Ventilation and chemoreflexes during enflurane sedation and anaesthesia in man, *Can Anaesth Soc J* 26:353-360, 1979.

91. Reitemeyer H, Klein HJ, Deegen E: The effect of sedatives on lung function in horses, *Acta Vet Scand* 82(suppl):111-120, 1986.

92. McCashin FB, Gabel AA: Evaluation of xylazine as a sedative and preanesthetic agent in horses, *Am J Vet Res* 36:1421-1429, 1975.

93. Marino PL: *The ICU book*, ed 3, Philadelphia, 2007, Lippincott Williams & Wilkins, 21-37.

94. Thurmon JC, Tranquilli WJ, Benson GJ: *Lumb & Jones' veterinary anesthesia and analagesia*, ed 4, Oxford, UK, 2007, Blackwell.

The Cardiovascular System

Colin C. Schwarzwald

John D. Bonagura

William W. Muir

Circulatory function in horses is markedly affected and significantly depressed by many sedative, tranquilizing, and anesthetic drugs.[1] The physiologic status of the cardiovascular system influences the choice and administration of the anesthetic technique chosen. Horses with a compromised (e.g., hemorrhage) or abnormal circulation (e.g., colic, endotoxemia) often require sedation or anesthesia. For these reasons a thorough cardiovascular examination should be performed before anesthesia, and the overall clinical significance of abnormal cardiac findings determined and treated when possible (see Chapter 6).

NORMAL CARDIOVASCULAR STRUCTURE AND FUNCTION

The interpretation of diagnostic techniques, including cardiac auscultation, electrocardiography, echocardiography, and cardiac catheterization, is predicated on an understanding of cardiac anatomy and function. Circulatory homeostasis and effects of drugs on the heart and circulation depend in part on the anatomic and functional relationships between the heart and blood vessels and integrated cardiovascular control mechanisms.[2-5]

The general arrangement of the cardiovascular system can be likened to two separate yet interdependent circulations, systemic and pulmonary, each with its own venous capacitance, atrioventricular (AV) pump, arterial distribution, mechanisms for altering vascular resistance, and microcirculatory bed (Table 3-1).[1,2] Because these two circulations are arranged in series and because the two ventricles share the same interventricular septum and a common pericardial sac, dysfunction of either circulation ultimately affects the other circulation (ventricular interdependence, see following paragraphs).

Cardiac Anatomy[6,7]

Pericardium

The pericardial space is formed by the reflection of the two pericardial membranes, the *parietal pericardium* and the *visceral pericardium (epicardium)* and normally contains a small amount of fluid. The pericardium, although not an essential structure, serves to restrain and protect the heart, acts as a barrier against contiguous infection, balances right and left ventricular output through diastolic and systolic interactions, limits acute chamber dilation, and exerts lubricant effects that minimize friction between cardiac chambers and surrounding structures.[8] Pericardial constraint limits chamber dilation at high filling volumes or in the presence of pathologic conditions such as pericardial effusion or constriction, particularly of the thinner-walled right atrium and ventricle; augments ventricular interdependence; and limits diastolic ventricular filling.[8]

Myocardium and Cardiac Chambers

The myocardium represents the mechanically active component of the cardiac pump and forms the bulk of the atrial and ventricular walls (Figure 3-1). The *right atrium* is located at the right craniodorsal aspect of the heart. It is separated from the right ventricle by the *right AV (tricuspid) valve* (see Figure 3-1). The *right ventricle* is crescent shaped on cross section but functionally is U shaped, with the inlet

Table 3–1. Comparative characteristics of the systemic and pulmonary circulations

Feature	Systemic circulation	Pulmonary circulation
Venous capacity	Relatively large	Relatively small
Arterial pressure	High pressure	Low pressure
Volume flow (cardiac output)	Equal	
Arterial resistance	High	Low
Origin of resistance	Arterioles	Arterioles, capillaries; left-atrial pressure (up to one third of total resistance)
Vascular innervation	Extensive in resistance vessels (arterioles); adrenergic	Primarily adrenergic
Local control of peripheral blood flow	Variable among regional circulations Adjusts local blood flow to metabolic demand of the tissues High oxygen (PO$_2$) is a vasoconstrictor	Serves to adjust local blood flow to ventilation (ventilation-perfusion-matching) Hypoxia (low PO$_2$) leads to vasoconstriction (hypoxic pulmonary vasoconstriction)

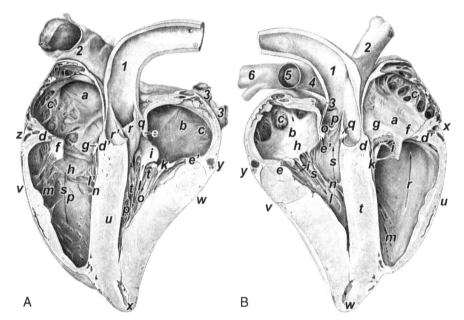

A   B

Figure 3–1. Sagittal section through the heart of a horse. **A,** Right half of the heart. *a,* Right atrium; *b,* left atrium; *c,* pectinate muscles; *d, d',* right atrioventricular ostium; *e, e',* left atrioventricular ostium; *f,* parietal cusp; *g,* septal cusp; *h,* angular cusp of the right atrioventricular (tricuspid) valve; *i,* septal cusp; *k,* parietal cusp of the left atrioventricular (bicuspid or mitral) valve; *l, l',* chordae tendineae; *m, n,* papillary muscles of the right ventricle; *o,* papillary muscle of the left ventricle; *p, p',* trabeculae septomarginalis (moderator bands, "false tendons") of the right and left ventricles; *q, r, r',* aortic valve in the aortic ostium (between *d'* and *e*); *q,* its left semilunar valve; *r,* its right semilunar valve; *r',* its septal semilunar valve; *s,* inflow tract of the right ventricle; *t, t,* inflow and outflow tracts of the left ventricle; *u,* interventricular septum; *v,* right ventricular free wall; *w,* left ventricular free wall; *x,* apex of the heart; *y, z,* coronary sulcus with coronary vessels; *1,* aortic arch; *2,* cranial vena cava entering the right atrium; *3,* pulmonary veins entering the left atrium. **B,** Left half of the heart. *a,* Right atrium with view into the right auricle; *b,* left atrium with view into the left auricle; *c,* pectinate muscles; *d, d',* right atrioventricular ostium; *e, e',* left atrioventricular ostium; *f,* parietal cusp, *g,* septal cusp of the right atrioventricular (tricuspid) valve; *h,* parietal cusp of the left atrioventricular (bicuspid or mitral) valve; *i, i,* chordae tendineae; *k,* papillary muscle of the right ventricle; *l,* papillary muscle of the left ventricle; *m,* carneous trabeculae; *n,* trabecula septomarginalis; *o, p, q,* aortic valve in the aortic ostium (between *e'* and *d*); *o,* its left semilunar valve; *p,* its right semilunar valve; *q,* its septal semilunar valve; *r,* outflow tract of the right ventricle; *s, s,* inflow and outflow tract of the left ventricle; *t,* interventricular septum; *u,* right ventricular free wall; *v,* left ventricular free wall; *w,* apex of the heart; *x, y,* coronary sulcus with coronary vessels; *1,* aortic arch; *2,* brachiocephalic trunk; *3,* origin of the left coronary artery; *4,* main pulmonary artery (trunk); *5, 6,* right and left pulmonary artery. Note the relationship of the interventricular septum (*u*A, *t*B) to the pulmonary and aortic outflow tracts. (From Schummer A et al: *The circulatory system, the skin, and the cutaneous organs of the domestic mammals,* Berlin, 1981, Verlag Paul Parey.)

at the right hemithorax and the outlet, *pulmonic valve*, and main *pulmonary artery* located at the left side of the chest. This arrangement is clinically relevant to understanding the areas for cardiac auscultation (aortic and pulmonic heart sounds are auscultated on the left side of the chest) and thoracic imaging (see Figure 3-1). The approximately three times thicker *left ventricle* is spherical in cross section and is functionally V shaped with an inlet and outlet separated by the septal (cranial or "anterior") leaflet of the *left Av (mitral) valve*. The mitral valve separates the *left atrium*, located at the left caudodorsal base of the heart, from the left ventricle (see Figure 3-1). The *aorta* originates in the left ventricular outlet, is continuous with the ventricular septum cranially and the septal mitral leaflet caudally, and exits from the center of the heart and to the right of the main pulmonary artery. The *atrial and ventricular septa* separate the right and left sides of the heart. Embryologic openings may persist in the septa as congenital defects; ventricular septal defects are the most common cardiac anomaly in the horse (see following paragraphs).

Endocardium and Valves

The cardiac chambers are lined by the *endocardium*. This layer also covers the AV and semilunar valves and is continuous with the endothelium of the great veins and arteries. The *inlet valves (tricuspid and mitral)* are anchored by the collagenous chordae tendineae, papillary muscles (three to five in the right ventricle and two in the left ventricle), valve annulus, and caudal atrial walls (see Figure 3-1). Disruption of any portion of this support apparatus can cause valvular insufficiency. The *outlet valves (pulmonic and aortic)* are trileaflet in nature. The coronary arteries originate within the aortic valve sinuses (of Valsalva). The right coronary artery is often dominant in the horse.

Impulse-Forming and Conduction Systems

The specialized cardiac tissues consist of the sinoatrial (SA) node, internodal pathways, AV node, bundle of His, bundle branches, fascicles, and Purkinje system (Figures 3-2 and 3-3). The *SA node* represents the physiological pacemaker. In the adult horse it consists of a relatively large crescent-shaped structure located subepicardially in the region of the terminal sulcus at the junction of the cranial vena cava and right atrium. Bachmann's bundle is one of the four conduction tracts that make up the atrial conduction system of the heart, which is responsible for transmitting the pacemaking impulses of the SA node. This bundle of specialized muscle fibers originates in the SA node and is the only tract that innervates the left atrium. The atrial conducting tracts are extremely important for rapidly transmitting electrical activity throughout the atria and to the atrioventricular node, especially during acid-base and electrolyte (hyperkalemia) disturbances. The *AV node* is situated in the atrial septum, close to the orifice of the coronary sinus and at or slightly above the level of the septal tricuspid leaflet. The *His-Purkinje system* extends from the AV node to the ventricular septum and ventricular myocardium. The horse has relatively complete penetration of Purkinje fibers into the ventricular free walls, except for a small portion of the left ventricular free wall. This anatomic feature causes the large ventricular mass of the horse's heart to be activated relatively quickly and simultaneously (in about 110 to 120 msec).[9]

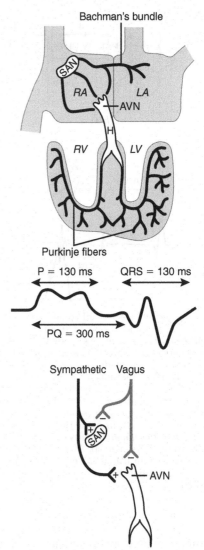

Figure 3–2. Impulse-forming and conduction systems of the heart. The impulse originates in the sinoatrial node *(SAN)* and is propagated across the right atrium *(RA)* and left atrium *(LA)*, generating the P wave. Specialized internodal and interatrial (Bachmann's bundle) pathways facilitate impulse conduction. The impulse is delayed in the atrioventricular node *(AVN)* and rapidly conducted through the bundle of His *(H)*, bundle branches and Purkinje network *(top)*. Electrical activation of ventricular myocytes generates the QRS complex. The automaticity of the SA node and conduction across the AV node are modulated by the autonomic nervous system (Courtesy Dr. Robert L. Hamlin.)

The electrical activation of the atria and ventricles and subsequent repolarization of the ventricles are responsible for the body surface electrical potentials recognized as the P-QRS-T complex. An atrial repolarization wave (Ta wave) is frequently observed in the electrocardiogram (ECG) of horses because of the large muscle mass of the horses atria compared to other species.

Ultrastructural Anatomy

The majority of cardiac tissue is made up of striated muscle cells (*cardiomyocytes*) that are responsible for the contractile function of the heart. The rest consists of specialized muscle cells (nodal and conducting tissues), blood vessels, nerves, and extracellular matrix. Neighboring

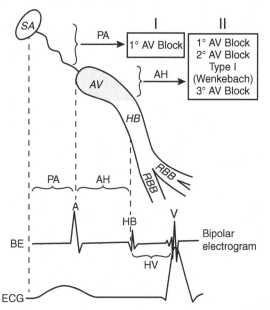

Figure 3–3. The surface electrocardiogram, intracardiac bipolar (His bundle) electrogram, and associated anatomical structures. The impulse spreads from the sinoatrial *(SA)* node to the AV node. Atrial depolarization generates a P wave and an atrial *(A)* spike on the electrogram. An electrical wave of depolarizations spreads across the atrioventricular *(AV)* node, the bundle of His (HB), the right *(RBB)*, and left *(LBB)* bundle branches, and finally ventricular Purkinje cells and myocardium. The PQ interval can be subdivided into atrial *(PA;* from SA node to lower atrium), nodal *(AH;* from the low atrium to the His bundle) and infranodal *(HV;* from the His bundle to the ventricle) intervals. AV block may develop from delay or interruption of conduction in the atrial muscle (PA interval), AV node (AH interval), or His bundle (HV interval). (From Narula OS et al: Atrioventricular block: localization and classification by His bundle recordings, *Am J Med* 50(2):147, 1971.)

cardiomyocytes possess tight end-to-end connections, also referred to as *intercalated disks*, containing large membrane-spanning protein complexes that serve as anchoring points for cytoskeletal proteins and ensure transmission of mechanical forces produced by the individual cells throughout the myocardium. *Gap junctions (connexons)*, primarily located in the intercalated disks, ensure rapid electrical communication between cells and allow the myocardium to act as a functional syncytium. The contractile units of the cardiomyocytes are the *myofibrils*, consisting of *actin* (thin filaments); *myosin* (thick filaments); and a variety of regulatory proteins, including *tropomyosin* and the *cardiac troponin complex*. The myofibrils are in close association with a variety of *cytoskeletal proteins*. The latter provide spatial stability, transmit mechanical forces, may act as molecular "sensors," and contribute to intracellular signaling. *Mitochondria*, interspersed in large numbers between the myofibrils, are the main source of energy supply in the cardiomyocytes and may serve as calcium buffers in conditions of intracellular calcium overload. The *sarcoplasmatic reticulum (SR)* consists of a large network of longitudinal tubules and subsarcolemmal cisternae. It serves as a calcium reservoir, contributes to intracellular calcium cycling, and is essential in excitation-contraction coupling (see following paragraphs). The terminal cisternae of the SR are in close contact with so-called *T tubules* or sarcolemmal transverse invaginations that are the main site of calcium entry into the cells during electrical

activation (see Cardiac Excitation-Contraction Coupling later in the chapter). Pacemaker cells and conducting cells are larger than contractile myocytes, contain fewer myofilaments, and show very prominent intercalated disks with abundant gap junctions to allow fast transmission of electrical impulses.[3,4,10]

Cardiac Electrophysiology

Cardiac myocytes form a functional syncytium, which is excitable and able to conduct electrical impulses in response to stimulation by a natural or artificial pacemaker. Some specialized regions within the heart are capable of spontaneous depolarization and impulse formation (automaticity) independent of extrinsic stimulation or neural input. The *SA node* is the physiologic pacemaker (fastest rate of spontaneous depolarization) of the heart; whereas atrial specialized fibers, the AV node, and the Purkinje fibers can act as *subsidiary (slower) pacemakers* if the SA nodal activity becomes disturbed (sinus arrest) or impulse conduction to the ventricles becomes disrupted (third-degree AV block, see following paragraphs).

The processes responsible for generation of electrical activity in the heart are caused by ion fluxes across the cell membrane (Table 3-2; Figures 3-4 and 3-5, *A*). The sum of the electrical activity of all cardiac myocytes can be recorded noninvasively on the body surface as an ECG. A general understanding of cellular electrical activity, generation and spread of the cardiac electrical impulse, and the effects of autonomic modulation is required for an appreciation of the horse's unique ECG and the recognition, interpretation, clinical relevance, and treatment of cardiac arrhythmias in horses.[3,4,11-14]

Normal Cellular Electrophysiology

Cardiac cellular electrical activity and intracellular potential (negative intracellular potential) are determined by the activity membrane-bound ion channels, exchangers, and pumps and depend on the time-dependent selective permeability (conductance) of the cardiac cell membrane and variations in the concentration gradients (voltage-dependent changes) of several electrolytes, notably K^+, Na^+, and Ca^{+2}, across the cell membrane. The extracellular fluid contains high concentrations of sodium ion compared to intracellular fluid, and the intracellular fluid contains a high concentration of potassium compared to extracellular fluid. Intracellular proteins contribute to the development of a significant intracellular negative electrical charge. Although there is a chemical (concentration) gradient for sodium influx and potassium efflux, such movements are modulated by time- and voltage-dependent changes in cardiac cell membrane conductance to the respective ions. Energy-dependent ion pumps and exchangers (Na^+-K^+ ATPase; adenosine triphosphate (ATP)–dependent Ca^{+2}; Na^+/ Ca^{+2} exchanger) help to maintain the transmembrane ionic gradients and resting membrane potential. The Na^+-K^+ ATPase pump exchanges sodium for potassium ions at a 3:2 ratio (electrogenic) and helps to maintain resting membrane potential. Sudden changes in cell membrane conductance to sodium, potassium, and calcium are responsible for the processes of depolarization, muscular contraction, and repolarization. These in turn are affected by the serum electrolyte concentration (K^+), acid-base status, autonomic modulation, myocardial perfusion and oxygenation, inflammatory processes, heart disease, and drugs.

Table 3–2. The cardiac action potential

Phase	Ions	Characteristics/Comments
0: Rapid depolarization	Na$^+$	Fast Na$^+$ (I$_{Na}$) inward channel; determines conduction velocity
1: Transient early repolarization	K$^+$	Transient outward channel (I$_{to}$)
2: Plateau	Ca^{+2}	L-type (I$_{Ca}$) channel; slow inward, long-lasting current; phase 2 of myocytes and phases 4 and 0 of SA and AV nodal cells
3: Repolarization	K$^+$	Delayed rectifier (I$_{Kr}$) channel; principal outward repolarizing current
4: Resting membrane potential	K$^+$	Inward rectifier (I$_{K1}$) channel; maintains negative potential in phase 4; closes with depolarization; its decay contributes to pacemaker currents
*Phase 4 pacemaker currents	Na$^+$	Slow inward Na$^+$ (I$_f$) channel; contributes to phase 4 pacemaker current in SA and AV nodal cells
	Ca^{+2}	T-type (I$_{Ca}$) channel; transient inward current; contributes to phas.acemaker current in SA and AV nodal cells

AV, Atrioventricular; *SA,* sinoatrial.

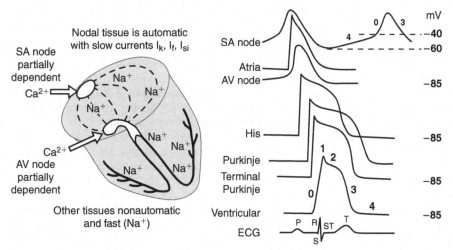

Figure 3–4. The algebraic sum of all the action potentials generated by the heart is responsible for the surface ECG. Action potentials are conducted more slowly in the SA and AV nodes because the resting membrane potential is less negative (–60 mV vs. –85 mV) and depends on slow inward (calcium) currents (I_{si} or I_{Ca-L}) for depolarization. Cardiac muscle cells are depolarized by activation of fast sodium channels. The duration of the action potential varies among cardiac tissues and partially accounts for differences in cell refractory periods. I_k, potassium current; I_f, pacemaker ("funny") current. (From Hoffman BF, Cranefield PF: Electrophysiology of the heart, New York, 1960, McGraw-Hill.)

The cardiac action potential. The cardiac cellular action potential generally is described in terms of five distinct phases representing the resting membrane potential (phase 4), rapid depolarization (phase 0), early (transient) repolarization (phase 1), a plateau (phase 2), and late repolarization (Phase 3) phase (see Table 3-2 and Figures 3-4 and 3-5, A).[4,5,11,12,15,16]

Resting membrane potential (phase 4). The membrane of normal cardiac myocytes is relatively impermeable to sodium and calcium ions at rest (Phase 4). Therefore the resting membrane potential of nonautomatic cells is determined primarily by the activity of the electrogenic Na$^+$-K$^+$ pump and a background inward rectifying outward potassium current (I$_{K1}$or I$_{Kir}$). Potassium ions leak out of the cells because of the high concentration gradient of K$^+$ across the membrane and the high K$^+$ conductance of the membrane at rest until an equilibrium between electrical and chemical forces (concentration gradient) is reached. The resting membrane potential of most cardiac cells is very close to the potassium equilibrium potential, which can be determined by the Nernst equation[5,10] and is approximately –90 mV in atrial and ventricular myocytes and Purkinje fibers.

Depolarization phase (phase 0). Electrical stimulation of cardiac cells by neighboring cells or an artificial pacemaker depolarizes the cell. An all-or-none electrical potential (action potential) ensues if the depolarization exceeds a threshold potential of approximately –55 mV. The rapid upstroke of the action potential (phase 0) is produced by

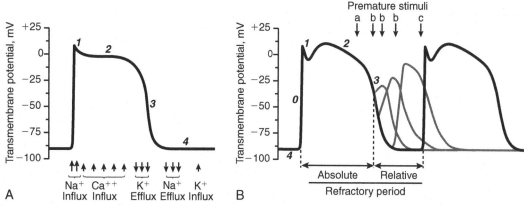

Figure 3–5. A, Phases of cellular action potentials and major associated currents in ventricular myocytes. The initial phase zero spike and overshoot *(1)* are caused by a rapid inward Na current, the plateau phase *(2)* by a slow Ca current through L-type Ca channels, and the repolarization phase *(3)* by outward K currents. The resting potential phase *(4)* (Na efflux, K influx), is maintained by Na-K-ATPase. The Na-Ca exchanger is mainly responsible for Ca extrusion. In specialized conduction system tissue, spontaneous depolarization takes place during phase 4 until the voltage resulting in opening of the Na channel is reached. **B,** Absolute (ARP) and relative refractory periods (RFP). Cardiac cells cannot be activated if stimulated during the ARP but can generate smaller slower conduction electrical potentials when activated during the RRP. The later abnormal potentials may be responsible for conduction delay or block and the development of reentrant circuits in the heart. (From LeWinter MM, Osol G: Normal physiology of the cardiovascular system. In Fuster V, editor: *Hurst's the heart*, ed 10, New York, 2001, McGraw-Hill, pp 63-94.)

Na^+ entering the cell (rapid Na^+ current: I_{Na}) secondary to activation of fast Na^+ channels. The entry of Na^+ into cardiac myocytes is responsible for rapid depolarization of the cell membrane (see Figure 3-5, A). The rate of change of the membrane potential (dV/dt) and the amplitude of the action potential (mV) are direct determinants of the conduction velocity of the electrical impulse. Both dV/dt and amplitude of the action potential depend on the availability of resting Na^+ channels, which in turn depend on the value of the resting membrane potential and the amount of time that has passed since the previous action potential. Membrane depolarization (i.e., hyperkalemia, hypoxia, ischemia) causes voltage-dependent inactivation of the Na^+ channels, leading to a slowing of impulse conduction (decreased dV/dt) and potentially conduction block.[11] Atrial myocytes seem to be especially sensitive to hyperkalemia, which can lead to cessation of normal atrial muscle cell activation, little-to-no effective atrial contraction, and a lack of P waves on the surface ECG.[17] Fast sodium channels are blocked by many drugs (i.e., quinidine, procainamide, lidocaine, high doses of injectable, and inhalant anesthetics).[12,18]

Transient repolarization phase (phase 1). Following phase 0 a short and rapid initial repolarization phase occurs (phase 1) as a result of the increase of a potassium-based transient outward rectifier current (I_{to}). The magnitude of phase 1 varies among different areas of the heart and different species (see Figure 3-5, A). The I_{to} current may be absent in equine ventricular myocytes.[15]

Plateau phase (phase 2). The transient partial repolarization is followed by the plateau phase (phase 2), during which the cardiac cells remain depolarized. Phase 2 is determined primarily by the inward movement of calcium through long-lasting (slow) voltage-gated L-type Ca^{+2} channels (I_{Ca-L}) once the membrane depolarizes to about –40 mV. The I_{Ca-L} is influenced by late Na^+ currents, repolarizing K^+ currents, and the activity of the Na^+-Ca^{+2} exchanger (see following paragraphs) and is blocked by calcium chan-

nel blockers (verapamil, diltiazem, nifedipine). The duration of phase 2 varies among different cardiac tissues. It is shortest in nodal and atrial tissues and longest in Purkinje fibers (see Figure 3-5, A). The duration of the plateau phase also varies between subendocardial and subepicardial ventricular myocardium.[4,12] The calcium entering the myocardial cells during the plateau phase is essential for induction of cardiac contraction, acting as a trigger for the release of calcium from calcium stores in the sarcoendoplasmatic reticulum (calcium-induced calcium release). The initiation of myocardial contraction by the electrical impulse is referred to as excitation-contraction coupling (see Cardiac Excitation-Contraction Coupling later in the chapter). Both injectable and inhalant anesthetics interfere with I_{Ca-L}, resulting in vasodilation and decreases in the force of cardiac contraction.[12,18]

Repolarization phase (phase 3). The repolarization phase (phase 3) leads to reconstitution of the resting potential. It is initiated by a decrease in the cell membrane conductance to sodium and calcium and an opening of potassium channels, allowing the movement of intracellular potassium out of the cell (see Figure 3-5, A). Repolarizing potassium currents are also referred to as delayed rectifier currents (I_K or I_{Kv}).[19] The opening probability of these channels is modulated by autonomic input and antiarrhythmic drugs (potassium channel blockers) and decreased by inhalant anesthetics.[12,18] Furthermore, several ligand-operated potassium channels exist, which also influence the cellular action potential duration (i.e., I_{KAch}, activated by acetylcholine).[4] In some species the ultra-rapid rectifier current (I_{Kur}) is responsible for the short action potential duration of atrial cardiomyocytes. The I_{Kur} is not limited to the atrial tissue but also contributes to ventricular repolarization in horses and may contribute to the rate-related adaptation of the action potential duration required for the wide range of heart rates exhibited by horses at rest and during exercise.[15] Hypoxia and abnormalities in serum potassium or calcium may alter the repolarization process. Hypoxia, in particular, is known to activate cardiac ATP-sensitive potassium (K[ATP]) channels in sarcolemma and mitochondria. Drugs that modulate the K(ATP) channels (as activators or blockers) have been used as useful experimental tools for basic studies on ischemia and increased resistance to ischemia. On the other hand, K(ATP) openers are viewed as possible therapeutic agents for limiting the myocardial injury and cardiac arrhythmias caused by ischaemic episodes. The clinical role and relevance of K(ATP) channels in horses, other than shortening action potential duration during periods of ischemia, require further investigation. Hyperkalemia increases membrane conductance to potassium, thereby accelerating (shortening) repolarization, decreasing the action potential duration, shortening the QT interval, and increasing the amplitude of the T wave (peaked T waves) on the surface ECG.[11,17] Note that, even in the presence of hyperkalemia, the high intracellular potassium (exceeding 100 mmol/L) is more than adequate to drive potassium out of the cell (because extracellular potassium rarely exceeds 10 mmol/L).

Refractory periods and action potential duration.
Refractoriness serves to prevent rapid repetitive or tonic activation of the heart from initiating new action potentials (i.e., arrhythmias).[4,11] Normally the refractory period is closely related to the cellular action potential duration and depends on the rate of recovery of inactivated sodium channels. On a cellular level the *absolute refractory period* defines the time during which the heart cells cannot be excited; thus no premature action potential can be initiated. This phase extends from the start of the action potential (phase 0) to the first part of the repolarization phase (phase 3) (see Figure 3-5, *B*). The time window from the start of phase 3 until early phase 4 is referred to as the *relative refractory period (RRP)*. Sodium channels partially recover from the inactivated state during the RRP and enter the resting state, such that a normal or supranormal stimulus can elicit an electrical, albeit diminutive, potential that is characterized by a slow phase 0 depolarization and a low amplitude (see Figure 3-5, *B*). If a propagated impulse is generated by the premature potential, the conduction velocity of the resulting impulse is low. However, in the whole heart an abnormal action potential may remain a local event that is unable to initiate a propagated response and therefore cannot be recorded by a surface ECG. The time during which a premature stimulus does not result in a propagated response is referred to as the *effective refractory period.*

The duration and dispersion of cardiac myocyte action potentials and refractoriness throughout the myocardium are important determinants in the genesis of cardiac arrhythmias (see following paragraphs). For example, high vagal activity may predispose to atrial fibrillation (AF) by decreasing atrial action potential duration and refractoriness. Conversely, many antiarrhythmic drugs (i.e., quinidine, procainamide) prolong action potentials, repolarization (slow phase 3), and the refractory period, thereby decreasing the likelihood for arrhythmia.[12,18] Injectable and inhalant anesthetics interfere with potassium currents, thereby shortening the action potential and refractoriness. These actions can be antiarrhythmic in some instances and proarrhythmic in others, depending on the differential pattern and onset of anesthetic drug effects and the type of electrophysiologic abnormalities produced by preexisting cardiac disease.

Nodal tissues (sinoatrial node, atrioventricular node).
Phase 0 of the action potential is determined primarily by the slow L-type calcium (I_{Ca-L}) and slow Na$^+$ (I_f) currents in SA and AV nodal cells.[4,5,11] Slower phase 0 depolarization is caused by a somewhat lower (less negative) resting potential in nodal tissues, which causes inactivation of the majority of the fast Na$^+$ channels. Similarly, ischemic muscle cells have a less negative membrane potential and are more dependent on the slow inward current carried by calcium. Since the conduction velocity of the electrical impulse is related to the upstroke velocity of phase 0 (dV/dt), nodal cells and ischemic myocardial tissues conduct electrical impulses (action potentials) at a much slower rate than normal healthy myocardium. Slow conduction is one of the prerequisites for reentrant arrhythmias in the atrial and ventricular myocardium (see following paragraphs). Sympathetic stimulation and catecholamines (epinephrine, dopamine, dobutamine) accelerate AV nodal conduction by increasing L-type calcium currents in nodal tissues. High doses of injectable and inhalant anesthetics can prevent impulse initiation and conduction in both the SA and AV nodes because of their depressive effects on calcium channels.

Pacemaker activity. Tissues with inherent automatic activity (automaticity) show somewhat different electrophysiologic characteristics, especially during phase 4 of the action potential.[4,5,11] Automatic tissues (SA node; around the AV node; Purkinje network) demonstrate slow spontaneous depolarization during phase 4 (phase 4 depolarization) independent of a prior electrical stimulus. Phase 4 diastolic depolarization is caused by spontaneous slow inactivation of potassium currents (I_{Kv}), activation of "funny" currents (I_f; slow Na$^+$ current) and T-type Ca^{+2} currents (I_{Ca-T}), and possible contribution of a Na$^+$-based background current (I_b) (see Table 3-2). The inward rectifier current (I_{K1}) is missing in nodal tissues. The automatic tissue with the fastest inherent spontaneous depolarization serves as the pacemaker for the heart. The SA node has the fastest rate of phase 4 depolarization and is the pacemaker in normal healthy horses. Subsidiary pacemakers may compete with or usurp the role of the SA node as pacemaker in sick horses or horses with cardiac disease. Changes in autonomic tone, electrolyte concentrations (K$^+$; Ca^{+2}), and drugs influence the rate of spontaneous depolarization. An increase in parasympathetic tone decreases automaticity, and an increase in sympathetic tone increases automaticity (Figures 3-6 and 3-7). Small increases in extracellular potassium activate potassium channels, increasing repolarizing potassium currents, thereby depressing pacemaker activity. Clinically relevant doses of opioids and α_2-agonists may decrease pacemaker activity by increasing vagal tone. High concentrations of injectable and inhalant anesthetic drugs depress pacemaker activity. Lower anesthetic concentrations may increase pacemaker activity secondary to increases in sympathetic tone caused by light planes of anesthesia, pain, or hypotension.

Restoration of electrolyte homeostasis. The production of a cardiac action potential changes intracellular electrolyte homeostasis, resulting in relatively small increases in intracellular sodium and calcium and a small increase in extracellular potassium. Normal intracellular and

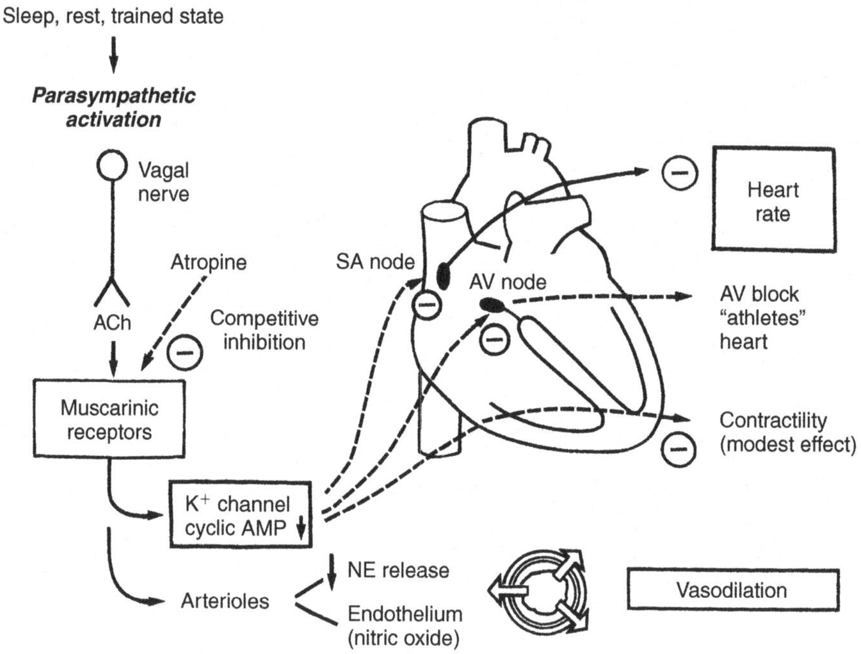

Figure 3–6. The parasympathetic nervous system produces inhibitory effects on the heart via muscarinic (M_2) receptors. Parasympathetic nerve stimulation decreases adenylate cyclase activity and opens potassium channels, decreasing SA node automaticity and slowing AV node conduction. Parasympathetic activity also dilates coronary arteries and has modest inhibitory effects on the force of ventricular contraction. (From Opie LH: *Control of the circulation. Heart physiology—from cell to circulation*, Philadelphia, 2004, Lippincott Williams & Wilkins, p 18. Figure copyright LH Opie, ©2004.)

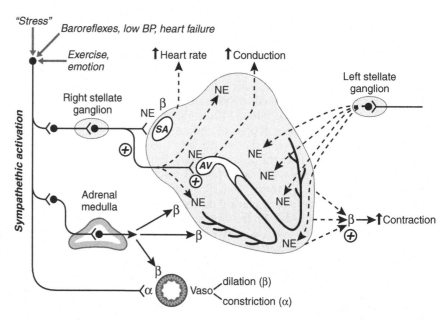

Figure 3–7. Activation of the sympathetic nervous system releases norepinephrine (NE), which increases cyclic AMP and activates calcium channels. The cardiac receptors primarily stimulated by sympathetic stimulation are β_1-adrenergic receptors. The vascular receptors are the α-adrenergic (α_1; α_2) vasoconstrictive receptors and the β_2-adrenergic vasodilatory receptors. Sympathetic stimulation increases the heart rate (+ chronotrope) and the conduction of the electrical impulse through the AV node and conduction system (+ dromotrope). The force of cardiac contraction and the rate of relaxation increase (+ inotrope; + lusitrope). Sympathetic stimulation also increases the myocardial excitability (+ bathmotrope) and therefore may increase arrhythmogenesis. (From Opie LH: *Control of the circulation. Heart physiology—from cell to circulation*, Philadelphia, 2004, Lippincott Williams & Wilkins, p 17. Figure copyright LH Opie, ©2004.)

extracellular concentrations of these principal electrolytes are restored and maintained by a variety of energy-consuming pumps, exchangers, and channels. Sodium and potassium gradients are primarily restored by the activity of the membrane-bound Na^+-K^+-ATPase. Calcium is removed from the cytoplasm by extrusion through the Na^+-Ca^{+2} exchanger and (to a minor extent) the Ca^{+2} pump. Intracellular calcium is also subject to reuptake by the sarcoendoplasmatic reticulum (SER) through an SER Ca^{+2}-ATPase (SERCA) mechanism (see following paragraphs; Figure 3-8). High doses of injectable and inhalant anesthetics interfere with all phases of the cardiac action potential most noticeably with phase 0 rapid depolarization and phase 2 and phase 3 delayed repolarization. This gives the cardiac action potential the appearance of an abbreviated triangle and results in a slow-

ing of conduction of electrical impulses; the potential for conduction block and cardiac arrhythmias; and decreases in transmembrane calcium flux, resulting in decreases in the force of cardiac contraction.

Cardiac activation. Intercellular connections within the myocardium, so-called gap junctions (connexons), allow ionic currents to pass rapidly from cell to cell. Electrically activated (depolarized) cells act to stimulate and depolarize adjacent cells, resulting in a rapid dispersion of electrical activity throughout the heart and causing the myocardial cells to act as a functional syncytium. Impulse conduction depends on active (action potential, ion currents) and passive properties (resistance, capacitance) of the conducting tissue, all of which can be influenced by physiologic regulatory

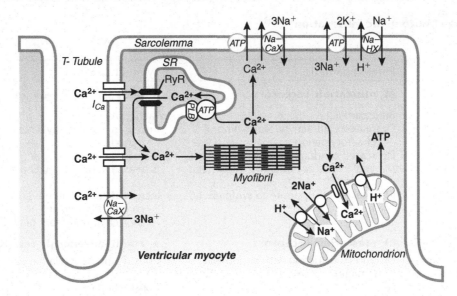

Figure 3–8. Depolarization of the cardiac cell membrane opens calcium (Ca^{+2}) channels, resulting in a calcium current (I_{Ca}), and increases in intracellular Ca^{+2}. Increases in intracellular Ca^{+2} trigger the release of calcium from SR via the RyR receptor. Additional calcium enters via the sodium-calcium exchanger. Increases in intracellular Ca^{+2} promote actin-myosin interaction and mitochondrial function (oxidative phoshorylation). Relaxation is initiated by uptake of Ca^{+2} into the SR. *RyR,* Ryanodine receptor (calcium-release channel); *SR,* sarcoplasmic reticulum; *Myofil,* myofilaments (actin and myosin; associated with tropomyosin and the troponin complex); *PLB,* phospholamban (associated with sarcoendoplasmatic reticulum Ca^{+2}-ATPase); *Na-CaX,* Na^+/Ca^{+2} exchanger (NCX); *ATP,* ATPase; *Na-HX,* Na^+/H^+ exchanger; *Mito,* mitochondrium. (From Bers DM: *Excitation—contraction coupling and cardiac contractile force,* ed 2, Dordrecht, 2001, Kluwer Academic Publishers, p 40.)

systems (e.g., autonomic tone, pH and electrolytes, circulating hormones) or by pathologic processes.[13]

The cardiac pacemaker, the *SA node,* located at the junction of the cranial vena cava and right auricle, initiates cardiac muscle depolarization and subsequent contraction across the right atrium. Specialized atrial muscle cells comprising *internodal pathways* and *Bachmann's bundle* facilitate transmission across the atria (see Figures 3-2 and 3-3).[20] Electrical conduction across the *AV nodal cells,* between the low right atrium and bundle of His, is very slow and subject to physiologic blockade from vagal efferent activity (see Figure 3-3).[21,22] Conduction delay in the AV node provides time for a coordinated, sequential AV contraction process and efficient cardiac pumping function. Conduction of electrical impulses through the *His bundle, bundle branches,* and *Purkinje system* proceeds at a faster velocity than through the ventricular muscle cells, ensuring a coordinated ventricular activation process.[9,23]

Terms such as *interatrial, atrioventricular, intraventricular,* and *interventricular synchronization* refer to the normal process of atrial and ventricular activation and contraction. Normal impulse conduction causes sequential contraction and relaxation of the atria and synchronized activation of the ventricles, ensuring synchronized and efficient cardiac pump function. Cardiac arrhythmias, especially those causing AV dissociation or abnormal ventricular activation, can result in a decrease in stroke volume. Large doses or rapid intravenous administration of almost any drug used for equine anesthesia can potentially cause sudden decreases in heart rate and, when combined with negative cardiac contractile effects and vasodilation, results in decreases in cardiac output and hypotension.

Autonomic Modulation of Cardiac Activation and Heart Rate

Activation of the SA node and therefore heart rate is modulated by the autonomic nervous system.[24] *Parasympathetic activity* depresses SA nodal activity and slows AV nodal conduction (Table 3-3; see Figure 3-6). The normal *resting heart rate* is usually lower than the *intrinsic heart rate* (observed under complete autonomic blockade), suggesting a predominance of the vagal over the sympathetic tone in resting unstressed horses.[25] Alterations in vagal tone control SA and AV nodal activity on a beat-by-beat basis in normal resting horses.[5] Acute changes in arterial blood pressure cause *baroreceptor reflex*–mediated inverse changes in heart rate secondary to changes in parasympathetic tone (see following paragraphs).[24] Parasympathetic stimulation also decreases conduction velocity and shortens the effective refractory period of the atrial tissue. Both slow conduction and a short refractory period predispose the heart to reentrant arrhythmias such as supraventricular tachycardias, including atrial flutter and AF. Injectable and inhalant anesthetic drugs, particularly halothane, may predispose anesthetized horses to supraventricular anrrhythmias, including AF caused by altered conduction and shortened refractoriness.

Sympathetic activity increases heart rate and shortens AV conduction time (see Table 3-3 and Figure 3-7). Sympathetic activity also increases cellular excitability, predisposes to cardiac arrhythmias, and increases myocardial oxygen consumption by augmenting the force of cardiac contraction, heart rate, and myocardial wall tension (see following paragraphs). Increases in sympathetic activity generally are more gradual than vagally mediated effects.[5] Sympathetic modulation is relatively unimportant in determining heart

Table 3–3. Effects of autonomic innervation[4,288,289]

Tissue	Response	
	Parasympathetic	**Sympathetic**
Heart	**M_2 muscarinic receptors**	**β_1 (and β_2) adrenergic receptors**
Sinoatrial node	Bradycardia	Tachycardia
Atrial tissue	Decreased contractility/Shortening of refractory period	Increased contractility/Shortening of refractory period
Atrioventricular (AV) node	Decreased conduction velocity, AV block	Increased automaticity and conduction velocity
His-Purkinje	Minimal effects opposite to sympathetic effects	Increased automaticity and conduction velocity
Ventricular myocardium	Minimal effects opposite to sympathetic effects	Increased contractility, relaxation, automaticity, conduction velocity, and O_2 consumption; shortened refractory period
Arterioles	**M_3 muscarinic receptors**	**α_1 and β_2 adrenergic receptors**
Coronary vessels	Dilation (constriction with endothelial damage)	Constriction (α_1); dilation (β_2)*
Skin and mucosa	—	Constriction (α_1)
Skeletal muscle	—	Constriction (α_1); dilation (β_2)*
Cerebral	—	Constriction (α_1; slight)
Pulmonary	—	Constriction (α_1) < dilation (β_2)*
Abdominal viscera	—	Constriction (α_1) > dilation (β_2)†
Renal	—	Constriction (α_1) > dilation (β_2)†
Veins	**M_3 muscarinic receptors**	**α_1 and α_2 adrenergic receptors**
Systemic	—	Constriction (α_1), dilation (β_2)
Bronchial smooth muscle	**M_3 muscarinic receptors**	**α_2 adrenergic receptors**
	Bronchoconstriction	Bronchodilation

— No effect.
*Dilation predominates in situ as a result of local metabolic autoregulation.
†Also dilation mediated by specific dopaminergic receptors.
Signaling pathways:
M_2: G_i-protein mediated inhibition of adenylyl-cyclase, decrease of cyclic adenosine monophosphate (cAMP); inhibition of L-type Ca^{2+} channels; activation of K^+ channels.
M_3: Phospholipase C–mediated formation of diacylglycerol (DAG) and inositol-triphosphate (IP_3); Ca^{2+} release from sarcoplasmatic reticulum (SR).
α_1: Phospholipase C–mediated formation of diacylglycerol (DAG) and inositol-triphosphate (IP_3); Ca^{2+} release from sarcoplasmatic reticulum (SR).
β_1: G_s-protein mediated stimulation of adenylyl-cyclase, increase of cAMP; stimulation of L-type Ca^{2+} channels, SERCA, troponin I, K^+ channels, and pacemaker currents (I_f).
β_2: G_i-protein mediated inhibition of adenylyl-cyclase, decrease of cAMP; inhibition of L-type Ca^{2+} channels [Heart: G_s and G_i-protein mediated effects].

rate in normal resting horses but becomes dominant during periods of stress or exercise.[24] Most drugs used to produce sedation and anesthesia produce some effect on autonomic tone in addition to their inherent direct effects on either parasympathetic or sympathetic nervous system activity. α_2-Agonists, opioids, and low doses of halothane can increase parasympathetic activity, leading to sinus bradycardia; sinus block or arrest; AV block; and AV dissociation, including isorhythmic dissociation.

Low doses of ketamine or tiletamine increase central sympathetic tone output, potentially resulting in sinus tachycardia. Most other injectable and inhalant anesthetics (thiopental, propofol, isoflurane, sevoflurane) depress sympathetic nervous system activity, resulting in sinus bradycardia, a slowing of AV conduction, and slow idioventricular rhythms.

Baroreceptor (pressure)–mediated reflexes are important in regulating heart rate primarily via alterations in para-sympathetic tone. The *Bainbridge reflex* is a baro (pressure) reflex that results in an increase in heart rate in response to a rise in atrial pressure. The Bainbridge reflex is most important when blood volume is raised above normal. In addition, arterial baroreceptors found in the arch of the aorta and bifurcation of the external and internal carotid arteries help to regulate arterial blood pressure by increasing parasympathetic tone and inhibiting sympathetic tone when arterial blood pressure increases, thereby decreasing heart rate, systemic vascular resistance (SVR) (vessel tone) and cardiac output (decreased cardiac contractile force). The arterial baroreceptor reflex predominates over the Bainbridge reflex even when the blood volume is diminished.[5] The physiologic relevance of the Bainbridge reflex in conscious or anesthetized horses is unknown. Furthermore, rhythmic changes in heart rate related to the respiratory cycle (*respiratory sinus arrhythmia*) are not very prominent in horses. Other reflexes, including *chemoreceptor reflexes, ventricular (stretch) receptor reflexes,* and *vasovagal mediated reflexes* are poorly defined in normal healthy horses and may play only a minor role in the regulation of the heart rate.[5]

Mechanical Function of the Heart

Normal cardiac activation is a prerequisite for normal heart function. Electrical excitation of the cardiac myocytes has to be transformed into mechanical activity for the heart to contract. This process is commonly referred to as *electromechanical coupling* or *excitation-contraction coupling.*

Electromechanical dissociation (EMD) describes a pathologic condition wherein electrical activation of the heart is not transformed into mechanical function. EMD is caused by severe metabolic derangements in myocardial metabolism and contractile element interaction. Clinically EMD is one cause for *pulseless electrical activity* (PEA), which may or may not be caused by a myocardial metabolic disturbance (Box 3-1). PEA is characterized by the presence of any recordable (normal or abnormal) cardiac electrical activity in the absence of a detectable heartbeat or pulse. The absence of a detectable heartbeat is usually the result of a combination of abnormal heart rate and/or rhythm, poor contractility, and abnormal ventricular loading conditions, resulting in inadequate stroke volume and cardiac output. The most common cause is hypovolemia, although it is important to remember that anesthetic overdose, particularly inhalant anesthetic overdose, can result in PEA and EMD that may be minimally responsive or unresponsive to large doses of epinephrine (200 µg/kg).

Cardiac Excitation-Contraction Coupling

Excitation-contraction coupling is the process whereby cardiac electrical activity (action potential) is converted to mechanical activity, resulting in cardiac contraction. Calcium ions entering the myocyte through L-type calcium channels during the plateau phase of the action potential trigger the release of intracellular calcium stored in the SR via calcium release channels (ryanodine receptors, RyR) (see Figure 3-8). This process is referred to as *calcium-induced calcium release.* The free calcium binds to the regulatory troponin-tropomyosin complex. Once calcium binds to

troponin-C (TN-C), a conformational change in the regulatory complex is induced such that troponin-I (TN-I) exposes a site on the actin molecule that is able to bind to the myosin ATPase located on the myosin head. This initiates cycling of contractile protein (actin-myosin) cross-bridges, leading to contraction of the myofilaments. Development of muscle tension and contraction follow the plateau of the action potential, with peak contraction occurring during late phase 3 or early phase 4 of the action potential.[4,5,26-28]

Myocardial *relaxation* requires removal of calcium from the cytoplasm by reuptake into the SR (through the SERCA) and by extrusion of calcium through the sarcolemma (through the sodium-calcium exchanger [NCX] and calcium ATPase) (see Figure 3-8). Note that myocardial relaxation is an active, energy-dependent process that, similar to myocardial contraction, depends on adequate energy and oxygen supply.

Inhalant anesthetics cause dose-dependent depression of myocardial contractility and relaxation by interfering with intracellular calcium cycling and decreasing the sensitivity of contractile filaments to calcium. Administration of calcium (calcium gluconate, calcium chloride) and catecholamines (dobutamine, dopamine) enhances the concentration of myocyte cytosolic calcium, increasing the amount of ATP metabolism, thereby attenuating the anesthetic-induced depression of ventricular function in horses anesthetized with halothane, isoflurane, and sevoflurane.[29]

The cardiac cycle (Wiggers' cycle). The relationship between electrical (ECG) and mechanical (pressure) events in the heart and their relation to heart sounds was first described by Carl J. Wiggers in the early 20th century.[30] Modifications of the Wiggers' diagram have since become the most frequently used descriptors of the temporal relationship among cardiac electrical, mechanical, and acoustic events (Figure 3-9, *A*).[3,5] Electrical activity precedes (and is a prerequisite of) mechanical activity; therefore arrhythmias can have important deleterious hemodynamic effects, especially during anesthesia.

The *P wave* of the ECG occurs as a result of electrical activation of the atria, late in ventricular diastole, and after passive filling of the ventricles. Atrial contraction (atrial pump) generates an *atrial sound (fourth heart sound,* S_4) filling the ventricle to a slightly greater extent (the *end-diastolic volume*). The increase in atrial pressure associated with atrial contraction generates the atrial *a* wave that is reflected into the systemic venous system, causing a normal *jugular pulse* in the ventral cervical region. The jugular pulse becomes particularly noticeable in horses that have right heart disease (tricuspid valve disease), are volume overloaded, or are recumbent. The magnitude of the atrial contribution to ventricular filling is greatest at high heart rates. Horses with AF and flutter lose the atrial contribution to ventricular filling (atrial priming effect) and therefore do not generate optimal cardiac output at higher heart rates (e.g., exercise).

The *QRS complex* signals *ventricular systole.* Depolarization of the ventricular myocardium initiates shortening of the myofilaments and increases in cardiac wall tension intraventricular pressure. The AV valves close once ventricular pressure exceeds atrial pressure, causing oscillations of the cardiohemic structures that generate the high-frequency *first heart sound* (S_1). This coincides with the beginning of *isovolumetric*

Box 3–1   Clinical Causes for Pulseless Electrical Activity

- Hypoxia
- Hypovolemia
- Trauma (hypovolemia from blood loss)
- Acidosis
- Hyperkalemia
- Hypoglycemia
- Hypocalcaemia
- Hyponatremia
- Hypothermia
- Overdose of calcium antagonist
- Drug (anesthetic) overdose
- Cardiac tamponade

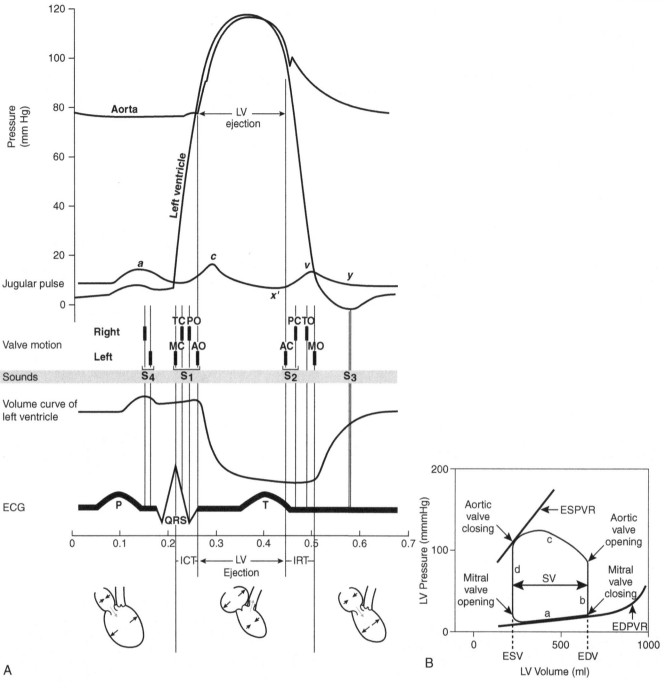

Figure 3–9. A, The cardiac cycle (Wiggers' diagram) illustrates the temporal relationship among the mechanical (pressure, volume), electrical (ECG), and acoustic (heart sounds) events that occur during each heart beat. Systolic ventricular events begin with the QRS complex and can be divided into periods of *isovolumetric contraction* (ICT; from mitral/tricuspid valve closure [MC/TC] to aortic/pulmonic valve opening [AO/PO]), *ventricular ejection* (from AO/PO to aortic/pulmonic valve closure [AC/PC]), and *isovolumetric relaxation* (IRT; from AC/PC to mitral/tricuspid valve opening [MO/TO]). During the ejection period the ventricular volume decreases from maximum (end-diastolic) to minimal (end-systolic) volume. The end-diastolic ventricular volume is an estimate of ventricular *preload*. The difference between the end-diastolic and the end-systolic volume is the *stroke volume*, which correlates to the area under the aortic time-velocity profile of the echocardiogram (not shown). The atrial pressure changes include the a, c, and v waves and the x' and y descents. Atrial contraction causes an increase in atrial pressure (a wave) with a resultant end-diastolic increment in ventricular filling. The x' wave is caused by atrial expansion resulting from ventricular contraction; the v wave represents the peak of venous return just before tricuspid or mitral valve opening; and the y descent represents emptying of atrial blood into the ventricles (rapid ventricular filling). The jugular pulse wave parallels the atrial pressure changes. The S_1 and S_2 heart sounds are caused by oscillations of cardiohemic structures associated with the closure of the atrioventricular and semilunar valves, respectively. The S_3 occurs during rapid ventricular filling. The S_4, or atrial sound, is related to vibrations that occur during atrial contraction and resultant filling of the ventricle. **B,** Cartoon of the left ventricular pressure-volume curve illustrating ventricular filling *(a)*, isovolumic contraction *(b)*, ventricular ejection *(c)*, isovolumic relaxation *(d)*, and associated heart valve opening and closing. The stroke volume *(SV)* is determined by the change in ventricular volume. The slope of the end-systolic pressure-volume relationship *(ESPVR)* is a load-independent index of ventricular contractility. (**A** Modified from Schlant: Normal physiology of the cardiac system, part I, chapter 3. In Hurst JW: The heart, vol I, ed 9, New York, 1998, McGraw-Hill.)

contraction. Once the intraventricular pressure exceeds the pressure in the great arteries (pulmonary artery, aorta), the semilunar valves (pulmonic, aortic) open, and the *ejection phase* begins. The contracting heart twists slightly during systole, and the left ventricle strikes the chest wall caudal to the left olecranon, causing the *cardiac impulse* or "apex beat" (a useful timing clue for cardiac auscultation). The delay between the onset of the QRS and the opening of the semilunar valves is termed the *preejection period.* During the ejection phase blood is ejected into the pulmonary and systemic arteries with an initial velocity generally peaking between 1 and 1.6 m/sec. Both the preejection period and aortic root velocity are useful measures of ventricular myocardial contractility. A *functional systolic murmur (ejection murmur),* likely caused by minor flow turbulences in the large vessels during the ejection phase, is often heard over the outlet valves and great vessels at the left base of the heart on the left chest wall. The *arterial pulse* can be palpated during systole, but the actual timing of the pulse depends on the proximity of the palpation site relative to the heart. Changes in ventricular volume during the ejection period (end-diastolic minus end-systolic ventricular volume) define the *stroke volume.* The ratio of the stroke volume to the end-diastolic volume is the *ejection fraction,* a common index of global systolic ventricular function (Box 3-2). The atria fill during ventricular systole, generating a positive-pressure wave (the *v wave*) in the atrial pressure curves (see Figure 3-9, *A*).

At the end of the ejection period, as ventricular pressures fall below that in the pulmonary artery and aorta, the semilunar valves close, resulting in the cardiohemic events that generate the high-frequency *second heart sound(s)* (S_2) and the incisura of the arterial pressure curve. The pulmonary valve may close either earlier or later than the aortic valve in horses. Asynchronous valve closure may lead to audible splitting of S_2, which can be extreme in some horses with

lung disease and pulmonary hypertension.[31] Closure of the semilunar valves defines the beginning of *ventricular diastole.* Ventricular diastole can be subdivided into four phases: isovolumetric relaxation, rapid ventricular filling, diastasis, and atrial contraction (see Figure 3-9, *A*).

The time interval between aortic valve closure and mitral valve opening is referred to as *isovolumetric relaxation phase.* Ventricular muscle tension decreases during this phase without lengthening so that ventricular volume remains unaltered. Once the ventricles have relaxed so that atrial pressure exceeds corresponding ventricular pressure, the AV valves open, and *rapid ventricular filling* ensues, with a peak inflow velocity of between 0.5 and 1 m/sec. The ventricular pressures increase only slightly during this phase, whereas the ventricular volume curves change dramatically. The changes in ventricular pressure and volume can be displayed as a ventricular pressure-volume curve, which in turn is used to determine the ventricular end-systolic pressure volume relationship (ESPVR), a load-independent index of ventricular contractility (see Figure 3-9, *B*). Rapid filling may be associated with a *functional protodiastolic murmur* heard best on either the right or left side of the chest wall over the ventricular inlet. Rapid ventricular filling is concluded by the *third heart sound* (S_3), which is caused by low-frequency vibrations generated by sudden cessation of rapid filling. The loss of atrial volume after the AV valves open results in a decrease in atrial pressure (the *y descent*) that can be reflected in the jugular furrow as the vein collapses. Rapid ventricular filling is followed by a period of markedly reduced low-velocity filling (diastasis). This period may last for seconds in the horse because of its slow heart rate and is accentuated in horses with sinus bradycardia or pronounced sinus arrhythmia. The last phase of diastole is the ventricular filling caused by the *atrial contraction.* Functional *presystolic murmurs* can be heard between the fourth and first heart sounds during this period in some horses (Figure 3-10).

Determinants of ventricular function. Systolic and diastolic ventricular function in conjunction with heart rate and rhythm determine the ability of the heart to pump blood (Figure 3-11). Measurements used to assess cardiac and circulatory function in horses include heart rate (HR) and heart sounds, pulse character and quality, arterial blood pressure (ABP), cardiac output (CO), stroke volume (SV), ejection fraction (EF), central venous pressure (CVP), pulmonary capillary wedge pressure (PCWP), and arteriovenous oxygen difference ($C_{a-v}O_2$). The advent of ultrasonography and use of first m-mode and then two-dimensional (2D) color flow echocardiography has added a whole new approach to the evaluation, diagnosis, and treatment of cardiovascular disease in horses.

Cardiac output, the amount of blood pumped by the left (or right) ventricle in 1 min (L/min), is the product of ventricular *stroke volume* (ml/beat) and heart rate (beats/min). *Cardiac index* refers to the cardiac output divided by (indexed) body surface area (see Box 3-2). The cardiac output is most often indexed to body weight in horses because of the lack of accurate estimates of body surface area. Cardiac output and *mean arterial blood pressure* (MAP) are used to calculate systemic vascular resistance (SVR) (SVR = MAP/CO); note that SVR and cardiac output are inversely related (see Box 3-2).

Box 3–2 Hemodynamic Associations

Stroke volume* = End-diastolic volume – End-systolic volume

$$\text{Ejection fraction} = \frac{\text{Stroke volume}}{\text{End diastolic volume}}$$

Cardiac output = Stroke volume × Heart rate

$$\text{Cardiac index} = \frac{\text{Cardiac output}}{\text{Body surface area}^\dagger}$$

Systemic vascular resistance [index] =
$$\frac{\text{Mean arterial pressure-Central venous pressure}}{\text{Cardiac output [index]}} \times 80$$

Pulmonary vascular resistance [index] =
$$\frac{\text{Mean pulmonary artery pressure-Left atrial pressure}^\ddagger}{\text{Cardiac output [index]}} \times 80$$

Blood pressure = Cardiac output × Vascular resistance

---

* Stroke volume is determined by heart rate, preload, afterload, and contractility.
† Cardiac output indexed to body weight (ml/min/kg).
‡ Pulmonary capillary wedge pressure is used as an estimate of left atrial pressure.

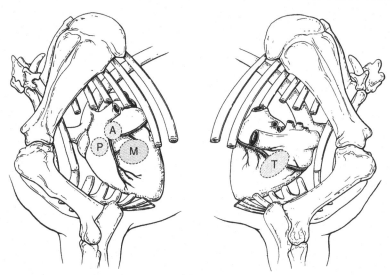

Figure 3–10. Note the size and anatomical position of the heart within the thorax (**A**, left; **B**, right). The cardiac apex (apical area) is usually slightly above the level of the olecranon and can be identified by palpation of the apical beat. The cardiac base (basilar area) is located more cranially at the level of the scapulohumeral joint. The shaded areas represent the respective valve areas (*P*, pulmonic; *A*, aortic; *M*, mitral; *T*, tricuspid). The right atrium (above T), tricuspid valve, and right ventricular inlet (inflow region, below T) are located on the right side of the thorax. Most (but not all) murmurs of tricuspid valve disease are heard best over the right chest wall, usually more dorsally as they radiate into the right atrium (above T). The right ventricular outflow projects to the left side of the thorax and continues into the pulmonary artery, which is located at the left dorsal cardiac base (above P). Thus murmurs originating in the right ventricular outlet (such as murmurs from subpulmonic ventricular septal defects), diastolic murmurs of relative pulmonic stenosis, and functional pulmonary arterial murmurs are heard best over the left chest wall (P). The aortic valve is located centrally within the chest; and diastolic murmurs of aortic insufficiency may be heard at either hemithorax, although they are usually loudest on the left (**A**). Functional murmurs generated in the pulmonary artery and ascending aorta are heard at the left base. The systolic murmur of mitral regurgitation radiates to the left apex of the heart and is usually heard across the left ventricular inlet (area caudoventral of M). The functional protodiastolic murmurs associated with ventricular filling are usually evident over the ventricular inlets and may be heard on either side of the thorax. (From Orsini JA, Divers TJ, editors: *Manual of equine emergencies: treatment and procedures*, ed 2, Philadelphia, 2003, Saunders, pp 130-188.)

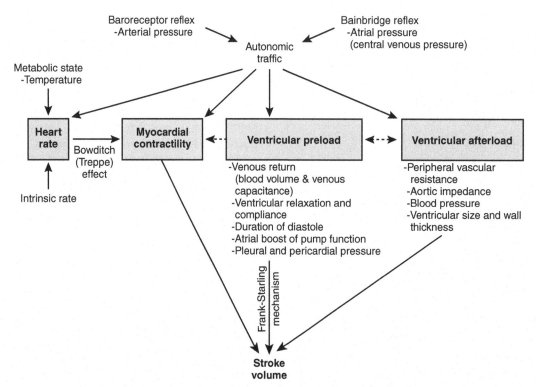

Figure 3–11. Determinants of cardiac output and blood pressure.

Ventricular systolic function. Ventricular systolic function is the principal determinant of stroke volume and depends on myocardial contractility (inotropy), relaxation (lusitropy), preload, and afterload (see Figure 3-11).[2,4,5,32] All of these factors are interrelated and coupled in the normal healthy heart. Myocardial *inotropy* is the inherent ability of cardiac contractile proteins, actin and myosin, to interact, contract, and develop force.[33] Autonomic tone, preload, and heart rate are the three most important mechanisms that acutely regulate cardiac contractile function under physiologic conditions.[33] β-Adrenergic stimulation enhances calcium cycling and sensitizes contractile proteins, thereby increasing the rate and force of contraction (and relaxation). Increases in preload stretch contractile proteins, sensitizing myosin heads to calcium (Frank-Starling mechanism, see following paragraphs); whereas an increase in heart rate produces a rate-dependent accumulation of cytosolic calcium (Bowditch or "treppe" effect), which helps to regulate the contractile state under physiologic conditions (see Figure 3-11). Dopamine, dobutamine, and digitalis glycosides increase cardiac contractility by a variety of mechanisms, including increases in intracellular calcium and sensitization of contractile proteins to calcium (see Chapters 22 and 23).[34] Conversely, inotropism is depressed by hypoxia, metabolic acidosis, hypothermia, endotoxemia and most anesthetic drugs.

Contractility is difficult to quantify in the clinical setting because inotropy, preload, and afterload are interrelated in such a way that a change in one variable will simultaneously alter the others (see Figure 3-11).[32,33] Put in more general terms, cardiac contractility is load dependent. Nonetheless it is useful to attempt to identify which variables are responsible for changes in cardiac contractility and cardiac output. A classical invasive index of cardiac contractility is the maximum rate of pressure change during isovolumetric contraction ($+dp/dt_{max}$; Figure 3-12 and Table 3-4).[35,36] Commonly used noninvasive indices determined by echocardiography (i.e., fractional shortening, ejection fraction, the ratio of pre-ejection period to ejection time) are strongly load dependent

and generally represent overall systolic function rather than contractility. A variety of other invasive and noninvasive indices are used in clinical and experimental settings.[32,33,36]

Ventricular *preload* (volume or pressure) is a positive determinant of ventricular systolic function, stretching the ventricular myofilaments before ejection. The relationship between end-diastolic ventricular volume and systolic ventricular performance (force or pressure development) is known as the *Frank-Starling mechanism* or *Starling's law of the heart*.[33,37] Normal ventricles are strongly preload dependent. Hypovolemia and subnormal venous filling pressures are two common causes of reduced cardiac output during anesthesia. Cardiac arrhythmias, anesthetic drugs, and drugs administered as preanesthetic medication increase vascular compliance, thereby decreasing venous return and cardiac output (see Chapters 10, 11, and 15).[38] α_2-Agonists increase venous tone and decrease venous capacitance early after administration, thereby increasing venous filling pressures and pressures in the right atrium. However, the long-term effect of α_2-agonists causes vasodilation, a decrease in venous return, and a potential decrease in cardiac contractile force and cardiac output. Noxious stimuli during light planes of anesthesia may increase venous return by causing sympathetic-induced venoconstriction. Conversely, venodilation (e.g., anesthetic drug overdose; endotoxemia) with pooling of blood decreases ventricular preload and cardiac output. Decreases in ventricular filling pressures are typically counteracted by infusion of intravenous crystalloid or colloid solutions (see Chapter 7). Preload can be estimated by determining ventricular end-diastolic volume or size (by echocardiography or impedance catheter) or by measuring venous filling pressures (e.g., CVP). Venous filling pressures (central venous, pulmonary diastolic, or PCWP) are accurate gauges of acute changes in preload only if heart rate and ventricular compliance (distensibility) are normal and do not change during the anesthetic period.

Ventricular *afterload* is a term used to describe the forces that resist the ejection of blood into the aorta and is closely related to the tension (or stress) in the ventricular wall during systole. Afterload can be thought of in terms of vascular resistance and reactance (stiffness). Standard formulas used to calculate vascular resistance (SVR = MAP/CO) do not account for the pulsatile nature of blood flow and the dynamic aspects of afterload (aortic input impedance and stiffness). However, they demonstrate that SVR and therefore afterload increase with arterial blood pressure. High afterload limits ventricular systolic performance and decreases stroke volume, thereby reducing cardiac output. The failing ventricle or the ventricle depressed by anesthetic drugs is more sensitive to afterload than the normal ventricle. One potential disadvantage of infusing vasoconstricting drugs to increase arterial blood pressure is the accompanying increase in left ventricular afterload; such drugs should only be used in situations in which volume loading and inotropic support of ventricular systolic function are insufficient to maintain perfusion pressures and in conditions in which hypotension is the result of extensive peripheral vasodilation (i.e., vascular hyporeactivity, severe sepsis, septic shock). Conversely a decrease in MAP (as a result of vasodilation) decreases afterload and ventricular wall stress and, providing ventricular inotropy is not impaired, can result in an increase in cardiac output.

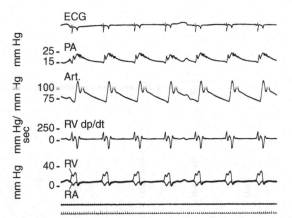

Figure 3–12. Blood pressure traces obtained from an anesthetized adult horse. *ECG,* surface electrocardiogram; *PA,* pulmonary arterial pressure; *Art.,* systemic arterial pressure; *dp/dt,* right ventricular rate of change of pressure, with the positive peaks corresponding to $+dp/dt_{max}$ occurring during isovolumetric contraction and the negative peaks corresponding to $-dp/dt_{max}$ occurring during isovolumetric relaxation; *RV,* right ventricular pressure; *RA,* right atrial pressure.

Table 3–4. Hemodynamic data from healthy resting horses

		Standardbred	Swedish Standardbred	Thoroughbred (Thb)	Quarter Horse (QH)	Pony	Various or n/d	QH and Thb foals
References		73 35	290	43 291 292 293	294	77 295 104 296	78 90 54	79
n		7 15	30 (20[i])	6 9 12 (7[i]) 7	5	7 8 18 5	8 39 14	2 9 4
Age	Years	6 to 23 3 to 30	5 to 18	2 to 4 3 to 6 2 to 16 3 to 6	2	Adult Adult 2 to 4 2 to 3	2 to 10 n/d n/d	2h 2d 2wk
Body weight	Kg	426 to 531 380 to 600	465 to 637	440 to 500 415 to 525 228 to 505 389 to 523	418 ± 30 442 ± 26	130 to 195 170 to 232 75 to 264 170 to 296	470 to 550 386 to 521 431 to 545	45.4 ± 3.4 48.3 ± 7.2 70.6 ± 12.2
Recording conditions		**Standing, conscious, unsedated**						**Lateral recumbency**
Heart rate	Min⁻¹	35 ± 3 34 ± 3	45 ± 10	33[h] 42 ± 6 39 ± 4 37 ± 2	47 ± 7 43 ± 2	56 ± 3 49 ± 2 58.8 ± 23 44[h]	37 ± 6 — —	83 ± 14 95 ± 18 95 ± 10
Systolic SBP	mm Hg	118 ± 13^{a,d} —	144 ± 17^{b,e}	142 ± 11.8^{b,e} 168 ± 6^{b,e}		131 ± 16^{b,d}		95.7 ± 17^{d,c} 91.4 ± 13.5^{d,c} 100.3 ± 6.4^{d,c}
Mean SBP	mm Hg	95 ± 12^{a,d} —	124 ± 13^{b,e}	114 ± 10.8^{b,e} 133 ± 4^{b,e}	121 ± 7^{b,e} 99 ± 5^{b,e}	110 ± 10^{b,d}		
Diastolic SBP	mm Hg	76 ± 10^{a,d} —	98 ± 14^{b,e}	99 ± 10.6^{b,e} 116 ± 4^{b,e}		86 ± 8^{b,d}		
Systolic PAP	mm Hg	45 ± 9^b	45 ± 9^b	37 ± 1^b 35^{b,h}		34 ± 5^{b,d}	42 ± 8^a 42 ± 5^b	
Mean PAP	mm Hg	23 ± 4^b —	30 ± 8^b	34 ± 5.8^b 29 ± 2^b	20 ± 4^b 22 ± 2^b	25.3 ± 2.1^a 22.7 ± 3^{b,d}	31 ± 6^a 26 ± 4^b	40.3 ± 6.6^c 27.8 ± 6.9^c 27.4 ± 6.0^c

(Continued)

Parameter	Units					
Diastolic PAP	mm Hg	22 ± 8			24 ± 6[a]; 18 ± 4[b]	
PCWP	mm Hg	16 ± 4[b]	22 ± 2[b]	19 ± 2[a]; 14.5 ± 3[b,d]	18 ± 6[a]; 13 ± 2[b]	7.5 ± 3.5[c]; 8.7 ± 2.4[c]; 8.1 ± 1.4[c]
Systolic LVP	mm Hg			125 ± 5.3[a]		
LVEDP	mm Hg	17 ± 7[a]			155 ± 9[b]; 29 ± 2.6[a]	
LV +dp/dt$_{max}$	mm Hg/sec	1241 ± 224[a]			12 ± 2[b]; 1361 ± 161[a]	
LV -dp/dt$_{max}$	mm Hg/sec	1756 ± 200[a]			1600[b]	
LV *Tau*	msec	41 ± 12[a]				
Mean RAP	mm Hg	5 ± 3[b]	10 ± 4[b]	5.3 ± 1.2[a]	8 ± 6[a]; 6 ± 3[b]	3.1 ± 0.9[c]; 4.1 ± 3.3[c]; 4.6 ± 1.8[c]
Systolic RVP	mm Hg	51 ± 9[b]	59 ± 6.9[b]	35 ± 2[a]	46 ± 6[b]	
Mean RVP	mm Hg		25 ± 4.0[b]	21 ± 4[a]; 21 ± 2[a]		
RVEDP	mm Hg	22 ± 4.8[a]	11 ± 6[b]; 15 to 19[a,h]; 7 ± 6[a]; 13 ± 4.4[b]		6 ± 4[b]	
RV +dp/dt$_{max}$	mm Hg/sec	477 ± 84[a]	560 ± 120[a]	670 ± 105[a]; 567 ± 14[a]		
RV -dp/dt$_{max}$	mm Hg/sec		680[a,h]; 380 ± 90[a]			

Table 3-4. Hemodynamic data from healthy resting horses—Cont'd.

Parameter	Units					
RV *Tau*	msec			39 ± 4[a] / 65 ± 10[a]		
CO	L/min	28 ± 4[f]	40 ± 11[g]			
CI	ml/min/kg	58 ± 9[f]	76 ± 19[g]	32.1 ± 7.1[g] / 32.23 ± 0.97[g]	10.9 ± 3.4[g] / 21[h,g]	155.3 ± 11.5[f] / 204 ± 35.4[f] / 222.1 ± 43.2[f]
SV	ml	854 ± 160[f]	864 ± 232[g]	69 ± 16[g] / 69 ± 3[g] / 820 ± 158[g] / 889 ± 55[g]	217 ± 103[g] / 72.6 ± 8.2[f]	
SI	ml/kg	1.8 ± 0.4[f]	1.6 ± 0.4[g]	1.8 ± 0.4[g]		1.89 ± 0.18[f] / 2.06 ± 0.27[f] / 2.3 ± 0.7[f]
SVR	Dynes·s·cm^{-5}	262.4 ± 63.4	265 ± 81		(807)[k]	1027 ± 246 / 723 ± 150 / 497 ± 174
PVR	Dynes·s·cm^{-5}	21.2 ± 21.0	68 ± 23	333 ± 18	(167)[k]	363 ± 59.4 / 167 ± 72 / 104 ± 42

CI, cardiac index; *CO*, cardiac output; $LV \pm dp/dt_{max}$, left ventricular positive and negative maximum rate of pressure change; *LVEDP*, left ventricular end-diastolic pressure; *LVP*, left ventricular pressure; *LV Tau*, left ventricular time constant of isovolumetric relaxation; *mm Hg*, millimeters of mercury; *n*, number; *PAP*, pulmonary artery pressure; *PCWP*, pulmonary capillary wedge pressure; *PVR*, pulmonary vascular resistance; *RAP*, right atrial pressure; *RVP*, right ventricular pressure; *RVEDP*, right ventricular end-diastolic pressure; $RV \pm dp/dt_{max}$, right ventricular positive and negative maximum rate of pressure change; *RV Tau*, right ventricular time constant of isovolumetric relaxation; *SBP*, systemic blood pressure; *SI*, stroke index; *SV*, stroke volume; *SVR*, systemic vascular resistance.

All data reported as mean ± SD unless stated otherwise.
[a]High-fidelity microtip pressure transducer (Millar or similar).
[b]Fluid-filled systems (zero-pressure reference point at level of shoulder [olecranon[292]]).
[c]Fluid-filled systems (zero-pressure reference point midthoracic level).
[d]Aortic pressures.
[e]Carotid artery pressures.
[f]Thermodilution.
[g]Dye dilution (indocyanine green).
[h]Mean derived from reported graphs.
[i]For CO and related parameters.
[k]Estimated from mean values (SVR = mean SBP×80/CO; PVR = mean PAP×80/CO).

Afterload is difficult to measure clinically. The SVR (see following paragraphs) only reflects peripheral vasomotor tone and does not allow adequate assessment of vascular stiffness. Sometimes SVR and afterload show discordant changes during pharmacologic interventions.[39] The diastolic aortic blood pressure and thus the pressure the left ventricle has to generate to initiate ejection of blood into the aorta can be used as a surrogate of left-ventricular afterload. Echocardiography can be used to assess the ventricular components of afterload such as ventricular size and wall thickness. However, the dynamic aspects of afterload that occur during the cardiac cycle are not easily quantified and therefore are not routinely monitored.[40]

The common septum (interventricular septum) and close anatomic association of the two ventricles within a common pericardial sack ensures that the function of one ventricle directly influences the function of the other ventricle. This interaction between the two ventricles is referred to as *ventricular interdependence*.[41,42] Direct interaction is caused by forces transmitted through the interventricular septum and by pericardial constraint. Series interaction is equally important and refers to the fact that over time cardiac output from the left ventricle has to equal that of the right ventricle because ventricular filling depends on venous return and output from the contralateral ventricle. Ventricular interdependence is responsible for the respiratory variations in stroke volume and systemic blood pressure observed in quiet resting horses and spontaneously breathing horses. These variables can change markedly during anesthesia and mechanical ventilation in horses that are volume depleted, have pericardial disease, or develop heart failure (see Chapters 17 and 22).[41,42]

Structural and functional competency of the cardiac valves and ventricular septa influence ventricular systolic function. Mitral or tricuspid valve insufficiency reduce the forward flow of blood and stroke volume and can result in either pulmonary or systemic venous and hepatic congestion, respectively. Aortic valve stenosis (rare) or insufficiency (common in old horses) may seriously reduce ventricular stroke volume unless there is adequate compensation from ventricular dilation and hypertrophy or increase in heart rate. Most atrial and ventricular septal defects are well tolerated at rest; however, large defects decrease ventricular stroke volume.

Ventricular diastolic function. Coronary perfusion occurs during diastole when the myocardium is relaxing and the intramural pressures are low. Large, thick-walled noncompliant ventricles are hard to perfuse, especially when heart rate is elevated. Diastolic function and ventricular filling are affected by ventricular wall thickness and compliance (passive ventricular filling in mid-to-late diastole), atrial rhythm and mechanical function (atrial contribution to ventricular filling), heart rate and rhythm (filling time), sympathetic activity (improves active relaxation and increasing filling pressures), venoconstriction and venous return (filling and preload), coronary perfusion (oxygen and energy supply), pericardial disease (restraining cardiac filling), and intrapleural pressure (opposing ventricular filling pressures). Generally horses with abnormal diastolic function depend more on heart rate and require higher filling pressures to distend the ventricles and to maintain cardiac output.

Myocardial *relaxation* or *lusitropy*, is an *active*, energy-consuming process linked to reuptake of calcium from the cytoplasm into the SER and extrusion of calcium through the cell membrane (see Figure 3-8). Lusitropy is closely linked to inotropy on the basis of its dependency on calcium cycling. Sympathetic stimulation exerts a positive lusitropic effect. Conversely ventricular relaxation is impaired by hypoxia; acidosis; and cardiac diseases, including ventricular hypertrophy and ischemia. The effects of anesthetic drugs on diastolic function in horses have not been systematically evaluated. However, inhalant anesthetics have been shown to impair right ventricular relaxation in horses.[43] Myocardial *compliance* is defined as the change in ventricular volume produced by a change in ventricular filling pressure (dV/dP). Alterations in ventricular compliance primarily affect passive filling during mid-to-late diastole. Myocardial fibrosis, ventricular hypertrophy, pericardial disease, or severe ventricular dilation reduce compliance. Passive ventricular filling is also impeded by elevated intrapleural pressure (i.e., with mechanical ventilation and positive end-expiratory pressure (see Chapter 17).

Atrial booster pump function or *contractile function* is responsible for late-diastolic ventricular filling and contributes to ventricular end-diastolic volume (see Figure 3-11).[44-46] Volatile anesthetic drugs decrease atrial contractility and relaxation.[44] AF leads to a loss of organized atrial contractile function, thereby reducing the effects of atrial contraction (priming) on ventricular preload and decreasing ventricular systolic performance. The loss of atrial pump function is not very important, is not associated with a deterioration of hemodynamics at resting or slow heart rates in horses, and is usually clinically irrelevant if no other cardiac diseases coexist.[47] Similarly, AF is well tolerated during anesthesia, providing the ventricular rate does not become elevated. Occasionally the acute onset of AF during anesthesia can result in increases in ventricular rate and a decrease in arterial blood pressure.[47] A sudden failure of atrial function can cause acute hemodynamic decompensation in patients with failing ventricular function, impaired ventricular relaxation, and reduced ventricular compliance.[44]

Several methods have been used to evaluate diastolic ventricular function in animals, including horses.[32,48] Invasive methods involve cardiac catheterization using high-fidelity catheter-tip pressure transducers (i.e., Millar catheters). The time constant of isovolumetric relaxation (*tau*) and the maximum rate of negative pressure change during the isovolumetric relaxation phase ($-dp/dt_{max}$) are considered the most reliable and least load-dependent indices of ventricular relaxation (see Table 3-4).[43,48] Evaluation of ventricular compliance and atrial mechanical function requires simultaneous recording of ventricular and atrial pressure and volume changes over time. Noninvasive methods, including echocardiography, are clinically more applicable but are less reliable, are generally more load dependent, and have not been adequately evaluated in horses.

Myocardial Oxygen Balance. *Myocardial oxygen demand* (MVO_2) is determined primarily by heart rate, myocardial inotropic state (contractility), and afterload (ventricular wall stress [affected by arterial blood pressure, ventricular size, and wall thickness]).[4,10] According to Laplace's law, *wall stress* (σ) in a thin-walled sphere is defined as:

$$\sigma = \frac{p \times r}{2d}$$

where p is pressure, r is radius, and d is wall thickness.[5] Alternatively wall stress can be calculated as $\sigma = p \times \sqrt[3]{V}/2d$ since r is proportional to $\sqrt[3]{V}$. The product of peak systolic pressure and heart rate (heart rate pressure product [RPP]) is commonly used as a clinical index of myocardial oxygen demand and represents an estimate of the external work performed by the cardiac pump (Table 3-5). Internal work caused by tension development, although equally important, is not routinely quantified. Nonetheless it should be noted that ventricular enlargement augments MVO$_2$ by increasing wall stress, even if heart rate, stroke volume, and blood pressure are unchanged. The failing ventricle is unable to maintain a normal stroke volume and evokes a compensatory increase in ventricular preload and peripheral vascular resistance to maintain arterial blood pressures; the ratio of external to internal work decreases, and the efficiency of work declines at the cost of a greater oxygen consumption.[4] Generally the work efficiency of the myocardium can be improved by decreasing the afterload and increasing the preload imposed on the ventricle.

An imbalance between myocardial oxygen demand and delivery can impair ventricular systolic and diastolic function and may affect cardiac rhythm. *Myocardial oxygen delivery (MDO$_2$)* depends on coronary blood flow and arterial oxygen content. The oxygen extraction in the myocardium is very high, and increased oxygen demands must be met primarily by an increase in coronary blood flow. *Coronary blood flow* depends on diastolic aortic blood pressure, diastolic (coronary perfusion) time, sympathetic tone, and local metabolic factors.[4,5] Increases in ventricular diastolic filling pressure appose coronary blood flow. Coronary vascular tone is predominantly under local, nonneural control, mediated by a variety of vasodilator substances (i.e., adenosine and nitric oxide) released during episodes of increased metabolic activity. Normally coronary perfusion is effectively *autoregulated,* even at high heart rates (up to 200/min in ponies); however, coronary autoregulation is not as effective if diastolic perfusing pressure in the aorta decreases.[4,49] Coronary flow is highest in the ventricular myocardium, ventricular septum, and left ventricular free wall.[50] The immediate subendocardial layer of myocardium is probably most vulnerable to ischemic injury[51] and may account in part for the ST-T depression and changes in the T waves observed in normal horses during tachycardia and hypotension. The combination of hypotension and tachycardia, which develops in some anesthetized horses, is deleterious to coronary perfusion and frequently leads to ST segment elevation or depression in the ECG.

The Circulation—Central Hemodynamics, Peripheral Blood Flow, and Tissue Perfusion

The circulation is divided into systemic and pulmonary components (Figure 3-13). The pressure generated by the left ventricle distributes the cardiac output to the tissues via large conduit arteries, smaller distributive arteries, local resistance arteries, and capillaries. Blood flow distribution and SVR are functions of the resistance arteries or arterioles. The low-pressure systemic veins are the major capacitance vessels for the circulation. The right ventricle pumps as much blood as the left ventricle, but at much lower systolic pressures, into the pulmonary artery. The pulmonary microcirculation is constructed to facilitate nutrient and gas exchange. Oxygen-rich pulmonary venous blood returns to the systemic circulation via the left atrium. Critical aspects of circulatory function and tissue perfusion include blood volume, SVR, blood pressure, cardiac output, regional blood flow, functional capillary density, and venous return (see Figures 3-9 and 3-13).

Central Hemodynamics

Hemodynamic variables that can be measured or calculated include arterial blood pressure, pulmonary artery pressure and pulmonary artery occlusion (capillary wedge) pressure, intracardiac pressures, CVP, cardiac output, systemic and pulmonary vascular resistances, arteriovenous oxygen difference, and oxygen extraction ratio (see Table 3-5, Figures 3-9 and 3-13, and Box 3-2; Box 3-3).[1,52-54] Normal values for these variables depend on the methods used for measurement; the head and body position of the horse (e.g., dorsal versus lateral recumbency); and the effects of administered tranquilizers, sedatives, or anesthetic drugs. Technical aspects of intravascular pressure recordings are important in the interpretation of pressure data.[52] For example, the difference in placement of the transducer relative to the heart ("zero reference") may account for differences in hemodynamic values reported in horses.[55]

Systemic Arterial Blood Pressure

Arterial blood pressure can be measured directly by arterial puncture or cannulation or indirectly using a variety of auscultatory, Doppler, or oscillometric techniques (see Chapter 8).[56-65] Percutaneous placement of an arterial catheter

Table 3–5. Calculation of myocardial oxygen demand[4]

Indices of MVO$_2$	Comment	Determinants of MVO$_2$		
		HR	Wall stress	Contractility
HR	Noninvasive, very easy	x	—	—
HR × SBP (Double product)	Noninvasive, easy	x	(x)	—
HR × SBP × ET (Triple product)	Noninvasive, more difficult (i.e., determination of ET or SV by echocardiography)	x	(x)	(x)
HR × SBP × SV (Pressure-work index)				
Pressure-volume area	Invasive; requires cardiac catheterization to record pressure-volume loops	x	x	x

ET, Ejection time; *HR,* heart rate; *MVO2,* myocardial oxygen demand; *SBP,* systolic blood pressure; *SV,* stroke volume, *x,* allowance for; *(x),* partial allowance for; —, no allowance for; principle determinants of MVO$_2$ are heart rate, contractility, wall stress (afterload; preload) and metabolic activity.

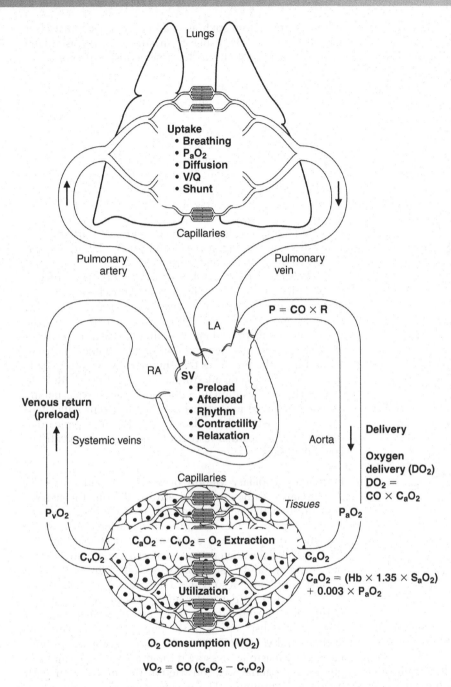

Lungs

Uptake
- **Breathing**
- **P_aO_2**
- **Diffusion**
- **V/Q**
- **Shunt**

Capillaries

Pulmonary
artery

Pulmonary
vein

$P = CO \times R$

LA

RA

SV
- **Preload**
- **Afterload**
- **Rhythm**
- **Contractility**
- **Relaxation**

**Venous return
(preload)**

Systemic veins

Aorta

Delivery

**Oxygen
delivery (DO_2)**
$DO_2 =$
$CO \times C_aO_2$

Capillaries

Tissues

P_vO_2

P_aO_2

$C_aO_2 - C_vO_2 = O_2$ **Extraction**

C_vO_2

C_aO_2

Utilization

$C_aO_2 = (Hb \times 1.35 \times S_aO_2)$
$+ 0.003 \times P_aO_2$

O_2 **Consumption (VO_2)**

$VO_2 = CO (C_aO_2 - C_vO_2)$

Figure 3–13. The uptake, delivery, extraction, and use of oxygen (O_2) by metabolizing tissues depend on the integrated function of multiple organ systems, including lung function, cardiac pump function, oxygen-carrying capacity, blood viscosity, vascular tone, global and regional distribution of blood flow, and tissue metabolism. $\dot{V}/\dot{Q}$, ventilation-perfusion matching; CO, cardiac output; P, pressure; R, resistance; PaO_2, partial pressure of oxygen in the arterial blood; PvO_2, partial pressure of oxygen in the venous blood; Hb, Hemoglobin; % Sat Hb, percent hemoglobin saturation; CaO_2, arterial oxygen concentration; CvO_2, venous oxygen concentration; DO_2, oxygen delivery; VO_2, oxygen uptake. (From Muir WW, Wellman ML: Hemoglobin solutions and tissue oxygenation, *J Vet Intern Med* 17:127-135, 2003.)

in the facial or dorsal metatarsal artery is frequently used to monitor the effects of anesthesia (see Chapter 7). Indirect methods have been used successfully to monitor pressure in the coccygeal artery; however, these methods are relatively insensitive during significant hypotension and may lag in response during rapid changes in blood pressure.[56,65,66] The width and placement of the occluding cuff when indirect methods are used are extremely important in obtaining accurate recordings.[61,67] The optimal width of the cuff (bladder) is approximately one third to one half of the circumference of the tail when measuring pressure in the middle coccygeal artery.[67-69] The arterial pulse wave itself varies, depending on the site of measurement; the distal arterial systolic pressure may be higher, and the diastolic pressure lower than the corresponding aortic pressures when the mean pressures are similar. This phenomenon is caused by summation of

the primary pressure waves with reflected waves returning from the peripheral circulation.[52]

Arterial blood pressure monitoring includes determination of systolic, diastolic, and mean pressures and pulse pressure (Figure 3-14). Arterial pressure depends on the interplay between cardiac output and vascular resistance (i.e., they are mathematically coupled). Therefore arterial pressure is not a reliable index of blood flow if vascular resistance is abnormal or changes over time. Normal reported values for indirect arterial systolic and diastolic pressures are 111.8 ± 13.3 (mean ± SD) and 67.7 ± 13.8, respectively.[70] Values for direct measurement of arterial pressure are higher than indirectly determined values (see Table 3-4). Arterial pressures fluctuate slightly with ventilation if there is positive-pressure ventilation or cyclic changes in heart rate (see Chapter 8). The systolic pressure is generated by the

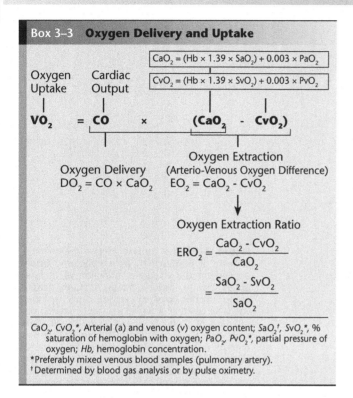

Box 3–3   Oxygen Delivery and Uptake

$$CaO_2 = (Hb \times 1.39 \times SaO_2) + 0.003 \times PaO_2$$
$$CvO_2 = (Hb \times 1.39 \times SvO_2) + 0.003 \times PvO_2$$

Oxygen Uptake		Cardiac Output			

$$VO_2 \quad = \quad CO \quad \times \quad (CaO_2 - CvO_2)$$

Oxygen Delivery
$DO_2 = CO \times CaO_2$

Oxygen Extraction
(Arterio-Venous Oxygen Difference)
$EO_2 = CaO_2 - CvO_2$

Oxygen Extraction Ratio

$$ERO_2 = \frac{CaO_2 - CvO_2}{CaO_2}$$

$$= \frac{SaO_2 - SvO_2}{SaO_2}$$

CaO_2, CvO_2,* Arterial (a) and venous (v) oxygen content; SaO_2,[†] SvO_2,* % saturation of hemoglobin with oxygen; PaO_2, PvO_2,* partial pressure of oxygen; *Hb,* hemoglobin concentration.
*Preferably mixed venous blood samples (pulmonary artery).
[†]Determined by blood gas analysis or by pulse oximetry.

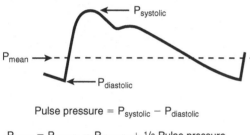

Pulse pressure = $P_{systolic} - P_{diastolic}$

$P_{mean} = P_{systolic} - P_{diastolic} + 1/3$ Pulse pressure

Figure 3–14. Pressure pulse within the aorta. The pulse pressure is the difference between the maximum pressure (systolic) and the minimum pressure (diastolic). The mean pressure is approximately equal to the diastolic pressure plus one third the pulse pressure.

left ventricle and is affected by stroke volume, aortic/arterial compliance, and the previous diastolic blood pressure. Arterial *pulse pressure,* the difference between systolic and diastolic values, is highly dependent on stroke volume and the peripheral arteriolar resistance. The pulse pressure is the primary determinant of the intensity of the palpable peripheral arterial pulse. Ventricular failure reduces pulse pressure (hypokinetic, weak pulse), whereas abnormal diastolic run-off resulting from aortic insufficiency or generalized vasodilation widens the pulse pressure (hyperkinetic, bounding, or water-hammer type pulse). Posture imposes a significant influence on arterial pressure, because raising the head from the feeding position necessitates a higher aortic pressure to maintain constant perfusion pressure at the level of the brain. MAP measured in the middle coccygeal artery varied by approximately 20 mm Hg with variable head position.[71]

Diastolic and mean pressures are better estimates of tissue perfusion pressure than systolic pressures. Tissue perfusion pressure can be increased by administering: (1) crystalloid or colloid fluids to improve filling pressures and ventricular loading; (2) catecholamines dobutamine or dopamine; or (3) vasoconstrictors such as α-adrenoceptor agonists (see Chapters 22 and 23). Drugs or anesthetics with vasodilator or cardiodepressant effects decrease perfusion pressure.

Left ventricular pressure.   Left ventricular pressure can be evaluated by inserting a fluid-filled or microtip manometer catheter (Millar) through the carotid artery and advancing the catheter into the left ventricle.[72,73] Left ventricular systolic pressure must exceed the aortic diastolic pressure for blood to be ejected from the ventricle. The first derivative of left or right ventricular pressure change during isovolumetric contraction, LV or RV $+dp/dt_{max}$, is a commonly used index of ventricular systolic function (see previous paragraphs).[35,36,73,74] It is largely determined by ventricular contractility (inotropic state) but also depends on loading conditions (heart rate, preload, afterload; see Figures 3-11 and 3-12).[75] LV $+dp/dt_{max}$ is decreased by most anesthetic drugs.[55,76]

Left ventricular diastolic pressure reflects ventricular compliance and the ability of the ventricle to empty its stroke volume. The reported diastolic pressure is usually the end-diastolic pressure (LVEDP), which is higher than the early (often subatmospheric) minimum diastolic left ventricular pressure. Horses and ponies have higher ventricular end-diastolic pressures than humans or dogs (see Table 3-5).[55,72,73,75,77] General anesthesia increases LVEDP by 10 to 15 mm Hg.[55,76] Elevation of end-diastolic pressures generally indicates reduced myocardial contractility, ventricular failure, volume overload, cardiac constriction (i.e., pericardial disease), or myocardial restriction and increasing ventricular wall stiffness.

Pulmonary capillary wedge pressure.   A balloon-tipped (Swan-Ganz) catheter can be advanced from the jugular vein through the right atrium and ventricle into the pulmonary artery to measure pulmonary artery pressure. A branch of the pulmonary artery may be occluded, and the "wedged" distal catheter tip can be used to estimate pulmonary capillary and venous pressures.[52,54,78] The pulmonary occlusion pressure, also commonly referred to as PCWP, is an estimate of left ventricular filling pressure and correlates to the left atrial and left ventricular end-diastolic pressure if there are no obstructions in the pulmonary vasculature or at the mitral valve. PCWP can be estimated by the pulmonary artery diastolic pressure if the heart rate is normal and pulmonary arterial vasoconstriction (as might occur with hypoxia) is minimal. The wedge pressure is reduced by hypovolemia and increased during left-sided heart failure, by severe mitral regurgitation, after excessive fluid administration, and by anesthetic overdose or anesthetics that depress left ventricular function.

Pulmonary artery pressures.   Systolic, diastolic, and mean pulmonary arterial pressures and waveforms can be assessed in a manner similar to that described for aortic pressures (see Table 3-4 and Figure 3-12).[54,72] Mean pulmonary artery pressure is higher in the newborn foal and decreases significantly during the first 2 weeks of life because of decreasing pulmonary arteriolar resistance (see Table 3-4).[79] Pulmonary arterial pressures (and all other pressures on the right side of the heart) are strongly affected by breathing and positive-pressure ventilation (see Chapter 17); pressures decrease during normal inspiration, but they increase during the inspiratory phase in a horse receiving positive-pressure ventilation. Unlike the systemic circulation, the pulmonary artery pressure not only depends on cardiac output and pulmonary arteriolar resistance but also on the downstream resistance produced by the pulmonary capillaries and the left atrial pressures. Alveolar hypoxia and acidosis can cause reactive pulmonary vasoconstriction, which raises pulmonary pressures.[80,81] Alveolar hypoxia is particularly important in producing pulmonary hypertension and can result in acute-onset pulmonary edema in horses recovering from anesthesia. This reaction may be particularly important in newborn foals.[82] Hypoxic pulmonary vasoconstriction (HPV) with or without concurrent structural vascular changes may be important in horses with recurrent airway obstruction or with pulmonary disease, causing various degrees of pulmonary hypertension.[83,84] Horses with congenital left-to-right shunts caused by a ventricular septal defect or with chronic mitral regurgitation or left-heart failure can undergo structural remodeling, causing the pulmonary vascular resistance and pulmonary artery pressure to increase.[85] Left ventricular failure invariably leads to secondary pulmonary hypertension.

Right ventricular pressure. Right ventricular pressure in horses is comparable to that in other species but is generally mildly elevated in anesthetized horses because of positioning effects and decreases in ventricular function (see Table 3-4 and Figure 3-12). Pathologic elevations in right ventricular diastolic pressure are encountered with pericardial disease, pulmonary hypertension, and right ventricular failure.[84] Elevated right ventricular systolic pressure has been recorded in pulmonary hypertension from hypoxia (see preceding paragraphs), large ventricular septal defects, and right ventricular outflow obstruction such as that caused by vegetative endocarditis at the pulmonic valve.

Systemic venous pressure. Central venous blood pressures vary with the horse's weight and exert a significant influence on ventricular end-diastolic pressure because the right ventricle is in direct continuity with the systemic venous system and right atrium.[86,87] Changes in central venous blood pressure cause corresponding alterations in the right ventricular end-diastolic pressure. The atrial pressure wave consists of two or three positive waves (*a wave* from atrial contraction, sometimes *c wave* following tricuspid valve closure, and *v wave* from atrial filling during ventricular systole) and two negative waves or "descents" (*x' descent* from downward displacement of the tricuspid valve annulus during ventricular systole and *y descent* from emptying of the atrial blood into the ventricle after opening of the tricuspid valve; see Figure 3-9). The pulsations vary with the phase of ventilation and are dramatically influenced by positive-pressure ventilation during anesthesia (see Chapter 17).

CVP is a balance between blood volume, venomotor tone, heart rate, and heart function and is influenced by drugs that change venous smooth muscle tone (acepromazine decreases CVP; xylazine increases CVP) and body position (see Chapters 10 and 21).[88] The CVP increases significantly in recumbent horses during general anesthesia. It frequently doubles from that in standing horses, and CVP values of 20 to 30 cm H_2O (15 to 22 mm Hg) are not uncommon.[87,88] The CVP may range from subatmospheric to values of about 10 cm H_2O (7.36 mm Hg) in anesthetized horses in lateral recumbency.

A single measurement of CVP in anesthetized horses is of little value. Changes or trends (increases or decreases) should be monitored closely (see Chapter 8). Changes in CVP reflect changes in blood volume, venous tone and capacitance, venous return, right ventricular systolic and diastolic function, and heart rate. Plasma volume contraction or venous pooling lower CVP. Right heart failure from any cause, pericardial disease, and overinfusion of fluid volume increase CVP. The *x' descent* of the pressure waveform may be replaced by a positive c-v wave in horses with tricuspid regurgitation.

Cardiac output. The determination of cardiac output is used as a global indicator of tissue perfusion and to assess the effects of drugs on the circulation. A change in either ventricular stroke volume or heart rate changes cardiac output (see Figure 3-11). Normal cardiac output values in resting adult horses (400 to 500 kg) are reported to range from between 28 and 40 L/min, corresponding to a cardiac index of approximately 60 to 80 ml/kg/min (see Table 3-4).[73,89] The cardiac index is higher in foals (2 hours and 2 weeks) and ranges between 150 and 220 ml/kg/min.[79] Cardiac output in the horse traditionally has been determined by indicator dilution (thermodilution; indocyanine green dye; lithium) techniques and the Fick method.[53,89,90-95] Lithium dilution has been used successfully in adult horses[96,97] and foals,[98] eliminating the need for right heart catheterization. Lithium dilution has been combined with pulse contour analysis to provide a noninvasive method for continuous cardiac output monitoring in horses during anesthesia.[97] Other noninvasive (but generally less accurate) methods that determine cardiac output in conscious and anesthetized horses include transthoracic and transesophageal echocardiography.[95,99-102] Additional noninvasive techniques have been reported recently, including partial carbon dioxide rebreathing[102] and electrical impedance dilution.[103] Their potential advantages and limitations have been described.[53,89]

Vascular resistance. The relationship between blood flow, pressure, and vessel resistance is described by *Poiseuille's law.* Resistance (R) to blood flow is determined by the radius (r) and the length (L) of the blood vessels and the viscosity (η) of blood.[5,53] The corresponding hydraulic resistance equation, $R = 8\eta L/\pi r^4$, indicates that resistance varies with the fourth power of vessel radius. Therefore small alterations in vascular tone can cause significant changes in the resistance to blood flow.

Systemic and pulmonary vascular resistances cannot be measured directly in the intact animal but are calculated using a variation of Ohm's law (see Box 3-2).[53] The cardiac output is usually measured in liters per minute, and pressures are expressed in millimeters of mercury. Correction values are added to convert resistance to cgs (centimeters-gram-second; dynes·sec·cm^{-5}) units (see Box 3-2 and Table 3-4).[104] Inasmuch as MAP is very similar in horses of different sizes, total cardiac output is lower, and vascular resistance is proportionally higher in smaller horses and ponies.[104] Both cardiac output and vascular resistance can be indexed to body size by multiplication with body surface area or (more commonly in veterinary medicine) body weight (see Box 3-2 and Table 3-4).

Mechanisms that increase SVR include increases in sympathetic nervous system activity, activation of the renin-angiotensin system, and the release of arginine vasopressin (antidiuretic hormone), epinephrine, or endothelin.[2]

Many pathological conditions are associated with elevated or reduced SVR. For example, shock may be associated with an abnormally high (hemorrhagic shock) or low (septic shock) SVR. Systemic hypotension generally is associated with an abnormally low (hemorrhagic shock) and, less frequently, high (septic shock) cardiac output. however, this example emphasizes that systemic arterial blood pressure should not be used as a single surrogate for cardiac output or tissue perfusion. Therapeutic interventions can influence SVR. Norepinephrine, phenylephrine, arginine vasopressin, dopamine, dobutamine, and ketamine increase vascular resistance; whereas acepromazine, calcium channel blockers, and inhalant anesthetics decrease vascular resistance.

Peripheral Circulation and Microcirculation

One of the main functions of the cardiovascular system is the transport of oxygen to the tissues in amounts that are adequate to meet the respective oxygen demands of each individual organ at any time and under all metabolic conditions (within physiological limits). Adequate oxygen delivery to tissues depends on the oxygen-carrying capabilities of blood and a high degree of integration between ventilation, myocardial performance, systemic and pulmonary hemodynamics and an appropriate distribution of peripheral blood flow based on need. Blood vessels provide the channels whereby blood is delivered to tissues and are classified as elastic, resistance, terminal sphincter, exchange, capacitance, and shunt vessels. Large arteries are elastic and serve as relatively low-resistance blood conduits that deliver blood to peripheral small arteries. The aorta is so elastic that it is actually responsible for a compressive ("Windkessel") effect that converts the phasic systolic inflow produced by ventricular ejection into a smoother, more continuous outflow to peripheral vessels. Large veins serve as conduits but also as capacitance vessels that can store and (if constricted) mobilize large amounts of blood, thereby influencing venous return to the heart (see Figure 3-13). The peripheral vascular network includes arterioles (sphincter), capillaries (exchange), and venules (capacitance or blood reservoirs) and collectively is considered as the *microcirculation*. The capillaries are the site for diffusion and filtration of gases, water, and solutes between the vascular and interstitial fluid compartments.[5] Regional blood flow is controlled by the *arterioles (precapillary sphincters)*, which represent the major resistance vessels in the systemic circulation. Arteriolar tone is modulated by central (mainly sympathetic) stimuli, circulating vasoactive substances (i.e., catecholamines, angiotensin, and vasopressin), and local (metabolic, endothelial, and/or myogenic) factors.[2,5] Central regulation of blood flow by the autonomic nervous system predominates in some areas such as the skin, the splanchnic tissues, and the resting skeletal muscle; whereas local factors are dominant in other areas such as the myocardium, brain, kidneys, lungs, and working skeletal muscle. Generally blood flow through vital organs such as the heart, brain, and kidneys (vessel-rich group tissues) is tightly controlled by a variety of autoregulatory mechanisms and therefore (within physiologic limits) relatively independent of perfusion pressures. Shunt vessels are particularly prominent in the skin and important in thermoregulation.

Arteriolar smooth muscle tone regulates the vessel diameter and the resistance to blood flow, thereby determining the distribution of blood flow to the capillaries and arterial

perfusion pressures. Intrinsic myogenic activity in response to an elevation in transmural pressure is partly responsible for the basal vascular tone independent of central neural input, thereby providing an autoregulatory mechanism independent of endothelial function. High oxygen tension may further contribute to basal vascular tone, and a decrease in oxygen supply or an increase in metabolic activity (hence oxygen consumption) results in local vaso*dilation* and increased blood flow. Conversely hypoxia exerts potent *vasoconstriction* effects in the pulmonary vasculature (HPV), an effect that helps maintain optimum blood flow distribution and ventilation-perfusion ratio in the lungs (see Chapter 2). An increase in vascular shear stress (which is proportional to blood flow velocity and viscosity) can cause vasodilation and capillary recruitment, presumably by release of nitric oxide from the endothelium.[105] Blood viscosity and flow velocity are important determinants of capillary perfusion, and tissue *functional capillary density* is a prime determinant of tissue survival during resuscitation from hypotension and hypovolemia. The viscosity of the blood is mainly determined by the concentration of red blood cells (hematocrit), cell-to-cell interactions, red cell deformability, plasma proteins, and shear rate (an estimate of relative velocity of fluid movement).[5,105,106]

The hematocrit and more precisely hemoglobin concentration determine the oxygen-carrying capacity of blood (see Figure 3-13). Generally maximum oxygen delivery can be achieved in most healthy horses at a packed cell volume (PCV) of approximately 30%.[105,106] A PCV greater than 60% dramatically increases blood viscosity and reduces blood flow to smaller vessels, thereby decreasing oxygen delivery. Decreases in PCV generally are better tolerated and may improve microvascular blood flow by decreasing blood viscosity and peripheral resistance. Moderate-to-severe anemia causes peripheral vasodilation, sympathetic activation, and compensatory increases in cardiac output, all of which help to maintain oxygen delivery to tissues.[2,107]

The *endothelium* plays an active role in regulating the microcirculation. Nitric oxide and prostaglandins are important vasodilators released by the endothelium in response to a variety of stimuli and mediators. Other vasodilator agents that may play a role in local metabolic control of tissue perfusion include histamine, serotonin, adenosine, hydrogen ions (pH), carbon dioxide, and potassium. Vasoconstrictors such as endothelin, angiotensin II, and vasopressin counteract these effects and become important during pathologic conditions such as pulmonary hypertension or congestive heart failure.[4,5] The capillary endothelium also exchanges water and solutes by diffusion, filtration, and pinocytosis. The role of hydrostatic and oncotic (colloid-osmotic) forces in regulating passive fluid passage across the capillary endothelium is described by *Starling's law of the capillary*. Fluid movement (Q_f) is determined by:

$$Q_f = k[(P_c + \pi_i) - (P_i + \pi_p)]$$

where k is filtration constant, P_c is capillary hydrostatic pressure, π_i is interstitial oncotic pressure, P_i is interstitial hydrostatic pressure, and π_p is plasma oncotic pressure.[2,5] Decreased capillary hydrostatic pressure (hypotension, hypovolemia) promotes an intravascular shift of interstitial fluid (autotransfusion), which restores a significant amount of the intravascular volume in a relatively short period of time. The administration of hypertonic saline or colloids or both during emergency situations can produce a rapid increase in intravascular osmotic pressure, drawing interstitial fluid into (autotransfusion) the vascular space (see Chapter 7).[108,109] Administration of colloids or plasma is also indicated in states of severe hypoproteinemia in which intravascular volume may be difficult to maintain because of decreased plasma oncotic pressure and transcapillary fluid losses.[109,110]

Restoration and maintenance of intravascular volume and oxygen-carrying capacity is crucial to maintaining hemodynamics and tissue perfusion in anesthetized horses as both the central and local mechanisms controlling peripheral blood flow and blood flow distribution. General anesthesia, particularly inhalant anesthetics, blunts autoregulatory (compensatory) responses to a decrease in MAP. Depressed autoregulatory responses combined with vasodilation and hypotension can result in a maldistribution of blood flow, inadequate tissue perfusion, tissue hypoxia, and lactic acidosis during general anesthesia (Figure 3-15).

Extrinsic Control of Blood Pressure and Peripheral Blood Flow

Vasomotor centers. The *vasomotor centers* in the medulla are responsible for central regulation of cardiac electrical activity, myocardial performance, and peripheral vascular tone.[4,5] Central regulation of peripheral blood flow in horses is accomplished primarily by integration and modulation of sympathetic and parasympathetic tone. Rhythmic changes in tonic activity of the vasomotor centers are responsible for slight oscillations of arterial pressures.

Vascular reflexes. The *baroreceptors* are high-pressure stretch receptors located in the carotid sinus and the aortic arch. They are especially responsive to acute changes in pulsatile flow close to the physiological range but are less sensitive to nonpulsatile sustained pressure changes or pressures changes far outside the physiologic range.[5,111] The baroreceptor reflex is mainly responsible for rapid, short-term regulation of blood pressure; whereas long-term control depends on alterations of blood volume and fluid balance by the kidneys (renin-angiotensin-aldosterone system).[2,4] An increase in arterial blood pressure stimulates baroreceptors, which then send nerve impulses to the medullary vasomotor centers and cause central inhibition of

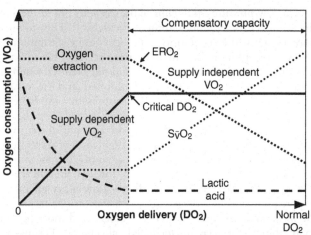

Figure 3–15. Relationship between oxygen delivery *(DO₂)*, oxygen consumption *(VO₂)*, and oxygen extraction in the systemic circulation. Tissues compensate for decreases in DO_2 (either because of a decrease in cardiac output or arterial oxygen concentration) by increasing oxygen extraction, thereby maintaining VO_2 constant *(continuous line)*. Consequently the mixed-venous oxygen saturation *(S$\bar{v}$O₂)* decreases, the arteriovenous oxygen difference widens, and the oxygen extraction ratio *(ERO₂)* increases. Once the compensatory capacity is exceeded *(shaded area)*, VO_2 becomes blood flow (DO_2)–dependent. Anaerobic metabolism ensues, leading to accumulation of lactic acid and metabolic acidosis. Venous (mixed venous) PO_2 and oxygen saturation, blood pH, and blood lactate concentration are clinically useful end points for assessing oxygen delivery and oxygen extraction in the tissues.

sympathetic tone and increases in parasympathetic tone. Conversely a decrease in arterial pressure causes baroreceptor reflex-mediated withdrawal of vagal tone and sympathetic activation, leading to cardiac acceleration, improved myocardial performance, constriction of arterial resistance and venous capacitance vessels, and increase in venous return. Fluctuations in vagal activity in response to blood pressure changes are the predominant cause for altering heart rate in the resting horse.[24] The pronounced sinus arrhythmia and second-degree AV block often encountered in normal horses are caused by modulation of vagal tone and likely serve to regulate arterial blood pressure in horses at rest (Figure 3-16).

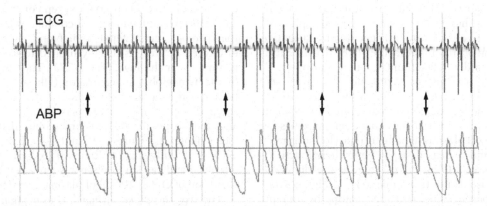

Figure 3–16. Base-apex electrocardiogram *(ECG)* and arterial blood pressure *(ABP)* recorded simultaneously in a standing, unsedated horse with a heart rate of 30 beats/min. Second-degree AV block *(arrows: P waves not followed by QRS complexes)* is triggered by an increase in arterial blood pressure and a baroreceptor reflex-mediated increase in vagal tone. Vagally induced AV blocks are thought to be one mechanism (together with sinus arrhythmia and sinus arrest) for controlling blood pressure in horses and can be eliminated by the administration of an anticholinergic (e.g., atropine, glycopyrrolate).

The *low-pressure cardiopulmonary receptors* are located in the atria, ventricles, and pulmonary vessels.[5,111] They mainly play a role in the regulation of blood volume. Stimulation of these receptors results in an increase in renal blood flow, urine production, and heart rate (*Bainbridge reflex*); whereas central vasoconstrictor centers are inhibited, and the release of angiotensin, aldosterone, and vasopressin (antidiuretic hormone) is reduced.

Chemoreceptors, located in the aortic arch and the carotid bodies, are involved primarily in the regulation of respiratory activity but also influence vasomotor centers. They are stimulated by decreases in oxygen tension, low pH, and increases in carbon dioxide tension. The direct stimulatory effects of hypercapnia and hydrogen ions on *chemosensitive regions of the medullary vasomotor centers* are considered more potent than the chemoreceptor-mediated effects.[5,111] Permissive mild-to-moderate hypercapnia ($PaCO_2$ 60 to 75 mmg Hg) and acidemia may be beneficial for maintenance of cardiac output and arterial perfusion pressures in horses under anesthesia. Restoration of normocapnia after a period of hypercapnia may suppress tonic activity from medullary centers and can be associated with a deterioration of blood pressures, cardiac output, and blood flow, particularly in horses that are already hemodynamically compromised.[112] It is important to note that injectable and in particular inhalant anesthetic drugs depress centrally and peripherally mediated acute homeostatic reflex responses. Intravenous anesthesia produces mild-to-moderate depression of homeostatic reflexes in horses, whereas most homeostatic reflex responses are totally obliterated by inhalant anesthetics administered at concentrations (1.3 MAC) necessary to produce surgical planes of anesthesia. This effect has important implications for choice of anesthetic technique in high-risk or emergency surgical patients (see Chapter 24).

Autonomic control. The autonomic nervous system extensively innervates the cardiovascular system. Interplay between the sympathetic and parasympathetic branches of the autonomic nervous system is modulated by a variety of reflexes (see previous paragraphs) that regulate cardiac performance and blood pressure in the horse.[113] The *heart* receives efferent traffic from both parasympathetic and sympathetic branches of the autonomic nervous system (see Table 3-3 and Figures 3-6 and 3-7). The vagus innervates supraventricular tissues and probably exerts effects on proximal ventricular septal tissues. Vagal influence is generally depressive to heart rate (negative chronotropic), AV conduction (negative dromotropic), excitability (negative bathmotropic), myocardial contractile state (negative inotropic), and myocardial relaxation (negative lusitropic).

The sympathetic nervous system provides extensive innervation throughout the heart, producing effects opposite those of the parasympathetic system. β-Adrenoceptors dominate in the heart. The increase in heart rate that attends exercise is related to withdrawal of parasympathetic tone (for heart rates up to 110/min) and increased sympathetic efferent activity (for heart rates above 110/min).[24] α-Adrenoceptors dominate in the systemic vasculature (see Table 3-3 and Figure 3-7).[4] Stimulation of postsynaptic α_1-adrenoceptors by norepinephrine, epinephrine, or other drugs with α-adrenoceptor agonistic activity (i.e., phenylephrine; dopamine) causes systemic arterioles and veins to constrict. These effects generally increase systemic arterial blood pressure and increase venous

return to the heart; however, vascular constriction can cause difficulties. For example, intense arterial vasoconstriction increases left ventricular afterload, whereas pronounced large vein constriction can cause venous pooling.[2] Furthermore, increases in vascular tone, vascular resistance, and arterial blood pressure do not ensure an increase in functional capillary density and tissue perfusion. Vascular α_2-adrenoceptors may cause differential vasoconstriction when stimulated, depending on the vascular bed. A reduction of tonic sympathetic efferent activity causes vasodilation as an autonomic reflex function for controlling systemic blood pressure. The presence of vasodilator β_2-adrenoceptors is clinically relevant, insofar as infused β_2-agonists (dopexamine) cause positive inotropic activity in horses and vasodilation in circulatory beds that contain high β_2-agonist adrenoceptor density.

Many vascular beds dilate in response to acetylcholine or after production of local vasodilator substances released during exercise, stress, or metabolic activity (see previous paragraphs).[2,4] Stimulation of histamine or serotonin receptors causes arteriolar dilation, venular constriction, and increased capillary permeability. There is significant variation of postsynaptic receptor subtypes throughout the regional circulatory beds, with varying density of α-, β-, histamine, and dopaminergic receptors and varying ability of vascular smooth muscle to respond to local vasodilator stimuli and autacoids. The macro hemodynamic effects of most common catecholamines (epinephrine, norepinephrine, dopamine, dobutamine, phenylephrine, ephedrine, dopexamine; see Chapter 22) have been described in horses; but their differential effects on specific organs (brain, heart, liver, kidney, lung) remain to be resolved.

Acid-base and electrolyte disturbances, hypoxemia, ischemia, and, most important, exposure to anesthetic (particularly inhalant) drugs blunt or abolish baroreceptor and chemoreceptor reflexes and diminish the vascular response to sympathetic stimulation, thereby reducing the compensatory capacity for restoration and maintenance of adequate tissue perfusion. Continuous monitoring of hemodynamic status is required in horses if arterial blood pressure, cardiac output, and tissue oxygenation are to be optimized (see Chapter 22).

Oxygen Delivery, Oxygen Uptake, Arteriovenous Oxygen Difference, and Oxygen Extraction Ratio

The *oxygen delivery (or supply)* to the tissues (DO_2) depends on cardiac output (CO), arterial oxygen content (CaO_2), microcirculatory hemodynamics (functional capillary density), and the rheologic characteristics of blood. Clinical assessment of oxygen delivery is usually limited to estimates of global parameters, including CO and CaO_2. The CaO_2 is determined by the hemoglobin concentration (Hb) and the saturation of hemoglobin in arterial blood (SaO_2), which is determined by the partial pressure of oxygen in the arterial blood (PaO_2) and the shape of the oxyhemoglobin dissociation curve (see Chapter 2: Figures 2-18 and 2-19; Box 3-3, and Figure 3-13).[105,114] Only small volumes of oxygen can be physically dissolved and carried in plasma, even when PaO_2 is elevated (0.003 ml of O_2 per 100 ml of plasma for each 1 mm Hg).

The *oxygen uptake (demand, consumption)* of the tissues (VO_2) can be quantified as the product of cardiac output and the difference between the arterial and venous oxygen content, also referred to as *arteriovenous oxygen difference* ($Ca\text{-}vO_2$) or *oxygen extraction* (EO_2) (see Box 3-3 and Figure 3-15).

The ratio between VO_2 and DO_2 is also referred to as the *oxygen extraction ratio (ERO$_2$)* (see Box 3-3). The ERO_2 normally ranges between 20% and 30% (i.e., $ERO_2 = (100 - 75)/100 = 25$%, when $SaO_2 = 100$% and $SvO_2 = 75$%) and increases with increases in metabolic rate and VO_2. Mixed venous samples obtained from pulmonary arterial catheters are superior to venous samples obtained from either the jugular or peripheral veins for assessment of global oxygen extraction.

Decreases in cardiac output or the oxygen content of blood (i.e., anemia) result in an increase in oxygen extraction from the blood to meet the oxygen demand (VO_2) of the tissues.[53,114] Consequently the venous oxygen content (CvO_2), the venous oxygen saturation (SvO_2), and the venous partial pressure of oxygen (PvO_2) decrease. Therefore CvO_2, SvO_2, and PvO_2 can be used as indirect measures of cardiac output (see Figure 3-15; Figure 3-17).[53,115,116] When DO_2 is decreased below a critical level (or when VO_2 is increased concurrently), the degree of oxygen extraction from the blood cannot be increased further, and the oxygen uptake by the tissue decreases parallel to the oxygen supply (supply-dependent oxygen uptake; see Figure 3-15). The resulting anaerobic metabolism leads to accumulation of lactate and causes metabolic acidosis.[114,117] Ultimately tissue hypoxia and limited metabolic capacity of the affected tissue can lead to tissue damage and organ failure.[118] The critical DO_2 is determined by the maximum ERO_2, which usually ranges between 50% and 60% (corresponding to an $SvO_2 <40$% to 50% when $SaO_2 = 100$%).

Most parameters used to assess tissue oxygenation (i.e., cardiac output, blood pressure, Hb, SaO_2, SvO_2, $Ca-vO_2$, and ERO_2) only provide an estimate of global oxygen delivery and oxygen extraction. They do not provide direct evidence on actual *use of oxygen* by metabolic pathways within the cells. Indeed, oxygen use can be severely disturbed in conditions such as endotoxemia, sepsis, and circulatory shock when the ability of the mitochondria to efficiently generate ATP via oxidative phosphorylation is severely impaired.[114] The direct assessment of cellular oxygen use is not feasible in clinical practice. Surrogate signs of organ dysfunction and hemodynamic deterioration such as pH, base deficit, SvO_2, strong ion gap (SIG), and blood lactate concentration are used as indicators of inadequate oxygen delivery.

RECOGNITION AND MANAGEMENT OF HEART DISEASE

Overview of Heart Disease in the Horse

Congenital and acquired cardiac disorders of the horse can be classified by anatomic lesion, pathophysiologic mechanism, and etiology (Box 3-4).[119,120] *Pathophysiologic mechanisms* of cardiac dysfunction can be grouped into the following categories: (1) myocardial contractility failure; (2) hemodynamic (volume or pressure) overload; (3) diastolic dysfunction; and (4) cardiac arrhythmia. Cardiovascular diseases can be *congenital* or *acquired* and are classified as *primary disorders* when the heart or vasculature is primarily diseased or *secondary disorders* when other underlying (often systemic) diseases directly or indirectly affect cardiovascular function.

Evaluation of Cardiovascular Function

The cardiovascular system of the horse should be examined thoroughly and carefully before anesthesia.[121-123] The initial evaluation should include a history, physical examination, and careful auscultation (see Chapter 6). Electrocardiography, thoracic radiography, ultrasonography, and clinical laboratory tests may be required, depending on the results of the initial evaluation.

History and Physical Examination

The history should include information regarding the horse's fitness and performance, exercise capacity, previous health issues, and presenting complaints. Poor performance and weight loss, although nonspecific, are common complaints often associated with cardiac disease and early heart failure, even in the absence of other clinical signs. Conversely, normal

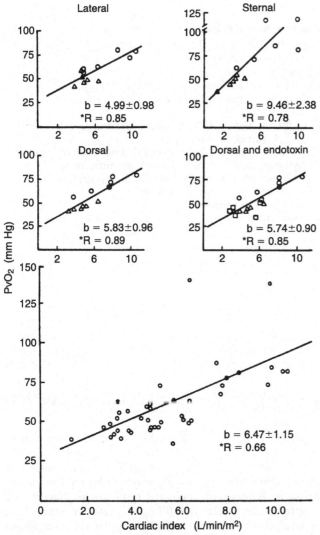

Figure 3–17. Relationship between mixed venous O_2 tension (PvO_2) and cardiac index in horses in lateral, sternal, and dorsal recumbencies and after endotoxin administration *(upper panels)*. Cumulative data on lower panel. Note that PvO_2 decreases as cardiac index decreases, regardless of the horse's position. (From Wetmore LA et al: Mixed venous oxygen tension as an estimate of cardiac output in anesthetized horses, *Am J Vet Res* 48:973, 1987.)

Box 3–4   Causes of Cardiovascular Disease in Horses

Congenital Cardiac Malformations

Left-to-right shunts
  Ventricular (most common) and atrial septal defects
  Patent ductus arteriosus (normal up to 72 hr postpartum)
Valvular dysplasia or atresia (rare)
Complex congenital defects (rare)

Valvular Heart Disease Causing Valve Insufficiency

Degenerative disease (most commonly aortic and mitral
  valve in middle-age to older horses)
Nonbacterial valvulitis (sometimes suspected in
  young horses; etiology unknown, possibly viral or
  immune-mediated)
Bacterial endocarditis (most commonly aortic and mitral valve)
Ruptured chordae tendineae (sudden onset of murmur and
  clinical signs)

Pulmonary Hypertension and Cor Pulmonale—Right-sided Ventricular Overload Secondary to Pulmonary Disease

Primary bronchopulmonary disease
Acute alveolar hypoxia with secondary reactive pulmonary
  arterial vasoconstriction
  Severe acidosis
Pulmonary thromboembolism

Myocardial Disease

Idiopathic dilated cardiomyopathy
Myocarditis
  Viral or bacterial (e.g., secondary to respiratory tract
  infection?)
Myocardial degeneration/necrosis
  Toxic injury (e.g., monensin)
  Nutritional deficiencies (e.g., selenium deficiency)
  Acute ischemia, thromboembolic events, infarction
Myocardial fibrosis (often incidental finding postmortem)
Myocardial depression
  Metabolic or systemic disease (e.g., acidosis, electrolyte
  disturbances, endotoxemia, septicemia)

Hypoxia, mild (transient) ischemia
Administration of sedatives/tranquilizing drugs and
  inhalation anesthetics

Pericardial Disease

Pericarditis, pericardial effusion (cardiac tamponade),
  constrictive pericarditis
Idiopathic
  Infectious (bacterial)
Traumatic

Diseases of the Great Vessels

Aortic aneurism, aortocardiac fistula

Diseases of the Peripheral Vessels

Venous thrombosis, thrombophlebitis (most commonly
  jugular veins)
Thrombosis of the mesenteric root (strongyles), mesenteric
  thromboembolism
Aortic thrombosis

Cardiac Arrhythmias

Supraventricular arrhythmias (especially atrial
  fibrillation/flutter)
Ventricular arrhythmias
Conduction disturbances (most are physiologic)
Arrhythmias caused by acid-base and electrolyte
  disturbances
Arrhythmias associated with metabolic disorders,
  endotoxemia, or septicemia
Arrhythmias resulting from myocardial ischemia or hypoxia
Arrhythmias resulting from autonomic imbalances
Cardiac arrhythmias associated with administration of:
  Sedatives and tranquilizing agents
  Inhalation anesthetics
  Antiarrhythmics
  Electrolytes (e.g., potassium, calcium)
  Other drugs

---

performance and body condition precludes the presence of severe cardiac disease. Heart murmurs and some types of cardiac arrhythmias are common in athletic horses and must be evaluated in relation to the history and physical examination findings; they may not be clinically relevant in the absence of additional clinical signs of heart disease.[124-127] Horses with severe systemic disease, including but not limited to gastrointestinal disease, endotoxemia, or septicemia, are likely to demonstrate some degree of circulatory compromise (e.g., prolonged capillary refill time). Assessment of the horse's volume status and cardiovascular function determines the anesthetic drugs, monitoring techniques, and circulatory support selected.

The *physical examination* should use methodologies and techniques that identify poor cardiopulmonary function, lung disease, or heart failure.[123-125] The surface temperature of the ears and limbs, the turgor of the skin, jugular vein filling, the color of the mucous membranes, and the capillary refill time provide important information on the horse's fluid volume status, peripheral vascular perfusion, blood pressure, and vascular reactivity. Capillary

refill time is prolonged during hypotension or peripheral vasoconstriction; conversely, it may be shortened when there is vasodilation (see Chapter 6). Peripheral edema may indicate right heart failure, vascular occlusion, severe hypoproteinemia, vascular disease, or impaired lymphatic drainage; whereas cough, nasal discharge, and abnormal thoracic auscultation may indicate left heart failure or respiratory disease.

Jugular pulsations are normally observed in the ventral third of the neck and are reflections of right atrial pressure changes (see Figure 3-9). Pronounced jugular venous pulsations that collapse normally may be observed in excited horses or horses with increased sympathetic tone. A lack of appropriate *jugular vein filling* is consistent with severe hypovolemia or venous occlusion. Jugular vein thrombosis or thrombophlebitis must be ruled out by careful inspection and palpation of both jugular veins before catheter placement and intravenous drug administration. Abnormal jugular pulses are observed in horses that have cardiac arrhythmias, diseases of the tricuspid valve, and right ventricular failure.

Irregularities in heart rate and rhythm and abnormalities in pulse quality can be identified by palpating the facial artery. The *arterial pulse* can be described as normal, hypokinetic (weak), hyperkinetic (bounding or water-hammer pulse), or variable. Irregularity in pulse rate or palpable changes in pulse quality suggests cardiac arrhythmia (see preceding paragraphs). Palpation of a peripheral pulse wave provides an estimation of pulse pressure (difference between systolic and diastolic pressure), but neither provides an accurate estimate of absolute pressures or corresponds to blood flow or tissue perfusion, although poor pulse quality is an excellent sign of low arterial blood pressure and low cardiac output.

Auscultation requires an understanding of anatomy, physiology, pathophysiology, and physics of sound and is a very accurate method for cardiac diagnosis.[128-132] The first prerequisite of auscultation is knowledge of the areas for

auscultation and appreciation of normal heart and lung sounds in horses (Tables 3-6 to 3-8, Box 3-5; see Figure 3-10).

Auscultation of the heart and lungs in a horse in good physical condition and with exercise tolerance suggests normal function and negates the need for additional diagnostic cardiac studies. The diagnostic sensitivity of cardiac auscultation is fairly high, and most serious cardiac disorders can be detected by physical examination and careful auscultation. Auscultation should include assessment of (1) heart rate, (2) cardiac rhythm, (3) intensity and character of the heart sounds, and (4) heart murmurs or "extra sounds." The *heart rate* in the horse can change rapidly and dramatically, varying with autonomic efferent traffic and the level of physical activity. The normal resting heart rate generally ranges between 26 and 48 beats/min, with an average rate of 40 beats/min. Anxiety may cause sudden increases in resting

Table 3–6. Identification of heart sounds and common cardiac murmurs

Auscultatory finding	Timing°		Point of maximal intensity (valve area)*
Normal Heart Sounds			
First heart sound (S_1)	Onset S		Left apex (mitral valve)
Second heart sound (S_2)	End S		Left base (aortic valve)
Pulmonic component	End S	S_4 S_1 $S_2 S_3$	Left base (pulmonic valve)
Third heart sound (S_3)	Early D		Left apex (mitral valve)
Fourth (atrial) sound (S_4)	Late D		Ventricular inlet or base (Left)
Functional Murmurs†			
Systolic ejection murmur	S		Left base (Aortic/pulmonary valves)
Early (proto-)diastolic	D		Ventricular inlets (Left/Right)‡
Late diastolic (presystolic)	D		Ventricular inlets (Left/Right)‡
Valvular Regurgitation§			
Mitral regurgitation	S		Left apex (mitral valve)
Tricuspid regurgitation	S		Right hemithorax (tricuspid valve)
Aortic regurgitation	S		Left base (aortic valve)
Pulmonary insufficiency	D		Left base (pulmonic valve)
Ventricular Septal Defect¶	S		Right sternal border/left cardiac base
Patent Ductus Arteriosus	S + D		Dorsal left base over pulmonary artery

°S, Systole, the interval between S_1 and S_2; D, diastole, the interval between S_2 and S_1.

*"Apex" refers to the ventral part of the heart, at the point of the palpable cardiac impulse (apex beat, see Figure 3-1); "base" refers to the craniodorsal area over the outlet valves (aortic, pulmonic) where the second heart sound is most intense.

†The systolic ejection murmur, which begins after the first heart sound and ends before the second heart sound, is the most commonly identified murmur in the horse; the protodiastolic murmur extends from the second to the third heart sound; the presystolic murmur is quite short, spanning the fourth and first heart sounds. Functional murmurs may be musical.

‡Ventricular inlets refer to thoracic area overlying the ventricular inflow tracts.

§Murmurs of atrioventricular valve insufficiency are generally heard over the affected valve, radiate dorsally, and project toward the apex of their respective ventricle. Some regurgitant murmurs are evident throughout systole or diastole and extend into the second heart sound (holosystolic or pansystolic) or first heart sound (holodiastolic or pandiastolic); however, late systolic murmurs, which can be related to valve prolapse, have been identified with mitral or tricuspid valve insufficiency, and the murmur of aortic insufficiency may not always be holodiastolic.

¶Murmurs caused by defects in the right ventricular inlet septum (paramembranous ventricular septal defect [VSD], common) are heard best above the right sternal border; murmurs from defects in the right ventricle outlet septum (subpulmonic VSD, rare) may be loudest over the pulmonic valve; increased flow across the pulmonic valve can cause left-basilar systolic murmurs of relative pulmonic stenosis in the absence of pulmonic valve pathology; flow across very large nonrestrictive defects can be relatively soft.

Table 3–7. Causes of cardiac murmurs

Cardiac murmur	Lesion identified by echocardiography, cardiac catheterization, or necropsy
Functional murmurs*	No identifiable lesions
Congenital heart disease murmurs	Defect(s) in the atrial or ventricular septa; patent ductus arteriosus; atresia/stenosis of tricuspid or pulmonic valve; valve stenosis; complex malformations of the heart
Mitral regurgitation[†]	Degenerative thickening of the valve; bacterial endocarditis; mitral valve prolapse into the left atrium; rupture of a chorda tendineae; dilated, hypokinetic ventricle (dilated cardiomyopathy, severe aortic regurgitation)
Tricuspid regurgitation[†]	Same as mitral regurgitation; also pulmonary hypertension from severe left heart failure or chronic respiratory disease
Aortic regurgitation[†]	Degenerative thickening and/or prolapse of the valve; congenital fenestration of the valve; bacterial endocarditis[‡]; aortic prolapse into a ventricular septal defect
Pulmonary insufficiency[†]	Bacterial endocarditis[‡]; pulmonary hypertension

*Functional murmurs may be innocent (unknown cause) or physiologic (suspected physiologic cause); functional murmurs are common in foals, trained athletes (athletic murmur), and horses with high sympathetic nervous system activity (pain, stress, sepsis); are associated with fever; and produced by anemia. Functional murmurs become more prominent at higher heart rates.

[†]"Silent" trivial or mild regurgitation across right-sided (most common) or left-sided (less common) cardiac valves; can be identified in some horses by Doppler echocardiography; this is probably a normal finding of no clinical significance. Pulmonary insufficiency is often silent. Many (up to 30%)[124-126] trained athletes have audible murmurs of tricuspid and/or mitral regurgitation that are not associated with poor performance or signs of heart disease (by physical examination and echocardiography) and are not considered clinically relevant.

[‡]Large valvular vegetations may result in anatomic stenosis, causing a systolic murmur, which is associated with a diastolic murmur of valve insufficiency; increased flow across a normal valve may generate a murmur of relative valve stenosis (e.g., with aortic regurgitation, there may be a systolic ejection murmur resulting from an increased stroke volume).

Table 3–8. Auscultation of cardiac arrhythmias

Rhythm	Typical heart rate	Heart sounds*	Auscultatory features
Sinus rhythms	26-50/min	S4-1-2 (3)	Rate and rhythm depend on autonomic tone
Sinus arrest/block	<26/min	S4-1-2 (3)	Irregular, long pauses
Sinus bradycardia	<26/min	S4-1-2 (3)	Generally regular unless escape rhythm develops
Sinus arrhythmia	26-50/min	S4-1-2(3)	Irregular, cyclic change in heart rate, usually variable interval between S_4-S_1, often associated with second-degree block
Sinus tachycardia	>50/min	S4-1-2-3	Typically regular, but second-degree atrioventricular (AV) block may develop if vagal tone also increases (e.g., recovery phase after exercise)
Atrial tachyarrhythmias			
Atrial tachycardia	AR: variable[†] VR: >30/min	Sl-2 (3)	Ventricular regularity/rate depends on AV conduction sequence and sympathetic tone; S_4 inconsistent or absent; variable intensity S_1
Atrial flutter	AR: 200-300/min[†] AR:	Sl-2 (3)	Ventricular response is irregular; ventricular
Atrial fibrillation	250-500/min[†] VR: >30/min		rate depends on sympathetic tone but is often normal (30-54/min); heart rates consistently above 60/min suggest significant underlying heart disease or heart failure; S_4 is absent; variable intensity S_1
Ectopic junctional and ventricular rhythms			
Escape rhythm: junctional	>25/min	S1-2 (3)	Heart rate usually regular during ectopic
Escape rhythm: ventricular	< 25/min		rhythm; heart rate depends on mechanism
Accelerated idioventricular rhythm (slow VT)	60-80/min		and sympathetic tone; inconsistent S_4; variable intensity and split heart sounds
Ventricular tachycardia (VT)	>60/min		

(Continued)

Table 3–8. Auscultation of cardiac arrhythmias—Cont'd.

Rhythm	Typical heart rate	Heart sounds*	Auscultatory features
Atrioventricular block			
Incomplete (first-degree, second-degree)	<50/min	S4-1-2 (3) S4/S1-2 (3)	Heart rate variable; cyclical arrhythmia, variable S_4-S_1 interval; some variation in heart sounds; isolated S_4 without following S_1-S_2 in second-degree AV block
Complete (third-degree)	AR: 28-60/min VR: <25/min	S4//S1-2 (3)	Ventricular escape rhythm, usually regular; independent atrial (S_4) sounds; variable intensity heart sounds
Premature complexes			
Supraventricular (atrial) Ventricular	—	Premature S1-2	Intensity of S_1 may be louder or softer than normal

*( ) = may be evident.
†Exact rate limits are not established in horses.

Box 3–5   Characterization of Heart Murmurs

Timing and Duration (see Figures 3-10 and 3-18 and Table 3-6)
Systolic, diastolic, or continuous
Early, mid, or late systolic or diastolic
Holosystolic (S1 to S2), holodiastolic (S2 to S1)

Grade
Grade 1/6: very quiet, only heard over a very localized area after careful auscultation in quiet environment, may be inconsistent
Grade 2/6: Quiet, heard consistently over the point of maximum intensity
Grade 3/6: Moderately loud, heard immediately and consistently, small area of radiation
Grade 4/6: Loud, radiating over a wider area, no palpable thrill
Grade 5/6: Very loud, radiating over widespread area, palpable precordial thrill
Grade 6/6: Extremely loud, also heard with the stethoscope held just above the skin surface

Point of Maximal Intensity
Apical: Location of the thoracic wall cardiac impulse (apical beat), approximately at or slightly above the level of the elbow (ventral region of the left ventricular inlet)
Basilar: Area above the elbow and slightly more cranial, below the triceps muscle (region of the ventricular outflow tracts, semilunar valves, and great vessels)
Mitral, aortic, pulmonic, tricuspid valve area (Figure 3-18)

Radiation
Dorsal-ventral, cranial-caudal, left-right

Quality
Frequency of sound: High pitch, low pitch, mixed pitch
Character of murmur: Harsh, coarse, rumbling, musical, honking, blowing

---

heart rate, often doubling it in a matter of seconds. The resting normal horse with high vagal tone may exhibit *physiologic arrhythmias* such as sinus block, sinus arrest, sinus arrhythmia, and incomplete Av block and may have an average heart rate of less than 30 beats/minute. Reducing vagal tone usually causes the arrhythmia to abate. This might be achieved by turning the horse in three or four quick circles or by examining the horse after exercise. Sustained or recurrent cardiac arrhythmias are easily discovered through cardiac auscultation and palpation of the facial artery pulse. If an arrhythmia persists after exercise or if the auscultatory findings suggest another arrhythmia (Table 3-8), an ECG should be obtained. It is worthwhile to concentrate on the individual *heart sounds* when assessing the cardiac rhythm because sound generation is closely associated with the systolic and diastolic events of the cardiac cycle and depends on the underlying rhythm (see preceding paragraphs and Figures 3-9 and 3-10; Figure 3-18).

Heart murmurs are common in horses, especially very young horses; however, some murmurs are indicative of

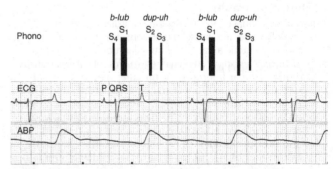

Figure 3–18. Relationship of normal heart sounds *(Phono)* to a surface electrocardiogram *(ECG)* and arterial blood pressure tracing *(ABP)* recorded from the transverse facial artery. *S1,* first (systolic) heart sound; *S2,* second (diastolic) heart sound; *S3,* third heart sound; *S4,* fourth (atrial) heart sound. Phono: *b(S4)-lub(S1) dup(S2)-uh(S3)* describes the sounds heard on auscultation. Note the timing of the heart sounds relative to the ECG and the (peripheral) pulse pressure wave.

cardiac disease.[120-126,128-130,132-137] Significant myocardial disease may result in arrhythmias and a cardiac murmur, especially in advanced cases in which ventricular dilation causes secondary mitral or tricuspid valve insufficiency.[129] Heart murmurs should be characterized on the basis of timing and duration, grade, point of maximum intensity, radiation, and quality (see Box 3-5). Most murmurs can be distinguished through careful auscultation (see Table 3-6), including evaluation of the effect of changing heart rate on the heart murmurs (i.e., by jogging or turning the horse in a tight circle). The assessment of the clinical relevance of an organic heart murmur may require ancillary tests (Box 3-6).[72,138-140]

Low-grade (innocent; 1 to 2/6) cardiac murmurs generally can be heard with careful auscultation at the left base of the heart (see Figure 3-10). Most innocent or physiologic cardiac murmurs are caused by vibrations that attend the ejection of blood from the heart during systole or the rapid filling of the ventricles during diastole. Typically these murmurs are soft (grade 1 to 2/6), localized, and labile. The most common physiologic murmur is the systolic ejection murmur heard at the left cardiac base over the aortic and pulmonic valves (see Figures 3-10 and 3-18 and

Table 3-6). Diastolic murmurs are also common, especially in Thoroughbred horses. Functional murmurs may be associated with sympathetic stimulation or decreased blood viscosity (i.e., associated with anemia). The detection of a loud murmur (>2 to 3), the development of a cardiac murmur in a horse that previously did not have a murmur, or the detection of a murmur at locations other than the left base suggests acquired cardiac (valvular) disease or a congenital cardiac malformation.[120,122,128] Causes of pathologic murmurs include incompetent cardiac valves, septal defects, vascular lesions, and (rarely) valve stenosis (see Tables 3-6 and 3-7). The continuous murmur of patent ductus arteriosus is normally present in full-term foals for up to 3 days postparturition.[79,135-137]

Besides the heart sounds and classical murmurs, *"extra sounds"* are sometimes detected and warrant consideration. Systolic clicks occasionally can be heard over the left apex and may indicate mitral valve disease or prolapse (especially when associated with a midsystolic to end-systolic murmur or mitral regurgitation). Ventricular knocks are loud ventricular filling sounds (correlating to S_3) heard with constrictive pericardial disease. Pericardial friction rub typically is a

---

Box 3–6 Diagnosis of Heart Disease in Horses

History*

Signalment, presenting complaints, general medical history, past illnesses, past and current medications, weight loss, work history and exercise tolerance

Physical Examination*

Body condition, heart rate, rhythm, arterial and venous pulses, venous distention, mucous membrane color and capillary refill time, subcutaneous edema, auscultation of the heart (heart sounds, heart murmurs, rhythm) and lungs

Electrocardiography*

Resting electrocardiogram: Heart rate, rhythm, P-QRS-T configuration, association of P and QRS-T, time intervals, and electrical axis

Exercise and postexercise electrocardiography (treadmill examination)†

24-hour Holter electrocardiography†

Echocardiography

Two-dimensional echocardiography: Cardiac anatomy, chamber size, and vessel dimensions; valve anatomy and motion; systolic atrial and ventricular function; identification of cardiac lesions or free fluid; estimation of cardiac output

M-mode echocardiography: Ventricular dimensions and systolic ventricular function; cardiac anatomy and valve motion; estimation of cardiac output

Doppler echocardiography: Identification of normal and abnormal flow; estimation of intracardiac pressures and pressure gradients; estimation of cardiac output; assessment of systolic and diastolic ventricular function

Thoracic Radiography

Evaluation of pleural space, pulmonary parenchyma, lung vascularity, and heart size

Clinical Laboratory Tests

Complete blood count and fibrinogen to identify anemia and inflammation

Serum biochemical tests, including electrolytes (particularly K^+, Mg^{+2}, Ca^{+2}), renal function tests, and muscle enzymes for assessment of arrhythmias; identification of low cardiac output (azotemia); and recognition of myocardial cell injury (CK and AST [unspecific] and cardiac troponin T or I [specific])

Serum proteins to identify hypoalbuminemia and hyperglobulinemia

Arterial blood gas analysis to evaluate pulmonary function (alternatively: pulse oximetry)

Venous blood gas analysis to assess acid-base status, oxygen delivery, and oxygen extraction in the tissues

Blood lactate to identify anaerobic metabolism associated with poor tissue oxygenation or impaired oxygen use in the tissues

Blood cultures in cases of thrombophlebitis or suspected endocarditis

Urinalysis to identify renal injury from heart failure or endocarditis

Serum/plasma assays for digoxin, quinidine, and other cardioactive drugs

Cardiac Catheterization and Angiocardiography‡

Diagnosis of abnormal blood flow and identification of abnormal intracardiac and intravascular pressures

Radionuclide Studies‡

Detection of abnormal blood flow or lung perfusion; assessment of ventricular function

---

*Most important part of the cardiac evaluation.
†May be needed to identify paroxysmal arrhythmias.
‡Not routinely performed.

triphasic sound (systole, early diastole, late diastole) indicating pericarditis. Pericarditis and cardiac tamponade usually are characterized by muffled heart sounds and pericardial friction rub and can result in right ventricular failure with jugular distention and subcutaneous edema.

Electrocardiography

The ECG is a graphic representation of the average electric potential generated by the heart over time. It is recorded throughout the different phases of the cardiac cycle and graphed in terms of voltage and time. Time is displayed along the x axis, and electrical potential is inscribed on the y axis. Generation of the various ECG waveforms (P-QRS-T) can be accounted for by considering the anatomical cardiac activation process.

The principles of recording and interpreting the ECG in horses are similar to those for humans, dogs, and other species, although some modified leads ("base-apex" lead; Box 3-7) have been developed for horses (Figure 3-19, A).[9,20,120,141-150] The base-apex lead accentuates the P wave in horses. The ECG waveforms observed in the base-apex

lead are temporally similar to those recorded in other leads, although the magnitude and polarity are different (Figure 3-19, B). They include P wave (atrial depolarization), PQ, or PR interval (mainly caused by slow AV nodal conduction), QRS complex (ventricular depolarization), and ST segment T wave (ST-T wave; ventricular repolarization; see Figures 3-3 and 3-4; Figure 3-20). A prominent atrial repolarization wave (T_a wave) is often noted in the PR (P-Q) segment of the equine ECG, particularly at faster heart rates (see Figures 3-19 and 3-20). Consistent lead positioning (e.g., base-apex lead), paper speed (e.g., 25mm/sec), and voltage calibration (e.g., 1cm/mV) facilitate rapid recognition of normal and abnormal electrocardiographic patterns. Paper speed, voltage calibration (Figure 3-21), and (in selected cases) leads may then be adjusted as necessary to optimize the quality and diagnostic value of the recording. A systematic approach to ECG analysis should be undertaken (Box 3-8), and quantitative measures should be compared with normal values (Table 3-9).

The sequential relationship of the normal ECG waveforms—P wave, the QRS complex, and the ST-T wave—must be understood to diagnose arrhythmias and detect other electrical

Box 3–7 Electrocardiographic Lead Systems

Base-Apex Monitor Lead (Most Commonly Used in Horses)
[+] Electrode over the left apex (left chest, at the level of the olecranon)
[–] Electrode over the right jugular furrow
 The most common method to obtain the base-apex lead is to place the left arm (LA) electrode over the left apex, the right arm (RA) electrode over the jugular furrow, and select 'lead I' on the electrocardiograph. This lead is the preferred choice for monitoring cardiac rhythm because it accentuates the P wave.

Bipolar Leads (Einthoven)*
Lead I = Left foreleg (LA) [+]; right foreleg (RA) [–]
Lead II = Left rearleg (LL) [+]; right foreleg (RA) [–]
Lead III = Left rearleg (LL) [+]; left foreleg (LA) [–]

Unipolar Augmented Limb Leads (Goldberger)*
Lead aVR = Right foreleg [+]; left foreleg and left rearleg [–]

Lead aVL = Left foreleg [+]; right foreleg and left rearleg [–]
Lead aVF = Left rearleg [+]; right foreleg and left foreleg [–]

Unipolar Precordial Chest Leads
[+] Electrode over selected precordial site
[–] Electrode composed of a compound electrode of left and right foreleg and left rearleg (Wilson central terminal)
The lead is named based on the location of the exploring (V or C) electrode.
V_{10} = [+] over the dorsal spine. Precordial leads other than V_{10} are not commonly used.

Modified orthogonal lead system
Lead X = Lead I, right [–] to left [+]
Lead Y = Lead aVF, cranial [–] to caudal [+]
Lead Z = Lead V_{10}, ventral [–] to dorsal [+]

*Frontal plane leads.

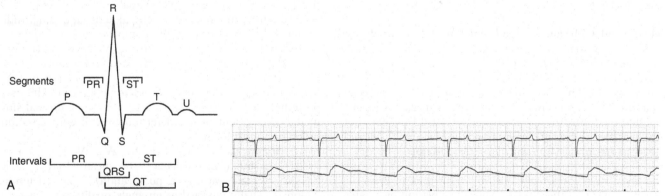

Figure 3–19. A, Cartoon of an idealized single, normal electrocardiographic cycle with waves, segments, and intervals identified. **B,** A base-apex ECG is obtained by placing the –electrode of lead 1 on the right jugular furrow and the +electrode of lead 1 on the left thoracic wall in the area of the left ventricular apex. An arterial pressure waveform is illustrated for timing purposes.

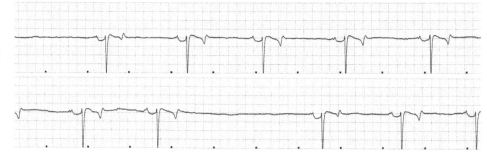

Figure 3–20. Base-apex ECGs from a mature horse. A normal bifid P wave can be observed. There is prominent downward deviation of the PR segment, indicative of atrial repolarization (T_a) wave.

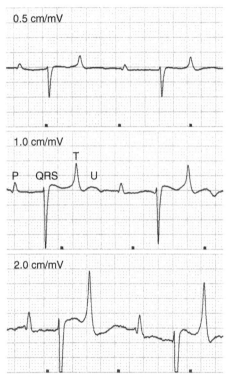

Figure 3–21. The gain (calibration) of the ECG determines the size of the ECG deflections (base-apex lead). The standard calibration of 1 cm/mV (middle) results in an ECG tracing of good diagnostic quality. Decreases in gain *(top)* lead to overall reduction in the size of the ECG complexes, which may mask deflections of small amplitude (e.g., first peak of the P wave or U wave). Conversely increases in gain *(bottom)* may complicate interpretation of the ECG by amplifying baseline deviations and artifacts. Generally ECGs should initially be recorded at standard calibration (1 cm/mV), and the gain adjusted as necessary for the individual horse.

abnormalities. The amplitude and duration of these waveforms depend on many factors, including lead position, body size, and age of the horse (see Table 3-9); size of the cardiac chambers; and the pattern of electrical activation.[137,151,152] The ECG is an excellent method for determining rhythm abnormalities in horses but is less sensitive for detecting cardiomegaly, especially mild-to-moderate heart enlargement. A normal ECG does not exclude heart disease in the horse, and the ECG cannot be used to assess mechanical function of the myocardium.

P wave. Electrical activation of the atria is responsible for generation of the P wave. Normal activation originates within the SA node (see preceding paragraphs) and proceeds from right to left and cranial to caudal, producing positive P waves in leads I, II, and aVF.[20,143,149] The normal P wave in horses is notched or bifid; however, single-peaked, diphasic, and polyphasic P waves may be encountered in normal horses.[20,142] A negative/positive P wave (coronary sinus P wave) is often recorded in the base-apex lead if the origin of pacemaker activity shifts to the caudal right atrium near the coronary sinus. The P wave morphology may differ among breeds and can change in a cyclic manner with waxing and waning of vagal (parasympathetic) tone during sinus arrhythmia in horses (*wandering pacemaker*). The P wave shortens and becomes more peaked during tachycardia and is often followed by a prominent *atrial repolarization (T_a) wave*. These electrocardiographic features make it difficult to identify atrial enlargement by ECG in horses.

PQ interval. The PQ interval (*PR interval*) represents the time for conduction from the SA node across the AV node and His-Purkinje system. Normal values for the PQ interval in horses vary considerably because of high resting parasympathetic tone. PQ interval values that persistently exceed 500 ms are probably abnormal in horses. The PQ interval depends on body size and is shorter in smaller horses, ponies, and foals (see Table 3-9). The atrial repolarization wave (T_a wave) is often observed between the end of the P wave and the onset of the QRS complex. Alterations in the horses breathing pattern and arterial blood pressure, heart rate, and autonomic tone can change the duration of the PQ interval.[153,154]

QRS complex. The ventricles of horses are activated simultaneously with a burst of depolarization caused by complete penetration of the conduction system into the ventricular free walls. Simultaneous activation of the ventricles results in cancellation of many of the divergent electromotive forces, producing a highly variable QRS pattern.[9,150,155] Consequently the normal electrical axis and amplitude (often of low mV) of the QRS complex vary considerably in the frontal plane leads I, II, III, aV$_R$, aV$_L$, and aV$_F$ (Figure 3-22, *A*). A prominent dorsally oriented vector causes a positive terminal deflection iitive terminal deflection in lead V$_{10}$, whereas the commonly used base-apex lead exhibits a prominent S wave (see Figure 3-20).[142,155] The normal slur in the ST segment makes determination of QRS duration difficult in most horses.[156]

The frontal (X-Y) leads (I, II, III, aV$_R$, aV$_L$, aV$_F$) can be used to quantitatively calculate the mean electrical axis (MEA; "average" wave of depolarization).[148] This determination is usually reported as an angle or direction, using a quadrant orientation (right or left; cranial or caudal) (lead I = 0°; II = 60°; aV$_F$ = 90°; III = 120°; aV$_R$ = –150°; aV$_L$ = –30°). The general direction of the QRS axis can be estimated

---

Box 3–8 Evaluation of the Electrocardiogram

Technical Aspects

Paper speed: Standard: 25 or 50 mm/s
Calibration: Standard: 1 cm/mV
Lead(s): see Box 3-5

Artifacts

Electrical, motion, twitching, muscle tremor, equipment (ventilator)

Heart Rate

Atrial and ventricular rate

Cardiac Rhythm

Regular, regularly irregular, irregularly irregular
Atrial, arteriovenous conduction sequence, ventricular, ventricular conduction
Arrhythmias

Site or chamber of abnormal impulse formation, myocardial fibrillation, or conduction
Rate of abnormal impulse formation
Conduction of abnormal impulses
Patterns or repeating cycles

Waves and Complexes

P wave: Morphology, duration, amplitude, variation
PQ interval: Duration, variation, conduction block (of P wave)
QRS: Morphology, duration, amplitude frontal plane mean electrical axis
ST segment: Depression or elevation
T wave: Changes in morphology or size
QT interval: Duration (consider heart rate)

Miscellaneous

Electrical alternans, synchronous diaphragmatic contraction

Table 3–9. Normal heart rates and ECG time intervals for horses at rest

Breed	HR (/min)	PQ (ms)	QRS (ms)*	QT (ms)
Adults[142,145,148,154,161,297,298]				
Large breeds	26-50	200-500	80-140	360-600
Small breeds, Ponies	30-54	160-320	60-120	320-560
Foals[151,299,300]				
Large breeds				
1-7 d	100-140	100-180	50-80	200-350
14 d	80-130	100-190	60-80	230-350
Ponies				
1-30 d	70-145	90-130	25-70	180-370
60 d	60-95	110-150	30-70	220-420
90 d	50-85	130-170	50-80	310-390

*QRS duration is often difficult to determine because of the normal slur in the ST segment.

quickly by surveying the height (mV) of the R waves in the frontal leads and selecting the lead with the greatest net-positive QRS complex (Figure 3-22, *B*). The MEA in foals and yearlings is variable and frequently cranial oriented; the frontal axis in most normal horses is directed leftward and caudally.[142] Abnormal axis deviations occur in horses with cardiomegaly, cor pulmonale, conduction disturbances, and electrolyte imbalance.[146] The conformation and MEA of the QRS complex also facilitates assessment of ventricular activation from ventricular ectopic foci.[155] The duration of the QRS complex is determined by the propagation velocity of the impulse in the ventricular myocardium. Ectopic impulse formation, aberrant impulse conduction, partial membrane depolarization in diseased tissue, hyperkalemia, and drug-induced Na^+ channel blocking drugs (e.g., quinidine, procaineamide) can slow impulse conduction and widen the QRS complex.

ST-T wave. Repolarization of the ventricles begins at the end of the QRS complex ("J point") and extends to the end of the T wave.[157] The T wave vector is generally directed toward the left leg, leading to a positive T wave in lead III and a negative or isoelectric T wave in lead I in most resting horses. Although some authors have suggested that abnormalities of the ST-T indicate cardiac dysfunction, marked variability of the ST segment and increased amplitude of the T wave occurs in normal horses after exercise or when excited.[157,158] Progressive J point or ST deviation in an anesthetized horse usually indicates myocardial hypoxia or ischemia; increasing amplitude of the T wave during anesthesia suggests myocardial hypoxia or hyperkalemia.[17]

QT interval. The QT interval represents the total electrical depolarization-repolarization time and is the algebraic sum of all of the cellular action potential durations (APDs) generated throughout the ventricular myocardium (see Figure 3-4). The upper limit for the QT interval at resting heart rates is approximately 600 ms in adult horses and 350 to 400 ms in foals (see Table 3-9). The QT interval shortens at higher heart rates and is influenced by changes in autonomic tone. A variety of population- or individual-based methods have been used in other humans, dogs, and cats to correct for heart rate–related changes in the QT interval (QT_c).[159,160] Although some data are available for horses,[154,161] QT correction methods are highly dependent on the recording conditions used to determine correction formulas (e.g., resting ECG or 24-hour Holter, exercise, cardiac pacing, or pharmacologic interventions to alter autonomic tone). Thus QT correction formulas have been difficult to apply to different populations or individual horses.[162] The diagnosis of QT prolongation in horses is further complicated by the commonly encountered problem of accurately detecting the end of the T wave.

Prolongation of the QT interval indicates delayed ventricular repolarization in a part (dispersion of repolarization) or all of the ventricles. Congenital (caused by ion channel mutations) or acquired (caused by drug effects on repolarizing currents) *long QT syndrome (LQTS)* is associated with life-threatening cardiac arrhythmias and sudden death in humans but has not been documented in horses. However, repolarizing currents in horses are similar to those in other species, and it has been suggested that horses may be at risk for acquired LQTS.[19] Many drugs that prolong cardiac repolarization (QT interval)

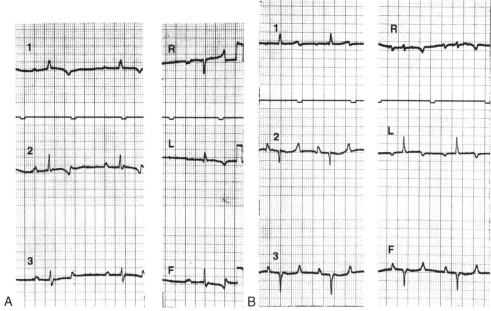

Figure 3–22. A, Normal frontal plane leads from a mature Standardbred horse. The frontal (I, II, III, aVr, aVl, aVf) lead axis is directed left and caudal. Paper speed, 25 mm/sec; lead calibrations of 1 mV at right. **B,** Normal frontal plane leads from mature Standardbred horse. Frontal axis is left and cranial, causing prominent R waves in leads I and aVL. Paper speed, 25 mm/sec; 1 cm/mV. (From Bonagura JD, Miller MS: Electrocardiography. In Jones WJ, editor: *Equine sports medicine,* Philadelphia, 1989, Lea & Febiger.)

in other species are administered to horses, including quinidine, procainamide, flecainide, amiodarone, cisapride, metoclopramide, erythromycin, clarithromycin, fluconazole, trimethoprim-sulfamethoxazole, sevoflurane, and isoflurane.[15] Quinidine-induced torsades de pointes, potentially related to drug-induced QT prolongation, has been reported in horses.[163] Furthermore, a slow resting heart rate and hypokalemia, commonly associated with gastrointestinal disease in horses, theoretically enhances the risk of drug-induced arrhythmias. therefore it is advisable to consider the potential proarrhythmic effects of medications, particularly QT-prolonging drugs before administering them to horses.

U wave.   The U wave is a small, low-frequency deflection that is sometimes seen after the T wave (see Figure 3-19, *A*). The electrophysiologic basis and clinical relevance of the U wave remains controversial but is likely related to delayed repolarization of ventricular muscle cells (dispersion of repolarization) or within the ventricular conducting system (Purkinje network).[164]

Echocardiography

Diagnostic ultrasonography is used to visualize the beating heart and identify specific cardiac lesions, detect abnormal blood flow patterns, assess the hemodynamic consequences of heart disease and drug therapy, and estimate the severity of cardiac disease (Figure 3-23). Clinically echocardiography is frequently used to accurately determine the source significance (heart size; function) of cardiac murmurs. A normal echocardiogram in a horse with a cardiac murmur is a favorable finding in a horse scheduled to be anesthetized. Conversely identification of a loud murmur (>2/6), significant cardiomegaly, and abnormal ventricular function indicates increased anesthetic risk.

Echocardiography may also be used to monitor cardiac performance and hemodynamic events during anesthesia. Transesophageal echocardiography (TEE) can be used to estimate cardiac output in adult horses under general anesthesia and to assess drug effects.[99,100,122,165,166] The velocity-time integral of the aortic blood flow (measured by Doppler echocardiography) multiplied by vessel area (determined by 2D echocardiography) provides an estimate of stroke volume. The velocity or acceleration of blood cells into the aorta indirectly assesses left ventricular contractile function. General anesthesia increases the time to peak velocity and decreases peak velocity, and both are changed toward normal by positive inotropic agents such as dobutamine.[165,166]

Detailed evaluation and quantitative assessment of equine echocardiograms should precede anesthesia in horses with evidence of cardiovascular disease.[167-175]

Structural Heart Disease

General anesthesia in horses with heart disease can be challenging and requires careful consideration of the pathophysiological processes and hemodynamic consequences produced, the influence of other confounding diseases, and the effects of anesthetic drugs. Most, if not all, anesthetic drugs produce cardiovascular effects that can be accentuated in horses with cardiovascular disease. Severe cardiovascular disease leading to congestive heart failure is not common in horses, but, if present, is usually associated with a poor prognosis. However, many horses requiring anesthesia for elective surgical procedures have physiologic heart murmurs and inconsequential cardiac arrhythmias and display echocardiographic images suggestive of mild-to-moderate structural heart disease. These horses can be safely anesthetized after careful evaluation and goal-directed selection of the appropriate anesthetic drugs and technique. Horses with

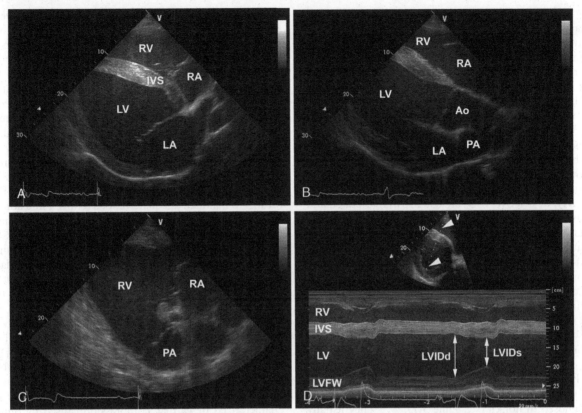

Figure 3–23. Two-dimensional echocardiograms obtained from the right side of the chest (**A** to **C**). The ECG is recorded simultaneously for timing purposes. **A,** Four-chamber view. **B,** Left-ventricular outflow tract view. **C,** Right-ventricular inflow and outflow tract view. The images, recorded in a right-parasternal long-axis view, allow subjective assessment of cardiac structures and myocardial function and measurement of selected cardiac dimensions. **D,** M-mode echocardiogram of the normal left ventricle performed in a right-parasternal short-axis view at the level of the chordae tendineae. The myocardial wall motion (y-axis) along the cursor line *(arrowheads)* is displayed over time (x-axis). An ECG is recorded simultaneously for timing. This view allows subjective assessment of right- and left-ventricular dimensions and left-ventricular systolic function, determination of left-ventricular internal dimensions in systole and diastole, and calculation of the left-ventricular fractional shortening (FS) (% change in the internal dimension; FS = [LVIDd – LVIDs] / LVIDd x 100). The latter provides an index of systolic left-ventricular function. *LV,* left ventricle; *LA,* left atrium; *RV,* right ventricle; *RA,* right atrium; *IVS,* interventricular septum; *Ao,* Aorta; *PA,* pulmonary artery; *LVFW,* left-ventricular free wall; *LVIDd,* left-ventricular internal diameter at end-diastole; *LVIDs,* left-ventricular internal diameter at peak systole.

advanced cardiovascular dysfunction generally lack sufficient cardiac reserve to compensate for anesthetic-induced depression.[176,177] Every effort should be made to maintain cardiac output and peripheral perfusion while avoiding extremely rapid heart rates, hypovolemia or hypervolemia, or an increase in afterload (peripheral vasoconstriction). Horses with cardiovascular disease may be predisposed to acute (hypotension) or insidious (low blood flow) hemodynamic deterioration and cardiac arrhythmias.[120,122,123] Vigilant monitoring of indices of cardiovascular function is required in all anesthetized horses.

Congenital cardiovascular disease. The most common congenital diseases in horses involve shunting of blood (see Box 3-4).[120] *Ventricular septal defects (VSDs)* are the most common congenital defect diagnosed in horses.[120]*Patent ductus arteriosus (PDA)* is uncommon in foals. The ductus arteriosus is sensitive to oxygen tension and functionally closes in most foals within 72 to 96 hours after birth. Surgical correction of PDA is possible and performed relatively easily within the first 3 to 4 months of life. Other congenital defects are relatively rare. Complex congenital

defects often lead to fetal death, birth of a nonviable foal or rapid hemodynamic deterioration early after birth.

Both VSDs and PDA result in systemic-to-pulmonary (left-to-right) shunting of blood. The shunt volume depends on the size of the defect (opening) and the relative resistance of the systemic and pulmonary vasculature. Pulmonary vascular resistance is still relatively high immediately after birth, and systemic pressures are low, limiting left-to-right shunting. Over the first few weeks of life significant shunting may develop as a result of a gradual decline in pulmonary vascular resistance and rise in systemic pressures (see Table 3-7). Left-to-right shunting of blood increases pulmonary blood flow and pulmonary venous return to the left heart and results in compensatory left atrial and ventricular enlargement and hypertrophy. Left-sided volume overload may be severe when the shunt is large, leading to left-sided or biventricular congestive heart failure. Pulmonary hypertension may occur secondary to increased transpulmonary flow, left-ventricular failure, and flow-related pulmonary vascular changes. A rise in pulmonary vascular and right ventricular pressures decreases the shunt volume and protects the left heart from severe volume overload while the workload of the right ventricle increases. Rarely severe pulmonary hypertension may result in reversed (right-to-left) shunting of blood and the development of arterial hypoxemia (Eisenmenger's physiology).

A thorough history and physical examination in conjunction with echocardiographic evaluation (2D and Doppler echocardiography) provide useful information for assessing the hemodynamic consequences and severity of the malformation.[120,168] VSDs are termed restrictive when their diameter is less than one third the diameter of the aorta (<2.5 cm in large-breed adult horses) with a peak shunt flow velocity greater than 4 m/s, equaling a left-to-right pressure gradient of at least 64 mm Hg (modified Bernoulli equation: $V^2 \times 4$ ($4^2 \times 4 = 64$). Restrictive VSDs are usually well tolerated and have a favorable prognosis, even for athletic performance.

Inhalation anesthesia (decreases SVR) and positive-pressure ventilation (increases pulmonary vascular resistance) limit left-to-right shunting of blood producing minimum hemodynamic impact in normal horses with mild-to-moderate heart disease but are not well tolerated in horses with heart failure.[177] Conversely, large increases in SVR (e.g., elevated sympathetic tone) should be avoided. Continuous invasive monitoring of arterial blood pressures is recommended in all horses with cardiovascular disease.

Valvular heart disease.   *Tricuspid and mitral regurgitation* and *aortic insufficiency* are the most common valvular cardiac diseases diagnosed in horses (see Table 3-7).[178-180] They usually result from chronic, degenerative valve disease and can be classified on the basis of clinical and echocardiographic findings as trivial (potentially physiologic), mild, moderate, and severe. Potential causes for valvular insufficiency include valvulitis, endocarditis,[181,182] mitral valve prolapse caused by rupture of the chordal tendinae,[183-185] and (rarely) congenital valve dysplasia.[186,187] Valvular insufficiency eventually produces ventricular volume overload, increased myocardial oxygen demand, heart failure, and decreases in cardiac output. The cardiovascular system is able to compensate for the hemodynamic consequences of valvular insufficiency in early stages of disease, and clinical signs of heart failure (exercise intolerance, poor performance, weight loss, ventral edema) do not occur until ventricular dysfunction is advanced. Eventually myocardial dysfunction and congestive heart failure may ensue from chronic volume overload. The anesthetic risk associated with valvular heart disease in horses is unknown but is logically related to the severity of ventricular enlargement, impairment of ventricular function, and the presence of cardiac arrhythmias. Minor procedures in horses with asymptomatic valvular disease are unlikely to impose a significant risk.

Ventricular stroke volume, ejection fraction, and cardiac output are strongly dependent on heart rate, myocardial contractility, and afterload in horses with advanced valvular disease. The volume of blood regurgitated backward through an incompetent aortic valve depends directly on the duration of diastole (determined by heart rate) and the pressure gradient across the aortic valve (arterial blood pressure and peripheral vascular resistance). Changes in heart rate, increases in SVR, and anesthetic drug-induced myocardial depression should be minimized in horses with reduced ventricular function. Conversely modest increases in heart rate and decreases in SVR associated with the administration of volatile anesthetics may minimize the deleterious hemodynamic effects of light inhalant anesthesia, providing myo-

cardial contractility is not significantly affected. Decreases in SVR and afterload reduce the mitral regurgitant volume and the forward flow of blood (stroke volume) in horses with mitral regurgitation.

However, cardiac inotropes such as dopamine or dobutamine may be used to increase myocardial contractility when ventricular contractile force is impaired. Dopamine is preferred for treating bradycardia and hypotension; dobutamine is preferred for treating hypotension without bradycardia. Positive inotropes should be used cautiously since larger doses can produce undesired vasoconstrictive and arrhythmogenic effects. Furthermore, respiratory rate should be minimized during mechanical ventilation to allow sufficient time between breaths to maintain adequate venous return. Fluid administration should be monitored carefully to maintain adequate ventricular filling pressures and avoid fluid overload (see Chapters 7 and 22). Invasive monitoring of venous and arterial pressure, cardiac output, and calculation of peripheral vascular resistance is not required in most horses with valvular heart disease but should be considered in horses with advanced valvular disease and compromised ventricular function.

Pericardial disease.   Pericardial diseases are rare and usually manifest as *fibrinous pericarditis, pericardial effusion,* or *constrictive pericarditis.*[120,188-193] Pericardial disease can be idiopathic or caused by bacterial or viral infections, trauma, or tumors. Pathophysiologically pericardial disease is usually characterized by cardiac compression caused by fluid accumulation within the pericardial space (*cardiac tamponade*) or *constriction* of the heart caused by fibrosis of the epicardium or pericardium. Both conditions impair diastolic filling of the ventricles, reduce preload and cardiac output, and eventually result in congestive heart failure with a predominantly right-sided component. Development of clinical signs depends on the volume and rate of pericardial fluid accumulation, compliance of the pericardium, and etiology of the effusion. The severity of pericardial disease should be assessed by clinical examination of pericardial fluid and echocardiography.

Sedation, general anesthesia, and positive-pressure ventilation in the presence of cardiac tamponade cause significant hemodynamic deterioration and hypotension as a result of bradycardia, peripheral vasodilation, a further decrease in venous return, and associated decrease in cardiac output. A pericardiocentesis should be performed in horses with significant cardiac tamponade before anesthesia. The procedure is performed relatively easily with ultrasonographic guidance under local anesthesia and often results in dramatic improvement of cardiac output.[120,194] Arterial blood pressure should be monitored if sedation is required to perform pericardiocentesis in severely affected horses. Severe hypotension should be treated with shock doses (40+ ml/kg) of crystalloid or colloid fluids to increase intravascular volume. High right atrial pressures may be necessary to offset the effects of pericardial effusion on ventricular filling and to improve cardiac output. Catecholamines (dopamine, dobutamine) increase myocardial contractility. Furosemide is contraindicated before pericardiocentesis since diuresis may reduce ventricular filling, cause hypotension, and result in syncope. The same principles apply for stabilization of patients with constrictive pericarditis.

Pulmonary hypertension and cor pulmonale.   *Pulmonary hypertension* can develop in horses secondary to mitral valve disease or chronic left-sided heart failure, an increase in pulmonary blood flow caused by congenital left-to right shunts, or an increase in pulmonary vascular resistance secondary to pulmonary vascular or parenchymal disease. *Cor pulmonale* is characterized by pulmonary hypertension caused by pulmonary parenchymal or vascular disease in the absence of left ventricular dysfunction with resultant right ventricular hypertrophy and dilation. Diagnosis of cor pulmonale requires evidence of pulmonary hypertension and exclusion of primary cardiac disease.[195,196] Cor pulmonale is uncommon in horses.[197-199]

Pulmonary hypertension is characterized hemodynamically by pulmonary artery pressures exceeding the upper normal limit by more than 10 mm Hg.[196] Pulmonary artery pressures can be estimated echocardiographically by Doppler flow imaging of tricuspid or pulmonic regurgitation velocities (modified Bernoulli equation). Enlargement of the pulmonary artery (exceeding the aortic root diameter) is considered a fairly specific (but not sensitive) indicator of pulmonary hypertension. Cardiac catheterization allows invasive measurement of pulmonary artery pressures and PCWPs and may aid in the diagnosis of pulmonary hypertension and cor pulmonale.

Pulmonary hypertension is diagnosed occasionally in foals and adult horses with severe respiratory disease.[199] A low alveolar oxygen tension is considered a very potent trigger of (reversible) pulmonary vasoconstriction, leading to an increase in pulmonary vascular resistance.[200,201] Hypoxia is known to be a contributing factor leading to (relatively mild) pulmonary hypertension in horses with recurrent airway obstruction.[83,84,202]

Anesthesia for elective surgical procedures is usually postponed in the presence of severe respiratory disease to allow adequate treatment and functional improvement of lung function. When anesthesia is required in horses with pulmonary hypertension, adequate alveolar and arterial oxygenation (preoxygenation, ventilation) is critical to minimize functional hypoxic vasoconstriction. Oxygenation can be improved by administration of increased inspiratory oxygen (FiO_2) concentrations and positive-pressure ventilation (see Chapter 17). Administration of nitrous oxide is not recommended and may produce pulmonary vasoconstric-

tion, further increasing pulmonary vascular resistance and pulmonary blood flow.[177] Continuous monitoring of arterial oxygen saturation (e.g., by pulse oximetry) and end-tidal CO_2 is recommended for assessment of pulmonary gas transport. Fluid therapy should aim at maintaining adequate filling pressures while avoiding volume overload. Positive inotropes may be used to improve myocardial function.

Congestive heart failure. Congestive heart failure is uncommon in horses. Most cardiac diseases (see preceding paragraphs) are not severe enough to lead to the elevation of venous pressures and the renal retention of sodium and water that characterize the congestive state.[203,204] Pathophysiologic abnormalities associated with heart failure are similar to those encountered in humans and dogs[205,206] but have not been studied extensively in horses.[122] The clinical signs of advanced *biventricular heart failure* in horses are straightforward and easy to recognize.[120,207] Important clinical findings include tachycardia, arrhythmia, weak pulses, jugular venous distention and pulsation, fluid retention (subcutaneous ventral edema, pleural effusion, pulmonary edema), cough, exercise intolerance, weight loss, and loss of body condition. Acute *left-ventricular failure* causes pulmonary venous congestion and pulmonary edema. Pulmonary edema caused by pure left-sided congestive heart failure can be misdiagnosed as pneumonia. Signs of *right-sided congestive heart failure* are commonly observed even when the primary cardiac lesion is on the left side of the heart (e.g., mitral insufficiency). This is because of the right-ventricular dilation and failure that develops secondary to pulmonary venous hypertension and pulmonary edema.

Therapy for congestive heart failure is possible in selected cases, although euthanasia is often elected because of the poor prognosis at the time of diagnosis. Acute heart failure or acute worsening of chronic heart failure is treated with diuretics (furosemide), positive inotropes (dopamine, dobutamine), and intranasal oxygen (Table 3-10). Vasodilators such as the arterial dilator hydralazine or the venodilator nitroglycerin have been administered, although the efficacy of these drugs in horses with

Table 3–10. Drug therapy for heart disease[122,194,301,302]

Indications	Drug or method*	Dose	Adverse effects
Congestive heart failure	Furosemide	0.5 to 2.0 mg/kg intravenously (IV) q12h or as needed. Usually start at higher/more frequent doses and then reduce to minimum effective dose	At high doses risk of hypovolemia, renal failure, electrolyte imbalances (Na+, K+, Ca+2)
	Digoxin	Intravenous loading dose: 0.0022 mg/kg q12h for 24 to 36 hr. PO maintenance dosage: 0.011 mg/kg q12h, adjusted to maintain therapeutic concentrations (therapeutic range: 0.8-1.2 ng/ml, trough level at 12 to 24 hours)	Depression, anorexia, abdominal pain; supraventricular and ventricular arrhythmias, bigeminy, atrioventricular (AV) block

(Continued)

Table 3–10.   Drug therapy for heart disease—Cont'd.

Indications	Drug or method*	Dose	Adverse effects
Cardiogenic shock, hypotension	Dobutamine [or] dopamine	1-5 µg/kg/min IV continuous-rate infusion	Dose-dependent effects Vasoconstriction, tachycardia, ventricular arrhythmias
Sinus arrest/bradycardia, high-grade or complete AV block, vagally induced bradyarrhythmias	Atropine [or] Glycopyrrolate	0.01-0.02 mg/kg IV 0.005-0.01 mg/kg IV	Ileus, abdominal pain, tachycardia
	Dobutamine [or] dopamine	1-5 µg/kg/min IV continuous-rate infusion	Dose-dependent effects Vasoconstriction, tachycardia, ventricular arrhythmias
Sinus tachycardia	Treat underlying disorder		
Atrial standstill and ventricular conduction disturbances resulting from hyperkalemia	0.9% NaCl	10-40 mL/kg/h IV	
	Sodium bicarbonate	1-2 mEq/kg IV over 15 min	At high doses metabolic alkalosis, hypernatremia, volume overload
	23% Ca gluconate in 5% dextrose	0.2-0.4 mL/kg IV 6 mL/kg IV	Proarrhythmic effects during rapid administration
	Regular insulin and 10% dextrose	0.1 U/kg IV 5-10 ml/kg IV	Hypoglycemia; monitor blood glucose concentration
Atrial/supraventricular arrhythmias	Quinidine Procainamide Digoxin (ventricular rate control)	See Box 3-10 See below	
	Diltiazem (rate control and interruption of sinoatrial (SA)/AV nodal-dependent supraventricular tachycardia (SVT)	0.125 mg/kg over 2 min IV, repeated every 10 minutes to effect, up to 1.25 mg/kg total dosage; doses above 0.5-1.0 mg/kg should be used with caution	At high doses hypotension, sinus arrhythmia and sinus arrest, AV block, neg. inotropic effect; monitor ECG and blood pressure
	Propranolol (rate control and unresponsive SVT)	0.03-0.16 mg/kg IV 0.38-0.78 mg/kg PO q8h	Bradycardia, AV block, hypotension, negative inotropism, worsening of heart failure, weakness, bronchoconstriction
Atrial fibrillation/flutter	See Box 3-9		
Ventricular arrhythmias	Lidocaine	0.25-0.5 mg/kg slow IV, repeat in 5-10 min, up to 1.5 mg/kg total dosage; followed by 0.05 mg/kg/min continuous-rate infusion	Overdoses may lead to muscle tremors, ataxia, central nervous system (CNS) excitement, seizures; hypotension, ventricular tachycardia, sudden death
	Magnesium sulfate (especially torsades)	2-6 mg/kg/min IV to effect, up to a total dosage of 55(-100) mg/kg	Overdoses may lead to CNS-depressant effects, muscular weakness, trembling, bradycardia, hypotension, respiratory depression, cardiac arrest
	Procainamide	25-35 mg/kg PO q8h 1 mg/kg/min IV to a maximum of 20 mg/kg	Hypotension, QRS and QT prolongation, negative inotropism, supraventricular/ ventricular arrhythmias
Ventricular asystole	Epinephrine	0.01-0.05 mg/kg IV 0.1-0.5 mg/kg intratracheally	Note different concentrations: 1:1,000 = 1 mg/ml 1:10,000 = 0.1 mg/ml

*Also reevaluate oxygenation, fluid and electrolyte status (K, Mg), acid-base balance and adjust level of anesthetic, if appropriate.

heart failure is poorly documented.[208,209] Drug therapy for chronic heart failure is commonly limited to furosemide and digoxin.[210-212] Doses and dose intervals are titrated to effect, the horse's renal function, electrolyte status, and serum digoxin concentrations. Angiotensin-converting enzyme inhibitors can be administered, although their effects and efficacy in horses with heart failure have not been studied extensively, and their benefits are largely unknown.[213-217] Antiarrhythmic drugs are effective for the treatment of some arrhythmias (e.g., ventricular tachycardia, AF), but the potential for adverse effects has to be weighed against the potential benefits of treatment. Antibiotics are used to treat cardiac infections. Pericardiocentesis is used for initial management of cardiac tamponade, and tube or surgical drainage of the effusion can also be considered.

Horses in congestive heart failure are generally unacceptable risks for general anesthesia. A complete physical examination and hematologic and blood chemistry profile should be completed before attempting anesthesia. Special diagnostic tests, including thoracic radiographs and echocardiogram, should be performed. Ventricular function should be evaluated thoroughly and stabilized before surgical procedures are contemplated. The failing heart is characterized by a poor myocardial contractility, a decrease of preload reserve, and an increased sensitivity to ventricular afterload. Anesthetic drugs and techniques must be chosen with the goal of optimizing cardiac output and oxygenation if general anesthesia becomes unavoidable. Ketamine and ketamine drug combinations are useful for induction and for maintenance during short procedures (see Chapters 12, 13, and 18). Barbiturates and volatile anesthetics cause dose-dependent cardiac and respiratory depression and should be administered carefully. When properly applied, positive-pressure ventilation may be beneficial by decreasing ventricular wall stress (afterload) and pulmonary congestion and improving arterial oxygenation, but it can reduce venous return and cardiac output in horses that are hypovolemic or have poor ventricular function (see Chapter 17). Fluid therapy must be administered carefully to maintain adequate preload while avoiding fluid overload and congestion. Cardiac output and arterial blood pressure should be augmented by the administration of positive inotropic agents when necessary, while refraining from excessive use of vasoconstrictors that lead to an increase in afterload and impose an increased workload on the failing heart. Invasive monitoring of arterial pressures is mandatory; and direct monitoring of cardiac output, vascular resistance, and filling pressures is recommended whenever possible (see Chapter 8).

Cardiac Rhythm Disturbances

Cardiac arrhythmias are common in horses at rest, during and after exercise, and during general anesthesia. Cardiac rhythm disturbances can be reliably diagnosed using surface electrocardiography, telemetric electrocardiography (during exercise), or 24-hour Holter electrocardiography (for detection of paroxysmal dysrhythmias). The ECG is an important diagnostic tool and is easily obtained before anesthesia as part of the preanesthetic examination and during general anesthesia. A variety of physiologic (e.g., AV block, sinus arrhythmia, sinus arrest) and pathologic arrhythmias (e.g.,

atrial flutter/fibrillation, atrial and ventricular premature complexes, accelerated idioventricular rhythm) can occur associated with the administration of anesthetic drugs in horses. Their causes and consequences determine the most appropriate therapy.

Electrophysiologic Mechanisms of Common Arrhythmias

Both atrial and ventricular arrhythmias are believed to be caused by three fundamental mechanisms: (1) increased automaticity, (2) reentry circuits, and (3) triggered activity caused by afterdepolarizations.[4,11-13,38]

Increased automaticity. Increased automaticity is caused by *enhanced normal automaticity* (i.e., SA node) or *abnormal automaticity* in pathologically altered conductive or myocardial tissue (i.e., from ischemia). Increased sympathetic nervous system activity increases automaticity caused by acceleration of phase 4 depolarization, resulting in sinus or junctional tachycardia.

Reentry. Reentrant excitation resulting from circus movement of electrical impulses is considered one of the most important mechanisms responsible for cardiac arrhythmias. Reentry requires an adequate structural and/or functional substrate. Normal (e.g., AV node) or abnormal (e.g., accessory pathways) conducting pathways can serve as part of a reentrant circuit. A decrease in conduction velocity (e.g., in partially depolarized ischemic tissue), a shortening of action potential duration and refractory period (e.g., high vagal tone), and an increase in myocardial mass (e.g., atrial enlargement caused by mitral regurgitation) predispose to reentrant arrhythmias. Furthermore, myocardial damage, ion channel abnormalities, or alterations in distribution and function of gap junctions (connexins) increase the risk of reentrant arrhythmias.

Reentry is responsible for some forms of supraventricular and ventricular tachyarrhythmia, including AV nodal–dependent supraventricular tachycardia, atrial flutter, or AF. Reentry is considered the most important cause for chronic AF (whereas ectopic activity and afterdepolarizations may be important triggers for the initiation and early persistence of AF).[218] Ventricular arrhythmias, including coupled ventricular depolarizations, ventricular tachycardia, and ventricular flutter/fibrillation, can be caused by reentrant.

Triggered activity. Triggered activity is the result of early or late *afterdepolarizations* that occur in association with normal electrical activation of heart muscle cells. Triggered activity is commonly characterized by a fixed coupling interval between the triggering beat and the triggered beat. *Early afterdepolarizations (EADs)* develop during repolarization of the action potential (phase 3) and are most common during slow heart rates or after long pauses. EADs can induce ventricular arrhythmias such as torsades de pointes. *Delayed afterdepolarizations (DADs)* occur after complete repolarization (phase 4) of the action potential. DADs are caused by intracellular calcium overload that results in activation of the Na^+-Ca^{+2} exchanger (NCX) and membrane depolarization through large inward Na^+ currents. Congestive heart failure activates NCX and predisposes to triggered activity.[218] Digoxin-induced (typically ventricular bigeminy) and certain catecholamine-dependent atrial and ventricular tachycardias are likely the result of DADs.

Common Cardiac Arrhythmias

Cardiac arrhythmias are recognized on the basis of their rate, regularity, morphology, and locus of origin.[219] A wide variety of cardiac arrhythmias have been recognized in horses, some of which are physiologic, and others that are potentially dangerous, particularly during anesthesia when the responses of cardiovascular control mechanisms may be blunted (Box 3-9).[220] Pathologic arrhythmias often develop in association with high sympathetic tone, fever, endotoxemia, sepsis, hypotension, electrolyte disorders, acidosis, hypoxemia, gastrointestinal disease, or severe pulmonary disease; following administration of proarrhythmic drugs (e.g., digoxin, quinidine) or agents known to sensitize the heart to catecholamines (e.g., thiobarbiturates, halothane); and infrequently after injectable or inhalant anesthetic drugs. The two most important considerations in evaluation of a cardiac arrhythmia are the *hemodynamic consequences* (pressure, cardiac output, perfusion; Figure 3-24) and the potential for further *electrical destabilization* (myocardial fibrillation).

Supraventricular Rhythms

Sinus rhythms. A number of hemodynamically inconsequential sinus rhythms can be recognized in horses. Normal resting horses frequently demonstrate vagally mediated sinus bradycardia, sinus arrhythmia, and sinus block/arrest; yet fear or sudden stimuli may provoke rapid withdrawal of vagal tone, sympathetic activation, and sinus tachycardia (Figures 3-25 and 3-26, *A* and *B*). Atrioventricular conduction generally tends to follow sinus activity: during sinus tachycardia AV nodal conduction is faster, and the PQ interval shortens; whereas during periods of progressive sinus arrhythmia slowing AV nodal conduction is prolonged, and the PQ interval increases, potentially resulting in second-degree AV block (Figure 3-27). Sinus arrhythmia, sinus arrest, and second-degree AV block may occur in normal standing horses, immediately after submaximum exercise, or shortly after being excited as heart rate returns to normal values.

Sinus rate and rhythm must be monitored carefully in anesthetized horses because heart rate is a major determinant of cardiac output and arterial blood pressure (see Figures 3-11 and 3-24, *C*). Many sedative (α_2-agonists) and anesthetic drugs (isoflurane, sevoflurane) and some antiarrhythmics slow automaticity in the sinus node, producing *sinus bradycardia*, which can progress to sinus arrest (see Figures 3-24, *C,* and 3-27; Figure 3-28). Anesthetic drugs or hypoxia, traction on abdominal viscus, ocular manipulation, hypothermia, hyperkalemia, and increased intracranial pressure can decrease sinus node activity. Sinus bradycardia generally is a benign rhythm in standing horses; however, during sedation or anesthesia sinus bradycardia may significantly reduce cardiac output and produce significant hypotension (see Figure 3-11). Treatment of symptomatic sinus bradycardia includes reduction or reversal of the anesthetic drug, when possible; administration of an anticholinergic (atropine, glycopyrrolate); and infusion of a catecholamine (dopamine, dobutamine, epinephrine; see Table 3-10 and

---

Box 3–9 Cardiac Rhythms in the Horse

Physiologic Rhythms

Sinus Rhythms*
Normal sinus rhythm
Sinus arrhythmia
Sinoatrial block/arrest
Sinus bradycardia
Sinus tachycardia

Conduction Disturbances*
Atrioventricular block (AV block)
　First-degree (long PQ or PR interval)
　Second-degree (P wave not followed by a QRS complex; commonly Mobitz type I, Wenckebach)

Pathologic Rhythms

Atrial Rhythm Disturbances
Atrial escape complexes[†]
Atrial premature complexes*
Atrial tachycardia, nonsustained and sustained
Reentrant supraventricular tachycardia
Atrial flutter, atrial fibrillation*

Junctional Rhythm Disturbances
Junctional escape complexes[†]
　Junctional escape rhythm[†] (idionodal rhythm)

Junctional premature complexes*
Junctional ("nodal") tachycardia
Reentrant supraventricular tachycardia

Ventricular Rhythm Disturbances
Ventricular escape complexes[†]
Ventricular escape rhythm[†] (idioventricular rhythm)
Ventricular premature complexes*
Accelerated idioventricular rhythm (idioventricular tachycardia, slow ventricular tachycardia)*
Ventricular tachycardia
Ventricular flutter
Ventricular fibrillation

Conduction Disturbances
Sinoatrial block (high grade or persistent)
Atrial standstill (sinoventricular rhythm caused by hyperkalemia)
AV block
　Second-degree (high-grade or persistent)
　Third-degree (complete)
Ventricular conduction disturbances
　Ventricular preexcitation

*Most common rhythms and arrhythmias.
[†]Escape complexes develop secondary to another rhythm disturbance.

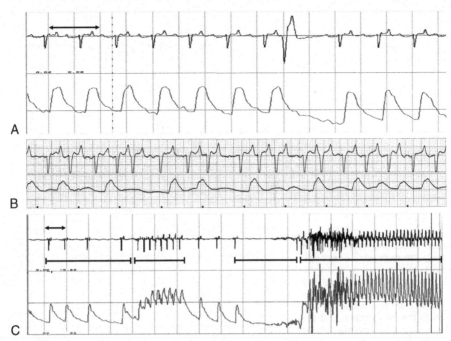

Figure 3–24. The ECG tracings are shown on top, concurrent arterial blood pressure tracings are displayed below. **A,** Ventricular premature depolarization (beat) in a standing, nonsedated horse (heart rate 52 beats/min). The premature beat stops the following sinus impulse from penetrating the AV node, resulting in a *compensatory pause*. Note the transient decrease in arterial blood pressure. **B,** Atrial fibrillation during general anesthesia. The ECG tracing shows a regularly irregular rhythm with a ventricular rate of 102 beats/min. The amplitudes of the pulse waves vary from beat to beat and are generally smaller after short R-R intervals (because of reduced ventricular filling). Note that not every QRS complex is associated with a distinct pulse wave; the pulse rate averages 72 pulse waves/min *(pulse deficit)*. Vigilant monitoring of the hemodynamic status is critical in this patient. **C,** Severe sinus arrhythmia and sinus arrest in a standing, nonsedated horse treated with the calcium channel antagonist diltiazem. High doses of diltiazem (>1 mg/kg intravenously) can cause hypotension (as a result of bradycardia and peripheral vasodilation) and severe SA node and/or AV node depression. The arterial pressure recording demonstrates the strong dependence of blood pressure on heart rate. An increase of the heart rate from 17 beats/min *(a)* to 60 beats/min *(b)* transiently increased blood pressure. A 10-second period of sinus arrest *(c)* caused arterial pressure to decrease dramatically, and the horse showed clinical signs of severe weakness. Intense reflex-mediated sympathetic activation increased the heart rate to 105 beats/min *(d)* and restored arterial blood pressures within a few seconds. This arrhythmia was considered clinically relevant and prompted immediate treatment with calcium gluconate, dobutamine, and intravenous fluids.

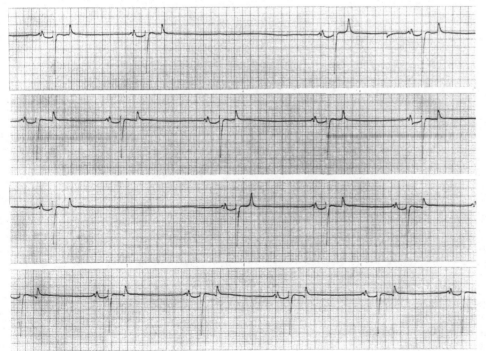

Figure 3–25. Sinus arrhythmia in an adult horse (paper speed 25 mm/sec, base-apex lead). The bottom trace was taken after administration of atropine.

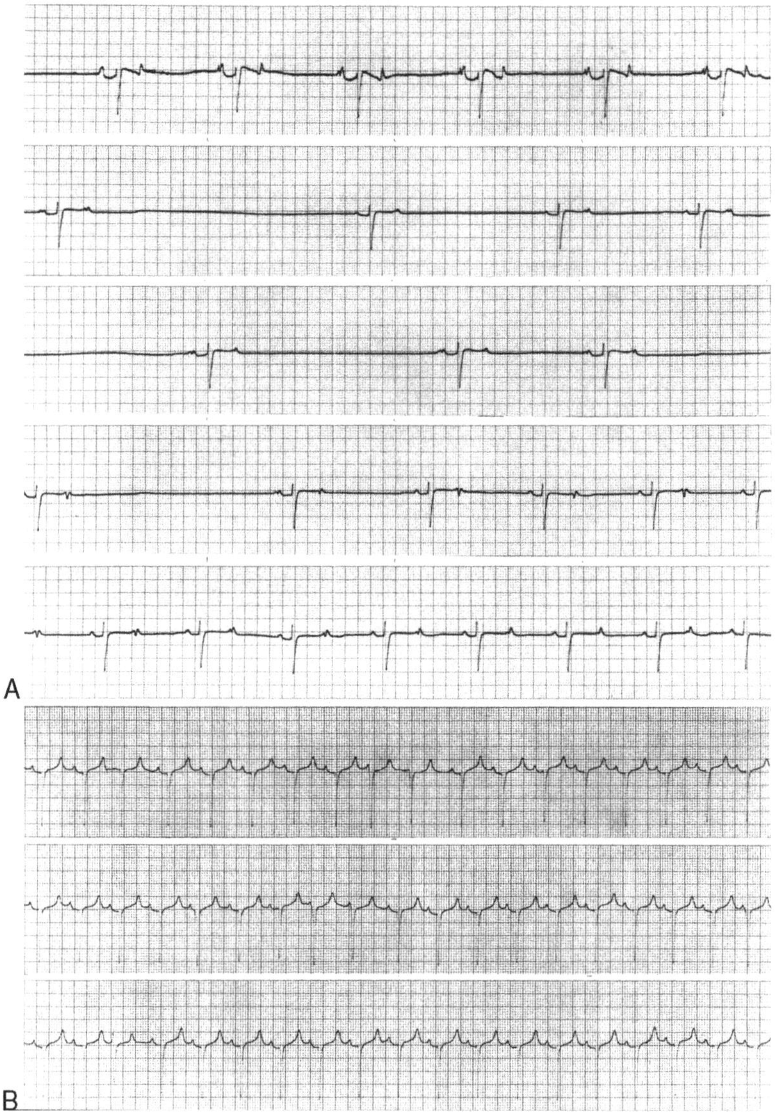

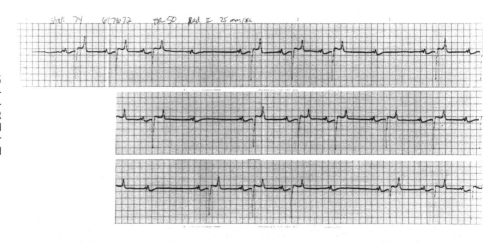

Figure 3–26. A, Base apex lead from an adult horse recorded before anesthesia, indicating normal sinus rhythm (top trace; 25 mm/sec). Pronounced sinus arrhythmia and sinus bradycardia occurred during general anesthesia (traces 2 and 3), which responded to atropine (last two traces) reestablishing normal sinus rhythm. **B,** Sinus tachycardia. Note the shortening of the P wave, PR, and QT intervals; the depression of the PR segment; and the elevation of the ST-T wave—all of which are physiologic changes observed with tachycardia.

Figure 3–27. Base apex lead ECG recorded from a 7-year-old Thoroughbred. Sinus arrhythmia and second-degree AV block are shown. The PR interval varies slightly in conducted complexes. Note the Ta wave after most blocked P waves (paper speed 25 mm/sec).

Figure 3-28). Anticholinergic drugs may not be effective in the setting of excessive direct anesthetic-induced depression of SA node function. Dopamine and dobutamine can be infused to increase heart rate and arterial blood pressure; however, the administration of intravenous epinephrine may be required in horses with severe bradycardia (see Chapters 22 and 23).[221] Excessive administration of catecholamines can cause sinus tachycardia, ectopic beats, and ventricular fibrillation. Epinephrine is reserved for acute and severe sinus arrest (see Chapter 23).

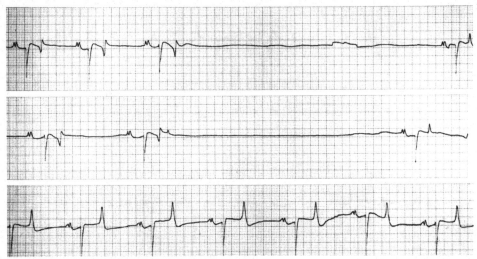

Figure 3–28. Sinus arrest (*top* and *middle* tracings) in a horse. Administration of atropine produces normal sinus rhythm (*bottom trace*).

Sinus tachycardia is common in nervous, excitable, or agitated horses and is associated with pain, hypotension, hypovolemia, hypercarbia, hypoxemia, anemia, endotoxemia, or excessive catecholamine administration in anesthetized horses. The underlying cause of sinus tachycardia must be sought and managed appropriately. The depth of anesthesia and the type and dose of all drugs administered should be evaluated continuously in the anesthetized horse and adjusted if necessary. Specific therapy for sinus tachycardia is rarely required because it represents a physiologic response to stress (see Chapters 4 and 23). It should be recognized that anesthetized horses are not as capable of increasing sinus rate in response to systemic hypotension as conscious horses because of the depressant effects of inhalant anesthetics on baroreceptor reflexes.[220] Increases in heart rate during anesthesia most frequently suggest increases in sympathetic tone caused by inadequate anesthesia, pain, hypotension, hypercarbia, or hypoxia.

Atrial arrhythmias. Cardiac arrhythmias originating in the atria are common in horses (see Box 3-9). Atrial arrhythmias may develop as functional disorders or can accompany structural lesions of the valves, myocardium, or pericardium. Atrial arrhythmias can develop in association with hypoxia, anemia, drugs (catecholamines, anesthetics), electrolyte disorders, cor pulmonale, fever, high sympathetic tone (accelerates ectopic foci), high vagal tone (favors reentry mechanism), or autonomic imbalance or from atrial muscle disease (dilation, fibrosis, inflammation, or ischemia). Mitral or tricuspid insufficiency, endocarditis, myocarditis, and cardiac (atrial) enlargement predispose to the development of atrial arrhythmias.

Single premature atrial depolarizations that arise within the atria but outside of the SA node are designated *atrial premature complexes*. The premature P (often referred to as P′) wave usually differs from the normal P wave in size and morphology. The P′ wave may be followed by a relatively normal QRS-T complex because the impulse uses normal conducting pathways in the AV node to activate the ventricles (Figure 3-29, *A* and *C*). Occasionally a P′ wave is not

conducted (blocked), especially if the atrial impulse occurs early in diastole and arrives at the AV node before it has completely repolarized (Figure 3-29, *B*). Premature atrial depolarizations can be delayed as they traverse the AV node (long PR interval; first-degree AV block) or conducted aberrantly through the ventricle as a result of lingering refractoriness of the AV or ventricular conducting tissues from the previous QRS-T complex. Abnormal (aberrant) ventricular conduction of an atrial premature complex causes the QRS-T complex to be wider than normal and atypical in configuration (see Figure 3-29, *A* and *C*). Occasional isolated atrial premature complexes are clinically inconsequential if they occur infrequently (e.g., less than one premature beat per minute). Frequent atrial premature complexes suggest excessive stress, inflammation, or structural cardiac disease and may precede the development of atrial flutter/fibrillation.

The ECG diagnosis of *sustained atrial arrhythmias* requires an ECG (Figure 3-30).[222-226] *Atrial tachycardia* is characterized by rapid and regular but abnormal atrial complexes typified by multiple, regular P′ waves that can be positive, negative, or diphasic in the base-apex lead, depending on the origin of the ectopic focus (see Figure 3-30, *A*). The atrial arrhythmia may show gradual onset ("warm-up") and offset when abnormal automaticity is the cause. *AV node–dependent supraventricular tachycardias* include reentrant tachycardias that are confined within the AV node or the AV junction or use the AV node as part of the reentrant pathway. This type of arrhythmia is typically paroxysmal and characterized by sudden onset and offset. Because of retrograde activation of the atria, the P′ waves can precede or follow the QRS complex and are sometimes hidden in the QRS-T complex. AV node–dependent supraventricular tachycardia is not very common in horses.

Atrial flutter causes regular "saw-toothed" cyclic variations of various magnitide in the isoelectric ECG (F waves; see Figure 3-30 *B*). AF is characterized by an absence of P waves and irregular, often prominent fibrillation F waves (see Figure 3-30, *C* and *D*; Figure 3-31, *A*).[227-230] The atrial flutter rate and activation process can vary in horses, producing a "coarse"

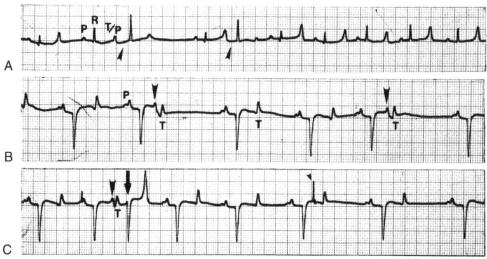

Figure 3–29. A, Lead II: the rhythm is sinus arrhythmia, and two atrial premature complexes are evident *(arrowheads)*. Premature P waves are superimposed on the T wave of the previous sinus complexes *(T/P)*. The atrial premature complexes are conducted with mild 1° AV block and with ventricular aberrancy as indicated by the varying morphology of the QRS complex. **B,** Two nonconducted atrial premature complexes *(arrowheads)* are buried in the ST segment of the previous sinus complex and are not conducted through the AV node (base-apex lead). **C,** A single atrial premature complex *(arrowhead)*; the associated QRS is nearly normal *(large arrow)*, although the T wave is different, indicating that the impulse was conducted with some aberration. A muscle twitch artifact *(small arrowhead)* is indicated and is not a premature complex (paper speed: 25 mm/sec). (From Bonagura JD, Miller MS: Electrocardiography. In Jones WJ, editor: *Equine sports medicine*, Philadelphia, 1989, Lea & Febiger.)

(flutter) and "fine" (fibrillation) baseline ECG. Occasionally the ECG shows alternating atrial flutter and fibrillatory activity, a rhythm also referred to as *atrial flutter/fibrillation*. Flutter-like activity is most frequently observed early after the onset of AF and generally progresses into fibrillatory activity with time, possibly indicating arrhythmia-induced changes in the electrical properties of the atrial tissue. Atrial flutter and AF are treated similarly in horses. Some horses develop paroxysmal (occurring suddenly, lasting from seconds to days, and ending spontaneously) AF, but most present with either a persistent (terminating only after treatment) or permanent (established and resistant to therapy) AF rhythm. The term *lone AF* refers to AF occurring in the absence of any detectable underlying cardiac disease, although there may well be some predisposing risk factors that cannot be easily detected by routine diagnostic measures. Recurrent episodes of AF are not uncommon and are more likely in the presence of concurrent structural or functional cardiac disease.

Atrial tachyarrhythmias generally produce variable AV conduction patterns; although periodicity of AV nodal conduction has been observed in horses with AF.[231,232] Some impulses are blocked and never enter the ventricles when the AV node is rapidly stimulated by atrial impulses. Consequently atrial tachyarrhythmias usually are characterized by atrial rates more rapid than ventricular rates. The ventricular response is usually irregular ("regularly irregular") in horses with AF because of the differential penetration through the AV node caused by varying AV nodal refractoriness (see Figures 3-30 and 3-31, A and B). This physiologic AV refractoriness is influenced by many factors, including but not limited to concealed (incomplete) conduction, vagal and sympathetic tone, and the atrial flutter/fibrillatory rate (see Figure 3-30, E). Drugs such as atropine

or quinidine reduce vagal tone and can enhance the ventricular rate.[163,231] Conversely digitalis, β-blockers (e.g., propranolol, atenolol), and the calcium-channel blocking drug (e.g., diltiazem) decrease the ventricular response to atrial tachyarrhythmias.[18,210,233] Injectable and inhalant anesthetics may predispose susceptible horses to both atrial and ventricular arrhythmias on the basis of their effects on autonomic nervous system activity and direct electrophysiologic effects to differentially alter or shorten cardiac muscle refractoriness.

Atrial arrhythmias are considered benign and inconsequential when atrial premature complexes are infrequent and their effects on arterial blood pressure are minimal.[234] Sustained atrial tachyarrhythmias are abnormal and indicate transient or progressive heart disease. Rapid or repetitive atrial arrhythmias that result in rapid ventricular rates are likely to reduce ventricular filling time, leading to a decrease in cardiac output that can result in a decrease in exercise tolerance, hypotension, syncope, or congestive heart failure. The ability of the horse to tolerate repetitive bouts of atrial arrhythmias such as atrial tachycardia, atrial flutter, or AF depends on preexistent ventricular function and the integrity of cardiovascular reflexes. The risk of anesthesia in horses with atrial arrhythmias is unknown and primarily depends on ventricular function. Isolated premature beats are not a contraindication for anesthesia but require vigilant ECG monitoring during the induction and maintenance of anesthesia. Frequent atrial premature complexes may be a harbinger of more serious atrial arrhythmias, although most horses with AF or atrial flutter and without underlying cardiac disease are hemodynamically stable at rest and during general anesthesia. Nevertheless, affected horses should be evaluated carefully, and treatment considered before anesthesia.[47,235]

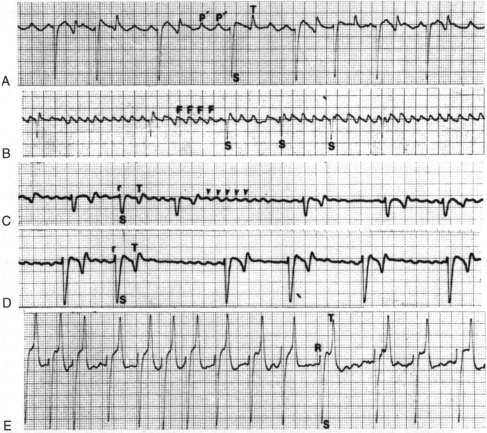

Figure 3–30. A, Atrial tachycardia in 12-year-old Quarter horse gelding. Atrial rate is approximately 215/min; ventricular response is 60/min (recorded at 25 mm/sec). Regular abnormal P waves *(P')* are evident throughout the strip, with many superimposed on the QRS and T complexes. Most of ectopic P waves are blocked in the AV node and are not conducted to the ventricles. **B,** Atrial flutter in 11-year-old Quarter Horse gelding. Atrial rate is approximately 307/min; ventricular response is 40 to 65/min. Atrial activity is characterized by saw-toothed flutter waves *(F)* occurring at a rapid rate and regular intervals. Flutter waves are blocked in the refractory AV node. **C** and **D,** Lead II **(C)** and base apex lead **(D)** ECGs from a 7-year-old female Thoroughbred with aortic regurgitation. Atrial fibrillation is evident, with coarse fibrillation waves *(small arrowheads)* noted throughout the trace. Atrial rhythm is irregular, chaotic, and quite rapid. The ventricular response is irregular, which is typical of atrial fibrillation. **E,** Atrial fibrillation with a rapid ventricular response in a 29-year-old Arab stallion with aortic and mitral regurgitation and congestive heart failure. The ventricular response is irregular and varies between 80 and 115/min. The QRS complexes are increased in amplitude, probably a result of left ventricular enlargement. The ST segment deviation may indicate subendocardial ischemia caused by the rapid heart rate (base-apex lead). (From Bonagura JD, Miller MS: Electrocardiography. In Jones WJ, editor: *Equine sports medicine,* Philadelphia, 1989, Lea & Febiger.)

Digoxin and quinidine are the drugs most commonly used in horses for controlling the ventricular rate (digoxin) and converting atrial tachyarrhythmias to normal sinus rhythm (quinidine).[163,223,230,235-241] Oral or intravenous quinidine is effective (efficacy 83% to 92%) for the treatment of AF, particularly when no other signs of heart failure are evident (Box 3-10).[163,223,235,239,241] However, quinidine has a narrow therapeutic window, and adverse effects may occur, even when plasma quinidine concentrations are within the therapeutic range (2 to 5 μg/ml). Common adverse effects include depression, inappetence, nasal edema, diarrhea, colic, a decrease in arterial blood pressure, and rapid supraventricular tachycardia caused by acceleration of the ventricular response rate (see Figure 3-31, A to C).[163,231] Quinidine may also exert proarrhythmic effects, leading to ventricular tachycardia or torsades de pointes (see Figure 3-31, D). The QRS may be prolonged after conversion of AF to sinus

rhythm (see Figure 3-31, E). A prolongation of the QRS duration of more than 25% compared to pretreatment values is considered a sign of quinidine toxicity (Figure 3-32, C and D). In rare cases paraphimosis, urticaria, convulsions, laminitis, and sudden death may occur. The development of laminitis associated with quinidine administration is more likely the result of drug overdose. Quinidine may worsen heart failure by transiently increasing the ventricular rate and reducing cardiac contractility. Some horses with AF are refractory to quinidine and do not convert to sinus rhythm.

Intravenous quinidine can be used to convert AF to normal sinus rhythm in anesthetized horses if the hemodynamic consequences of AF warrant immediate treatment (see Box 3-10).[47,241] Electrolyte abnormalities (particularly hypokalemia and hypomagnesemia) should be corrected. Suitable fluid volume replacement should be administered to maintain arterial blood pressure. Catecholamines may be required

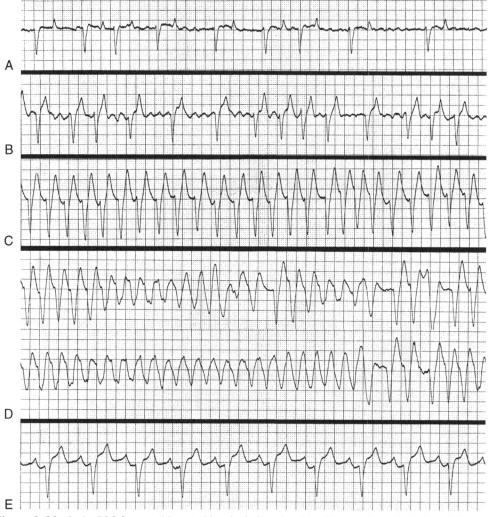

Figure 3–31. A, An ECG from an 11-year-old male draft mule with a history of exercise-induced dyspnea and collapse (base-apex, 25 mm/sec). The rhythm is atrial fibrillation with a ventricular response rate of 60 beats/min. **B,** After two doses of quinidine sulfate (22 mg/kg PO q2h), the ventricular response rate increased to 90 beats/min; and the atrial rhythm has a more regular, flutter-like appearance. The increase in T wave amplitude is likely related to the increase in heart rate. **C,** The ventricular rate increased to 156 beats/min after the sixth dose of quinidine sulfate. Orientation, morphology, and duration of the QRS complexes are similar to the previous recording. The changes in T wave morphology and QT interval are likely related to tachycardia. **D,** Five minutes after **C** the ECG shows transition to ventricular flutter with a rate of 186 beats/min. The rhythm has a torsade de pointes–like appearance, characterized by polymorphic ventricular complexes with undulation of the QRS axis. At this point immediate treatment with sodium bicarbonate, magnesium sulfate, and lactated Ringer's solution was initiated. **E,** Conversion to sinus rhythm 30 minutes later. The heart rate is still slightly elevated at 66 beats/min. All medications were discontinued. The mule was released from the clinic a few days later.

to maintain arterial blood pressure but should be administered cautiously since they may increase AV nodal conduction, leading to a rapid, irregular ventricular response and inadequate cardiac filling time. Antiarrhythmic therapy may be delayed to the postanesthetic period if the horse tolerates the arrhythmia (maintaining normal intraoperative hemodynamics).

Other pharmacologic and nonpharmacologic treatment options for AF in horses include amiodarone, flecainide, and procainamide and transvenous electrical cardioversion.[242-253] The efficacy and safety of these therapies have not been established in horses. Prognosis is guarded in

horses with AF or atrial tachyarrhythmias and underlying myocardial disease.[235,239]

Transvenous electrical cardioversion has been attempted as an effective alternative to quinidine therapy for the treatment of supraventricular arrhythmias and AF in horses, especially when quinidine is either ineffective or not well tolerated (Figure 3-33).[242-244] However, there is still limited experience with this new technique in horses, and adverse effects are possible (lung injury, hypotension, sudden death).[245] Furthermore, electrical cardioversion requires general anesthesia, special equipment, and expertise.

Box 3–10 Management of Atrial Fibrillation[194,303]

Preparation Before Treatment

Intravenous catheter for rapid venous access in case of an emergency

Nasogastric tube/transnasal feeding tube for quinidine administration

(Telemetric) ECG for continuous monitoring of heart rate, rhythm, and conduction times

Ensure adequate hydration and correct electrolyte and acid-base disturbances

Horse Without Heart Failure

Quinidine sulfate PO (by nasogastric tube):

22 mg/kg q2h until (1) conversion to sinus rhythm, (2) adverse or toxic effects occur, or (3) a total of 4 (to 6) doses have been administered

Plasma quinidine concentration should be measured if (1) conversion has not occurred 1 hour after the fourth dose, or (2) the patient exhibits adverse or toxic effects

Therapeutic concentration: 2-5 μg/ml, toxic concentration: >5 μg/ml

Treatment intervals should be increased to every 6 hours if:

(1) Plasma quinidine concentration is >4 μg/ml, or

(2) After the fourth dose if concentrations cannot be measured

Treatment every 6 hours can be continued, until:

(1) Conversion to sinus rhythm

(2) Adverse or toxic effects occur

(3) A total cumulative dose of 80 to 90 g is reached

Quinidine gluconate intravenously (IV):

During anesthesia: 1 to 2 mg/kg IV as a slow bolus, every 10 min to effect

Total dosages exceeding 8 mg/kg usually are not recommended; higher doses can result in adverse effects (hypotension, proarrhythmic effects)

Horse with Heart Failure

Cardioversion using quinidine is usually not attempted: stabilization of congestive heart failure and ventricular rate control. Treat with *furosemide* to control edema and *digoxin* to control heart rate and treat heart failure (see Table 3-10).

Monitoring

Monitor for response to treatment and adverse/toxic effects (see text)

Ensure adequate fluid intake during prolonged quinidine treatment

Monitor serum electrolytes and blood urea nitrogen/creatinine in horses with heart failure and during prolonged treatment with quinidine

Management of Quinidine-Induced Adverse and Toxic Effects

Accelerated ventricular response rate—may occur within therapeutic range:

If rate is <100 beats/min and horse is hemodynamically stable, continue treatment with close monitoring

If rate is persistently >100 beats/min, administer *digoxin* (0.0022 mg/kg IV; may repeat dose once)

If rate is sustained in excess of 150 beats/min and/or pressures are poor, administer *digoxin* and $NaHCO_3$ (1 mEq/kg IV)

Other options for rate control include *diltiazem* or *propranolol* (see Table 3-10; administer to effect, monitor ECG and direct blood pressures).

Prolongation of QRS (>25%): Indication of toxicity, discontinue quinidine

Severe hypotension: Administer *phenylephrine* (0.1-0.2 μg/kg/min to effect, up to 0.01 mg/kg total dosage)

Ventricular arrhythmia (ventricular tachycardia, torsades de pointes): Discontinue quinidine, administer *lidocaine* (0.25-0.5 mg/kg slow IV, repeat in 5-10 min, up to 1.5 mg/kg total dosage) and $MgSO_4$ (2-6 mg/kg/min IV to effect, up to a total dosage of 55-100 mg/kg)

Alternative Treatment Options

Procainamide: Potentially effective, may be used at a dose of 1 mg/kg/min IV to a maximum of 20 mg/kg when atrial fibrillation occurs during anesthesia; efficacy for conversion of AF unknown[194,253]

Transvenous biphasic electrical cardioversion: Transvenous catheter placement in standing, conscious horse; cardioversion under general anesthesia; may be used as first-line treatment or in horses with previous treatment failure or adverse/toxic effects to quinidine[243,244]

Junctional and ventricular arrhythmias. Cardiac arrhythmias that originate in or below the AV node are classified as junctional (AV node or bundle of His) or ventricular (ventricular conducting tissues or myocardium), respectively. Determining the exact origin of the abnormal impulse can be difficult but occasionally may be achieved by careful inspection of the QRS complex. *Junctional* impulses are more likely to result in a narrow, relatively normal-appearing QRS complex (Figure 3-34). Complexes that originate in the ventricles, by contrast, are conducted abnormally and more slowly, resulting in wide, morphologically abnormal QRS and abnormal T waves (Figures 3-35 and 3-36). Some junctional tachycardias may be conducted *aberrantly*, resulting in wide and morphologically bizarre QRS complexes. Junctional and ventricular ectopic rhythms may produce abnormal ventricular activation patterns that can be electri-cally destabilizing deteriorating ventricular flutter or fibrillation (see Figure 3-36, *E*).

The normal heart contains latent (subsidiary) cardiac pacemakers within the AV and ventricular specialized tissues. The activity of these potential pacemakers may become manifest during periods of sinus bradycardia (see previous paragraphs) or AV block (see following paragraphs), leading to *escape complexes* or *escape rhythms*. Escape rhythms are characterized by slow ventricular rates, often between 15 to 25 beats/min (see following paragraphs and Figure 3-34, *B*). Specific antiarrhythmic drug suppression of escape rhythms generally is not necessary and is contraindicated because these rhythms may serve as the only rescue mechanism for the initiation of ventricular contraction. Management of escape rhythms should be toward determination of the cause of sinus bradycardia or AV block.

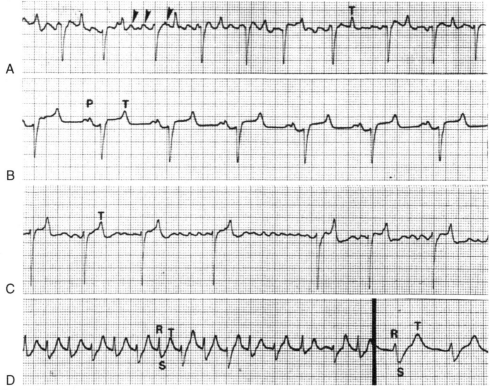

Figure 3–32. A, ECG from treatment of a 6-year-old Standardbred racehorse with sudden onset of poor performance (base-apex 25 mm/sec). The rhythm is atrial fibrillation with prominent fibrillation waves *(arrowheads)* and irregular ventricular response. **B,** The rhythm is converted to normal sinus rhythm 6 hours after administration of 40 g of quinidine sulfate. **C,** Atrial fibrillation in a 7-year-old working cattle horse. The irregular ventricular response averages about 55 beats/min. **D,** The horse remained in atrial fibrillation 10 hours after administration of 65 g of quinidine, but the ventricular response increased as a result of enhanced AV conduction. Evidence of quinidine toxicosis is manifested by widening of the QRS complex. No further quinidine was administered. (**C,** Base-apex lead; **D,** lead II ECG; both recorded at 25 mm/sec except for the lower right panel strip, recorded at 50 mm/sec paper speed.) (From Bonagura JD, Miller MS: Electrocardiography. In Jones WJ, editor: *Equine sports medicine,* Philadelphia, 1989, Lea & Febiger.)

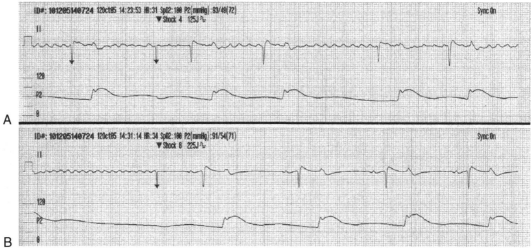

Figure 3–33. Transvenous electrical cardioversion for treatment of atrial fibrillation in a 2-year old Standardbred racehorse under general anesthesia. A surface ECG (25 mm/sec) and an arterial blood pressure tracing are displayed. The QRS complexes are automatically detected by the defibrillator unit and marked by small triangles. Biphasic electrical shocks (larger triangles on top) are applied at increasing energy levels. Delivery of the shocks is synchronized to the QRS complex to avoid the vulnerable period (T wave) and prevent induction of ventricular arrhythmias. **A,** Unsuccessful attempt at an energy level of 125 J. **B,** Successful cardioversion at an energy level of 225 J. The baseline ECG signal flattens immediately after the shock, and normal sinus rhythm resumes.

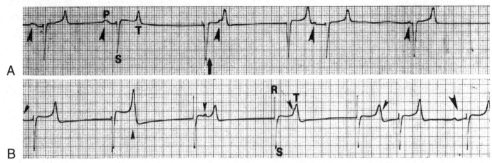

Figure 3–34. A, Junctional (or high-ventricular) rhythm (note the morphology of the ventricular activation process) in a horse under general anesthesia. Two sinus complexes are seen at the beginning of the trace. The third, fourth, and last QRS-T complexes are the result of an ectopic pacemaker *(large arrow)*. Underlying sinus arrhythmia and P waves are noted throughout the tracing *(arrowheads)*. Some P waves are nonconducted because the junctional focus depolarized AV tissues, rendering it refractory. The last QRS complex, although preceded by a P wave, is probably not a sinus-conducted impulse because the PQ interval is too short for normal AV transmission (base-apex lead recorded at 25 mm/sec). **B,** ECG from a horse anesthetized with xylazine, halothane, and oxygen. The first, sixth, and last QRS complexes are sinus and are preceded by a P wave *(arrowheads)*. A normal PQ interval *(large arrowhead)* is noted in the last complex. Two different ventricular waveforms are evident (second complex versus third, fourth, and fifth complexes). P waves are present throughout the tracing *(arrowheads)*, but are not transmitted across the AV junctional region because the tissues have been depolarized by the ectopic complex. (Base-apex ECG recorded at 25 mm/sec.) (From Bonagura JD, Miller MS: Electrocardiography. In Jones WJ, editor: *Equine sports medicine*, Philadelphia, 1989, Lea & Febiger.)

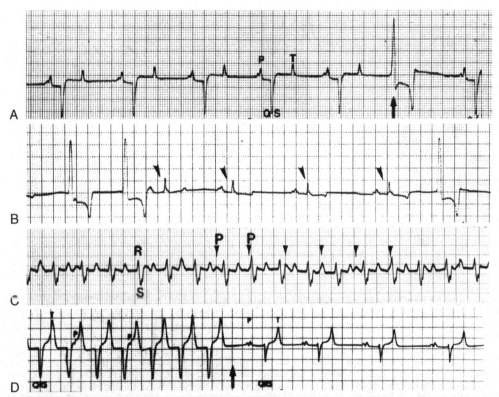

Figure 3–35. A, The ventricular ectopic complex *(arrow)* is wide and bizarre when compared with sinus-conducted impulses (base-apex ECG recorded at 25 mm/sec). **B,** Three ventricular ectopic complexes are evident. The QRS complex is much larger and wider than normal sinus complexes *(arrowheads;* lead II ECG recorded at 25 mm/sec.) **C,** Sustained ventricular tachycardia with a regular rate of about 120/min in an adult horse. QRS complexes are slightly widened, and there is AV dissociation, with an atrial rate of 96/min. P waves are indicated *(arrowheads;* lead II ECG recorded at 25 mm/sec.) **D,** There is a wide and bizarre QRS-T configuration, with dissociated P waves buried in QRS-T complexes at the left in a horse with ventricular tachycardia. Spontaneous conversion to normal sinus rhythm occurs *(arrow)*, resulting in the expected wave base-apex QRS morphology (recorded at 25 mm/sec). (ECG from The OSU Teaching Files courtesy of Dr. R. W. Hilwig.)

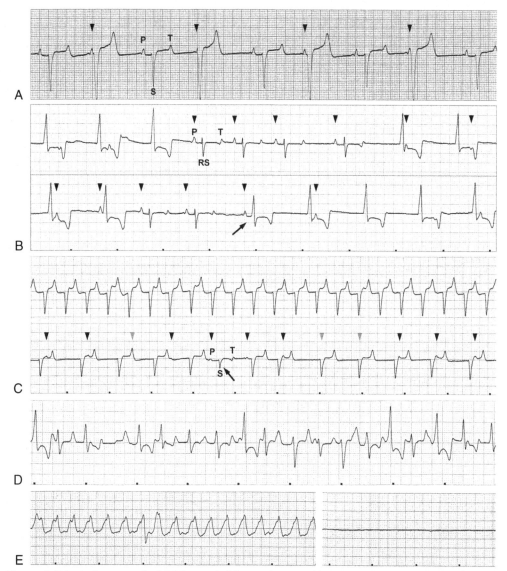

Figure 3–36. A, Base-apex lead ECG recorded from a 15-year-old Arab mare with ventricular bigeminy. Normal sinus beats alternate with slightly larger and wider ventricular ectopic beats. The SA node discharge is not affected by the ectopic beats, as indicated by the presence of nonconducted P waves immediately before the ectopic beats (*arrowheads*) (paper speed 25 mm/sec). **B,** Base-apex lead ECG recorded from an 18-year old Arab mare recovering from acute diarrhea and endotoxemia. The ECG shows an intermittent accelerated idioventricular rhythm at a rate of 50 beats/min. P wave intervals are indicated (*arrowheads*). The recording demonstrates that the ectopic focus is suppressed at higher rates of SA node discharge. The ventricular rhythm only becomes manifest when the SA rate drops below the rate of the ventricular pace-maker. SA node discharge is not affected by the ectopic rhythm, resulting in AV dissociation. A fusion beat is present (*arrow*), resulting from summation of a conducted sinus impulse with an ectopic ventricular beat (paper speed 25 mm/sec, voltage calibration 0.5 cm/mV). **C,** Base-apex lead ECG recorded from a 3-year old Clydesdale gelding with a regular tachycardia at a rate of 120 beats/ min. The appearance of the QRS-T complexes does not allow conclusive distinction between a supraventricular rhythm with rapid ventricular response and a ventricular rhythm. However, as the rate slows (bottom trace), AV dissociation caused by ventricular tachycardia becomes apparent. P waves (*arrowheads*) and a capture beat (*arrow*) are indicated (paper speed 25 mm/sec, voltage calibration 0.25 cm/mV). **D,** Base-apex ECG recorded from a 5-year old Clydesdale stallion with acute myocardial necrosis of unknown etiology. The serum cardiac troponin I con-centrations were elevated (404 ng/ml; normal <0.15 ng/ml). The ECG shows multiform ventricular tachy-cardia at a rate of 120 beats/min (paper speed 25 mm/sec, voltage calibration 0.5 cm/mV). **E,** Lead II ECG recorded from a 3-week old Danish Warmblood filly with botulism supported by mechanical ventilation. The rhythm *(left)* is consistent with ventricular flutter. Cardiac arrest occurred shortly thereafter *(right)* despite resuscitative attempts (paper speed 25 mm/sec).

Occasionally the normal subsidiary pacemakers may be enhanced and discharge at a rate that is equal to or slightly above the SA rate (usually between 60 and 80 beats/min). The resulting rhythm is commonly referred to as *accelerated idionodal* or *idioventricular rhythm* or *slow ventricular tachycardia* (see Figure 3-36, *B*). Conditions that favor the development of accelerated idioventricular rhythms include endotoxemia, autonomic imbalance, acid-base disturbances, and electrolyte abnormalities.[254] Some combinations of preanesthetic drugs such as xylazine and detomidine and anesthetic drugs (halothane) suppress SA function, potentially resulting in sinus bradycardia while enhancing the effects of catecholamines on latent junctional and ventricular pacemakers.[255] Idioventricular rhythms are often quite regular and can be misdiagnosed as sinus tachycardia during auscultation or palpation of peripheral pulses. Persistent, unexplained mild–to-moderate tachycardia should prompt an ECG evaluation to correctly determine cardiac rhythm. Most idioventricular rhythms generally are of little clinical (electrophysiologic and hemodynamic) significance and resolve spontaneously with appropriate treatment or resolution of the underlying disease. Electrolyte supplementation (potassium, magnesium) and correction of fluid deficits and acid-base disturbances may be beneficial. Lidocaine therapy is sometimes administered as an intraoperative adjunct to general anesthesia or as a prokinetic drug in the management of postoperative ileus (see Chapter 22).

Junctional and ventricular complexes that arise early relative to the next normal cardiac cycle are designated as *premature junctional or ventricular complexes* (see Figures 3-34, *A*, and 3-35, *A*). They are often associated with administration of drugs (i.e., catecholamines, digoxin, halothane), sympathetic stimulation, electrolyte disturbances (i.e., hypokalemia, hypomagnesemia), acid-base disorders, ischemia, or inflammation. Premature complexes may occur as *single* events, *couplets* (pairs), *triplets*, or short *runs*. A cardiac rhythm characterized by sinus beats followed at a fixed coupling interval by premature ventricular beats is referred to as *ventricular bigeminy* (see Figure 3-36, *A*). Repetitive ectopic complexes that occur in short bursts or runs are termed *nonsustained* or *paroxysmal ventricular tachycardias*. *Sustained junctional* and *ventricular tachycardias* may also occur (see Figures 3-35, *C* and *D*, and 3-36, *C*). Ventricular tachycardias are referred to as *uniform (monomorphic)* if the QRS-T morphology of the ectopic beats is consistent throughout the recording and as *multiform (polymorphic)* if two or more abnormal QRS-T configurations can be identified (see Figure 3-36, *D*). *Torsades de pointes* represent a specific form of polymorphic ventricular tachycardia characterized by progressive changes in QRS direction, leading to a steady undulation in the QRS axis. *Ventricular flutter* and *fibrillation* are characterized by a chaotic ventricular activation pattern, leading to uncoordinated undulations of the electrical baseline (Figure 3-36, *E*).

Ventricular premature complexes and junctional arrhythmias are usually considered abnormal in the horse, although isolated ventricular ectopic complexes may be more common than recognized from routine ECG studies.[127,256] The clinical significance of an occasional junctional or ventricular premature complex in the horse is difficult to ascertain. Persistent or repetitive junctional or ventricular rhythms are indicative of heart disease, systemic disease, or a drug-induced abnormality of cardiac rhythm. Ventricular tachycardia may be life threatening if the arrhythmia is rapid (e.g., above 180 beats/min), multiform (polymorphic, including torsades de pointes), or characterized by a short coupling interval and R-on-T phenomenon (R-on-T refers to premature complexes occurring on the peak of the preceding T wave). Ventricular tachycardia can progress into ventricular flutter or ventricular fibrillation, rhythms that commonly indicate terminal events (see Figure 3-36, *E*).

Accelerated idionodal or idioventricular rhythms and junctional or ventricular tachycardias usually cause interference with AV conduction of normal SA impulses while leaving atrial activation unaffected. The resulting (independent) coexistence of the SA activity (P wave) and the ectopic ventricular activity (QRS-T) is commonly referred to as *AV dissociation* (see Figures 3-34, *A* and *B*, 3-35, *C* and *D*, and 3-36, *B*). The P waves may appear to "march in and out" of the QRS complex when the independent atrial and ventricular pacemaker foci discharge at similar rates. This phenomenon is called *isorhythmic AV dissociation* and is occasionally observed in adult horses during inhalation anesthesia; it rarely requires therapy because the ventricular rate is maintained near normal values. It is important to note that escape rhythms associated with sinus bradycardia or complete AV block also cause AV dissociation (Figure 3-37, *C*). Thus *AV dissociation* is a purely descriptive term of an ECG finding and neither characterizes the type and pathophysiologic mechanism of the arrhythmia nor determines the therapeutic approach.

The identification of nonconducted P waves is common during sustained junctional or ventricular tachycardias (see Figure 3-36). Some P waves may be buried in the ectopic QRS-T complexes (especially during faster heart rates), making their identification difficult. The use of ECG calipers helps determine the P-P interval and can greatly facilitate the identification of P waves. Occasionally atrial impulses may be conducted normally, leading to capture beats or fusion beats. *Capture beats* are characterized by a normal P-QRS-T configuration, resulting from normal ventricular activation occurring before the ectopic focus discharges (see Figure 3-36, *C*). *Fusion beats* are seen when both the conducted impulse and an ectopic impulse cause simultaneous ventricular activation. The QRS-T morphology of a fusion beat represents the summation of a normal and an ectopic beat (see Figure 3-36, *B*).

The ECG should be monitored closely during induction and throughout the maintenance of anesthesia in horses with junctional or ventricular arrhythmias (see Chapter 8). Sedatives and anesthetic drugs should be chosen carefully to avoid administration of proarrhythmic drugs (e.g., halothane). Antiarrhythmic drugs should be available (see Table 3-10).[194,211,257] Junctional and ventricular arrhythmias that develop intraoperatively should be treated when premature complexes are frequent, multiform (polymorphic), or rapid (>100 to 120 beats/min); they show R-on-T characteristics; or there is evidence of hypotension. Lidocaine is commonly used as treatment for junctional or ventricular arrhythmias in horses. Lidocaine is usually well tolerated, but bolus doses should not exceed 2 mg/kg intravenously. Excessive doses of lidocaine can

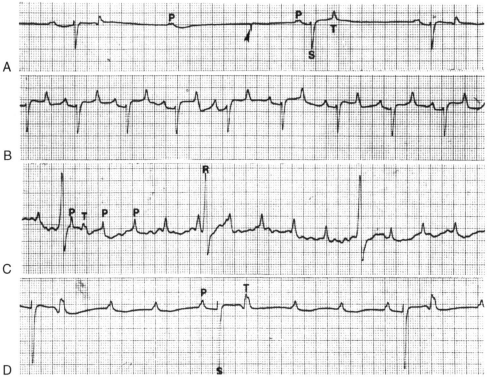

Figure 3–37. A, A single nonconducted P wave is evident (top trace; second-degree AV block. The PQ interval for conducted beats varies. A muscle twitch artifact *(arrowhead)* is also evident. **B,** The heart rate is 63/min after exercise, and sinus rhythm is regular with no evidence of AV block (base-apex lead ECG recorded at 25 mm/sec). **C,** Third-degree (complete) AV block in 3-year-old Quarter horse mare. Atrial rate is rapid (approximately 105/min); none of the P waves are conducted to the ventricles. The QRS complexes are wide and probably originate from the ventricular conduction system. **D,** The ECG suggests high-grade, second-degree AV block (>2 P consecutive waves are not conducted). The horse did not respond to intravenous atropine therapy. Thus the AV block may not be vagal induced but instead is caused by organic heart disease. The horse later reverted to third-degree AV block. (From Bonagura JD, Miller MS: Electrocardiography. In Jones WJ, editor: *Equine sports medicine*, Philadelphia, 1989, Lea & Febiger.)

produce neurotoxic side effects (disorientation, muscle fasciculations, and convulsions) or hypotension in anesthetized horses. Fluid therapy and especially maintenance of normal serum potassium concentration (4 to 5 mEq/L) are essential for antiarrhythmic therapy to be effective. Magnesium supplementation (e.g., 25 to 150 mg/kg/day intravenously, diluted in polyionic isotonic solution) may be beneficial. Therapeutic doses of magnesium are considered the treatment of choice for torsades de pointes (see Table 3-10). Procainamide or quinidine gluconate is potentially effective therapy for the treatment of ventricular tachyarrhythmias resistant to lidocaine and magnesium. Both drugs can cause hypotension and reduced myocardial contractility and must be administered cautiously. The risk-benefits of preoperative or intraoperative antiarrhythmic treatment should be considered carefully before initiating therapy.[120,122,194]

Prognosis is favorable for infrequent single ectopic ventricular complexes, particularly in the absence of other signs of cardiac disease. The prognosis for sustained junctional or ventricular tachycardia is usually guarded, especially when there is evidence of significant structural heart disease or congestive heart failure. The prognosis for multiform ventricular tachycardia or torsades de pointes is usually poor.

Conduction disturbances. The sequence of cardiac electric activation is usually dictated by the specialized conducting tissues in the atria, AV node, bundle of His, bundle branches, and the Purkinje network (see Figures 3-2 and 3-3). This conduction system permits orderly and sequential activation of the atria and ventricles, providing the stimulus for mechanical activation of the heart. A variety of electrical *conduction disorders* have been observed in horses, including SA nodal exit block, atrial standstill (usually caused by hyperkalemia), AV block, bundle branch block, and ill-defined ventricular conduction disturbances (see Figure 3-37; Figures 3-38 through 3-40).

SA block (SA nodal exit block) is considered physiological in horses and is associated with a high vagal tone. Sinoatrial exit block is often seen with sinus bradycardia and AV block. Electrocardiographically it is characterized by a normal sinus rhythm interrupted by occasional pauses without detectable P-QRS-T activity. The differentiation between sinus arrest and SA nodal exit block may be difficult based on a surface ECG and is clinically irrelevant in horses.

Delays in AV conduction are the most common conduction disorders in the horse. These are classified as first, second, and third degree (or complete). *First-degree AV block* produces prolongation of the PQ (PR) interval (see Table 3-9). The atrial impulse still transmits through the AV conduction

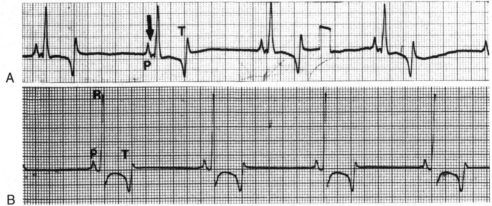

Figure 3–38. Lead II ECG (**A**) and base-apex ECG (**B**) obtained from a Standardbred stallion with ventricular preexcitation. Sinus rhythm, short PQ interval *(arrow)*, and initial abnormal activation of ventricle are evidenced by the small deflection in the PQ segment and a slurred upstroke of the QRS complex (delta wave). The base-apex lead shows abnormal ventricular conduction characterized by an atypical, positive waveform in this lead (which is normally negative). PQ interval is about 0.14 to 0.18 sec. (From Bonagura JD, Miller MS: Electrocardiography. In Jones WJ, editor: *Equine sports medicine*, Philadelphia, 1989, Lea & Febiger.)

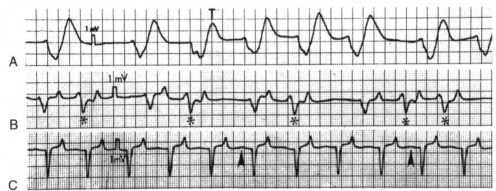

Figure 3–39. A, Hyperkalemia in a 14-day-old foal with a patent urachus produced atrial standstill, a ventricular conduction disturbance (wide QRS), and ST-T abnormalities. The serum potassium was 9.3 mmol/L, and sodium was 107 mmol/L. Traces **B** and **C** were obtained after intravenous fluids, sodium bicarbonate, and oxygen therapy. **B,** The ECG trace indicates improvement of ventricular conduction and possible appearance of coupled premature complexes (*). **C,** The bottom trace indicates normalization of ventricular conduction and suggests the reappearance of P waves *(arrowheads; base-apex lead; 25 mm/sec).* (From OSU Teaching Files courtesy Dr. R.W. Hilwig.)

system and activates the ventricle, causing a QRS complex. Some P waves are not conducted to the ventricles during *second-degree AV block,* resulting in occasional P waves not followed by a QRS-T complex (see Figure 3-27, *A*). Progressive prolongation of the PQ interval is classified as *Mobitz type I (Wenckebach)* second-degree AV block. The PQ (PR) interval may vary in duration in horses with second degree AV block (see Figure 3-27). A constant PQ interval preceding a blocked P wave is termed *Mobitz type II* second-degree AV block. Occurrence of two or more consecutive P waves not followed by a QRS complex in the presence of a normal or slow SA rate is called *high-grade (advanced) AV block* (see Figure 3-37, *D*).

First- and second-degree AV block are considered normal variations in the horse. These rhythms are most often associated with high vagal tone and are common in horses with sinus bradycardia and sinus arrhythmia during the recovery phase immediately after exercise or following the administration of α_2-agonists (e.g., xylazine, detomidine,

romifidine). Second-degree AV block can be eliminated by light exercise (spinning round, jogging, lunging, riding) or by administering vagolytic drugs (e.g., atropine, glycopyrrolate; see Figure 3-37, *A* and *B*). Persistent high-grade second-degree AV block may progress into complete AV block in some horses (see Figure 3-37, *C*). If second-degree AV block persists despite exercise or vagolytic drugs, structural AV node disease should be suspected (see Figure 3-37, *D*). *Third-degree* or *complete AV block* is characterized by complete dissociation of atrial and ventricular electrical activity. A junctional or ventricular escape rhythm must develop to prevent ventricular asystole,. The resulting ventricular activity (manifested by QRS complexes) is considerably slower than the atrial activity (manifested by P waves), and P waves are not related to QRS complexes (see Figure 3-37, *C*). Complete AV block usually indicates organic heart disease or severe drug toxicity.

Life-threatening AV block and other bradyarrhythmias occasionally occur in horses or foals with severe metabolic

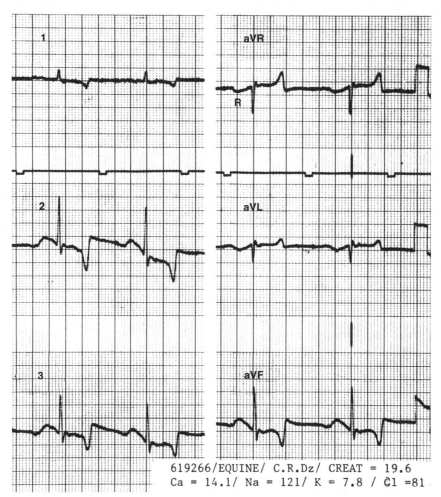

Figure 3–40. ECG from a horse with chronic renal disease and mild-to-moderate hyperkalemia (7.8 mmol/L). The P waves are abnormally wide, and there are ST-T segment changes characterized by deviation and increased amplitude of the T waves. (Leads recorded at 25 mm/sec.)

diseases. The development of second-degree or third-degree AV block during anesthesia suggests sensitivity to the direct depressant effects of anesthetic drugs. Initial treatment should include atropine or glycopyrrolate, particularly if hypotension develops (see Table 3-10). Dopamine or dobutamine may be required if the horse does not respond to anticholinergic therapy or develops significant hypotension (see Chapters 22 and 23).[258] Sudden development of complete AV block may require administration of epinephrine or the placement of a transvenous pacing wire into the right ventricle.[245,259] Persistent complete AV block in horses has been treated by implanting a permanent transvenous pacing catheter.[260-262]

Intraventricular conduction disturbances or *conduction blocks* are uncommon in horses, are difficult to diagnose, and produce widening of the QRS complex and abnormalities in the mean electrical axis.[263] They generally occur in horses with severe metabolic diseases that are poisoned or following accidental drug overdose.

Ventricular preexcitation or *accelerated AV conduction* can occur in horses.[264] Ventricular preexcitation in humans and dogs is caused by an anomalous atria-to-ventricular conducting pathway that bypasses the AV node, resulting in

early excitation of the ventricles and predisposing to reentrant supraventricular tachycardias. The ECG is characterized by an extremely short PQ interval, early excitation of the ventricle and slurring of the initial portion of the QRS complex (a delta wave), and an overall widening of the QRS complex (see Figure 3-38).

Hyperkalemia is a life-threatening disorder that can occur in foals with uroperitoneum and in adult horses with acute renal failure and oliguria, during shock, after severe strenuous exercise, following excessive intravenous potassium replacement, and in Quarter horses with hyperkalemic periodic paralysis. The cardiovascular manifestations of hyperkalemia include hypotension, depression of atrial, AV, and ventricular conduction and shortening of ventricular repolarization. ECG changes become evident when serum potassium concentrations are greater than 6 mEq/L and become severe when serum potassium concentrations are between 8 to 10 mEq/L.[17,265] Broadening and flattening of the P wave are the most consistently observed ECG changes (see Figures 3-39 and 3-40). The PQ interval prolongs, and bradycardia develops, eventually producing atrial standstill (sinoventricular rhythm) characterized by complete absence of P waves. The T waves may become inverted or increase in

Table 3–11. Hemodynamic effects of clinically relevant doses of drugs used to produce chemical restraint and anesthesia*

Drug	Rate of rhythm	Arterial blood pressure	Cardiac output	Cardiac contractility	Other Important effects
Tranquilizer/sedative					
Phenothiazine	↑	↓	—↑	—	α₁-Antagonist
α₂-Agonist	↓	↑—↓	↓	—	Vagal effects Respiratory depression
Opioid	—↑	—↑	—↑	—	Respiratory depression
Central muscle relaxants					
Benzodiazepines	—	—	—	—	
Guaifenesin	—	—↓	—↓	—	
Intravenous anesthetic					
Barbiturates	—↑↓	↓	↓	↓	Respiratory depression
Cyclohexylamines (ketamine, tiletamine)	↑	↑	↑↓	—↓	Respiratory depression, poor muscle relaxation
Inhalation anesthetics					
Halothane	—↓	↓	↓↓	↓↓	Sensitization to catecholamines
Sevoflurane	—↓	↓	↓	↓	Respiratory depression
Isoflurane	—↓	↓	↓	↓	Respiratory depression
Desflurane	—↓	↓	↓	—↓	Respiratory depression

*Effects observed when safe and effective anesthetic doses are used; ↑, increase; ↓, decrease; —, minimal change or no effect.

magnitude (tenting) as the QT interval shortens.[266] Marked widening of the QRS complex suggests near-lethal concentrations of potassium. Cardiac rhythm generally deteriorates to ventricular asystole or fibrillation if untreated.[17] Therapy for hyperkalemia includes correction of the underlying problem and administration of 0.9% NaCl, sodium bicarbonate, 23% calcium gluconate in 5% dextrose, and catecholamines. Regular insulin with dextrose may be added to the treatment if the previous measures are unsuccessful (see Table 3-10).

GENERAL EFFECTS OF ANESTHETIC DRUGS ON CARDIOVASCULAR FUNCTION

Sedative, tranquilizing, and anesthetic drugs exert profound effects on the cardiovascular system and cardiovascular function (see Chapters 10 to 13, 15, 18, and 19). These effects are generally but not invariably depressant to the electrical and mechanical activity of the heart and vascular system and the homeostatic mechanisms that regulate them (Table 3-11).[267] The cardiovascular effects of anesthetic drugs can be direct (i.e., the result of drug action on cardiac and vascular tissues) or indirect (i.e., mediated through changes in autonomic tone, endocrine function, or patterns of blood flow). Metabolic disturbances brought about by recumbency, hypoxia, hypercarbia, or acidosis may exacerbate anesthetic drug effects.[268] The cardiovascular effects

of most preanesthetic and anesthetic drugs on cardiovascular function, especially heart rate, cardiac output, arterial blood pressure, and gas exchange, have been evaluated in horses.[269-280] The effects of positioning, mechanical ventilation, and disease all contribute to tissue ischemia and hypoxia; and, when they are combined with the horse's temperament, anatomy, and size, they contribute to a greater potential for anesthetic-related morbidity and mortality than any other commonly anesthetized species.[281-287]

REFERENCES

1. Holmes JR: Sir Frederick Smith Memorial Lecture: a superb transport system—the circulation, *Equine Vet J* 14:267-276, 1982.
2. Guyton AC, Hall JE: Unit IV: The circulation. In Guyton AC, Hall JE, editors: *Textbook of medical physiology*, ed 11, Philadelphia, 2006, Elsevier Saunders, pp159-288.
3. Guyton AC, Hall JE: Unit III: The heart. In Guyton AC, Hall JE, editors: *Textbook of medical physiology*, ed 11, Philadelphia, 2006, Elsevier Saunders, pp. 101-157.
4. Opie LH: *Heart physiology: from cell to circulation*, ed 4, Philadelphia, 2004, Lippincott Williams & Wilkins.
5. Berne RM, Levy MN: *Cardiovascular physiology*, ed 8, St Louis, 2001, Mosby.
6. Schummer A et al: *The circulatory system, the skin, and the cutaneous organs of the domestic mammals*, Berlin, 1981, Verlag Paul Parey.
7. Dyce KM, Sack WO, Wensing CJG: The cardiovascular system. In Dyce KM, Sack WO, Wensing CJG, editors: *Textbook of veterinary anatomy*, ed 3, Philadelphia, 2002, Elsevier Saunders, pp 217-258.

8. Goldstein JA: Cardiac tamponade, constrictive pericarditis, and restrictive cardiomyopathy, *Curr Probl Cardiol* 29: 503-567, 2004.

9. Hamlin RL, Smith CR: Categorization of common domestic mammals based upon their ventricular activation process, *Ann N Y Acad Sci* 127:195-203, 1965.

10. Katz AM: *Physiology of the heart*, ed 3, Philadelphia, 2001, Lippincott Williams & Wilkins.

11. Spooner PM, Rosen MR: *Foundations of cardiac arrhythmias: basic concepts and clinical approaches*, New York, 2001, Marcel Dekker.

12. Task Force of the Working Group on Arrhythmias of the European Society of Cardiology: The Sicilian gambit: a new approach to the classification of antiarrhythmic drugs based on their actions on arrhythmogenic mechanisms. Task Force of the Working Group on Arrhythmias of the European Society of Cardiology, *Circulation* 84:1831-1851, 1991.

13. Kleber AG, Rudy Y: Basic mechanisms of cardiac impulse propagation and associated arrhythmias, *Physiol Rev* 84:431-488, 2004.

14. Roden DM: Cardiac membrane and action potentials. In Spooner PM, Rosen MR, editors: *Foundation of cardiac arrhythmias: basic concepts and clinical approaches*, New York, 2001, Marcel Dekker, pp 21-41.

15. Finley MR et al: Structural and functional basis for the long QT syndrome: relevance to veterinary patients, *J Vet Intern Med* 17:473-488, 2003.

16. Nerbonne JM, Kass RS: Molecular physiology of cardiac repolarization, *Physiol Rev* 85:1205-1253, 2005.

17. Glazier DB, Littledike ET, Evans RD: Electrocardiographic changes in induced hyperkalemia in ponies, *Am J Vet Res* 43:1934-1937, 1982.

18. Opie LH, Gersh BJ: *Drugs for the heart*, ed 6, Philadelphia, 2005, Saunders.

19. Finley MR et al: Expression and coassociation of ERG1, KCNQ1, and KCNE1 potassium channel proteins in horse heart, *Am J Physiol Heart Circ Physiol* 283:H126-H138, 2002.

20. Hamlin RL et al: Atrial activation paths and P waves in horses, *Am J Physiol* 219:306-313, 1970.

21. Yamaya Y, Kubo K, Amada A: Relationship between atrioventricular conduction and hemodynamics during atrial pacing in horses, *J Equine Sci* 8:35-38, 1997.

22. Yamaya Y et al: Intrinsic atrioventricular conductive function in horses with a second-degree atrioventricular block, *J Vet Med Sci* 59:149-151, 1997.

23. Smith CR, Hamlin RL, Crocker HD: Comparative electrocardiography, *Ann N Y Acad Sci* 127:155-169, 1965.

24. Hamlin RL et al: Autonomic control of heart rate in the horse, *Am J Physiol* 222:976-978, 1972.

25. Matsui K, Sugano S: Relation of intrinsic heart rate and autonomic nervous tone to resting heart rate in the young and the adult of various domestic animals, *Nippon Juigaku Zasshi* 51:29-34, 1989.

26. Bers DM: Cardiac excitation-contraction coupling, *Nature* 415:198-205, 2002.

27. Loughrey CM, Smith GL, MacEachern KE: Comparison of Ca^{2+} release and uptake characteristics of the sarcoplasmic reticulum in isolated horse and rabbit cardiomyocytes, *Am J Physiol Heart Circ Physiol* 287:H1149-H1159, 2004.

28. Bers DM: *Excitation-contraction coupling and cardiac contractile force*, ed 2, Dordrecht, 2001, Kluwer Academic Publishers.

29. Grubb TL et al: Hemodynamic effects of ionized calcium in horses anesthetized with halothane or isoflurane, *Am J Vet Res* 60:1430-1435, 1999.

30. Wiggers CJ: *Circulation in health and disease*, ed 2, Philadelphia, 1923, Lea & Febiger.

31. Welker FH, Muir WW: An investigation of the second heart sound in the normal horse, *Equine Vet J* 22:403-407, 1990.

32. Grossman W: Evaluation of systolic and diastolic function of the ventricles and myocardium. In Baim DS, editor: *Grossman's cardiac catheterization, angiography, and intervention*, ed 7, Philadelphia, 2006, Lippincott Williams & Wilkins, pp 315-332.

33. Opie LH, Perlroth MG: Ventricular function. In Opie LH, editor: *Heart physiology: from cell to circulation*, ed 4, Philadelphia, 2004, Lippincott Williams & Wilkins, pp 355-401.

34. Poole-Wilson PA, Opie LH: Digitalis, acute inotropes, and inotropic dilators: acute and chronic heart failure. In Opie LH, Gersh BJ, editors: *Drugs for the heart*, ed 6, Philadelphia, 2005, Elsevier Saunders, pp 149-183.

35. Nollet H et al: Use of right ventricular pressure increase rate to evaluate cardiac contractility in horses, *Am J Vet Res* 60:1508-1512, 1999.

36. Schertel ER: Assessment of left-ventricular function, *Thorac Cardiovasc Surg* 46(suppl)2:248-254, 1998.

37. Fuchs F, Smith SH: Calcium, cross-bridges, and the Frank-Starling relationship, *News Physiol Sci* 16:5-10, 2001.

38. Opie LH: Electricity out of control: arrhythmias. In Opie LH, editor: *The heart*, ed 4, Philadelphia, 2004, Lippincott Williams & Wilkins, pp 599-623.

39. Lang RM et al: Systemic vascular resistance: an unreliable index of left ventricular afterload, *Circulation* 74:1114-1123, 1986.

40. Nichols W et al: Input impedance of the systemic circulation in man, *Circ Res* 40:451-458, 1977.

41. Belenkie I, Smith ER, Tyberg JV: Ventricular interaction: from bench to bedside, *Ann Med* 33:236-241, 2001.

42. Santamore WP, Gray L: Significant left-ventricular contributions to right-ventricular systolic function—mechanism and clinical implications, *Chest* 107:1134-1145, 1995.

43. Grubb TL et al: Techniques for evaluation of right ventricular relaxation rate in horses and effects of inhalant anesthetics with and without intravenous administration of calcium gluconate, *Am J Vet Res* 60:872-879, 1999.

44. Pagel PS et al: Mechanical function of the left atrium: new insights based on analysis of pressure-volume relations and Doppler echocardiography, *Anesthesiology* 98:975-994, 2003.

45. Stefanadis C, Dernellis J, Toutouzas P: A clinical appraisal of left atrial function, *Eur Heart J* 22:22-36, 2001.

46. Hoit BD: Left atrial function in health and disease, *Eur Heart J* 2(suppl):K9-K16, 2000.

47. Muir WW, McGuirk SM: Hemodynamics before and after conversion of atrial fibrillation to normal sinus rhythm in horses, *J Am Vet Med Assoc* 184:965-970, 1984.

48. Constable P, Muir WW, Sisson D: Clinical assessment of left ventricular relaxation, *J Vet Intern Med* 13:5-13, 1999.

49. Parks C, Manohar M, Lundeen G: Regional myocardial blood flow and coronary vascular reserve in unanesthetized ponies during pacing-induced ventricular tachycardia, *J Surg Res* 35:119-131, 1983.

50. Reddy VK et al: Regional coronary blood flow in ponies, *Am J Vet Res* 37:1261-1265, 1976.

51. Hamlin RL, Levesque MJ, Kittleson MD: Intramyocardial pressure and distribution of coronary blood flow during systole and diastole in the horse, *Cardiovasc Res* 16:256-262, 1982.

52. Grossman W: Pressure measurement. In Baim DS, editor: *Grossman's cardiac catheterization, angiography, and intervention*, ed 7, Philadelphia, 2006, Lippincott Williams & Wilkins, pp 133-147

53. Grossman W: Blood flow measurement: cardiac output and vascular resistance. In Baim DS, editor: *Grossman's cardiac catheterization, angiography, and intervention*, ed 7, Philadelphia, 2006, Lippincott Williams & Wilkins, pp 148-162.

54. Milne DW, Muir WW, Skarda RT: Pulmonary arterial wedge pressures: blood gas tensions and pH in the resting horse, *Am J Vet Res* 36:1431-1434, 1975.
55. Hillidge CJ, Lees P: Studies of left ventricular isotonic function in conscious and anaesthetised horse, *Br Vet J* 133:446-453, 1977.
56. Ellis PM: The indirect measurement of arterial blood pressure in the horse, *Equine Vet J* 7:22-26, 1975.
57. Glen JB: Indirect blood pressure measurement in anesthetised animals, *Vet Rec* 87:349-354, 1970.
58. Kvart C: An ultrasonic method for indirect blood pressure measurement in the horse, *J Equine Med Surg* 3:16-23, 1979.
59. Muir WW, III, Wade A, Grospitch B: Automatic noninvasive sphygmomanometry in horses, *J Am Vet Med Assoc* 182:1230-1233, 1983.
60. Ostlund C, Pero RW, Olsson B: Reproducibility and the influence of age on interspecimen determinations of blood pressure in the horse, *Comp Biochem Physiol A* 74:11-20, 1983.
61. Parry BW, Anderson GA: Importance of uniform cuff application for equine blood pressure measurement, *Equine Vet J* 16:529-531, 1984.
62. Will JA, Bisgard GE: Cardiac catheterization of unanesthetized large domestic animals, *J Appl Physiol* 33:400-401, 1972.
63. Nout YS et al: Indirect oscillometric and direct blood pressure measurements in anesthetized and conscious neonatal foals, *J Vet Emerg Crit Care* 12:75-80, 2002.
64. Giguere S et al: Accuracy of indirect measurement of blood pressure in neonatal foals, *J Vet Intern Med* 19:571-576, 2005.
65. Franco RM et al: Study of arterial blood pressure in newborn foals using an electronic sphygmomanometer, *Equine Vet J* 18:475-478, 1986.
66. Fritsch R, Hausmann R: Indirect blood pressure determination in the horse with the Dinamap 1255 research monitor, *Tierarztl Prax* 16:373-376, 1988.
67. Parry BW et al: Correct occlusive bladder width for indirect blood pressure measurement in horses, *Am J Vet Res* 43:50-54, 1982.
68. Latshaw H et al: Indirect measurement of mean blood pressure in the normotensive and hypotensive horses, *Equine Vet J* 11:191-194, 1979.
69. Geddes LA et al: Indirect mean blood pressure in the anesthetized pony, *Am J Vet Res* 38:2055-2057, 1977.
70. Johnson JH, Garner HE, Hutcheson DP: Ultrasonic measurement of arterial blood pressure in conditioned Thoroughbreds, *Equine Vet J* 8:55-57, 1976.
71. Parry BW, Gay CC, McCarthy MA: Influence of head height on arterial blood pressure in standing horses, *Am J Vet Res* 41:1626-1631, 1980.
72. Brown CM, Holmes JR: Haemodynamics in the horse: 2. Intracardiac, pulmonary arterial, and aortic pressures, *Equine Vet J* 10:207-215, 1978.
73. Schwarzwald CC, Bonagura JD, Luis-Fuentes V: Effects of diltiazem on hemodynamic variables and ventricular function in healthy horses, *J Vet Intern Med* 19:703-711, 2005.
74. Manohar M, Bisgard GE, Bullard V: Blood flow in the hypertrophied right ventricular myocardium of unanesthetized ponies, *Am J Physiol* 240:H881-H888, 1981.
75. Brown CM, Holmes JR: Assessment of myocardial function in the horse. 2. Experimental findings in resting horses, *Equine Vet J* 11:248-255, 1979.
76. Muir WW, Bonagura JD: Cardiac performance in horses during intravenous and inhalation anesthesia, unpublished observations.
77. Rugh KS et al: Left ventricular function and haemodynamics in ponies during exercise and recovery, *Equine Vet J* 21:39-44, 1989.
78. Manohar M: Pulmonary artery wedge pressure increases with high-intensity exercise in horses, *Am J Vet Res* 54:142-146, 1993.
79. Thomas WP et al: Systemic and pulmonary haemodynamics in normal neonatal foals, *J Reprod Fertil Suppl* 35:623-628, 1987.
80. Bisgard GE, Orr JA, Will JA: Hypoxic pulmonary hypertension in the pony, *Am J Vet Res* 36:49-52, 1975.
81. Benamou AE, Marlin DJ, Lekeux P: Endothelin in the equine hypoxic pulmonary vasoconstrictive response to acute hypoxia, *Equine Vet J* 33:345-353, 2001.
82. Drummond WH et al: Pulmonary vascular reactivity of the newborn pony foal, *Equine Vet J* 21:181-185, 1989.
83. Dixon PM: Pulmonary artery pressures in normal horses and in horses affected with chronic obstructive pulmonary disease, *Equine Vet J* 10:195-198, 1978.
84. Littlejohn A, Bowles F: Studies on the physiopathology of chronic obstructive pulmonary disease in the horse. II. Right heart haemodynamics, *Onderstepoort J Vet Res* 47:187-192, 1980.
85. Rich S: Pulmonary hypertension. In Braunwald E, editor: *Heart disease*, ed 6, Philadelphia, 2001, Saunders, pp 1908-1935.
86. Sheridan V, Deegen E, Zeller R: Central venous pressure (CVP) measurements during halothane anaesthesia, *Vet Rec* 90:149-150, 1972.
87. Hall LW, Nigam JM: Measurement of central venous pressure in horses, *Vet Rec* 97:66-69, 1975.
88. Klein L, Sherman J: Effects of preanesthetic medication, anesthesia, and position of recumbency on central venous pressure in horses, *J Am Vet Med Assoc* 170:216-219, 1977.
89. Corley KT et al: Cardiac output technologies with special reference to the horse, *J Vet Intern Med* 17:262-272, 2003.
90. Muir WW, Skarda RT, Milne DW: Estimation of cardiac output in the horse by thermodilution techniques, *Am J Vet Res* 37:697-700, 1976.
91. Dunlop CI et al: Thermodilution estimation of cardiac output at high flows in anesthetized horses, *Am J Vet Res* 52:1893-1897, 1991.
92. Amend JF et al: Hemodynamic studies in conscious domestic ponies, *J Surg Res* 19:107-113, 1975.
93. Hillidge CJ, Lees P: Cardiac output in the conscious and anaesthetised horse, *Equine Vet J* 7:16-21, 1975.
94. Fisher EW, Dalton RG: Determination of cardiac output of cattle and horses by the injection method, *Br Vet J* 118:143-151, 1961.
95. Mizuno Y et al: Comparison of methods of cardiac output measurements determined by dye dilution, pulsed Doppler echocardiography, and thermodilution in horses, *J Vet Med Sci* 56:1-5, 1994.
96. Linton RA et al: Cardiac output measured by lithium dilution, thermodilution, and transesophageal Doppler echocardiography in anesthetized horses, *Am J Vet Res* 61:731-737, 2000.
97. Hallowell GD, Corley KTT: Use of lithium dilution and pulse contour analysis cardiac output determination in anaesthetized horses: a clinical evaluation, *Vet Anaesth Analg* 32:201-211, 2005.
98. Corley KT, Donaldson LL, Furr MO: Comparison of lithium dilution and thermodilution cardiac output measurements in anaesthetised neonatal foals, *Equine Vet J* 34:598-601, 2002.
99. Young LE et al: Measurement of cardiac output by transoesophageal Doppler echocardiography in anaesthetized horses: comparison with thermodilution, *Br J Anaesth* 77:773-780, 1996.
100. Young LE et al: Feasibility of transoesophageal echocardiography for evaluation of left ventricular performance in anaesthetised horses, *Equine Vet J* (suppl):63-70, 1995.

101. Blissitt KJ et al: Measurement of cardiac output in standing horses by Doppler echocardiography and thermodilution, *Equine Vet J* 29:18-25, 1997.

102. Giguere S et al: Cardiac output measurement by partial carbon dioxide rebreathing, 2-dimensional echocardiography, and lithium-dilution method in anesthetized neonatal foals, *J Vet Intern Med* 19:737-743, 2005.

103. Wilkins PA et al: Comparison of thermal dilution and electrical impedance dilution methods for measurement of cardiac output in standing and exercising horses, *Am J Vet Res* 66:878-884, 2005.

104. Orr JA et al: Cardiopulmonary measurements in nonanesthetized resting normal ponies, *Am J Vet Res* 36:1667-1670, 1975.

105. Muir WW, Wellman ML: Hemoglobin solutions and tissue oxygenation, *J Vet Intern Med* 17:127-135, 2003.

106. Birchard GF: Optimal hematocrit: theory, regulation, and implications, *Am Zool* 37:65-72, 1997.

107. Marino PL: Erythrocyte transfusions. In Marino PL, editor: *The ICU book*, ed 2, Philadelphia, 1998, Lippincott Williams & Wilkins, pp 691-708.

108. Muir WW: Small volume resuscitation using hypertonic saline, *Cornell Vet* 80:7-12, 1990.

109. Rudloff E, Kirby R: The critical need for colloids: administering colloids effectively, *Compend Contin Educ Pract Vet* 20:27-43, 1997.

110. Rudloff E, Kirby R: The critical need for colloids: selecting the right colloid, *Compend Contin Educ Pract Vet* 19:811-825, 1997.

111. Heesch CM: Reflexes that control cardiovascular function, *Am J Physiol* 277:S234-S243, 1999.

112. Wagner AE, Bednarski RM, Muir WW: Hemodynamic effects of carbon dioxide during intermittent positive-pressure ventilation in horses, *Am J Vet Res* 51:1922-1929, 1990.

113. Slinker BK et al: Arterial baroreflex control of heart rate in the horse, pig, and calf, *Am J Vet Res* 43:1926-1933, 1982.

114. Mellema M: Cardiac output, wedge pressure, and oxygen delivery, *Vet Clin North Am Small Anim Pract* 31:1175-1205, 2001.

115. Wetmore LA et al: Mixed venous oxygen tension as an estimate of cardiac output in anesthetized horses, *Am J Vet Res* 48:971-976, 1987.

116. Weber JM et al: Cardiac output and oxygen consumption in exercising Thoroughbred horses, *Am J Physiol* 253:R890-R895, 1987.

117. Marino PL: Respiratory gas transport. In Marino PL, editor: *The ICU book*, ed 2, Philadelphia, 1998, Lippincott Williams & Wilkins, pp 19-31.

118. Kumar A, Parrillo JE: Shock: classification, pathophysiology, and approach to management. In Parrillo JE, Dellinger RP, editors: *Critical care medicine: principles of diagnosis and management in the adult*, ed 2, St Louis, 2001, Mosby, pp 371-420.

119. Bonagura JD: Equine heart disease: an overview, *Vet Clin North Am Equine Pract* 1:267-274, 1985.

120. Bonagura JD, Reef VB: Disorders of the cardiovascular system. In Reed SM, Bayly WM, Sellon DC, editors: *Equine internal medicine*, ed 2, St Louis, 2003, Saunders, pp 355-459.

121. Gerring EL: Clinical examination of the equine heart, *Equine Vet J* 16:552-555, 1984.

122. Marr CM: *Cardiology of the horse*, London, 1999, Saunders.

123. Patteson M: *Equine cardiology*, Oxford, 1995, Blackwell Science.

124. Patteson MW, Cripps PJ: A survey of cardiac auscultatory findings in horses, *Equine Vet J* 25:409-415, 1993.

125. Kriz NG, Hodgson DR, Rose RJ: Prevalence and clinical importance of heart murmurs in racehorses, *J Am Vet Med Assoc* 216:1441-1445, 2000.

126. Young LE, Wood JL: Effect of age and training on murmurs of atrioventricular valvular regurgitation in young Thoroughbreds, *Equine Vet J* 32:195-199, 2000.

127. Ryan N, Marr CM, McGladdery AJ: Survey of cardiac arrhythmias during submaximal and maximal exercise in Thoroughbred racehorses, *Equine Vet J* 37:265-268, 2005.

128. Patteson M, Blissitt K: Evaluation of cardiac murmurs in horses 1. Clinical examination, *In Pract* 18:367-373, 1996.

129. Brown CM: Acquired cardiovascular disease, *Vet Clin North Am Equine Pract* 1:371-382, 1985.

130. Patterson DF, Detweiler DK, Glendenning SA: Heart sounds and murmurs of the normal horse, *Ann N Y Acad Sci* 127:242-305, 1965.

131. Smetzer DL, Hamlin RL, Smith CR: Cardiovascular sounds. In Swenson MJ, editor: *Dukes' physiology of domestic animals*, ed 8, Ithaca, 1970, Comstock Publishing, pp 159-168.

132. Smith CR, Smetzer DL, Hamlin RL: Normal heart sounds and heart murmurs in the horse. In Proceedings of the Eighth Annual American Association of Equine Practitioners Convention, Chicago, 1962, pp 49-64.

133. Reef VB: The significance of cardiac auscultatory findings in horses: insight into the age-old dilemma, *Equine Vet J* 25:393-394, 1993.

134. Reef VB: Heart murmurs in horses: determining their significance with echocardiography, *Equine Vet J* (suppl):71-80, 1995.

135. Machida N, Yasuda J, Too K: Auscultatory and phonocardiographic studies on the cardiovascular system of the newborn Thoroughbred foal, *Jpn J Vet Res* 35:235-250, 1987.

136. Machida N et al: A morphological study on the obliteration processes of the ductus arteriosus in the horse, *Equine Vet J* 20:249-254, 1988.

137. Rossdale PD: Clinical studies on the newborn Thoroughbred foal. II. Heart rate, auscultation and electrocardiogram, *Br Vet J* 123:521-532, 1967.

138. Carlsten J, Kvart C, Jeffcott LB: Method of selective and nonselective angiocardiography for the horse, *Equine Vet J* 16:47-52, 1984.

139. Carlsten J: Imaging of the equine heart: an angiocardiographic and echocardiographic investigation, Thesis, University of Agricultural Sciences, Uppsala, Sweden, 1986.

140. Koblik PD, Hornof WJ: Diagnostic radiology and nuclear cardiology: their use in assessment of equine cardiovascular disease, *Vet Clin North Am Equine Pract* 1:289-309, 1985.

141. Detweiler DK: Electrocardiogram of the horse, *Fed Proc* 11:34, 1952.

142. Fregin GF: The equine electrocardiogram with standardized body and limb positions, *Cornell Vet* 72:304-324, 1982.

143. Hamlin RL et al: P wave in the electrocardiogram of the horse, *Am J Vet Res* 31:1027-1031, 1970.

144. Landgren S, Rutqvist L: Electrocardiogram of normal cold blooded horses after work, *Nord Vet Med* 5:905-914, 1953.

145. Lannek N, Rutqvist L: Normal area of variation for the electrocardiogram of horses, *Nord Vet Med* 3:1094-1117, 1951.

146. White NA, Rhode EA: Correlation of electrocardiographic findings to clinical disease in the horse, *J Am Vet Med Assoc* 164:46-56, 1974.

147. Senta T, Smetzer DL, Smith CR: Effects of exercise on certain electrocardiographic parameters and cardiac arrhythmias in the horse: a radiotelemetric study, *Cornell Vet* 60:552-569, 1970.

148. Fregin GF: Electrocardiography, *Vet Clin North Am Equine Pract* 1:419-432, 1985.

149. Illera JC, Hamlin RL, Illera M: Unipolar thoracic electrocardiograms in which P waves of relative uniformity occur in male horses, *Am J Vet Res* 48:1697-1699, 1987.

150. Illera JC, Illera M, Hamlin RL: Unipolar thoracic electrocardiography that induces QRS complexes of relative uniformity from male horses, *Am J Vet Res* 48:1700-1702, 1987.

151. Tovar P, Escabias MI, Santisteban R: Evolution of the ECG from Spanish-bred foals during the post natal stage, *Res Vet Sci* 46:358-362, 1989.

152. Ayala I et al: Morphology and amplitude values of the P and T waves in the electrocardiograms of Spanish-bred horses of different ages, *J Vet Med Assoc* 46:225-230, 1999.

153. Miller PJ, Holmes JR: Interrelationship of some electrocardiogram amplitudes, time intervals, and respiration in the horse, *Res Vet Sci* 36:370-374, 1984.

154. Deegen E, Reinhard HJ: Electrocardiographic time patterns in the healthy Shetland pony, *Dtsch Tierarztl Wochenschr* 81:257-262, 1974.

155. Hamlin RL, Smetzer DL, Smith CR: Analysis of QRS complex recorded through a semiorthogonal lead system in the horse, *Am J Physiol* 207:325-333, 1964.

156. Grauerholz H, Jaeschke G: Problems of measuring and interpreting the QRS duration in the ECG of the horse, *Berl Munch Tierarztl Wochenschr* 99:365-369, 1986.

157. Holmes JR, Rezakhani A: Observations on the T wave of the equine electrocardiogram, *Equine Vet J* 7:55-62, 1975.

158. Persson SGB, Forssberg P. Exercise tolerance in Standardbred trotters with T-wave abnormalities in the electrocardiogram. In Proceedings of the Second International Conference on Equine Exercise Physiology, San Diego, 1986, pp 772-780.

159. Davey P: How to correct the QT interval for the effects of heart rate in clinical studies, *J Pharmacol Toxicol Methods* 48:3-9, 2002.

160. Funck-Brentano C, Jaillon P: Rate-corrected QT interval: techniques and limitations, *Am J Cardiol* 72:17B-22B, 1993.

161. Buss DD, Rwalings CA, Bisgard GE: The normal electrocardiogram of the domestic pony, *J Electrocardiol* 8:167-172, 1975.

162. Boyle NG, Weiss JN: Making QT correction simple is complicated, *J Cardiovasc Electrophysiol* 12:421-423, 2001.

163. Reef VB, Reimer JM, Spencer PA: Treatment of atrial fibrillation in horses: new perspectives, *J Vet Intern Med* 9:57-67, 1995.

164. Ritsema van Eck HJ, Kors JA, van Herpen G: The U wave in the electrocardiogram: a solution for a 100-year-old riddle, *Cardiovasc Res* 67:256-262, 2005.

165. Young LE et al: Haemodynamic effects of a sixty minute infusion of dopamine hydrochloride in horses anaesthetised with halothane, *Equine Vet J* 30:310-316, 1998.

166. Young LE et al: Temporal effects of an infusion of dopexamine hydrochloride in horses anesthetized with halothane, *Am J Vet Res* 58:516-523, 1997.

167. Boon JA: *Manual of veterinary echocardiography*, Baltimore, 1998, Williams & Wilkins.

168. Reef VB: Cardiovascular ultrasonography. In Reef VB, editor: Equine diagnostic ultrasound, Philadelphia, 1998, Saunders, pp 215-272.

169. Bonagura JD, Blissitt KJ: Echocardiography, *Equine Vet J* 19(suppl):5-17, 1995.

170. Otto CM: *Textbook of clinical echocardiography*, ed 3, Philadelphia, 2004, Elsevier Saunders.

171. Blissitt KJ, Bonagura JD: Colour flow Doppler echocardiography in horses with cardiac murmurs, *Equine Vet J* 19(suppl): 82-85, 1995.

172. Long KJ, Bonagura JD, Darke PG: Standardised imaging technique for guided M-mode and Doppler echocardiography in the horse, *Equine Vet J* 24:226-235, 1992.

173. Bonagura JD, Pipers FS: Diagnosis of cardiac lesions by contrast echocardiography, *J Am Vet Med Assoc* 182:396-402, 1983.

174. O'Callaghan MW: Comparison of echocardiographic and autopsy measurements of cardiac dimensions in the horse, *Equine Vet J* 17:361-368, 1985.

175. Bonagura JD, Herring DS, Welker F: Echocardiography, *Vet Clin North Am Equine Pract* 1:311-333, 1985.

176. Paddleford RR, Harvey RC: Anesthesia for selected diseases: cardiovascular dysfunction. In Thurmon JC, Tranquilli WJ, Benson GJ, editors: *Lumb and Jones' veterinary anesthesia*, ed 3, Baltimore, 1996, Williams & Wilkins, pp 766-771.

177. Stoelting RK, Dierdorf SF: *Anesthesia and co-existing disease*, ed 4, New York, 2002, Churchill Livingstone.

178. Miller PJ, Holmes JR: Observations on seven cases of mitral insufficiency in the horse, *Equine Vet J* 17:181-190, 1985.

179. Reef VB, Bain FT, Spencer PA: Severe mitral regurgitation in horses: clinical, echocardiographic, and pathological findings, *Equine Vet J* 30:18-27, 1998.

180. Reef VB, Spencer P: Echocardiographic evaluation of equine aortic insufficiency, *Am J Vet Res* 48:904-909, 1987.

181. Maxson AD, Reef VB: Bacterial endocarditis in horses: ten cases (1984-1995), *Equine Vet J* 29:394-399, 1997.

182. Buergelt CD et al: Endocarditis in six horses, *Vet Pathol* 22:333-337, 1985.

183. Holmes JR, Miller PJ: Three cases of ruptured mitral valve chordae in the horse, *Equine Vet J* 16:125-135, 1984.

184. Marr CM et al: Confirmation by Doppler echocardiography of valvular regurgitation in a horse with a ruptured chorda tendinea of the mitral valve, *Vet Rec* 127:376-379, 1990.

185. Reef VB: Mitral valvular insufficiency associated with ruptured chordae tendineae in three foals, *J Am Vet Med Assoc* 191:329-331, 1987.

186. Schober KE, Kaufhold J, Kipar A: Mitral valve dysplasia in a foal, *Equine Vet J* 32:170-173, 2000.

187. McGurrin MK, Physick-Sheard PW, Southorn E: Parachute left atrioventricular valve causing stenosis and regurgitation in a Thoroughbred foal, *J Vet Intern Med* 17:579-582, 2003.

188. Worth LT, Reef VB: Pericarditis in horses: 18 cases (1986-1995), *J Am Vet Med Assoc* 212:248-253, 1998.

189. Hardy J, Robertson JT, Reed SM: Constrictive pericarditis in a mare: attempted treatment by partial pericardiectomy, *Equine Vet J* 24:151-154, 1992.

190. Freestone JF et al: Idiopathic effusive pericarditis with tamponade in the horse, *Equine Vet J* 19:38-42, 1987.

191. Bernard W et al: Pericarditis in horses: six cases (1982-1986), *J Am Vet Med Assoc* 196:468-471, 1990.

192. Wagner PC et al: Constrictive pericarditis in the horse, *J Equine Med Surg* 1:242-247, 1977.

193. Buergelt CD, Wilson JH, Lombard CW: Pericarditis in horses, *Compend Contin Educ Pract Vet* 12:872-877, 1990.

194. Reef VB: Cardiovascular system. In Orsini JA, Divers TJ, editors: *Manual of equine emergencies: treatment and procedures*, ed 2, Philadelphia, 2003, Saunders, pp 130-188.

195. Bonagura JD, Reef VB: Cardiovascular diseases. In Reed SM, Bayly WM, editors: *Equine internal medicine*, Philadelphia, 1998, Saunders, pp 290-370.

196. Oh JK, Seward JB, Tajik AJ: Pulmonary hypertension. In Oh JK, Seward JB, Tajik AJ, editors: *The echo manual*, Philadelphia, 1999, Lippincott Williams & Wilkins, pp 215-222.

197. Spörri H, Schlatter C: Blutdruckerhöhungen im Lungenkreislauf, *Schweiz Arch Tierheilkd* 101:525-541, 1959.

198. Davis JL et al: Congestive heart failure in horses: 14 cases (1984-2001), *J Am Vet Med Assoc* 220:1512-1515, 2002.

199. Schwarzwald CC et al: Cor pulmonale in a horse with granulomatous pneumonia, *Equine Vet Educ* 18:182-187, 2006.

200. Atkins CE: The role of noncardiac disease in the development and precipitation of heart failure, *Vet Clin North Am Small Anim Pract* 21:1035-1080, 1991.

201. Rhodes J: Comparative physiology of hypoxic pulmonary hypertension: historical clues from brisket disease, *J Appl Physiol* 98:1092-1100, 2005.

202. Dixon PM et al: Chronic obstructive pulmonary disease anatomical cardiac studies, *Equine Vet J* 14:80-82, 1982.

203. Else RW, Holmes JR: Cardiac pathology in the horse. 2. Microscopic pathology, *Equine Vet J* 4:57-62, 1972.

204. Else RW, Holmes JR: Cardiac pathology in the horse. 1. Gross pathology, *Equine Vet J* 4:1-8, 1972.

205. Dyer GSM, Fifer MA: Heart failure. In Lilly LS, editor: *Pathophysiology of heart disease*, ed 3, Philadelphia, 2003, Lippincott Williams & Wilkins, pp 211-236.

206. Colucci WS, Braunwald E: Pathophysiology of heart failure. In Zipes DP et al, editors: *Braunwald's heart disease: a textbook of cardiovascular medicine*, ed 7, Philadelphia, 2005, Saunders, pp 509-538.

207. Marr CM: Heart failure. In Marr CM, editor: *Cardiology of the horse*, London, 1999, Saunders, pp 289-311.

208. Bertone JJ: Cardiovascular effects of hydralazine HCl administration in horses, *Am J Vet Res* 49:618-621, 1988.

209. Manohar M, Goetz TE: Pulmonary vascular pressures of strenuously exercising Thoroughbreds during intravenous infusion of nitroglycerin, *Am J Vet Res* 60:1436-1440, 1999.

210. Brumbaugh GW, Thomas WP, Hodge TG: Medical management of congestive heart failure in a horse, *J Am Vet Med Assoc* 180:878-883, 1982.

211. Muir WW, McGuirk SM: Pharmacology and pharmacokinetics of drugs used to treat cardiac disease in horses, *Vet Clin North Am Equine Pract* 1:335-352, 1985.

212. Staudacher G: Individual glycoside treatment by means of serum concentration determination in cardiac insufficiency in horses, *Berl Munch Tierarztl Wochenschr* 102:1-3, 1989.

213. De Luna R et al: ACE-inhibitors in the horse: renin-angiotensin-aldosterone system evaluation after administration or ramipril (preliminary studies), *Acta Med Vet* 41:41-50, 1995.

214. Guglielmini C et al: Use of an ACE inhibitor (ramipril) in a horse with congestive heart failure, *Equine Vet Educ* 14:297-306, 2002.

215. Gehlen H, Vieht JC, Stadler P: Effects of the ACE inhibitor quinapril on echocardiographic variables in horses with mitral valve insufficiency, *J Vet Med Assoc* 50:460-465, 2003.

216. Gardner SY et al: Characterization of the pharmacokinetic and pharmacodynamic properties of the angiotensin-converting enzyme inhibitor, enalapril, in horses, *J Vet Intern Med* 18:231-237, 2004.

217. Muir WW et al: Effects of enalaprilat on cardiorespiratory, hemodynamic, and hematologic variables in exercising horses, *Am J Vet Res* 62:1008-1013, 2001.

218. Nattel S: New ideas about atrial fibrillation 50 years on, *Nature* 415:219-226, 2002.

219. Hilwig RW: Cardiac arrhythmias in the horse, *J Am Vet Med Assoc* 170:153-163, 1977.

220. Hellyer PW et al: Effects of halothane and isoflurane of baroreflex sensitivity in horses, *Am J Vet Res* 50:2127-2134, 1989.

221. Trim CM, Moore JN, White NA: Cardiopulmonary effects of dopamine hydrochloride in anaesthetised horses, *Equine Vet J* 17:41-44, 1985.

222. Amada A, Kiryu K: Atrial fibrillation in the race horse, *Heart Vessels* 2(suppl):2-6, 1987.

223. Deem DA, Fregin GF: Atrial fibrillation in horses: a review of 106 clinical cases, with consideration of prevalence, clinical signs, and prognosis, *J Am Vet Med Assoc* 180:261-265, 1982.

224. Detweiler DK: Auricular fibrillation in horses, *J Am Vet Med Assoc* 126:47-50, 1955.

225. Glazier DB, Nicholson JA, Kelly WR: Atrial fibrillation in the horse, *Irish Vet J* 13:47-55, 1959.

226. Bonagura JD, Miller MS: Electrocardiography. In Jones WE, editor: *Equine sports medicine*, Philadelphia, 1985, Lea & Febiger, pp 89-106.

227. Holmes JR, Darke PGG, Else RW: Atrial fibrillation in the horse, *Equine Vet J* 1:212-222, 1969.

228. Holmes JR et al: Paroxysmal atrial fibrillation in racehorses, *Equine Vet J* 18:37-42, 1986.

229. Bentz BG, Erkert RS, Blaik MA: Evaluation of atrial fibrillation in horses, *Compend Contin Educ Pract Vet* 24:734-738, 2002.

230. Blissitt KJ: Diagnosis and treatment of atrial fibrillation, *Equine Vet Educ* 11:11-19, 1999.

231. Gelzer ARM et al: Temporal organization of atrial activity and irregular ventricular rhythm during spontaneous atrial fibrillation: an in vivo study in the horse, *J Cardiovasc Electrophysiol* 11:773-784, 2000.

232. Meijler FL et al: Nonrandom ventricular rhythm in horses with atrial fibrillation and its significance for patients, *J Am Coll Cardiol* 4:316-323, 1984.

233. Schwarzwald CC et al: Atrial, SA nodal, and AV nodal electrophysiology in standing horses: reference values and electrophysiologic effects of quinidine and diltiazem. In the 24th Annual Forum of the ACVIM, Louisville, Ky, 2006.

234. Miller PJ, Holmes JR: Effect of cardiac arrhythmia on left ventricular and aortic blood pressure parameters in the horse, *Res Vet Sci* 35:190-199, 1983.

235. Morris DD, Fregin GF: Atrial fibrillation in horses: factors associated with response to quinidine sulfate in 77 clinical cases, *Cornell Vet* 72:339-349, 1982.

236. Glendinning SA: The use of quinidine sulphate for the treatment of atrial fibrillation in twelve horses, *Vet Rec* 77:951-960, 1965.

237. Guthrie AJ et al: Sustained supraventricular tachycardia in a horse, *J S Afr Vet Assoc* 60:46-47, 1989.

238. McGuirk SM, Muir WW, Sams RA: Pharmacokinetic analysis of intravenously and orally administered quinidine in horses, *Am J Vet Res* 42:938-942, 1981.

239. Reef VB, Levitan CW, Spencer PA: Factors affecting prognosis and conversion in equine atrial fibrillation, *J Vet Intern Med* 2:1-6, 1988.

240. Bentz BG, Erkert RS, Blaik MA: Atrial fibrillation in horses: treatment and prognosis, *Compend Contin Educ Pract Vet* 24:817-821, 2002.

241. Muir WW, III, Reed SM, McGuirk SM: Treatment of atrial fibrillation in horses by intravenous administration of quinidine, *J Am Vet Med Assoc* 197:1607-1610, 1990.

242. McGurrin MK et al: Transvenous electrical cardioversion in equine atrial fibrillation: technique and successful treatment of 3 horses, *J Vet Intern Med* 17:715-718, 2003.

243. McGurrin MKJ, Physick-Sheard PW, Kenney DG: How to perform transvenous electrical cardioversion in horses with atrial fibrillation, *J Vet Cardiol* 7:109-119, 2005.

244. McGurrin MK et al: Transvenous electrical cardioversion of equine atrial fibrillation: technical considerations, *J Vet Intern Med* 19:695-702, 2005.

245. van Loon G et al: Transient complete atrioventricular block following transvenous electrical cardioversion of atrial fibrillation in a horse, *Vet J* 170:124-127, 2005.

246. Trachsel D et al: Pharmacokinetics and pharmacodynamic effects of amiodarone in plasma of ponies after single intravenous administration, *Toxicol Appl Pharmacol* 195:113-125, 2004.

247. De Clercq D et al: Intravenous amiodarone treatment in horses with chronic atrial fibrillation, *Vet J* 172:129-134, 2006.

248. De Clercq D et al: Evaluation of the pharmacokinetics and bioavailability of intravenously and orally administered amiodarone in horses, *Am J Vet Res* 67:448-454, 2006.

249. Ohmura H et al: Safe and efficacious dosage of flecainide acetate for treating equine atrial fibrillation, *J Vet Med Sci* 62:711-715, 2000.

250. Ohmura H et al: Determination of oral dosage and pharmacokinetic analysis of flecainide in horses, *J Vet Med Sci* 63:511-514, 2001.

251. van Loon G et al: Use of intravenous flecainide in horses with naturally occurring atrial fibrillation, *Equine Vet J* 36:609-614, 2004.

252. Risberg AI, McGuirk SM: Successful conversion of equine atrial fibrillation using oral flecainide, *J Vet Intern Med* 20:207-209, 2006.

253. Ellis EJ et al: The pharmacokinetics and pharmacodynamics of procainamide in horses after intravenous administration, *J Vet Pharmacol Ther* 17:265-270, 1994.

254. Cornick JL, Seahorn TL: Cardiac arrhythmias identified in horses with duodenitis/proximal jejunitis: six cases (1985-1988), *J Am Vet Med Assoc* 197:1054-1059, 1990.

255. Taylor PM, Browning AP, Harris CP: Detomidine-butorphanol sedation in equine clinical practice, *Vet Rec* 123:388-390, 1988.

256. Reef VB: Frequency of cardiac arrhythmias and their significance in normal horses. In the Seventh American College of Veterinary Internal Medicine Forum, San Diego, 1989, pp 506-508.

257. McGuirk SM, Muir WW: Diagnosis and treatment of cardiac arrhythmias, *Vet Clin North Am Equine Pract* 1:353-370, 1985.

258. Whitton DL, Trim CM: Use of dopamine hydrochloride during general anesthesia in the treatment of advanced atrioventricular heart block in four foals, *J Am Vet Med Assoc* 187:1357-1361, 1985.

259. Van Loon G, Laevens H, Deprez P: Temporary transvenous atrial pacing in horses: threshold determination, *Equine Vet J* 33:290-295, 2001.

260. Van Loon G et al: Dual-chamber pacemaker implantation via the cephalic vein in healthy equids, *J Vet Intern Med* 15:564-571, 2001.

261. van Loon G et al: Implantation of a dual-chamber, rate-adaptive pacemaker in a horse with suspected sick sinus syndrome, *Vet Rec* 151:541-545, 2002.

262. Reef VB et al: Implantation of a permanent transvenous pacing catheter in a horse with complete heart block and syncope, *J Am Vet Med Assoc* 189:449-452, 1986.

263. Glazier DB, Littledike ET, Cook HM: The electrocardiographic changes in experimentally induced bundle branch block, *Irish Vet J* 37:71-76, 1983.

264. Muir WW, McGuirk SM: Ventricular preexcitation in two horses, *J Am Vet Med Assoc* 183:573-576, 1983.

265. Epstein V: Relationship between potassium administration, hyperkalaemia, and the electrocardiogram: an experimental study, *Equine Vet J* 16:453-456, 1984.

266. Hardy J: ECG of the month: hyperkalemia in a mare, *J Am Vet Med Assoc* 194:356-357, 1989.

267. Staddon GE, Weaver BMG, Webb AI: Distribution of cardiac output in anaesthetised horses, *Res Vet Sci* 27:38-40, 1979.

268. Gillespie JR, Tyler WS, Hall LW: Cardiopulmonary dysfunction in anesthetized laterally recumbent horses, *Am J Vet Res* 30:61-72, 1969.

269. Aitken MM, Sanford J: Effects of tranquillizers on tachycardia induced by adrenaline in the horse, *Br Vet J* 128:vii-ix, 1972.

270. Alitalo I et al: Cardiac effects of atropine premedication in horses sedated with detomidine, *Acta Vet Scand* 82(suppl):131-136, 1986.

271. Dunlop CI et al: Temporal effects of halothane and isoflurane in laterally recumbent ventilated male horses, *Am J Vet Res* 48:1250-1255, 1987.

272. Grandy JL et al: Arterial hypotension and the development of postanesthetic myopathy in halothane-anesthetized horses, *Am J Vet Res* 48:192-197, 1987.

273. Harvey RC et al: Isoflurane anesthesia for equine colic surgery: comparison with halothane anesthesia, *Vet Surg* 16:184-188, 1988.

274. Nilsfors L, Kvart C: Preliminary report on the cardiorespiratory effects of the antagonist to detomidine, MPV-1248, *Acta Vet Scand* 82(suppl):121-129, 1986.

275. Nilsfors L et al: Cardiorespiratory and sedative effects of a combination of acepromazine, xylazine, and methadone in the horse, *Equine Vet J* 20:364-367, 1988.

276. Serteyn D et al: Circulatory and respiratory effects of ketamine in horses anesthetized with halothane, *Can J Vet Res* 51:513-516, 1987.

277. Steffey EP, Howland D: Cardiovascular effects of halothane in the horse, *Am J Vet Res* 39:611-615, 1978.

278. Steffey EP, Howland D: Comparison of circulatory and respiratory effects of isoflurane and halothane anesthesia in horses, *Am J Vet Res* 41:821-825, 1980.

279. Steffey EP, Kelly AB, Woliner MJ: Time-related responses of spontaneously breathing, laterally recumbent horses to prolonged anesthesia with halothane, *Am J Vet Res* 48:952-957, 1987.

280. Steffey EP et al: Cardiovascular and respiratory effects of acetylpromazine and xylazine on halothane-anesthetized horses, *J Vet Pharmacol Ther* 8:290-302, 1985.

281. Manohar M, Goetz TE: Cerebral, renal, adrenal, intestinal, and pancreatic circulation in conscious ponies and during 1.0, 1.5, and 2.0 minimal alveolar concentrations of halothane-O_2 anesthesia, *Am J Vet Res* 46:2492-2497, 1985.

282. Manohar M, Gustafson R, Nganwa D: Skeletal muscle perfusion during prolonged 2.03% end-tidal isoflurane-O_2 anesthesia in isocapnic ponies, *Am J Vet Res* 48:946-951, 1987.

283. Manohar M et al: Systemic distribution of blood flow in ponies during 1.45%, 1.96%, and 2.39% end-tidal isoflurane-O_2 anesthesia, *Am J Vet Res* 48:1504-1510, 1987.

284. Stegmann GF, Littlejohn A: The effect of lateral and dorsal recumbency on cardiopulmonary function, *J South Afr Vet Assoc* 58:21-27, 1987.

285. Beadle RE, Robinson NE, Sorenson PR: Cardiopulmonary effects of positive end expiratory pressure in, *Am J Vet Res* 36:1435-1438, 1975.

286. Hodgson DS et al: Effects of spontaneous assisted and controlled ventilatory modes in anesthetized geldings, *Am J Vet Res* 47:992-996, 1986.

287. Weaver BM, Walley RV: Ventilation and cardiovascular studies during mechanical control of ventilation in horses, *Equine Vet J* 7:9-15, 1975.

288. Hardman JG, Limbird LE: *Goodman & Gilman's The pharmacological basis of therapeutics*, ed 10, New York, 2001, McGraw-Hill.

289. Guyton AC, Hall JE: The autonomic nervous system and the adrenal medulla. In Guyton AC, Hall JE, editors: *Textbook of medical physiology*, ed 11, Philadelphia, 2006, Elsevier Saunders, pp 748-760.

290. Bergsten G: Blood pressure, cardiac output, and blood-gas tension in the horse at rest and during exercise, *Acta Vet Scand* 48(suppl):1-88, 1974.

291. Durando MM, Reef VB, Birks EK: Right ventricular pressure dynamics during exercise: relationship to stress echocardiography, *Equine Vet J* 34(suppl):472-477, 2002.

292. Eberly VE, Gillespie JR, Typler WS: Cardiovascular parameters in the Thoroughbred horse, *Am J Vet Res* 25:1712-1716, 1964.

293. Steffey EP et al: Cardiovascular and respiratory measurements in awake and isoflurane-anesthetized horses, *Am J Vet Res* 48:7-12, 1987.

294. Sexton WL, Erickson HH, Coffman JR: Cardiopulmonary and metabolic responses to exercise in the Quarter Horse: effects of training. In Proceedings of the Second International Conference on Equine Exercise Physiology, San Diego, 1986.

295. Goetz TE, Manohar M: Pressures in the right side of the heart and esophagus (pleura) in ponies during exercise before and after furosemide administration, *Am J Vet Res* 47:270-276, 1986.

296. Hillidge CJ, Lees P: Left ventricular systole in conscious and anesthetized horses, *Am J Vet Res* 38:675-680, 1977.

297. Reinhard HJ, Zichner M: Evaluation of telemetrically derived stress electrocardiograms of the horse using an electronic computer, *Dtsch Tierarztl Wochenschr* 77:211-217, 1970.

298. Schwarzwald CC, Hamlin RL: Normal electrocardiographic time intervals in horses of various sizes, unpublished observations, 2006.

299. Lombard CW et al: Blood pressure, electrocardiogram, and echocardiogram measurements in the growing pony foal, *Equine Vet J* 16:342-347, 1984.

300. Lombard CW: Cardiovascular diseases. In Koterba AM, Drummond WH, Kosch PC, editors: *Equine clinical neonatology*, Philadelphia, 1990, Lea & Febiger, pp 240-261.

301. Marr CM: Treatment of cardiac arrhythmias and cardiac failure. In Robinson NE, editor: *Current therapy in equine medicine 4*, Philadelphia, 1997, Saunders, pp 250-255.

302. Plumb DC: *Veterinary drug handbook*, ed 3, Ames, 1999, Iowa State University Press.

303. Reef VB: Arrhythmias. In Marr CM, editor: *Cardiology of the horse*, London, 1999, Saunders, pp 179-209.

Stress Associated with Anesthesia and Surgery

Ann E. Wagner

1. Horses develop a stress response to anesthesia and surgery.
2. Total intravenous anesthesia in horses causes less stress than inhalation (halothane) anesthesia.
3. Major surgical procedures increase the stress response.
4. Judicious use of select preanesthetic medications, particularly α_2-agonists, reduces the stress response.
5. Adequate analgesia and maintenance of an appropriate depth of anesthesia, optimum cardiorespiratory function, and goal-oriented fluid therapy minimize the stress response in anesthetized horses.
6. The influence of the stress response on perianesthetic morbidity and mortality in horses is unknown but likely contributes to altered immune function and an increased potential for infection.

Animals respond to noxious stimuli such as physical manipulation, pharmacologic restraint, anesthesia, and accidental or surgical trauma through a variety of neural, humoral, and metabolic changes designed to restore or maintain homeostasis. Physical trauma or surgical insult results in local inflammation, a component of healing. In addition to this local response, there is a more generalized response comprised of various endocrine-metabolic changes—the so-called stress response (Figure 4-1). As editorialized by Muir, "Although generally considered as something that should be avoided, stress prepares the animal for the immediate future by activating the adrenocortical system, which increases and redistributes blood flow (fight or flight), mobilizes body resources to provide substrates such as glucose and free fatty acids, and activates the immune system. Why then should we be concerned about stress? Although stress may produce beneficial effects that could help the animal to respond to exogenous or endogenous deleterious forces, it also produces significant neuroendocrine and metabolic effects that may result in undesirable hemodynamic changes, limit the availability of glucose to tissues, depress the immune system and prolong healing and tissue repair."[1] In other words, a certain amount of stress may be beneficial, but too much stress (distress) may be harmful, and the transition from one state to the next has yet to be defined clearly (Boxes 4-1 and 4-2). To date no correlation has been made between the stress response in horses and their perianesthetic morbidity or mortality.

In humans, anesthesia alone causes little stress, as evidenced by minimum changes in plasma cortisol. Cortisol does increase with surgery, and the magnitude and duration of the change depends on the severity of the procedure (Table 4-1).[2]

Horses respond differently, in that inhalation anesthesia alone is associated with a marked increase in plasma cortisol.[3] Minor surgery has little additional effect on the stress response to anesthesia, but major abdominal surgery causes significantly higher plasma cortisol concentrations (Table 4-2).[3] Several studies have indicated that total intravenous anesthesia (TIVA) in horses does not produce an increase in plasma cortisol or catecholamines, leading to speculation that TIVA might be advantageous in obtunding the stress response and possibly improving surgical outcome.[4,5]

The degree of stress imposed by anesthetic drugs or surgery in horses is difficult to determine because there is no single index or variable or combination of variables that specifically or consistently defines stress. Traditional approaches to assessing stress include measuring discrete physiologic and blood chemical responses such as heart rate and plasma cortisol concentration. Additional measures could include assessments of long-term effects of stress on functions such as immunity, metabolism, and reproduction.[6]

Horses are one of the most challenging of domestic species to anesthetize, with the potential for major complications before, during, and after anesthesia and surgery (see Chapter 22). Studies of the equine stress response to anesthetic drugs, mechanical ventilation, and surgery require continued investigation.

MARKERS OF THE STRESS RESPONSE

Corticosteroids

Increases in circulating corticosteroid concentrations are frequently used as an index of stress, but there are stressful conditions to which the adrenal gland does not respond.[6,7] Stress causes plasma glucocorticoids to increase most of the time. Glucocorticoids produce hyperglycemia by increasing hepatic gluconeogenesis, inhibiting glucose uptake by cells, and enhancing lipid-protein catabolism. These glucocorticoid effects may lead to ketosis, hyperlipemia, hyperaminoacidemia, and metabolic acidosis. Glucocorticoids also stimulate tissue cells to produce lipocortins (i.e., peptide hormones that interact with the immune system to decrease production of prostaglandins, thromboxanes, and leukotrienes) and decrease migration of inflammatory cells into tissues.[1] T lymphocytes, monocytes, and eosinophils are lysed or marginated along the walls of blood vessels, whereas normally marginated neutrophils go into the circulating pool of blood leukocytes. This gives rise to the classic stress leukogram of mature neutrophilia, lymphopenia, eosinopenia, and monocytosis. The long-term effects of increased circulating glucocorticoids may include delayed wound healing,

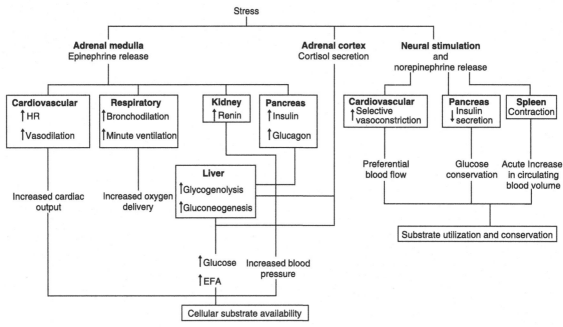

Figure 4–1. Diagrammatic representation of the stress response.

muscle wasting, immune deficiencies, and increased susceptibility to infection. Lipocortin also inhibits prostaglandin production in the gastrointestinal tract, which may promote gastrointestinal ulceration.[8]

Plasma concentrations of the glucocorticoid hormone cortisol vary widely in anesthetized horses, resulting in an inability to detect significant changes.[9,10] Nevertheless, plasma cortisol concentration is frequently determined in studies of the equine stress response to anesthesia and surgery (Figure 4-2). In addition, blood glucose and lactate concentrations have been determined (Figure 4-3).

Catecholamines

Adrenergic responses are an integral component of the general stress response. The basal adrenergic state influences the adrenergic response to anesthesia in that animals with elevated norepinephrine tend to demonstrate no change or decreases after anesthesia and those with low sympathetic tone have increases after anesthesia.[3-7,11] Side effects of anesthesia (hypercapnia, hypotension) and surgery (pain, blood loss) may be responsible for increases in plasma cathecholamines.[12] Individual variation in equine catecholamine concentrations has made detection of significant increases or decreases challenging.[13]

Insulin and Glucose

Plasma insulin concentrations are variably affected by anesthetic drugs. Xylazine causes hyperglycemia because it inhibits insulin release by stimulating α_2-adrenoceptors in pancreatic β cells.[14] Combinations of various preanesthetic and induction drugs increase, decrease, or have no effect on plasma insulin.[9,10] Food intake also affects insulin levels, and fasting tends to suppress insulin release, whereas refeeding enhances insulin release.[10,13,15]

Surgery in humans generally causes a hyperglycemic response, which is proportional to the degree of trauma

Table 4–1. Principal hormonal responses to surgery

Endocrine gland	Hormones	Changes in secretion
Anterior pituitary	ACTH	Increases
	GH	Increases
	TSH	May increase or decrease
	FSH and LH	May increase or decrease
Posterior pituitary	AVP	Increases
Adrenal cortex	Cortisol	Increases
	Aldosterone	Increases
Pancreas	Insulin	Often decreases
	Glucagon	Usually small increases
Thyroid	Thyroxine, tri-iodothyronine	Decreases

ACTH, Adrenocorticotropic hormone (corticotropin); *AVP*, arginine vasopressin; *FSH*, follicle-stimulating hormone; *GH*, growth hormone; *LH*, luteinizing hormone; *TSH*, thyroid-stimulating hormone.

Table 4–2. Endocrine-metabolic factors influenced by anesthesia

Type of response	Inhibition or improvement	No important effect	No data
Pituitary	ACTH	T_3 and T_4	Gastrointestinal peptides
	β-Endorphin	Coagulation and	Testosterone
	GH	fibrinolysis	Estradiol
	AVP	Acute-phase proteins	
	TSH	Water and sodium	
	LH and FSH	balance	
	Prolactin		
Adrenal/renal/nervous system	Cortisol		
	Aldosterone		
	Adrenaline		
	Renin		
	Noradrenaline		
Metabolic	Hyperglycemia and glucose tolerance		
	Lipolysis		
	Muscle amino acids		
	Nitrogen balance		
	Oxygen consumption		
	Urinary potassium excretion		

ACTH, Adrenocorticotropic hormone (corticotropin); *AVP*, arginine vasopressin; *FSH*, follicle-stimulating hormone; *GH*, growth hormone; *LH*, luteinizing hormone; *TSH*, thyroid-stimulating hormone.

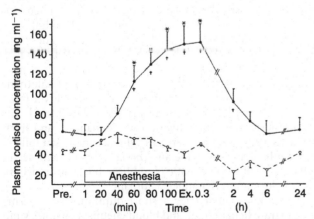

Figure 4–2. Plasma cortisol concentration (ng/ml) during 2 hr of thiopentone-halothane anesthesia (●) versus mock anesthesia (O) in six ponies. *Different from "pre" values; †different from mock anesthesia (P<0.05). (From Taylor PM: Equine stress response to anaesthesia, *Br J Anaesth* 63:705, 1989.)

inflicted and not the anesthetic used.[16] In horses the hyperglycemic response varies with the anesthetic regimen used and may be prominent in foals.[10] $α_2$-Agonists (e.g., xylazine), as previously mentioned, are associated with increased blood glucose, whereas other drugs or combinations of drugs may decrease blood glucose (Figure 4-4).[10,13,15]

Nonesterified Fatty Acids

The nonesterified fatty acids (NEFAs) are affected by the hormonal changes associated with stress and excitement. Lipolysis is mediated by β-adrenoceptors in the horse;[17] thus the increased sympathetic activity associated with pain or fear may cause NEFAs to rise. Decreased sympathetic activity produced by sedation or anesthesia has the opposite effect. Suppression of insulin may also affect plasma NEFAs. Suppression of insulin tends to cause increased NEFAs because insulin is antilipolytic. Hypoxemia can also elevate plasma NEFAs by inhibiting metabolism.[9] It is

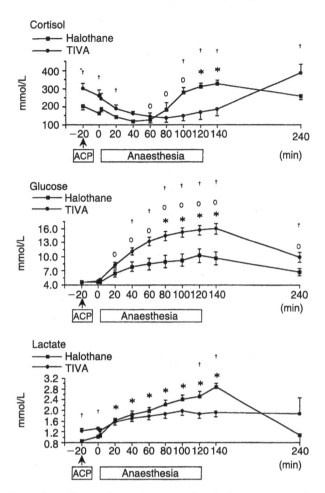

Figure 4–3. Plasma glucose, lactate, and cortisol concentrations during halothane and TIVA (detomidine-ketamine-guaifenesin; mean ± SEM). *Significant change from preanesthetic value (halothane anesthesia); °significant change from preanesthetic value (TIVA); †significant difference between groups. (From Luna SPL, Taylor PM, Wheeler MJ: Cardiorespiratory, endocrine, and metabolic changes in ponies undergoing intravenous or inhalation anaesthesia, *J Vet Pharmacol Ther* 19:251-258, 1996.)

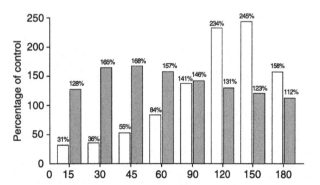

Figure 4–4. Percent (%) of control in plasma glucose *(white bar)* and serum insulin *(shaded bar)* compared to control in Thoroughbred horses administered intravenous xylazine hydrochloride. (From Thurmon JC et al: Xylazine hydrochloride-induced hyperglycemia and hypoinsulinemia in Thoroughbred horses, *J Vet Pharmacol Ther* 5:243, 1982.)

probably desirable to prevent large increases in NEFAs from occurring in the horse because in humans increased NEFAs are associated with cardiac problems (decreased contractility, increased incidence of cardiac dysrhythmias). NEFAs in horses tend to be increased with preoperative fasting and apprehension but fall once the horse is sedated and may be decreased or normal in the immediate postoperative period.[10,15] Whether or not increased NEFAs cause any cardiac abnormalities in anesthetized horses is unknown.

Hematology and Clinical Chemistry

Certain clinical pathologic changes occur in horses after anesthesia, but these are relatively minor and predictable. Hematocrit (packed cell volume; PCV) and total white blood cell (WBC) count are significantly increased at 1 hr and after 5 to 6 hr of halothane anesthesia but return to normal 1 day after anesthesia (Table 4-3).[18] A similar duration of isoflurane anesthesia produces no change in PCV, but WBC count is increased significantly 1 day after anesthesia (Table 4-4).[19] The suggestion that these small changes in blood cells are attributable to the effects of increased circulating catecholamines or cortisol is supported by the accompanying increase in mature and band neutrophils and decrease in lymphocytes and eosinophils (the classic "stress leukogram").[19]

The PCV in ponies decreased after induction to anesthesia with acepromazine, thiopental, and halothane, indicating low sympathetic activity with uptake of red blood cells into the spleen.[13] Platelet numbers and aggregation declined during 5.5 hr of halothane anesthesia in adult horses.[20] Platelet aggregation remained depressed for up to 4 days after anesthesia, but hyperaggregability was noted on the seventh day.[20]

Renal function in horses apparently is only minimally and transiently impaired by anesthesia with halothane, isoflurane, or sevoflurane. Urea nitrogen, creatinine, and inorganic phosphate were increased 1 hr after halothane or isoflurane anesthesia without intravenous fluid administration but returned to normal or below normal by the next day.[18-20] Presumably treatment of anesthetic-induced hypotension and appropriate fluid replacement help to prevent these changes.

Serum concentrations of certain enzymes may increase at any time from 1 hr to 4 days after anesthesia. Poor perfusion of skeletal muscle, resulting from anesthesia-induced hypotension or pressure on muscle tissue during recumbency, is the probable reason for increases in creatine phosphokinase and aspartate aminotransferase following inhalant anesthesia in horses (Table 4-5).[18-20] Hypoxemia during anesthesia may exacerbate increases in muscle enzymes.[21] However, ponies anesthetized with acepromazine, thiopental, and halothane had no significant changes in muscle enzymes.[13] Liver function in ponies or horses is not greatly affected by 2 to 5 hours of anesthesia. Bilirubin excretion was enhanced, and liver-derived serum enzymes were only slightly increased following halothane or isoflurane anesthesia.[22-24] Isoflurane seems to have less effect on hepatic blood flow, bile acid transport, and bile formation than does halothane.[24]

Horses anesthetized for a short duration (1 to 1.5 hr) demonstrate hematologic and blood chemical changes similar to horses anesthetized for a prolonged period (5 to 6 hr), but the changes are of smaller magnitude and duration after shorter anesthetic periods (see Chapter 15).[18,19] Horses

Table 4–3. Summary of PCV, TP, and WBC count in horses anesthetized with halothane (n = 6)*

	Normal (min-max)	Baseline	Hour 1	Day 1	Day 2	Day 3-4	Day 7
PCV (%)	32-53	33 ± 6	40 ± 4[†]	35 ± 5	35 ± 6	33 ± 7	33 ± 5
Plasma protein (g/dl)	5.8-8.7	7.7 ± 0.6	8.0 ± 0.8	8.1 ± 0.7[†]	8.0 ± 0.7	7.9 ± 0.6	7.8 ± 0.7
Total WBC count (/µl)	5,400-14,300	10,383 ± 2798	14,700 ± 4653*	14,617 ± 2784	14,440 ± 2772	11,283 ± 4293	9,817 ± 3741

Modified from Steffey EP et al: Alterations in horse blood cell count and biochemical values after halothane anesthesia, *Am J Vet Res* 41:934, 1980.
PCV, Packed cell volume; *TP,* total plasma protein; *WBC,* white blood cell.
*Values given are mean ± SD.
[†]Indicates significant difference from baseline.

Table 4–4. Summary of PCV, TP, and WBC count in horses anesthetized with isoflurane (n = 6)*

	Normal (min-max)	Baseline	Hour 1	Day 1	Day 2	Day 3-4	Day 7
PCV (%)	32-53	34 ± 4	36 ± 3	34 ± 4	33 ± 4	33 ± 7	32 ± 6
Plasma protein (g/dl)	5.8-8.7	7.7 ± 0.3	7.3 ± 0.5	7.4 ± 0.4	7.4 ± 0.4	7.8 ±0.5	7.8 ± 0.5
Total WBC count (/µl)	5,400-14,300	9,808 ± 3474	10,033 ± 5857	13,033 ± 3626[†]	11,483 ± 3142	9,733 ± 3646	11,183 ± 4709

Modified from Steffey EP, Zinkl J, Howland D: Minimal changes in blood cell counts and biochemical values associated with prolonged isoflurane anesthesia of horses, *Am J Vet Res* 40:1646, 1979.
PCV, Packed cell volume; *TP,* total plasma protein; *WBC,* white blood cell.
*Values given are mean ± SD.
[†]Indicates significant difference from baseline.

Table 4–5. Muscle enzymes in horses anesthetized with halothane[18,19,50]

	Baseline	Hour 1	Day 1	Day 2	Day 3-4	Day 7
AST (U/L)						
HAL	329 ± 107	337 ± 92	503 ± 30*	501 ± 34*	631± 296*	438 ± 94
ISO	246 ± 71	238 ± 29	447 ± 93*	439 ± 116*	411± 117*	370 ± 130
SEVO	212 ± 26	209 ± 26	803 ± 261*	830 ± 249*	701 ± 213*	ND
CPK (U/L)						
HAL	37 ± 27	286 ± 179*	320 ± 159*	241± 228	181 ± 209	102 ± 113
ISO	31 ± 16	152 ± 88*	394 ± 243*	220 ± 173*	153 ± 218	83 ± 52*
SEVO	227 ± 42	941± 324*	4,435 ± 1,595*	2,392 ± 880*	716 ± 183*	ND
LDH (U/L)						
HAL	321 ± 131	393 ± 139*	744 ± 249*	651 ± 238*	495 ± 179	414 ± 158
ISO	287 ± 118	299 ± 94	684 ± 462	528 ± 312	436 ± 124	393 ± 279

AST, Aspartate aminotransferase; *CPK,* creatine phosphokinase; *HAL,* halothane, n = 6; *ISO,* isoflurane,[18] n = 6; *LDH,* lactate dehydrogenase; *ND,* no data; *SEVO,* sevoflurane,[50] n = 5. Values given are mean ± SD.
*Indicates significant difference from baseline.

anesthetized on 3 consecutive days for approximately 1 hr each day, demonstrated leukogram changes indicative of stress (increased neutrophils and decreased lymphocytes, as mentioned previously), which persisted for 3 to 4 days, leading to the conclusion that multiple anesthetic exposures are more stressful than single, short-duration exposures.[20] However, no study has demonstrated that repeated or prolonged anesthesia in normal horses has clinically important long-term effects on organ function or the stress response.

EFFECT OF ANESTHESIA WITHOUT SURGERY

Total Intravenous Anesthesia Without Surgery

Ponies anesthetized briefly with thiopental or anesthetized and maintained for up to 2 hours with pentobarbital exhibited no significant increase in the markers of stress (except increased cortisol and adrenocorticotropic hormone

[ACTH] associated with struggling during recovery), leading the investigator to conclude that "stress-free anesthesia can be achieved in the horse."[4] However, marked respiratory depression and poor-quality recoveries preclude the sole use of short-acting barbiturates for clinical anesthesia in horses.[4] Ponies anesthetized for 2 hours with a combination of detomidine, ketamine, and guaifenesin had no change in catecholamines and a decrease in plasma cortisol.[5,25] Recoveries are long but uneventful, suggesting that this drug combination might be clinically useful. A similar anesthetic protocol composed of the same drugs but a lower infusion rate of guaifenesin produced no change in catecholamines but decreased cortisol and is associated with improved recoveries, encouraging further refinement of TIVA as a substitute for inhalation anesthesia (see Chapters 12-13).[26]

In support of the concept that TIVA is less stressful than inhalation anesthesia, perioperative fatalities have been reported to be less common when horses are anesthetized with TIVA (0.31%) compared to horses induced by intravenous drugs and maintained on halothane or isoflurane (0.99%).[27] However, most TIVA episodes were less than 90 minutes in duration, which may partially explain the lower mortality rate since risk of death in horses increases with the duration of anesthesia and surgery time.[27]

Inhalation Anesthesia Without Surgery

Numerous studies describe the hormonal and metabolic response to halothane anesthesia.[28-37] All have demonstrated a twofold to threefold rise in plasma cortisol, although the onset of the stress response varies with the type of premedication and injectable anesthetic drugs used; acepromazine and thiopental administered before halothane or isoflurane anesthesia produce significant increases in plasma cortisol at 40 minutes, whereas the administration of xylazine and ketamine delay the increase in cortisol until 80 minutes.[13,38] Cortisol levels are highest at about 2 hr.[13,38] Substituting isoflurane for halothane after induction with either acepromazine-thiopental or xylazine-ketamine apparently does not mitigate the stress response.[39] To date the equine stress response to sevoflurane or desflurane requires investigation.

The exact reason for the development of a stress response to inhalation anesthesia is not yet known. It is not thought to be a direct effect of the anesthetic itself, nor does varying the depth of anesthesia affect the degree of stress.[40] A variety of possible inciting causes have been investigated (Box 4-3). Because hypotension is much more common during inhalation anesthesia compared to TIVA, there is speculation that low arterial blood pressure elicits the stress response.[13] Therefore a variety of preventions or treatments for hypotension have been studied, including dopamine, dobutamine, a modified gelatin plasma expander, and the α_1-agonist methoxamine.[29,31-33] A low infusion of dopamine does not prevent the increase in plasma cortisol associated with halothane anesthesia, whereas a high infusion does.[29] Hypotension does not seem to be the primary stimulus responsible for the stress response since blood pressures were similar in the two groups.[29] Plasma cortisol still increased when dobutamine was administered to halothane-anesthetized ponies to maintain their blood pressures at awake values, suggesting that blood pressure alone is not

> **Box 4-3** **Systemic Responses to Surgery**
>
> - Sympathetic nervous system activation
> - Endocrine "stress response"
>   - Pituitary hormone secretion
>   - Insulin resistance
> - Immunological and hematological changes
>   - Cytokine production
>   - Acute phase reaction
>   - Neutrophil leukocytosis
>   - Lymphocyte proliferation

the stimulus for the stress response during anesthesia.[31] A modified gelatin plasma expander administered (48 ml/kg) to halothane-anesthetized ponies maintained mean arterial blood pressure close to preanesthetic values and was not associated with significant changes in cortisol or ACTH; however, complications (prolonged bleeding times) were associated with this dose of plasma expander. In the same study a lower dose of the plasma expander (10 ml/kg) combined with an infusion of dobutamine resulted in no increase in cortisol or ACTH.[33] Maintenance of normal arterial blood pressure by administering methoxamine during halothane anesthesia in ponies attenuates but does not prevent increases in cortisol concentration, suggesting that hypotension is an important stimulus of stress.[32] Therefore hypotension may contribute to stress during halothane anesthesia because of an effect on tissue perfusion.[33]

The possible effects of hypoxemia and hypercapnia on the stress response to halothane anesthesia have been investigated.[34] Blood glucose and lactic acid increased 20 minutes after establishing an arterial oxygen tension of approximately 40 mm Hg during 2 hours of halothane anesthesia, but no further increase in cortisol occurred compared to normoxemic anesthetized horses.[34] Forty minutes of hypercapnia ($PaCO_2$ approximately 75 mm Hg) in halothane-anesthetized ponies was associated with a slight amelioration of hypotension and lactic acidemia, but cortisol concentrations were similar to those of normocapnic ponies.[35] Therefore neither hypoxemia nor hypercapnia seems to be the stimulus for the stress response during inhalation anesthesia.

Infusion of glucose during 2 hours of halothane anesthesia prevents the usual increase in plasma cortisol, ACTH, and catecholamines.[36] The reduced stress response occurs despite cardiorespiratory depression similar to that of previous studies investigating the stress response to halothane anesthesia, leading to speculation that metabolism and availability of energy are important cofactors in the equine stress response.[36]

EFFECT OF ANESTHESIA WITH SURGERY

Anesthesia without surgery does not elicit a stress response in humans, but surgery does cause an increase in cortisol concentration.[2] The magnitude and duration of increased cortisol depends on the severity of the procedure.[2] Arthroscopic surgery in halothane-anesthetized horses produces only minor and relatively short-lived (6 hours) increases in

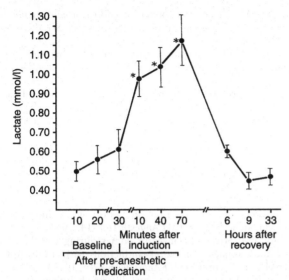

Figure 4–5. Changes (mean ± SEM) in blood lactate (mmol/L) associated with surgery in halothane-anesthetized horses. *Different from other values (P<0.05). (From Robertson SA: Some metabolic and hormonal changes associated with general anesthesia and surgery in the horse, *Equine Vet J* 19:288, 1987.)

plasma β-endorphin and cortisol after surgery.[15] Surgery to relocate a carotid artery to a subcutaneous position results in only slightly greater increases in plasma cortisol and lactate concentrations and slightly lower glucose values compared to anesthesia without surgery (Figure 4-5).[41] Abdominal surgery in ponies produces a tenfold increase in plasma cortisol.[42] Further evidence that the surgical procedure and the severity of surgical intervention influences the stress response is provided by a report of plasma cortisol levels in two groups of halothane-anesthetized clinical cases: horses anesthetized for abdominal (colic) surgery compared to horses anesthetized for soft tissue or orthopedic surgery.[43] The only difference in anesthetic technique was that the nonabdominal surgery patients received acepromazine as part of their premedication. Preoperative plasma cortisol was markedly higher in the abdominal group than in the nonabdominal group, decreased after induction or anesthesia, increased slightly during surgery, and took approximately 60 hours to return to normal values.[43] Plasma cortisol started at a lower level in the abdominal group, increased during surgery, but decreased to normal within 48 hours, despite the fact that some of these horses had painful conditions.[43] Therefore abdominal surgery induces only a slight increase in the stress response above that already incited by abdominal pathology and anesthesia, suggesting that the stress response associated with colic may already be maximum.

EFFECT OF HYPOTHERMIA ON THE STRESS RESPONSE TO ANESTHESIA

Horses, like other animals, are susceptible to hypothermia during anesthesia and surgery.[44] Without external warming devices, mean core body temperature of anesthetized adult horses decreases by about 0.37° C/hr.[44] The possible influence of hypothermia on the stress response to anesthesia has not been investigated in horses but has been studied in humans.[45] Several studies have reported increases in plasma

norepinephrine levels in hypothermic human patients, which may reflect the attempt of the body to vasoconstrict and minimize further heat loss.[45-47] Plasma epinephrine may be unchanged or increased during hypothermia, but cortisol concentration is generally no different between normothermic and hypothermic human patients.[45,46,48,49] Whether or not hypothermia significantly alters the equine stress response to anesthesia remains undetermined.

CONCLUSION AND CLINICAL RELEVANCE

The exact cause of the equine stress response to anesthesia and surgery is multifactorial. Pain, tissue perfusion, and energy availability may be important determinants of stress. Further research is needed to define what the optimal tolerable stress response can be in horses and to develop anesthetic protocols that modulate the stress response in a desirable way. The impact of modulating the stress response will have an important impact on anesthetic morbidity and potentially mortality (see Chapter 22). Currently TIVA seems to hold promise as a technique for reducing stress and potentially improving outcomes for anesthetized horses.

REFERENCES

1. Muir WW: The equine stress response to anaesthesia, *Equine Vet J* 3:302-303, 1990.
2. Traynor C, Hall GM: Endocrine and metabolic changes during surgery: anaesthetic implications, *Br J Anaesth* 53:153-160, 1981.
3. Taylor PM: Changes in plasma cortisol concentration in response to anesthesia in the horse. In Proceedings of the Second International Congress of Veterinary Anesthesiologists, Sacramento, 1985, p 165.
4. Taylor PM: The stress response to anaesthesia in ponies: barbiturate anaesthesia, *Equine Vet J* 3:307-331, 1990.
5. Taylor PM, Luna SPL: Total intravenous anaesthesia in ponies using detomidine, ketamine, and guaiphenesin: pharmacokinetics, cardiopulmonary and endocrine effects, *Res Vet Sci* 59:17-23, 1995.
6. Moberg GP: Biological response to stress: key to assessment of animal well-being? In Moberg GP, editor: *Animal stress*, Bethesda, 1985, American Physiological Society, pp 27-49.
7. Moberg GP: Problems in defining stress and distress in animals, *J Am Vet Med Assoc* 191:3107-3130, 1987.
8. Breazile JE: Physiologic basis and consequences of distress in animals, *J Am Vet Med Assoc* 191:1212-1215, 1987.
9. Robertson SA: Metabolic and hormonal responses to neuroleptanalgesia (etorphine and acepromazine) in the horse, *Equine Vet J* 19:214-217, 1987.
10. Robertson SA: Some metabolic and hormonal changes associated with general anaesthesia and surgery in the horse, *Equine Vet J* 19:288-294, 1987.
11. Reves JC, Knopes KD: Adrenergic component of the stress response, *Anesth Report* 1:175-191, 1989.
12. Wagner AE, Bednarski RM, Muir WW: Hemodynamic effects of carbon dioxide during intermittent positive-pressure ventilation in horses, *Am J Vet Res* 51:1922-1929, 1990.
13. Taylor PM: Equine stress response to anaesthesia, *Br J Anaesth* 63:702-709, 1989.
14. Thurmon JC et al: Xylazine hydrochloride-induced hyperglycemia and hypoinsulinemia in thoroughbred horses, *J Vet Pharmacol Ther* 5:241-245, 1982.
15. Robertson SA, Steele CJ, Chen C: Metabolic and hormonal changes associated with arthroscopic surgery in the horse, *Equine Vet J* 22:313-316, 1990.

16. Clarke RSJ: Anaesthesia and carbohydrate metabolism, *Br J Anaesth* 45:237-241, 1973.
17. Snow DH: Metabolic and physiological effects of adrenoceptor agonists and antagonists in the horse, *Res Vet Sci* 27:372-378, 1979.
18. Steffey EP et al: Alterations in horse blood cell count and biochemical values after halothane anesthesia, *Am J Vet Res* 41:934-939, 1980.
19. Steffey EP, Zinkl J, Howland D: Minimal changes in blood cell counts and biochemical values associated with prolonged isoflurane anesthesia of horses, *Am J Vet Res* 40:1646-1648, 1979.
20. Stover SM et al: Hematologic and serum biochemical alterations associated with multiple halothane anesthesia exposures and minor surgical trauma in horses, *Am J Vet Res* 49:236-241, 1988.
21. Whitehair KJ et al: Effects of inhalation anesthetic agents on response of horses to three hours of hypoxemia, *Am J Vet Res* 57:351-360, 1996.
22. Lees P, Mullen PA, Tavernor WD: Influence of anaesthesia with volatile agents on the equine liver, *Br J Anaesth* 45:570-577, 1973.
23. Engelking LR et al: Effects of halothane anesthesia on equine liver function, *Am J Vet Res* 44:607-615, 1984.
24. Engelking L et al: Effects of isoflurane anesthesia on equine liver function, *Am J Vet Res* 45:616-619, 1984.
25. Taylor PM, Watkins SB: Stress responses during total intravenous anaesthesia in ponies with detomidine-guaiphenesin-ketamine, *J Vet Anaesth* 19:13-17, 1992.
26. Luna SP, Taylor PM, Wheeler MJ: Cardiorespiratory, endocrine, and metabolic changes in ponies undergoing intravenous or inhalation anaesthesia, *J Vet Pharmacol Ther* 19:251-258, 1996.
27. Johnston GM et al: The confidential enquiry into perioperative equine fatalities (CEPEF): mortality results of phases 1 and 2, *Vet Anaesth Analg* 29:159-170, 2002.
28. Luna SPL, Taylor PM: Pituitary-adrenal activity and opioid release in ponies during thiopentone/halothane anaesthesia, *Res Vet Sci* 58:35-41, 1995.
29. Robertson SA, Malark JA, Steele CJ: Metabolic, hormonal, and hemodynamic changes during dopamine infusions in halothane anesthetized horses, *Vet Anesth* 25:88-97, 1996.
30. Luna SPL, Taylor PM, Massone F: Midazolam and ketamine induction before halothane anaesthesia in ponies: cardiorespiratory, endocrine, and metabolic changes, *J Vet Pharmacol Ther* 20:153-159, 1997.
31. Taylor PM: Adrenocortical and metabolic responses to dobutamine infusion during halothane anaesthesia in ponies, *J Vet Pharmacol Ther* 21:282-287, 1998.
32. Brodbelt DC, Harris J, Taylor PM: Pituitary-adrenocortical effects of methoxamine infusion on halothane anaesthetized ponies, *Res Vet Sci* 65:119-123, 1998.
33. Taylor PM: Endocrine and metabolic responses to plasma volume expansion during halothane anaesthesia in ponies, *J Vet Pharmacol Ther* 21:485-490, 1998.
34. Taylor PM: Effects of hypoxia on endocrine and metabolic responses to anaesthesia in ponies, *Res Vet Sci* 66:39-44, 1998.
35. Taylor PM: Effects of hypercapnia on endocrine and metabolic responses to anaesthesia in ponies, *Res Vet Sci* 65:41-46, 1998.
36. Luna SPL, Taylor PM, Brearley JC: Effects of glucose infusion on the endocrine, metabolic, and cardiorespiratory responses to halothane anaesthesia of ponies, *Vet Rec* 145:100-103, 1999.
37. Luna SPL, Taylor PM: Cardiorespiratory and endocrine effects of endogenous opioid antagonism by naloxone in ponies anaesthetized with halothane, *Res Vet Sci* 70:95-100, 2001.
38. Taylor PM: Stress response in ponies during halothane or isoflurane anaesthesia after induction with thiopentone or xylazine/ketamine, *J Vet Anaesth* 18:8-14, 1991.
39. Taylor PM: Stress responses in ponies during halothane or isoflurane anaesthesia after induction with thiopentone or xylazine/ketamine, *J Vet Anaesth* 18:8-14, 1991.
40. Lacoumenta S et al: Effects of two differing halothane concentrations on the metabolic and endocrine response to surgery, *Br J Anaesth* 58:844-850, 1986.
41. Taylor PM: Effects of surgery on endocrine and metabolic responses to anaesthesia in horses and ponies, *Res Vet Sci* 64:133-140, 1998.
42. Taylor PM: Changes in plasma cortisol concentrations in response to anaesthesia in the horse. In Proceedings of the Second International congress of Veterinary Anesthesiologists, Sacramento, 1985, pp 165-166.
43. Stegmann GF, Jones RS: Perioperative plasma cortisol concentration in the horse, *J S Afr Vet Assoc* 69:137-142, 1998.
44. Tomasic M: Temporal changes in core body temperature in anesthetized adult horses, *Am J Vet Res* 60:556-562, 1999.
45. Frank SM et al: The catecholamine, cortisol, and hemodynamic responses to mild perioperative hypothermia—a randomized clinical trial, *Anesthesiology* 82:83-93, 1995.
46. Frank SM et al: Adrenergic, respiratory, and cardiovascular effects of core cooling in humans, *Am J Physiol Regul Integr Comp Physiol* 272:R557-R565, 1997.
47. Frank SM et al: Threshold for adrenomedullary activation and increased cardiac work during mild core hypothermia, *Clin Sci* 102:119-125, 2002.
48. Motamed S et al: Metabolic changes during recovery in normothermic versus hypothermic patients undergoing surgery and receiving general anesthesia and epidural local agents, *Anesthesiology* 88:1211-1218, 1998.
49. Chi OZ et al: Intraoperative mild hypothermia does not increase the plasma concentration of stress hormones during neurosurgery, *Can J Anaesth* 48:815-818, 2001.
50. Steffey EP et al: Effects of sevoflurane dose and mode of ventilation on cardiopulmonary function and blood biochemical variables in horses, *Am J Vet Res* 66:606-614, 2005.

Physical Restraint

James T. Robertson
William W. Muir

KEY POINTS

1. Physical restraint and restraining devices can be used to restrict movement, modify behavior, and facilitate medical and surgical treatment.
2. No more physical restraint than is necessary should be applied.
3. Sedation and anesthesia should be considered as preferred alternatives to physical restraint when appropriate.
4. Alternate plans to offset potential handler-horse altercations should be formulated before attempting physical restraint.
5. Familiarity with equine behavior and horsemanship increases the confidence of owners and attendants, improves interactions with the horse, and helps to avoid accidents and injury.

Physical restraint techniques are necessary for the everyday handling of horses. The choice of technique is based on the horse's temperament, age, size, and physical condition; the procedure to be performed; the equipment available; the qualifications of assistants; and the type of facilities available. Procedures as minor as physical examination and intramuscular injection of drugs require some form of restraint. It is impractical to sedate every horse for brief, relatively pain-free procedures that they might resist. Furthermore, sedation may be contraindicated in many instances such as regional anesthesia for diagnostic nerve blocks during lameness examinations.

Horses are capable of inflicting serious injury to themselves and attendants. They should be adequately restrained at all times because unexpected events beyond the attendant's control may startle a horse and endanger the horse and handler. The owner may sometimes be the most capable of restraining the horse. However, enlisting the owner's help is not advisable for medico-legal reasons. Mastery of the techniques described in the following paragraphs is essential for anyone who wishes to work with horses.

Horses by nature tend to be inquisitive, apprehensive, and excitable. They are apprehensive of strange surroundings and the devices of humans. If possible, interaction with horses should occur in familiar surroundings. Ideally the site chosen should be quiet and free of distractions or obstacles that could endanger the horse or attendant. The footing should be secure to prevent the horse from slipping and injuring itself (Figure 5-1).

The attendant should be familiar with proper horsemanship, experienced with horses, and confident of his or her ability.

The most basic forms of restraint, from simply holding a lead shank attached to a halter to more elaborate procedures

necessary for anesthesia should be mastered (Box 5-1).[1-3] Using the least restraint possible may be the best management technique because many horses resent any form of restraint. Regardless of the technique used, the handler should always remain attentive and in control of the horse. Unless contraindicated, sedatives should be used when necessary because they decrease apprehension (see Chapter 10) and make the horse easier to work with and more cooperative. The goal of physical restraint is to accomplish the intended procedure without jeopardizing the safety of the horse or attendants.

HALTER AND LEAD

A halter and lead are essential equipment for controlling any horse. The halter should fit snugly to prevent objects in the environment from inadvertently being entangled and to keep the halter from slipping off. Halters typically are made of nylon or strong leather, and the lead preferably is made of a soft material that will not burn the attendant's hands.

Horses are customarily approached from the left side. Handlers should talk to the horse in calm, reassuring tones to alert it to their presence. This helps prevent a "startle" response, which could result in the horse jumping or kicking. It is wise to approach near the horse's shoulder because this is the location toward which the horse is least likely to be able to direct a kick or strike. Horses are customarily led from the left side, and the handler should remain on the left side of the horse unless the operator is working on the right side, in which case the handler should stand on the same side as the operator. The assistant should hold the horse on a short lead and remain attentive to the horse and operator throughout the procedure. A horse should not be tied unless it is accustomed to this and should never be tied during any procedure. Tying a horse for an examination or procedure increases the risk of injuring the horse should it panic. Owners or trainers may frequently tie their horses, but the veterinarian should not.

Use of the Chain Lead

Lead ropes with a chain affixed to the most proximal portion have many applications in restraint of horses. The chain may be placed over the nose, under the lower jaw, through the mouth, or over the upper incisors between the lip and teeth (Figure 5-2). One word of caution: some horses are unfamiliar with these forms of restraint, and their use may make the horse more unmanageable.

Lip or nose chains exert their effect by gentle, abrupt tugs on the lead that inflict pain and divert the horse's attention away from the operator. This method of restraint is used as negative reinforcement. The chain is given an abrupt tug (when the horse misbehaves) to punish the undesired

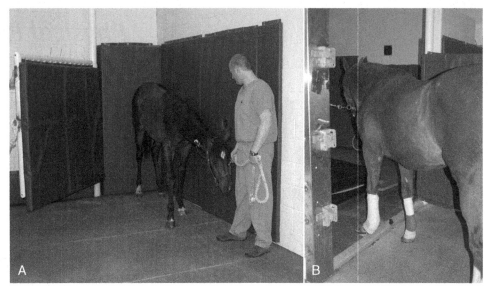

Figure 5–1. Secure footing is paramount when working with normal or sedated horses. **A,** Rough surfaced flooring in hallways and firm but compressible rubberized mats in anesthetic induction boxes are ideal. **B,** Note that the horse has been bathed and the limb to be operated on has been surgically prepared and completely bandaged before anesthesia. This minimizes contamination and total anesthesia time, respectively.

Box 5–1   **Methods of Restraint**
• Ropes
• Halters
• Lead shanks
• Hobbles
• Twitches
• Stockades
• Harnesses
• Slings

behavior. Chains should be used judiciously because they can injure the horse if used maliciously. A horse should never be tied with a chain. Lip and nose chains are useful for coaxing an unwilling horse into stocks, anesthetic induction stalls, or trailers. The horse is led forward with the chain in place over the nose or under the lip. The chain is tightened in an abrupt manner only if the horse attempts to back up. The pressure is released when the horse stops. Caution should be taken not to exert continuous pressure on the chain because this usually produces the opposite effect and causes the horse to resist more vigorously and flee the source of pain. Nose and lip chains are forms of negative reinforcement, and the chain should be tightened only in response to malicious or truly undesired behavior. Continuous pressure on the chain causes continuous pain and does not allow the horse to distinguish between acceptable and unacceptable behavior.

TWITCHES

Most twitches are fashioned from a strong wooden handle with either a chain or rope loop attached through the end (Figure 5-3, *A*). The so-called humane twitch is constructed of a pair of short aluminum rods hinged at the center, which may be tightened around the lip by a string and then clipped to the horse's halter (Figure 5-3, *B*). The humane twitch is no more or less humane than a conventional twitch, but many owners prefer its use. The humane twitch does have the advantage of being self-retaining, which frees the hands of the assistant. Many horses that object to conventional twitches do not readily recognize the humane twitch, making it easier to apply.

A twitch is applied by grasping the horse's upper lip, sliding the chain around the portion of the lip held, and twisting the chain tight. Twitches exert their beneficial effect by a combination of mechanisms. A twitch causes pain, which serves to distract the horse from the objectionable stimulus. In addition, the twitch may cause endorphin release from stimulation of acupuncture points located in the upper lip.[4] Gently tapping the twitch with a finger or shaking it further distracts the horse's attention from the procedure or operator. The twitch should not be applied until needed because its effect is attenuated with time. Furthermore, the handler should not overtighten the chain because this may lacerate the horse. The assistant holding the twitch should remain attentive and observe all other precautions because the twitch in no way incapacitates the horse.

Twitches customarily are applied to the upper lip but may also be used on the lower lip or the ear. If no twitch is available, it may suffice to grasp the lip with a firm hand grip, although this is not as secure or as efficacious (Figure 5-4, *A*).

Ear and shoulder twitches and grasping the lip can be used when restraint is needed for a brief period only. These forms of restraint are not usually as efficacious as a chain twitch applied to the upper lip but are adequate when temporary restraint is needed for an injection, venipuncture, suture removal, or short procedures. Both procedures are helpful in fractious horses when a chain twitch alone is inadequate. It may be necessary for an assistant to grasp an ear or the shoulder to enable another individual to apply a chain twitch to an apprehensive horse.

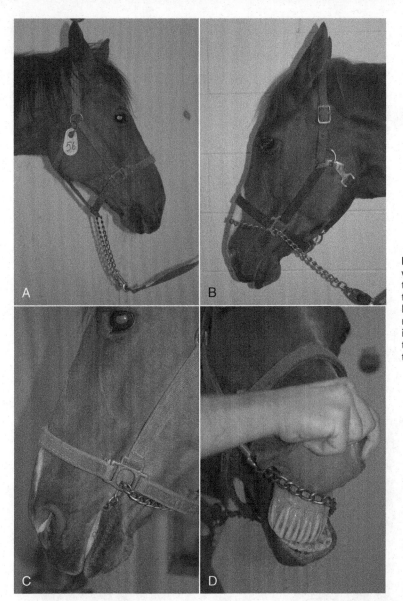

Figure 5–2. A, Horse with halter and lead shank. **B,** Horse with chain lead in place over the nose. Lead is clipped to the side ring on the halter. **C,** Horse with chain lead through the mouth. The lead is threaded through the side ring of the halter, through the mouth, and clipped to the opposite side ring of the halter. **D,** Horse with lip chain in place. The chain is passed through the side ring of the halter, threaded over the upper arcade, and clipped to the opposite side ring on the halter.

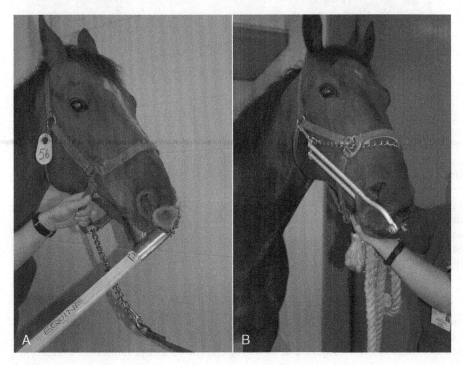

Figure 5–3. A, Proper application of the chain twitch. **B,** Humane twitch in use. The twitch may also be handheld.

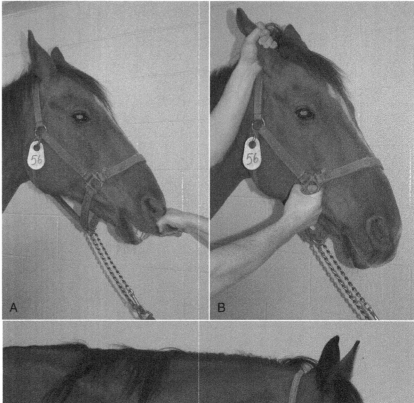

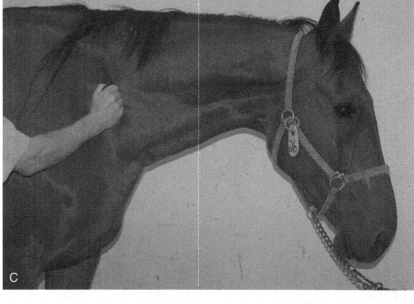

Figure 5–4. A, Hand twitch on the upper lip. The lip is grasped firmly and squeezed. **B,** Use of an ear twitch. The ear is twisted but not pulled down. The forearm of the arm twisting the ear can be used to keep the horse at a proper distance. **C,** Shoulder twitch. Note the chain lead in place.

The ear twitch is accomplished by grasping the ear and twisting it (Figure 5-4, *B*). The ear should not be pulled down as it is twisted because this may damage the nerves supplying motor function to the ear. Ear twitches inflict pain, which distracts the horse. Head-shy horses are not the best candidates for ear twitches because the benefits are outweighed by apprehension, making the horse more difficult to restrain. The shoulder twitch is performed by grasping the loose skin cranial to the scapula and rolling the skin into the fist by flexing the wrist (Figure 5-4, *C*). The technique is more efficacious in young horses.

PICKING UP A FOOT

Picking up a foot is often helpful for immobilizing a horse or when weight bearing on the contralateral limb is desired (Figure 5-5). This technique may be used in conjunction

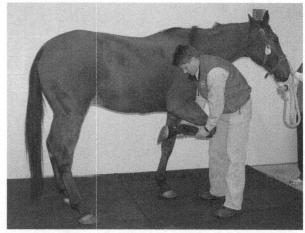

Figure 5–5. Picking up the right front foot to immobilize a horse.

with any of the previously described forms of restraint. Picking up a front or a hind foot forces the horse to stand on the other three limbs and eliminates some avoidance response to noxious stimuli. Raising a foot is used for regional anesthesia, suturing of lower leg wounds, arthrocentesis, and other procedures that require the limb to be stationary. Either the contralateral or the considered limb can be raised, depending on the situation and the procedure to be performed. The assistant holding the limb should be cautious of his or her own foot placement because sudden attempts by the horse to escape may cause the horse's foot to land forcefully on top of the handler's feet.

STOCKS

Stocks are used to confine the horse and produce a stationary patient (Figure 5-6). Stocks confine the horse's movement; they do not immobilize the limbs. Thus caution should be exercised when working near the limbs. Horses are capable of jumping over the front or side of stocks and can jump up and kick over the back door with both hind feet. Stocks present hazards not present when working on an unconfined horse. Persons working near stocks should be careful not to interpose arms or legs between the horse and the rigid frame or doors of the stocks.

If ropes are used to enclose the horse in stocks, they should be tied securely with knots that can be quickly untied ("quick release" slip knots) if the horse falls down or panics. Slip knots that can be untied with a single pull of the loose end are preferred (Figure 5-7).[2] An attentive assistant should remain at the horse's head throughout the procedure. Use of stocks reduces the number of assistants needed but does not eliminate their need. Putting cotton in

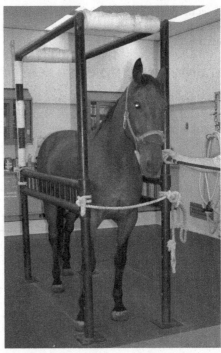

Figure 5–6. Horse in stock with an attendant (not shown) at the head. Ropes in front and back are tied with a quick-releasing slip knot.

some horses' ears makes them more manageable. If standing surgical procedures are performed in stocks, the horse usually requires a combination of sedation and application of a local anesthetic (see Chapters 10 and 11). If an epidural anesthetic is required, the horse's tail should be tied with a quick release knot, and the rope pulled over the back of the

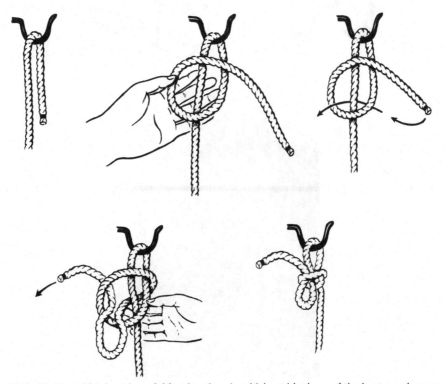

Figure 5–7. Slip knot. This knot is useful for situations in which rapid release of the knot may be necessary if the horse should panic.

stocks and secured to provide support if the horse becomes weak in the hind limbs. The tail rope may prevent the horse from falling down.

LEADING UNWILLING HORSES

Many horses are reluctant to follow where they are led. Changes in floor color or texture, doors, odors, sounds, unfamiliar equipment and smells, and confined spaces (induction stalls, stocks) can produce apprehension in a horse. As a general rule, confined spaces should be devoid of objects that may be dangerous or agitating to the horse. Usually gentle coaxing and reassurance by a confident handler are all that is required for patient compliance. Offering the horse grain, standing at a safe distance behind the horse and clapping, shaking a broom, or gesturing with a whip may get the horse to move. When appropriately used, lip or nose chains may achieve the desired effect (see Figure 5-2). Many horses can be backed into an area that they may not walk into because the horse's attention is diverted to the handler's pushing and its own foot placement instead of the avoided area.

Blindfolding and then circling the horse to disorient it may allow the handler to lead the horse into an objectionable area. The blindfold can be made from a towel tucked under the sides of the halter (Figure 5-8). The towel should be placed in such a manner that it may be hastily removed should the horse panic and try to escape.

Two assistants may be used to coax an unwilling horse by locking their arms behind the horse's rump and pushing (Figure 5-9). The assistants should be careful to stand to the side with only their arms behind the horse to minimize the chance of being kicked. This latter technique is reserved for horses that have shown no willingness to sit down or kick and should be abandoned after the first such attempt by the horse.

FOAL RESTRAINT

Foals generally are more easily restrained than adult horses because of their smaller size and comparatively lesser strength. Most foals have never been disciplined, and restraint is purely physical. Disciplinary devices such as lip or nose chains are not used because many foals will not respond to their use.

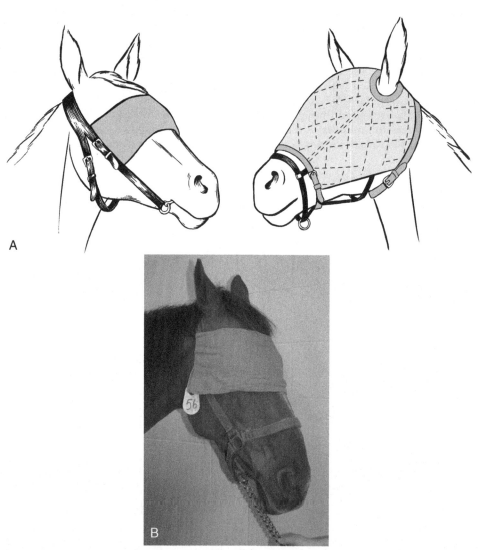

Figure 5–8. A, Horse with a blindfold in place. **B,** A simple blindfold consists of a towel tucked under the side band of the halter.

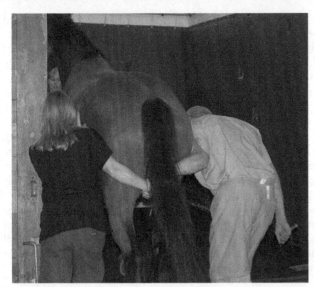

Figure 5–9. Assistants coaxing a horse into an induction stall. The arms are locked behind the horse, and the assistants attempt to remain at the horse's side.

Young foals may not be wearing a halter and do not respond well to it. The foal is caught as it walks around the mare. The holder cradles one arm under the foal's neck, and the other hand is used to grasp the tail. The tail is pulled up over the foal's back without twisting (Figure 5-10, *A*). Some foals may squat or refuse to bear weight on their rear legs when the tail is held. This problem can be corrected by decreasing the amount of pull on the tail. Shoulder twitches work well in foals. Holding the foal by both ears and exerting a steady upward pull serves to immobilize the foal similar to an ear twitch in an adult horse and removes the assistant's arm from under the neck, allowing access to the jugular veins for venipuncture (Figure 5-10, *B*). This latter technique is very effective. Another useful technique is to grasp the foal over its dorsum just cranial to the withers with one or both hands and squeeze (Figure 5-10, *C*). It may be more expedient to physically lay very active or resistant foals down and work from a more secure, controlled position (Figure 5-10, *D*).

Restraint of recumbent foals is indicated for some procedures. The assistant may accomplish this by placing a fore-

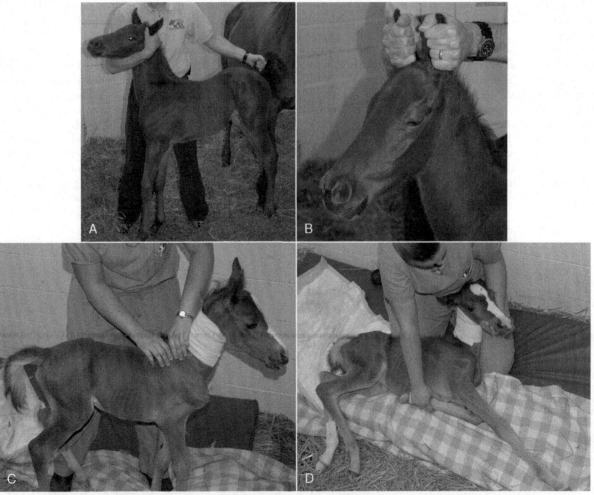

Figure 5–10. A, Proper restraint of a foal, with one hand holding the tail over the foal's back and the other arm cradled under the foal's neck. **B,** Holding the foal by the ears, the ears are pulled upward. An additional assistant may hold the foal's tail. This affords more restraint than other methods. **C,** Squeezing the foal over the dorsum cranial to the withers for standing restraint. **D,** Proper restraint of the recumbent foal. Holding the down leg prevents the foal from rolling into sternal recumbency. The other hand restrains the foal's head.

arm across the foal's neck and simultaneously holding the down front leg folded underneath the foal. By pulling up on the down leg, the handler prevents the foal from rolling into sternal recumbency and rising (see Figure 5-10, *D*).

Mares are often protective of their foals and become excited and anxious if they think the foal is being threatened. This protective behavior may be directed toward the attendants; the mare may unexpectedly bite or kick the attendants. An additional assistant is always required to restrain the mare, or the mare may be placed in stocks, and the foal restrained within view of the mare. Alternatively a "foal bed" can be placed in the doorway at the front of the stall and in full view of the mare. This allows the foal to be restrained and treated while the mare is able to observe. Sedation for the mare is indicated when the foal is removed from the mare's sight.

RESTRAINT FOR INDUCTION TO ANESTHESIA

Anesthetic drugs are administered to produce sedation, hypnosis, muscle relaxation, and analgesia rapidly, safely, and predictably. The horse can injure itself and bystanders if these conditions are not met. Such restraint is best accomplished by a swinging door with a rope in front to prevent the horse from falling forward (Figure 5-11, *left*). A minimum of two attendants are required. One attendant restrains the animal's head to prevent the horse from falling forward or backward or flailing on induction and injuring the head. The second attendant holds the rope in front of the horse and uses body weight against the door to contain the horse (Figure 5-11, *right*). Both assistants should remain alert and aware of their own and the horse's foot placement. The horse could panic and strike with its feet as it falls. The jugular catheter may be dislodged by the restraining rope if improperly secured. The attendants should be aware of this and allow the rope to loosen as the horse falls.

Many short term surgical procedures can be performed with the horse in its own stall (e.g., sternothyroid tenectomy). The stall should be examined carefully for any protruding objects such as eye hooks or nail heads and these should be removed. A tarp should be placed against the wall and on the floor to minimize debris and injury to the horse. The horse is placed parallel to a wall in the stall, and an assistant controls the head while the veterinarian administers the anesthetic drugs. When the horse begins to slump from the anesthetic, one assistant continues to control the head while two other assistants push the body of the horse against the wall. Generally the horse will slump backwards and into sternal recumbency. The horse is then pulled into position for surgery. In some horses it takes a few minutes for the anesthetic drugs to produce the relaxation required to allow moving the horse (Figure 5-12). Firm control of the head using a heavy leather halter and lead shank can be used during field procedures (Figure 5-13).

RESTRAINT DURING ANESTHESIA

Restraint during anesthesia may not be necessary if anesthetic depth is appropriate. The halter should be removed once the horse is recumbent to prevent damage to branches of the facial nerve. A small pillow can be placed under the horse's head to further prevent facial nerve damage (see Chapter 22).

Horses may wake up unexpectedly and begin paddling their limbs. Tying the front limbs helps to prevent the horse from injuring itself and contaminating the surgery site (Figure 5-14). Large-diameter soft cotton rope should be used. A tomfool knot is tied near the end of a rope with an eye and placed under the horse.[2] The loops of the tomfool knot are placed over each foot around the pastern of the horse and secured (see Figure 5-14). Tying horses in this fashion provides an extra handle around the horse's midsection for moving the horse during surgery. Care should be taken not to tie the rope too tight because this can restrict

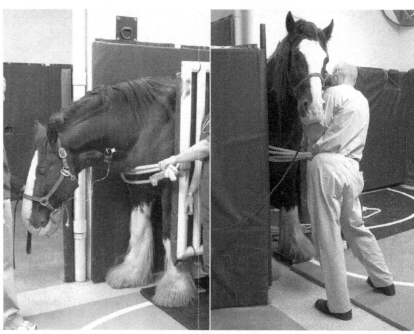

Figure 5-11. Horse restrained behind a swinging door for anesthetic induction. The assistant holding the horse's head (not shown) is the key to safe induction of anesthesia.

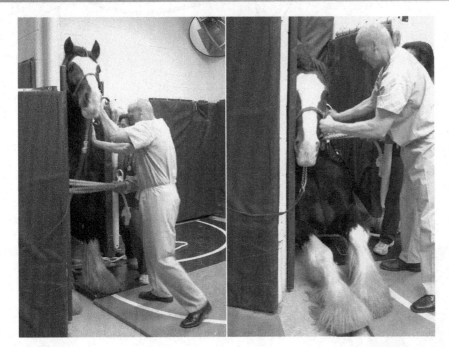

Figure 5–12. Anesthetic induction accomplished behind a swinging door. The assistant on the side restrains the horse's head and prevents the horse from falling backward or forward. The assistant holding the front rope keeps the horse contained behind the door. The front rope should be allowed to loosen as the horse falls to prevent dislodging the intravenous catheter.

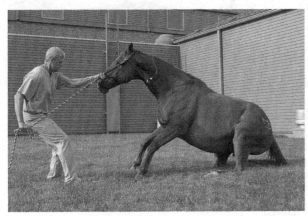

Figure 5–13. Field anesthesia.

breathing. It is not necessary to tie the rear legs. It is often tempting to pull the hind limbs caudally and tie them to prevent the horse from kicking should the anesthetic plane become inadequate. This should not be done because tying the rear legs in an extended position puts the horse at great risk for developing femoral nerve paralysis. Variations in positioning from lateral or dorsal recumbency may also create a need for special padding.

Occasionally the need to tie a horse's hind legs arises, such as during castration performed under intravenous anesthesia with the horse in lateral recumbency. To do so, the upper limb can be tied forward (Figure 5-15). A bowline on a bight knot (nonslip knot) is tied, using a long piece of soft cotton rope (Figure 5-16).[2] This creates a doubled loop of rope that fits over the horse's head and around the shoulders. The hind limb is pulled forward and tied to the loop of rope around the neck.[1,3] The loop of rope around the neck should be of sufficient diameter that it slides easily on the neck and does not occlude the jugular vein or airway at the

thoracic inlet. Other procedures may be performed during intravenous anesthesia with the horse in dorsal recumbency. An assistant can straddle the sternum of the horse. keeping it in dorsal recumbency and holding the folded forelimbs for very short procedures (e.g., sternothyroid tenectomy). The operator and the assistant straddling the horse need to be acutely aware that even a seemingly anesthetized horse can react adversely to pain by suddenly extending one or both of its forelimbs.

RESTRAINT DURING ANESTHETIC RECOVERY

The time period beginning with emergence from the effects of anesthesia to full standing recovery is when a horse is most likely to sustain serious injury.[5] Horses can be temporarily restrained during recovery by turning the head back along the neck (Figure 5-17). Semiconscious horses are easily controlled using this technique. Delaying the horse's attempts to roll to a sternal position and stand provides more time for drug elimination, thereby decreasing the severity of disorientation and ataxia when the horse does attempt to stand. Assisting the horse to a standing position during recovery from anesthesia can decrease the incidence of complications, particularly if the recovery stall flooring does not provide good traction (see Chapter 21).

Head and tail ropes can be used for helping horses to a standing position. A rope is tied to an appropriately fitted halter and to the tail (tail tie, sheet bend knot; Figure 5-18).[2] A soft cotton rope is less likely to burn the assistant's hands and should never be wrapped around the wrists or arms as the horse is helped to its feet. The head and tail ropes are threaded through rings placed high on the walls of the recovery stall (Figure 5-19). One or two persons pull on the tail rope as the horse attempts to stand. Tension is maintained on the ropes until the horse is able to support

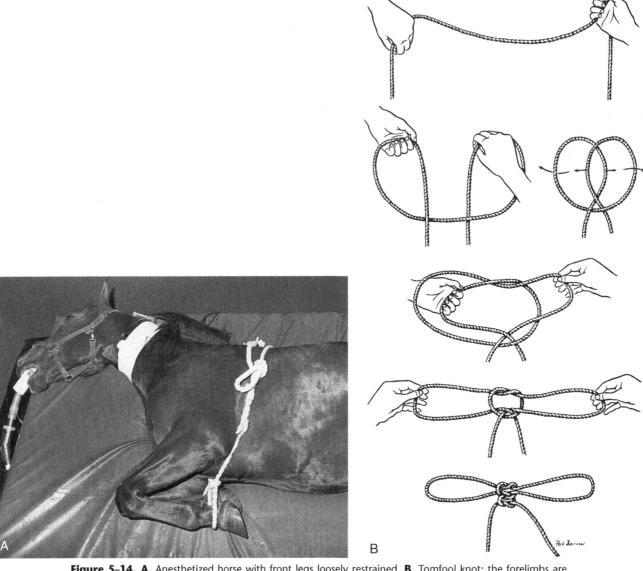

Figure 5–14. A, Anesthetized horse with front legs loosely restrained. **B,** Tomfool knot: the forelimbs are restrained using a tomfool knot. The two loops are placed over each front foot and secured around the pasterns. The ends of the rope are tied around the horse's girth to restrain the front legs.

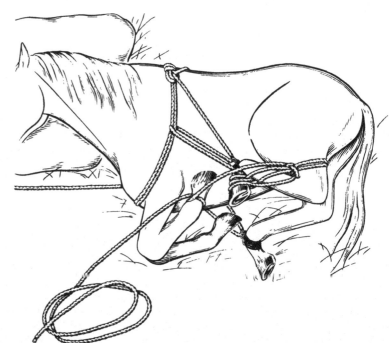

Figure 5–15. Illustration of a horse restrained as if for castration with the right hind leg tied forward. The knot is a bowline on a bight.

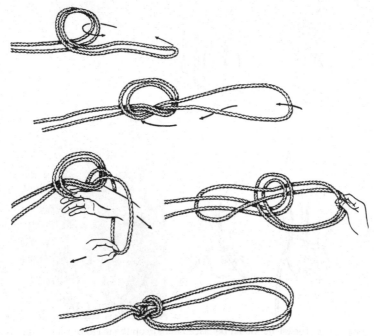

Figure 5–16. Bowline on a bight. This knot forms a doubled loop of rope to place around the horse's neck.

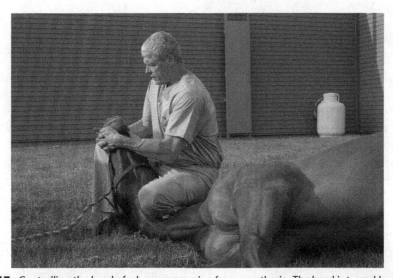

Figure 5–17. Controlling the head of a horse recovering from anesthesia. The head is turned back along the neck and held firmly. The assistant's knee is placed across the horse's neck for added restraint and balance.

its weight. The tail rope provides stability and helps to prevent the horse from falling or crashing into a wall. The head rope must be left loose while the horse is rolling into sternal recumbency because the horse requires unrestrained movement of its head for balance during this phase of recovery. The head rope is gradually tightened as the horse stands facing the wall of the recovery stall. If the horse loses its balance, the head rope may be tightened to prevent the horse from injuring its head. The ropes should remain on the horse, keeping it stationary until it can move with minimum ataxia. Horses are permitted to drink but not eat because of the possibility of pica and choke during this time. A muzzle

can be attached to the horse's halter and will ensure that the horse cannot eat bedding material or feed during this period (Figure 5-20).

Horses that have had short procedures performed that do not interfere with locomotion can recover on their own without assistance. These horses should not be encouraged to stand until they are ready. A towel can be placed over their eyes, the light reduced, and the area kept as silent as possible to minimize environmental stimulation that could stimulate the horse to stand. The towel will fall off when the horse first attempts to stand. Occasionally slings are used to assist recovery in horses that are unable to stand (see Chapter 21).

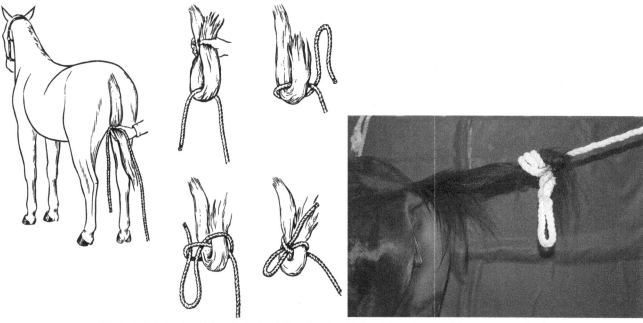

Figure 5–18. Tail tie in place. The tail tie should be placed as high on the tail as possible to prevent slipping. It is wise to test the security of the tie before the horse's recovery.

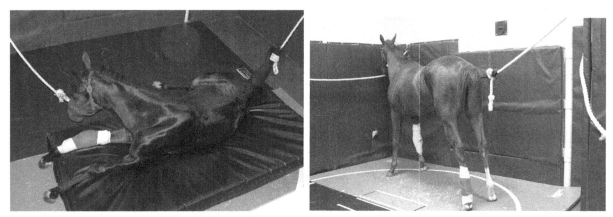

Figure 5–19. Horses restrained for anesthetic recovery with head and tail ropes.

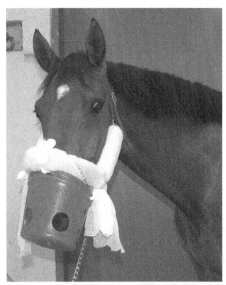

Figure 5–20. A simple plastic muzzle that clips to the halter is used to prevent the horse from eating hay or straw immediately before and after anesthesia.

REFERENCES

1. Frank ER: *Veterinary surgery*, ed 7, Minneapolis, 1964, Burgess Publishing, pp 13-38.
2. Leahy JR, Barrow P: *Restraint of animals*, ed 2, Ithaca, NY, 1953, Cornell Campus Store, pp 38-85.
3. Vaughn JT, Allen R: Physical and chemical restraint. In Mansmann RA, McAllister ES, Pratt PW, editors: *Equine medicine and surgery*, ed 3, vol 1, Santa Barbara, Ca, 1982, American Veterinary Publishers, pp 219-226.
4. Lagerweij E et al: The twitch in horses: a variant of acupuncture, *Science* 225:1172-1174, 1984.
5. Bidwell LA, Bramlage LR, Rood WA: Equine perioperative fatalities associated with general anaesthesia at a private practice—a retrospective case series, *Vet Anaesth Analg* 34:23-30, 2007.

6

Preoperative Evaluation: General Considerations

James T. Robertson

Claire Scicluna

KEY POINTS

1. A thorough evaluation of the history, signalment, physical condition, past and current medications, and the anticipated type and duration of anesthesia/surgery to be performed should be completed and documented before preparing for anesthesia.
2. The owner/agent should be informed and consent in writing to the risks associated with anesthesia and surgery.
3. The physical examination should emphasize neurologic, musculoskeletal, cardiovascular, and respiratory function.
4. Laboratory tests are supplemental and should be tailored to the results of the history and physical examination. A hemogram, including packed cell volume (PCV) and total protein, should be performed on all horses before surgery. Additional ancillary tests should be considered as needed.
5. A systematized, standardized, and prioritized protocol (standard operating procedure) should be developed for the evaluation, preparation, and conduct of anesthesia and recovery.
6. The maxim, "If it wasn't written down, it didn't happen," is a valuable admonition.

HISTORY

A detailed, accurate history should be considered an essential part of a preoperative evaluation (Box 6-1). In retrospect, lack of a complete history looms as a serious omission when a horse develops a postoperative problem related to a preexisting condition. A horse's previous and current diseases, medications, or previous anesthetic experiences may be difficult to obtain. The owner may have little knowledge of the horse's medical history, and information elicited from the trainer or groom is usually from memory and not documented. Important facts are often forgotten or overlooked. If a racehorse has been claimed recently, the medical history may be unknown or vague at best. Previous disease conditions take on significance when their residual effects compromise the horse while under anesthesia or become exacerbated as a result of the stress of anesthesia and recovery (see Chapters 4 and 22).

A special effort should be made to detect horses with chronic lung infection or cardiovascular disease. Frequently these horses have a history of poor performance. Exercise intolerance or reduced appetite may be the only clinical sign of lung or heart disease. Although horses that have minimum airway or lung disease may not pose an anesthetic management problem, they are at higher risk for developing postoperative complications, including pleuritis and pleuropneumonia. A horse with a history of pleuropneumonia should be auscultated carefully using a rebreathing bag and have radiographic and ultrasound examinations of the chest for evidence of lung consolidation or abscessation and pleural fluid accumulation (Figure 6-1). The owner and insurance carrier should be made aware of the increased risks. If significant abnormalities are discovered and the horse must be anesthetized, broad-spectrum antibiotic treatment should start the day before the procedure and continue for 5 days. Horses with a history of recent respiratory infection should be allowed at least 3 weeks' convalescence before general anesthesia is considered again.

Horses with myocarditis may have atrial or ventricular rhythm disturbances that increase anesthetic risks. Horses with a history or physical findings of a cardiac rhythm disturbance or heart murmur should be auscultated carefully and have preoperative electrocardiogram and echocardiographic examinations performed (see Chapter 3).

Horses that have a history of recurrent episodes of exertional rhabdomyolysis may be at higher risk for developing postoperative myositis. A preoperative serum chemistry screen for elevated muscle enzymes, creatinine phosphokinase, and serum glutamate oxaloacetate transaminase aid in diagnosis (see Laboratory Tests). Preoperative administration of dantrolene sodium may help prevent postoperative myositis in some horses.[1] The history should include pertinent information regarding previous drug therapy and whether the horse had adverse reactions or sensitivity to medication. Penicillin is the most likely antibiotic to produce an adverse reaction in horses. Signs can range from mild (head shaking, hyperactivity) to severe (falling down, seizures) and can be potentially fatal. No form of penicillin should be administered to a horse with a history of a penicillin reaction. Sedatives or tranquilizers that have previously produced an unexpected response (excitement for example) should be avoided.

Hyperkalemic periodic paralysis (HYPP), a rare syndrome in Quarter Horses that produces intermittent episodes of muscle weakness or collapse, can be provoked by perioperative medications and the stress of anesthesia (see Chapter 22). Horses with HYPP should be medicated before anesthesia to reduce the chance of a hyperkalemic episode (see Chapter 22). Most horses with HYPP can be identified before surgery by obtaining a complete history, performing a blood test that confirms that the horse is carrying the defective gene that causes the disease, and identifying myopathy based on electromyography and in vitro muscle electrode studies.[2]

| Box 6–1 | **Preoperative Considerations** |

- History (disease, drugs, reactions, surgery)
- Signalment
- Physical status
- Attitude, behavior
- Current medications
- Special considerations (e.g., lame, pregnant, recumbent)
- Technical help
- Facilities
- Equipment

Occasionally a performance horse has been administered a substance that is forbidden by the rules of racing or showing, and the owner or trainer is reluctant to divulge this information. This is likely of little consequence in healthy horses presented for elective surgical procedures. However, the effects of the unknown drug may take on greater significance in highly stressed, fatigued, or sick horses that must undergo emergency surgery. It is difficult to control racehorses with sedatives and analgesics if they have suffered a severe orthopedic injury and may have been administered an illegal stimulant; and they are at greater risk for developing cardiovascular complications during induction and maintenance of anesthesia because of the arrhythmogenic effects of high concentrations of endogenous catecholamines and the effects of anesthetic drugs (see Chapter 22).

The medical and anesthetic record of a horse that has been anesthetized previously should be retrieved and reviewed carefully for any undesirable responses during induction, maintenance, or recovery from anesthesia (see Chapter 8).

PHYSICAL EXAMINATION

A thorough physical examination should be performed before general anesthesia (Table 6-1). All body systems should be examined. The axiom that "for every mistake that is made for not knowing, many more are made for not looking" applies. The physical examination is best performed in a quiet environment after the horse has become accustomed to its surroundings. Special attention should be paid to the cardiovascular and respiratory systems. The weight of the horse should be recorded to facilitate calculation of dosages of anesthetic drugs (see Figure 6-1). Methods of estimating body weight (Box 6-2) for horses are based on heart girth, height at the withers, and length (Figures 6-2 and 6-3).[3,4] Emaciation or obesity must be taken into consideration when determining

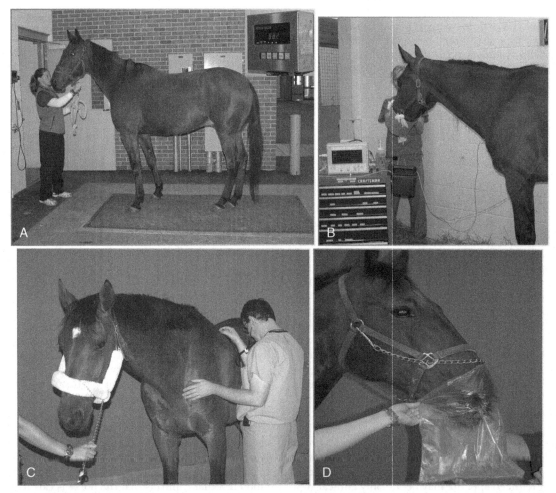

Figure 6–1. Preoperative evaluation of the surgical patient. **A,** Digital scale for determining the horse's weight. **B,** Base-apex electrocardiogram. **C,** Auscultation of heart and lungs. **D,** "Bagging" the horse before thoracic auscultation to initiate larger tidal volumes.

Table 6–1. Physical findings in normal horses and foals

	Adult	Foal
Temperature (° F)	99.5-101.0	100.5-101.5
Temperature (° C)	37.0-38.0	37.5-38.5
Pulse (beats/min)	30-45	50-70
Respiration (breaths/min)	8-20	15-30

Box 6–2 Formulas for Estimating Body Weight of Horses

$$\text{Body w (lb)} = \frac{\text{Heart girth (in)}^2 \times \text{length (in)}}{241}$$

$$\text{Body w (kg)} = \frac{\text{Heart girth (cm)}^2 \times \text{length (cm)}}{8717}$$

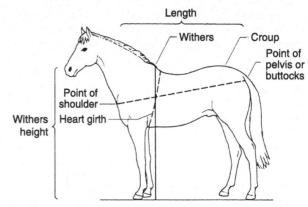

Figure 6–3. Linear body measurements used in estimating body weight of horses and ponies. (From Frape DL: *Equine nutrition and feeding*, ed 3, Oxford & ames, Iowa, 2004, Blackwell Publishing & Iowa State University Press.)

drug dosages. Heavy draft horses tend to require lower doses of sedative and anesthetic drugs on a dose/weight basis. Temperament, age, breed, and surgical procedure should be considered when determining drug dosages.

A horse's temperament, response to physical interaction, and overall body condition can be assessed by visual inspection at the onset of the physical examination. Some horses are tranquilized before transport and may be depressed for a few hours after arrival. Healthy horses are usually alert and responsive and often become nervous or apprehensive during the initial stages of the examination. Horses that are ill, dehydrated, debilitated, or in pain are frequently depressed. Horses presented for elective surgical procedures that appear depressed should be

examined and scrutinized closely for signs of impending illness that could be stress-related (Box 6-3).

A horse's heart rate and temperature are often elevated to above 40 beats/min and 101° F (38° C) after transport, particularly on a hot day. The temperature should return to normal by the following morning in healthy adult horses. A temperature of 101° F (38° C) or greater should be considered elevated in adult horses and should result in patient reevaluation and postponement of elective procedures requiring general anesthesia. Foals tend to have a slightly higher normal temperature range than adults (up to 101.5° F or 38.5° C).

The cardiovascular system can be assessed initially by palpating the facial artery pulse, observing the color of the oral mucous membranes, estimating capillary refill time, and checking skin elasticity. Palpation of the facial artery pulse provides an estimate of heart rate and indicates cardiac rhythm abnormalities. The strength of the pulse is related to the force of myocardial contraction, cardiac valve competency, and vascular fluid volume. Mucous membrane color is an index of the tissue perfusion and oxygen-carrying capacity of the blood. The oral mucous membranes are pink and moist in a healthy horse, and capillary refill should be less than 2.5 sec. A prolonged capillary refill time indicates a poor tissue perfusion and suggests decreased cardiac output, hypotension, reduced vascular volume, or an increase in peripheral vascular resistance. Both jugular veins should be checked for patency. A jugular vein that is difficult to raise or that feels thickened or thrombosed should not be used for venipuncture or catheterization.

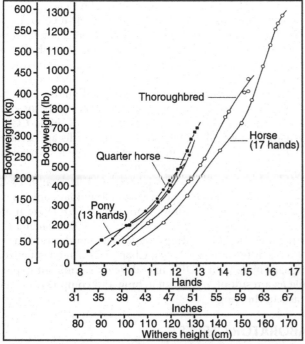

Figure 6–2. Relationship between body weight and withers height in normally growing horses and ponies (1 hand = 10.16cm). (From Frape DL: *Equine nutrition and feeding*, ed 3, Oxford & Ames, Iowa, 2004, Blackwell Publishing & Iowa State University Press.)

Box 6–3 Signs of Disease

- Depression
- Sweating at rest (unless weather is very hot)
- Rapid respiration when at rest, coughing
- Not eating or drinking
- Weight loss
- Poor hair coat
- Spending too much time lying down
- Lying in an abnormal position
- Displaying unusual posture or stretching (e.g., carrying most of the weight on hind legs)
- Shifting weight
- Reluctant to move
- Deviating from usual personality or behavior

The heart should be auscultated from both sides of the chest to determine heart rate and to detect the presence of murmurs or cardiac rhythm disturbances (see Chapter 3). Heart rate will range from 30 to 45 beats/min or less in healthy adult horses. An electrocardiogram should be performed on all horses before anesthesia, and a representative electrocardiogram should be preserved in the medical record (see Figure 6-1).

The respiratory rate, pattern of breathing, and respiratory effort should be observed when the horse is relaxed (see Table 6-1).[5] Body mass, thoracic dimensions, and body shape influence PaO_2 in anesthetized horses and ponies.[5a,5b] Pulmonary auscultation is best performed in a quiet room or stall. The horse should be made to breathe deeply by manual occlusion of the nostrils or by placing a rebreathing bag over the nose during auscultation (see Figure 6-1). Deep breathing increases the flow velocity and accentuates the lung sounds, making it much easier to evaluate breath sounds. Normal breath sounds are loudest on inspiration over the ventral portions of the lung and quietest over the diaphragmatic region. Abnormal lung sounds are produced by pathological changes in the lung. High-pitched wheezes can be heard during inspiration, particularly end inspiration, in horses with bronchopneumonia or chronic obstructive pulmonary disease (COPD). Abnormal lung sounds necessitate a complete lung evaluation to avoid anesthesia-associated exacerbation of pulmonary disease. Pleuritis produces pleural friction rubs and an absence of breath sounds if pleural fluid has accumulated. Lung consolidation produces increased bronchial sounds, which approximate the sounds heard over the trachea.[6] Deep breathing can induce coughing in a horse with tracheobronchial inflammation. Tracheal auscultation may reveal abnormal sounds if there is abundant tracheal mucus, and a tracheal squeeze is likely to induce a cough in a horse with a tracheitis. External palpation of the pharynx also produces a cough in horses with active pharyngitis. A horse with an active respiratory tract infection frequently has an elevated white blood cell (WBC) count and plasma fibrinogen concentration.

Thoracic radiography and scanning ultrasonography generally are performed before surgery on horses when lung sounds are abnormal, when the lungs are difficult to auscultate, or when there is a history or risk of developing pleuropneumonia or pleuritis. Radiographs are used to assess the pulmonary parenchyma for evidence of consolidation and abscessation and to assess the pleural cavity for fluid accumulation. Lung radiographs should be evaluated carefully by experienced individuals and not overinterpreted because almost all racehorses, even 2-year-olds, have a mild degree of diffuse, increased interstitial density and peribronchiolar infiltrates. Diagnostic ultrasonography is used to detect pleural fluid, fibrin formation in the pleural spaces, pleural thickening, adhesions, and lung consolidation. Pulmonary abscesses that extend to the lung surface can also be detected. Ultrasound scanning is useful for demonstrating small areas of lung consolidation at the surface of the lung, roughened visceral pleural surfaces, and low levels of pleural fluid accumulation in asymptomatic horses. These findings represent either a resolving inflammatory process or an active low-grade inflammation that is undetectable by physical examination.[7]

Two types of clinical scenarios are likely to present in horses with occult yet active respiratory infection: horses less than 1 year of age that have not been closely observed before transportation; and horses, particularly race horses (Thoroughbreds), that have been transported long distances. Horses that have been transported long distances should be examined carefully; and, if there is any suspicion of respiratory disease, they should be observed for a few days before a decision is made to anesthetize them. Horses incubating a respiratory infection may have a serous, ocular, or nasal discharge; increased respiratory rate; fever; submandibular lymphadenopathy; and increased lung sounds. Thoracic radiographs and ultrasonography performed in the early stages of a respiratory infection are often normal. Outbreaks of the neurologic form of equine herpes virus (EHV-1) are highly contagious and often fatal. Horses that have a fever, cough, and nasal discharge should be tested for the EHV-1 infection and dealt with according to the biosecurity guidelines of the individual hospital. Horses that have had a history of upper respiratory tract infection and start to show weakness, ataxia, or urinary incontinence should be isolated immediately from the main hospital population. Elective procedures should be postponed for at least 4 weeks after complete remission of signs of respiratory disease in horses that have a viral or bacterial respiratory tract infection. The added stress of anesthesia and surgery in sick or convalescing horses predisposes them to pleuropneumonia and pleuritis.

Some horses have chronic, low-grade bronchial infections that can be exacerbated by general anesthesia and surgery, particularly if invasive upper respiratory tract procedures are performed and the horse aspirates blood. The owner or trainer may relate a history of respiratory tract infection or recurring episodes of "throat infection," but most horses are asymptomatic. The diagnosis is made on the basis of the history, auscultation of the lung and upper airway, and observation of mucopurulent exudate in the trachea during a preoperative endoscopic examination. Occasionally these horses have abnormal inspiratory sounds in the cranial ventral lung fields. The abnormal lung sounds are often subtle enough to be missed on auscultation, particularly if the horse is not made to breathe deeply. A complete blood count (CBC) and thoracic radiographs may be within the normal range. A tracheobronchial aspirate should be obtained for cytologic and microbiologic examination. *Streptococcus* spp. and *Actinobacillus* spp. are frequently cultured. A positive bacterial culture necessitates antibiotic treatment for at least 3 days before an elective anesthetic procedure. A diagnosis of low-grade COPD ("heaves") is made if the bacterial culture results are negative and the cytologic findings are supportive. There is no need for preoperative antibiotic treatment in these horses.

Older horses with more advanced COPD exhibit expiratory dyspnea with an exaggerated abdominal component (lift) during quiet breathing. Horses with COPD are more likely to develop ventilation-perfusion ($\dot{V}/\dot{Q}$) mismatching during anesthesia, resulting in a lower than desirable arterial oxygen tension (PaO_2; see Chapter 2). An anesthetized pregnant mare with COPD may develop significant hypoxemia as a result of $\dot{V}/\dot{Q}$ mismatching and compression atelectasis of the lung.

LABORATORY TESTS

A CBC and total plasma protein determination should be performed on all horses before general anesthesia (Table 6-2). Blood should be obtained when the horse is relaxed because

Table 6–2. Normal hematologic values in the adult horse

	Normal range	Interpretation
Packed cell volume (%)	32-52	Increase: splenic contraction, dehydration Decrease: anemia/blood loss
Total plasma protein (g/dl)	6.0-8.5	Increase: dehydration Decrease: blood loss, gastrointestinal or renal loss
Fibrinogen (mg/dl)	100-400	Increase: acute or chronic infection, dehydration
Total white blood cell count (WBC/μl)	5,500-12,500	Increase: stress, infections Decrease: extreme demand—enteritis

excitement produces marked elevation in PCV as a result of splenic contraction.

The normal range for PCV in adult hot-blooded horses is 32% to 52%; PCV in cold-blooded horses ranges from 24% to 44%.[8] Chronic blood loss such as that encountered from an ethmoid hematoma or a bleeding intestinal ulcer causes a progressive decrease in PCV. Severe blood loss produces a rapid heart rate and pale mucous membranes. The volume of blood lost can be estimated by assessing the PCV deficit, although the PCV may not accurately reflect the magnitude of blood loss following acute surgical blood loss because of inadequate time for body fluids (interstitial) to reequilibrate and the effects of anesthesia. Acute blood loss usually cannot be assessed until 24 to 48 hours after hemorrhage.[9]

Both PCV and total protein are elevated in horses that are dehydrated. Horses in severe pain can become dehydrated as a result of decreased water intake and sweating. Gastrointestinal diseases that cause obstruction or diarrhea can produce severe fluid and electrolyte loss, elevated PCV, and acid-base disturbances. Attempts should be made to correct vascular (blood, plasma) volume deficits, electrolyte disturbances, pH, and blood gas (PaO_2, $PaCO_2$) abnormalities before anesthetizing horses that require emergency surgery. By contrast, generalized dehydration requires 18 to 24 hours to be corrected. The PCV should be lowered to below 50% to prevent blood sludging and achieve adequate tissue perfusion before anesthesia.[10]

Normal total plasma protein values range from 6 to 8.5 g/dl in normal horses.[8] Plasma or hetastarch can be administered before surgery to increase vascular oncotic pressure in horses with an adequate PCV, but the plasma protein level may drop to below 3.5 g/dl as a result of a severe inflammatory condition (peritonitis, pleuritis, protein-losing enteropathy). Continued protein loss in combination with crystalloid fluid therapy (endotoxemia) predisposes the horse to hypoproteinema, pulmonary edema, and $\dot{V}/\dot{Q}$ mismatch.

Elevated total protein concentration in a horse that is not dehydrated can be caused by a high globulin fraction resulting from chronic infection. These horses generally have a history of fever and an elevated white blood cell count, and they frequently demonstrate an increased plasma fibrinogen (>300 mg/dl). Plasma fibrinogen concentration is elevated in horses with inflammatory, neoplastic, and traumatic disorders.[11]

The WBC count (leukogram) of most horses should be within a range of 5,500 to 12,500 in healthy horses but typically reflects a mild leukocytosis, neutrophilia, and lymphopenia, indicative of the stress and excitement associated with transportation and hospitalization.[8] Foals generally exhibit more of a physiologic leukocytosis in response to stress than adults.[11] The stress leukogram is more elevated in painful or injured horses. Values outside the normal WBC count range or an abnormal differential count should be evaluated carefully before anesthetizing any horse. Leukocytosis and marked neutrophilia suggest the presence of an infection and may occur before a fever develops. Leukopenia and marked neutropenia with a left shift (immature cells) are associated with severe gastrointestinal disease such as salmonellosis or endotoxemia. Elective surgery should be postponed in horses that have an abnormal WBC count, fever (>101° F, 38° C) or both. Occasionally horses with a WBC count that is consistently on the low or high end of normal are encountered. Surgery is reconsidered in 1 to 2 days if the horse remains afebrile and appears healthy on repeated physical examinations. It is not necessary to obtain a complete preoperative blood chemistry profile in healthy, elective surgical patients unless there is some specific indication (Table 6-3).

Complete blood chemistry profiles are performed routinely on all horses that are sick. Total protein and serum electrolyte values, specifically Na, K, Cl, and Ca, should be determined in dehydrated horses before anesthesia

Table 6–3. Serum chemistry values in the adult horse[17]

Blood urea nitrogen	10-25 mg/dl
Creatinine	1-2.4 mg/dl
Glucose	70-130 mg/dl
Total bilirubin	1-5 mg/dl
Cholesterol	100-189 mg/dl
Alkaline phosphatase	84-128 U/L
SGOT	157-253 U/L
Lactic dehydrogenase	100-191 U/L
Creatine phosphokinase	97-188 U/L
Sorbitol dehydrogenase	1-6 U/L
Sodium	130-143 mEq/L
Chloride	98-109 mEq/L
Potassium	2.2-4.1 mEq/L
Calcium	10.3-13.3 mg/dl

SGOT, Serum glutamic oxaloacetic transaminase.

because serious electrolyte disturbances can contribute to the development of muscle weakness, cardiac rhythm disorders, and acid-base disturbances during anesthesia that can lead to postoperative weakness during recovery. Horses that have been fasted for at least 12 hours in preparation for anesthesia generally have increased plasma bilirubin concentrations as a result of decreased bilirubin excretion.[11]

ANESTHETIC RISK AND PHYSICAL STATUS

Although anesthetic risk, operative risk, and the physical status of the horse are interrelated, they are not the same.[12] The knowledge and skill of the anesthetist, the type of anesthetic drugs used, and the duration of anesthesia are factors to consider when determining anesthetic risk (see Chapter 22). Operative risk takes into consideration anesthetic risk, physical status, the skill of the surgeon, and the type of surgical procedure. The physical status of the patient can be categorized, and generally there is a correlation between the horse's physical status and increased morbidity and mortality (Table 6-4). Physical rating systems are useful when planning anesthetic management and determining prognosis. There is less margin for error in horses that have an American Society of Anesthesiologists category of III or greater (see Table 6-4).

PREOPERATIVE CONSIDERATIONS ASSOCIATED WITH SPECIFIC CONDITIONS OR DISEASES

Colic

Horses with colic from strangulating obstructions represent one of the greatest anesthetic risks encountered. Numerous factors, including hypovolemia, acid-base and electrolyte disturbances, endotoxemia, metabolic acidosis, and abdominal distention, contribute to serious cardiovascular and respiratory compromise.

Pain relief is the first preoperative consideration in most instances. Repeated doses of α_2-agonists (xylazine, detomidine, romifidine) as needed may be useful for control of pain (see Chapter 10). The analgesia produced by xylazine may last only 10 to 15 minutes in horses with severe pain. α_2-agonists may produce increases in arterial blood pressure followed by hypotension, second-degree heart block,

and ileus but produce safe and effective preanesthetic analgesia. Xylazine can be administered repeatedly and is used as an indicator of when to perform surgery in horses with unresponsive unrelenting colic. A combination of xylazine and butorphanol provides analgesia and is safe as a preanesthetic (see Chapter 10). Most colic patients have received some type of nonsteroidal antiinflammatory drug (NSAID) such as flunixin meglumine before arriving at a surgical facility. Some horses that have received repeated doses and have been overdosed may no longer show signs of abdominal pain but are depressed, even in the face of a strangulating bowel lesion. The serum creatinine concentration should be determined in horses referred for colic surgery that have a history of multiple treatments (α_2-agonists; NSAIDs) to assess renal function.

A nasogastric tube should be placed and secured before producing anesthesia to allow gastric decompression, which relieves gastric distention and pain and prevents gastric rupture. There is also less likelihood of nasogastric reflux and potential aspiration of stomach contents during induction to anesthesia after decompression. The nasogastric tube should be as large (inside diameter) as possible, sutured to the nostril or affixed to the halter, and kept in place during anesthesia, even if there is little or no reflux of fluid.

A large-diameter sterile catheter should be placed in the jugular vein for fluid administration (see Chapter 7). The objective of preoperative fluid therapy is rapid correction of volume deficits and normalization of electrolyte and acid-base abnormalities. Fluid requirements are guided by heart rate, mucous membrane color, capillary refill time, PCV, total plasma protein, and arterial blood pressure (see Chapter 8). The PCV and total protein values may range from 45% to >60% and 7 to >9 g/dl, respectively, with mild-to-severe dehydration. The fluid volume deficit represents about 4% of the body weight in mild dehydration and 10% or greater with severe dehydration. The deficit can range from 18 to >45 L of fluid in a 450-kg horse. Attempts should be made to lower the PCV below 50% before anesthesia by rapid fluid (balanced electrolyte solution) replacement. If the total plasma protein falls below 3.5 g/dl, the rate of fluid administration should be decreased.

Most horses with strangulating obstruction of the bowel have metabolic acidosis. Although it may not be possible to normalize blood pH, the arterial pH (pHa) should be maintained above 7.2. A pHa below 7.2 with a normal or decreased $PaCO_2$ suggests significant nonrespiratory acidosis and can interfere with tissue metabolism and myocardial contractility and the response of the myocardium to supportive catecholamines (see Chapter 23).[13] Not all horses with surgical colic have nonrespiratory metabolic acidosis. Some horses with large colon displacements and nonstrangulating large bowel obstructions and those with duodenal obstruction may have a hypochloremic metabolic alkalosis. The electrolyte disturbances associated with a strangulating obstruction are usually relatively mild because of isotonic fluid loss. Serum sodium, potassium, chloride, and calcium values are determined routinely in most colic patients. If possible, the ionized fraction of the total serum calcium should be determined to assess the biologically active calcium deficit.[14] Hypokalemia and hypocalcemia both can contribute to the development of hypotension

Category	Description
I	Healthy patient
II	Mild systemic disease: no functional limitation
III	Severe systemic disease: definite functional limitation
IV	Severe systemic disease that is a constant threat to life
V	Moribund patient unlikely to survive 24 hr with or without operation

Table 6–4. **American Society of Anesthesiologists (ASA) physical status classification**

and dysrhythmias under anesthesia, and serious deficits (K^+ <3 mEq/L) should be corrected before induction to anesthesia.[15]

Distended large intestine can produce bloat, which causes severe respiratory and hemodynamic compromise as a result of pressure on the diaphragm and circulatory compromise as a result of reduced venous return. Every effort should be made to decompress a horse with abdominal distention before producing anesthesia. Using simultaneous auscultation and percussion, the gas-filled bowel, usually the cecum, can be identified and decompressed using a 6-inch, 14-gauge needle inserted through the right flank. This procedure can result in some leakage of bowel contents with peritoneal contamination; thus the procedure should be limited to emergency situations with severe distention. Horses with severe abdominal distention should not be ventilated mechanically until decompressed unless they are apneic. The veterinary surgeon must be prepared to provide positive-pressure ventilation to ensure adequate ventilation during surgery.

Prophylactic antibiotics should always be administered before colic surgery. Peritoneal contamination can result from bowel trocharization, paracentesis, leakage of bacteria from devitalized bowel, intestinal resection and anastomosis, enterotomy, needle punctures of the intestine for decompression, and breaks in sterile technique. Other sites of potential sepsis include the catheterized jugular veins and the lungs as a result of aspiration of gastric reflux before or during surgery. Broad-spectrum antibiotics effective against both aerobic and anaerobic bacteria are indicated. Penicillin (20,000 U/kg intramuscularly [IM]) and gentamicin (0.8 mg/lb IM) are commonly selected for prophylactic therapy. Although gentamicin has the potential to enhance neuromuscular blockade and cardiovascular depression, particularly in anesthetized horses, this problem is rare unless peripheral neuromuscular blocking drugs (e.g., atracurium) are used during anesthesia (see Chapter 19).

Uroperitoneum

Foals with uroperitoneum (most commonly from a ruptured bladder) become progressively hyperkalemic, hyponatremic, hypochloremic, and acidotic. Serious hypotension and potentially fatal arrhythmias can develop before or during anesthesia because the hyperkalemia potentiates vasodilation and the cardiotoxicity of anesthetic drugs.[15] Before surgery every effort should be made to restore circulating blood volume, correct electrolyte abnormalities (hyponatremia, hyperkalemia), and decrease abdominal pressure. A cannula or peritoneal dialysis catheter can be placed into the abdominal cavity to drain urine while NaCl is given intravenously to elevate the serum sodium and chloride and lower potassium. The serum potassium should be decreased significantly (i.e., from >7 mEq/L to ≤6 mEq/L) before the foal is anesthetized. Insulin and glucose can be added to the intravenous fluids to lower the serum potassium level.[15]

Pleural fluid accumulation, possibly as a result of extravasation of urine across the diaphragm, is a common finding in foals with uroperitoneum of prolonged duration. Thoracic radiographs help to determine if there is a significant accumulation of pleural fluid and the need to perform pleurocentesis and drainage before and during anesthesia. The foal should be placed on controlled mechanical ventilation.

Orthopedic Injuries

Horses that have serious orthopedic trauma such as a long bone fracture or other breakdown injuries are stressed and painful. The horse may have and should be treated with various combinations of sedative or analgesic drugs. Every effort should be made to provide adequate fracture stabilization by bandaging, splinting, or casting the injured limb before and during anesthetic induction. Anesthesia and surgical repair should be delayed while intravenous fluids and analgesic drugs are administered if the horse is in great distress or showing signs of shock. There is minimum likelihood of further injury at the fracture site during induction of anesthesia, regardless of the method used (most fractures occur during recovery from anesthesia), if the fracture has been stabilized adequately, and appropriate drugs are used in a controlled environment (see Chapter 24). There may be some benefit in using a technique in which the horse does not slump or fall to the ground if the fracture is located above the carpus or hock where it is impossible to cast or splint and bandage securely. This can be accomplished by inducing the horse in a standing position while suspended in a sling or securing the horse in a standing position to a tilt table (see Chapter 16). If applicable, a standing preparation of the surgical site can significantly reduce anesthesia time. Every effort should be made to prevent the horse from falling on the injured limb. however, it is possible for a horse to complete a long bone stress fracture located above the hock or carpus during the induction process.

A horse with a comminuted pelvic fracture is at risk of having the internal iliac artery severed by a sharp bone fragment. Although pelvic radiographs might be useful for evaluating the fracture, the diagnosis generally can be made by rectal examination. Anesthesia is contraindicated in these horses because there is no surgical treatment and there is a great risk associated with induction and recovery. Similarly, if a horse is suspected of having a spinal fracture and is still standing, anesthesia should not be performed.

Injuries or Diseases Causing Blood Loss

Hemorrhaging horses that require surgery may show signs of shock and require immediate acute fluid volume replacement while a compatible blood donor is identified. Fluids should be administered until the horse is stabilized; and, if the PCV drops below 20%, 4 to 8 L of blood from a compatible donor should be administered (see Chapter 7). A severely anemic (PCV <15%) horse under general anesthesia could suffer tissue hypoxia. A horse that has chronic blood loss and has a PCV of less than 15% should also be transfused with whole blood before anesthesia.

Horses with a PCV, platelet count, and blood clotting profile should be evaluated in preparation for a procedure in which massive blood loss is a possibility. An intraoperative transfusion may be necessary, and rapid fluid volume replacement may be needed to counter hypotension. The administration of 2 L of hypertonic saline (7% NaCl) and 4 L of hetastarch (Hextend) helps reverse the hypotension and produces an improvement in hemodynamics that allows time for adequate volume replacement and the transfusion of blood (see Chapter 22).[16]

Upper Respiratory Tract Obstruction

Obstructive diseases of the upper airway that are severe enough to cause respiratory stridor at rest may require a tracheostomy to allow adequate oxygenation before producing anesthesia. An endotracheal tube (at least 26 mm inside diameter) can be passed into the trachea through an incision made between the tracheal rings either with the horse standing or after induction of anesthesia (see Chapter 14). Surgical procedures such as arytenoidectomy or cleft palate repair necessitate tracheal intubation to remove the tube from the surgical area; however, the tracheostomy generally is performed after anesthetic induction. Surgery of the nasal passages and maxillary and frontal sinuses is often accompanied by Seton bandages, effectively occluding the airway and necessitating a tracheotomy. The need for a tracheotomy should be anticipated before surgery. An endotracheal tube with an inflated cuff should be used to prevent aspiration of blood from the upper airway. The endotracheal tube tip should be positioned proximal to the carina (see Chapter 14).

Pregnancy

Elective procedures should be limited in pregnant mares during the first trimester of pregnancy because of the potential risks of some anesthesia. The mare is at greater anesthetic risk for premature delivery or abortion during the last trimester because of compromise of maternal ventilation and circulation from the additional weight of the gravid uterus. Extra precaution should be taken to prevent hypotension and hypoxemia in anesthetized pregnant mares. Expediency is a prime concern.

Foals

Preoperative evaluation of the foal encompasses the same concerns as evaluation of the adult. A thorough physical examination should be performed in the neonate to identify any congenital defects that may increase anesthetic risk (e.g., patent ductus arteriosus; ventricular septal defect). Evaluation of serum IgG concentration should be performed to screen for failure of passive transfer of maternal antibodies. Serum IgG values of <800 mg/dl and <400 mg/dl indicate partial or complete failure, respectively. Plasma transfusion should be considered in both instances. Serum glucose determination should be performed in neonatal foals. Foals that have been deprived of nursing or are septicemic are frequently hypoglycemic. The mare's milk is not usually withheld from foals before anesthesia.

PREPARATION OF THE HORSE FOR ANESTHESIA AND SURGERY

The technical and medical aspects of preparing the adult horse or foal for anesthesia and surgery must be emphasized with a focus on the horse's physical status and the availability of trained and knowledgeable personnel (Box 6-4). Specific procedures used to prepare a horse for surgery vary, depending on the medical or surgical procedure to be performed and the facilities, equipment, and personnel available. Generally food but not water is withheld for at least 6 hours. Appropriate examinations should be performed, and the horse should be bathed and have its shoes removed and feet thoroughly cleaned before surgery (Figure 6-4). Appropriate grooming, surgical scrubbing and bandaging (when possible), and placement of protective padding (protective hoods, leg wraps) should be completed before administration of anesthetic drugs. The horse's mouth should be rinsed thoroughly, and a jugular catheter placed and secured using aseptic technique (see Box 6-4; Figure 6-5).

Box 6–4   Preparation of the Horse for Anesthesia and Surgery

- Withhold food but not water for 6 hr
- Physical examination
- Laboratory evaluation (PCV, TP, WBC count)
- Electrocardiogram
- Pull shoes, bathe, clean feet, rinse mouth,
- Standing surgical prep (when possible)

PCV, Packed cell volume; *TP*, total protein; *WBC*, white blood cell.

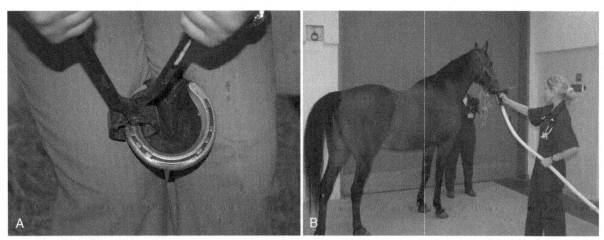

Figure 6–4. Preparation of the horse for surgery. **A,** Remove shoes or bandage feet in plastic bags to minimize contamination. **B,** Bathe horse.

(Continued)

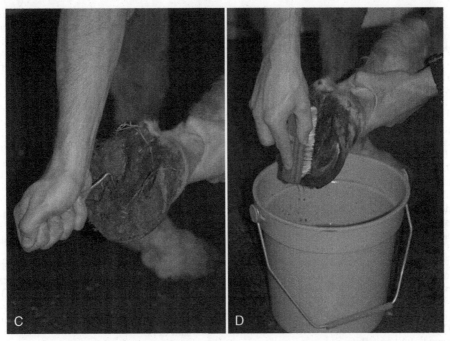

Figure 6–4—Cont'd. C, Pick out soles of feet. **D**, Scrub hoof with a brush.

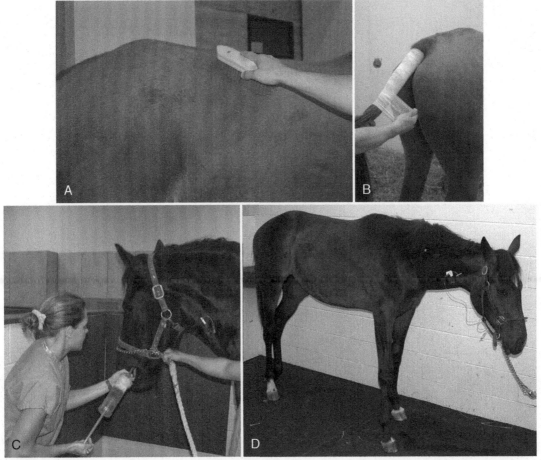

Figure 6–5. Preparation of horse for surgery. **A**, Brush horse to remove dander and loose hair. **B**, Wrap tail. **C**, Rinse mouth with clean water to remove debris. **D**, Place a jugular venous catheter. Determine and administer appropriate preanesthetic medication.

REFERENCES

1. Hodgson DR: Exertional rhabdomyolysis. In Robinson NE, editor: *Current therapy in equine medicine 2*, Philadelphia, 1987, Saunders.
2. Spier SJ et al: Hyperkalemic periodic paralysis in horses. In Proceedings of the Seventh Annual Veterinary Medical Forum, San Diego, 1989, ACVIM, pp 499-500.
3. Milne J, Hewitt D: Weight of horses: improved estimate based on girth and length, *Can Vet J* 10:314-317, 1969.
4. Reavell DG: Measuring and estimating the weight of horses with tapes, formulae, and by visual assessment, *Equine Vet Educ* 11:314-317, 1999.
5. Derksen FJ: Evaluation of the respiratory system: diagnostic techniques. In Robinson NE, editor: *Current therapy in equine medicine 2*, Philadelphia, 1987, Saunders.
5a. Moens Y et al: Distribution of inspired gas to each lung in the anaethetised horse and influence of body shape, *Equine Vet J* 27:110-116, 1995.
5b. Mansel JC, Clutton RE: The influence of body mass and thoracic dimensions on arterial oxygenation in anaesthetised horses and ponies, *Vet Anaesth Analg* 15:392-399, 2008.
6. Curtis RA et al: Lung sounds in cattle, horses, sheep, and goats, *Can Vet J* 27:170-172, 1986.
7. Rantanen NW: Disease of the thorax, *Vet Clin North Am (Diagnostic Ultrasound)* 2:49-66, 1986.
8. Brobst DF, Parry BW: Normal clinical pathology data. In Robinson NE, editor: *Current therapy in equine medicine 2*, Philadelphia, 1987, Saunders.
9. Becht JL, Gordon BJ: Blood and plasma therapy. In Robinson NE, editor: *Current therapy in equine medicine 2*, Philadelphia, 1987, Saunders.
10. McDonell WN: General anesthesia for equine gastrointestinal and obstetric procedures, *Vet Clin North Am (Large Anim Pract)* 3:163-194, 1981.
11. Jain NC: The horse: normal hematology with comments on response to disease. In Feldman BF et al, editors: *Schalm's veterinary hematology*, ed 4, Philadelphia, 1986, Lea & Febiger.
12. Lumb WV, Jones EW: Statistics and records. In Lumb WV, Jones EW, editors: *Veterinary anesthesia*, ed 2, Philadelphia, 1984, Lea & Febiger.
13. Trim CM: Anesthesia of the horse with colic. In Robinson NE, editor: *Current therapy in equine medicine 2*, Philadelphia, 1987, Saunders.
14. Chew DJ, Carothers M: Hypercalcemia, *Vet Clin North Am (Small Anim Pract)* 19:265-287, 1989.
15. Klein L: Anesthesia for neonatal foals, *Vet Clin North Am (Equine Pract)* 1:77-89, 1985.
16. Schmall LM, Muir WW, Robertson JT: Hemodynamic effects of small volume hypertonic saline in experimentally induced hemorrhagic shock, *Equine Vet J* 22:273-277, 1990.
17. Krehbiel JD: Normal clinical pathology data. In Robinson NE, editor: *Current therapy in equine medicine*, Philadelphia, 1983, Saunders.

7

Venous and Arterial Catheterization and Fluid Therapy

Joanne Hardy

KEY POINTS

1. Water is the universal diluent in the body. Approximately 60% of the horse's body weight is water. The extracellular fluid volume (approximately 25% body weight) is composed of the blood volume (7% to 8% body weight) and the interstitial volume.
2. Sodium is the principal extracellular cation and is critical for determination of osmolality.
3. Chloride is the principal extracellular anion and is usually linked to acid-base disturbances (hypochloremic alkalosis, hyperchloremic acidosis).
4. Potassium is the principal intracellular cation and determines the electrical potential across cell membranes. Increases or decreases in extracellular potassium can produce abnormalities in skeletal muscle function, skeletal muscle weakness, and cardiac arrhythmias.
5. Calcium is the key ion responsible for muscle contraction and is usually decreased by general, particularly inhalant, anesthesia.
6. Glucose is an important energy source and may require supplementation following prolonged surgical procedures, particularly in foals.
7. Total protein is a key component of fluid distribution between the intravascular and insterstitial fluid compartments and is critical for the determination of colloid osmotic pressure.
8. Nonrespiratory (metabolic) acidosis in anesthetized horses is caused by hypotension, reduced cardiac output, maldistribution of blood flow, and poor tissue perfusion.
9. A secure intravenous catheter should be placed in every horse before producing general anesthesia.
10. A secure arterial catheter should be placed in all horses requiring emergency surgery or extended periods of general anesthesia.
11. Fluid therapy should be tailored to the horse's needs as determined by hydration, electrolyte, acid-base, total protein, and hemoglobin status.
12. The rate of fluid therapy should be determined by the horse's physical condition, the surgical procedure, the duration of anesthesia, and the amount of blood loss.

PURPOSE OF VASCULAR CATHETERIZATION

Vascular catheters are placed in veins or arteries to provide rapid access to vessels for: (1) injecting fluids, (2) obtaining blood samples, (3) monitoring blood pressure, or (4) administering drugs. Intravenous catheters are recommended when large volumes of fluids are administered, repeated injections are required, tissue toxic drugs are administered, drug infusions are required, or the collection of blood samples is anticipated. A properly placed and secured intravenous catheter ensures that solutions are not injected perivascularly, an important consideration when irritating anesthetic drugs (e.g., thiopental) are used.

METHODS OF INTRAVENOUS CATHETERIZATION

Several veins are accessible for catheterization in horses (Figure 7-1). The jugular veins are large, easily visualized, and palpable in horses. They are: (1) accessible; (2) large in diameter and have a relatively rapid blood flow, thereby reducing the risk of thrombosis; and (3) long enough to allow multiple catheters to be placed either consecutively or concurrently in the same vein. Thrombophlebitis or venous occlusion after prolonged jugular vein catheterization may preclude the use of the jugular vein. The cephalic, saphenous, median, and lateral thoracic veins are alternatives; the lateral thoracic veins may have some advantage because they are less affected by movement than are the others.[1] Lower blood flow in smaller veins compared with that of the jugular vein makes them more susceptible to thrombosis and thrombophlebitis and less satisfactory for the administration of irritating solutions.[2]

Procedures for proper intravenous catheter placement must be developed and strictly followed to minimize adverse events (see Chapter 22; Box 7-1 and Figure 7-2). The skin (10-cm square) should be clipped and aseptically prepared. Sterile

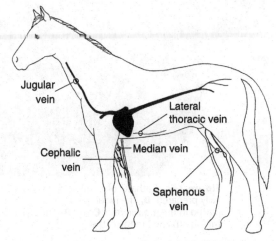

Figure 7–1. Veins commonly catheterized in the horse.

Box 7–1   Procedure for Intravenous Catheter Placement in the Horse

1. Clip or shave a 10-cm square area of skin over the vessel.
2. Perform a surgical preparation of the area.
3. Inject 1 to 2 ml of local anesthetic subcutaneously at the site or apply 5% lidocaine (LMX) cream.
4. (Optional for short-term catheters) Put on sterile gloves.
5. (Optional) Make a small hole or stab incision over the vessel through the skin only, using 14-gauge needle or scalpel blade.
6. Remove catheter cap and/or sleeve, keeping the catheter sterile.
7. Raise the vein by occluding the vein. (An assistant may do this to prevent the person performing the catheterization from contamination.)
8. Push catheter and stylet through the skin at an appropriate 45-degree angle to the vessel. Maintain this slight angle while puncturing the vessel wall. Blood should appear in the hub of the catheter.

9. With the vein still occluded, decrease the angle of the catheter so that it is nearly parallel to the vessel, and advance both catheter and stylet at least 5 mm into the vessel to ensure that the tip of the catheter itself is within the vessel.
10. Release pressure on the vein.
11. Holding the stylet completely still, slide the catheter over the stylet until the catheter is completely inserted into the vessel. Remove the stylet.
12. Attach a male adapter cap or fluid-filled extension set to the catheter hub, and flush the catheter assembly with heparinized saline.
13. Secure the catheter to the skin with glue, tape, or sutures.
14. Apply antibiotic ointment at the catheter insertion site and secure with elastic bandage.
15. Tape the extension set or administration set tubing to the bandage to prevent unnecessary traction on the catheter during fluid administration.

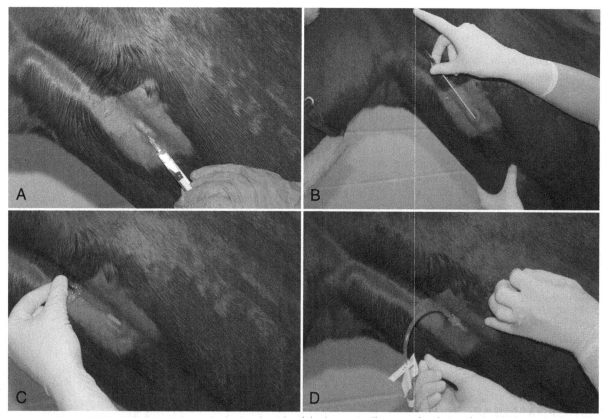

Figure 7–2. Catheter placement in the jugular vein of the horse. **A,** The area of catheter placement is surgically prepared. **B,** The jugular is occluded (left hand), and an over-the-needle (OTN) catheter (12- to 14-g) is placed in the jugular vein. **C** and **D,** The stylet is removed from the OTN catheter, and a short fluid extension tube is attached to the catheter.

(Continued)

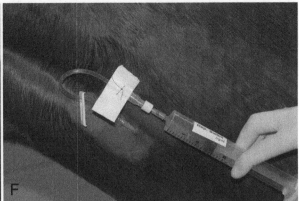

Figure 7–2—Cont'd. E and **F,** One-inch tape is placed around the catheter extension ("butterfly") and used to secure (suture) the tube to the horse's neck. The extension tubing is flushed with sterile saline.

gloves are not necessary if the catheter is protected, sterile, and remains in the vein for only a short time. Care should be taken to keep the catheter from becoming contaminated during insertion; it should be handled by the hub only. Sterile gloves should be worn if the catheter is to be left in a vein for more than a few hours. Infiltration of the skin and subcutaneous tissues with 1 to 2 ml of a local anesthetic or 5% lidocaine (LMX cream) may facilitate catheter placement in young foals or horses with nervous temperaments. A 22- or 25-gauge needle is recommended for infiltration of local anesthetic.

The intravenous catheter should be connected to an injection cap or an intravenous fluid extension set and flushed with heparinized saline (5 to 10 USP units of sodium heparin per milliliter of normal saline) as soon as the catheter is threaded in the vein (see Chapter 6). Heparinized saline should be prepared, handled aseptically, and discarded within 72 hours to minimize possible contamination. The venous catheter should be flushed at least every 4 to 6 hours if no fluids are being administered. A continual slow infusion of heparinized saline (2 USP units/ml, 60 ml/hr) is advisable if a small vein is used or to maintain an arterial catheter.[3] Occluded catheters should be removed and replaced. Forcible flushing of an occluded catheter to restore patency can result in the release of emboli into the pulmonary circulation, obstructing blood flow and potentially seeding bacteria into the lungs and systemically.

Intravascular catheters should be secured to minimize catheter movement, potential kinking, and loss of vascular access. The application of cyanoacrylate tissue glue to the catheter hub is a simple and fast method for securing a catheter. The glue will hold for 2 to 3 days as long as the skin and catheter hub are dry when the glue is applied. Sutures can be placed through the skin and around the hub of the catheter to help minimize catheter movement. A "butterfly" of adhesive tape can be placed around the extension set (the extension set must be dry before the tape is placed), with the skin sutures placed through the tape (see Figure 7-2).

In general, catheters are not bandaged in adult horses unless the horse is recumbent for prolonged periods of time. This facilitates examination of the catheter site before and during injection of drugs and rapid identification of catheter-related problems. Covering the catheter site with a bandage is recommended in recumbent horses, horses that rub their catheters, or foals. A small amount of antiseptic or antibiotic ointment

such as povidone-iodine or nitrofurazone can be applied to the catheter insertion site. Once inserted, the catheter is covered with sterile gauze sponges and secured with an elastic adhesive bandage. The bandage should be changed at least once a day or replaced if it becomes wet or soiled. The length of time that a catheter is left in place is determined by the catheter material, catheter configuration, and clinical signs of inflammation. Polytetrafluoroethylene (Teflon) catheters are suitable for short-term catheterization and should be replaced every 2 to 3 days. Polyurethane and silastic catheters can be left in place for 2 weeks or more.[4] Over-the-wire catheters generally are less thrombogenic than over-the-needle catheters because they are more flexible.[4]

Catheter removal is performed by cutting the retaining sutures and pulling on the catheter hub in a direction parallel to the catheter. Finger pressure can be applied to the venous puncture site; but if continued bleeding persists, a pressure bandage can be placed over the venipuncture site for a few hours. Pressure should be applied immediately to the vein below the catheter insertion site if the catheter fractures during removal (Figure 7-3). Ultrasound can be used to locate the catheter within the vein; and, if retrievable, the catheter should be surgically removed. A fibrin sleeve may be mistaken for the actual catheter (Figure 7-4).[5]

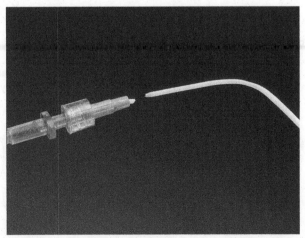

Figure 7–3. Illustration of a catheter after removal showing common site of breakage of over-the-needle catheters.

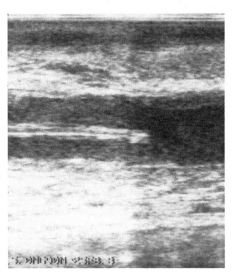

Figure 7–4. Ultrasound of the jugular vein of a horse, performed using a 7.5 Mhz probe showing a fibrin sleeve that commonly forms around catheters after prolonged intravenous catheterization.

METHODS OF ARTERIAL CATHETERIZATION

Arterial catheters are placed for collection of arterial blood samples (pHa, PaO_2, $PaCO_2$), to facilitate measurement of arterial blood pressure, and to determine cardiac output using lithium dilution.[6] Any palpable superficial artery large enough to accommodate a catheter can be used (Figure 7-5). The facial artery with its branches is one of the most commonly catheterized arteries in horses and is accessible along the cranial border of the masseter muscle or more distally where it branches into the lateral nasal and angularis oculi arteries. The facial artery is most easily catheterized at the point where it crosses the ventral aspect of the mandible when the horse is in dorsal recumbency (see Figure 7-5). The transverse facial artery is generally catheterized in horses that are laterally recumbent, and the dorsal metatarsal artery on the lateral aspect of the hind limb is catheterized when the horse's head is inaccessible (see Figure 7-5).

An 18- to 20-gauge through-the-needle or over-the-needle catheter is used for routine clinical cases (Figure 7-6 and Table 7-1). Generally a needle stylet penetrates the vessel and is advanced a small distance to ensure that the catheter tip enters the vessel lumen. The catheter is advanced over the needle into the vessel lumen until the catheter hub reaches the skin. The stylet is held stationary in its original position in the vessel until the catheter is fully threaded into the vessel; premature withdrawal of the stylet may cause the catheter to burr, bend, or kink and prevent complete insertion of the catheter. The disadvantage of the through-the-needle style catheter is that it is more likely to cause hematoma formation when the needle is withdrawn from the artery because the catheter is smaller in diameter than the hole through which it is passed. Arterial puncture is associated with a greater risk of hematoma formation because the arterial blood pressure is higher than venous blood pressure. Muscular arterial walls contract around the catheter, limiting hemorrhage if digital pressure is maintained for 15 to 30 seconds.

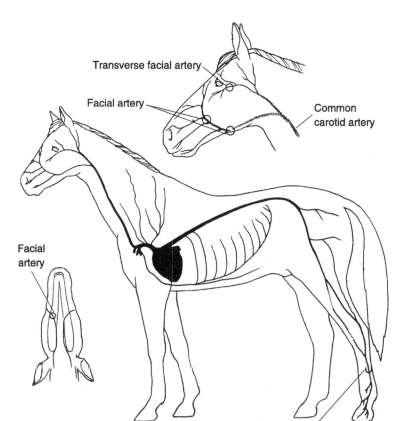

Figure 7–5. Arteries that are easily catheterized in the horse.

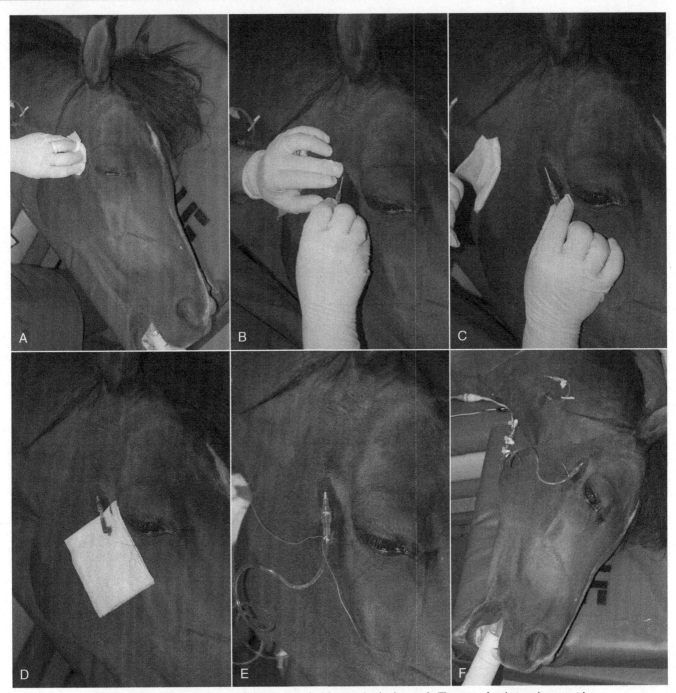

Figure 7–6. Catheterization of the transverse facial artery in the horse. **A,** The area of catheter placement is surgically prepared. **B** and **C,** A branch of the facial artery is located, and an over-the-needle (OTN) catheter (20-g) is placed. **D,** The stylet is removed from the OTN catheter. Blood should flow freely. **E** and **F,** A short fluid extension tube is attached to the catheter. A loop is placed in the extension tubing, and the catheter and extension tubing are sutured to the horse's face (*middle*). This helps to prevent direct tension on the arterial catheter. The extension tubing is flushed with sterile saline and connected to a pressure transducer.

Over-the-wire catheters are preferred for long-term arterial catheterization or for arterial catheterization of small and/or hypotensive horses (see Table 7-1). Over-the-wire catheters are inserted using the Seldinger technique (Figure 7-7). The transverse facial artery is the most common site for long-term arterial catheterization in adult horses (Figure 7-8). The dorsal metatarsal artery is the preferred site in foals. Rolled gauzes are placed on either side of the catheter to stabilize the catheter, and elasticized adhesive bandage is applied.

Catheter site–related infections can be serious.[7] Arterial catheters may be fixed in place with cyanoacrylate tissue glue, tape, or sutures. Arterial catheters need to be flushed with heparinized saline solution more often than venous catheters. Slight pressure on the plunger of the flush syringe while closing the stopcock prevents blood from advancing into the catheter. Automatic, continual flushing devices are available commercially (see following paragraphs). Special attention should be paid to ensure that all connections are

Table 7–1. Advantages and disadvantages of various catheters

Type	Advantages	Disadvantages
Butterfly	Simple to use Self-contained extension tubing	Needle may lacerate vessel Needle may come out of vessel Not appropriate for long-term use
Over-the-needle (OTN)	Available in large diameters Needle is removed after insertion Catheter is same diameter as puncture	Diameter is limited Catheter tip may fray during skin puncture Needle tip may puncture catheter if catheter tip gets ahead of needle
Through-the-needle (TTN)	Catheter can be of any length	Diameter is limited by trochar size Trochar must be removed or covered with guard Hole in skin and vessel is larger than catheter diameter, predisposing to hematoma formation
Over-the-wire (OTW)	Puncture site snug around catheter Flexible, best suited for short necks Can be placed in tortuous or collapsed vessels Multilumen available Material has low thrombogenicity	Technically challenging Cost

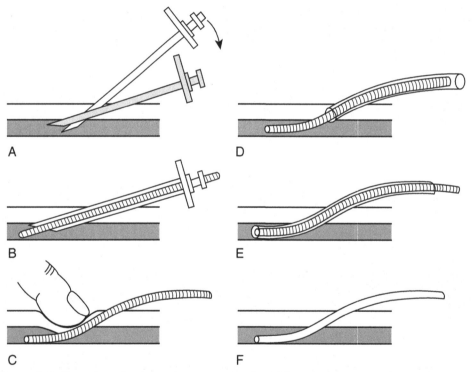

Figure 7–7. Illustration of catheter placement using the Seldinger technique. **A,** The vessel is punctured using a needle, making sure that the tip of the needle is completely inserted in the vessel. **B,** The guide wire is inserted in the vessel through the needle; for venipuncture a J wire is used to prevent obstruction of passage by the venous valves; for arterial puncture a soft-tip straight wire is used. **C,** The wire has been advanced into the vessel, and the hollow needle removed; with arterial puncture, pressure is placed on the vessel to prevent excessive bleeding during the procedure. **D,** The catheter is placed over the wire and advanced into the vessel; it is important to hold the wire during advancement of the catheter; if advancement of the catheter is difficult because of poor skin distensibility, a dilator may be used before catheter placement. **E,** The catheter is positioned within the vessel. **F,** The wire is removed, and the catheter is secured in place.

secure to prevent blood loss because of the high pressures in the arterial system. Digital pressure should be applied to all catheter sites (30 seconds, veins; 3 minutes, arteries) after the catheter is removed to prevent the development of hematomas.

TYPES OF CATHETERS

Selection of catheter type and size depends on the patient's size and the intended use for the catheter. The advantages and disadvantages of various catheter types should be considered (see Table 7-1).

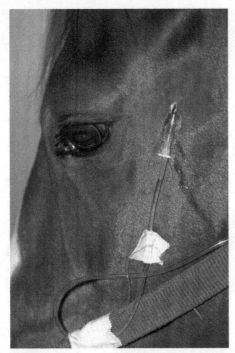

Figure 7–8. Adult, standing, conscious horse with an arterial catheter placed in the transverse facial artery for serial arterial blood collection and measurement of cardiac output using a lithium dilution method. The local application of 5% lidocaine (LMX) cream facilitates this procedure.

Butterfly Catheters

Butterfly catheters (Figure 7-9) consist of butterfly-like wings attached to the needle and then to a length of flexible tubing. The butterfly wings facilitate placement and fixation after needle placement. Butterfly catheters are suitable for short-term venous access when movement at the puncture site is limited. The needle remains in the vessel; thus the risk of puncture through the vessel, laceration of the vessel wall, or inadvertent withdrawal must be considered.

Over-the-Needle Catheters

Over-the-needle catheters (see Figure 7-9) are relatively short (usually 14 cm or less) and stiff. They are available in various gauges (10- to 22-gauge). The needle (stylet) protrudes slightly past the tip of the catheter. Occasionally the tip of the catheter becomes frayed as it penetrates the skin,

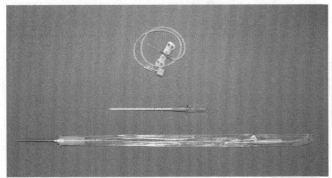

Figure 7–9. The common types of catheters—butterfly *(top)*, over-the-needle *(middle)*, and through-the-needle *(bottom)*—used in horses.

which makes puncture of the vessel wall more difficult and traumatic (see Table 7-1). A small hole made in the skin by a large needle or with a scalpel blade minimizes damage to the catheter. The catheter should never be pulled back onto the needle because the sharp tip of the needle could sever the catheter. If the catheter cannot be advanced, the needle and catheter should be withdrawn from the vessel as a single unit. The catheter should be examined for kinks or other defects and flushed with heparinized saline before attempting placement. Once the catheter is successfully threaded into the vessel, the needle is removed; and the catheter is flushed with sterile saline, capped, and secured.

Through-the-Needle Catheters

Through-the-needle (TTN) catheters (see Figure 7-9) are available commercially and can be improvised by placing polyethylene tubing through hypodermic needles (Table 7-2). The advantage of the improvised TTN catheter is that the catheter can be made to any length and is more flexible than most over-the-needle catheters. The major disadvantages of TTN catheters are that the catheter diameter is limited by the size of the needle through which it passes and the hole left by the needle (needle diameter) is larger than the catheter diameter. The larger puncture wound predisposes to seepage of blood around the catheter and hematoma formation (see Table 7-1). TTN catheters should not be withdrawn if resistance occurs during catheter insertion because of the possibility of shearing off the catheter tip by the needle. The needle and catheter should be withdrawn as a single unit, and the procedure for catheter placement repeated.

Over-the-Wire Catheters

Over-the-wire catheters are made of flexible polyurethane or silastic material and are less thrombogenic (Figure 7-10). They are preferred for long-term catheterization in foals and small horses. Over-the-wire catheters can have single, double, or multiple lumens and vary in length. A catheter clamp is provided, allowing selection of variable insertion lengths, depending on the size of the patient. The Seldinger technique is performed for catheter placement (see Figure 7-7).

CATHETER MATERIALS AND SIZES

Vascular catheters are made from a variety of materials. Polyethylene tubing is inexpensive, inherently flexible, and elastic but thrombogenic. Polytetrafluroethylene (Teflon) is less thrombogenic but kinks easily. Siliconized rubber (silastic) tubing is very nonreactive and nonthrombogenic, but it is so flexible that it tends to "whip" within the vessel and kinks

Table 7–2.	Catheter supplies for home-made catheter systems*		
Polyethylene tubing size (90 cm long)	**Needle for venipuncture (reusable)**		**Needle for threading into tubing**
160	14 gauge (thin wall)		18 gauge
205	12 gauge		16 gauge
240	10 gauge		14 gauge

*All of these catheters require caps or three-way stopcocks.

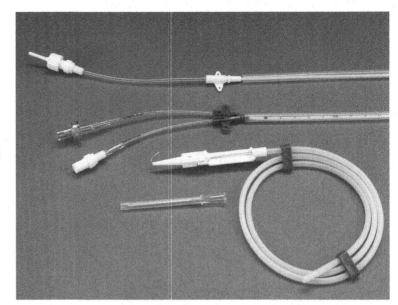

Figure 7–10. Over-the-wire catheters: single lumen *(top)*, double lumen *(middle)*, J wire within sheath *(bottom)*, and insertion needle.

easily. Polyurethane is flexible, resistant to collapsing or kinking, relatively nonthrombogenic, and currently the most common catheter material used for long-term catheterization.

Selection of the appropriate catheter size (internal diameter) depends on the size of the vessel and the animal's fluid requirement. Fluid flow is proportional to the internal diameter of the catheter raised to the fourth power; halving the diameter decreases flow rate by a factor of 16.[8] Smaller catheters create less tissue trauma and allow relatively undisturbed blood flow past the catheter. Large internal–diameter catheters should be used in situations in which large volumes of fluid must be administered rapidly. Currently the largest commercially made over-the-needle catheter is 10 gauge (ID). A 14-gauge catheter generally is adequate for routine fluid administration in horses. Most foals' jugular veins can easily accommodate a 14-gauge catheter, although an 18-gauge catheter is often sufficient.

Extension Sets, Coil Sets, Injection Caps, and Administration Sets

Catheter extension tubing sets are used to connect the catheter to the fluid administration tubing. They can be sewn to the horse's skin and help to prevent the catheter from being pulled out of the vessel during fluid administration. Some catheter extension sets contain access ports that facilitate the intravenous administration of drugs. Extension sets are available in several lengths and diameters. For large-volume fluid delivery, a large diameter or "high-flow" extension set should be used. Long extension sets are preferred in anesthetized horses so that fluids and drugs can be administered at a distance from the horse. Various configurations of T ports, dual or triple ports with separate injection ports, are available. Luer-lock connections are preferred to male/female connectors to prevent disconnected catheters. Long "coiled" extension sets are used for fluid administration in stalls since they allow the horse to move, lie down, or eat. An overhead pulley system with a rotating hook prevents fluid lines from getting tangled (Figure 7-11).

Injection caps are used to seal the catheter between drug administrations. Antireflux valves prevent accidental air

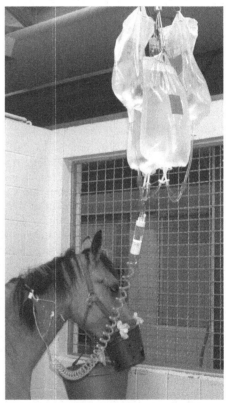

Figure 7–11. In-stall pulley and coil fluid administration set helps prevent the horse from becoming tangled in the intravenous extension tubing and allows the horse free movement in the stall.

aspiration or blood loss if the fluid line becomes disconnected. Needleless injection caps prevent accidental needle punctures of the horse or attendant.

Standard fluid administration sets that deliver 10, 20, and 60 drops/ml are used for short-term fluid or drug administration. Foal coil sets are available that deliver 15 drops/ml. Care should be taken to use the appropriate fluid administration set when fluid pumps are used. Long coiled extension sets can then be used to connect fluids to the horse.

Fluid Pumps

Calibrated fluid pumps facilitate the accurate delivery of fluids or drugs. Most fluid pumps have alarms that signal if air is in the line, the fluid bag is empty, or the pressure required to infuse fluids is increasing or too great (kinked or plugged catheters). The maximum rate of fluid administration for most fluid pumps is 999 ml/hour, which is insufficient for fluid replacement in adult horses. Peristaltic (pulsatile) pumps can deliver up to 40 L an hour but must be monitored since they will continue to run even if the fluid reservoir (bag) is empty. Large-bore catheters should be used when fluids are administered at rapid rates to avoid vascular endothelial trauma from catheter whip.

COMPLICATIONS ASSOCIATED WITH VENOUS OR ARTERIAL CATHETERIZATION

Trauma to the vessel wall during catheter placement, turbulent blood flow at the catheter tip, and the introduction of foreign material (the catheter) into the vessel contribute to thrombosis of cannulated veins. Additional risk factors for the development of catheter-associated jugular thrombophlebitis include systemic illness, hypoproteinemia, enterocolitis, endotoxemia, large intestinal disease, and salmonellosis.[9] Complications associated with arterial catheterization in horses are relatively rare because of the high pressures, rapid blood flow in the arteries, and the fact that arterial catheters are not maintained for long periods of time. Infection, arterial thrombosis, and hematoma formation are potential complications (Table 7-3). Osteomyelitis following dorsal metatarsal artery catheterization has occurred, emphasizing the importance of aseptic technique during catheter placement.[7]

FLUID THERAPY

Successful fluid therapy is based on an applied knowledge of the fluid compartments of the body, osmosis, osmolality, tonicity, and colloid osmotic (oncotic) pressure in relation to the wide variety of fluids that are available and the horse's fluid, electrolyte, hematologic, and acid-base status. It is important to remember that all commercially available

Table 7–3. Complications of catheterization		
Problem	**Signs**	**Causes**
Thrombophlebitis/infection/ catheter sepsis	Pain at catheter site Swelling Edema Fever	Inadequate preparation Poor patient hygiene Poor antiseptic technique Leaving catheter in too long Irritating or hypertonic solutions Contaminated solutions Poor patient immune status
Extravasation of intravenous fluids into subcutaneous tissue	Pain Swelling Edema Decreased infusion rate Failure to get blood back on aspiration Possible tissue necrosis	Dislodgement of catheter Manual pushing of drug Use of high-volume infusion pumps
Pyrogenic reactions	Abrupt onset of fever and chills Hives, wheals Hypotension Cyanosis	Foreign proteins in solution or administration set
Air embolism	Anxiety Malaise Ataxia Collapse Cyanosis Loss of consciousness	Catheter open to room air Air-pressurized fluid bottles
Exsanguination	Blood loss from catheter Internal blood loss	Catheter not capped Excessive heparinization
Arterial thrombosis/occlusion	Tissue necrosis, slough	Same as thrombophlebitis/ infection/catheter sepsis
Hematoma	Localized swelling Bleeding	Laceration or multiple punctures High pressure (arteries) Accidental arterial puncture during placement of venous catheters
Catheter breakage	Catheter sleeve absent during catheter removal Localized pneumonia Arrhythmia Endocarditis	Use of stiff over-the-needle catheters

fluids and most horse-derived colloidal solutions other than blood are dilutional to some component of blood and therefore may exacerbate one problem while correcting another. Water is the predominant universal diluent for all fluids in the body and is an essential ingredient in almost all chemical reactions. Water represents approximately 60% of the adult horse's body weight and up to 80% in neonates (Box 7-2).[10-13]

Fluid therapy can be divided into two broad categories based on the primary reason (goal) for administering fluids. One goal of fluid therapy is directed toward the restoration and maintenance of normal hydration or, said another way, the treatment of dehydration. Many horses requiring emergency surgery (trauma, colic, lacerations) may not have had adequate access to water for several hours or may have developed significant dehydration associated with their disease process. These horses frequently demonstrate signs of dehydration (dry mucous membranes, tented skin, sunken eyes, increased packed cell volume [PCV]). The restoration and maintenance of normal hydration can be successfully accomplished by administering crystalloids, the term commonly used to describe solutions that contain various concentrations of inorganic (salts, e.g., Na^+, Cl^-) or small organic molecules (glucose) in water (Table 7-4 and Box 7-3). Commercially available crystalloids are isotonic (similar osmolality), hypotonic, or hypertonic to plasma and are usually selected on the basis of the horse's electrolyte concentrations and need for water. Large volumes of crystalloid are frequently administered to dehydrated horses in an attempt to expand the circulating blood volume and restore normal levels of hydration. This approach to fluid therapy (replacement and maintenance) generally is well tolerated in horses that are mild to moderately dehydrated and when treatment regimens can be administered for extended periods of time (6 to 24 hours). However, the rapid administration of large volumes of crystalloids to horses that are dehydrated and hypovolemic often results in the accumulation of fluid in the interstitial fluid compartment (<10% to 20% of a crystalloid is retained in the vascular compartment after 1 hour). Overhydration with crystalloids dilutes critical blood components (proteins, hemoglobin, platelets) and predisposes the horse to tissue ischemia, hypoxia, and bleeding disorders. Horses that

are moderately to severely volume depleted or hypotensive derive greater benefit from the administration of fluids (resuscitative) that contain large ultramicroscopic particles (>30,000 Daltons), termed *colloids*, that are retained within the vascular compartment and dependent on their concentration (colloid osmotic pressure) to draw fluid from the interstitium (autotransfuse) into the vascular compartment, even in dehydrated horses. Colloids vary in their magnitude and duration of plasma volume expansion, hemodynamic benefits (arterial blood pressure, cardiac output), hemostatic and hemorheologic effects, potential to produce adverse effects, and cost. All currently available semisynthetic colloids (dextrans, hydroxyethyl starches) are polydisperse (consist of molecules of different sizes) and have the potential to produce impairment of hemostasis, although this has not been a problem for newer colloids and has been largely attributed to hemodilution. Resuscitative fluids (colloids, blood, blood substitutes) are administered with the primary goal of restoring the vascular volume to the extent necessary to improve tissue perfusion and tissue oxygenation. Colloids are more effective than crystalloids in restoring normal hemodynamics and must be dosed (milliliters per kilogram; 20 to 40 ml/kg/day) to avoid vascular fluid overload, hemostatic impairment, and excessive dilution of plasma proteins and hemoglobin. Some colloids produce antiinflammatory effects and help to reduce capillary leak associated with tissue hypoxia. Colloids of smaller molecular weights or that contain smaller molecules can accumulate in the interstitial fluid compartment and may induce tissue edema in horses that are severely ill or have locally compromised tissue blood flow patterns. Most horses requiring surgery and anesthesia derive greater benefit from the judicious use of crystalloids (lactated Ringer's solution: 3 to 5 ml/kg/hr) in conjunction with colloids (6% hetastarch; 5 to 10 ml/kg) to restore the effective circulating blood volume and maintain normal hemodynamics than the use of crystalloids alone. Indeed, there is little evidence that the acute administration of crystalloids to anesthetized horses requiring elective, and in particular, emergency surgical procedures does little more than provide venous access and transient improvement in hemodynamics and induce diuresis. Less than 10% to 20% of a crystalloid is retained within the vascular compartment after 60 minutes of discontinuing their administration (<100 to 200 ml of every liter). By contrast, colloids produce a sustained increase in plasma volume that increases with time (autotransfusion) dependent on the solution's colloid osmotic (oncotic) pressure.

Body solutes are not distributed equally throughout the body. Sodium is the main cation in plasma, and chloride and bicarbonate are the main anions; proteins contribute to the total negative charge and provide protein osmotic (oncotic) pressure. Albumin or molecules of similar size (>30,000 Daltons) are the main contributors to the development of oncotic pressure. Interstitial space is highly compliant; comprises about 75% of extracellular fluid volume (ECFV); and is composed mainly of sodium, chloride, and bicarbonate; but the concentration of protein is low compared to blood. The slightly increased concentration of anions and decreased concentration of cations in blood occurs because of the greater concentration of negatively charged proteins in plasma (Gibbs-Donnan equilibrium). This difference is small enough in horses that the measured concentration

---

Box 7–2   Percent Body Water in Horses

The extracellular fluid volume (ECFV) is approximately 20% to 25% of total body weight (TBW) in adult horses and up to 40% of BW in neonates. Experimental estimates of fluid distribution in adult horses are reported to be 0.67 L/kg (67%) for total body water (TBW), 0.21 L/kg (21%) for ECFV, and 0.46 (46%) for intracellular fluid volume (ICFV; TBW = ECFV + ICFV).[10,11] The ECFV (interstitial fluid + blood) is approximately 40% of TBW in neonates, decreasing to approximately 30% by 24 weeks of age.[12] Generally estimated values of 30% (0.3 × TBW) for adults and 40% (0.4 × TBW) for foals are used for calculating fluid requirements. Blood volume in sedentary horses represents approximately 8% (8 ml/kg) of TBW and can reach 14% of TBW in fit horses.[13] Blood volume in neonates can be 15% of TBW, decreasing to adult values by 12 weeks of age.[12]

Table 7–4. Composition and principal uses of common intravenous fluid replacements

	pH	Osmolality mOsmol/L	Na mEq/L	K mEq/L	Ca mEq/L	Mg mEq/L	Cl mEq/L	Buffer mEq/L	Use
Dextrose 5%	3.5–6.5	252	—	—	—	—	—	—	Primary water deficit; Hypoglycemia
Lactated Ringer's	6.2–6.7	273	130	4	3	—	109	Lactate 28	Routine maintenance and rehydration
Lactated Ringer's and 5% dextrose	5	525	130	4	3	—	109	Lactate 28	Rehydration and hypoglycemia
Plasmalyte A	7.4	294	140	5	—	3	98	Acetate 27 Gluconate 23	Rehydration, indicated with liver disease
Plasmalyte 148	5.5	294	140	5	—	3	98	Acetate 27 Gluconate 23	Rehydration, indicated with liver disease
Plasmalyte 56	5.5	111	40	13	—	3	40	Acetate 16	Maintenance
Normosol R	7.4	296	140	5	—	3	98	Acetate 27 Gluconate 23	Rehydration, indicated with liver disease
Normosol M	5.5	111	40	13	—	3	40	Acetate 16	Maintenance; Hyperkalemia; Hyponatremia; Hypochloremia
Normal saline	5.0	308	154	—	—	—	154		
Ringer's	5.8–6.1	309	147	4	4.5	—	156		Routine maintenance and rehydration
Dextran-40	3.5–7	Hypertonic	154	—	—	—	154		Acute treatment of hypoproteinemia
Dextran-70	3–7	Hypertonic	154	—	—	—	154		Acute treatment of hypoproteinemia
Hetastarch in 0.9% saline	3.5–7.0	Hypertonic	154	—	—	—	154		Acute treatment of hypoproteinemia, volume expansion
Hextend (6% hetastarch in LRS)	5.9	307	143	3	5	0.9	124		Acute treatment of hypoproteinemia, volume expansion
3% NaCl	5.0	Hypertonic	513	—	—	—	513		Acute blood loss (see Chapter 22)
7% NaCl	5.0	Hypertonic	1198	—	—	—	1198		Acute blood loss, shock (see Chapter 22)

—, Not present.

Box 7–3   Administering Glucose to Horses

Calories: 5% dextrose can be administered at a rate of 1 to 2 mg/kg/min in adults or 4 to 8 mg/kg/min in foals.

---

of solutes in plasma is thought to reflect the concentration of solutes throughout the ECFV. The composition of the intracellular fluid volume (ICFV) is different; the principal cations are potassium and magnesium, and the important anions are phosphates and proteins.

Transfer of fluid between compartments is an important issue during administration of large volumes of fluids. *Osmolality* is the concentration of osmotically active particles in solution per kilogram of solvent (mOsm/kg). *Osmolarity* is the number of particles of solute per unit (L) of solvent (mOsm/L). The difference between the two concentrations in plasma is negligible, and the two terms are often used interchangeably. Normal plasma osmolality in adult horses ranges from 275 to 312 mOsm/kg; it varies slightly between breeds.[14] Lower values are reported for normal foals.[15] The effective osmolality (tonicity) is the osmotic pressure generated by the difference in osmolality between two compartments. The osmotic pressure generated by proteins, mainly albumin (oncotic pressure), can be determined by a colloid osmometer (Wescor, Logan, Utah). Normal values range from 19.2 to 31.3 mm Hg in adult horses and 15 to 22.6 mm Hg in foals.[16,17] Water and ionic solute exchange between the vascular and interstitial compartment occurs at the capillary level and is rapid; equilibrium is reached within 15 to 30 minutes. The rate of exchange or net filtration that occurs between the plasma and interstitial fluid is controlled by a balance between the forces that favors filtration (capillary hydrostatic pressure and tissue oncotic pressure) and forces that tend to retain fluid within the vascular space (plasma oncotic pressure and tissue hydrostatic pressure) as described by Starling's law of the capillary (Box 7-4). Fluid transfer between plasma and interstitial fluid is relatively rapid (minutes), depending on prevailing "Starling" forces and the capillarity (porosity) of the tissue bed.

Fluid exchange between the interstitial fluid compartment and the intracellular fluid compartment is governed by the number of osmotically active particles within each space. Sodium is the most abundant cation in the extracellular fluid (ECF) and consequently accounts for most of the osmotically active particles in the ECF. Other osmotically active compounds that contribute to ECF osmolality are glucose and urea (Box 7-5).[18]

The *osmolar gap* is the difference between measured osmolarity and calculated osmolarity; an increased osmolar

---

Box 7–4   Starling's Law of the Capillary

$$\text{Net filtration} = K_f [(P_{cap} - P_{int}) - \sigma (\pi_p - \pi_{int})]$$

Where K_f is the filtration coefficient, which varies depending on surface area available for filtration and permeability of the capillary wall; P_{cap} and P_{int} are the hydrostatic pressure within the capillary or interstitium; π_p and π_{int} are the oncotic pressures within the plasma or interstitial fluid; and σ is the reflection coefficient of proteins across the capillary wall.

Box 7–5   Serum Osmolality

$$\text{ECF osmolality} = 2[Na^+] + \frac{Glucose}{18} + \frac{Urea}{2.8}$$

Cell membranes are permeable to urea and K. Therefore the effective osmolarity is calculated by:

$$\text{ECF osmolality} = 2[Na^+] + \frac{Glucose}{18}$$

ECF, Extracellular fluid.

---

gap exists when unmeasured solutes such as mannitol are present in the plasma.[19] Fluid exchange between the extracellular and intracellular compartments is comparatively slow, taking 18 to 24 hours to reach equilibrium.

Fluid Administration

Dehydration is the loss of solute and water from the body. Hypovolemia is a form of dehydration resulting from the loss of fluid from the vascular compartment. This distinction is important since a lack of water intake may not change heart rate and parameters of perfusion (capillary refill time) but hypovolemia exists (see Chapter 6). Dehydration should be treated, and ICFV replenished relatively slowly to allow time for compensatory fluid shifts to occur between the plasma and interstitial fluid compartments and subsequently into the intracellular fluid compartment. Parameters that can be used for estimation of dehydration include serial body weights, heart rate, mucous membrane color, skin elasticity (skin tenting), cool extremities, decreased arterial blood pressure, and decreased urine output. Useful laboratory parameters include PCV, total protein, creatinine concentration, and urine specific gravity. Increases in PCV and total plasma protein concentration (TP) indicate reduced plasma and ECF volume from dehydration (Tables 7-5 and 7-6). These variables differ considerably among horses and may be difficult to interpret unless initial values are available for comparison; a PCV of 40% and TP of 7.5 g/dl may be normal in one horse but indicate severe dehydration in a horse with initial normal PCV and TP of 30% and 5.7 g/dl. The capacity of the equine spleen to release erythrocytes into the circulation (sympathetic stimulation) makes PCV less reliable as an indicator of dehydration. Blood or protein losses also complicate interpretations. By contrast, acute loss of circulating blood volume generally alters cardiovascular parameters that are typified by increased heart rate, increased capillary refill time, poor perfusion, pale mucous membranes, and decreased pulse quality. Hypovolemia can be treated by rapid restitution of effective circulating blood volume. Measurement of lactate is now routine for assessing tissue oxygenation and tissue perfusion in horses and can be determined by most chemistry and point-of-care analyzers (Accutrend Lactate, www.Lactate.com) (see Chapter 8).[20] When possible, blood samples should be analyzed immediately after collection to avoid in vitro lactate production by erythrocytes; or the blood should be collected in tubes containing fluoride (after plasma separation) and stored on ice. Increases in blood lactate concentration are most often the result of poor tissue perfusion or hypoxia. Inadequate oxygen delivery to tissues can occur as a result of hypovolemia,

Table 7–5. Parameters useful to estimate the degree of hypovolemia in adult horses, assuming a normal PCV of 35% and total protein of 6.5 g/dl

% Loss in effective circulation volume	Heart rate (beats/min)	CRT (sec)	PCV/TP (%/g/dl)	Creatinine (mg/dl)
6	40-60	2	40/7	1.5-2
8	61-80	3	45/7.5	2-3
10	81-100	4	50/8	3-4
12	>100	>4	>50/>8	>4

CRT, Capillary refill time; *PCV,* packed cell volume; *TP,* total plasma protein concentration.

Table 7–6. Interpretation of packed cell volume and total protein values

PCV(%)	Total plasma proteins (g/dl)	Interpretation
Increased	Increased	Dehydration
Increased	Normal or decreased	Splenic contraction
		Polycythemia
		Dehydration with preexisting hypoproteinemia
Normal	Increased	Normal hydration with hyperproteinemia
		Anemia with dehydration
Decreased	Increased	Anemia with dehydration
		Anemia with preexisting hyperproteinemia
Decreased	Normal	Nonblood loss anemia with normal hydration
Normal	Normal	Normal hydration
		Dehydration with preexisting anemia and hypoproteinemia
		Acute hemorrhage
		Dehydration with secondary compartment shift
Decreased	Decreased	Blood loss
		Anemia and hypoproteinemia
		Overhydration

PCV, Packed cell volume.

decreased blood oxygen content, or reduced blood flow caused by impaired myocardial function resulting in hyperlactatemia. Hypermetabolic states or impaired oxygen use caused by mitochondrial dysfunction (relative hypoxia) can also increase blood lactate concentration. Less commonly increased lactate can result from impaired clearance as a result of liver dysfunction, thiamine deficiency, or increased catecholamine production.[21] Normal blood lactate concentrations in resting adult horses are generally less than 2 mmol/L; concentrations above this value indicate inadequate tissue oxygenation. Neonates (<24 hrs) have higher blood lactate concentrations (3 to 5 mmol/L) that decrease to adult values by 24 hours of age.[22,23] Serial measurements of lactate are useful for monitoring the response of global tissue perfusion to fluid therapy.

Evaluating total body electrolyte imbalances in horses is difficult because plasma electrolyte concentrations do not always reflect overall body abnormalities. Increases in serum sodium concentration can result from actual sodium excess or water deficit (dehydration). Serum potassium abnormalities are extremely important because of their potential effects on cardiac rate, rhythm, and conduction; yet potassium is a poor indicator of total body potassium because less than 2% of total body potassium is located in the ECF (because most potassium is inside cells).[24] It is important to note that total body potassium deficits may be present in sick horses, even when serum potassium is normal or increased. The functional pool of calcium and magnesium is best assessed by measurement of ionized calcium and ionized magnesium concentrations. These cations are critical for skeletal and smooth muscle function and play an important role in vascular tone and intestinal motility. Low concentrations of these electrolytes are frequently present in endotoxic horses.

Acute (minutes to hours) fluid administration is directed toward increasing vascular volume to support arterial blood pressure and maintain tissue perfusion. The administration of 3 to 10 ml/kg/hr of a "balanced" (similar to plasma) polyionic salt solution is adequate for most routine elective equine surgical procedures (Box 7-6).

TYPE OF FLUIDS

Selection of the "best" fluid for administration to anesthetized horses is determined by PCV, TP, electrolyte concentrations, acid-base status, and hemodynamics. The first step is to select a fluid; and the second step is to decide which additives will be used, depending on specific deficits or excesses such as hyponatremia/hypernatremia, hypokalemia/hyperkalemia, hypocalcemia/hypercalcemia, hypomag-

Box 7-6   Fluid Replacement

- Initial minimum rates of fluid administration: 3-10 ml/kg/hr LRS for 3 hours, then reevaluate.

- Increase this rate if significant hypotension develops: 20-30 ml/kg/hr.

- Fluid challenge: 20 to 40 ml/kg

- Monitor PCV and TP for hemodilution

  - If PCV <20% or TP <3.5 g/dl, consider giving a colloid, plasma, or blood.

- Estimate total blood loss and administer 3-5 ml of crystalloid solution for each milliliter of blood lost (unless blood transfusion is indicated) over and above the initial minimum rate of fluid administration.

  - Crystalloids are rapidly redistributed from the blood (approx. 8% body weight) vascular compartment into the interstitial compartment (15% to 25% body weight), which is approximately three times larger than the blood volume.

- Maximum rate of fluid that is administered during shock therapy varies considerably; the rule of thumb is 90 ml/kg/hr.

LRS, Lactate Ringer's solution; *PCV*, packed cell volume; *TP*, total plasma protein.

nesemia/hypermagnesemia, hypoglycemia, and acid-base abnormalities.

Two types of crystalloids are commonly used for replacement fluid therapy: 0.9% saline and balanced electrolyte solutions (BESs; see Table 7-4). In general, BESs are preferred when serum electrolytes and hemodynamics are near normal values. Lactate, acetate, and gluconate are used as bicarbonate precursors in BESs. Lactate is converted to bicarbonate in the liver, whereas acetate and gluconate are metabolized to bicarbonate in the plasma and other tissues. All BESs contain potassium (see Table 7-4). Saline (0.9%) contains physiologic Na$^+$ concentrations (154 mEq/L) but much higher chloride concentrations (154 mEq/L) than normally found (105 to 110 mEq/L) in plasma and is administered when Na is lower than 125 mEq/L or to dilute potassium [K$^+$] during hyperkalemia, hyperkalemic periodic paralysis, or renal failure. Horses with a metabolic (nonrespiratory) acidosis can become hyperkalemic. Potassium supplementation is indicated if horses are not eating or drinking and fluid therapy is continued for more than 24 hours. Horses should not receive more than 0.5 mEq of potassium per kilogram per hour to avoid hyperkalemia and associated cardiovascular complications (bradycardia, muscle weakness, vasodilation, hypotension). Most horses benefit from the addition of 12 mEq of potassium chloride per liter of fluids (80 mEq/5-L bag).

The use of a BES for prolonged periods (>4 to 5 days; maintenance fluid therapy) results in hypernatremia, hypokalemia, hypomagnesemia, and hypocalcemia. Hypokalemia can also develop because of lack of intake, diuresis, and gastrointestinal disease. The administration of half-strength BES, to which potassium, calcium and, magnesium are added, should be considered for this purpose (see Table 7-4).

Calcium, potassium, and *magnesium supplementation* are included in fluid replacement regimens when oral intake has stopped because of gastrointestinal disease (Box 7-7). Low serum ionized calcium (iCa) and magnesium (iMg) concentrations are common in horses with surgical gastrointestinal disease, particularly in horses with small intestinal or large and small colon nonstrangulating infarction, strangulation, or postoperative ileus.[25,26] Horses with enterocolitis also have low iCa and iMg and a decreased fractional clearance of calcium.[27] Total calcium and magnesium concentrations are not reliable for identification of calcium and magnesium imbalances; thus ionized concentrations are preferred.[25,26,28] Measurement of total calcium can be misleading when total protein is low (ionized calcium may still be normal) or if the horse becomes alkalotic (total calcium may be normal with a low ionized fraction). Recently fractional excretion of magnesium has been suggested as a diagnostic tool for the assessment of magnesium status in horses.[29] Supplementation of calcium and magnesium appears beneficial for fluid therapy in horses (see Box 7-7). Some crystalloid fluids such as Plasmalyte-A and Normosol-R contain 3 mEq/L of elemental magnesium. This amount may be insufficient to replace increased losses in sick horses.

Fluids Used for Severe Hypotension, Hypovolemia, and Resuscitation

Isotonic crystalloids

Isotonic (osmotically similar to plasma) crystalloids are administered intravenously and can restore circulating volume transiently if administered rapidly (40 to 90 ml/kg/hr). Balanced electrolyte (electrolyte concentration similar to plasma) solutions (e.g., lactated or acetated Ringer's) are preferred as routine fluid therapy in anesthetized horses to maintain normal plasma electrolyte concentrations and provide base replacement. However, all crystalloids distribute into the

Box 7-7   Calcium and Magnesium Therapy

- Addition of 50 to 100 ml of 23% calcium gluconate to every 5 L of intravenous fluid is usually sufficient to maintain normocalcemia. In the presence of severe hypocalcemia (iCa <4 mg/dl), addition of 500 ml of calcium gluconate to 5 L of BES is indicated.

- Hypocalcemia that is refractory to calcium therapy suggests hypomagnesemia, and concurrent magnesium (Mg) replacement is required.

- Maintenance requirements of Mg in horses are estimated at 13 mg/kg/day of elemental Mg, which can be provided by 31 mg/kg/day of MgO, 64 mg/kg/day of MgCO$_3$ or 93 mg/kg/day of MgSO$_4$.[30] These requirements may be increased in critically ill patients as indicated by the high prevalence of hypomagnesemia in hospitalized patients.[28]

- The concentration of elemental Mg in the compound should be determined when considering Mg supplementation.

- Administration of 150 mg/kg/day of MgSO$_4$ (0.3 ml/kg of a 50% solution) is equivalent to 14.5 mg/kg/day or 1.22 mEq/kg/day of elemental Mg and provides the daily requirements for the horse.[30] MgSO$_4$ can be diluted in saline, dextrose, or a balanced polyionic fluid.

interstitial fluid compartment in a short time (<30 min), limiting their value as a treatment for hypovolemia. Many texts suggest that, since the ECF compartment is at least three times the volume of the vascular (blood) compartment, a minimum of three times as much isotonic crystalloid as estimated blood lost should be administered to restore plasma volume and theoretically improve the effective circulating blood volume. For example, if blood loss is estimated at 6 L for a 500-kg horse, 18 L of a crystalloid should be required at a rate of 40 to 80 ml/kg/hr. This rationale, although logical, rarely provides adequate hemodynamics or successfully restores tissue perfusion and, when applied to horses that have suffered severe blood loss (>25 ml/kg), usually leads to hemodilution (decreased hemoglobin, hypoproteinemia), impaired clotting, and activation of neutrophils (systemic inflammatory response). Horses that are hypotensive (systolic blood pressure [BP] <80 to 90 mm Hg; mean BP <50 to 60 mm Hg) or have suffered severe blood loss are more appropriately treated with colloids, a mixture of colloids and crystalloids, or blood (PCV <15% to 20%), depending on the horse's disease, hemodynamics, electrolyte, and acid-base status.

Hypertonic (7.2% NaCl) Saline

Hypertonic (7.2% NaCl) saline (HS) is approximately eight times the tonicity of plasma and ECF (composition: Na, 1200 mosmol/L; Cl, 1200 mosmol/L) and is used in emergency situations as a "bridging" solution to rapidly restore vascular volume and improve hemodynamics. Hypertonic solutions expand the vascular volume by redistributing fluid from the interstitial and intracellular spaces. Each liter of 7.2% HS expands the plasma volume by 3 to 4.5 L, producing immediate and at times dramatic increases in arterial blood pressure, cardiac output, and tissue perfusion. However, this effect is short lived (30 to 90 minutes in horses) because the electrolytes (Na$^+$; Cl$^-$) are not constrained by the capillary wall and redistribute into the interstitial fluid compartment. Eventually the excess salt and water shifts back into the plasma and is eliminated via the kidney. Because the principal effect of HS is fluid redistribution, a total body fluid deficit may still persist that will require replacement. The duration of effect of hypertonic solutions is directly proportional to the tonicity and distribution constant of the solution, which is the indexed cardiac output. The intravenous administration of 4 ml/kg of 7.2% HS produces beneficial hemodynamic effects that persist for at least 45 minutes in most horses. This effect can be exaggerated and prolonged by administering 7.2% HS in a colloid (see following section). An effective resuscitative fluid that produces a sustained effect can be made by mixing 1 L of 23.4% NaCl (American Regent) with 2 L of 6% hetastarch and dosing at 4 ml/kg intravenously.

Colloids

Colloids are fluids that contain molecules that are too large (>30,000 Daltons) to cross the capillary wall. Some of the molecules eventually redistribute into the interstitial fluid compartment but at a much slower rate than crystalloids, thereby prolonging the duration of vascular volume expansion (see Table 7-4). Hetastarch (hydroxy ethyl starch) is a commonly used colloid for volume expansion in horses. The colloid osmotic pressure of 6% hetastarch (approximately 40 mm Hg versus equine plasma approx-

imately 20 mm Hg) suggests that the circulating blood volume expands by approximately one additional liter for each liter of hetastarch administered, resulting in a total volume expansion of approximately 2 L. The administration of 5 to 10 ml/kg of 6% hetastarch produces immediate and sustained beneficial hemodynamic effects in anesthetized horses, which may persist for up to 18 to 24 hours.[16] The combination of hypertonic saline and hetastarch (4 ml/kg) produces a more pronounced and prolonged beneficial hemodynamic effect than either fluid alone or the administration of a crystalloid.[31,32] The preoperative administration of a hydroxyethyl starch, pentastarch, to horses with colic improves cardiac index to a greater extent than that of 7.2% hypertonic saline.[33]

BICARBONATE REPLACEMENT

Poor tissue perfusion and tissue hypoxia are the most common causes of nonrespiratory acidosis and lactic (metabolic) acidosis in sick hypovolemic, hypotensive, and anesthetized horses. Fluid replacement should be the first and principal means for correcting this problem. Sodium *bicarbonate* supplementation may be required in horses when *metabolic acidosis* produces a pH value less than 7.2 (Box 7-8).

Most methods for determining sodium bicarbonate replacement therapy are based on the plasma bicarbonate concentration (mEq/L) or base deficit (mEq/L) and an estimation of the horse's ECFV (e.g., 500 kg × 0.3 [30%] = 15 L; see Boxes 7-2 and 7-8 and Table 7-6).

Horses that have developed an acute metabolic acidosis during anesthesia are administered one-half of the calculated dose (e.g., 500 × 0.3 × base deficits [10] = 150 mEq × ½ = 75 mEq) and reassessed before administering the remaining amount. Horses that are severely acidotic or continue to lose bicarbonate (e.g., diarrhea) generally require the full calculated amount of sodium bicarbonate because the body's buffering capabilities have been depleted. Oral sodium bicarbonate administration is a practical method of treating

---

Box 7–8 Rules of Thumb for Bicarbonate Supplementation in *Acute* Metabolic Acidosis

Guidelines for Base Replacement in Anesthetized Horses

- Administration of half of the calculated amount of HCO$_3^-$, rapidly followed by the remainder over 12-24 hours.
- Intravenous bicarbonate should not be given with calcium-containing solutions.

$$HCO_3^- (mEq) = 0.3 \times BW (kg) \times Base\ deficit\ (mEq/L)$$

or

$$HCO_3^- (mEq) = \frac{BW\ (lb)}{7} \times Base\ deficit\ (mEq/L)$$

Note: 12 mEq HCO$_3^-$/g NaHCO$_3$

Therefore:

$$\frac{mEq\ of\ HCO_3^-\ needed}{12} = Total\ grams\ of\ NaHCO_3 required$$

ongoing sodium bicarbonate losses in conscious horses with diarrhea. Bicarbonate can be administered orally as a powder: 1 g $NaHCO_3$ = 12 mEq of HCO_3^-. Excess bicarbonate administration can result in hypernatremia or hypokalemia and may cause or worsen respiratory acidosis because bicarbonate and water produce carbon dioxide. Carbon dioxide can enter the cerebrospinal fluid or cells and produce paradoxical central nervous system and intracellular acidosis. Other potential problems include a decrease in the plasma concentrations of ionized calcium and an increase in hemoglobin affinity for oxygen (left shift in the oxyhemoglobin dissociation curve), thereby decreasing the amount of oxygen carried and available for tissue metabolism.

Blood Component Therapy

Blood or blood component fluid therapy is indicated when there has been a significant loss of whole blood or its components (Box 7-9). Blood or plasma loss may be caused by severe lacerations, as a result of surgery, or in horses with chronic gastrointestinal diseases. Transfused red blood cells survive for 2 to 4 days in horses, and incompatibility may lead to anaphylactic reactions, despite compatible cross-matching.[34] Whole blood or packed red cells are indicated only when blood loss is life threatening (i.e., PCV falls below 12% to 15% or the hemoglobin falls below 4 to 5 g/dl). Plasma replacement is indicated when the plasma TP is less than 3 g/dl (or 4 g/dl if signs of edema are present[35]) or the albumin is less than 1.5 g/dl. The PCV and TP may remain essentially unchanged after acute blood loss for up to 6 to 12 hours, depending on the amount of blood loss (spleen contracts). The decision to transfuse after acute blood loss must be based on clinical signs of hypovolemia (increased heart rate, decreased blood pressure, pale mucous membranes) and estimates of total blood losses (>20% blood volume), in addition to PCV and TP.

The three most important antigenic blood groups in horses are responsible for most cases of equine neonatal isoerythrocytolysis. Although anti-Ca antibodies are common, they do not seem to produce clinical reactions. Therefore a suitable equine blood donor should be healthy; Coggins test negative; and negative for Aa and Qa antigens, common antierythrocyte antibodies and, if possible, Ca antigens.[36]

Blood compatibility (cross-matching) in horses is best evaluated using tests for hemolysis rather than agglutination. Major and minor cross-matching may fail to demonstrate all incompatibilities that could become evident on transfusion of the patient. Prior blood typing of prospective donors is recommended to avoid the common reactive blood groups.[36] A gelding of the same breed that has never been transfused is the best choice for a blood donor when tests for compatibility cannot be done. Acid-citrate-dextrose (ACD), citrate-phosphate-dextrose (CPD), and citrate-phosphate-dextrose-adenine (CPDA-1) are the recommended anticoagulants for collecting and storing blood. The ratio of anticoagulant to whole blood should be 1:9.[36] Kits are available commercially that contain sodium citrate as the anticoagulant, but they should not be used for storage of red blood cells. Blood may be collected into glass bottles or intravenous solution bags that contain an appropriate amount of anticoagulant. Blood should not be collected in glass bottles for platelet preservation. Whole blood or erythrocytes can be refrigerated (4° C) up to 21 days in ACD or CPD, and up to 35 days in CPDA-1.[37] Plasma may be separated from erythrocytes by centrifugation or sedimentation; equine erythrocytes usually sediment within 2 hours if undisturbed. Separated plasma should be frozen and can be kept for up to 1 year.

The donor's PCV and TP should be checked before blood collection. Blood must be collected aseptically to minimize the risk of bacterial contamination. The area over the donor's jugular vein should be clipped, surgically prepared, and locally anesthetized with 1 to 2 ml of 2% lidocaine. A 10- to 12-gauge, 2- to 3-inch needle or bleeding trochar is inserted cranial into the jugular vein and connected by sterile tubing to the bottle or bag containing anticoagulant. The jugular vein may be occluded distally to promote blood collection. The collection bottle or bag should be rocked gently to ensure adequate mixing of blood and anticoagulant. A total volume of up to 20 ml/kg (approximately 8 to 9 L in a 450-kg horse) can safely be collected from a donor every 3 weeks.[38,39]

Blood Replacement

Whole blood transfusions are recommended only when necessary (PCV <15%; hemoglobin <5 g/dl) to save the horse's life because transfused erythrocytes survive only about 4 to 6 days even when cross-matching tests indicate compatibility. Horses can increase their PCV at a rate of about 0.67% per day after a single incident of blood loss. The change in PCV and TP following acute blood loss may not be measurable for

---

Box 7–9   Amount of Blood and Plasma Needed

Fresh whole blood or blood substitutes should be administered to replace acute blood loss (>20% loss of blood volume) and improve oxygen delivery to tissues.

$$\text{Amount of donor blood needed (ml)} = \text{Recipient blood volume (ml)} \times \frac{\text{Desired PCV} - \text{Actual PCV (patient)}}{\text{PCV of anticoagulated donor blood}}$$

A general rule is that 2 to 3 ml of whole blood per kilogram of recipient body weight (assuming donor PCV of 40%) will raise the recipient's PCV by 1%.

$$\text{Amount of donor plasma needed (ml)} = \text{Recipient plasma volume (ml)} \times \frac{\text{Desired TP} - \text{Actual TP (patient)}}{\text{TP of anticoagulated donor plasma}}$$

12 to 24 hours. Administration of shock doses of crystalloids and/or colloids helps to restore circulating blood volume but not oxygen-carrying capacity (requires hemoglobin). If improvements in tissue perfusion do not occur or if the PCV drops to <20% and TP to <4.5 g/dl during fluid administration, a blood transfusion may be necessary (see Box 7-9).

Hemoglobin-Based Oxygen Carriers

Oxyglobin, a hemoglobin-based oxygen carrier (HBOC), is a glutaraldehyde polymerized bovine hemoglobin solution that has been administered safely to horses for restoration of oxygen-carrying capacity.[40-43] Volume expansion occurs following Oxyglobin administration because of the colloidal nature of the solution. Administration of 15 ml/kg at the rate of 10 ml/kg/hr improved hemodynamics and oxygen transport parameters without adverse renal or coagulation effects in ponies with experimentally induced normovolemic anemia; however, one pony suffered an anaphylactoid reaction during infusion.[43] The half-life of Oxyglobin is relatively short; therefore the patient may require additional tranfusions.[43]

Plasma Replacement

Whole blood or blood components should be warmed to near body temperature before administration. Blood should not be exposed to temperatures greater than 40° C during this warming process. Plasma should be thawed in warm water. Equine plasma should not be thawed in a microwave.

Blood or plasma should be administered using a blood administration set with a filter to prevent clots from entering the patient's vascular system. Whole blood should be administered slowly for the first 5 min, if possible, to minimize the risk of a significant transfusion reaction. Blood may be administered at a rate of up to 20 ml/kg/hr if no adverse signs (e.g., hypotension, skin wheals) occur. Plasma should be administered at 10 ml/kg/hr for the treatment of hypoproteinemia to avoid volume overload.

References

1. Spurlock GH, Spurlock SL: A technique of catheterization of the lateral thoracic vein in the horse, *Equine Pract* 9:33-35, 1987.
2. Deem D: Complications associated with the use of intravenous catheters in large animals, *Calif Vet* 35:19-24, 1981.
3. Bayly WM, Vale B: Intravenous catheterization and associated problems in the horse, *Compend Contin Educ* 4:S227-S237, 1982.
4. Spurlock SL et al: Long-term jugular vein catheterization in horses, *J Am Vet Med Assoc* 196:425-430, 1990.
5. Warmerdam EP: Ultrasound corner: "pseudo-catheter-sleeve" sign in the jugular vein of a horse, *Vet Radiol Ultrasound* 39:148-149, 1998.
6. Corley KT et al: Cardiac output technologies with special reference to the horse, *J Vet Intern Med* 17:262-272, 2003.
7. Barr ED et al: Destructive lesions of the proximal sesamoid bones as a complication of dorsal metatarsal artery catheterization in three horses, *Vet Surg* 34:159-166, 2005.
8. Fulton RB, Hauptman JG: In vitro and in vivo rates of fluid flow through catheters in peripheral veins of dogs, *J Am Vet Med Assoc* 198:1622-1624, 1991.
9. Dolente BA et al: Evaluation of risk factors for development of catheter-associated jugular thrombophlebitis in horses: 50 cases (1993-1998), *J Am Vet Med Assoc* 227:1134-1141, 2005.
10. Fielding CL et al: Pharmacokinetics and clinical utility of sodium bromide (NaBr) as an estimator of extracellular fluid volume in horses, *J Vet Intern Med* 17:213-217, 2003.
11. Fielding CL et al: Use of multifrequency bioelectrical impedance analysis for estimation of total body water and extracellular and intracellular fluid volumes in horses, *Am J Vet Res* 65:320-326, 2004.
12. Spensley MS, Carlson GP, Harrold D: Plasma, red blood cell, total blood, and extracellular fluid volumes in healthy horse foals during growth, *Am J Vet Res* 48:1703-1707, 1987.
13. Persson SG, Funkquist P, Nyman G: Total blood volume in the normally performing standardbred trotter: age and sex variations, *Zentralbl Veterinarmed A* 43:57-64, 1996.
14. Brownlow MA, Hutchins DR: The concept of osmolality: its use in the evaluation of "dehydration" in the horse, *Equine Vet J* 14:106-110, 1982.
15. Edwards D, Brownlow M, Hutchins D: Indices of renal function: value in eight normal foals from birth to 56 days, *Aust Vet J* 67:251-254, 1990.
16. Jones PA, Tomasic M, Gentry PA: Oncotic, hemodilutional, and hemostatic effects of isotonic saline and hydroxyethyl starch solutions in clinically normal ponies, *Am J Vet Res* 58:541-548, 1997.
17. Runk DT et al: Measurement of plasma colloid osmotic pressure in normal thoroughbred neonatal foals, *J Vet Intern Med* 14:475-478, 2000.
18. Rose B, Post T: The total body water and the plasma sodium concentration. In Rose BD, Post T: *Clinical physiology of acid-base and electrolytes disorders*, ed 5, New York, 2000, McGraw-Hill, pp 241-257.
19. Guglielminotti J et al: Osmolar gap hyponatremia in critically ill patients: evidence for the sick cell syndrome? *Crit Care Med* 30:1051-1055, 2002.
20. Evans D, Golland L: Accuracy of Accusport for measurement of lactate concentrations in equine blood and plasma, *Equine Vet J* 28:398-402, 1996.
21. Friedrich C: Lactic acidosis update for critical care clinicians, *J Am Soc Nephrol* 12:S15-S19, 2001.
22. Corley KT, Donaldson L, Furr MO: Arterial lactate concentration, hospital survival, sepsis, and SIRS in critically ill neonatal foals, *Equine Vet J* 37:53-59, 2005.
23. Silver M et al: Sympathoadrenal and other responses to hypoglycaemia in the young foal, *J Reprod Fertil* 35(suppl):607-614, 1987.
24. Rose RJ: A physiological approach to fluid and electrolyte therapy in the horse, *Equine Vet J* 13:7-14, 1981.
25. Dart A et al: Ionized concentration in horses with surgically managed gastrointestinal disease 147: cases (1988–1990), *J Am Vet Med Assoc* 201:1244-1248, 1992.
26. Garcia-Lopez J et al: Prevalence and prognostic importance of hypomagnesemia and hypocalcemia in the equine surgical colic patient, *Am J Vet Res* 62:7-12, 2001.
27. Toribio RE et al: Comparison of serum parathyroid hormone and ionized calcium and magnesium concentrations and fractional urinary clearance of calcium and phosphorus in healthy horses and horses with enterocolitis, *Am J Vet Res* 62:938-947, 2001.
28. Johansson A et al: Hypomagnesemia in hospitalized horses, *J Vet Intern Med* 17:860-867, 2003.
29. Stewart AJ et al: Validation of diagnostic tests for determination of magnesium status in horses with reduced magnesium intake, *Am J Vet Res* 65:422-430, 2004.
30. Stewart A: Magnesium disorders. In Reed S, Bayly W, Sellon D, editors: *Equine internal medicine*, St Louis, 2004, Saunders, pp1365-1379.
31. Prough DS et al: Hypertonic/hyperoncotic fluid resuscitation after hemorrhagic shock in dogs, *Anesth Analg* 73:738-744, 1991.

32. Vollmar B et al: Hypertonic hydroxyethyl starch restores hepatic microvascular perfusion in hemorrhagic shock, *Am J Physiol* 266:H1927-1934, 1994.

33. Hallowell GD, Corley KT: Preoperative administration of hydroxyethyl starch or hypertonic saline to horses with colic, *J Vet Intern Med* 20:980-986, 2006.

34. Kallfelz FA, Whitlock RH, Schultz RD: Survival of 59 Fe-labeled erythrocytes in cross-transfused equine blood, *Am J Vet Res* 39:617-620, 1978.

35. Morris DD: Blood products in large animal medicine: a comparative account of current and future technologies, *Equine Vet J* 9:272-275, 1987.

36. Schmotzer WB: Time-saving techniques for the collection, storage, and administration of equine blood and plasma, *Vet Med* 80:89-94, 1985.

37. Mudge MC et al: Comparison of 4 blood storage methods in a protocol for equine pre-operative autologous donation, *Vet Surg* 33:475-486, 2004.

38. Malikides N et al: Cardiovascular, haematological, and biochemical responses after large volume blood collection in horses, *Vet J* 162:44-55, 2001.

39. Malikides N et al: Haematological responses of repeated large volume blood collection in the horse, *Res Vet Sci* 68:275-278, 2000.

40. Belgrave RL et al: Effects of a polymerized ultrapurified bovine hemoglobin blood substitute administered to ponies with normovolemic anemia, *J Vet Intern Med* 16:396-403, 2002.

41. Maxson AD et al: Use of a bovine hemoglobin preparation in the treatment of cyclic ovarian hemorrhage in a miniature horse, *J Am Vet Med Assoc* 203:1308-1311, 1993.

42. Perkins G, Divers T: Polymerized hemoglobin therapy in a foal with neonatal isoerythrolysis, *J Vet Emerg Crit Care* 11:141-143, 2001.

43. Soma LR et al: The pharmacokinetics of hemoglobin-based oxygen carrier hemoglobin glutamer-200 bovine in the horse, *Anesth Analg* 100:1570-1575, 2005.

8

Monitoring Anesthesia

John A.E. Hubbell
William W. Muir

KEY POINTS

1. Monitoring consciousness and the "depth of anesthesia" is the key to safe anesthetic practice.
2. Producing "ideal anesthesia" is not a single pharmacological process but a balance between hypnosis (unconsciousness), analgesia (pain relief), and muscle relaxation to produce nonresponsiveness to surgical stimuli.
3. Vigilance, awareness, and timely response to clinical signs and stimulus-response pairs is particularly important in horses because external cardiac massage is of limited value and resuscitation therapies are limited.
4. Knowledge and familiarity with the pharmacology of drugs used to produce anesthesia, including their side effects, is the basis for safe anesthesia.
5. The type of monitoring required for anesthesia depends on the patient, the procedure, and the anticipated duration of anesthesia.
6. Monitoring depth of anesthesia, respiratory rate, mucous membrane color and perfusion time, and arterial blood pressure is of particular importance.
7. Direct arterial blood pressure monitoring should be used in sick horses, those undergoing major surgical procedures, or that involve significant blood loss. The maintenance of mean arterial blood pressures in excess of 60-70 mm Hg reduces the incidence of postoperative complications.
8. Objective, accurate, and precise data should be recorded at frequent (5-minute) intervals.
9. The legal maxim, "If it wasn't written down, it didn't happen," is a guide for anesthetic record keeping.
10. No piece of monitoring equipment exists that can replace a knowledgeable, trained, experienced, and attentive anesthetist.

All animals respond somewhat differently to anesthetic drugs, and horses are not unique in this regard. Safe anesthesia is predicated on knowledge of the appropriate drugs and dosages required to produce anesthesia in horses on the basis of their physical characteristics and condition; the scale and duration of surgery; and the ability to detect, recognize, and correct abnormalities before they become problems (see Chapter 6). The identification and interpretation of the nuances associated with equine anesthesia are learned skills that improve with practice and clinical experience and are complimented by a variety of technological devices. Regardless, a trained and skilled anesthetist is required to identify and elucidate the various physical, physiological, and technological signs that occur during anesthesia to avoid complications and prevent adverse outcomes. Toward this end, emphasis has been placed on the assessment of factors that suggest changes in vital processes that are most closely linked to the horses' immediate survival and most commonly includes evaluation of central nervous system and cardiovascular and respiratory functions. Changes in other organ system functions, although important (e.g., renal, liver) generally are considered preoperatively or in decisions regarding long-term care.

Both subjective (qualitative) and objective (quantitative) data are used to monitor (describe) anesthesia. Qualitative data generally are obtained by categorically recording visual, tactile, and auditory data. For example, a horse recovering from anesthesia may be tearing, relaxed, with pink mucous membranes, exhibiting inspiratory stridor, and snoring. A specific value cannot be placed on any of the aforementioned variables, but they can be described and categorized (e.g., minimum versus maximum; pale pink versus reddish; quiet versus loud). Quantitative data can be obtained by indirect (noninvasive) or direct (invasive) methods and are recorded as a numerical value that is limited only by the precision and accuracy of the measurement process.

Monitoring methods are divided into physical and technological techniques. Physical monitors parallel skills involved in performing a physical examination but also include assessment of muscle tone and reflexes, particularly those involving the horse's eye reflexes and movements. Technological methods use instruments to quantify various aspects of homeostasis, physiological variables, and the depth of anesthesia. Technologic monitoring provides important information regarding responses to drugs and trends in physiological variables. Technological devices that use indirect methods for assessing physiological function are less precise (good agreement between repeated observations) and less accurate (observed value agrees with the true value) than direct methods because the data obtained are influenced (biased) by more technical factors and demonstrate a greater inherent variability.

Anesthetic monitoring in horses encompasses an integrated, qualitative, and quantitative assessment of central nervous system and cardiovascular and respiratory functions to produce the safest anesthetic experience possible and ensure the most favorable outcome.

The American College of Veterinary Anesthesiologists has developed guidelines for equine anesthesia that include recommendations for the level of monitoring (Box 8-1).[1] The physical status of the patient, the anesthetic technique chosen, the procedure to be performed, and, most important, the anticipated duration of the anesthetic period are key factors used to determine the sophistication of monitoring techniques. Once again, despite technological advances in monitoring, there is no substitute for a skilled, attentive, vigilant anesthetist.

Box 8–1   American College of Veterinary Anesthesiologists Monitoring Guidelines for Horses

Monitoring of the Cardiovascular System

- Digital pulse palpation
- Capillary refill time, mucous membrane color
- Electrocardiogram, if indicated
- Arterial blood pressure, if indicated (strongly recommended whenever inhalation anesthesia is used)

Monitoring of the Respiratory System

- Observation or respiratory rate and rhythm
- Pulse oximetry, if indicated
- Capnometry, if indicated
- Arterial blood gas analysis, if indicated

THE ANESTHESIA RECORD

The anesthesia record provides key information regarding the anesthetic experience, helps to ensure that all appropriate steps are performed, and provides a framework for organizing anesthetic procedures (Figure 8-1). Computer-based digital note/graphic pads are available for recording key data and can be transferred immediately to computer-based hospital data storage systems (Figure 8-2). The anesthesia record is a legal document that verifies the preanesthetic evaluation, outlines the drugs and equipment used, records responses to those drugs, and identifies and documents the types and frequency of significant events (onset of surgery, tourniquet placement, position changes). Most important, the anesthesia record prompts the anesthetist to regularly observe, evaluate, and record information concerning the horse's status. The minimum information that the anesthesia record should contain includes patient identification, a brief history, a summary of the preanesthetic examination, the anesthetic drugs administered with dose and time, and regular recording of heart rate and respiratory rate (Box 8-2). It is good anesthetic practice to record significant events such as the beginning and ending of surgery, the administration of ancillary drugs (antibiotics), and the type and quantity of intravenous fluids administered. The sophistication of the anesthesia record should increase as the level of monitoring increases (see Box 8-2).

Frequent recording of physiologic variables facilitates recognition of trends and adjustments to the anesthetic protocol. For example, an anesthetized foal with a heart rate of 50 beats/min may not be remarkable, but a foal with a heart rate of 50 10 minutes ago that is currently 70 beats/min requires evaluation.

MONITORING THE DEPTH OF ANESTHESIA

The level of consciousness or depth of anesthesia is a key concern during equine anesthesia. Horses that are too "light" may respond to surgical stimulation, resulting in excessive stress, movement, and contamination of the surgical site and injury to themselves and operating room personnel (see Chapter 4). Horses that are too "deep" may suffer excessive cardiorespiratory depression, predisposing to a poor recovery and myopathy (see Chapter 22). Historically the depth of anesthesia has been categorized into stages and planes for both descriptive and academic purposes (Table 8-1). These stages and planes were developed on the basis of the physical signs produced by increasing concentrations of inhalant (ether) anesthesia but have been modified and applied to describe the effects of both inhalant and intravenous anesthetic drugs (see Chapters 12 and 15). More sophisticated methods for monitoring anesthetic depth have evolved in human anesthesia. Most of these methods depend on determination of drug plasma concentrations, exhaled (end-tidal) inhalant anesthetic concentration, or alterations in the electroencephalogram (EEG).

Physical Signs

Anesthesia depth generally is assessed by physical signs, including movement, the position of the eye, the degree of depression of the protective reflexes (palpebral; corneal) of the eye, the loss of the swallowing reflex, the rate and depth of breathing, and the horse's response to surgical stimulation (see Table 8-1). Other indicators of a "light" plane of anesthesia include shivering, tightening of muscles in the neck and shoulders, or occasional stretching in foals. Adequately anesthetized horses generally are relaxed, do not respond to surgical stimulation, and have eyes that are ventromedially or centrally located with reduced reflex responses (Box 8-3; see Table 8-1). The anal reflex (contraction of the anal sphincter when the anus is stimulated) is a crude index of anesthesia depth if the head is not accessible. Absence of the anal reflex indicates an excess depth of anesthesia. Reflex responses generally become more depressed and less reliable during prolonged anesthetic procedures. The administration of neuromuscular blocking drugs (atracurium) and dissociative anesthetics (ketamine and tiletamine) produces special exceptions. Neuromuscular blocking drugs prevent motor responses, obviating the use of movement and reflex motor responses. Monitoring the depth of anesthesia and the magnitude of neuromuscular blockade when using skeletal muscle relaxants requires special techniques (see Chapter 18). Alternatively, ketamine or tiletamine increases muscle tone, limiting the use of muscle relaxation and eye signs as reliable indicators of anesthesia depth during dissociative total intravenous anesthesia (TIVA) (see Chapter 13).

Eye Signs

Lateral nystagmus, tearing, and unstimulated closure of the eyelids are frequently observed during light planes of anesthesia and disappear as the effects of the anesthetic drugs intensify to a surgical plane. The eyeball rotates ventromedially ("forward") during "light" planes of anesthesia and returns to a central location as the level of anesthesia deepens (Figure 8-3; see Table 8-1). The palpebral reflex (closure of the lids when the cilia are stimulated) and the corneal reflex (closure of the lids when pressure is applied to the cornea) are two key reflexes used to evaluate anesthetic depth. The usual response to palpebral stimulation is rapid closure of the eyelids. The palpebral response is

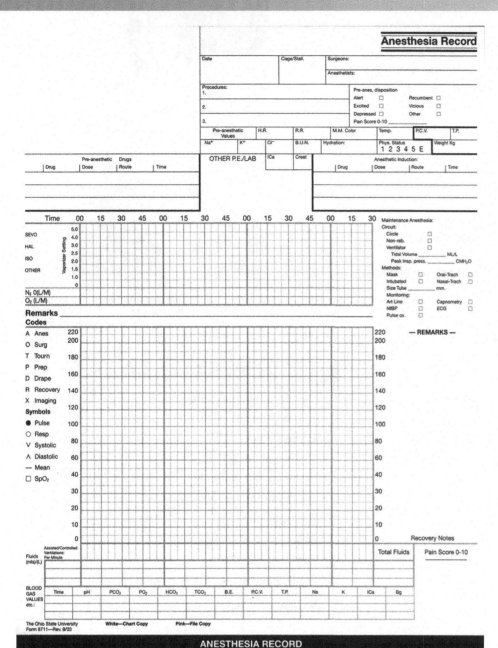

Figure 8–1. Example of an anesthesia record used to monitor key anesthetic, physiological, surgical, and therapeutic events associated with anesthesia. (See also Appendix C.)

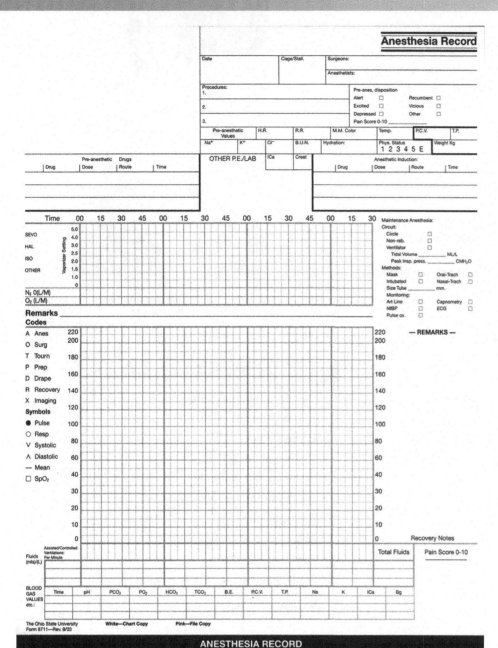

Figure 8–2. Computer-based digital note pads facilitate the collection and transfer of monitored data to hospital computer data storage files.

progressively depressed as anesthetic drug effects intensify. Horses induced to anesthesia with ketamine or tiletamine maintain active palpebral reflexes during the transition from injectable to inhalant anesthesia. Furthermore, the eye is usually centrally located in the globe in horses administered dissociative anesthetics and often exhibits unstimulated blinking, lacrimation, and oculogyric activity. A progressive reduction in reflex activity can be used as an index of the onset of inhalant anesthetic effects. The palpebral response is depressed significantly and may be absent during surgical levels of inhalant anesthesia in some horses. The corneal reflex should always be present. Absence of the corneal reflex suggests an excessive anesthesia depth and central nervous system depression during either inhalant anesthesia or TIVA. Changes in the depth of anesthesia produced by inhalant anesthetics are dose dependent.

Box 8–2   The Anesthesia Record

Minimum Information

- Patient identification
- Key physical and laboratory data
- Medical or surgical procedure performed
- Timing, dose, and route of anesthetic drugs administered
- Time line: recording of heart rate and respiratory rate (5-minute intervals)
  - Arterial blood pressure should be monitored during inhalant anesthesia and prolonged (>45 minute) procedures
- Significant events (apnea, blood loss, position changes)
- Additional therapies (intravenous fluids, antibiotics, emergency drugs)
- Specific equipment used (endotracheal tubes, monitors, fluid pumps, ventilator)

Optional Information

- Arterial blood pressure (direct or indirect)
- pH and blood gas values
  - Pulse oximetry values
  - End-tidal carbon dioxide tension values
- Temperature
- Ventilation values (tidal volume, peak inspiratory pressure, I:E ratio)
- Central venous pressure
- Cardiac output
- Other (e.g., inhalant anesthetic conc.)

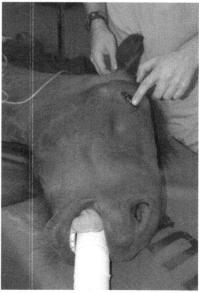

Figure 8–3. "Eye" signs, including the palpebral (eyelid) and corneal responses to touch, eye position, and tearing can also be used to judge the depth of anesthesia. Palpebral and corneal reflexes are less reliable in horses administered neuromuscular blocking drugs and dissociative anesthetics (ketamine, tiletamine).

Box 8–3   Physical Signs of Anesthesia Depth

- Muscle tone/movement
- Palpebral reflex
- Corneal reflex
- Position of the eyeball
- Lacrimation/nystagmus
- Swallowing/ear movement
- Anal sphincter tone
- Response to surgical stimulation
- Shivering, stretching
- Respiratory rate, heart rate and arterial blood pressure are less reliable indictors and may be depressed during surgical anesthesia (Stage 3; plane 2 & 4)

Table 8–1.   Monitoring anesthesia depth: modified for horses from Guedel's stages and planes of anesthesia

Stage	Pupil position/size	Eye reflex	Respirations/heart rate/ blood pressure
One (analgesia)	Central/small	P/C active	
Two (delirium)	Central (active)/large	P/C active	Variably increased
Three			
Plane 1 ("light")	**Ventromedial/small**	**P mildly depressed C active**	**Normal or elevated** (occasional swallowing)
Plane 2 (medium)	**Ventromedial/medium**	**P depressed C mildly depressed**	**Normal or minimally depressed**
Plane 3 (medium-deep)	**Central/medium**	**P depressed C depressed**	**Minimally to moderately depressed**
Plane 4 ("deep")	Central/large	P absent C markedly depressed	Markedly depressed
Four (overdose)	Central full dilation	P/C absent	Collapse

P/C, Palpebral/corneal; *ventromedial,* eyes are forward.
Ideal anesthetic depths are in bold.

Assessment of physical signs (purposeful movement and eye signs) as measures of adequate anesthesia depth can be problematic in some horses. Some purposeful movements may be reflexive in nature without conscious control, and occasional horses have markedly depressed eye signs at lighter planes of anesthesia. The degree of responsiveness generally depends on the degree of analgesia, the depth of hypnosis, and the type and magnitude of the noxious stimulus. Analgesia depends on drug-induced depression of ascending pain (nociceptive) pathways before or after they reach the level of the dorsal horn of the spinal cord, brainstem reticular formation, thalamic nuclei, and cerebral cortex (see Chapter 20). Inhibition of nociceptive transmission helps to prevent activation of the cerebral cortex and the conscious perception of pain. Inadequate analgesia results in cortical arousal and a greater likelihood of a purposeful response. thus assessment of consciousness is a dynamic process dependent on the functional integrity of sensory pathways that transmit pain signals to the brain. therefore arousal from an apparent unconscious state can occur in an otherwise adequately anesthetized horse if the pain-inducing stimulus is sufficient.

Electroencephalography

Electroencephalography is the monitoring of brain electrical activity. Alterations in the EEG waveform have a weak correlation with anesthetic depth, and the EEG alone is not considered a sensitive or specific index of anesthetic depth because of subtle variations in the EEG patterns generated during anesthesia and the large number of variables that can affect these patterns.[2,3] Increasing doses of anesthetic produce different EEG patterns, depending on the anesthetic administered. Computer-enhanced encephalography (compressed spectral analysis, fast Fourier transformation) generates frequency spectra that have been used to develop monitors that are advocated as means to predict the depth of anesthesia.[2] Processed EEG variables such as the spectral edge frequency and the median frequency are used clinically to monitor anesthetic depth in humans.[2-6] The bispectral index or BIS is a dimensionless EEG parameter derived from Fourier and bispectral calculations derived from an algorithm that relates the degree to which EEG waveforms are in phase (biocoherence), the amount of EEG power, and the proportion of the EEG that is isoelectric. The degree of biocoherence is inversely related to the derived BIS (more biocoherence–lower BIS). The BIS could potentially be useful as an indicator of anesthesia depth and as an index of cerebral perfusion in horses similar to other species.[1] The effect of isoflurane on BIS values has been evaluated in 16 horses before, during, and after castration.[4] Horses were premedicated with detomidine and butorphanol followed by detomidine, ketamine, and diazepam. BIS values obtained after detomidine-butorphanol premedication were extremely variable, and mean BIS values during 1.4% (n = 8) and 1.9% (n = 8) end-tidal isoflurane concentrations were not significantly different from values in sedated horses (n = 16). Mean BIS values did show a downward trend in isoflurane-anesthetized horses, and the variability of measurements was considerably less than in sedate horses.[4] The authors concluded that the BIS was not a good indicator of level of consciousness and, although potentially useful, of little use for routine clinical use at this time.

Monitoring the Concentration of Anesthetic Drugs

The plasma concentration of injectable drugs or the end-tidal concentration (partial pressure, %) of inhaled anesthetic drugs can be monitored to determine the dose-response effects that ensure adequate anesthetic depth (see Chapter 9). Inhalation anesthetic concentration can be monitored by analyzing an end-tidal gas sample from the airway (Figure 8-4). The end-tidal partial pressure or percentage of the anesthetic gas is an index of the partial pressure of the gas in the alveoli and brain and serves as a measure of the quantity of anesthetic being delivered. The partial pressure or percent of the anesthetic gas in the end-tidal sample can be determined by mass spectrometry, infrared or ultraviolet absorption, silicone rubber relaxation, or crystal oscillation. The percent concentration of inhaled anesthetic required to produce and maintain anesthesia is decreased by sedatives, the presence of preexisting diseases, and the coadministration of anesthetic adjuncts, particularly analgesic drugs (see Chapters 10 to 13). Future technological advances may become available that relate plasma or end-tidal gas concentrations to a physical sign (skeletal muscle tone), thereby providing a pharmacodynamic assessment of anesthetic effect.

MONITORING RESPIRATORY AND CARDIOVASCULAR VARIABLES

Maintaining adequate pulmonary and cardiovascular function is a primary goal of successful equine anesthesia (Boxes 8-4 and 8-5; Table 8-2). These two organ systems are responsible for maintaining adequate delivery of oxygenated blood to peripheral tissues and the removal of waste products (see Chapters 2 and 3). Tissue oxygenation depends on the volume of oxygen delivered to (oxygen transport; DO_2) and consumed by (oxygen consumption; VO_2) the tissues (Figure 8-5). This supply-demand relationship is determined by five principal factors, including the hemoglobin concentration, the percentage of hemoglobin

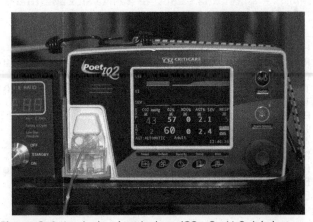

Figure 8–4. Inspired and expired gas (CO_2, O_2, N_2O, inhalant anesthetics) concentration can be monitored continuously. Note the end-tidal CO_2 (43 mm Hg) and inspired concentration of sevoflurane (2.4%) in this horse breathing 60% O_2. The ability to monitor circuit inhalant anesthetic concentrations ensures that the vaporizer is functioning properly.

Box 8–4   Monitoring Respiratory Status

- Respiratory rate and pattern
  - Chest wall and abdominal movement
  - Air movement at nostrils
  - Intermittent breathing
- Depth of respiration
  - Degree of chest wall movement
  - Small and large volume breaths
  - Rebreathing bag volume changes
- Mucous membrane color
- Inspiratory effort
- Technological monitors
  - Arterial blood gases
  - Capnometry (end-tidal carbon dioxide tension)
  - Pulse oximetry
  - Arterial oxygen content

Box 8–5   Monitoring Cardiovascular Status

Physical Monitors

- Heart rate
  - Auscultation
  - Palpation of the pulse
- Pulse strength
- Capillary refill time
- Mucous membrane color

Technological Monitors

- Electrocardiography
- Arterial blood pressure (direct and indirect)
- Central venous pressure
- Cardiac output
- Pulse oximetry
- Arterial and venous blood gases
- Echocardiography

in the arterial blood that is saturated with oxygen, the affinity of hemoglobin for oxygen, the cardiac output, and oxygen consumption (Figure 8-5). All of these variables or their determinants can be monitored in some way. For example, mean arterial blood pressure values in excess of 60 to 70 mm of Hg usually indicate adequate cardiac output (CO) since cardiac output is directly related to arterial blood pressure (ABP = CO × systemic vascular resistance). Arterial blood pressure values above 60 mm Hg are known to reduce anesthetic-related morbidity and the incidence of postoperative complications, even though some horses may have low cardiac output values because of high systemic vascular resistance.[8]

The respiratory system is monitored to ensure adequate gas (O_2, CO_2) exchange, oxygenation of hemoglobin, and drug delivery if an inhalant anesthetic is being used. The key components of respiratory function are minute volume and arterial oxygen content (CaO_2; see Chapter 2). Respiratory minute volume is the product of the breathing frequency (f) and the volume of gas (tidal volume, VT) exchanged during each breathing cycle. Respiratory rate is easily obtained by observing chest wall movements and the passage of air at the nostrils or by visualizing changes

Table 8–2. Routine values for awake and anesthetized horses*		
	Awake	Anesthetized
Heart rate (beats/min)	30-45 (60-80)	30-45 (35-60)
Respiratory rate (breaths/min)	8-20 (30-40)	6-20 (spontaneous)
Capillary refill time (sec)	<2	<2.5
Temperature (° F)	99.5-101.0 (100.5-101.5)	
Temperature (° C)	36.5-38	
Packed cell volume (%)	32-50	25-45
Total plasma protein (g/dl)	6.0-7.5	5.0-7.0
Arterial pH	7.4 ± 0.2	7.30-7.45
$PaCO_2$ (mm Hg)	40 ± 3	40-60
PaO_2 (mm Hg)	94 ± 3 (room air)	100-500 (100% O_2)
Base excess (mEq/L)	0 ± 1	0 ± 1
End-tidal CO_2 (mm Hg)	40-50	30-50
Central venous pressure (cm H_2O)	5-10	10-25 lateral recumbency 5-10 dorsal recumbency
Mean arterial blood pressure (mm Hg)	80-120	60-70
Cardiac output (ml/kg/min)	60-80 (70-90)	30-50 (40-60)

* When different, values for foals are in parentheses.

The Fick Equation

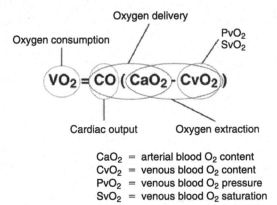

$$VO_2 = CO \, ((CaO_2 - CvO_2))$$

Oxygen consumption — Oxygen delivery — PvO_2 SvO_2 — Cardiac output — Oxygen extraction

CaO_2 = arterial blood O_2 content
CvO_2 = venous blood O_2 content
PvO_2 = venous blood O_2 pressure
SvO_2 = venous blood O_2 saturation

Figure 8–5. Oxygen consumption, cardiac output, oxygen delivery, and oxygen extraction are all components of the Fick equation. This equation is used to determine aerobic capacity and the capacity of the cardiovascular system to transport and use oxygen.

in volume of the rebreathing bag if an anesthetic machine is used. Tidal volume is not as easily assessed unless the rebreathing bag is housed in a graduated cylinder (see Chapter 17). Arterial oxygen content cannot be assessed by physical means, but mucous membrane color can be used as a subjective indicator of whether or not hemoglobin has been oxygenated. Hemoglobin desaturation to the point of blue mucous membranes (cyanosis) suggests the presence of at least 5 g/100 ml of unoxygenated (desaturated) hemoglobin. Supplementing inspired air with oxygen can decrease the likelihood of cyanosis and low CaO_2, providing that hemoglobin concentrations remain within normal limits.

The cardiovascular system is monitored to ensure adequate blood flow, blood pressure, and oxygen delivery to tissues. The most important components of cardiovascular function are cardiac output, blood pressure, and the distribution of blood flow to tissues. Cardiac output can be determined by indicator dilution techniques (thermodilution, indocyanine green, lithium), although this monitoring modality is not commonly used in horses.[9-11] Cardiac output is the product of heart rate and stroke volume (see Chapter 3). Heart rate is easily determined, but stroke volume is not easily obtained. Determination of the arterial blood pressure in conjunction with capillary refill time (CRT) and the strength of the peripheral pulse (pulse pressure) provides subjective information regarding cardiac output and tissue perfusion as previously inferred. However, tissue perfusion can become critical as the duration of anesthesia lengthens because of changes in blood flow distribution, particularly to muscles of dependent limbs.

Respiratory Monitoring

The respiratory system is evaluated initially by auscultating the thorax, feeling the passage of air at the nostrils, visualizing the rate and degree of chest wall or rebreathing bag movement, and checking the color of the mucous membranes (see Box 8-4). Auscultation of breath sounds in the recumbent horse is difficult because of positioning and extraneous background noise. Respiratory rate, normally

between 5 and 15 breaths/min in adult horses, can be assessed by feeling the passage of air at the nostril or watching chest and abdominal wall movement (see Table 8-2). however, the volume of gas exchanged during each breath is difficult to determine. Chest wall movement suggests that gas is inhaled, but the volume of gas exchanged may be small, particularly when abdominal distention is present. A subjective assessment of the volume of air passing the nostrils is of limited use. The degree of collapse of the rebreathing bag with each breath when using inhalant anesthetics is a crude but better indicator of tidal volume. The degree of respiratory center depression or respiratory effort can be assessed crudely by placing a hand over the rebreathing bag port on the anesthetic machine (if used) and watching the pressure gauge attached to the anesthetic circuit. Horses should be able to generate 15 to 20 cm of H_2O of negative pressure on inhalation. The rate and pattern of respiration varies with the depth of anesthesia and the anesthetics used. Breathing may slow or cease after inadvertent anesthetic overdose or at excessive anesthesia depth. An exaggerated (abdominal lift) apneustic (breath-holding) or "agonal" (gasping) pattern of ventilation suggests poor perfusion of the brain and an emergency situation. Ketamine, tiletamine, and overdoses of guaifenesin can cause an apneustic pattern of breathing (see Chapter 12).

The presence of cyanosis is the classic sign of respiratory insufficiency (Figure 8-6). However, the absence of cyanosis does not ensure normal arterial oxygenation or normal arterial blood gases. As stated previously, the appearance of cyanosis indicates that a horse has at least 5 g/100 ml of unoxygenated (desaturated) hemoglobin. Thus anemic horses may never become cyanotic, despite severe respiratory embarrassment.

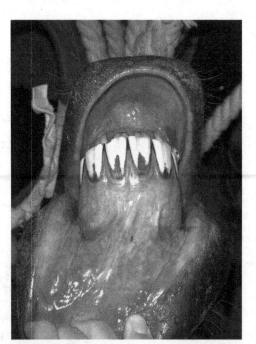

Figure 8–6. Mucous membrane color is a subjective indicator of the arterial blood oxygenation. Bluish (cyanotic) colored mucous membranes suggest that at there is at least 5 g/100 ml of unoxygenated (desaturated) hemoglobin.

Noninvasive (Indirect) Methods for Monitoring Respiratory Function

Capnometry. Carbon dioxide (CO_2) is a by-product of tissue metabolism, transported to the lungs by blood returning to the heart, and exhaled into the atmosphere (Figure 8-7). Capnometry is the measurement and display of airway CO_2 tension (mm Hg) and is most frequently assessed as end-tidal CO_2 ($ETCO_2$, mm Hg) in numeric form. Capnography is the comprehensive measurement and display of the real-time CO_2 waveform (Figure 8-8). Exhaled carbon dioxide tensions can be analyzed continuously, or a gas sample can be withdrawn from the endotracheal tube at the end of exhalation.[12-14] Theoretically the CO_2 tension within the endotracheal tube at the end of expiration should be in equilibrium with the CO_2 tension in the blood leaving the alveoli (the arterial blood). Thus, by measuring $ETCO_2$, information can be inferred about arterial blood CO_2 tension ($PaCO_2$). The $ETCO_2$ is used to assess ventilation (hypoventilation, hyperventilation), verify endotracheal tube placement, and ensure airway and anesthetic/ventilator circuit integrity (see Figure 8-8). The accuracy of using the $ETCO_2$ concentration to predict $PaCO_2$ in horses is somewhat controversial.[14,15] $ETCO_2$ tends to be 10 to 15 mm Hg lower than $PaCO_2$. Comparison of an initial value for $ETCO_2$ to $PaCO_2$ can be used to determine this difference but requires the use of a blood gas machine. Furthermore, the $PaCO_2$-$ETCO_2$ difference is influenced by ventilation and body position and increases as the anesthetic period lengthens or with decreases in cardiac output.[16] Nevertheless, the $ETCO_2$ and the $PaCO_2$-$ETCO_2$ generally are stable from measurement to measurement within the same horse and can be used to identify trends or sudden changes in ventilatory status. Increases in $PaCO_2$-$ETCO_2$ suggest increases in alveolar dead space ventilation, incomplete alveolar emptying, ventilation-perfusion mismatch or a leak (dilution by room air) in the sampling system (Table 8-3; see Chapter 2). Capnometers do not replace the measurement of $PaCO_2$ but can reduce the number of arterial blood gas samples analyzed.

Pulse oximetry. Pulse oximeters display heart rate and are used to obtain and indirectly estimate the percentage of the arterial blood hemoglobin that is saturated with oxygen (SaO_2) by measuring the degree of absorption or reflectance of emitted light by tissues and correlating that value to derived values of hemoglobin saturation (Figure 8-9).[17-19] Their function depends on a reasonable peripheral pulse

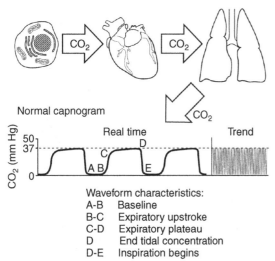

Normal capnogram

Waveform characteristics:
A-B   Baseline
B-C   Expiratory upstroke
C-D   Expiratory plateau
D   End tidal concentration
D-E   Inspiration begins

Figure 8–7. Carbon dioxide (CO_2) is produced in the tissues, carried to the lungs by blood, and breathed into the atmosphere. The cyclical variations in the CO_2 concentration during breathing is called a *capnogram* and can be used as an index of arterial blood CO_2 concentration.

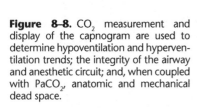

Figure 8–8. CO_2 measurement and display of the capnogram are used to determine hypoventilation and hyperventilation trends; the integrity of the airway and anesthetic circuit; and, when coupled with $PaCO_2$, anatomic and mechanical dead space.

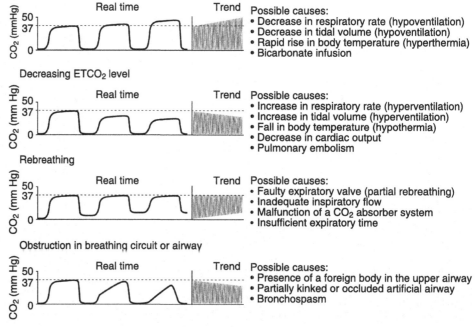

Increasing ETCO2 level

Possible causes:
• Decrease in respiratory rate (hypoventilation)
• Decrease in tidal volume (hypoventilation)
• Rapid rise in body temperature (hyperthermia)
• Bicarbonate infusion

Decreasing ETCO2 level

Possible causes:
• Increase in respiratory rate (hyperventilation)
• Increase in tidal volume (hyperventilation)
• Fall in body temperature (hypothermia)
• Decrease in cardiac output
• Pulmonary embolism

Rebreathing

Possible causes:
• Faulty expiratory valve (partial rebreathing)
• Inadequate inspiratory flow
• Malfunction of a CO_2 absorber system
• Insufficient expiratory time

Obstruction in breathing circuit or airway

Possible causes:
• Presence of a foreign body in the upper airway
• Partially kinked or occluded artificial airway
• Bronchospasm

Table 8–3.	Blood gas variables used to determine cardiopulmonary status
Variable	**Indication**
↑ $PAO_2 - PaO_2$	Efficiency of pulmonary gas exchange
↑ $PaCO_2$	Adequacy of ventilation
↑ $PaCO_2$-$ETCO_2$	Dead space ventilation; ventilation/perfusion mismatch; anesthetic circuit leak
↓ PvO_2	Cardiac output
↑ $PvCO_2$	Cardiac output
↑ $PvCO_2 - PaCO_2$	Cardiac output
↑ $PaCO_2 - PACO_2$	Ventilation-perfusion mismatching
↑ $PaCO_2 - PACO_2$	Cardiac output; arterial blood pressure
↑ $PaO_2 - PvO_2$	Cardiac output; arterial blood pressure
↓ $PaCO_2$	Cardiac output

↑, Increase; ↓, decrease.

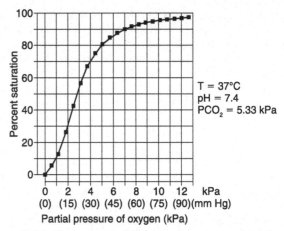

Figure 8–10. The oxyhemoglobin dissociation curve relates the percent saturation of hemoglobin (% Hb Sat) to the partial pressure of oxygen ($PaO2_2$) in arterial blood. Pressure is often reported in kPa (1 kPa = 7.5 mm Hg).

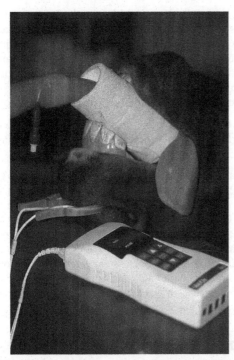

Figure 8–9. Pulse oximeters are used to determine the percent saturation of hemoglobin with oxygen (SpO_2). They depend on a detectable peripheral pulse and therefore provide heart rate and serve as an indirect measure of peripheral perfusion. High SpO_2 values do not ensure adequate O_2 delivery to tissues when hemoglobin concentrations are low (<5 g/100 ml).

(thus the name) to produce a measurement (SpO_2 value) and therefore serve as an index of tissue perfusion. SpO_2 values greater than 90% generally indicate adequate hemoglobin saturation and oxygenation, providing that hemoglobin concentration is within normal values (>7 g/dl; see Table 8-2; Figure 8-10). Most pulse oximeters underestimate hemoglobin saturation in horses and lose precision as tissue perfusion or saturation decreases. They do not measure oxygen content because hemoglobin concentration is not measured, nor do they assess the adequacy of ventilation (see Chapter 2 and calculation of CaO_2).[20] Pulse oximeters

are easily applied; but, as suggested, the signal depends on identification of a peripheral pulse and is frequently lost because of the inability of the sensors to detect an adequate peripheral pulse and vasoconstriction.[15] The signal usually returns when peripheral blood flow improves or the probe is repositioned.

Transcutaneous and conjunctival oxygen measurement. Transcutaneous and surface oximetry provides an index of arterial and tissue oxygenation, respectively.[21-23] Signal detection and technical issues have precluded their routine clinical application.

Invasive (Direct) Methods for Monitoring Respiratory Function

pH and blood gases (PO_2, PCO_2). Determination of blood hemoglobin concentration and arterial pH and blood gas tensions is the standard method of evaluating ventilatory adequacy and acid-base abnormalities. A sample of arterial blood is anaerobically drawn into a syringe coated with heparin. Care should be taken so that blood does not enter the syringe and mix with the blood. The sample is maintained airtight and analyzed as soon as possible. It should be cooled if analysis is delayed. Analysis of arterial blood samples (PaO_2, $PaCO_2$) is required when evaluating ventilatory adequacy. The normal value for arterial pH ranges between 7.30 and 7.45 (see Table 8-2). Maintenance of arterial pH in the normal range is important to preserve the integrity of tissue metabolism and cellular homeostasis.

The $PaCO_2$ is used to assess the adequacy of breathing (hypoventilation, hyperventilation) because it reflects the balance between the metabolic production of carbon dioxide and its elimination by the lungs (see Figure 8-7). Production of carbon dioxide generally decreases during anesthesia; thus alterations in $PaCO_2$ almost always indicate changes in ventilation. Increases in $PaCO_2$ indicate a decrease in alveolar ventilation (hypoventilation), and decreases in $PaCO_2$ indicate the opposite (hyperventilation; see Chapter 2). The normal range for $PaCO_2$ is 35 to 45 mm Hg (see Table 8-2). The concentration at which increases in $PaCO_2$ become detrimental is somewhat controversial.[24-27]

Moderate increases in $PaCO_2$ (50 to 70 mm Hg) may augment cardiac output and tissue blood flow via vasodilation and epinephrine release.[28] More severe increases (>70 to 80 mm Hg) can cause increases in arterial blood pressure but negatively affect blood pH, predispose to cardiac rhythm disturbances, and increase intracranial pressure. Most horses are ventilated when $PaCO_2$ levels are greater than 70 to 80 mm Hg because arterial pH approaches 7.20 (pH decreases approx. 0.5 units for every increase of 10 mm Hg in $PaCO_2$). Controlled ventilation also stabilizes and ensures the delivery of inhalant anesthetics (see Chapter 17).

The PaO_2 is used to determine if arterial blood is oxygenated adequately. The PaO_2 is not linearly related to hemoglobin saturation or the arterial oxygen content because of the sigmoid shape of the oxyhemoglobin dissociation curve; however, PaO_2 values greater than 90 mm Hg generally are associated with SaO_2 and SpO_2 values greater than 90% to 100% (see Figure 8-10). Increases in PaO_2 values above 100 mm Hg do not substantially increase the oxygen content (CaO_2) of the blood dramatically since the majority of the hemoglobin is already saturated, but they do cause more oxygen (0.3 ml/100 mm Hg/100 ml) to be carried in physical solution in the plasma. The percent saturation of hemoglobin and thus the oxygen content of blood decrease rapidly at PaO_2 values below 60 mm Hg in anesthetized horses. Given the issues associated with the horse's size, weight, and hemodynamic status during anesthesia and anesthetic-induced alterations in the distribution of blood flow, it is advisable to maintain PaO_2 values above 200 mm Hg in anesthetized horses whenever possible (see Chapters 2, 3, and 22).

Arterial and venous blood pH and blood gas values provide important information regarding the acid-base and cardiorespiratory status of acutely ill horses requiring surgery and anesthesia (see Table 8-3). A variety of bench-top and point-of-care machines are available to measure pH and blood gas tensions. Portable point-of-care analyzers allow rapid determination of blood gas values, with accuracies sufficient to direct clinical therapy (Figure 8-11).[29,30]

Arterial oxygen content. Arterial blood oxygen content (CaO_2) is measured by a co-oximeter after anaerobic collec-

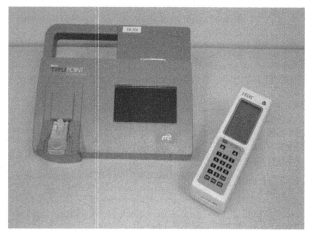

Figure 8–11. Point of care pH and blood gas analyzers (ERMA Trupoint; 1-Stat) facilitate the immediate acid-base analysis of arterial and venous blood samples. Most analyzers also determine electrolyte and lactate values.

tion of a heparinized arterial blood sample. Arterial oxygen content is the sum of oxygen bound to hemoglobin and oxygen carried in physical solution in the blood. The equipment required to determine CaO_2 requires frequent calibration and provides little additional information other than that produced by measuring hemoglobin concentration and PaO_2. Arterial oxygen content can be calculated using the equation:

Arterial oxygen content/100 ml blood = 1.39 ml oxygen/g hemoglobin/100 ml blood at 100% saturation + PaO_2 × 0.003 ml oxygen/mm Hg[31]

Thus a horse with a PaO_2 of 100 mm Hg and 15 g of saturated hemoglobin has a potential arterial oxygen content of 15 × 1.39 ml O_2/g + 100 mm Hg × 0.003 ml O_2/mm Hg = 21.15 ml O_2/100 ml of blood. A key point requiring emphasis is that the CaO_2 depends primarily on the hemoglobin concentration and horses that are anemic (Hb <5 to 7 g/dl) may be suffering from inadequate oxygen delivery to tissues, regardless of adequate PaO_2 and SpO_2 values (Box 8-6). The CaO_2 also decreases when the hemoglobin oxygen saturation decreases (low PaO_2; see Figure 8-10).

Box 8–6   Effects of Hemoglobin Concentration and Inspired Oxygen on Oxygen Content

Arterial oxygen content (CaO_2)/100 ml blood = 1.39 ml oxygen/g hemoglobin/100 ml blood at 100% saturation (% Sat) + PaO_2 × 0.003 ml oxygen/mm Hg

Arterial oxygen content with normal hemoglobin levels (15 g/100 ml) breathing room air

CaO_2/100 ml = 1.39 × 15 g × % Sat (100%) + 0.003 × 100 mm Hg (PaO_2) = 20.8 + 0.3 = 21.1 ml

Arterial oxygen content during anemia (hemoglobin = 6 g/100 ml) breathing room air

CaO_2/100 ml = 1.39 × 6 g × % Sat (100%) + 0.003 × 100 mm Hg (PaO_2) = 8.3 + 0.3 = 8.6 ml

Arterial oxygen content with normal hemoglobin levels (15 g/100 ml) breathing 100% oxygen

CaO_2/100 ml = 1.39 × 15 g × % Sat (100%) + 0.003 × 500 mm Hg (PaO_2) = 20.8 + 1.5 = 22.3 ml

Arterial oxygen content during anemia (6 g/100 ml) breathing 100% oxygen

CaO_2/100 ml = 1.39 × 6 g × % Sat (100%) + 0.003 × 500 mm Hg (PaO_2) = 8.3 + 1.5 = 9.8 ml

Cardiovascular Monitoring

The cardiovascular system can be evaluated by thoracic auscultation, assessment of mucous membrane color and CRT, palpation of a peripheral pulse, and a variety of indirect and direct technologies (see Box 8-5).

Auscultation permits the assessment of heart and lung sounds, the determination of heart rate and rhythm, and the identification of cardiac murmurs (see Chapters 3 and 5). Auscultation of the heart in the recumbent horse is often problematic because the normal relationship of the heart to the chest wall is distorted, particularly in supine horses. The position of the heart and noise from ventilatory assist devices make it difficult to hear heart sounds consistently.

CRT and the color of the mucous membranes provide subjective information regarding hemoglobin concentration and oxygenation, peripheral vascular tone, and tissue perfusion. Prolonged CRT (longer than 2 to 3 seconds) is indicative of poor perfusion and low cardiac output. The gingiva, eyelids, and vulva are sites where CRT and mucous membrane color can be evaluated. CRT is variably affected by the anesthetic drugs administered. For example, xylazine and detomidine increase CRT by causing vasoconstriction, whereas acepromazine shortens CRT by causing vasodilation. Therefore the presence of a normal CRT may not be a reliable indicator that tissue perfusion is adequate, although markedly prolonged (>3 seconds) CRTs are significant. Many anesthetic drugs (thiopental, isoflurane) cause vasodilation, resulting in pink mucous membranes and normal CRTs during the early stages of anesthesia, even though cardiac output and arterial blood pressure are reduced. The mucous membranes become more pale, and CRT increases as anesthetic depth is increased or during prolonged surgical procedures. The color of mucous membranes is an indicator of respiratory and cardiovascular status. Pale mucous membranes suggest peripheral vasoconstriction or decreased circulating red cells. Pale mucous membranes may not be associated with poor hemodynamic status. Brick-red mucous membranes and a prolonged CRT usually indicate poor gas exchange and sludging of blood in the capillaries.

Digital palpation of a peripheral arterial pulse is a reliable method for determining cardiac rate and rhythm in recumbent horses. A decrease in pulse rate is indicative of the depressant effects of anesthetic drugs but is not a reliable indicator of anesthetic depth in adult horses. Pulse rate usually decreases with anesthetic depth in foals but remains remarkably constant in adult horses until anesthetic depth is pronounced. Palpation of the peripheral pulse provides a qualitative assessment of the pulse pressure, in addition to the ability to determine pulse rate and rhythmicity. Cardiac arrhythmias are often discovered by palpating irregular pulses of variable intensities (Figure 8-12). Pulse pressure or "strength" is the difference between systolic and diastolic (systolic-diastolic) arterial blood pressure (see Figure 8-14). Pulse pressure does not indicate perfusion pressure and should not be overinterpreted in anesthetized horses because anesthetic drugs generally decrease peripheral vascular tone, thereby increasing pulse pressure and consequently pulse strength even when perfusion pressure (mean arterial blood pressure) is decreased. for example, isoflurane and sevoflurane produce vasodilation, resulting in an increase in pulse pressure but a decrease in perfusion pressure. Digital evaluation of the pulse may suggest an increase in

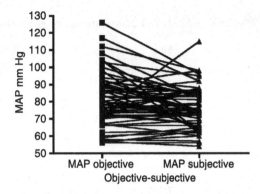

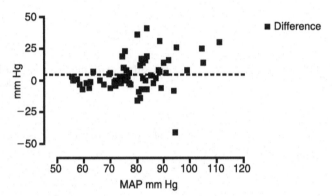

Figure 8–12. Digital assessment of arterial blood pressure is a learned skill. Subjective assessment of arterial blood pressure correlates (reduced bias and difference) with objective measurements as the assessor's skill improves.

pulse strength even when the tissue perfusion pressure is reduced. Conversely ketamine administration may result in vasoconstriction and a reduction in pulse pressure (systolic-diastolic) even though perfusion pressure increases. The digital assessment of perfusion pressure (estimate of mean arterial pressure) is a valuable skill that, once learned, can provide important, reasonably accurate, albeit subjective, information regarding the quality and magnitude of the arterial blood pressure (see Figure 8-12). The subjective nature and technical errors associated with physically monitoring arterial blood pressure have resulted in recommendations for more quantitative measurements and ultimately the direct monitoring of arterial blood pressure in horses, particularly when they are anesthetized with inhalant anesthetics or for extended periods of time.

The quantitative determination of arterial blood pressure is a key element in the clinical management of anesthetized horses. Both original research reports and retrospective studies of anesthetic complications indicate that mean arterial blood pressures below 60 mm Hg are associated with an increased incidence of complications, particularly the development postoperative rhabdomyolysis.[8,32-36] Arterial blood pressure is directly related and correlated with cardiac output in anesthetized horses, although a number of factors, especially the effects of anesthetic drugs on vascular tone (preload, afterload; see Chapter 3) and cardiac contractile force, affect this relationship.[33,34] Arterial blood pressure can be estimated indirectly (noninvasive) using Doppler or oscillometric methods and directly (invasive) using methods that require cannulation of an artery (Table 8-4).

Table 8–4.   Methods of arterial blood pressure measurement

Method	Site	Advantages	Disadvantages
Auscultation (Korotkoff)	Radial artery	Inexpensive Noninvasive	Systolic pressure only Not automatic Overestimates systolic pressure Not useful during hypotension Accuracy depends on cuff size Requires training
Doppler	Tail, other extremities	Noninvasive Simple to use Relatively inexpensive Portable, battery-operated	Not automatic Accuracy depends on cuff size Inaccurate during hypotension Only systolic pressure is measured
Oscillometric	Tail, other extremities	Easily applied Noninvasive Automatic	Accuracy depends on cuff size Inaccurate during hypotension, bradycardia, or arrhythmias
Electronic sphingomanometry	Tail, other extremities	Noninvasive	Not automatic May be inaccurate during hypotension Requires training Underestimates systolic and diastolic pressures
Direct measurement	Facial artery Transverse facial artery Dorsal metatarsal artery	Can obtain systolic, diastolic, and mean pressures continuously Most accurate and repeatable method Automatic once in place Requires frequent flushing to maintain patency	Invasive (potential for hematoma) Catheter placement requires some skill Expensive (other than aneroid) Infection

Noninvasive (Indirect) Methods for Monitoring Cardiovascular Function

Electrocardiography. The electrocardiogram (ECG) is used to evaluate the electrical activity of the heart. The primary goals of electrocardiography in the anesthetized horse are to determine the timing and morphology of cardiac electrical events to determine heart rate and rhythm (Figures 8-13 and 8-14). The ECG can also be used to indicate whether or not myocardial perfusion and oxygenation are adequate or if electrolyte abnormalities exist.[35] The base-apex lead is used routinely to monitor the ECG in anesthetized horses (see Chapter 3). This lead is useful because it is easily applied and characteristically accentuates the P wave, making it easier to identify changes in P-QRS-T timing and morphology (see Chapter 3 and Figure 8-14). Artifacts can make the evaluation of the ECG more difficult (Figure 8-15). A normal ECG suggests normal cardiac electrical activity but does not indicate normal hemodynamics or normal cardiac contraction.

Korotkoff sounds. Arterial blood pressure can be estimated by using a stethoscope to hear characteristic (Korotkoff)

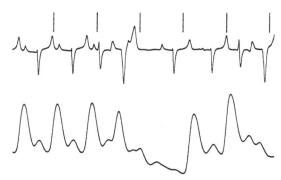

Figure 8–13. Electrocardiogram *(top)* and corresponding arterial pressure waveform *(bottom)* from a horse anesthetized with halothane. Note the effect of the premature ventricular depolarizations on the arterial pressure pulse and presence of a compensatory pause.

sounds produced by arterial blood flow through an artery as pressure is released from an occlusive cuff. The method can be used to assess trends in systolic blood pressure in horses but is critically dependent on cuff width and is inaccurate at low arterial pressures. The technique is relatively inaccurate and hampered by interference from background noise.

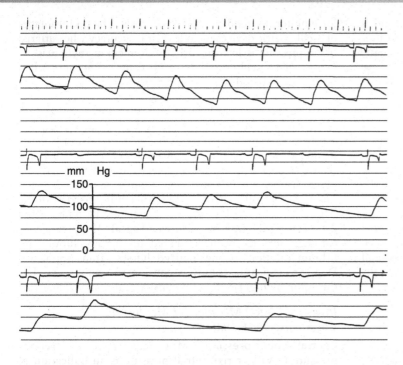

Figure 8–14. Electrocardiogram *(top)* and corresponding arterial pressure waveform from a horse with second-degree atrioventricular block *(middle and bottom traces)*. Note the absence of the arterial pressure pulses and the decrease in diastolic arterial pressure following the blocked P waves.

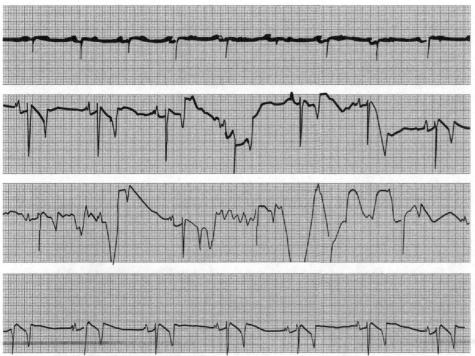

Figure 8–15. Electrocardiogram artifacts: inappropriate trace calibration *(top trace)*; 60-cycle electrical noise *(second trace)*; movement artifact *(third trace)*; electrical bias (DC offset) or incorrect positioning *(bottom trace)*.

Doppler-ultrasound. Arterial blood pressure can be estimated using Doppler-ultrasound devices.[36-38] Doppler techniques detect blood flow through an artery as pressure is released from an occlusive cuff. They provide reasonably accurate estimates of systolic arterial blood pressure but are not reliable for determining diastolic arterial blood pressure.[39] Doppler-ultrasound devices detect blood flow by transmitting, receiving, and amplifying the characteristic changes (Doppler shift) in an emitted frequency when blood flows through a vessel. Systolic arterial blood pressure is estimated by applying the Doppler transducer distal to an occlusive cuff that is attached to a sphygmomanometer. The occlusive cuff usually is placed

at the tail base in adult horses or on a limb in foals. The cuff is inflated until the Doppler device indicates that blood flow has stopped (no sound). The occlusive cuff pressure is released gradually to the point at which blood flow is detected (sound returns), and the pressure value displayed on the sphygmomanometer is recorded as an estimate of systolic arterial blood pressure. The accuracy of this technique depends on the width of the occlusive cuff used to stop blood flow (bladder width to tail girth ratio of approximately 0.2-0.4) and recumbency.[38-40] Doppler-ultrasonic measurements recorded from a cuff placed around the tail of supine adult horses usually exhibit unacceptably large measurement errors.

The ease of application and the fact that the method is noninvasive are the principal advantages of Doppler-ultrasonic devices. Doppler-ultrasonic devices are not automatic (they require an operator to inflate and release the occlusive cuff), lose accuracy when the horse is in dorsal (supine) recumbency, and are not dependable when systolic blood pressures are low. They may have some value for determining trends in arterial blood pressure.

Oscillometric devices. Oscillometric methods for determining arterial blood pressure detect the magnitude and frequency of arterial pulsations induced in an air-filled cuff.[41,42] Similar to Doppler-ultrasonic techniques, the cuff is placed around an extremity (usually the tail; Figure 8-16). The cuff is inflated to a preset pressure in excess of systolic arterial pressure and then slowly released. Arterial pressure pulsations cause pressure oscillations within the cuff as the cuff pressure falls. These oscillations are superimposed over the declining pressure curve. The pressure oscillations increase until a maximum value is reached and then decrease in magnitude as the cuff pressure deflates further. The systolic pressure is taken at the point where the pressure fluctuations begin to increase in size. The mean arterial pressure is taken at the point where the fluctuations are the largest. Diastolic arterial blood pressure is estimated as the point when cuff oscillations no longer decline. Most oscillometric devices also measure heart rate. The ideal bladder width to tail girth ratio ranges between 0.2 and 0.4 in horses.[43,44] Increasing this ratio leads to underestimation of systolic arterial blood pressures, and decreases in the ratio lead to overestimation. Most oscillometric devices are automatic and are useful for monitoring trends, especially in foals. The disadvantages of oscillometric devices include their inaccuracy when arterial blood pressure is low or during movement, arrhythmias, or bradycardia. Oscillometric devices become less accurate when mean arterial blood pressure is less than 65 mm Hg.[43]

Transesophageal Doppler echocardiography. Transesophageal Doppler echocardiography generates a noninvasive estimate of cardiac output by determining blood flow velocity in a major vessel (aorta; pulmonary artery) of known cross-sectional area and multiplying the obtained value by the heart rate (see Chapter 3).[45] The Doppler probe is advanced into the esophagus via the nose until a long axis view of the left ventricular outflow tract and aorta are obtained using 2-D echocardiography. Transesophageal Doppler echocardiography has been compared to thermodilution and lithium dilution in anesthetized horses. Transesophageal Doppler echocardiography is considered noninvasive, but the equipment generally is expensive and not available.

Invasive (Direct) Methods for Monitoring Cardiovascular Function

Central venous pressure. Measurement of central venous pressure (CVP) or right atrial pressure is an indication of the filling pressure of the right side of the heart and vascular fluid volume (see Chapter 3).[46] CVP can be altered by heart rate, myocardial contractility, blood volume, intrathoracic pressure, and the tone of the peripheral venous vasculature.[46] In addition, the choice of anesthetic drug and body position influences CVP (Figure 8-17). Horses in lateral recumbency have CVPs that range from 15 to 25 cm

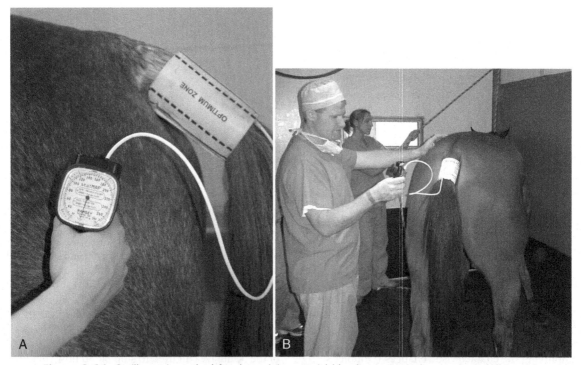

Figure 8–16. Oscillometric method for determining arterial blood pressure in horses. **A,** A cuff is positioned at the base of the tail and inflated to a pressure greater than the arterial blood pressure **B,** As the cuff is deflated, the magnitude of the pulsations in the air-filled cuff are used to determine systolic, diastolic, and mean arterial blood pressure. (LA-MAP, Ramsey Medical Inc; **A** and **B** Courtesy Dr Paul Rothaug, Woodland Run Equine Veterinary Facility.)

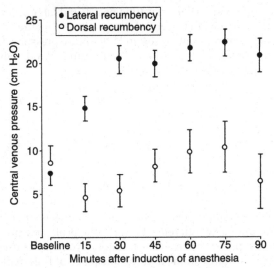

Figure 8–17. The central venous pressure is elevated in horses positioned in lateral or dorsal (supine) recumbency and is a rudimentary and often inaccurate indicator of blood volume changes in horses.

cannulating an artery and attaching a pressure-sensing device to measure the pressures within the vessel (see Chapter 7; Figure 8-19). Arterial catheterization is a learned skill and, if improperly performed, can result in hematoma formation, infection, arteriospasm, or tissue necrosis; although these problems are rare in horses if aseptic techniques are performed properly.[51,52] Methods of measuring arterial blood pressure after the cannulation of a peripheral artery include the use of simple aneroid manometers and pressure transducers with electronic displays (Figure 8-20).

Standard aneroid manometers are inexpensive and can be adapted to attach to most catheters using a length of noncompliant tubing and a three-way stopcock. The noncompliant tubing should be long enough that the manometer can be centered at the level of the heart. A stopcock is attached to a catheter filled with heparinized saline, and the mean arterial blood pressure is estimated by noting the upper deflection as the needle swings on the dial of the manometer. Fluid and potentially blood occasionally back up into the tubing and should be eliminated by frequent flushing with heparinized saline. The manometer can be contaminated or ruined if blood or fluid reaches the internal mechanism. A fluid trap can be added to the system to protect the aneroid manometer. Fluid traps tend to dampen the pressure response somewhat but allow measurement of mean arterial pressure.

More sophisticated methods for measuring arterial blood pressure incorporate pressure transducers and electronic recorders (see Figure 8-20). Changes in arterial blood pressure distort a pressure-sensitive diaphragm, which changes the electrical conductivity through the diaphragm. The magnitude of the change in conductivity is proportional to the changes in the arterial blood pressure. Systolic and diastolic blood pressures are measured directly. Mean arterial blood pressure (MAP) is usually calculated by measuring the area under the pulse pressure curve. MAP can be estimated from the systolic (SAP) and diastolic (DAP) blood pressure using the formula:

$$(SAP-DAP)/3 + DABP = MAP \text{ (see Figure 3-14)}$$

Pressure transducers and recorders allow beat-to-beat determination of heart rate, arterial blood pressure, and

H_2O, whereas horses in dorsal recumbency have pressures that range from 5 to 10 cm H_2O (see Chapter 3).[47,48] The periodic measurement of CVP is of little clinical value unless an initial baseline value has been recorded and changes in CVP are recorded for an extended period of time as trends. The reference points (zero) for CVP measurement are the point of the shoulder in standing or dorsally recumbent horses and the sternum in laterally recumbent horses.

Arterial blood pressure. Arterial catheterization is the most accurate and reliable method for measuring arterial blood pressures.[49,50] The measurement and display of systolic, diastolic, and mean arterial pressure values and the arterial pressure waveform provide important information regarding cardiovascular function and status. The use of constant flow systems or periodic flushing of catheters with heparinized saline is required to maintain patency of arterial catheters (Figure 8-18). Arterial catheters also provide convenient access ports for sampling of arterial blood gases. Direct measurement of arterial blood pressure is accomplished by

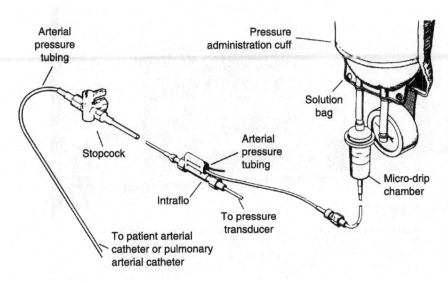

Figure 8–18. A continuous arterial line flushing system can be assembled by attaching a solution administration set connected to a pressurized bag of fluids to the blood pressure transducer. Many pressure transducers include an arterial flush valve.

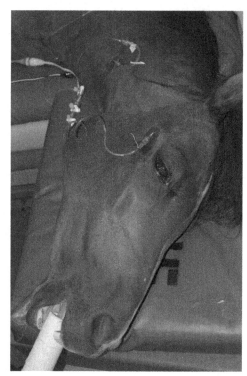

Figure 8–19. Arterial catheters are frequently placed in branches of the facial artery. Note that the catheter is sutured to the skin to help prevent its dislodgement.

assessment of the arterial pressure waveform configuration. Instruments with digital displays cycle automatically and update the information every few seconds.

Arterial blood pressure waveform. The principal determinants of arterial blood pressure and the arterial pressure waveform are the distensibility of the vessel wall (compliance), cardiac stroke volume, cardiac output, peripheral vascular resistance, and the distance from the heart to the sampling point (Table 8-5). Blood volume and heart rate modify these determinants. The distensibility of the arteries decreases with age and is greater in peripheral arteries than in the central aorta. Peripheral pulse waveforms have

steeper upstrokes, higher systolic peaks, and later or absent diacrotic notches than central artery pulses (Figure 8-21). Slow heart rates usually result in larger pulse pressures (systolic-diastolic) when cardiac function and blood volume are normal because of a longer time for peripheral drainage ("runoff") of blood (see Figure 8-14). Tachycardia produces the opposite effect. One and sometimes two additional pulsations are frequently palpable and observed in peripheral arterial recordings in horses.

The shape of the arterial pressure waveform can be analyzed subjectively (Box 8-7). Changes in the arterial pressure waveform are particularly apparent in horses that are mechanically ventilated. Typically the highest systolic pressures occur at the peak of the inspiratory cycle, and the lowest systolic pressures occur immediately after peak inspiration.[53] The difference between the peak pressure and the lowest pressure across a respiratory cycle can be used as an index of fluid volume and the adequacy of fluid replacement (see Chapter 17).[54] The normal arterial pressure waveforms depict a relatively rapid initial rate of pressure rise (inotropic phase) and a gradual descent. Increases in the force of cardiac contraction (inotropy) and vasodilation usually increase the rate of pressure rise. however, peripheral vasodilation generally increases the pulse pressure and causes the arterial pressure waveform to rise and fall rapidly. Decreases in force of contraction and stroke volume decrease the rate of rise of the arterial pressure waveform. Acute blood loss (>25 ml/kg) may increase the rate of rise of the arterial pressure because inotropy increases to compensate for blood loss. Rapid heart rates make the previous generalizations regarding the arterial pressure waveform more difficult to interpret but still worth noting. Arterial pressure waveforms are variable among patients but offer valuable insight regarding the emergence of cardiovascular complications and trends in cardiovascular function.

Cardiac output. Cardiac output can be determined by indicator dilution (temperature, dye, lithium) and Doppler echocardiographic techniques (see Chapter 3).[45,55-58] The determination of cardiac output by thermodilution requires that a thermistor-tipped flow-directed (Swan-Ganz) catheter is introduced into the jugular vein and advanced through

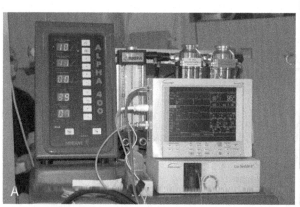

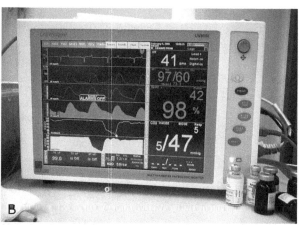

Figure 8–20. **A,** Multiparameter physiological recording monitors (Datascope; Life Windows) permit the simultaneous display and recording of the ECG, heart rate, arterial blood pressure, SpO_2, $ETCO_2$, and body temperature. **B,** Some are equipped to monitor inspired and expired (O_2, inhalant anesthetic, N_2O) gas concentrations. (**A** Courtesy Dr. Claire Scicluna: clinvetplessis@wanadoo.fr **B** Courtesy Dr. Paul Rothaug, Woodland Run Equine Veterinary Facility.)

Table 8–5. Pulse type and arterial pressure waveform observations

Pulse type and waveform	Description
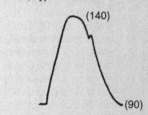 Pulse pressure 1. Stroke volume 2. Arterial compliance Systolic pressure (120) Dicrotic notch Mean pressure (94) 1. Cardiac output 2. Peripheral resistance Diastolic pressure (80) Inotropic phase / Volume displacement phase Systole / Diastole	The normal arterial blood pressure (ABP) waveform: arterial pressures (systolic, diastolic, and mean), and pulse pressure (PP; $ABP_{systolic} - ABP_{diastolic}$) depend on cardiac output (CO), systemic vascular resistance (SVR), stroke volume (SV), arterial compliance (stiffness), and heart rate (HR). Decreases in CO lower ABP; decrease the rate of rise, and prolong the inotropic phase. Decreases in SVR increase the rate of rise and shorten the inotropic phase, decrease the pulse width, lower the dicrotic notch, and increase PP. Decreases in SV only decrease PP, whereas decreases in arterial compliance increase PP. Age and drugs (α_2-agonists) decrease arterial compliance.
Normal, hypertensive (140) (90)	Usually caused by increased CO, SV, and SVR. The PP is increased (50). Systolic, diastolic, and mean ABP are elevated. The inotropic phase is rapid. The dicrotic notch occurs early in diastole. Associated with light levels of anesthesia or the administration of vasopressors. Occasionally seen as a response to pain from tourniquet placement.
Hyperkinetic, bounding 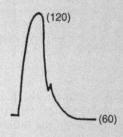 (120) (60)	Usually caused by an increased SV and decreased SVR. Systolic arterial pressure is usually elevated, whereas mean and diastolic arterial pressures are decreased. The PP is increased (60). The upstroke (inotropic phase) is rapid as is the downstroke. The dicrotic notch is very low or may not be observed. Indicative of a hyperkinetic state caused by arteriovenous shunts, fever, and anemia or rapid runoff of blood from the arterial system caused by vasodilators (acepromazine), early endotoxemia, and septicemia.
Hypokinetic, thready 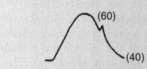 (60) (40)	Usually caused by decreased CO and SV and increased SVR. The systolic, diastolic, and mean arterial pressures generally are decreased. PP is reduced (20).[20] The inotropic phase is prolonged, and the dicrotic notch is high or normally located. The diastolic phase is usually abbreviated during increased HR. Hypokinetic pulses are indicative of myocardial depression (anesthesia), shock (hemorrhage, endotoxemia), or conditions that increase HR and cause peripheral artery vasoconstriction (late endotoxemia).
Ventilator effect 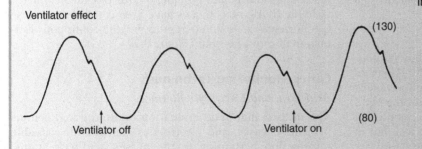 Ventilator off / Ventilator on (130) (80)	Intermittent positive-pressure ventilation (IPPV) can decrease venous return and CO, resulting in a decrease in ABP and an increase in SVR. The arterial pressure waveform may not change, but the PP may decrease, and cyclic alterations in arterial pressures are frequently observed associated with inspiration and expiration. ABP, especially systolic pressure, increases during the inspiratory cycle; the opposite occurs during the expiratory phase. Marked changes in ABP caused by mechanical ventilation are an indication for fluid therapy or inotropic support (see Chapter 17).

(Continued)

Table 8–5. Pulse type and arterial pressure waveform observations—Cont'd

Pulse type and waveform	Description
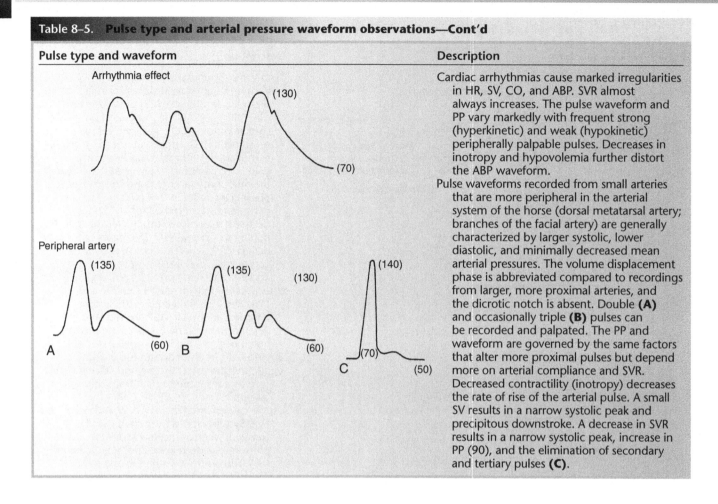	Cardiac arrhythmias cause marked irregularities in HR, SV, CO, and ABP. SVR almost always increases. The pulse waveform and PP vary markedly with frequent strong (hyperkinetic) and weak (hypokinetic) peripherally palpable pulses. Decreases in inotropy and hypovolemia further distort the ABP waveform. Pulse waveforms recorded from small arteries that are more peripheral in the arterial system of the horse (dorsal metatarsal artery; branches of the facial artery) are generally characterized by larger systolic, lower diastolic, and minimally decreased mean arterial pressures. The volume displacement phase is abbreviated compared to recordings from larger, more proximal arteries, and the dicrotic notch is absent. Double **(A)** and occasionally triple **(B)** pulses can be recorded and palpated. The PP and waveform are governed by the same factors that alter more proximal pulses but depend more on arterial compliance and SVR. Decreased contractility (inotropy) decreases the rate of rise of the arterial pulse. A small SV results in a narrow systolic peak and precipitous downstroke. A decrease in SVR results in a narrow systolic peak, increase in PP (90), and the elimination of secondary and tertiary pulses **(C)**.

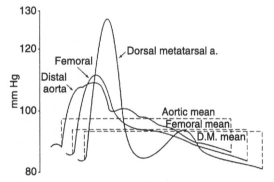

Figure 8–21. Representative arterial pressure waveforms from the distal aorta, femoral, and dorsal metatarsal arteries. Note the narrower pulse, increased systolic blood pressure, and lower diastolic and mean arterial pressures in the metatarsal artery. Also note the presence of a second pulse waveform in the dorsal metatarsal artery. (From Remington JW, Wood EH: *Am J Physiol* 9:440; 1956.)

the heart until the tip lies in the pulmonary artery (as confirmed by characteristic pressure waveforms).[10,56] A second catheter is introduced into the jugular vein and advanced until its tip lies in the right atrium; it is used for the rapid injection of iced fluids. The technique can be accomplished with just the thermistor-tipped catheter in the foal, but in adult horses a second catheter is required because of the large volume of fluid injected. A known volume of iced isotonic fluid is injected and mixes with blood. The administration

of iced fluids changes the temperature of the blood as it flows through the heart. The temperature change is detected by the thermistor in the pulmonary artery. The magnitude and duration of the temperature change are inversely proportional to the cardiac output. Proprietary computer algorithms integrate the area under the temperature change curve and calculate cardiac output. Thermodilution is not difficult but does require the placement of a second catheter; thus it is not used routinely.

Alternatively lithium chloride solution can be administered via a central venous catheter.[10,55] Cardiac output is derived from the magnitude and duration of the arterial plasma lithium concentration.[10] The lithium dilution technique is simple because it can be performed using a jugular catheter and a catheter placed in any peripheral artery (catheterization of the pulmonary artery is not required). Lithium dilution techniques have been coupled with pulse contour analysis in an attempt to provide continuous estimation of cardiac output (Figure 8-22).[10]

Other Monitoring Techniques

Acid-Base and Electrolyte Balance

The measurement and evaluation of arterial and venous pH, blood gases, and electrolytes can provide valuable information pertaining to the horse's acid-base status, peripheral blood flow, and pulmonary gas exchange (see Chapter 7 and Table 8-6). There is a positive correlation

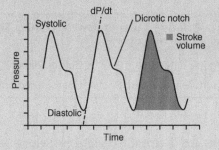

Myocardial Contractility

The upstroke of the arterial pulse pressure wave (inotropic phase) depends on left ventricular dP/dt. A steep upstroke generally indicates good left ventricular function.

Stroke Volume

The area under the systolic ejection phase (volume phase) of the pulse pressure tracing is proportional to stroke volume.

Systemic Vascular Resistance

A low dicrotic notch and a steep downstroke indicate rapid diastolic runoff and a low peripheral vascular resistance.

Heart Rate, Rhythm, and Other Factors of Hemodynamic Significance

Knowledge of the sweep speed or the paper speed permits an immediate estimation of heart rate.

Cardiac arrhythmias can be identified by comparing the electrocardiogram to the arterial pulse waveform (premature atrial or ventricular beats).

The hemodynamic significance of rate and rhythm changes is indicated by alterations in arterial blood pressure and contour on a beat-to-beat basis.

Ventilation modifies the pulse contour by augmenting the arterial blood pressure.

Positive-pressure ventilation increases the stroke volume of the first beat or two and then decreases the stroke volume of subsequent beats.

Circulating Blood Volume

Exaggerated beat-by-beat changes in blood pressure in relation to ventilation suggest hypovolemia.

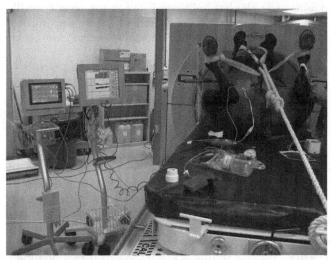

Figure 8–22. Lithium dilution determination of cardiac output (Lidco Ltd.) in a sevoflurane anesthetized horse. The lithium dilution monitor *(right)* can be coupled to an arterial blood pressure monitor *(left)* for the continuous assessment of trends in cardiac output by arterial pulse wave analysis.

between PvO_2 and cardiac output (as cardiac output falls, PvO_2 falls; see Chapter 3 and Figure 3-17).[58] Decreases in cardiac output (anesthetic drugs, circulatory failure, shock, or cardiac arrest) prolong capillary transit time, thereby producing a greater time for oxygen extraction and lower PvO_2 values. A similar rationale can be used to explain why $PvCO_2$ and the $PvCO_2$-$PaCO_2$ difference are increased when cardiac output is decreased.[59] Blood returning to the heart from the tissues carries a bigger carbon dioxide load.[59] Ventilation maintains arterial carbon dioxide tension ($PaCO_2$) at its normal value, but venous carbon dioxide tension may increase. The measurement of $PaCO_2$-$ETCO_2$ has been advocated as an index of ventilation-perfusion mismatching ($\dot{V}/\dot{Q}$), cardiac output, and mean arterial blood pressure during clinical anesthesia (see Table 8-3).[60] The $PaCO_2$-$ETCO_2$ difference increases as $\dot{V}/\dot{Q}$ mismatching increases and cardiac output and mean arterial blood pressure decrease. This relationship is influenced significantly by body weight, indicating a weight-related maldistribution

Table 8–6.	Acid-base and associated pH, $PaCO_2$, and HCO_3^- changes			
	pH	$PaCO_2$	HCO_3^-	Other terms
Uncompensated				
Metabolic acidosis	↓	N	↓↓	Nonrespiratory (metabolic) acidosis
Metabolic alkalosis	↑	N	↑↑	Nonrespiratory (metabolic) alkalosis
Respiratory acidosis	↓	↑↑	N	Acute ventilatory failure
Respiratory alkalosis	↑	↓↓	N	Chronic alveolar hyperventilation
Compensated				
Metabolic acidosis	↓	↓	↓↓	Nonrespiratory (metabolic) acidosis
Metabolic alkalosis	↑	↑	↑↑	Nonrespiratory (metabolic) alkalosis
Respiratory acidosis	↓	↑↑	↑	Chronic ventilatory failure
Respiratory alkalosis	↑	↓↓	↓	Chronic alveolar hyperventilation

↑, Increase; ↓, decrease; N, normal range.

of blood flow relative to ventilation in larger recumbent, anesthetized horses. Similarly the measurement of $ETCO_2$ is indicative of changes in cardiac output when everything else is held constant.[61] Decreases in $ETCO_2$ suggest a decrease in the delivery of carbon dioxide from peripheral tissues because of reduced venous return and pulmonary blood flow and a reduced cardiac output.[62]

The accurate interpretation of acid-base abnormalities is based on the assessment of both arterial and venous blood samples. Arterial pH and blood gases are used to assess pulmonary gas exchange, and venous blood pH and blood gases are used to evaluate tissue acid-base status. Regardless of whether an arterial or venous blood sample is obtained, there are fundamental and key concepts that must be appreciated. First, acidemia or alkalemia is determined by the blood pH value. Values below 7.35 indicate acidosis, and values above 7.45 indicate alkalosis. Respiratory acidosis is considered to be present when the $PaCO_2$ value is in excess of 50 mm Hg. Respiratory alkalosis is present when the $PaCO_2$ value is below 35 mm Hg. Nonrespiratory acidosis is present when the pH is below 7.35 coupled with a plasma bicarbonate concentration below the accepted normal (25 mEq/L). Nonrespiratory alkalosis is when the pH is above 7.45 coupled with plasma bicarbonate above the accepted normal (see Table 8-2). Compensatory changes occur in an attempt to restore normal body pH values, but the primary problem can be determined by matching the pH change with either the respiratory or nonrespiratory component. For example, a horse with an arterial pH of 7.2 is acidemic. If this pH change is coupled with a $PaCO_2$ of 80 mm Hg and an arterial bicarbonate concentration of 32 mEq/L, the diagnosis is primary respiratory acidosis. The plasma bicarbonate concentration has increased in an attempt to compensate (return the pH to the normal range of 7.35 to 7.45) for the respiratory acidosis. In this case compensation has not occurred. Furthermore, this pH change is predictable since pH decreases an idealized value (7.40) by approximately 0.05 units for every increase of 10 mm Hg in the $PaCO_2$ above the ideal $PaCO_2$ (40 mm Hg). Therefore a $PaCO_2$ value of 80 mm Hg would be expected to produce a pH value of 7.20 ($0.05 \times [80-40] = 0.2$; $7.40 - 0.2 = 7.20$). If the pH value indicates extreme academia and both the $PaCO_2$ and the arterial bicarbonate values indicate acidosis, the interpretation is a mixed respiratory and metabolic acidosis. Using this simple approach, most clinical acid-base abnormalities can be diagnosed rapidly and accurately, and appropriate therapy can be determined (see Table 8-6). Occasionally a situation arises in which both the $PaCO_2$ and the bicarbonate values are deranged in opposite directions but the pH remains within normal limits. The question then arises: what is the primary problem and what is compensatory? The answer that is almost always correct is that the directionality of the pH change determines the primary problem. Stated another way, clinical acid-base abnormalities are rarely totally compensated, and overcompensation almost never occurs. It should be emphasized that pH (the hydrogen ion concentration) depends on a number of independent variables. The independent variables are the dissociation of water and, more specifically, the ion product of water (k_w, a constant); the $PaCO_2$ (discussed previously); the strong ion difference (SID); and the concentration of weak ions or buffers ([A tot]) in the plasma (Box 8-8).[63,64]

Box 8–8   Primary Independent Variables That Determine pH

- Strong ion difference
- Carbon dioxide (CO_2)
- A_{TOT} (sum of week acids)
- Unmeasured anions

Strong ions are electrically charged particles that are completely dissociated in water at physiological pH and are principally represented by both cations (Na^+ K^+, Ca^{+2}, Mg^{+2}) and anions (Cl^- and lactate). This charge difference generates a positive apparent strong ion difference (SIDa) under normal conditions and is counterbalanced by the negative charge produced by albumin (weak acid) and phosphates in the plasma, the strong ion difference effective (SIDe). The difference between the SIDa and SIDe is termed *the strong ion gab (SIG)* which, when equal to zero, generates a pH of 7.40 at a PCO_2 of 40 mm Hg. The presence of an SIG (SIDa ≠ SIDe) indicates the presence of unmeasured ions, positive or negative, depending on the value of the gap. The unmeasured ions alter pH because they contribute to charge in the plasma. The SIG has been correlated to the severity of illness and outcome in several species and requires further investigation as a prognostic indicator in horses (www.ccm.upmc.edu/education/resources/phorum.html).[63]

The production of lactic acid is a major and potentially important contributor to acid-base imbalance in anesthetized or hemodynamically compromised horses (see Chapter 7). Lactate is formed by glycolysis (the breakdown of glycogen and glucose to pyruvate) with no net change in hydrogen ions. Accumulation of lactate in the plasma indicates that it is being formed faster than it can be metabolized. During hypoxia, ischemia, and reductions in tissue perfusion, impaired delivery of oxygen results in the development of lactic acidosis.[65,65a,66] Lactic acid is a strong ion and in the dissociated state lowers the SIDe. Lactic acid and other strong anions are referred to as unmeasured anions because they are not routinely determined. It is helpful to calculate the SIG during acidemia. An increased SIG indicates the presence of unmeasured anions (usually lactate). Other strong ions (ketoacids) can be produced during disease and various pathologic states but are seldom a concern during equine anesthesia (Table 8-7).

Table 8–7.   Effects of independent variables on acid-base balance

Independent variable	Change	Suspect
PCO_2	↑	Respiratory acidosis
PCO_2	↓	Respiratory alkalosis
SIDa	↑	Nonrespiratory alkalosis
SIDa	↓	Nonrespiratory acidosis
TP	↑	Nonrespiratory acidosis
TP	↓	Nonrespiratory alkalosis
La⁻	↑	Nonrespiratory acidosis

↑, Increase; ↓, decrease; *SIDa*, apparent strong ion difference; *TP*, total protein; *La⁻* = lactate.

A multitude of shortcuts and rules of thumb have been applied to simplify the interpretation of clinical acid-base abnormalities. The determination of the respiratory component of a given pH change allows for rapid estimation of the patient's status during anesthesia. This information is helpful because hypoventilation and the development of respiratory acidosis are common in anesthetized horses and impact decisions regarding the need to assist or control ventilation. The CO_2 hydration equation ($CO_2 + H_2O \leftrightarrows H_2CO_3 \leftrightarrows H^+ + HCO_3^-$) indicates that obligatory changes in hydrogen ion concentration and thus pH occur anytime the $PaCO_2$ changes. As suggested previously, for each 10 mm Hg increase in $PaCO_2$ above 40 mm Hg, the pH value decreases 0.05 from the ideal normal value of 7.4. Conversely, for each 10 mm Hg decrease in $PaCO_2$ below 40 mm Hg, the pH increases approximately 0.1 units. Remembering these relationships allows the immediate determination of the respiratory component of a given pH change. For example, a horse with a $PaCO_2$ of 60 mm Hg would be expected to have a pH of 7.3. When the measured pH is above or below 7.3, a nonrespiratory acidosis or alkalosis, respectively, should exist (see Chapter 7). Treatment of acid-base abnormalities resulting in pH values between 7.25 and 7.55 generally is not required.

Temperature

Body temperature is usually monitored by rectal thermometer. Rectal and esophageal thermistor devices are available. Fecal material in the rectum and dilation of the anus may cause falsely low rectal temperature readings. Monitoring body temperature provides information regarding the horse's metabolic rate and its ability to dissipate heat. Significant hypothermia is uncommon in adult horses because of the large body mass and relatively low body surface area.[67,68] Sick and smaller horses and foals can become hypothermic, particularly when the anesthetic period is prolonged or a body cavity has been opened. Low ambient temperatures and wetting of body surfaces contribute to temperature loss, with externally applied heat partially effective in reducing temperature loss.[69] Hypothermia decreases the amount of anesthetic agent required to produce a given depth of anesthesia and can prolong the recovery period. Oxygen consumption can increase during the recovery period as the horse shivers. Malignant hyperthermia-like syndromes occur in horses but are extremely rare (see Chapter 22). Tachypnea, tachycardia, and increases in muscle tone usually precede the increases in temperature.

In conclusion, monitoring anesthesia and the consequences of anesthetic drugs is essential if anesthetic morbidity and mortality are to be minimized (see Chapter 25). Horses are especially predisposed to a variety of anesthetic-related complications based on their temperament, size, and weight. The maintenance of tissue blood flow, especially muscle perfusion, is critical to rapid and uneventful recovery from anesthesia. Hopefully future technological developments will evolve that permit the noninvasive assessment of this important issue. Toward this end it is essential that trained and experienced equine anesthetists use every physical and technological method that is relevant and feasible to assess and maintain optimal physiological values.

REFERENCES

1. The American College of Veterinary Anesthesiologists guidelines of anesthetic monitoring, *J Am Vet Med Assoc* 206:936-937; 1995. http://www.acva.org/diponly/action/Guidelines_Anesthesia_Horses_041227.htm
2. Otto K, Short CE: Electroencephalographic power spectrum analysis as a monitor of anesthetic depth in horses, *Vet Surg* 20:362-371, 1991.
3. Miller SM, Short CE, Ekstrom PM: Quantitative electroencephalographic evaluation to determine the quality of analgesia during anesthesia of horses for arthroscopic surgery, *Am J Vet Res* 56:374-379, 1995.
4. Haga HA, Dolvik NI: Evaluation of bispectral index as an indicator of degree of central nervous system depression in isoflurane-anesthetized horses, *Am J Vet Res* 63:438-442, 2002.
5. Murrell JC et al: Changes in the EEG during castration in horses and ponies anaesthetized with halothane, *Vet Anaesth Analg* 30:138-146, 2003.
6. Johnson CB, Bloomfield M, Taylor PM: Effects of midazolam and sarmazenil on the equine electroencephalogram during anaesthesia with halothane in oxygen, *J Vet Pharmacol Ther* 26:105-112, 2003.
7. Liu SS: Effects of bispectral index monitoring on ambulatory anesthesia, *Anesthesiology* 101:311-315, 2004.
8. Grandy JL et al: Arterial hypotension and the development of postanesthetic myopathy in halothane-anesthetized horses, *Am J Vet Res* 48:192-197, 1987.
9. Muir WW, Skarda RT, Milne DW: Estimation of cardiac output in the horse by thermodilution techniques, *Am J Vet Res* 37:697-700, 1976.
10. Hallowell GD, Corley KT: Use of lithium dilution and pulse contour analysis cardiac output determination in anaesthetized horses: a clinical evaluation, *Vet Anaesth Analg* 32:201-211, 2005.
11. Linton RA et al: Cardiac output measured by lithium dilution, thermodilution, and transesophageal Doppler echocardiography in anesthetized horses, *Am J Vet Res* 61:731-737, 2000.
12. Gaynor JS, Bednarski RM, Muir WW: Effect of hypercapnia on the arrhythmogenic dose of epinephrine in horses anesthetized with guaifenesin, thiamylal sodium, and halothane, *Am J Vet Res* 54:315-321, 1993.
13. Moens Y, DeMoor A: Use of infra-red carbon dioxide analysis during general anesthesia in the horse, *Equine Vet J* 13:229-234, 1981.
14. Geiser DR, Rohrbach BW: Use of end-tidal CO2 tension to predict arterial CO2 values in isoflurane-anesthetized equine neonates, *Am J Vet Res* 53:1617-1621, 1992.
15. Koenig J, McDonell W, Valverde A: Accuracy of pulse oximetry and capnography in healthy and compromised horses during spontaneous and controlled ventilation, *Can J Vet Res* 67:169-174, 2003.
16. Neto FJ et al: The effect of changing the mode of ventilation on the arterial-to-end-tidal CO2 difference and physiological dead space in laterally and dorsally recumbent horses during halothane anesthesia, *Vet Surg* 29:200-205, 2000.
17. Whitehair KJ et al: Pulse oximetry in horses, *Vet Surg* 19:243-248, 1990.
18. Matthews NS et al: Evaluation of pulse oximetry in horses surgically treated for colic, *Equine Vet J* 26:114-116, 1994.
19. Matthews NS, Hartke S, Allen JC: An evaluation of pulse oximeters in dogs, cats, and horses, *Vet Anaesth Analg* 30:3-14, 2003.
20. Watney GCG, Norman WM, Schumacher JP: Accuracy of a reflectance pulse oximeter in anesthetized horses, *Am J Vet Res* 54:497-501, 1993.
21. Warren RG, Webb AI, Kosch PC: Evaluation of transcutaneous oxygen monitoring in anaesthetized pony foals, *Equine Vet J* 16:358-361, 1984.

22. Webb AI, Daniel RT, Miller HS: Preliminary studies on the measurement of conjunctival oxygen tension in the foal, *Am J Vet Res* 46:2566-2569, 1985.

23. Snyder JR et al: Surface oximetry for intraoperative assessment of colonic viability in horses, *J Am Vet Med Assoc* 204:1786-1789, 1994.

24. Taylor PM: Effects of hypercapnia on endocrine and metabolic responses to anaesthesia in ponies, *Res Vet Sci* 65(1):41-46; 1998.

25. Cullen LK et al: Effect of high $PaCO_2$ and time on cerebrospinal fluid and intraocular pressure in halothane-anesthetized horses, *Am J Vet Res* 51:300-304, 1990.

26. Taylor PM: Effects of hypercapnia on endocrine and metabolic responses to anaesthesia in ponies, *Res Vet Sci* 65:41-46, 1998.

27. Khanna AK et al: Cardiopulmonary effects of hypercapnia during controlled intermittent positive pressure ventilation in the horse, *Can J Vet Res* 59:213-221, 1995.

28. Wagner AE, Bednarski RM, Muir WW: Hemodynamic effects of carbon dioxide during intermittent positive-pressure ventilation in horses, *Am J Vet Res* 51:1922-1929, 1990.

29. Mitten LA, Hinchcliff KW, Sams R: A portable blood gas analyzer for equine venous blood. *J Vet Intern Med* 9:353-356, 1995.

30. Grosenbaugh DA, Gadawski JE, Muir WW: Evaluation of a portable clinical analyzer in a veterinary hospital setting, *J Am Vet Med Assoc* 213:691-694, 1998.

31. Clerbaux T et al: Comparative study of the oxyhaemoglobin dissociation curve of four mammals: man, dog, horse and cattle, *Comp Biochem Physiol Comp Physiol* 106:687-694, 1993.

32. Klein L: A review of 50 cases of postoperative myopathy in the horse—intrinsic and management factors affecting risk. In *Proceedings of the Fourth Annual American Association of Equine Practitioners*, vol 24, 1978, pp 89-94.

33. Trim CM et al: A retrospective survey of anaesthesia in horses with colic, *Equine Vet J* 7 (suppl):84-90, 1989.

34. Lindsay WA et al: Induction of equine postanesthetic myositis after halothane-induced hypotension, *Am J Vet Res* 50:404-410, 1989.

35. Young SS, Taylor PM: Factors influencing the outcome of equine anaesthesia: a review of 1314 cases, *Equine Vet J* 25:147-151, 1993.

36. Hahn AW et al: Indirect measurement of arterial blood pressure in the laboratory pony, *Lab Anim Sci* 23:889-893, 1973.

37. Johnson JH, Garner HE, Hutcheson DP: Ultrasonic measurement of arterial blood pressure in conditioned thoroughbreds, *Equine Vet J* 8:55-57, 1976.

38. Parry BW et al: Correct occlusive bladder width for indirect blood pressure measurement in horses, *Am J Vet Res* 43:50-54, 1982.

39. Bailey JE et al: Indirect Doppler ultrasonic measurement of arterial blood pressure results in a large measurement error in dorsally recumbent anaesthetized horses, *Equine Vet J* 26:70-73, 1994.

40. Giguere S et al: Accuracy of indirect measurement of blood pressure in neonatal foals, *J Vet Intern Med* 19:571-576, 2005.

41. Geddes LA et al: Indirect mean blood pressure in the anesthetized pony, *Am J Vet Res* 38:2055-2057, 1977.

42. Muir WW, Wade A, Grospitch BS: Automatic noninvasive sphygmomanometry in horses, *Am J Vet Res* 182:1230-1233, 1983.

43. Porciello F et al: Blood pressure measurements in dogs and horses using the oscillometric technique, *Vet Res Commun* 28(suppl1):367-369; 2004.

44. Fritsch R, Hausmann R: Indirect blood pressure determination in the horse with the Dinamap 1255 research monitor, *Tierarztl Prax* 16(4):373-376, 1988.

45. Young LE et al: Measurement of cardiac output by transoesophageal Doppler echocardiography in anaesthetized horses: comparison with thermodilution, *Br J Anaesth* 77:773-780,1996.

46. Gelman S: Venous function and central venous pressure, *Anesthesiology* 108:735-748, 2008.

47. Hall LW, Nigam JM: Measurement of central venous pressure in horses, *Vet Rec* 97:66-69, 1975.

48. Klein L, Sherman J: Effects of preanesthetic medication, anesthesia, and position of recumbency on central venous pressure in horses, *J Am Vet Med Assoc* 170:216-219, 1977.

49. Riebold TW, Evans AT: Blood pressure measurements in the anesthetized horse: comparison of four methods, *Vet Surg* 14:332-337, 1985.

50. Taylor PM: Techniques and clinical application of arterial blood pressure measurement in the horse, *Equine Vet J* 13:271-275, 1981.

51. Barr ED et al: Destructive lesions of the proximal sesamoid bones as a complication of dorsal metatarsal artery catheterization in three horses, *Vet Surg* 34:159-166, 2005.

52. Schneider RK et al: A retrospective study of 192 horses affected with septic arthritis/tenosynovitis, *Equine Vet J* 24:436-442, 1992.

53. Tavernier B et al: Systolic pressure variation as a guide to fluid therapy in patients with sepsis-induced hypotension, *Anesthesiology* 89:1313-1321, 1998.

54. Bennett-Guerrero E et al: Comparison of arterial systolic pressure variation with other clinical parameters to predict the response to fluid challenges during cardiac surgery, *Mt Sinai J Med* 69:95-100, 2002.

55. Corley KT et al: Cardiac output technologies with special reference to the horse, *J Vet Intern Med* 17:262-272, 2003.

56. Dunlop CI et al: Thermodilution estimation of cardiac output at high flows in anesthetized horses, *Am J Vet Res* 52:1893-1897, 1991.

57. Valverde A et al: Comparison of noninvasive cardiac output measured by use of partial carbon dioxide rebreathing or the lithium dilution method in anesthetized foals, *Am J Vet Res* 68:141-147, 2007.

58. Wetmore LA et al: Mixed venous oxygen tension as an estimate of cardiac output in anesthetized horses, *Am J Vet Res* 48:971-976, 1987.

59. Bleich HL: The clinical implications of venous carbon dioxide tension, *N Eng J Med* 320:1345-1346, 1989.

60. Moens Y: Arterial-alveolar carbon dioxide tension difference and alveolar dead space in halothane anaesthetized horses, *Equine Vet J* 21:282-284, 1989.

61. Moens Y, DeMoor A: Use of infra-red carbon dioxide analysis during general anesthesia in the horse, *Equine Vet J* 13:229-234, 1981.

62. Gazmuri RJ et al: Arterial PCO_2 as an indicator of systemic perfusion during cardiopulmonary resuscitation, *Crit Care Med* 17:237-240, 1989.

63. Constable PD: Hyperchloremic acidosis: the classic example of strong ion acidosis, *Anesth Analg* 96:919-922, 2003.

64. Muir WW, deMorais HAS: Acid-base physiology. In Tranquilli WJ et al, editors: *Lumb & Jones veterinary anesthesia and analgesia*, ed 4, Ames, Iowa, 2007, Blackwell Publishing, pp 169-182.

65. Mizock BA: Controversies in lactic acidosis: implications in critically ill patients, *JAMA* 258:497-501, 1987.

65a. Magdesian KG et al: Changes in central venous pressure and blood lactate concentration in response to acute blood loss in horses, *J Am Vet Med Assoc* 229:1458-1462, 2006.

66. Rose RJ: Electrolytes: clinical applications, *Vet Clin North Am (Equine Pract)* 6:281-294, 1990.

67. Tomasic M: Temporal changes in core body temperature in anesthetized adult horses, *Am J Vet Res* 60:556-562, 1999.

68. Tomasic M, Nann LE: Comparison of peripheral and core temperatures in anesthetized horses, *Am J Vet Res* 60:648-651, 1999.

69. Mayerhofer I et al: Hypothermia in horses induced by general anesthesia and limiting measures, *Equine Vet Educ* 17:53-56, 2005.

9

Principles of Drug Disposition and Drug Interaction in Horses

Richard A. Sams

William W. Muir

KEY POINTS

1. Drugs act by binding to receptors. Receptor binding generates a sigmoid relationship between receptor occupancy and drug concentration.
2. The drug plasma concentration versus time relationship is used to determine key pharmacokinetic parameters: clearance and volume of distribution. These values are used to determine elimination half-life and calculate dosage regimens.
3. The elimination half-life is used to estimate the time to steady-state drug concentration during infusion and drug elimination. Approximately 90% of the steady-state plasma concentration (or elimination) of a drug is reached in 3.3 half-lives. Infusion of a drug with a long half-life is usually preceded by a loading dose.
4. The plasma concentration-versus-response relationship determines the potency and efficacy of the drug. The median effective dose (ED_{50}) is used to compare drug potencies.
5. The relationship between the median lethal dose (LD_{50}) and ED_{50} determines the therapeutic index (LD_{50}/ED_{50}) of a drug. The ratio between the LD_1 and ED_{99} is a much more clinically relevant relationship.
6. Variable responses to drugs are caused by age, disease, and the effects of other drugs.
7. Drug combinations can interact to produce additive, infraadditive, or synergistic actions.

PHARMACOKINETICS

Pharmacokinetics is the study of the rates of drug absorption, distribution, metabolism, and elimination from the body; whereas pharmacodynamics is the study of the relationship between drug concentrations and effects. Integrated pharmacokinetic-pharmacodynamic (PK/PD) studies in healthy animals can provide a fundamental understanding of these processes and form the basis for dosage regimens designed to produce plasma drug concentrations sufficient to elicit the desired clinical or pharmacological effect while avoiding toxicities.

On the other hand, clinical pharmacokinetics is the study of pharmacokinetics in injured or diseased animals. The effects of injury, disease, and general anesthesia on pharmacokinetic parameters are studied to establish dosage regimens appropriate for patient animals. Most anesthetic drugs have relatively low therapeutic indices and therefore must be administered with extreme care. Relatively small changes in the pharmacokinetics of drugs used for anesthesia in horses may result in drug failure or drug toxicity unless these changes are recognized and appropriate dosage adjustments are made.

RECEPTOR THEORY

Many drugs are believed to exert their pharmacologic and toxic effects as a result of reversible interaction with receptors as depicted:

[Drug] + [Receptor] ≈ [Drug-receptor complex] → Drug effect

Formation of the drug-receptor complex results in a cellular response such as release of an intracellular messenger (e.g., cyclic adenosine monophosphate by norepinephrine) or blockade of an ion pump (e.g., blockade of the sodium ion pump in nerve cell membranes by local anesthetics), which results in observable drug effects. The magnitude of the drug effect is proportional to the number of drug-receptor complexes formed. Therefore, low drug concentrations are associated with the formation of few drug-receptor complexes, and minimum drug effects are observed. As the drug concentration increases, the number of drug-receptor complexes increases, and the intensity of the drug effect increases until it reaches a maximum. Maximum effect (depending on the effect monitored) may be reached long before all the receptors are occupied. Therefore the intensity of the drug response assumes a sigmoidal shape as a function of drug concentration at the receptor site. Other types of receptors may interact with drug molecules as drug concentration increases so that other types of drug effects or toxicities may appear. Alternatively the drug may interact with the same receptors but in a different tissue, thereby eliciting a different effect.

Although estimates of the concentration of drug at the receptor site or the number of drug-receptor complexes formed would be useful in estimating the intensity of the drug response, neither of these values can be determined in clinical patients. However, the concentration of drug in the blood generally attains equilibrium with the concentration of drug at the receptor site. Consequently certain concentrations of drug in the blood are associated with no drug effect, whereas higher concentrations are associated with desired drug effects or even toxicities. Therefore it is possible to measure the concentration of drugs in blood (or plasma) to determine whether the concentration is within the range of concentrations associated with the desired clinical effect. Drug failures thought to result from refractoriness are often found to result from failure to attain a sufficiently high drug concentration because of incomplete drug delivery or higher than normal or expected rates of drug elimination. Horses that are extremely excited or stressed may also require larger than expected doses of anesthetic drugs to produce unconsciousness. On the other hand, toxicity may be shown to result from attainment of blood drug concentrations higher than those associated with the desired clinical response because of altered rates of drug elimination.

Therapeutic concentrations for most anesthetic drugs have been determined. The aim of clinical pharmacology is adjustment of the drug regimen to attain the desired blood drug concentration and clinical effect.

COMPARTMENTAL MODELS OF DRUG DISPOSITION

Models of drug disposition are used to describe drug concentration versus time data obtained after administration of a drug to an experimental animal. The simplest of these models is the one-compartment model of drug disposition, which is characterized by rapid distribution of drug from the blood to other tissues. Equilibration of a nonprotein-bound drug between the plasma and other tissues occurs so rapidly that changes in drug concentrations in the plasma and the tissues occur in parallel. Many drugs distribute more widely throughout the body, and multicompartmental models of drug disposition are used to characterize the slower distribution of drug from the plasma to other tissues. Distribution of some drugs to certain tissues is so slow that a substantial amount of the drug is eliminated before equilibration of the drug between blood and tissues occurs.

One-Compartment Models

The one-compartment model (Figure 9-1) is the simplest model of drug disposition but is encountered uncommonly with drugs used for anesthesia. The rate of change of drug concentration after intravenous drug administration in the one-compartment model is:

$$dC_p/dt = C_p \times k$$

where dC_p/dt is the rate of change of drug concentration, C_p is the plasma drug concentration, and k is the elimination rate constant. Rearrangement and integration of this equation result in the following expression for the concentration of drug at any time after drug administration:

$$C_p = C_p^0 \exp(-kt)$$

where C_p^0 is the plasma drug concentration immediately after drug administration, and exp is the base of the natural logarithms. If the logarithm of each side of this expression is obtained, the expression is transformed to:

$$\ln C_p = \ln C_p^0 - kt$$

where ln is the natural logarithm. This expression is most useful because it indicates that a plot of $\ln C_p$ versus time will be linear with a slope of k and an intercept of C_p^0 (Figure 9-2). Initial evaluation of intravenous drug concentration versus time data usually involves a plot of $\ln C_p$ versus time to determine whether a straight line is obtained. If the line is straight, a one-compartment model of drug disposition is inferred. On the other hand, curvature of this plot in the early time period after intravenous drug administration is indicative of a multicompartment model of drug disposition.

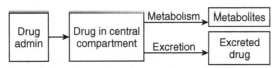

Figure 9–1. One-compartment model of drug distribution.

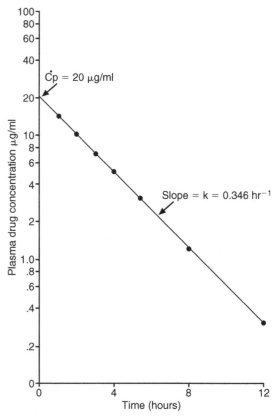

Figure 9–2. Plot of plasma drug concentration versus time data after intravenous administration. Note that the vertical axis is logarithmic. Linearity of this plot indicates a one-compartment model.

Multicompartmental Models

Distribution of drug from the blood to other tissues is slower in multicompartmental models of drug disposition than in the one-compartment model. As a consequence, the plot of $\ln C_p$ versus time is nonlinear during the early period after drug administration while drug is being distributed to the slowly equilibrating tissues (Figure 9-3). The plasma and rapidly equilibrating tissues are considered to be the central compartment in multicompartmental models of drug disposition (Figure 9-4), whereas the slowly equilibrating tissues are considered to be one or more peripheral compartments. The number of peripheral compartments that can be discerned is often one but can be two if the drug has an affinity for a tissue that slowly releases the drug back into the central compartment.

The plasma drug concentration after intravenous administration in a two-compartment model of drug disposition is given by the following expression:

$$C_p = A \exp(-\alpha t) + B \exp(-\beta t)$$

where A and B are preexponential terms with units of concentration (e.g., microgram per milliliter or nanogram per milliliter). A plot of the logarithms of intravenous drug concentrations versus time (see Figure 9-3) is curved in the early period after drug administration but becomes linear at later times. The slope during the terminal portion of drug distribution is equal to β, and the intercept of the line extrapolated to time equal to zero is B. A new straight line with slope equal to α and intercept of A will be obtained

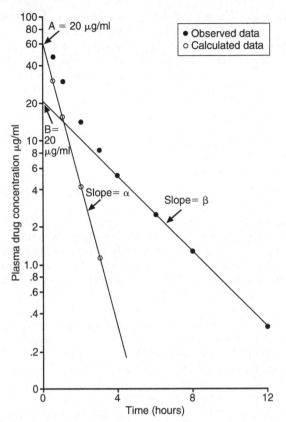

Figure 9–3. Plot of plasma drug concentration versus time data for a drug administered intravenously. Note that the vertical axis is logarithmic. Curvature of this plot (●) from 0 to 4 hr after dosing indicates a multicompartment model.

if the logarithms of the differences between observed drug concentrations and the extrapolated drug concentrations at each observation time are plotted versus time. If this new line is curved in the early period after drug administration, this process, known as *feathering* or *curve stripping*, is repeated until a straight line is obtained.

All of the pharmacokinetic parameters that are required to calculate dosages can be calculated directly from the slopes and intercepts (i.e., C_p^0 and k for a one-compartment model and A, α, B, and β for a two-compartment model) obtained from plots of logarithms of experimental drug concentration versus time after drug administration and the experimentally administered dose.

Drugs are reversibly distributed to the peripheral tissues in multicompartmental models of drug distribution and must return to the central compartment for elimination by

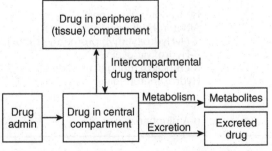

Figure 9–4. Two-compartment model of drug distribution.

metabolism or excretion. The concentration of drug in the plasma is high relative to that in other tissues in the period immediately after intravenous drug administration and provides the driving force for drug distribution to other tissues. As drug is eliminated from the plasma, it diffuses from the peripheral tissues back to the plasma.

PHARMACOKINETIC TERMINOLOGY

Clearance

Clearance is a measure of the body's ability to remove a drug by either metabolism or excretion. Clearance is defined as the proportionality constant between the rate of drug elimination and the drug concentration:

$$\text{Rate of drug elimination} = Cl \times C_p$$

where Cl is the total clearance and C_p is the drug concentration in blood or plasma. The units of clearance, like those of flow, are volume per unit time. Therefore, clearance represents that volume of blood (or plasma) from which the drug has been completely removed per unit time. For example, if drug concentration is 10 μg/ml and clearance is 100 ml/min, the rate of drug elimination is 1000 μg/min. The rate of drug elimination decreases until it eventually reaches zero as the drug concentration decreases because of clearance of the drug from the body. On the other hand, the clearance is generally constant and independent of drug concentration.

Because of the wide range of body weights of horses, it is customary to normalize the clearance by dividing it by the total weight of the animal. For example, if a horse weighing 400 kg has a clearance of 100 ml/min, the normalized clearance is 0.25 ml/min/kg of body weight. Similarly the total body clearance of a drug in a specific animal of known body weight is calculated from the normalized clearance of the drug and the total body weight of the animal. Therefore the clearance of a drug with a total body clearance of 0.020 ml/min/kg of body weight in a 300-kg horse is 6 ml/min.

The total body clearance of a drug is the sum of all individual organ clearances for that drug and is inversely proportional to the area under the blood (or plasma) drug concentration versus time curve:

$$\text{Total clearance} = \text{Dose}/\text{AUC}$$

where AUC is the area under the blood (or plasma) drug concentration versus time curve from the time of drug administration to infinity. The AUC is readily calculated as C_p^0/k for a one-compartment model drug and A/α + B/β for a two-compartment model drug.

The relationship between total clearance and AUC indicates that a drug with a higher total body clearance has a correspondingly lower area under the blood (or plasma) drug concentration versus time curve than another drug given at the same dose (Figure 9-5). Alternatively a drug administered to a horse with reduced total body clearance resulting from disease has a higher area under the plasma drug concentration versus time curve than the same drug administered to a horse with normal clearance. Therefore the diseased horse is exposed to higher drug concentrations for a longer period of time, and greater and more persistent drug effects would be expected unless the dose of the drug is reduced accordingly.

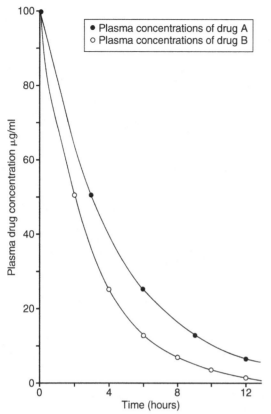

Figure 9–5. Plot of plasma drug concentration versus time data for two different drugs following intravenous administration of the same dose. Note that drug B (○), which has a lower area under the plasma drug concentration versus time curve, is cleared more rapidly than drug A (●).

The clearance of each organ of elimination for a specific drug is the product of the blood flow to the organ and the extraction ratio for the drug, a measure of the ability of the organ to remove the drug by metabolism or excretion. Because the extraction ratio ranges from 0.0 for a drug that is not eliminated by the organ to 1.0 for a drug that is completely eliminated by an organ, the clearance of a drug by any organ can range from a minimum value of zero to a maximum value equal to the blood flow rate

to the organ. Therefore the maximum clearances for the liver and kidneys, the major organs of elimination in the horse, are equal to the blood flow rates to these organs or approximately 20 to 30 ml/min/kg of body weight and 10 ml/min/kg of body weight, respectively. The actual clearance of an organ of elimination depends on a multitude of factors, including the physicochemical properties of the drug and the nature of the clearance processes involved. The influences of these factors on clearances of the major organs of elimination are reviewed in the following sections on hepatic and renal clearances.

Hepatic Clearance

Hepatic clearance is caused by metabolic transformation of drugs by hepatic microsomal enzymes and biliary excretion of drugs into the bile. Metabolic transformations known to occur in the horse include oxidation, hydrolysis, reduction, and conjugation (Table 9-1). Frequently a drug simultaneously undergoes metabolism by several different pathways, resulting in a mixture of metabolites. For example, phenylbutazone is oxidized simultaneously to oxyphenbutazone and hydroxyphenylbutazone in the horse. The relative amounts of the two metabolites depend on the relative rates of the parallel pathways. Furthermore, primary metabolites may undergo further metabolism. For example, oxidation, reduction, and hydrolysis are often followed by conjugation. Codeine is oxidized sequentially to morphine and then conjugated to form morphine-3-glucuronide. The water solubility of a drug metabolite is often greater than that of the parent drug; consequently the renal clearance of the metabolite is almost always greater than that of the parent drug.

Hepatic clearance is the product of the total hepatic blood flow from the hepatic artery and the portal system times the hepatic extraction ratio:

$$Cl_H = Q_H \times E_H$$

where Cl_H is the total hepatic clearance, Q_H is the total hepatic blood flow rate, and E_H is the hepatic extraction ratio. The hepatic extraction ratio depends on the plasma protein binding of a drug, the intrinsic clearance of the drug-metabolizing enzymes for the drug, and the hepatic blood flow rate:

$$E_H = \{(Q_H \times f_{up} \times Cl_{int})/(Q_H + f_{up} \times Cl_{int})\}$$

Drug	Active metabolite	Inactive metabolite
Phenylbutazone	Oxyphenbutazone	
Morphine	Morphine-6-glucuronide	Morphine-3-glucuronide
Butorphanol		Butorphanol glucuronide
Propranolol	4-Hydroxypropranolol	
Isoxsuprine		Isoxsuprine glucuronide
Albuterol		Albuterol sulfate
Acepromazine		2-(1-Hydroxyethyl) promazine sulfoxide
Lidocaine		3-Hydroxylidocaine
Methocarbamol	Guaifenesin	Methocarbamol glucuronide
Detomidine		Hydroxydetomidine
Ketamine	Norketamine	
Diazepam	Oxazepam, temazepam	
Procaine		p-Aminobenzoic acid

Table 9–1.   Metabolic transformations in horses*

*Classification: [O], oxidation; [R], reduction; [H], hydrolysis; [C], conjugation.

where f_{up} is the fraction of drug molecules not bound to plasma proteins, and Cl_{int} is the intrinsic clearance of the liver enzymes. When the hepatic blood flow rate is much greater than the product of the unbound fraction in plasma and the intrinsic clearance, the hepatic extraction ratio is low, and the hepatic clearance is approximated by:

$$Cl_H \approx f_{up} \times Cl_{int}$$

Under these conditions of low hepatic extraction, the hepatic clearance is highly dependent on the extent of plasma protein binding and the activity of the hepatic drug-metabolizing enzymes but is relatively independent of the hepatic blood flow rate. Therefore hepatic clearances of low–extraction ratio drugs such as phenylbutazone and theophylline are affected by changes in plasma protein binding and enzyme activity but not by changes in hepatic blood flow rate. Disease states such as inflammation, renal disease, and chronic liver disease, which may result in alterations in plasma protein binding or changes in hepatic enzyme activity, may affect the hepatic clearances of low hepatic extraction ratio drugs. Furthermore, concomitant administration of other drugs that compete for plasma protein-binding sites or that modify hepatic enzyme activity by inhibition or stimulation (e.g., induction of microsomal enzyme activity by barbiturates) may also affect hepatic clearances of low extraction ratio drugs. For example, the hepatic clearance of phenylbutazone is decreased by approximately 50% when chloramphenicol, a known enzyme inhibitor, is administered concurrently.[1] When these changes in clearance are significant, changes in dosages or dosing frequency may be necessary to maintain drug effects or to avoid unacceptable risks of toxicity.

The product of the fraction unbound in plasma and the intrinsic clearance is much greater than the hepatic blood flow for drugs that are highly extracted by the liver. The hepatic clearance of highly extracted drugs is approximated by:

$$Cl_H \approx Q_H$$

Therefore the hepatic clearances of highly extracted drugs depend on the hepatic blood flow rate but are relatively independent of changes in plasma protein binding and hepatic enzyme activity. Drugs such as detomidine, ketamine, lidocaine, propranolol, doxapram, fentanyl, morphine and most of the opiates, chloramphenicol, isoxsuprine, xylazine, and pyrilamine are highly extracted by the liver of the horse (Table 9-2). Hepatic clearances of these drugs are relatively large and account for most, if not all, of the total body clearance of the drug. Their hepatic clearances are highly dependent on changes in hepatic blood flow rate but are much less dependent on changes in plasma protein binding and hepatic enzyme activity. Because the hepatic blood flow rate is decreased by many drugs, including some of the gaseous and intravenous anesthetic drugs, clearances of highly extracted drugs often decrease when administered in conjunction with anesthetic agents. The clearance of lidocaine and fentanyl is less when administered during isoflurane anesthesia, presumably as a result of decreased hepatic blood flow during anesthesia (Figure 9-6).[2,3] Furthermore, drugs such as propranolol that significantly decrease hepatic blood flow reduce their own hepatic clearance, as well as that of other highly extracted drugs. Therefore drug failure

Table 9–2.	**Hepatic extraction ratios of representative drugs in horses**		
Low	**Intermediate**	**High**
Digitoxin	Dantrolene	Amphetamine
Phenylbutazone	Phenytoin	Diazepam
Phenobarbital		Doxapram
		Propranolol
		Pentazocine
		Lidocaine
		Isoxsuprine
		Procaine
		Acepromazine
		Xylazine
		Detomidine
		Ketamine
		Methocarbamol
		Morphine

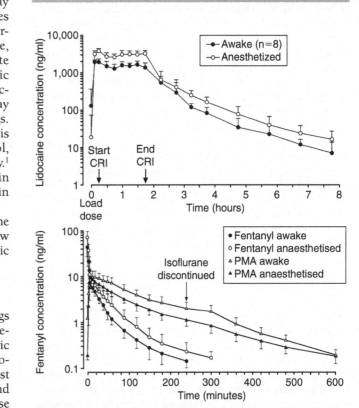

Figure 9–6. Plasma lidocaine *(top)* and fentanyl *(bottom)* concentrations versus time in awake and anesthetized horses. Fentanyl metabolite *(PMA)* is also shown. Note the decreased clearance of both drugs during isoflurane anesthesia. (From Feary DJ et al: Influence of general anesthesia on pharmacokinetics of intravenous lidocaine infusion in horse, *Am J Vet Res* 66(4):574-580, 2005 *[top]*; and Thomasy SM et al: Influence of general anaesthesia on the pharmacokinetics of intravenous fentanyl and its primary metabolite in horses, *Equine Vet J* 39(1):54-58, 2007 *[bottom]*.)

or toxicity while using highly extracted drugs may often be explained by abnormal values of hepatic clearance resulting from unanticipated alterations in the hepatic blood flow rate. Adjustments in drug dosage or rate of administration of highly extracted drugs frequently are necessary because hepatic clearance is high and is generally the major route of elimination for this group of drugs.

Renal Clearance

Renal clearance is a significant route of elimination of water-soluble drugs and drug metabolites. It is a measure of the ability of the kidneys to eliminate drugs and is the net result of glomerular filtration, tubular secretion, and tubular resorption:

$$\text{Renal clearance} = \frac{(\text{Filtration rate} + \text{Rate of secretion} - \text{Rate of resorption})}{C_p}$$

Drugs are removed from blood by the kidneys by way of filtration of unbound drug in plasma at the glomerulus. Therefore the filtration rate of a drug is:

$$\text{Filtration rate} = f_{up} \times C_p \times \text{GFR}$$

where f_{up} is the fraction unbound in plasma; C_p is the plasma drug concentration; and GFR is the glomerular filtration rate, which in the normal horse is approximately 1.92 ml/min/kg of body weight.[4] Therefore filtration is relatively unimportant for drugs such as phenylbutazone and propranolol, which are extensively bound to plasma proteins, but is important for drugs such as theophylline and caffeine, which are bound sparingly to plasma proteins in horses. The maximum renal clearance of a drug that is filtered but neither secreted nor resorbed is equal to the glomerular filtration rate or approximately 1.92 ml/min/kg of body weight in the normal horse.

Certain drugs are also excreted from the blood in the kidneys by tubular secretion. Separate secretory mechanisms exist for transporting acids (anions) and bases (cations), including quaternary ammonium compounds such as glycopyrrolate and succinylcholine, from the plasma into the tubular lumen. These mechanisms are relatively nonspecific, active processes that are saturable and subject to competitive and noncompetitive inhibition. High concentrations of drugs or drug metabolites may cause saturation of tubular transport processes; this occurs only rarely with normal drug dosages in horses but can occur with overdoses. Competitive inhibition of tubular secretion of penicillin by probenecid has been used clinically in persons to reduce the renal clearance and thereby prolong the duration of effect of penicillin. Although inhibition of tubular secretion of organic anions by probenecid has been observed in studies in horses, it has not been used clinically because of the high doses required.[5] Apparently the transport mechanisms are able to strip drugs from plasma proteins rapidly enough that plasma protein binding does not reduce tubular secretion. The maximum renal clearance for a drug that is both filtered and secreted but not resorbed is approximately 10 ml/min/kg of body weight in the normal horse.

Resorption of drugs is the third and perhaps most important factor controlling the renal handling of drugs. The rate and extent of tubular resorption of a drug depend on the physicochemical properties (e.g., pKa, lipophilicity, molecular size) of the drug, the pH of the urine, and the urine flow rate. Nonionized drugs with sufficient lipophilicity are passively resorbed from the urine as drug concentration in the urine increases relative to that in the plasma as water is resorbed. The concentrations of nonionized drug in plasma and urine are equal at equilibrium. Because the pH of the urine in normal resting horses is approximately 8.0 to 8.5, weak bases are relatively more ionized in plasma than in urine and tend to be extensively resorbed.[6] Therefore renal clearance of lipophilic weak bases such as detomidine, ketamine, xylazine, morphine and other opioids, lidocaine, acepromazine, and pyrilamine is a relatively unimportant route of elimination in the normal resting horse. On the other hand, weak organic acids are relatively more ionized in urine than in plasma and are much less likely to be resorbed. Therefore renal clearance of weak organic acids such as the penicillins, cephalosporins, phenylbutazone, naproxen, flunixin, and furosemide is generally of more significance than that of weak organic bases. However, reduction of urine pH as a result of exercise, administration of urinary acidifiers, and various disease processes (e.g., ischemia, hypoxia) can result in a decrease in the resorption of weak bases and an increase in the resorption of weak acids.

An increase in the urine flow rate caused by disease or by the administration of fluids or diuretics decreases the drug concentration gradient between urine and plasma, generally reduces the urine pH, and decreases the time available for attainment of equilibrium. The net effect of these factors is a decrease in the tubular resorption of both acids and bases, with an increase in their renal clearances. The significance of this increase in renal clearance depends on the magnitude of the renal clearance relative to the total clearance. Very large increases in renal clearance are required before significant changes in total clearance are observed if the renal clearance of a drug is normally a small fraction of its total body clearance.

Volume of Distribution

The volume of distribution of a drug is the proportionality constant between the amount of drug in the body and the plasma concentration of the drug:

$$\text{Vd} = X/C_p$$

where Vd is the volume of distribution, X is the amount of drug in the body at a particular time, and C_p is the plasma drug concentration at that time. In other words, the volume of distribution is the volume that drug would occupy if it were present throughout the body at the plasma concentration. Because drug is often sequestered or concentrated in certain tissues, the volume of distribution may be much larger than the volume of total body water. For example, if the amount of drug in the body is 2000 mg and the plasma concentration is 2 μg/ml, the volume of distribution is 1,000,000 ml or 1000 L, which is more than the total body water of an adult horse weighing about 500 kg (the total body water represents about 60% to 70% of the total body weight or 300 to 350 L in a 500-kg horse). For convenience, the volume of distribution is usually normalized to body weight because it is reasonable to expect that the volume of distribution will increase with body weight. In the above example, this volume of distribution in a horse weighing 500 kg could be expressed as 2 L/kg of body weight.

Drugs that are bound extensively to plasma proteins generally are not widely distributed. Therefore their volumes of distribution are relatively small (e.g., 0.1 to 0.4 L/kg of body weight). On the other hand, drugs with less extensive plasma protein binding but affinity for tissues such as muscle or adipose tissue often have large volumes of distribution (e.g., 1 to 5 L/kg of body weight). Digoxin, which is bound to skeletal muscle, and thiopental, which has high lipid solubility, both have relatively high volumes of distribution.

An instructive model for the volume of distribution after attainment of distribution equilibrium is:

$$Vd = Vp + \{f_{up}/f_{ut}\} \times Vt$$

where Vp is the volume of plasma water; f_{up} and f_{ut} are the fractions of the drug molecules not bound to plasma proteins and tissue proteins, respectively; and Vt is = the volume of tissue water. The volume of distribution equals the plasma water plus the tissue water for a drug that is not bound to either plasma or tissue proteins (i.e., f_{up} and f_{ut} = 1). This volume is the total body water and is approximately 600 to 700 ml/kg of body weight in adult horses.

If a drug is bound extensively to plasma proteins (i.e., f_{up} is very small), the volume of distribution is approximately equal to the volume of plasma water or about 50 ml/kg of body weight. Evans Blue dye is used to estimate plasma volume in horses because it is extensively bound to plasma proteins and therefore is limited in its distribution to the plasma volume.

Drugs that are more extensively bound to plasma proteins than to tissues have volumes of distribution between 50 and 700 ml/kg of body weight. Drugs that are more extensively bound to tissues than to plasma proteins have volumes of distribution greater than 700 ml/kg of body weight. Although there is no upper limit to the volume of distribution, few values higher than about 10 L/kg of body weight have been reported.

Variables affecting the volume of distribution are the volumes of plasma and tissue water, the binding of drug to plasma proteins and to the tissues, and the rate of blood flow to the tissues because reduced flow can result in failure of the drug to attain distribution equilibrium. Drug-drug or drug-disease interactions that alter binding in either plasma or tissues can affect the volume of distribution. Dehydration or reduced rates of blood flow to tissues of distribution can affect the magnitude of the volume of distribution.

The volume of distribution is used to calculate a loading dose (LD) of a drug if a target plasma drug concentration is known (Box 9-1):

$$LD = C_{target} \times Vd$$

For example, the LD of a drug with a volume of distribution of 0.3 L/kg of body weight and a target plasma drug concentration of 1 μg/ml is 0.3 mg/kg of body weight. The total dosage to be administered is 135 mg if the horse weighs 450 kg. Known or anticipated changes in the volume of distribution of drug in the horse being medicated require proportional changes in the LD.

Half-Life

The half-life of a drug is the time required for one half of the drug to be removed from the body (Box 9-2 and Table 9-3). Although frequently used as a measure of the efficiency of drug elimination processes, half-life is determined by both volume of distribution and clearance:

$$t\tfrac{1}{2} = 0.693\ Vd/Cl$$

where t½ is the drug half-life. The volume of distribution affects the half-life of a drug because the drug must be in blood to be delivered to the organs of elimination. A drug with a large volume of distribution (e.g., propranolol and acepromazine) is not exposed to the organs of elimination as extensively as a drug with a smaller volume of distribution (e.g., naproxen and phenylbutazone) and therefore has a longer half-life if the clearances are the same. The half-life of a drug can change without a change in organ clearance if there is a change in the volume of distribution.

Weak organic bases (e.g., lidocaine, fentanyl, oxymorphone, isoxsuprine, detomidine, ketamine) tend to have large volumes of distribution and large total clearances; weak organic acids (e.g., flunixin, phenylbutazone, furosemide, ampicillin) tend to have smaller volumes of distribution and smaller total clearances. However, half-lives of those drugs used clinically in horses tend to be rather similar in spite of these differences in volumes of distribution and clearances.

The administration of a drug at intervals equal to its half-life results in the maximum plasma drug concentration being 1.58 times the minimum plasma drug concentration. If the time between administration of a drug is increased relative to the half-life, the ratio of the maximum to the minimum plasma drug concentration increases. Increasing the dosing interval relative to the half-life can result in toxicity during part of the dosing interval and lack of effect during another part of the interval (Figure 9-7). The solution is to reduce the time interval between doses or, if the half-life is too short, to give the drug by constant intravenous infusion.

Bioavailability

The bioavailability of a drug is a measure of the rate and extent of drug entry into the systemic blood circulation

---

Box 9–1 Determining Loading and Maintenance Doses

Loading Dose (LD) = C_p × Vd

Example: C_p = 2 μg/ml, Vd = 2 L/kg

  Then LD = 2 μg/ml × 2000 ml/kg = 4000 μg/kg

  LD = 4 mg/kg

Maintenance Dose (MD) = C_p × Cl

Example C_p = 2 μg/ml, Cl = 20 ml/kg/min

  Then MD = 2 μg/ml × 20 ml/kg/min = 40 μg/kg/min

  MD = 28.8 mg/kg bid

Box 9–2 Time to Drug Steady State or Drug Elimination

Estimate the time required for removal of a drug from the body:

  1 × half-life: 50% eliminated

  2 × half-life: 75% eliminated

  3 × half-life: 87.5% eliminated

  3.3 × half-life: 90% eliminated

  4 × half-life: 93.75% eliminated

Estimate time required to approach steady-state value:

  1 × half-life: 50% of steady-state

  2 × half-life: 75% of steady-state

  3 × half-life: 87.5% of steady-state

  3.3 × half-life: 90% of steady state

Table 9–3. Examples of pharmacokinetic parameters for drugs in horses

Drug	Cl_T (ml/min/kg)	Vd (ml/kg)	t½ (min)	Elimination mechanism
Acepromazine[20]	26.3	6600	174	Metabolism
Dantrolene[21]	4.35	791	129	Metabolism
Detomidine[7]	6.7	740	76.5	Metabolism
Diazepam[22]	7.48	6280	582	Metabolism
Etodolac[23]	4.0	290	160	Metabolism/renal
Fentanyl[17]	16.4	840	48.5	Metabolism
Guaifenesin[12]	8.2	970	84.5	Metabolism
Ketamine[24]	31.1	2722	65.8	Metabolism
Lidocaine[13]	52.0	2858	39.6	Metabolism
Meperidine[25]	?	?	66	Metabolism
Methocarbamol[26]	11.7	880	60.8	Metabolism/renal
Morphine[27]	5.33	1980	257	Metabolism
Pentazocine[28]	28.8	2970	71.5	Metabolism
Pentobarbital[29]	7.64	833	75.6	Metabolism
Phenobarbital[30]	0.51	803	1098	Metabolism
Xylazine[31]	21.0	2456	81.0	Metabolism

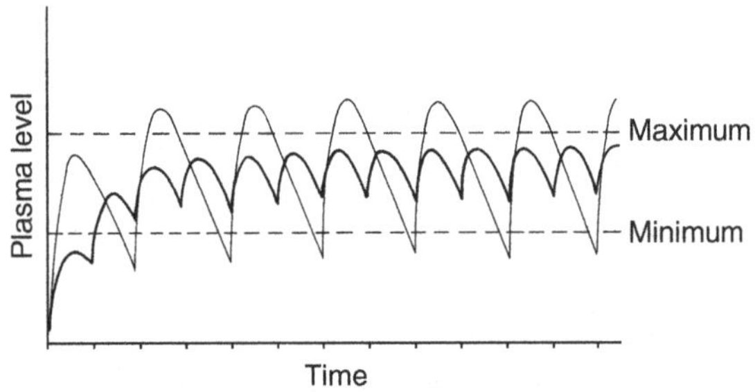

Figure 9–7. Plots of plasma drug concentration versus time. Note that drug concentrations are greater than the maximum therapeutic concentration and below the minimum therapeutic concentration when the same total dosage is administered less frequently *(light line)*.

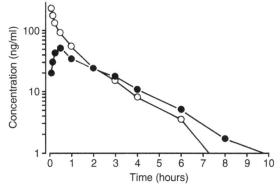

Figure 9–8. Plot of plasma detomidine concentration versus time data following intravenous (○) and intramuscular (●) administration of detomidine. Areas under the respective curves are nearly equal, indicating essentially complete bioavailability of the intramuscular dose. (From Salonen JS et al: Single-dose pharmacokinetics of detomidine in the horse and cow, *J Vet Pharmacol Ther* 12:65, 1982.)

after oral, intramuscular, subcutaneous, and other nonintravenous routes of drug administration. The extent of bioavailability is calculated from the relative areas under the plasma drug concentration versus time curves after nonintravenous (e.g., intramuscular, subcutaneous, and oral) and intravenous doses of the drug:

$$F = \{AUC_{niv}/AUC_{iv}\} \times \{Dose_{iv}/Dose_{niv}\}$$

where F is the extent of bioavailability; and niv and iv are nonintravenous and intravenous routes of administration, respectively. The bioavailability of intramuscularly administered detomidine has been shown to be essentially complete (Figure 9-8).[7]

The extent of bioavailability of an orally administered drug may be reduced because of incomplete absorption, degradation of the drug in the gastrointestinal tract, or metabolism during passage through the gut wall and liver. The extent of metabolism during passage through the liver is extensive for drugs with high extraction ratios and can be predicted by:

$$f = (1 - E_H)$$

where f is the fraction of drug escaping metabolism or excretion during passage through the liver. This effect, known as the first-pass effect because it occurs during the first pass of the drug through the liver, is considerable in the horse because of the large number of drugs with high hepatic extraction ratios. For some drugs the effect is so great that the drug is not effective when administered orally (e.g., lidocaine), whereas for other drugs the oral dose must be much larger than the parenteral dose to achieve a clinical effect (e.g., isoxsuprine, pyrilamine, propranolol).

The rate of drug absorption depends on the physicochemical properties of the drug, the dose form, drug formulation factors, the site of drug administration, and the blood flow rate to the site of administration. As a general rule, drugs in solution are absorbed faster than drugs not in solution. A large surface area to volume ratio, such as that in a suspension or rapidly disintegrating solid formulation, promotes rapid absorption. In addition, drugs are more rapidly absorbed from sites with higher blood flow rates. For example, the rate of absorption of lidocaine is slowed by the coadministration of epinephrine, which constricts blood vessels, thereby reducing the blood flow rate to the injection site.

Plasma Protein Binding

Many drugs are reversibly bound to plasma proteins such as albumin and acid glycoprotein (Figure 9-9). Only unbound drug can penetrate cell membranes. Albumin is quantitatively more important for acidic drugs such as the thiobarbiturates and

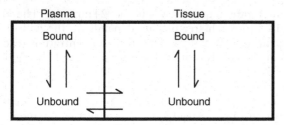

Figure 9–9. Schematic indicating reversible nature of drug binding to proteins in plasma and tissue compartments. Since only unbound drug can pass through cell membranes, the concentrations of unbound drug in plasma and tissue compartments are equal. (Reprinted with permission from Rowland M, Tozer TN: *Clinical pharmacokinetics: concepts and applications*, Philadelphia, 1980, Lea & Febiger.)

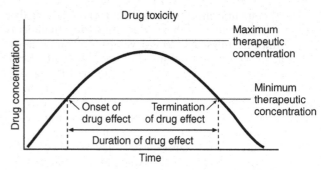

Figure 9–10. Plot of plasma drug concentration versus time after a nonintravenous drug dose indicating time to onset of drug effect, duration of drug effect, and termination of drug effect.

phenylbutazone; acid glycoprotein is more important for basic drugs such as lidocaine and ketamine. Bound drug is regarded as pharmacologically inactive, but drug assays generally measure the total drug concentration. Because the concentration of albumin decreases in various liver diseases, the fraction of drug bound to albumin may decrease under these conditions, thereby increasing the concentration of pharmacologically active drug in plasma without affecting the total drug concentration.

PHARMACODYNAMIC CONCEPTS

Relationship Between Drug Concentration and Drug Effect

Both the therapeutic and the toxic effects of many drugs result from reversible interaction of the drug with one or more receptor types within the body. These sites are located in the skeletal muscles, the kidneys, the brain, the lungs, the heart, and other tissues. Because these sites are not located in the blood and because drug concentrations throughout the body depend on a variety of factors such as plasma and tissue binding, the concentration of drug at the receptor site is usually not equal to the concentration of drug in blood. However, the drug concentration at the receptor site is proportional to the drug concentration in plasma once distribution equilibrium is complete. In fact, drug concentrations at receptor sites in rapidly equilibrating tissues reach equilibrium before distribution equilibrium has occurred.

Therefore drug concentrations in plasma can be related to the appearance of therapeutic and toxic effects of drugs. Generally plasma drug concentrations above a certain value are associated with therapeutic effects, and plasma drug concentrations above a higher value are associated with toxic effects (Figure 9-10). The *onset of drug action* coincides with the attainment of the plasma drug concentration referred to as the *minimum therapeutic concentration*. The *intensity of drug effect* increases with increasing plasma drug concentration until a plateau is reached, at which point the receptors are believed to be saturated. If plasma drug concentrations are allowed to increase until toxic effects are observed, the *maximum therapeutic concentration* can be determined (see Figure 9-10). The ratio of the maximum therapeutic concentration to the minimum therapeutic concentration is termed the *therapeutic index* and is a measure of the safety of the drug (Figure 9-11). Dosages of drugs with low therapeutic indices must be determined very carefully to produce a therapeutic effect without producing toxicity.

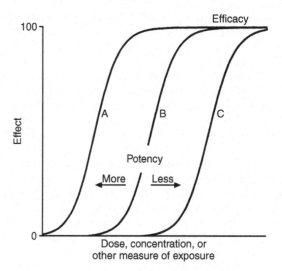

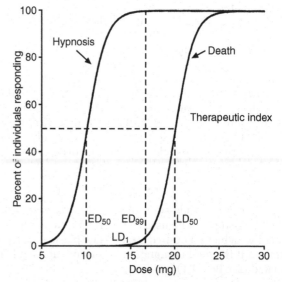

Figure 9–11. The dose or drug concentration versus effect relationship is sigmoidal *(top)*. The concentration-response curve is shifted to the left or right, with decreases or increases in potency, respectively (drug A is most potent; drug C is least potent). The median effective dose *(ED$_{50}$)* required to produce a desired effect (e.g., hypnosis) and the median lethal dose *(LD$_{50}$)* are used to determine the therapeutic index *(LD$_{50}$/ED$_{50}$)* of a drug. The LD$_{1}$/ED$_{99}$ is a much more clinically relevant number.

The therapeutic effect persists as long as the plasma drug concentration remains above the minimum therapeutic concentration, unless *tolerance* develops. Tolerance can be either acute or chronic and may be caused by a number of different factors, including down-regulation of receptors or increased drug clearance. *Acute tolerance* occurs when the intensity of drug effect is less than expected after a normal dose of the drug and may occur as a result of an increased rate of distribution of drug to peripheral tissues. For example, this could occur in an excited horse in which cardiac output is higher than normal, leading to more rapid distribution of the drug from central to peripheral tissues. *Chronic tolerance* occurs when the intensity of drug effect diminishes after repeated dosing of the drug to a horse. Chronic tolerance may result from increased rates of drug metabolism as a result of exposure to the drug or from a reduction in the number of drug receptors as a result of repeated exposure in a process called down-regulation.

The intensity of drug effects diminishes, and the drug effect terminates as the drug is distributed to more slowly equilibrating tissues if the drug receptors are located in rapidly equilibrating tissues. This *redistribution* of drug is often responsible for the termination of effects of anesthetic drugs that exert central effects and have high lipophilicity. Because the brain is rapidly perfused and highly lipophilic drugs cross the blood-brain barrier rapidly, drugs in blood rapidly equilibrate with receptor sites in the brain. However, as the drug is distributed from the blood to less rapidly equilibrated tissues such as the skeletal muscles and adipose tissues, drug in the brain rapidly reestablishes equilibrium with drug in the blood, resulting in rapidly decreasing concentrations of drug at the receptor site with early termination of drug effect. Caution must be observed when administering a second dose of these drugs, which will be eliminated from the plasma more slowly than the first dose because of the presence of drug in tissues from the earlier dose.

Repeated dosing of any drug before the earlier dose has been eliminated results in *accumulation* of the drug in a predictable manner. The drug accumulates until the rate of drug elimination equals the rate of drug administration. This occurs because the rate of drug elimination increases with increasing drug concentration and the rate of drug administration is constant. When the two rates are equal, *steady-state* plasma drug concentration is achieved. The concentration of drug at steady state is determined by the total clearance of the drug and its rate of administration:

$$C_{p_{ss}} = \text{Dosage rate/Cl}$$

where $C_{p_{ss}}$ is the steady-state plasma drug concentration. This relationship can be used to determine the dosage rate required to achieve a desired steady-state plasma drug concentration if the total clearance is known or can be reliably estimated (see Box 9-1):

$$\text{Dosage rate} = C_{p_{ss}} \times \text{Cl}$$

Therefore the intravenous infusion rate required to achieve a steady-state plasma drug concentration of 2 µg/ml for a drug with a total clearance estimated at 30 ml/min/kg of body weight is 60 µg/min/kg of body weight. If the body weight of the animal is 400 kg, the intravenous

infusion rate required would be 24 mg/min. The time required to reach steady state depends on the half-life of the drug (see Box 9-2). The drug concentration reaches 50% of the steady-state value after just one half-life, is at 75% after two half-lives, and is at 90% of the steady-state value after 3.3 half-lives (Figure 9-12). Many clinicians use the value of 3.3 times the half-life as the estimate of the time to reach steady state because there generally is no clinically significant difference between plasma drug concentrations that are 90% of steady state and those at steady state.

This relationship between clearance, steady-state drug concentration, and dosage rate can also be used when the drug is to be given as individual doses separated by a dosing interval. In this case the steady-state drug concentration is the average drug concentration during the dosing interval after steady state is achieved. For example, the dose required to produce an average drug concentration of 5 µg/ml for a drug with a total clearance estimated at 1 ml/min/kg of body weight is 5 µg/min/kg of body weight. If the dosing interval chosen for this drug is 6 hours, the dose to be administered is 1.8 mg/kg of body weight every 6 hours (5 µg/min × 360 min = 1800 µg/min). Drug concentrations rise and fall during each dosing interval. The maximum drug concentration is 1.58 times the minimum drug concentration when the dosing interval is equal to the half-life of the drug. As the dosing interval is increased relative to the half-life, the differences between maximum and minimum drug concentration increase. For example, if the dosing interval is twice the half-life, the maximum drug concentration is about 2.5 times the minimum drug concentration during each dosing interval at steady state. Therefore, if the drug has a relatively low therapeutic index, it is important to choose a dosing interval that is not much longer than the half-life, or drug concentrations during the dosing interval may reach toxic concentrations during the early part of the dosing interval and fall to ineffective concentrations during the latter part of the interval. For these reasons drugs with short half-lives and low therapeutic indices are administered by intravenous infusions to minimize fluctuations in drug concentrations (e.g., lidocaine, dopamine, dobutamine).

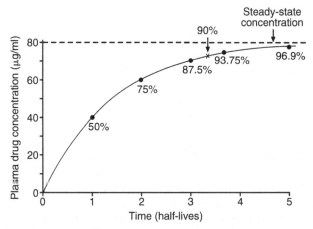

Figure 9–12. Plot of plasma drug concentration versus time following constant intravenous infusion of a drug for five half-lives.

EFFECTS OF VARIABLES ON DRUG PHARMACOKINETICS

Age

Age-related differences in receptor sensitivity and pharmacokinetic parameters affect drug response. In neonates, drugs are absorbed more rapidly from the gastrointestinal tract, they have a lower extent of plasma protein binding, they have an increased volume of distribution if they are drugs that are distributed into extracellular fluid or total body water, they have increased rates of entry into the central nervous system, and they are cleared more slowly.[8] Therefore dosages for neonates may need to be decreased or increased, depending on the parameters that exert the greatest influence. For example, greater absorption from the gastrointestinal tract, a lower extent of plasma protein binding, increased permeability into the central nervous system, and slower clearance would all require reductions in dose or dose frequency. On the other hand, an increased volume of distribution might require an increase in dose. The time required for these parameters to reach adult values depends on the nature of the processes involved. The half-life of erythromycin in a group of foals ranging in age from 1 to 12 weeks was equal to adult values, indicating that any maturation of hepatic processes had taken place during the first week after birth.[9] Volume of distribution and total body clearance estimates for phenobarbital in neonatal foals are 860 ml/kg and 0.94 ml/min/kg, respectively.[10] These values are similar to values reported for adult horses except for the clearance, which is almost twice as large in neonatal foals as it is in adult horses. The rate of maturation of renal mechanisms in foals apparently has not been studied. However, it should be noted that the urine of neonatal foals is acidic in contrast to that of most adult horses. Consequently, the renal clearance of weak bases may be higher in neonates than in adult horses. Very few studies of the rate of development of these and other parameters in horses have been conducted.

Aged horses can be expected to eliminate drugs more slowly because both renal and hepatic clearances decrease with age. For example, the total clearance of flunixin decreases with age in Thoroughbred horses.[11] Again, the rates of decline of these parameters in horses have not been investigated extensively.

For these reasons, caution should be exercised in the use of anesthetic agents in foals, particularly during the neonatal period and in elderly horses. Reductions in dose or dosage rate for these groups of horses are prudent until drug response has been determined.

Body Weight

Drug dosages generally are expressed on a body weight basis so that the appropriate dosage can be calculated merely by multiplying the dose by the estimated weight of the horse. This works reasonably well for horses of normal size and weight but may not work as well for very large (e.g., draft horses) or very small (e.g., ponies and miniature horses) horses because elimination processes do not increase linearly with body weight. Apparently the body surface area is better correlated with dose than is body weight. The ratio of body surface area to weight is larger in smaller animals compared with those of medium size, whereas it is smaller in larger animals compared with those of medium size. Therefore rates of elimination in smaller animals are generally underestimated, whereas those in larger animals are overestimated if dosages are based on body weights. However, dosages based on body surface area of the horse do not exist at this time.

Gender

Studies in other species have indicated that the gender of an animal sometimes affects the pharmacokinetics of certain drugs. This area of investigation has not been studied extensively in horses. The half-life of guaifenesin is greater in stallions than in mares.[12] The reason for this difference is unknown.

Breed

The effect of breed differences on the pharmacokinetics of drugs in horses has been largely ignored. Except for the anecdotal assertion that Thoroughbred and certain other breeds of horses are "hot blooded" and therefore better able to eliminate drugs, nothing has been reported concerning the effects of breed differences on the disposition of drugs in horses.

EFFECTS OF DISEASE

Blood Flow Rate

Diseases and other conditions affecting the blood flow rate to the organs of elimination affect the clearances of drugs that are highly extracted but have minimum effect on drugs that are poorly extracted. Several drugs, including the volatile anesthetics, are known to decrease the hepatic blood flow rate, thereby decreasing the hepatic clearances of other drugs that are highly extracted by the liver (e.g., fentanyl).[3] In addition, low cardiac output states resulting from cardiovascular disease or administration of certain drugs can result in greatly reduced hepatic blood flow rates and decreased hepatic clearance of high extraction ratio drugs.

Intrinsic Clearance

Liver disease or exposure of an animal to a drug or other substance that alters the intrinsic clearance of the liver may affect the hepatic clearance of drugs that are poorly extracted by the liver. Other conditions may also affect hepatic clearance of drugs. The total clearances of lidocaine, acetaminophen, and antipyrine declined in horses when feed was withheld for 3 days, but the volumes of distribution were not affected.[13] These changes were attributed to reductions in intrinsic hepatic clearances of these drugs because lidocaine, the drug with the highest hepatic extraction ratio, was the least affected.

Protein Binding

Drugs bind reversibly to plasma proteins (primarily albumin and α_1-acid glycoprotein):

$$[\text{Drug}] + [\text{Protein}] \approx [\text{Drug-Protein}]$$

The fraction of drug molecules bound to plasma proteins depends on both the affinity and the number of binding sites. Therefore any condition that decreases the plasma protein concentration decreases the number of binding sites and increases the fraction of drug molecules not bound to plasma protein. Liver disease, protein-losing enteropathy, colic, administration of fluids, and other conditions may cause decreased plasma protein concentrations. Administration of drugs to horses in these low protein states can result in greater intensity and longer duration of drug effects because drug action is related to the concentration of unbound drug in plasma rather than the total drug concentration. For example, horses that have received fluids often remain sedated for longer periods than expected after thiobarbiturate anesthesia. Several factors can affect physiologic variables, which in turn can affect pharmacokinetic parameters (Tables 9-4 and 9-5).

DRUG INTERACTIONS

Effects on Metabolism

Any drug that increases or decreases hepatic microsomal enzyme activity may affect the clearance of other drugs given concomitantly or soon after the first drug, particularly if hepatic extraction is low or intermediate. Chloramphenicol is a hepatic microsomal enzyme inhibitor that decreases the metabolic clearance of many other drugs. Administration of chloramphenicol to horses decreases the total clearance of phenylbutazone by approximately 50%.[14] Administration of chloramphenicol to horses 1 hour before thiamylal anesthesia increases the sleep time from 21.8 min to 36.0 min.[14]

Table 9-4. Some factors that affect physiological variables in horses

Physiological variable	Factors affecting variable
Hepatocellular enzyme activity	Drugs, plant toxins, pesticides, environmental factors
Hepatic blood flow	Cardiac output, posture, drugs, disease
Renal blood flow	Cardiac output, drugs, disease
Renal transport system	Drugs, disease
Urine pH	Exercise, diet, drugs, disease
Urine flow rate	Fluid intake, drugs, environmental factors, disease
Blood flow at absorption site	Cardiac output, drugs, posture, food, disease
Gastric motility	Food, drugs, disease (colic), electrolytes

Table 9-5. Dependence of primary pharmacokinetic parameters on physiological variables in horses

Pharmacokinetic parameter	Independent physiological variables
Hepatic clearance	Hepatic blood flow, binding of drug in blood, intrinsic hepatocellular activity
Renal clearance	Renal blood flow, binding of drug in blood, active secretion, resorption, urine pH, urine flow rate
Volume of distribution	Binding of drug in blood, binding of drug in tissues, body composition
Absorption rate constant	Blood flow at absorption site, rate of gastric movements

Organophosphate insecticides inactivate plasma cholinesterases, which are responsible for hydrolyzing succinylcholine and certain other depolarizing skeletal muscle relaxants. Because hydrolysis is the major route of inactivation and elimination of these drugs, their effects are prolonged if hydrolysis does not occur or if its rate is reduced. Therefore these drugs must be used with extreme caution in horses with recent exposure to organophosphate insecticides. Atracurium is a neuromuscular blocking drug that is metabolized by both ester hydrolysis and Hoffman elimination and therefore can be used somewhat more safely in horses with reduced plasma cholinesterase activity resulting from trichlorfon exposure without prolongation of neuromuscular blockade.[15]

Drugs such as barbiturates and rifampin that stimulate the synthesis of hepatic microsomal enzymes are known as hepatic microsomal enzyme inducers. Repeated administration of these drugs causes synthesis of hepatic microsomal enzymes, leading to increased clearance of the inducing agent and other drugs that are metabolized by the induced enzymes. The level of enzyme activity returns to preexposure values after the inducing agent is withdrawn. The time required for return to normal values appears to be less than 2 weeks. Administration of rifampin increases the total clearance of phenylbutazone in horses, and the clearance returns to normal values within 15 days after cessation of rifampin therapy.[14]

Effects on Renal Clearance

Drug interactions producing significant changes in renal clearance are rare in horses. There is no evidence that furosemide administration produces clinically significant changes in renal clearances of other substances.

DRUG ADDITIVITY AND SYNERGISM

Drug additivity, infraadditivity, and synergy are possibilities when drugs are coadministered. Drug combinations are considered additive when a proportional increase in one drug exactly compensates for a proportional decrease in the second drug. Synergy occurs when low dosages of the drug combination produce a much better effect than expected.[15a]

ROUTES OF ADMINISTRATION

Intravenous

The intravenous bolus route of administration involves delivery of the total drug dosage in solution directly to the blood over a short period of time (15 to 60 sec). Consequently, the onset of drug effects is more rapid, highest drug concentrations are observed, and the greatest drug response is seen after intravenous bolus dose administration. The bioavailability of drugs administered intravenously is complete (Table 9-6).

The intravenous infusion route of drug administration involves delivery of the drug dose in solution directly into the blood over a longer period of time (e.g., hours) to attain and maintain constant drug concentrations. Because of the slower delivery of drug, the onset of drug effects is delayed unless an LD is administered. The time required to reach the steady-state plasma drug concentration is determined solely by the half-life of the drug. The drug concentration in the plasma is equal to 90% of the steady-state value after 3.3 half-lives of constant infusion (see Figure 9-12). The actual value of the steady-state concentration is determined by the infusion rate of the drug

Table 9–6. Comparison of effects of routes of administration on drug effects

Route	Onset	Intensity	Duration	Bioavailability
Intravenous	Rapid	Greatest	Shortest	Complete
Intramuscular	Intermediate	Intermediate-low*	Intermediate-long*	Nearly complete
Subcutaneous	Intermediate	Intermediate-low*	Intermediate-long*	Nearly complete
Topical	Intermediate-slow*	Intermediate-low*	Intermediate-long*	Variable*
Oral	Slowest	Lowest	Longest	Variable*

*Formulation factors may exert large effects on intensity, duration, and bioavailability.

and its total clearance in the horse being treated. Bioavailability is complete because the drug is administered directly into the blood.

Intramuscular and Subcutaneous

Intramuscular and subcutaneous routes of administration involve drug administration in various formulations, including solids into the muscle tissue or directly under the skin. The rate of drug absorption from the site of administration is determined by the nature of the drug formulation, the physicochemical properties of the drug, the nature of the surrounding tissues, and the rate of blood flow to the injection site. Therefore the onset of drug action may be highly variable, and the intensity of drug response generally is less if these routes of administration are used (see Table 9-6). However, the duration of action may be longer because of slow and prolonged absorption from the site of administration. These routes provide pharmaceutical manufacturers with many opportunities for modifying the drug formulation to modify the rate of absorption and therefore the duration and intensity of effect. Incomplete bioavailability after these routes of administration are used is not uncommon and may result from precipitation of the drug at the site of administration, poor or nonideal formulation, local biodegradation, or diminished blood flow at the site of administration resulting from local drug effects.

Oral

The oral route of drug administration involves oral delivery of the drug in solution or in various solid, semisolid, or liquid dosage forms. The drug must be absorbed into the systemic circulation before it can exert a systemic effect. Therefore the onset of drug effects is delayed relative to most other routes of administration, and the intensity of drug effects is generally less (see Table 9-6). The duration of drug effects may be longer than that after intravenous bolus dose administration. Bioavailability of orally administered drugs may be incomplete because of complexation of the drug by the contents of the gastrointestinal tract, degradation of the drug in the gastrointestinal contents (e.g., penicillin), poor absorption because of low lipid solubility (e.g., neomycin and other aminoglycosides) or large size, first-pass metabolism by the gut wall or liver, high gastrointestinal motility that causes the drug to be eliminated in the feces before complete absorption can occur, and poor blood flow to the gastrointestinal tract (e.g., colic and cardiovascular disease).

Topical

Topically administered drugs are formulated in a variety of preparations that may affect the rate and extent of drug availability. Since the drug needs to dissolve before it can be absorbed, drugs that are applied as solids typically are absorbed more slowly than those that are in solution. Furthermore, drugs that are in solution in oily materials must partition into an aqueous phase before they can be absorbed; thus these substances generally are absorbed more slowly than drugs in water-based creams.

More recently, topically administered drugs in extended-release formulations or proprietary materials have been investigated experimentally in horses. Fentanyl-containing

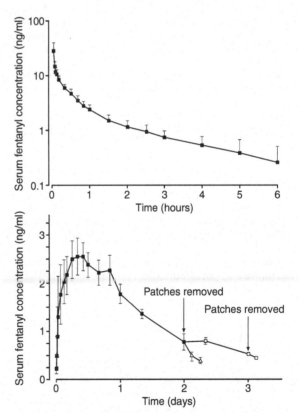

Figure 9–13. Serum fentanyl concentration (ng/ml) versus time curves for fentanyl following a 2-mg dose intravenously *(top)* and a 20 mg dose administered transdermally *(bottom)* for 48 hours. Note the rapid decline in serum concentration at 48 hours when the patch is removed. (From Maxwell LK et al: Pharmacokinetics of fentanyl following intravenous and transdermal administration in horses, *Equine Vet J* 35(5):484-490, 2003.)

patches that are formulated to release the drug at a constant rate for use as long-term analgesic drugs in humans have been investigated in horses (Figure 9-13).[16,17] This product has also been investigated for clinical efficacy in treating visceral and somatic pain in horses.[18,19] Whether these products release the drug at an appropriate rate to achieve clinically relevant concentrations in horses remains to be determined.

REFERENCES

1. Gerken DF, Sams RA: Inhibitory effects of chloramphenicol sodium succinate on the disposition of phenylbutazone and its metabolites in the horse, *J Pharmacokinet Biopharm* 13(5): 467-476, 1985.
2. Feary DJ et al: Influence of general anesthesia on pharmacokinetics of intravenous lidocaine infusion in horses, *Am J Vet Res* 66(4):574-580; 2005.
3. Thomasy SM et al: The effects of intravenous fentanyl administration on the minimum alveolar concentration of isoflurane in horses, *Br J Anaesth* 97:232-237, 2006.
4. Kohn CW, Strasser SL: 24-Hour renal clearance and excretion of endogenous substances in the mare, *Am J Vet Res* 47(6):1332-1337, 1986.
5. Juzwiak JS et al: Effect of probenecid administration on cephapirin pharmacokinetics and concentration in mares, *Am J Vet Res* 50(10):1742-1747, 1989.
6. Wood T et al: Equine urine pH: normal population distributions and methods of acidification, *Equine Vet J* 22(2):118-121, 1990.
7. Salonen JS et al: Single-dose pharmacokinetics of detomidine in the horse and cow, *J Vet Pharmacol Ther* 12:65-72, 1987.
8. Baggot JD, Short CR: Drug disposition in the neonatal animal, with particular reference to the foal, *Equine Vet J* 16(4): 364-367, 1984.
9. Prescott JF, Hoover DJ, Dohoo IR: Pharmacokinetics of erythromycin in foals and adult horses, *J Vet Pharmacol Ther* 6:67-74, 1983.
10. Spehar AM et al: Preliminary study of the pharmacokinetics of phenobarbital in the neonatal foal, *Equine Vet J* 16(4): 368-371, 1984.
11. Jensen RC, Fischer MC, Cwik MJ: Effect of age and training status on pharmacokinetics of flunixin meglumine in thoroughbreds, *Am J Vet Res* 51(4):591-594, 1990.
12. Davis LE, Wolff WA: Pharmacokinetics and metabolism of glyceryl guaiacolate in ponies, *Am J Vet Res* 31:469-473, 1970.
13. Engelking LR et al: Pharmacokinetics of antipyrine, acetaminophen, and lidocaine in fed and fasted horses, *J Vet Pharmacol Ther* 10:73-82, 1987.
14. Burrows GE et al: Interactions between chloramphenicol, acepromazine, phenylbutazone, rifampin, and thiamylal in the horse, *Equine Vet J* 21(1):34-38, 1989.
15. Hildebrand SV, Hill T, Holland M: The effect of organophosphate trichlorfon on the neuromuscular blocking activity of atracurium in horses, *J Vet Pharmacol Physiol* 12(3):277-282, 1989.
15a. Shager SL et al: Additivity versus synergy: a theoretical analysis of implications for anesthetic mechanisms, *Anesth Analg* 107:507-525, 2008.
16. Thomasy SM et al: Transdermal fentanyl combined with nonsteroidal anti-inflammatory drugs for analgesia in horses, *J Vet Intern Med* 18:550-554, 2004.
17. Maxwell LK et al: Pharmacokinetics of fentanyl following intravenous and transdermal administration in horses, *Equine Vet J* 35(5):484-490; 2003.
18. Wegner K: How to use fentanyl transdermal patches for analgesia in horses. In Proceedings of the American Association of Equine Practitioners, Orlando, 2002, vol 48, pp 291-294.
19. Sanchez LC et al: Effect of fentanyl on visceral and somatic nociception in conscious horses, *J Vet Intern Med* 21: 1067-1075, 2007.
20. Ballard S et al: The pharmacokinetics, pharmacological responses, and behavioral effects of acepromazine in the horse, *J Vet Pharmacol Ther* 5:21-31, 1982.
21. Court MH et al: Pharmacokinetics of dantrolene sodium in horses, *J Vet Pharmacol Ther* 10(3):218-226, 1987.
22. Muir WW et al: Pharmacodynamic and pharmacokinetic properties of diazepam in horses, *Am J Vet Res* 43(10):1756-1762, 1982.
23. Davis JL et al: Pharmacokinetics of etodolac in the horse following oral and intravenous administration, *J Vet Pharmacol Ther* 30:43-48, 2007.
24. Waterman AE, Robertson SA, Lane JG: Pharmacokinetics of intravenously administered ketamine in the horse, *Res Vet Sci* 42:162-166, 1987.
25. Alexander F, Collett RA: Pethidine in the horse, *Res Vet Sci* 17:136-137, 1974.
26. Muir WW, Sams RA, Ashcraft S: Pharmacologic and pharmacokinetic properties of methocarbamol in the horse, *Am J Vet Res* 45(11):2256-2260, 1984.
27. Combie JD, Nugent TE, Tobin T: Pharmacokinetic and protein binding of morphine in horses, *Am J Vet Res* 44(5):870-874, 1983.
28. Tobin T, Miller JR: The pharmacology of narcotic analgesics in the horse. I. The detection, pharmacokinetics and urinary "clearance time" of pentazocine, *J Equine Med Surg* 3:191-198, 1979.
29. Alexander F, Nicholson JD: The blood and saliva clearances of phenobarbital and pentobarbitone in the horse, *Biochem Pharmacol* 17:203-210, 1968.
30. Duran SH et al: Pharmacokinetics of phenobarbital in the horse, *Am J Vet Res* 48(5):807-810, 1987.
31. Garcia-Villar R et al: The pharmacokinetics of xylazine hydrochloride: an interspecific study, *J Vet Pharmacol Ther* 4:87-92, 1981.

10

Anxiolytics, Nonopioid Sedative-Analgesics, and Opioid Analgesics

William W. Muir

KEY POINTS

1. Many procedures can be performed on standing horses using combinations of sedative and analgesic drugs supplemented by appropriate local anesthesia and physical restraint.
2. The administration of reduced dosages of multiple drugs (multimodal therapy) to produce sedation and analgesia (neuroleptanalgesia) may be safer and more effective than administering larger doses of a single drug.
3. The practical goals of standing chemical restraint and preanesthetic medication are to produce a calm and sedate horse that is reluctant to move and indifferent to environmental or noxious stimulation and physical manipulation.
4. Adequate sedation and analgesia are the most important factors determining successful anesthesia in horses.
5. Acepromazine and α_2-adrenoceptor agonists are excellent anxiolytics and muscle relaxants in horses.
6. α_2-Adrenoceptor agonists produce sedation, muscle relaxation, and analgesia. They are administered before, during, or after anesthesia to enhance sedation and analgesia and to decrease the requirement for other anesthetic drugs.
7. Opioid analgesics produce analgesia and mild euphoria at low dosages; they produce excitement, agitation, sympathetic activation, and increased locomotor activity at high dosages.
8. α_2-Adrenoceptor agonists and opioid analgesics impair gastrointestinal motility and prolong transit time, predisposing to ileus and impaction colic.
9. Benzodiazepines produce minimum calming effects and excellent muscle relaxation but do not produce or enhance analgesia.
10. α_2-Adrenoceptor agonists, opioids, and benzodiazepines can be antagonized with selective antagonists.

Anxiolytic and analgesic drugs are administered to increase the efficacy and safety of general anesthesia and produce a stress-free and uneventful medical or surgical experience (see Box 10-1). The variety of drugs and drug combinations administered to produce a cooperative, calm horse is strong testimony to the diversity of opinions regarding which drugs and drug techniques are best suited for different clinical situations (see Table 10-1).[1-4] No one drug provides ideal anxiolytic or analgesic effects in every horse. Standardized sedation and preanesthetic protocols must be modifiable to meet each horse's individual requirements and frequently necessitate the administration of multiple drugs (multimodal therapy).

Most drugs used to produce sedation or analgesia are categorized on the basis of their chemical structure; pharmacological effects; or the mechanism by which they produce calming, muscle relaxation, and analgesia. *Tranquilizers* such as acepromazine, also referred to as *ataractics* or *neuroleptics,* are noted for their ability to produce calming (anxiolysis) and behavioral modification. *Sedatives* such as xylazine produce similar effects; whereas *hypnotics* such as chloral hydrate and thiopental reduce consciousness, induce sleep, and, when administered in large enough doses, produce unresponsiveness to noxious stimuli (i.e., anesthesia). Because of their similar clinical uses, the terms *tranquilizer* and *sedative* are used interchangeably in veterinary practice and connote central nervous system (CNS) depression, anxiolysis, decreased motor activity, and decreased arousal. The term *narcotic* is defined as a drug that produces stupor, insensibility, and sleep, but is commonly applied when referring to opiates (alkaloids of opium) or opioids (compounds related to opium; see Table 10-1). Most drugs used as preanesthetic medication in horses produce some degree of CNS depression in addition to their peripheral effects. Furthermore, many drug combinations have the potential to produce additive or synergistic effects. For example, the concurrent administration of a nonsteroidal antiinflammatory drug (NSAID) or an α_2-adrenoceptor agonist and an opioid produce synergistic analgesic effects.

The anticholinergic drugs atropine and glycopyrrolate are not routinely administered as preanesthetic medication to horses. Anticholinergic drugs block the effects of acetylcholine released from postganglionic parasympathetic nerves (muscarinic receptor antagonists), helping to prevent vagally induced bradycardia, reduce airway secretions, and produce bronchodilation.[5-7] The increases in heart rate produced by anticholinergic drugs (atropine, glycopyrrolate) result in improvement of hemodynamics (see Figure 10-1).[8] However, the rationale for their use as preanesthetic medication in horses is not readily apparent since horses do not salivate excessively and infrequently develop clinically relevant bradycardia during induction to or maintenance of inhalant anesthesia. Furthermore, both drugs are capable of producing ileus, intestinal distention, and impaction. Intestinal stasis, impaction, and signs of colic lasting for up to 24 hours have been produced in ponies and adult horses administered atropine or glycopyrrolate.[5,8] One study demonstrated that the administration of a specific muscarinic type-2 (M_2) antagonist (methoctramine) produced an increase in heart rate, cardiac output, and arterial blood pressure without affecting normal intestinal motility, an M_3 receptor function, and suggested that M_2 antagonists

Box 10–1   Qualities of an Ideal Preanesthetic or Perianesthetic Drug

- Rapid onset of action
- Produces calming and reduces stress
- Produces cooperation without excessive drowsiness or ataxia
- Produces predictable and prolonged analgesia
- Facilitates a rapid, uneventful induction and recovery from anesthesia
- Reduces the amount of anesthetic required (anesthetic-sparing effect)
- Minimizes or eliminates the undesirable side effects
- Predictable
- Potent, soluble in water; has a wide therapeutic index
- Compatible with other drugs
- Minimum no side effects or toxicity
- Reversible

Table 10–1.   Examples of drugs used as preanesthetic medication and for standing chemical restraint in horses

Drug category	Drug group	Generic name
Sedatives	Chloral derivatives	Chloral hydrate
	Phenothiazines*	Acepromazine
		Promazine
	Butyrophenones*	Azaperone
		Droperidol
		Haloperidol
	Benzodiazepines	Diazepam
		Midazolam
		Climazolam
		Zolazepam
Nonopioid analgesics	α_2-Adrenoceptor agonists	Xylazine
		Detomidine
		Romifidine
		Medetomidine
		Dexmedetomidine
Opioid analgesics	Opioid agonists	Morphine
		Meperidine
		Methadone
		Hydromorphone
		Fentanyl
		Etorphine
	Opioid partial agonists	Buprenorphine
	Opioid agonist/antagonists	Pentazocine
		Butorphanol
		Nalbuphine

*Also referred to as tranquilizers or neuroleptics.

provide a safe alternative for the treatment of intraoperative bradycardia in horses.[9] Because of their intestinal hypomotility effects, the administration of atropine or glycopyrrolate to horses should be reserved for the treatment of bradycardia and bradyarrhythmias.

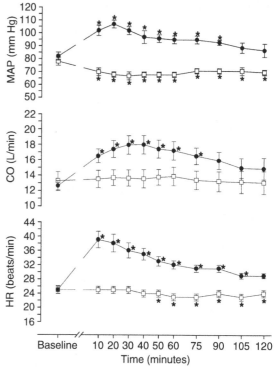

Figure 10–1. Effects of 0.9% saline (□) and glycopyrrolate (cumulative dose of 5 or 7.5 µg/kg to increase HR by >30%; ●) on heart rate *(HR)*, cardiac output *(CO)*, and mean arterial blood pressure *(MAP)* in six halothane anesthetized horses administered an infusion of xylazine (1 mg/kg/hr). (From Teixeira Neto FJ et al: Effects of glycopyrrolate on cardiorespiratory function in horses anesthetized with halothane and xylazine, *Am J Vet Res* 65:456-463, 2004.)

PHENOTHIAZINE TRANQUILIZERS

Phenothiazine tranquilizers include a large number of compounds recognized for their ability to alter behavior and calm and relax horses while maintaining arousability and avoidance behaviors should a significant event (sudden movement, loud noise) or painful stimulus occur.[10] Phenothiazine and butyrophenone tranquilizers are not considered to produce clinically relevant analgesia but do enhance the CNS depressant and analgesic effects of opioids and α_2-adrenoceptor agonists. They are frequently referred to as neuroleptics based on their calming effects and antagonism of dopamine, particularly D_2 receptors; the risk of extrapyramidal effects (abnormal postures, rigidity, catatonia) is increased when large doses are administered. Chlorpromazine is considered the prototypic phenothiazine tranquilizer and was one of the first tranquilizers to be used in horses.[11,12] The clinical use of chlorpromazine in horses has been abandoned because of its unpredictability and the frequency of adverse side effects, including excitement, severe ataxia, and prolonged depression. Propiopromazine, propionylpromazine, and promethazine have met similar fates for similar reasons, in addition to producing a high incidence of persistent penile prolapse.[13] Only promazine and acepromazine are administered as anxiolytic or preanesthetic medication to horses, and acepromazine is by far the more popular.[1] Acepromazine is a yellow, odorless, crystalline water-soluble powder with a bitter taste; it possesses very low toxicity when used in clinically relevant doses.

Injectable acepromazine is marketed in a brown bottle to prevent decomposition by light. Marked overdoses, exceeding 20 mg/kg intravenously, have not produced death. Acepromazine is more potent than chlorpromazine or promazine and is less likely to produce adverse side effects when administered intravenously or intramuscularly to horses.[14]

Mechanism of Action

Acepromazine and other phenothiazine tranquilizers produce calming, sedation, indifference, and reduced locomotor activity by depressing the basal ganglia and limbic system and modulating nervous system activity in the reticular activating system.[15] Their principal mechanism of action may be to interfere with the actions of dopamine as a synaptic neurotransmitter in the basal ganglia and limbic portions of the brain.[16] Dopamine is an important neurotransmitter in the basal ganglia, limbic system, and portions of the forebrain. Phenothiazines also modify the CNS activity of other catecholamines, including norepinephrine and epinephrine. Pharmacologically these effects have important clinical implications because phenothiazines are known to inhibit opioid-induced excitement and manic behavior in horses.[17] Opioids in general and morphine in particular are known to enhance the release of dopamine and norepinephrine in the CNS, resulting in increased locomotor activity and excitement in horses. Blockade of opioid-induced dopamine release by phenothiazine tranquilizers offers a rational alternative to inhibiting opioid-induced excitement in horses by administering an opioid antagonist and supports the long-standing practice of coadministering a phenothiazine tranquilizer and opioid (neuroleptanalgesia) to produce more predictable calming and pain relief. However, large doses of phenothiazines may produce extrapyramidal effects typified by abnormal behavior, reluctance to move, mild rigidity, muscle tremor, and restlessness.[16] These effects are caused by phenothiazine interference with the actions of dopamine in the basal ganglia and may resemble Parkinson's disease (dyskinesia tarda) in humans (dopamine deficiency in the basal ganglia). Other CNS effects produced by phenothiazine tranquilizers that are related to dopamine blockade include anticonvulsant and antiemetic effects and a loss of appetite. Low doses of phenothiazines may stimulate appetite. The CNS seizure threshold is lowered by the administration of phenothiazines in humans, and it is suggested that their use be avoided in epileptic patients.[16] However, the clinical relevance of this latter effect in horses remains undetermined. Peripherally phenothiazines block cholinergic, histaminic, adrenergic, and ganglionic activity. They are α_1-adrenoceptor blocking drugs and have antiarrhythmic (quinidine-like), antifibrillatory, antipyretic, antishock, and hypothermic effects. Acepromazine is compatible with other sedative-hypnotics, opioids, and nonopioid analgesics and is frequently coadministered with the latter drugs in reduced doses to produce more predictable and prolonged neuroleptanalgesia.

Applied Pharmacology

Phenothiazine tranquilizers typically produce calming, indifference, and decreased locomotor activity in horses. A decrease in arterial blood pressure is the most commonly reported hemodynamic effect. Clinically applicable doses (0.05 to 0.1 mg/kg) of acepromazine reduce arterial blood pressure 15 to 20 mm Hg (see Figure 10-2).[18] Heart rate, cardiac output, and cardiac contractility decrease minimally or remain unchanged because of decreases in sympathetic nervous system activity (see Figure 10-3).[18] The reduction in arterial blood pressure is dose dependent and may produce reflex tachycardia, which is pronounced in anxious or excited horses that have increased circulating concentrations of catecholamines as a result of fear or stress. Phenothiazine-induced hypotension is caused by depression of the hypothalamus, peripheral α_1-adrenoceptor blockade, and a direct vasodilatory effect on blood vessels.[19] Vasodilation and hypotension can result in hyperglycemia because of release of epinephrine from the adrenal medulla and hypothermia caused by cutaneous heat loss. Phenothiazine tranquilizers are partially effective in the treatment of malignant hyperthermia-like syndromes in "hot" horses.

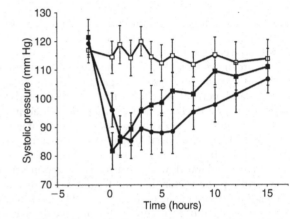

Figure 10–2. Effects of 0.15 mg/kg intramuscular (●) and 0.1 mg/kg intravenous (■) acepromazine on systolic blood pressure (mm Hg) in adult horses. (Control, □.) (From Parry PW, Anderson GA, Gay CG: Hypotension in the horse induced by acepromazine maleate, *Aust Vet J* 59:148, 1982.)

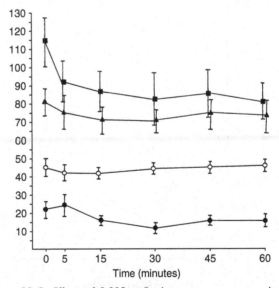

Figure 10–3. Effects of 0.009 mg/kg intravenous acepromazine on mean arterial blood pressure (mm Hg; ■), cardiac output (ml/kg/min; ▲), heart rate (beats/min; o), and respiratory rate (breaths/min; ●) in adult horses. (From Muir MW, Skarda RT, Sheehan WC: Hemodynamic and respiratory effects of a xylazine-acetylpromazine drug combination in horses, *Am J Vet Res* 40:1518, 1979.)

Decreases in arterial blood pressure may result in ataxia, sweating, hyperpnea, and tachycardia, prompting intravenous fluid therapy to prevent collapse ("fainting"). Phenothiazine tranquilizers produce antiarrhythmic and antifibrillatory effects similar to those of quinidine and inhibit the sensitization of the myocardium to catecholamine-induced cardiac arrhythmias facilitated by thiobarbiturate and halothane anesthesia.[20] Acepromazine caused a significant and sustained elevation in cardiac output via a rise in stroke volume in halothane-anesthetized horses.[21] All drugs depressing the CNS are capable of depressing breathing, but the effects of phenothiazine tranquilizers on arterial blood gases are minimal in conscious horses. Respiratory rate decreases after acepromazine administration; but tidal volume increases, thereby maintaining a relatively stable minute volume and normal pH and blood gas (PaO_2, $PaCO_2$) values.[22] The respiratory center response to an increase in $PaCO_2$ is decreased (decreased sensitivity), indicative of CNS depression, and the potential for respiratory compromise when administered in conjunction with general anesthetics (see Figure 10-4).

Phenothiazine tranquilizers produce a myriad of effects on various organ systems, including the gut, liver, and kidneys. They decrease esophageal and gastrointestinal secretions, tone, and peristalsis, effects that are attributed to their CNS depressant effects and peripheral anticholinergic actions.[14] These effects can predispose to esophageal obstruction ("choke"), delayed gastric emptying, and prolonged intestinal transit times in some horses. Decreases in liver and renal blood flow are secondary to hypotension and may prolong the metabolism and elimination of concurrently administered medications. Improved blood flow to these organs may facilitate the elimination of some drugs and promote diuresis. Phenothiazine tranquilizers are thought to depress the release of antidiuretic hormone or inhibit salt and water resorption in the renal tubules, inducing diure-

sis and decreasing the urinary concentrations ("masking" effects) of concurrently administered drug.[14] They can increase prolactin release, inhibit the estrous cycle, and prolong gestation in some mares.[14] The significance of all of these effects has not been thoroughly evaluated in horses.

Priapism and paralysis of the retractor penis muscle have been associated with the use of phenothiazine tranquilizers in colts, stallions, and geldings, regardless of dosage (see Figure 10-5).[23,24] The mechanism for these responses remains undetermined but is dose dependent and attributed to phenothiazine blockade of central and peripheral adrenergic and dopaminergic receptors. Conservative methods for treatment include massage to reduce edema, confining the penis to the preputial sheath, cold water hydrotherapy, and the administration of analgesics (e.g., xylazine, butorphanol).[24] The administration of various catecholamines and anticholinergic drugs to antagonize the process has had limited success. The intravenous administration of 0.01 to 0.02 mg/kg of benztropine has reversed priapism in a gelding.[25]

Acepromazine and other phenothiazine tranquilizers decrease packed cell volume and total protein concentration in horses.[26-29] Decreases in packed cell volume are the most sensitive indicator of the pharmacological response to acepromazine, followed by penile extension, decreases in respiratory rate, and locomotor responses.[30] The decreases in packed cell volume are believed to be dose dependent, may last in excess of 12 hours, and are attributed to sequestration of red blood cells in the spleen and dilution of red blood cells and protein by interstitial water entering the vascular compartment secondary to drug-induced hypotension. Splenectomy eliminates the decrease in packed cell volume.[31-33] White blood cell concentrations are minimally affected by phenothiazine administration and are believed to result from margination of white blood cells along vascular walls.[34,35] Phenothiazine tranquilizers decrease platelet activity and prolong clotting times.

Biodisposition

Phenothiazine tranquilizers are metabolized by the liver, and the metabolites are excreted in the urine (see Chapter 9).[30,36,37] Hydroxylation and glucuronidation are the predominant metabolic pathways for most phenothiazines, although rela-

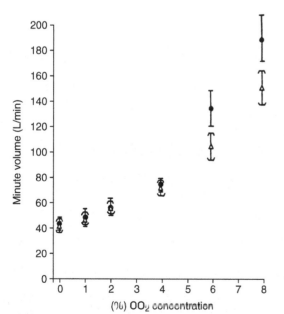

Figure 10–4. Changes in minute volume ($\dot{V}$; L/min) in horses before (o) and after (Δ) acepromazine administration (0.065 mg/kg intravenous) during increases in inspired CO_2. (From Muir WW, Hamlin RL: Effects of acetylpromazine on ventilatory variables in the horse, *Am J Vet Res* 36:1439, 1975.)

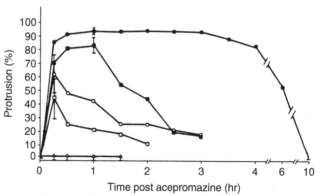

Figure 10–5. Effect of intravenous acepromazine 0.4 mg/kg (●), 0.1 mg/kg (■), 0.04 mg/kg (□), 0.01 mg/kg (o), and 0.004 mg/kg (Δ) on penile protrusion in geldings. Penile protrusion plotted as percent of maximum. (From Ballard S et al: The pharmacokinetics, pharmacological responses, and behavioral effects of acepromazine in the horse, *J Vet Pharmacol Ther* 5:21, 1982.)

tively large amounts of the nonconjugated metabolite promazine sulfoxide can be found in the urine after acepromazine administration.[36] The pharmacological and clinical activity of these metabolites remains undetermined. The elimination half-life for acepromazine ranges from 50 to 150 minutes in horses, and urinary metabolites can be found in the urine for longer than 3 days.[36] Acepromazine is rapidly absorbed after oral administration (bioavailability of approximately 55%) and has an elimination half-life of approximately 6 hours.[37,38] Plasma protein binding is usually greater than 90% for most phenothiazines, suggesting a prolonged duration of action and increased effects in hypoproteinemic horses resulting from increased circulating concentrations of active (unbound) drug. Frequent use of phenothiazine tranquilizers stimulates liver microsomal enzymes and cytochrome P-450, which may influence the metabolism of other drugs. The metabolism and elimination of phenothiazine tranquilizers in foals is expected to be prolonged, although this has not been studied.

Clinical Use and Antagonism

Acepromazine is the most frequently used phenothiazine tranquilizer in equine practice. Promazine is less effective, requires larger doses, is less predictable, and is more likely to produce side effects.[39,40] The relatively high potency and comparatively low incidence of side effects of acepromazine make it the best phenothiazine tranquilizer for use in horses. The administration of 0.02 to 0.1 mg/kg of intravenous acepromazine to adult horses produces calming, indifference to the surrounding environment, reluctance to move, and mild degrees of ataxia (see Table 10-2). Peak drug effects generally are reached within 10 minutes after intravenous administration, 20 to 40 minutes after intramuscular administration, and approximately 1 hour after oral administration. Protrusion of the flaccid penis is a sign of sedation in males (see Figure 10-5).[37] Sedated horses can be aroused with minor painful stimuli and may strike. The duration of sedation varies considerably after the administration of clinically recommended doses, and some horses demonstrate minimum effects or paradoxically become anxious and restless, whereas others remain markedly sedate and ataxic for prolonged periods (>6 hours). Acepromazine is additive with and capable of potentiating the effects of many other sedatives, opioid or nonopioid analgesics, and hypnotics, although it has little or no analgesic activity.[18,41,42] It is frequently coadministered with opioid or nonopioid analgesics to produce short-term standing sedation and analgesia in inactive or exercised horses.[18,41,42] The administration of acepromazine before induction to anesthesia has the potential to decrease the dose requirements for injectable or inhalant anesthetics and may reduce morbidity and mortality associated with equine anesthesia.[43-45] Acepromazine generally improved hemodynamics and reduced disturbances and falls in PaO$_2$ during tiletamine-zolazepam anesthesia in horses.[46] Phenothiazine tranquilizers do not provide sufficient sedation to be administered as single therapy before ketamine or as adjuncts during general anesthesia.[47]

There are no known antagonists for phenothiazine tranquilizers, although synthetic amphetamine analogs, fluids (diuresis), and drugs that increase arterial blood pressure (phenylephrine) may increase the level of consciousness and hasten drug elimination.[48]

Table 10–2. Intravenous doses of drugs used for equine chemical restraint*

Agent	Dosage range (mg/kg)	Dose when used before anesthesia (mg/kg)
Chloral derivatives†		
Chloral hydrate	2.0-6.0	3.0
Phenothiazines		
Acepromazine	0.025-0.15	0.05
Promazine	0.5-1.0	0.05
Benzodiazepines		
Diazepam	0.02-0.1	0.05
Midazolam	0.02-0.15	0.05
Benzodiazepine antagonists		
Flumazenil	0.01-0.05	0.025
Sarmazenil	0.025-0.1	0.04
α$_2$-Adrenoceptor agonists		
Xylazine	0.5-1.1	0.6
Detomidine	0.005-0.02	0.005
Romifidine	0.08-0.160	0.08
Medetomidine	0.005-0.02	0.005
α$_2$-Adrenoceptor antagonists		
Yohimbine	0.04-0.15	0.1
Tolazoline	2.0-6.0	4.0
Atipamezole	0.05-0.2	0.1
Opioid analgesics		
Morphine	0.05-0.1	0.08
Meperidine	0.5-1.0	.05
Hydromorphone	0.01-0.03	0.02
Methadone	0.05-0.1	0.07
Butorphanol	0.01-0.02	0.01
Pentazocine	0.5-1.0	0.7
Opioid antagonist		
Naloxone	0.01-0.05	0.025
Naltrexone	0.1-1.0	0.5
Nalmefene	0.5-1.0	0.5
Diprenorphine	0.02-0.05	0.03

*Intramuscular dosages are two times the intravenous dose.
†See Chapter 12 for description.

Complications, Side Effects, and Toxicity

The most disconcerting aspects associated with the routine clinical use of acepromazine are inadequate or unpredictable calming, a lack of analgesic activity, and the potential for side effects. Readministration or increasing the dose of acepromazine may not improve sedation and generally results in hypotension, a greater degree of ataxia, and other side effects. Ataxia, hypotension, and reflex tachycardia are the most common side effects and may be related because hypotension produces a feeling of heaviness and weakness. There is no way to predict which horses will become hypotensive, although the administration of a phenothiazine tranquilizer to a horse that is excited or stressed generally produces a profound decrease. Signs of impending collapse include profuse sweating, hyperpnea, tachycardia, and marked ataxia, usually within 5 minutes of intravenous drug administration. The administration of epinephrine is contraindicated since the blockade of α_1-adrenoceptors by the phenothiazine combined with the β_2-adrenoceptor vasodilating properties of epinephrine may result in "epinephrine reversal," resulting in a further decrease in arterial blood pressure. Anxious or stressed horses that are believed to have increased circulating concentrations of epinephrine (fear, stress) may be more susceptible to the hypotensive effects of phenothiazine tranquilizers.[49] Treatment of phenothiazine-induced hypotension is symptomatic, generally requiring little more than fluid replacement (20 ml/kg intravenously) and rarely the administration of phenylephrine, an α_1-adrenoceptor agonist (see Chapter 22).

Flaccid paralysis of the retractor penis muscle resulting in a fully extended penis priapism and paraphimosis is a devastating and potentially life-threatening side effect of phenothiazine administration (see Figure 10-5).[23,24,50] These side effects are believed to be less frequent after the administration of acepromazine compared to other phenothiazine tranquilizers but remain an important consideration when contemplating its administration to a valuable breeding stallion. Stallions successfully tranquilized on previous occasions may develop flaccid prolapse of the penis after acepromazine administration at a later date. The mechanism responsible for this effect is unknown, although phenothiazine-induced antiadrenergic and antidopaminergic effects are conjectured to be important.[25] Treatment is oriented toward protecting the penis and preventing or reducing swelling.[24] Failure of the penis to retract may necessitate amputation.[51] The incidence of this uncommon side effect is believed to be less than 1 in 10,000 and therefore does not contraindicate the general use of acepromazine in stallions or geldings.

Some horses become severely ataxic after acepromazine administration. They are reluctant to move and periodically stumble or relax their hind legs as if to sit down and then suddenly lunge forward. This response may trigger excitement and fear. Horses administered larger doses of acepromazine (>0.2 mg/kg IV) may demonstrate extrapyramidal effects and Parkinson-like symptoms typified by muscle rigidity, involuntary muscle twitching, and excitement.

Phenothiazine tranquilizers are known to augment hypothermia resulting from peripheral vasodilatory effects. Rarely, and although possessing antiarrhythmic properties, acepromazine may be responsible for the development of cardiac arrhythmias, including bradycardia and ventricular arrhythmias. The CNS actions of phenothiazines have been implicated as responsible for these latter effects.

The toxicity of organophosphate pesticides and anthelmintics is increased by phenothiazine tranquilizers. Like organophosphates, phenothiazine tranquilizers inhibit acetylcholinesterase and pseudocholinesterase. Inhibition of cholinesterase activity by phenothiazine tranquilizers is reversible.

Accidental intracarotid injection of promazine and acepromazine has been reported in horses.[52,53] Horses generally become excited, collapse, and develop uncontrollable paddling activity followed by seizures within seconds of intracarotid drug administration. Some horses literally "fall off the needle." Treatment is directed toward protecting the horse (paddling) and controlling seizures. Diazepam, 0.01 mg/kg intravenously, is an effective anticonvulsant and can be coadministered with thiopental to produce anesthesia. Accidental intracarotid injection can be avoided by prior placement of an intravenous catheter.

BUTYROPHENONES

Butyrophenone tranquilizers produce similar effects to those of phenothiazine tranquilizers but are less predictable and more likely to induce extrapyramidal side effects in horses (see Table 10-1).[54] Similar to the phenothiazines, they are believed to produce their pharmacological effects by depressing the reticular activating system and interfering with the CNS actions of dopamine and norepinephrine. Butyrophenones may also mimic the actions of gamma-aminobutyric acid (GABA), a CNS inhibitory neurotransmitter. The butyrophenone drugs that have been studied in horses include azaperone, droperidol, lenperone, and haloperidol.[55-57] As a group, these drugs are noted for their behavior-modifying and antiemetic effects. They produce minimum depression of respiration and cardiovascular function and are less likely to induce hypotension than phenothiazines.[54] Hypotension, although less pronounced, is caused by α_1-adrenoceptor blockade similar to that produced by the phenothiazines. This may contraindicate their use intraoperatively. Sedation is usually evident within 3 to 5 minutes of intravenous administration and is characterized by minimum behavior change. Some horses lower their head and neck and relax their lower lip, and the penis may protrude in males. The metabolism and elimination of butyrophenone tranquilizers has not been studied extensively in horses, although elimination may be prolonged based on the clinical duration of effects. Although potentially useful as preanesthetic medication, the administration of butyrophenone tranquilizers to horses is not recommended based on a lack of predictability and the potential for the development of bizarre or violent behavior patterns. Horses administered low doses (0.01 mg/kg intravenously) of droperidol and lenperone have shown minimal or no signs of calming and have refused to eat or drink water for periods in excess of 4 days (author's experience). Some horses suddenly become frightened and panic, either throwing themselves to the ground or attempting to escape by running backwards. Similar observations, although not as severe, have been observed after intravenous administration (0.1 to 0.3 mg/kg) of azaperone to adult horses.[55,58] Some horses sweat initially, followed by a period of sedation and ataxia. Others suddenly become excited, begin to vocalize, and then become stuporous. Occasionally horses relax in the rear quarters or dog-sit and then suddenly lunge forward, completing a forward somersault. This activity may be repeated for extended periods of time, endangering personnel and resulting in injury to the horse.

BENZODIAZEPINES

Benzodiazepines (diazepam, midazolam, climazolam) produce anxiolytic, muscle relaxant, and anticonvulsant effects and have the potential to enhance the sedative-hypnotic effects of injectable and inhalant anesthetics (see Table 10-1).

They are rarely administered as single drug therapy to horses but are combined with tranquilizers, opioid, and nonopioid analgesics to provide added sedation and muscle relaxation and reduce the amount of injectable or inhalant anesthetic required to maintain anesthesia. Benzodiazepine drugs are frequently coadministered with dissociative anesthetics and occasionally intraoperatively as an adjunct to general anesthesia to provide added muscle relaxation. Diazepam is the most popular benzodiazepine derivative used in equine practice. Diazepam is insoluble in water and formulated with propylene glycol to improve solubility. The amount of propylene glycol administered to horses during clinical dosing of diazepam is low and of little clinical relevance. Midazolam, a water-soluble benzodiazepine derivative, is more potent and shorter acting than diazepam.

Mechanism of Action

Benzodiazepines produce muscle relaxant, anticonvulsant, anxiolytic, and hypnotic effects by binding to inhibitory GABA receptor sites in the brainstem reticular formation and spinal cord.[59] Specific benzodiazepine binding sites (BZ receptors) have been identified throughout the brain and in peripheral tissues (heart, lung, liver, kidney). These binding sites are associated with a group of ionotropic $GABA_A$ receptors that modulate chloride entry into cells. Unlike barbiturates, benzodiazepines do not activate $GABA_A$ receptors directly but require GABA to produce their effects. Identification and categorization of benzodiazepine binding sites have resulted in the development of specific competitive benzodiazepine antagonists. Flumazenil and sarmazenil are benzodiazepine antagonists that competitively antagonize the effects of benzodiazepines on $GABA_A$ receptors (see Table 10-2). Benzodiazepines potentiate the CNS depressant effects of thiobarbiturates and other hypnotics (propofol, etomidate) that act on the $GABA_A$ receptors.[59] The mechanism responsible for this effect is uncertain, although increases in benzodiazepine receptor affinity have been suggested.[59]

Applied Pharmacology

Diazepam, midazolam, and climazolam produce little-to-no effect on cardiorespiratory variables in adult horses.[43,60,61] Clinical doses (0.05 to 0.1 mg/kg) do not change respiratory rate, tidal volume, pH and blood gases ($PaCO_2$, PaO_2), heart rate, cardiac output, mean arterial blood pressure, or the force of cardiac contraction.[43] Relatively large intravenous doses (0.6 mg/kg) reduce respiratory rate and cause insignificant decreases in arterial blood pressure, possibly because of a decrease in CNS sympathetic activity. Decreases in CNS activity may also be responsible for the antiarrhythmic effects of diazepam in humans and dogs.[62]

The effects of benzodiazepines on gut motility or uterine tone have not been investigated in horses. Fetal depression has not been reported but is a consideration if diazepam is administered to pregnant mares before parturition. Diazepam effectively blocks the negative effect of novel environment and experimentally suppressed precopulatory arousal and sexual response in stallions. Stallions that showed no interest in breeding returned to normal sexual behavior after diazepam administration.[63] Finally, diazepam and other benzodiazepines stimulate food intake in adult and weanling horses.[64]

Biodisposition

Benzodiazepines are metabolized by the liver, and the metabolites are excreted in urine (see Chapter 9).[65-67] Metabolites are not detectable in the plasma but N-desmethyldiazepam, oxazepam, temazepam, and N-methyloxazepam are detectable after glucuronide hydrolysis of urine, suggesting extensive metabolism (see Chapter 9). The plasma half-life in horses ranged from 7 to 22 hours, much longer than the duration of observable clinical effects, suggesting that repeated doses are cumulative.[65,66] Plasma protein binding for diazepam is greater than 80% in horses, and extrahepatic metabolism is suspected but has not been documented. Foals less than 1 month old demonstrate delayed metabolism and elimination.[67]

Clinical Use and Antagonism

Occasionally benzodiazepines are administered in combination with other sedative-hypnotics, opioids, and nonopioid analgesics to produce standing chemical restraint.[68] However, ataxia and muscle relaxation can be pronounced; thus this practice is not encouraged, particularly if the horse must be moved while tranquilized. Diazepam produces mild calming effects; reluctance to move; a fixed gaze; and muscle fasciculations on the face, neck, and thorax when intravenous doses of 0.05 mg/kg are administered (see Table 10-2). Ataxia and recumbency may occur when intravenous doses greater than 0.15 mg/kg are administered, although the horses appear to be aware of their surroundings and maintain normal cardiorespiratory function. Larger doses of diazepam, 0.2 mg/kg intravenously, produce pronounced ataxia or recumbency, which can persist for up to 50 minutes. Horses that become recumbent usually stand within 10 to 20 minutes but remain calm and mildly ataxic for 2 to 3 hours. Foals administered diazepam frequently become recumbent and can be restrained easily for nonpainful procedures.

Diazepam is frequently coadministered with ketamine to facilitate induction to anesthesia or as an adjunct to general anesthesia.[43,69,70] It reduces the requirement for inhalant anesthetics by 29% in ponies.[71] Similar effects are observed when diazepam is coadministered with other injectable or inhalant anesthetics, especially in sick adult horses and foals. The CNS sedative and peripheral pharmacological effects of diazepam can be antagonized with the specific benzodiazepine antagonists flumazenil or sarmazenil (see Table 10-2). Administration of a benzodiazepine antagonist produces rapid reversal of sedation and muscle relaxation and restores normal behavior. The potential for adverse effects (excitement, seizures) has been reported after intravenous administration of flumazenil to humans.[59] This problem has not been reported in horses.

Complications, Side Effects, and Clinical Toxicity

Diazepam produces minimum calming effects, is not an analgesic, and can produce pronounced ataxia and recumbency. It should not be administered as single therapy for standing immobilization or to provide chemical restraint before minor surgical procedures. Some horses become anxious, apprehensive, and mildly agitated within 5 to 10 minutes after intravenous administration of diazepam. This response generally is transient, lasting less than 15 minutes. Most horses return to a normal behavior pattern or become mildly depressed. Some horses develop pica for brief periods. No other serious side effects or toxicities have been reported after administration of diazepam, midazolam, or climazolam to horses.

NONOPIOID SEDATIVE-ANALGESICS

Nonopioid sedative-analgesics are represented by a large number of compounds that produce anxiolysis and skeletal muscle relaxation and relieve pain in horses. Xylazine, detomidine, romifidine, and medetomidine, collectively referred to as α_2-adrenoceptor agonists, are favored for this purpose and have been investigated extensively in horses (see Table 10-1).[72-74] Other α_2-adrenoceptor agonists, including dexmedetomidine and clonidine, have been demonstrated to produce sedative-analgesic effects in horses but have not become popular in equine practice.[75,76]

All α_2-adrenoceptor agonists are highly soluble in water and available as aqueous solutions for injection. They vary considerably in potency, depending on their α_2-adrenoceptor selectivity (Box 10-2).[77] Xylazine serves as the prototype and was the first α_2-adrenoceptor agonist approved for use in horses.[78] Detomidine and medetomidine are more potent than romifidine, and all three are more potent than xylazine in horses.[74,79] Interestingly, differences exist among species regarding the sedative effects of α_2-adrenoceptor agonists. Approximately one tenth the dose of xylazine is required to produce sedation in cattle and steers compared to horses; but similar doses of detomidine, medetomidine, and romifidine are used in both species.[80] The α_2-adrenoceptor agonists possess many of the qualities required for an ideal preanesthetic drug, including predictability, anxiolysis, marked sedation, stupor, and indifference to mildly painful procedures (see Box 10-1).[72-74] They are frequently administered as monotherapy or in conjunction with acepromazine or opioids to facilitate standing medical procedures and as preanesthetic medication.[74] They are also administered as sedative or analgesic adjuncts to intravenous or inhalant anesthesia to decrease anesthetic requirements (see Chapter 13).[81,82] Finally, α_2-adrenoceptor agonists can be administered by epidural or subarachnoid routes to produce local or segmental spinal analgesia (see Chapter 11).[83]

Mechanism of Action

Activation of α (α_1 and α_2)-adrenoceptors produces varied pharmacologic effects (see Table 10-3).[77,84] The α_2-adrenoceptor agonists produce sedation and analgesia and potentiate the effects of other sedative-hypnotic and anesthetic drugs by activating α_2-receptors in the locus ceruleus and spinal cord.[84] Stimulation of α_2-adrenoceptors in the CNS hyperpolarizes neurons and inhibits norepinephrine and dopamine storage and release. These effects decrease the discharge

rate of central and peripheral neurons, resulting in sedation, analgesia, and muscle relaxation. α_2-Adrenoceptor agonists decrease CNS sympathetic output and peripheral sympathetic tone.[85] Parasympathetic (vagal) tone is increased initially as a result of transient increases in arterial blood pressure and increases in baroreceptor sensitivity.[80] Most α_2-adrenoceptor agonists, especially xylazine, also produce some degree of α_1-adrenoceptor activation, although the more selective α_2-adrenoceptor agonists (detomidine, medetomidine, dexmedetomidine) are relatively devoid of this effect (see Box 10-2). Interestingly, large (pharmacological) doses of α_2-adrenoceptor agonists, including dexmedetomidine, produce minimum sedation initially, followed by a much longer period of pronounced sedation. This response is believed to be caused by activation of CNS α_1-adrenoceptors, which are known to functionally antagonize the hypnotic effects of α_2-adrenoceptor agonists.[86] Other neuromodulators, including endogenous opioids, purines, and cannabinoids, are speculated to be important contributors to the CNS effects of α_2-adrenoceptor agonists and are believed responsible for synergistic and additive interactions when α_2-adrenoceptor agonists are coadministered with opioid analgesics.[87] The α_2-adrenoceptor agonists can be antagonized by a variety of α_2-adrenoceptor antagonists, including atipamezole, tolazoline, and yohimbine (see Table 10-2).[88-90]

Applied Pharmacology

The α_2-adrenoceptor agonists produce relatively predictable sedation and muscle relaxation. They all produce dose-dependent sedation, increases in horses' tolerance to painful

Table 10–3. Location and function of α_1- and α_2-adrenoceptors

Receptor type and location	Function
α_1	
Central nervous system	Increase awareness and activity
Heart	Increase force of contraction and sensitization of the myocardium to catecholamines during halothane anesthesia
Smooth muscle	Vasoconstriction
Liver	Glycogenolysis; gluconeogenesis
α_2	
Central nervous system	Decreases norepinephrine and dopamine release causing sedation and cardiopulmonary depression
Sympathetic nerve terminal	Inhibition of norepinephrine release
Cholinergic neurons	Inhibition
Heart	Decrease norepinephrine release
Smooth muscle	Vasoconstriction
Gut	Reduced tone and propulsive activity
Pancreatic islet cells	Inhibition of insulin release
Platelets	Aggregation
Fat	Inhibition of lipolysis (clonidine)

Box 10–2 α_2:α_1-Selectivity

Drug	α_2:α_1
Xylazine	160:1
Detomidine	260:1
Medetomidine	1620:1
Romifidine	340:1
Clonidine	220:1

stimuli, and depression of cardiorespiratory function.[73,74,80] α_2-Agonists produce excellent relaxation of the muscles of the head, neck, and ears, followed by drooping of the head, ears, and lips (see Figure 10-6).[73,91] These effects are centrally mediated, are well correlated with degree of sedation, and have become widely accepted as objective methods for the assessment of the depth and duration of the sedation.[91,92] Dose-dependent sedation decreases respiratory rate, tidal volume, and minute volume and results in mild decreases in PaO_2 and increases in $PaCO_2$ values in conscious horses.[80,93,94] Decreases in PaO_2 are particularly noticeable after the administration of detomidine (see Figure 10-7). In addition, hemodynamic changes such as vasoconstriction and pulmonary redistribution of blood flow are considered to be responsible for the early onset of impaired oxygenation. The mucous membranes may become pale and pinkish-gray as a result of peripheral vasoconstriction and decreases in PaO_2.[94,95] Some horses may demonstrate signs of increased inspiratory effort (abdominal lift) or begin to snore as a result of a lowered head position and relaxation of muscles in the larynx and nares.[96] The respiratory depressant effects of xylazine and romifidine are less than those produced by medetomidine and detomidine and are clinically irrelevant in most conscious horses.

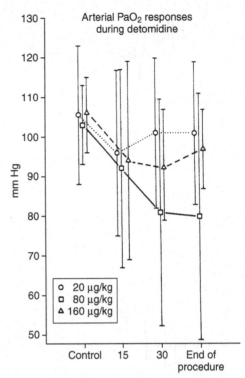

Figure 10–7. The effect of detomidine on arterial PaO_2 values in horses. (From Short CE: Cardiovascular and pulmonary function studies of a new sedative/analgetic (detomidine, domosedan) for use alone, in horses, or as a preanesthetic, *Acta Vet Scand* 82(suppl): 139-155, 1986.)

The α_2-adrenoceptor agonists decrease pulmonary dynamic compliance.[95,95] Breathing may become exaggerated and intrapleural pressure is increased, due to abnormal and asynchronous laryngeal movement.[93,97] Detomidine (and acepromazine) significantly alter laryngeal function by reducing the ability to abduct the left laryngeal cartilage; it has been suggested that horses that completely lose this ability when sedated are demonstrating early signs of recurrent laryngeal neuropathy.[98] α_2-Adrenoceptor agonists also produce marked relaxation of the alar muscles, predisposing to upper airway obstruction and respiratory stridor.[97] The cough reflex is suppressed, increasing the danger for the accumulation of mucus or foreign material in the trachea, an important consideration in horses recovering from nasal sinus or laryngeal surgery. The respiratory depressant effects of α_2-adrenoceptor agonists are enhanced when they are coadministered with injectable and inhalant anesthetics. α_2-Adrenoceptor agonists are noted for their potent and sometimes dramatic cardiovascular effects (see Figure 10-8).[18,80,94] All α_2-adrenoceptor agonists have the potential to produce rapid and significant decreases in heart rate and predispose to the development of first- and second-degree atrioventricular block and occasionally third-degree atrioventricular block (see Chapter 3; Figure 10-9).[72,73,94,99,100] Occasionally horses develop pronounced sinus bradycardia with ventricular escape beats (see Chapter 3). Stroke volume remains relatively unchanged or decreases minimally after intravenous administration of α_2-adrenoceptor agonists, but cardiac output (heart rate × stroke volume) is markedly decreased (see Figure 10-10).[94] Decreases in cardiac output parallel the

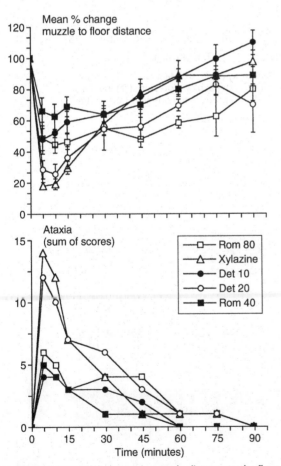

Figure 10–6. Percent (%) change in muzzle distance to the floor and degree of ataxia score in horses administered xylazine, detomidine, and romifidine. (From England GC, Clarke KW: α_2-adrenoceptor agonists in the horse: a review, *Br Vet J* 152(6): 641-657, 1996.)

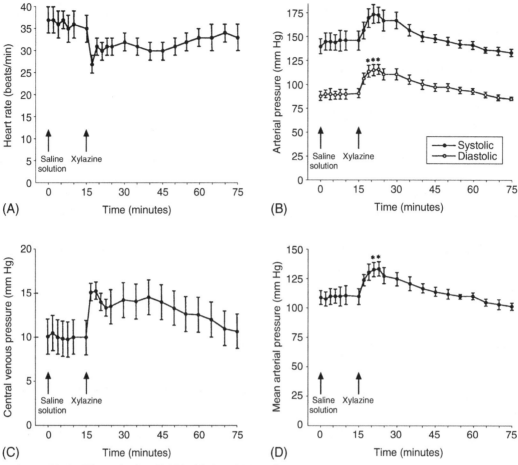

Figure 10–8. Effects of saline (0.011 ml/kg) and 1.1 mg/kg intravenous xylazine on heart rate **(A)**, central venous pressure **(B)**, systolic and diastolic arterial pressure **(C)**, and mean arterial blood pressure **(D)** in adult horses. (From Moore RM, Trim CM: Effect of xylazine on cerebrospinal fluid pressure in conscious horses, *Am J Vet Res* 53:1558-1563, 1992.)

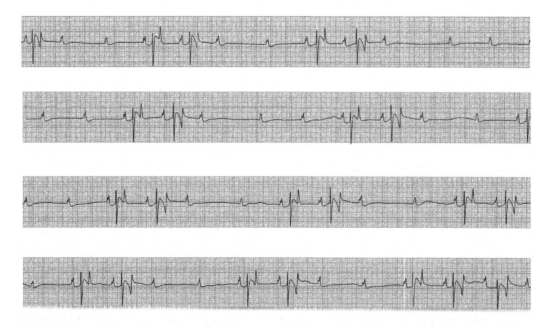

Figure 10–9. Effect of 1.1 mg/kg intravenous xylazine on heart rate and rhythm in an adult horse. Note the presence of first- (prolonged PR interval) and second- (P wave not followed by a ventricular complex) degree atrioventricular block. There are instances of multiple P waves not followed by ventricular complexes (high grade second-degree atrioventricular block).

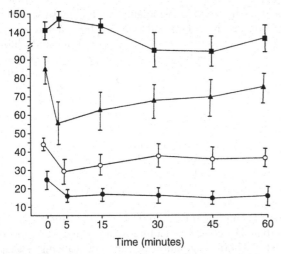

Figure 10–10. Effects of 1.1 mg/kg intravenous xylazine on mean arterial blood pressure (mm Hg; ■), cardiac output (ml/kg/min; ▲), heart rate (beats/min; o), and respiratory rate (breaths/min; •) in adult horses. (From Muir WW, Skarda RT, Sheehan WC: Hemodynamic and respiratory effects of a xylazine-acetylpromazine drug combination in horses, *Am J Vet Res* 40:1518, 1979.)

on vascular smooth muscle, resulting in both arteriolar and venular constriction. Venular constriction produces increases in central venous pressure.[103] Hypertension is less pronounced and may not occur after intramuscular administration. Subsequent hypotension is caused by bradycardia in conjunction with decreases in cardiac output and CNS sympathetic outflow. The administration of an anticholinergic (atropine, glycopyrrolate) can increase heart rate and cardiac output, resulting in large increases in arterial blood pressure, particularly in the presence of peripheral vasoconstriction.[99] The administration of an anticholinergic drug should be considered carefully in horses because of the potential to cause sinus tachycardia and increases in myocardial oxygen demand, intestinal stasis, and impaction, which may increase morbidity in aged, debilitated horses or horses requiring surgery for colic.[6,7]

α_2-Adrenoceptor agonists produce a marked reduction in myoelectrical activity, propulsive motility, and emptying times from the esophagus to the colon in ponies and horses, effects largely attributed to inhibition of postganglionic cholinergic activity.[104-112,119] These effects may last for up to 3 hours after xylazine administration and longer after detomidine or romifidine administration and can be antagonized by the administration α_2-adrenoceptor antagonists.[105,109] All α_2-adrenoceptor agonists can suppress or "mask" the signs of colic. This effect is particularly pronounced and prolonged following the administration of detomidine (see Figure 10-12). All α_2-adrenoceptor agonists induce hyperglycemia in adult horses but less so in foals (see Figure 10-13).[73,74,113] This effect may persist for more than 3 hours and is mediated by stimulation of α_2-adrenoceptors located on pancreatic β-cells, which inhibit insulin secretion. Increases in serum glucose and decreases in serum insulin concentrations have been reported in ponies and horses (see Figure 10-13).[114,115] Changes in other blood chemical values, red and white blood cell numbers, and platelet numbers have not been evaluated closely in controlled studies in horses, although small decreases in packed cell volume and total protein can develop 30 to 45 minutes after intravenous α_2-adrenoceptor agonist administration.[116,117]

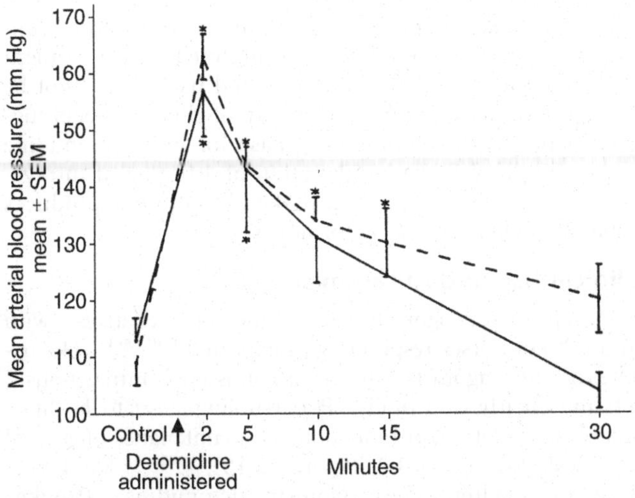

decreases in heart rate and can be restored to near normal values by administering drugs that increase heart rate (atropine, glycopyrrolate; see Figure 10-1).[99] Cardiac contractile performance is not changed after administration of α_2-adrenoceptor agonists, although small decreases can occur secondary to decreases in central sympathetic outflow.[101] Intravenous administration of an α_2-adrenoceptor agonist produces an initial and relatively short-lived (10 to 15 minutes) increase in arterial blood pressure followed by a decrease in arterial blood pressure, although arterial blood pressure rarely falls below 20% of baseline values (see Figures 10-8, 10-10, and 10-11).[79,80,94] The increase in arterial blood pressure is more prolonged after detomidine and romifidine.[94,102] Systolic blood pressures in excess of 200 mg Hg have been recorded from horses administered xylazine or detomidine. The hypertension is attributed to stimulation of α_1- and α_2-adrenoceptors

Figure 10–11. Effects of 10 (—) and 20 (---) µg/kg intravenous detomidine on mean arterial blood pressure in 114 adult horses of various breeds. (From Clarke KW, Taylor PM: Detomidine: a new sedative for horses, *Equine Vet J* 18:366, 1986.)

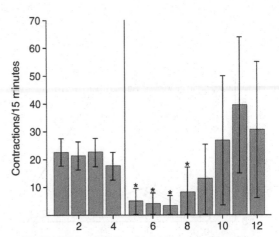

Figure 10–12. Effect of 12.5 µg/kg intravenous detomidine on contraction rate in the proximal portion of the duodenum in four horses. The x-axis periods are 15 minutes (epochs) in duration. (From Meritt AM, Burrow JA, Hartless CS: Effect of xylazine, detomidine and a combination of xylazine and butorphanol on equine duodenal motility, *Am J Vet Res* 59:619-623, 1998.)

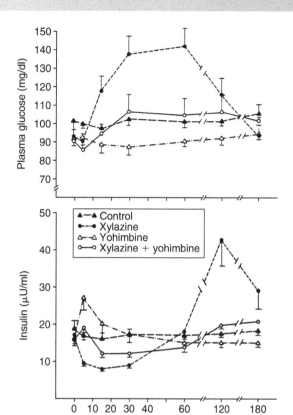

Figure 10–13. Plasma glucose (mg/dl, *top*) and serum insulin (μU/ml, *bottom*) concentrations in mares administered 1.1 mg/kg intravenous xylazine, 0.125 mg/kg intravenous yohimbine, or 0.125 mg/kg intravenous yohimbine followed in 5 minutes by 1.1 mg/kg intravenous xylazine. Control mares were administered saline. Yohimbine inhibited the increase in plasma glucose concentration caused by xylazine. (From Greene SA et al: Effect of yohimbine on xylazine-induced hypoinsulinema and hyperglycemia in mares, *Am J Vet Res* 48:676, 1987.)

α₂-Adrenoceptor agonists increase urine output in horses, with maximum flow occurring between 30 and 60 minutes after drug administration (see Figure 10-14). Although originally attributed to osmotic effects secondary to hyperglycemia, glucosuria has not been a consistent finding.[115,118,119]

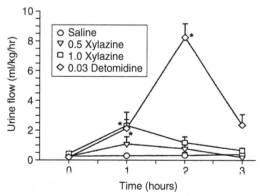

Figure 10–14. Effect of saline, xylazine, and detomidine on urine flow (nl/kg/hr) in six adult horses. (From Nunez E et al: Effects of α₂-adrenergic receptor agonists on urine production in horses deprived of food and water, *Am J Vet Res* 65:1342-1346, 2004.)

Urine specific gravity, osmolality, and glucose concentration decreased in horses and ponies administered xylazine; whereas the excretion of sodium, potassium, and chloride increased.[118,119] Similar responses, including increases in sodium excretion, are produced by detomidine and attributed to an increase in glomerular filtration rate, inhibition of antidiuretic hormone release and response by the renal tubules, and increased atrial natriuretic hormone release.[119] The increase in urine flow is not trivial and should be considered in anesthetic management decisions (see Figure 10-14). The placement of a urethral catheter before or after induction of anesthesia and before surgery helps to control bladder distention and reduce agitation during the recovery period. The increase in urine flow is directly related to dose and type of α₂-adrenoceptor agonist used. Dehydration in horses may be exacerbated by concurrent administration of α₂-adrenoceptor agonists. Thermoregulation is altered, causing sweating and transient increases in body temperature. Uterine tone increases in mares administered α₂-adrenoceptor agonists, but an increased incidence of abortion has not been demonstrated in healthy pregnant mares administered detomidine at 3-week intervals during the last trimester of pregnancy.[120,121] α₂-Adrenoceptor agonists are well tolerated by foals, which, in contrast to adults, demonstrate minimum changes in blood glucose values or plasma insulin. Sedation, recumbency, and hypothermia are common as are the other cardiopulmonary changes discussed previously.[122,123]

Biodisposition

α₂-Adrenoceptor agonists are metabolized extensively in the liver, and their metabolites are excreted in the urine (see Chapter 9). The pharmacological activity of most metabolites is unknown. Intravenous administration is followed by a rapid onset of effect resulting from their high lipophilicity and rapid entry into the brain. Peak effect is reached in 3 to 5 minutes after intravenous administration and 10 to 15 minutes after intramuscular administration. The plasma half-life after intravenous administration of α₂-adrenoceptor agonists in horses varies from less than 1 hour to over an hour for detomidine and roughly parallels the duration of their clinically useful sedative and analgesic effects.[124-127] The faster metabolism and shorter duration of action suggests that xylazine and medetomidine may be more clinically useful than detomidine or romifidine for the treatment of colic because the signs of stress and pain would not be "masked" for as long.[128] The duration of clinical effects suggests a prolonged elimination phase for both detomidine and romifidine. The administration of 40 μg/kg of intravenous detomidine or 80 to 120 μg/kg of romifidine produces behavioral changes lasting for hours.

Clinical Use and Antagonism

α₂-Adrenoceptor agonists are predictable sedatives, with over 80% of horses responding as expected.[73,92,129-131] The α₂-adrenoceptor agonists can be administered intravenously, intramuscularly, and orally (PO) (sublingually) to facilitate anxiolysis, sedation, or induction and maintenance of general anesthesia (see Box 10-3; Figure 10-15).[73,81,82,132] Sublingual doses of α₂-adrenoceptor agonists (detomidine: 60 μg/kg) produce sedation, analgesia, and muscle relaxation, resulting in horses that are easier to work with, reluctant to move, and uninterested in their surroundings.[132,133] Oral dosing is less

Uses of α₂-Adrenoceptor Agonists

- Anxiolysis-sedation
- Analgesia (systemically, epidural, subarachnoid)
- Muscle relaxation
- Preanesthetic medication
  - Coadministered with other sedatives, analgesics, hypnotics and dissociative anesthetics
- Reduce the amount of injectable or inhalant anesthetic
- Adjuncts to inhalation anesthesia
- Quiet and control recovery from anesthesia

("explode") with rapid and well-directed kicks, only to become sedated again when left alone. The lack of sedation and analgesia in some horses has resulted in the coadministration of α₂-adrenoceptor agonists and opioid agonists, especially butorphanol and acepromazine (see Figures 10-16 and 10-17). The combination of α₂-adrenoceptor agonists and butorphanol or acepromazine demonstrates greater efficacy than when either drug is used alone, without an increase in untoward or toxic effects.[135-137]

Repeating or administering large doses of α₂-adrenoceptor agonists may not increase the degree of sedation. Accidental administration of 5.5 mg/kg of intravenous xylazine and 500 μg/kg of romifidine did not produce sedation, most likely because of α₁-adrenoceptor opposition of α₂-adrenoceptor–mediated effects and may be a result

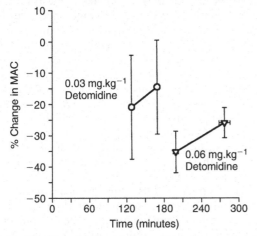

Figure 10–15. Effects of detomidine on the minimum alveolar concentration *(MAC)* of isoflurane. Note the reduction from baseline (0%) values. (From Steffey Ep, Pascoe PJ: Detomidine reduces isoflurane anesthetic requirement (MAC) in horses, *Vet Anaesth Analg* 29:223-227, 2002.)

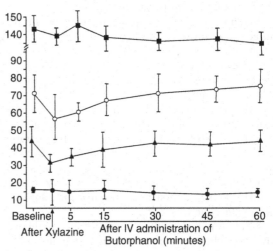

Figure 10–16. Effects of 0.5 mg/kg xylazine and 0.02 mg/kg intravenous butorphanol on mean arterial blood pressure (mm Hg; ■), cardiac output (ml/kg/min; o), heart rate (beats/min; ▲), and respiratory rate (breaths/min; ●) in adult horses. (From Robertson JT, Muir WW: A new analgesic drug combination in the horse, *Am J Vet Res* 44:1667, 1983.)

predictable and may require up to 45 minutes for maximum drug effect. Intravenous or intramuscular administration of α₂-adrenoceptor agonists produces more rapid and relatively more predictable effects than oral dosing. Most horses become clinically depressed within 3 to 5 minutes after intravenous administration (see Table 10-2). They are indifferent to their surroundings, drop their heads, and extend their necks (see Figure 10-6). The lower lip often becomes flaccid. Facial edema can occur following administration of detomidine and romifidine. The existence of facial edema is attributed to venous congestion that occurs when horses hold their head down after sedation; therefore its severity is correlated with the duration and degree of lowering of the head.[92,132] Nasal edema often accompanies facial edema and may lead to respiratory compromise.[132,134] Some horses assume a sawhorse stance or support themselves by leaning against a rope, railing, or wall. The knees or hind legs may buckle, and some horses stumble or become markedly ataxic. The penis becomes relaxed and is extended in males (see Chapter 6). Draft horses and foals are very susceptible to α₂-adrenoceptor agonist sedation; whereas hot-blooded, excited, or fearful horses may become only mildly sedated. Horses administered α₂-adrenoceptor agonists may startle and should be approached cautiously. Horses that appear profoundly sedated may react violently

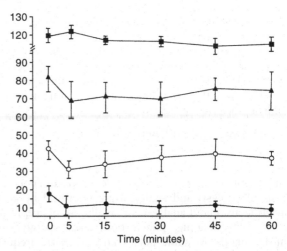

Figure 10–17. Effects of 0.55 mg/kg intravenous xylazine combined with 0.05 mg/kg intravenous acepromazine on mean arterial blood pressure (mm Hg; ■), cardiac output (ml/kg/min; ▲), heart rate (beats/min; o), and respiratory rate (breaths/min; ●) in adult horses. (From Muir WW, Skarda RT, Sheehan WC: Hemodynamic and respiratory effects of a xylazine-acetylpromazine drug combination in horses, *Am J Vet Res* 40:1518, 1979.)

of distribution of α_2-receptor subtypes and α_2: α_1 receptor selectivity binding ratio.[86,138] Mild sedation did occur 1 to 2 hours after drug administration. Similar observations have been made after intravenous administration of detomidine with 160 µg/kg, which produced a longer duration of action but similar sedative effects compared with 20 µg/kg.[139]

α_2-Adrenoceptor agonists can be administered safely to foals, although their effects may be much more pronounced than in adults.[122,123,140] Respiratory depression, bradycardia, and hypothermia can occur, which may produce cyanotic or pale mucous membranes and could require ventilatory support, oxygen therapy, or antagonism.[140] Many foals begin to sweat and become markedly ataxic and recumbent after α_2-adrenoceptor agonist administration. Increased urination may be noticed 60 to 90 minutes after administration.

α_2-Adrenoceptor drugs can be injected epidurally and intrathecally to produce localized and segmental analgesia in horses (see Chapter 11). Epidural or intrathecal administration produces localized sweating associated with regional analgesia, minimum ataxia, and analgesia lasting for approximately 3 and 5 hours, respectively.[83]

Recovery from anesthesia should be a quiet, coordinated, and uneventful process but can be prolonged, dangerous, and extremely stressful. The intravenous administration of reduced doses of α_2-adrenoceptor agonists immediately before or during the recovery process prolongs recovery but markedly improves the quality of recovery by reducing excitement, ataxia, and stress without significant cardiorespiratory consequences.[90,141]

α_2-Adrenoceptor agonists are antagonized rapidly and completely by α_2-adrenoceptor antagonists (see Table 10-2).[88-90,142] Yohimbine and tolazoline produce extremely variable effects and also antagonize α_1-adrenoceptors, producing hypotension in some horses.[143] The α_2-adrenoceptor atipamezole is much more selective for α_2-adrenoceptors and does not cause significant hypotension.[88,90,144] α_2-Adrenoceptor blocking drugs are administered occasionally to antagonize the CNS depressant effects of intravenous anesthetics and hasten recovery from inhalant anesthesia in horses that do not return to a standing position in a reasonable time (60 to 90 minutes) or are reluctant to stand. Alternatively, doxapram, a CNS and respiratory stimulant, antagonizes sedation produced by α_2-adrenoceptor agonists.[145] Doxapram is nonspecific but stimulates CNS activity, including the respiratory centers, resulting in arousal in mildly to moderately sedated horses.

Complications, Side Effects, and Clinical Toxicity

Inadequate sedation, analgesia, and ataxia are the most frequent complaints reported after use of α_2-adrenoceptor agonists. Anxiolysis and analgesia are improved by coadministering an opioid analgesic or small dose of acepromazine.[18,130,135,136] Sweating, piloerection, and hyperglycemia occur frequently in adult horses and are more frequent and pronounced after intravenous detomidine administration.[113-115] The volume and frequency of urination usually increase within 30 to 60 minutes of administration. All α_2-adrenoceptor agonists reduce or abolish gastrointestinal motility for at least 1 hour after intravenous adminis-

tration.[110-113] Gas distention and colic can occur following administration, particularly after repeated doses, and are generally responsive to the administration of α_2-adrenoceptor antagonists.[109] Accidental subcutaneous injections after attempts to administer intramuscular xylazine or detomidine can produce localized inflammatory responses. The cause for this response is unknown. Abortion can occur after xylazine or detomidine, although the evidence for this response is weak.[146]

Sinus bradycardia, first- and second-degree atrioventricular block, and respiratory depression are frequently observed after administration of α_2-adrenoceptor agonists.[99] Heart rates less than 30 beats/min are common, and heart rates less than 20 beats/min can occur.[94] Interestingly, the bradycardic effects of α_2-adrenoceptor agonists are not aggravated by intravenous or inhalant anesthesia. Heart rates usually return to the normal range once recumbency is produced. Heart rates less than 25 beats/min in anesthetized horses should be treated by administering an anticholinergic (atropine, glycopyrrolate) because of the associated marked decreases in cardiac output.[7-9] Respiratory depression combined with pronounced relaxation of the nasal alar and laryngeal muscles may lead to "snoring," respiratory stridor, and upper airway obstruction, which may require nasotracheal intubation and oxygen administration. Upper airway obstruction is particularly problematic during recovery from anesthesia and can trigger agitation, stress, and poor recovery. Treatment includes the placement of a nasotracheal or orotracheal tube during the recovery process (see Chapter 14). Some horses, particularly foals, hypoventilate and can become hypoxemic and develop cyanosis after α_2-adrenoceptor agonist administration.[122] Oxygen supplementation is required, particularly in aged horses or horses with respiratory disease.

Xylazine can potentiate and increase the sensitization of the myocardium to catecholamines during halothane anesthesia in dogs.[147] This effect is likely to be unique to xylazine and mediated by activation of α_1-adrenoceptors. It is important to note that similar studies in horses were unable to reproduce similar results, suggesting that the clinical relevance of this finding is likely to be of little or no consequence.[148] Sudden death resulting from ventricular fibrillation has been reported after administration of xylazine to conscious and halothane-anesthetized horses.[149] Death after administration of detomidine in horses has been attributed to cardiac sensitization and the concurrent use of potentiated sulfonamides.[150] Accidental intracarotid injection of α_2-adrenoceptor agonists produces excitement, disorientation, ataxia, recumbency, and paddling. Some horses may develop seizures. Treatment is symptomatic and supportive but usually involves the administration of an anticonvulsant (diazepam) or anesthetics (thiopental) and oxygenation. Prior placement of an intravenous catheter eliminates this problem (see Chapter 7).

α_2-Adrenoceptor agonists are very potent CNS and respiratory depressants in humans.[151] Near-fatal accidents have occurred after their intentional and inadvertent exposure in humans.[152] The self-administration of a xylazine overdose resulted in unconsciousness for 48 hours and required controlled ventilation for 3 days.[153] The administration of an α_2-adrenoceptor antagonist and controlled ventilation may be lifesaving.

OPIOID ANALGESICS

The terminology used in conjunction with opioid analgesics is confusing. Opioids are often referred to as *narcotics*, a term that can also be applied to any drug that produces sleep. *Narcosis*, a term originally used by Galen, refers to agents that deaden the senses, causing loss of feeling or paralysis. Today the term *narcotic* is generally used to refer to any substance that reduces pain, induces sleep, or alters mood but generally refers to substances derived from opium. The preferred term, *opioid*, refers to any exogenous substance that specifically binds to any of a variety of *opioid receptors* (endogenous opioid peptides and opiates produce their pharmacological effects by activating membrane-bound opioid receptors).[154,155] Although new opioid receptors and receptor subtypes continue to emerge, most opiates are described and discussed on the basis of their activation of OP_3 (μ; mu), OP_2 (κ; kappa), and OP_1 (δ; delta) opioid receptors (see Table 10-4).[155] Some substances bind to opioid receptors but initiate few or no agonistic effects; and others produce either partial agonistic or antagonistic actions, depending on the dose. The terms *opioid agonist, partial agonist, opioid agonist-antagonist,* and *opioid antagonist* are used to refer to drugs that possess opioid receptor activity.

Morphine is the prototypic opioid agonist. Thebaine and morphine are alkaloids of opium. Thebaine is the precursor of etorphine (M-99), a drug purported to have 1000 times or more the analgesic potency of morphine.[156] Morphine is used in the preparation of heroin, apomorphine, and oxymorphine. Other structurally distinct chemical classes of drugs have been produced that produce effects similar to morphine.[4,157] Regardless of derivation, the drugs generally share similar pharmacological effects, resulting from the ability to stimulate or block opioid receptors (see Table 10-4). The discovery of endogenous opioids (enkephalins and endorphins), which share many of the pharmacological properties of opioid agonists, has increased current understanding of the mechanisms responsible for pain but has complicated the clinical use of opioid antagonists. All opioids are white powders that are highly soluble in water. Opioids are frequently combined with sedative-hypnotics to produce neuroleptanalgesia. The term *neuroleptanalgesia* refers to the combination of a neuroleptic (tranquilizer or sedative) and an opioid analgesic (e.g., acepromazine/meperidine; xylazine/morphine).[4]

Mechanism of Action

Opioid agonists produce the majority, if not all, of their pharmacological effects by binding to saturable stereospecific opioid receptors that are widely dispersed but unevenly distributed throughout the CNS (brain, spinal cord, autonomic nervous system) and peripheral organs.[155-159] Biochemical studies have identified four clinically relevant types of opioid receptors and several receptor subtypes (see Table 10-4). The four receptors correspond to the pharmacologically defined μ,κ, and δ receptors and a fourth receptor that binds to a novel peptide termed *nociceptin* or *orphanin FQ*. Opioid agonists can bind to several opioid receptors, resulting in varied pharmacological activity profiles dependent on their receptor selectivity and affinity.[154,160] Alterations in autonomic tone and increases in dopamine release or brain dopamine receptor sensitivity are responsible for peripheral pharmacological effects, behavioral changes, increased locomotor activity, and stereotypic behavior.[157,161] The analgesic effects of opioids are believed to derive from their ability to inhibit ascending transmission of nociceptive information from the dorsal horn of the spinal cord and to activate descending pain control circuits from the midbrain via the rostral ventromedial medulla.[157] The location, density, and overlap (colocalization) of the various opioid receptors with other relevant receptors (i.e., α_2-adrenoceptor) in the CNS and periphery determine their behavioral, autonomic, and pain-modulating effects. Horses possess a unique opioid receptor profile and density compared to other species and are sensitive to opioid-induced CNS stimulatory and locomotor effects.

The clinical use of the sedative and anesthetic sparing effects of opioids in horses is controversial, although fentanyl produced a small (18%) decrease in the minimum alveolar concentration of isoflurane (see Figure 10-18).[162] Future research will lead to the discovery of new opioid receptors and more selective opioid receptor agonists and antagonists (see Table 10-2). Spiradoline, ethylketazocine, and U-50488H are specific kappa (κ) agonists that produce analgesia and mild sedation without significantly affecting cardiopulmonary function or increasing body temperature

Table 10–4.	Opioid receptor nomenclature	
Recommended nomenclature	**Old nomenclature**	**Examples of potential ligands***
μ (MOP)	OP_3	Morphine Fentanyl
κ (KOP)	OP_2	Butorphanol
δ (DOP)	OP_1	Methadone (?)
NOP	OP_4	Nociceptin

DOP, delta opioid; *KOP,* kappa opioid; *MOP,* mu opioid; *NOP,* nociceptor opioid.
*The opioid receptors can be activated by endogenous opioids (endorphin, enkephalin, dynorphin).
Nociceptin (orphanin FQ) is an endogenous peptide.

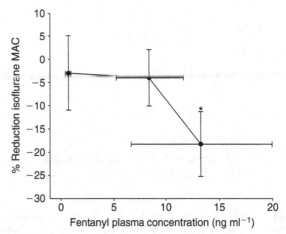

Figure 10–18. Percentage reduction in isoflurane MAC at three different plasma concentrations of fentanyl in eight adult horses. (From Thomasy SM et al: The effects of intravenous fentanyl administration on the minimum alveolar concentration of isoflurane in horses, *Br J Anaesth* 97:232-237, 2006.)

in the horse.[163,164] A great deal more research in horses is required before the full picture of the use and potential misuse of opioid agonists and agonists-antagonists can be appreciated.

Applied Pharmacology

Opioid agonists and agonist-antagonists produce their most clinically relevant pharmacological effects on the CNS and gastrointestinal tract.[4,165-167] These effects include analgesia, mild sedation or excitement, increases in locomotor activity, respiratory modulation, cardiovascular depression, decreased gastrointestinal propulsive motility, and mild increases in body temperature (see Figure 10-19).[4,167-172] Opioid agonists increase pain tolerance in horses when they are coadministered with α_2-adrenoceptor agonists or NSAIDs.[134-136] However, the relative analgesic potency and clinical efficacy of opioids are not well defined in horses, particularly in relation to optimum dosages and the treatment of superficial, deep, and visceral pain (see Table 10-5; Figure 10-20). Evidence suggests that opioids such as butorphanol that exert a greater κ-opioid effect may be efficacious for the treatment of visceral pain in horses.[163,164,173-176] Butorphanol significantly decreased plasma cortisol concentrations and improved recovery characteristics in horses undergoing abdominal surgery.[175,177] It produced minimum effects on sharp, immediate, A-delta-mediated superficial pain but did alter spinal processing and decreased the delayed sensations of pain.[178] Morphine may be a better analgesic than butor-

Table 10–5.	Relative analgesic potency of selected opioid agonists and agonist-antagonists in horses
Drug	**Relative potency**
Morphine	1
Methadone	1
Meperidine	0.5
Oxymorphone	2.0
Pentazocine	0.25
Butorphanol	2.5
Nalbuphine	1.0
Buprenorphine	1.0
Fentanyl	0.5-50?
Xylazine*	3.5
Detomidine*	10-15?

*Included for comparison.

phanol for the treatment of superficial and deep somatic pain but is more likely to predispose horses to the development of ileus and constipation (see Figures 10-20 and 10-21).[167,173] Notably, low doses of opioid agonists-antagonists and full opioid agonists have produced the most beneficial clinical

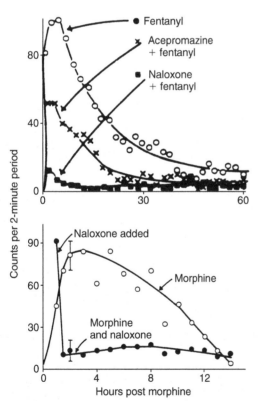

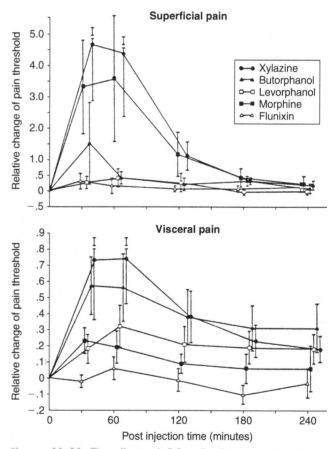

Figure 10-19. Effects of acepromazine (0.1 mg/kg intravenous) and naloxone (0.015 mg/kg intravenous, *top*; 0.02 mg/kg, *bottom*) in horses administered fentanyl (0.2 mg/kg intravenous, *top*) and morphine (2.4 mg/kg intravenous, *bottom*) on locomotor response. (From Combie J et al: Pharmacology of narcotic analgesics in the horse: selective blockade of narcotic-induced locomotor activity, *Am J Vet Res* 42:716, 1981.)

Figure 10-20. The effects of 2.2 mg/kg intramuscular xylazine; 0.66 mg/kg intramuscular morphine; 0.22 mg/kg intramuscular butorphanol; 0.033 mg/kg intramuscular levorphanol; 2.2 mg/kg intramuscular flunixin meglumine in adult ponies. (From Kalpravidh M et al: Effects of butorphanol, flunixin, levorphanol, morphine, and xylazine in ponies, *Am J Vet Res* 45:211, 1984.)

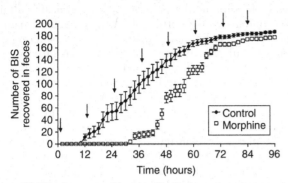

Figure 10–21. Recovery of barium-filled spheres from horses administered 0.5 mg/kg intravenous morphine every 12 hours for 6 days. Morphine reduced propulsive motility and moisture content. (From Boscan P et al: Evaluation of the effects of the opioid agonist morphine on gastrointestinal tract function in horses, *Am J Vet Res* 67:992-997, 2006.)

effects, including analgesia.[179-182] Morphine, administered at doses up to 0.15 mg/kg intravenously, produced analgesia, decreased anesthetic requirements, and improved recovery in halothane-anesthetized horses.[180-182] However, larger dosages of morphine (>0.25 mg/kg IV) diminish opioid-induced anesthetic sparing and beneficial recovery effects.[4,183] Fentanyl, a comparatively selective mu opioid agonist, believed to be 100 times more potent than morphine as an analgesic, can induce excitement and hyperresponsiveness to sound, touch, and environmental stimuli.[171,172] However, fentanyl infusions designed to produce clinically relevant analgesic effects (1 to 16 mg/ml) did not produce somatic or visceral analgesia and only minimally lowered inhalant anesthetic requirements in horses (see Figure 10-18).[184,185] Together these studies suggest that opioids produce qualitatively similar but quantitatively different effects in horses compared to other species and that analgesic activity is most prominent when opioids are administered at lower doses or coadministered with sedative-hypnotics (acepromazine) or nonopioid analgesics (xylazine, detomidine).

Opioid agonists and agonist-antagonists have the potential to depress ventilation in most species, but this effect may not be clinically relevant in conscious or anesthetized horses.[180,186] For example, morphine decreases respiratory rate when administered in low doses (<0.05 mg/kg) but induces tachypnea and hyperventilation with doses greater than 0.1 mg/kg intravenously.[168] Similarly, other opioid agonists may alter ventilation based on their opioid receptor specificity and potential to induce excitement (see Table 10-4). Tidal volume usually increases in horses in which the opioid agonist has reduced respiratory rate, thereby maintaining minute volume, arterial pH, and blood gases (PaO_2, $PaCO_2$). The potential respiratory depressant effects of opioid agonists are more likely to occur in horses that are heavily sedated and administered doses that do not produce CNS agitation or excitement. The administration of opioids to deeply anesthetized or severely compromised (sick, depressed, debilitated) dogs and humans has the potential to result in decreases in both respiratory rate and tidal volume. This effect has been attributed to reduced respiratory center responsiveness to carbon dioxide (decreased sensitivity) but has not been thoroughly evaluated in horses.[157] The potential respiratory depressant effects of adjunctive

opioid administration before or during general anesthesia in horses are likely to be of little clinical relevance in otherwise normal healthy or moderately ill horses (see Chapter 13). Opioid agonists are potent cough suppressants and could predispose to the accumulation of blood, secretions, or exudates in the trachea, which may be an important consideration in horses with respiratory disease or scheduled for laryngeal, sinus, or upper airway surgery.[157]

Clinical doses of most opioid agonists do not produce major effects on heart rate, cardiac output, arterial blood pressure, or cardiac contractility (see Table 10-2 and Figures 10-16 and 10-22).[168,186] Larger doses of morphine and butorphanol increase heart rate and arterial blood pressure for sustained periods of time, most likely secondary to their CNS excitatory effects.[168-170] Interestingly, and in contrast to the potential respiratory depressant effects of opioid agonists when used in conjunction with sedatives and anesthetics, opioid agonist drug combinations do not produce significant hemodynamic changes.[135-137] The administration of an opioid agonist to a previously sedated or anesthetized horse may produce a slight decrease in heart rate and arterial blood pressure. Opioid-induced decreases in heart rate are likely caused by CNS depression and increases in vagal tone.[157] Administration of an anticholinergic drug (atropine; glycopyrrolate) rapidly antagonizes opioid-induced bradycardia. Decreases in arterial blood pressure associated with lower doses of opioids are also likely to be caused by CNS depression and decreases in central sympathetic outflow, although this is uncommon in horses. The administration of naloxone reverses opioid-induced hypotension and, when administered in large doses, is partially effective in the

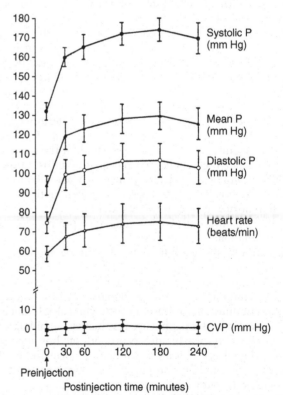

Figure 10–22. The effects of 0.1 mg/kg intravenous morphine on systolic, diastolic, and mean arterial blood pressure *(P)*, central venous *(CVP)*, and heart rate in six adult conscious horses.

treatment of hypotension associated with septic and endo-toxic shock, suggesting a possible role of opioid receptors in these diseases.[187] Other potential mechanisms believed responsible for opioid-associated hypotension include direct vasodilation of peripheral arteries and veins and the release of histamine. The importance of opioid-induced histamine release in producing hypotension in horses and the potential therapeutic antishock effects of selection of opioid antagonists remain to be investigated.[188]

The clinical importance of opioid agonists on gastrointestinal motility in horses is controversial, although pronounced and often prolonged decreases in propulsive motility can occur.[165-167,189,190] Characteristically, opioids inhibit the release of acetylcholine from the mesenteric plexus, increasing gastrointestinal muscle tone and reducing propulsive rhythmic contractions.[191] This initial period of intestinal hypermotility is often associated with restlessness and defecation and is followed by a decrease in intestinal motility, decreased gut sounds, delayed defecation, and fecal drying. Opioids also increase smooth muscle sphincter tone, predisposing to abdominal discomfort and constipation.[167,191] These effects are not common to all opioid agonists. Butorphanol, an opioid agonist-antagonist, produces minimum effect on intestinal transit time and gut sounds and does not delay the time to first defecation after treatment or alter fecal consistency.[177] One study demonstrated that morphine administered at 0.5 mg/kg twice daily decreased propulsive motility and moisture content in the gastrointestinal tract lumen and suggested that gastrointestinal effects may predispose treated horses to the development of ileus and constipation.[167] This dose is far in excess of clinical recommendations (0.05 to 0.1 mg/kg qid). Another study reported that morphine was associated with a fourfold increased risk of colic compared with the use of no opioid or butorphanol, although the number of horses evaluated and other confounding factors may have influenced the results.[192] Similar studies in a large number of horses with naturally occurring disease, including colic, have demonstrated that the clinical use of opioids, including morphine, may be responsible for an increased incidence of gastrointestinal side effects but suggested that other factors may be more important in determining gut motility.[193,194] Collectively the data suggest that the efficacy of opioid agonists other than butorphanol for the treatment of colic is not predictable and repeated administration of opioids should be considered against their potential to produce long-term alterations in gastrointestinal motility and a return to normal gastrointestinal function.

Opioid agonists and agonist-antagonists produce a variety of other pharmacological effects in dogs and humans, which have not been studied but are believed to be applicable to horses. Pruritus has been reported following the extradural administration of morphine to a horse.[195] Antidiuresis and urinary retention can occur secondary to opioid-induced antidiuretic hormone release, but the clinical relevance of these effects in horses has not been evaluated. Opioids inhibit stress-induced release of adrenocorticotropic hormone and depress the release of follicle-stimulating hormone, luteinizing hormone, and thyrotropin and can postpone or inhibit estrus in pony mares.[196]

The lack of controlled clinical trials and the inconsistency of results has led one group of investigators to conclude that "study results do not provide convincing, objective evidence to support the opinion that systemically administered opioids consistently and effectively relieve pain in horses.[4,167] Given this lack of evidence, and considering that opioids stimulate locomotor and other forms of unwanted excitant behavior, reduce propulsive gastrointestinal motility, decrease alveolar ventilation (especially in association with general anesthesia), and require regulatory and practical considerations for abuse potential in both humans and horses, we conclude that routine indiscriminate administration of opioids for pain relief in horses is not justified."[167] They further suggest that focused objective studies of selective beneficial opioid actions to provide guidance for appropriate clinical use are long overdue.[167]

Biodisposition

The metabolism and elimination of opioid agonists and agonist-antagonists is complex and dose related (see Chapter 9). Current evidence suggests that opioid agonists and agonist-antagonists are extensively metabolized by the liver, that some metabolites retain parent compound activity, and that metabolites are excreted in the urine.[197,198] The prolonged presence of some opioid agonists (morphine) in the plasma may represent related metabolites, the slow release of drug from tissues, or enterohepatic recirculation. Data on biliary excretion in horses are not available for most opioid agonists. The plasma half-lives of morphine, meperidine, and pentazocine in conjunction with the isolation in urine of both glucuronide conjugated and unconjugated metabolites suggest that opioid metabolites retain parent compound activity and that opioid effects may be prolonged. For example, morphine has a relatively short elimination half-life (40 to 60 minutes), but metabolites remain detectable in the plasma and urine of some horses for 5 to 6 and 144 hours, respectively (see Chapter 9).[183,184,197-199] Protein binding is variable and seemingly dose independent; it ranges from 20% to 40%.[197]

These data suggest that the metabolites of most opioid agonists and agonist-antagonists have the potential to be cumulative and that repeated dosing could produce untoward side effects.

Clinical Use and Antagonism

Opioids are generally administered intravenously or intramuscularly but can be administered transdermally or injected into the epidural and subarachnoid (intrathecal) space to produce localized or segmental analgesia (see Table 10-2 and Chapter 11).[4,83,200,201] Appropriate doses of morphine (0.1 mg/kg IV) improve analgesia and recovery from anesthesia.[181] Transdermal administration of fentanyl has been suggested as a relatively noninvasive method to provide analgesia for up to 48 hours, but analgesic efficacy has been questioned.[185] Epidural or subarachnoid (spinal) delivery of opioids facilitates drug binding to opioid receptors in the substantia gelatinosa of the dorsal horn of the spinal column. Drug clearance depends on dilution in cerebrospinal fluid, redistribution by bulk flow, binding to nervous tissue, and vascular absorption.[83] The intravenous administration of lower doses of opioid agonists (<0.1 mg/kg) to adult horses produces minimal changes in behavior, although decreased awareness, indifference, minor muscle tremors, and increased responsiveness to sound may occur. Some horses demonstrate moderate sedation by lowering their head. Others are reluctant to move and appear totally indifferent to their surroundings. They may begin to sweat or become noticeably ataxic. The quality of analgesia is highly variable and often unpredictable when opioids are administered as single therapy but is markedly improved by the coadministration of α_2-adrenoceptor agonists or acepromazine.[134-137,185,202-204] Repeated or large doses of opioid agonists or partial agonists (buprenorphine) frequently results in hyperresponsiveness, hyperexcitability, defecation, increased locomotor activity, sweating, tachycardia, hyperventilation, vocalization, and increases in body temperature in conscious horses.[179-172,204,205] These signs may persist for extended periods but can be diminished or abolished by administering an opioid antagonist or small doses of a tranquilizer or sedative-hypnotic.[170,206]

Opioid agonist, partial agonists, and agonist-antagonists are most useful when coadministered with sedative-hypnotic drugs to provide added analgesia for standing chemical restraint.[4] They can be administered alone for the treatment of pain, including colic (butorphanol); coadministered with α_2-adrenoceptor agonists; and infused as adjuncts to inhalation anesthesia, with strict adherence to dosage recommendations to avoid CNS excitatory effects (see Table 10-6; Chapter 13).[4] The use of the opioids to reduce inhalant anesthetic requirements continues to be controversial because of evidence suggesting either no or minimal effects on the inhalant anesthetic concentrations required to maintain anesthesia.[180,183,184] More controlled studies in horses are required to determine the efficacy of opioid agonists as adjuncts to anesthesia.

All known opioid agonists and agonist-antagonists are reversible with opioid antagonists (see Table 10-2). The intravenous administration of naloxone promptly reverses both the central and peripheral effects of opioid agonists, including behavioral and cardiorespiratory effects, locomotor activity, and analgesia.[206] The administration of naloxone also antagonizes endogenous opiates (enkephalins, endorphins), triggering pain, restlessness, and abdominal distress in some

horses.[207,208] Naloxone administration partially reverses the analgesia produced by sedative-hypnotics and inhalation anesthetics. This latter effect is worth considering in horses that have been administered an opioid agonist before or during surgery and demonstrate a significant degree of postoperative pain, require a long time to recover from anesthesia, or demonstrate marked ataxia during recovery. The use of opioid agonist-antagonists that possess minimal sedative but analgesic effects (butorphanol, buprenorphine) may be a more logical choice in such instances. Opioid antagonists may also inhibit stereotypic and self-mutilative behaviors in horses.[209] Intravenous administration of naloxone, naltrexone, nalmefene, and diprenorphine (opioid antagonists) completely abolished cribbing for periods lasting up to a week. Pawing was also abolished by narcotic antagonists.[209-210]

Complications, Side Effects, and Clinical Toxicity

The most common complications associated with the clinical use of opioid agonists and agonist-antagonists are disorientation, increased locomotor activity, hyperresponsiveness to touch and sound, and the development of ataxia (see Figure 10-19). Some horses appear sedate but can be aroused immediately (startled) by physical stimulation or a loud noise. Increasing doses of narcotics may worsen these responses and produce prolonged periods of increased locomotor activity and elevated body temperature. Constipation and impaction colic can occur after repeated administration of opioid agonists (see Figure 10-21). The feces become dry and hard. Stereotypic behavior such as pawing the floor, stall walking, or circling may develop and are believed to be caused by increased dopamine release in the brain or and increase in the sensitivity of dopamine receptors.[211] Extremely large doses of opioid agonists may produce seizures. The mechanism responsible for seizures is uncertain, but they can be controlled with sedative-hypnotic drugs and controlled ventilation. The administration of large (excessive) doses of opioid agonists or agonist-antagonists during intravenous or inhalant anesthesia can influence anesthetic requirements and may result in undesirable recovery. Most, if not all, of these complications can be antagonized by administering supportive hemodynamic therapies (fluids, dobutamine) or opioid antagonists (naloxone; see Figure 10-19). The administration of opioid antagonists that do not cross the blood-brain barrier (N-methylnaltrexone) has been suggested to prevent adverse gastrointestinal side effects without altering CNS-induced analgesic effects.[212] Naloxone may have to be readministered to conscious horses that have received longer-acting opioid agonists (morphine), although sedatives (acepromazine, α_2-adrenoceptor agonists) can be administered to horses demonstrating mild-to-moderate side effects. The administration of opioid agonists, agonist-antagonists, or partial agonists to foals usually produces stupor and analgesia but has not been investigated extensively.

SEDATIVE-HYPNOTIC, OPIOID, AND NONOPIOID DRUG COMBINATIONS

Lack of predictability, an inability to produce desired effects, and the development of side effects, particularly excitement and ataxia at higher doses, are the primary reasons why opioids are administered in combination with sedative-hypnotic

Table 10–6.	Sedative, nonopioid, and opioid drug combinations administered to horses	
Drug combination*	**Intravenous dose (mg/kg)**
Sedative-opioid	
Acepromazine-meperidine	0.04/0.6
Acepromazine-methadone	0.04/0.1
Acepromazine-hydromorphone	0.04/0.02
Acepromazine-butorphanol	0.04/0.02
Acepromazine-pentazocine	0.04/0.4
Xylazine-butorphanol	0.66/0.02
Xylazine-pentazocine	0.66/0.4
Xylazine-buprenorphine	0.6/0.01
Xylazine-morphine	0.6/0.3-0.66
Sedative-nonopioid	
Acepromazine-xylazine	0.02/0.5
Sedative-nonopioid-opioid	
Acepromazine-xylazine-butorphanol	0.02/0.66/0.03
Acepromazine-xylazine-pentazocine	0.02/0.66/0.3
Chloral hydrate-xylazine-morphine	2-6/0.66/0.3-0.66

*Detomidine can be substituted for xylazine in any listed drug combination at an intravenous dose of 2.5 to 5 µg/kg.

drugs (see Table 10-6). The practical benefits of adding a low dose of an opioid to a horse sedated with acepromazine or an α_2-adrenoceptor agonist to enhance sedation and produce analgesia have long been recognized. The combination of neuroleptics (acepromazine, promazine) and opioid analgesics (morphine, methadone, meperidine) has been popular in equine practice for decades. Regardless of personal opinion, there should be a logical and rational reason for combining drugs, particularly if cardiorespiratory depression or other side effects could be exacerbated. The goals for combining two or three drugs to produce standing sedation-analgesia in horses should be to increase predictability, enhance analgesia, and improve safety for the horse and attending personnel. Drugs that produce muscle relaxation as their primary effect (diazepam, midazolam) are of little benefit in standing horses because they may not improve sedation, are not analgesics, and can induce marked ataxia. Diazepam and midazolam are useful in combination with intravenous or inhalant anesthetics to improve muscle relaxation. Finally, clinical experience has demonstrated that some drug combinations are far superior to others for calming excited or fractious horses and improving analgesia. The simultaneous administration of the neuroleptic drug acepromazine and opioid analgesics (meperidine) was one of the first drug combinations ("lytic cocktail") to be used successfully as a sedative-analgesic horses.[213] Combinations of nonopioid and opioid analgesics (xylazine-morphine, xylazine-butorphanol, detomidine-butorphanol) are also considered as neuroleptanalgesics and are noted for their ability to produce profound sedation and analgesia. Clinically, the combination of reduced dosages of sedatives and nonopioid or opioid analgesics (acepromazine-xylazine, acepromazine-detomidine, xylazine-morphine) are known to produce better sedation and analgesia than either drug administered alone. Although some concern has been raised regarding the potential for hypotensive effects, no adverse side effects have been reported when used at recommended dosages (see Figure 10-17).

One potential advantage of drug combinations containing opioid or nonopioid analgesic effects is the potential to partially reverse side effects, should they occur (see Table 10-2). This may become important if sedation leads to severe ataxia, thus predisposing the horse or attending personnel to injury. Then again, α_2-adrenoceptor agonists should not be antagonized when administered in combination with moderate-to-large doses of opioid analgesics unless absolutely necessary. Reversal of their sedative effects could result in opioid-related CNS excitement, locomotor activity, and hyperthermia. The coadministration of multiple drugs for standing procedures in horses raises many unanswered questions regarding potential side effects, cardiopulmonary depression, and drug interactions. For these reasons the indiscriminate or random use of unexamined drug combinations is not recommended.

REFERENCES

1. Muir WW: Drugs used to produce standing chemical restraint in horses, *Vet Clin North Am (Large Anim Pract)* 3:17-44, 1981.
2. Taylor PM: Chemical restraint of the standing horse, *Equine Vet J* 17:269-273, 1985.
3. Taylor PM, Clarke KW: *Sedation and premedication: handbook of equine anaesthesia*, ed 2, Philadelphia, 2007, Elsevier, pp 17-32.
4. Bennett RC, Steffey EP: Use of opioids for pain and anesthetic management in horses. In Mama KR, Hendrickson DA, editors: *The veterinary clinics of North America (equine practice)*, Philadelphia, 2002, Saunders, pp 47-60.
5. Ducharme NG, Fubini SL: Gastrointestinal complications associated with the use of atropine in horses, *J Am Vet Med Assoc* 182:229-231, 1983.
6. Short CE et al: The use of atropine to control heart rate responses during detomidine sedation in horses, *Acta Vet Scand* 27:548-559, 1986.
7. Singh S et al: The effect of glycopyrrolate on heart rate and intestinal motility in conscious horses, *J Vet Anaesth* 241:14-19, 1997.
8. Teixeira Neto FJ et al: Effects of glycopyrrolate on cardiorespiratory function in horses anesthetized with halothane and xylazine, *Am J Vet Res* 65:456-463, 2004.
9. Teixeira Neto FJ et al: Effects of muscarinic type-2 antagonist on cardiorespiratory function and intestinal transit in horses anesthetized with halothane and xylazine, *Am J Vet Res* 65:464-472, 2004.
10. Gibb M: Acetylpromazine maleate, *Vet Rec* 102:291, 1978.
11. Martin JE, Beck JD: Some effects of chlorpromazine hydrochloride in horses, *Am J Vet Res* 17:678-686, 1956.
12. Hall LW: The effect of chlorpromazine on the cardiovascular system of the conscious horse, *Vet Rec* 72:85-87, 1960.
13. Wheat JD: Penile paralysis in stallions given propriopromazine, *J Am Vet Med Assoc* 148:405-406; 1966.
14. Booth NM: Psychotropic agents. In Booth NH, McDonald LE, editors: *Veterinary pharmacology and therapeutics*, ed 6, Ames, Ia, 1988, Iowa State University Press, pp 371-376.
15. Mysinger PW et al: Electroencephalographic patterns of clinically normal, sedated, and tranquilized newborn foals and adult horses, *Am J Vet Res* 46:36-41, 1985.
16. Baldessarini RJ Tarazi FI: Pharmacotherapy of psychosis and mania. In Goodman LS, Gilman S, editors: *The pharmacological basis of therapeutics*, ed 11, New York, 2006, McGraw-Hill, pp 461-481.
17. Combie J et al: Pharmacology of narcotic analgesics in the horse: selective blockade of narcotic-induced locomotor activity, *Am J Vet Res* 42:716-721, 1981.
18. Muir WW, Skarda RT, Sheehan WC: Hemodynamic and respiratory effects of a xylazine-acetylpromazine drug combination in horses, *Am J Vet Res* 40:1518-1522, 1979.
19. Walker M, Geiser D: Effects of acetylpromazine on the hemodynamics of the equine metatarsal artery, as determined by two-dimensional real-time and pulsed Doppler ultrasonography, *Am J Vet Res* 47:1075-1078, 1986.
20. Muir WW, Werner LL, Hamlin RL: Effects of xylazine and acetylpromazine upon induced ventricular fibrillation in dogs anesthetized with thiamylal and halothane, *Am J Vet Res* 36:1299-1303, 1975.
21. Steffey EP et al: Cardiovascular and respiratory effects of acetylpromazine and xylazine on halothane-anesthetized horses, *J Vet Pharmacol Ther* 8:290-302, 1985.
22. Muir WW, Hamlin RL: Effects of acetylpromazine on ventilatory variables in the horse, *Am J Vet Res* 36:1439-1442, 1975.
23. Gerring EL: Priapism after ACP in the horse, *Vet Rec* 109:64; 1981.
24. Nie GJ, Pope KC: Persistent penile prolapse associated with acute blood loss and acepromazine maleate administration in a horse, *Am J Vet Med Assoc* 211:587-589, 1997.
25. Sharrock AG: Reversal of drug-induced priapism in a gelding by medication, *Austral Vet J* 58:39-40, 1982.
26. Dalton RG: The significance of variations with activity and sedation in the hematocrit, plasma protein concentrations, and erythrocyte sedimentation rate of horses, *Br Vet J* 128:439-445, 1972.

27. DeMoor A et al: Influence of promazine on the venous haematocrit and plasma protein concentration in the horse, *Zentralbl Veterinarmed* 25:189-197, 1978.
28. Courtot D, Mouthon G, Mestries JC: The effect of acetyl-promazine medication on red blood cell metabolism in the horse, *Ann Rev Vet* 9:17-24, 1978.
29. Parry BW, Anderson GA: Influence of acepromazine maleate on the equine haematocrit, *J Vet Pharmacol Ther* 6:121-126, 1983.
30. Ballard S et al: The pharmacokinetics, pharmacological responses, and behavioral effects of acepromazine in the horse, *J Vet Pharmacol Ther* 5:21-31, 1982.
31. Persson SGB: The circulatory significance of the splenic red cells pool. In Proceedings of the First International Symposium on Equine Hematology, East Lansing, Michigan, 1975, pp 303-310.
32. Persson SGB et al: Circulatory effects of splenectomy in the horse. I. Effect on red cell distribution and variability of haematocrit in the peripheral blood, *Zentralbl Veterinarmed* 20:441-455, 1973.
33. Persson SGB et al: Circulatory effects of splenectomy in the horse. II. Effect of plasma volume and total circulating red cell volume, *Zentralbl Veterinarmed* 20:456-468, 1973.
34. Lumsden JH, Valli VEO, McSherry BJ: The comparison of erythrocyte and leukocyte response to epinephrine and acepromazine maleate in standardbred horses. In Proceedings of the First International Symposium on Equine Hematology, East Lansing, Michigan, 1975, pp 516-523.
35. Meagher DM, Tasker JB: Effects of excitement and tranquilization on the equine hemogram, *Mod Vet Pract* 53:41-43, 1972.
36. Marroum PJ et al: Pharmacokinetics and pharmacodynamics of acepromazine in horses, *Am J Vet Res* 55(10):1428-1433, 1994.
37. Hashem A, Keller H. Disposition, bioavailability, and clinical efficacy of orally administered acepromazine in the horse, *J Vet Pharamcol Ther* 16:359-368; 1093.
38. Chou CC et al: Development and use of an enzyme-linked immunosorbent assay to monitor serum and urine acepromazine concentrations in thoroughbreds and possible changes associated with exercise, *Am J Vet Res* 59(5):593-597; 1998.
39. Raker CW, English B: Promazine—its pharmacological and clinical effects in horses, *J Am Vet Med Assoc* 134:19-22, 1959.
40. Raker CW, Savers AC: Promazine as a preanesthetic agent in horses, *J Am Vet Med Assoc* 134:23-24, 1959.
41. Jacobsen CE: Morphine-promazine: a better preanesthetic, *Mod Vet Pract* 51:29-30, 1970.
42. Hubbell JA et al: Cardiorespiratory and metabolic effects of xylazine, detomidine, and a combination of xylazine and acepromazine administered after exercise in horses, *Am J Vet Res* 60:1271-1279, 1999.
43. Muir WW, Mason DE: Effects of diazepam, acepromazine, detomidine, and xylazine on thiamylal anesthesia in horses, *J Am Vet Med Assoc* 203:1031-1038, 1993.
44. Doherty TJ, Geiser DR, Rohrback BW: Effect of acepromazine and butorphanol on halothane minimum alveolar concentration in ponies, *Equine Vet J* 29:374-376; 1997.
45. Johnston GM et al: The confidential enquiry into perioperative equine fatalities (CEPEF): mortality results of phases 1 and 2, *Vet Anaesth Analg* 29:159-170, 2002.
46. Marntell S et al: Effects of acepromazine on pulmonary gas exchange and circulation during sedation and dissociative anaesthesia in horses, *Vet Anaesth Analg* 32(2):83-93, 2005.
47. Fuentes VO: Short-term immobilization in the horse with ketamine HCl and promazine HCl considerations, *Equine Vet J* 10:78-81, 1978.
48. Jones RS: Methylamphetamine as an antagonist of some tranquillizing drugs in the horse, *Vet Rec* 75:1157-1159, 1963.

49. Aitken MM, Sanford J: Effects of tranquilizers on tachycardia induced by adrenaline in the horse, *Br Vet J* 128:vii-ix, 1972.
50. Jones RS: Penile paralysis in stallions, *J Am Vet Med Assoc* 149:124, 1966.
51. Boyer K et al: Penile hematoma in a stallion resulting in proximal penile amputation, *Equine Pract* 17:8-11; 1995.
52. Christian RG, Mills JHL, Kramer LL: Accidental intracarotid artery injection of promazine in the horse, *Can Vet J* 15:29-33, 1974.
53. Gabel AA: The effects of intracarotid artery injection of drugs in domestic animals, *J Am Vet Med Assoc* 142:1397-1403, 1963.
54. Booth NM: Psychotropic agents. In Booth NH, McDonald LE, editors: *Veterinary pharmacology and therapeutics*, ed 6, Ames, Ia, 1988, Iowa State University Press, pp 382-385.
55. Lees P and Serrano L: Effects of azaperone on cardiovascular and respiratory functions in the horse, *Br J Pharmacol* 56:263-269, 1976.
56. Serrano L, Lees P: The applied pharmacology of azaperone in ponies, *Res Vet Sci* 20:316-323, 1976.
57. Serrano L, Lees P, and Hillidge CJ: Influence of azaperone/metomidate anaesthesia on blood biochemistry in the horse, *Br Vet J* 132:405-415, 1976.
58. Dodman NH, Waterman E: Paradoxical excitement following the intravenous administration of azaperone in the horse, *Equine Vet J* 11:33-35, 1979.
59. Charney DS, Mihic SJ, Harris RA: Hypnotics and sedatives. In Goodman LS, Gilman S, editors: *The pharmacological basis of therapeutics*, ed 11, New York, 2006, McGraw-Hill, pp 401-414.
60. Kaegi B: Anesthesia by injection of xylazine, ketamine, and the benzodiazepine derivative climazolam and the use of the benzodiazepine antagonist Ro 15-3505], *Schweiz Arch Tierheilkd* 132(5):251-257, 1990.
61. Bettschart-Wolfensberger R et al: Physiologic effects of anesthesia induced and maintained by intravenous administration of a climazolam-ketamine combination in ponies premedicated with acepromazine and xylazine, *Am J Vet Res* 57(10):1472-1477, 1996.
62. Muir WW, Werner LL, Hamlin RL: Antiarrhythmic effects of diazepam during coronary artery occlusion in dogs, *Am J Vet Res* 36:1203-1206, 1975.
63. McDonnell SM, Garcia MC, Kenney RM: Pharmacological manipulation of sexual behaviour in stallions, *J Reprod Fertil* 35(suppl):45-49, 1987.
64. Brown RF, Houpt KA, Schryver HF: Stimulation of food intake in horses by diazepam and promazine, *Pharmacol Biochem Behav* 5:495-497, 1976.
65. Muir WW et al: Pharmacodynamic and pharmacokinetic properties of diazepam in horses, *Am J Vet Res* 43:1756-1762, 1982.
66. Shini S, Klaus AM, Hapke HJ: Kinetics of elimination of diazepam after intravenous injection in horses, *Dtsch Tierarztl Wochenschr* 104(1):22-25, 1997.
67. Norman WM, Court MH, Greenblatt DJ: Age-related changes in the pharmacokinetic disposition of diazepam in foals, *Am J Vet Res* 58(8):878-880, 1997.
68. Klein LV, Klide AM: Central α₂-adrenergic and benzodiazepine agonists and their antagonists, *J Zoo Wildl Med* 20:138-153, 1989.
69. Muir WW et al: Comparison of four drug combinations for total intravenous anesthesia of horses undergoing surgical removal of an abdominal testis, *J Am Vet Med Assoc* 217(6):869-873, 2000.
70. Hubbell JA et al: Anesthetic, cardiorespiratory, and metabolic effects of four intravenous anesthetic regimens induced in horses immediately after maximal exercise, *Am J Vet Res* 61(12):1545-1552: 2000.

71. Matthews NS, Dollar NS, Shawley RV: Halothane-sparing of benzodiazepines in ponies, *Cornell Vet* 80:259-265, 1990.

72. England GC, Clarke KW, Goossens L: A comparison of the sedative effects of three α_2-adrenoceptor agonists (romifidine, detomidine and xylazine) in the horse, *J Vet Pharmacol Ther* 15(2):194-201, 1992.

73. England GC, Clarke KW: α_2-adrenoceptor agonists in the horse: a review, *Br Vet J* 152(6): 641-657; 1996.

74. Daunt DA, Steffey EP: α_2-Adrenergic agonists as analgesics in horses, *Vet Clin North Am (Equine Pract)* 18(1):39-46, 2002.

75. Bettschart-Wolfensberger R et al: Cardiopulmonary effects and pharmacokinetics of IV dexmedetomidine in ponies, *Equine Vet J* 37(1):60-64, 2005.

76. Dirikolu L et al: Clonidine in horses: identification, detection, and clinical pharmacology, *Vet Ther* 7(2):141-155, 2006.

77. Virtanen R, Ruskoaho H, Nyman L: Pharmacological evidence for the involvement of α_2-adrenoceptors in the sedative effect of detomidine, a novel sedative-analgesic, *J Vet Pharmacol Ther* 8:30-37, 1985.

78. Clarke KW, Hall LW: "Xylazine"—a new sedative for horses and cattle, *Vet Rec* 85:512-517, 1969.

79. Yamashita K et al: Cardiovascular effects of medetomidine, detomidine, and xylazine in horses, *J Vet Med Sci* 62(10):1025-1032, 2000.

80. LemkeKA: Anticholinergics and sedatives. In Tranquilli WJ, Thurmon JC, Grimm KA, editors: *Lumb & Jones veterinary anesthesia and analgesia*, ed 4, 2007, Ames, Iowa, Blackwell Publishing, pp 210-224.

81. Steffey EP et al: Effects of xylazine hydrochloride during isoflurane-induced anesthesia in horses, *Am J Vet Res* 61(10):1225-1231, 2000.

82. Steffey EP, Pascoe PJ: Detomidine reduces isoflurane anesthetic requirement (MAC) in horses, *Vet Anaesth Analg* 29:223-227, 2002.

83. Robinson EP, Natalini CC: Epidural anesthesia and analgesia in horses, *Vet Clin North Am (Equine Pract)* 18(1):61-82, 2002.

84. Doze VA, Chen B-X, Maze M: Dexmedetomidine produces a hypnotic-anesthetic action in rats via activation of central α_2-adrenoceptors, *Anesthesiology* 71:75-79, 1989.

85. Schmitt H, Fournadjiev G, Schmitt H: Central and peripheral effects of 2-(2,6-dimethylphenyl amino)-4-H-5,6-dihydro-1,3 thiazin (Bayer 1470) on the sympathetic system, *Eur J Pharmacol* 10:230-238, 1970.

86. Guo TZ et al: Central α_1-adrenoceptor stimulation functionally antagonizes the hypnotic response to dexmedetomidine, an α_2-adrenoceptor agonist, *Anesthesiology* 75 (2):252-256, 1991.

87. ThamSM et al: Synergistic and additive interactions of the cannabinoid agonist CP55,940 with mu opioid receptor and α_2-adrenoceptor agonists in acute pain models in mice, *Br J Pharmacol* 144(6):875-884, 2005.

88. Yamashita K et al: Antagonistic effects of atipamezole on medetomidine-induced sedation in horses, *J Vet Med Sci* 58(10):1049-1052, 1996.

89. Skarda RT, Muir WW III: Effects of intravenously administered yohimbine on antinociceptive, cardiorespiratory, and postural changes induced by epidural administration of detomidine hydrochloride solution to healthy mares, *Am J Vet Res* 60(10):1262-1270, 1999.

90. Hubbell JA, Muir WW: Antagonism of detomidine sedation in the horse using intravenous tolazoline or atipamezole, *Equine Vet J* 38(3):238-241, 2006.

91. Hoffman PE: Clinical evaluation of xylazine as a chemical restraining agent, sedative, and analgesic in horses, *J Am Vet Med Assoc* 164:42-45, 1974.

92. Freeman SL, England GC: Investigation of romifidine and detomidine for the clinical sedation of horses, *Vet Rec* 147:507-511, 2000.

93. Reitemeyer H, Klein HJ, Deegen E: The effect of sedatives on lung function in horses, *Acta Vet Scand* 82(suppl):111-120, 1986.

94. Wagner AE, Muir WW, Hinchcliff KW: Cardiovascular effects of xylazine and detomidine in horses, *Am J Vet Res* 52(5):651-657, 1991.

95. Lavoie JP, Phan ST, Blais D: Effects of a combination of detomidine and butorphanol on respiratory function in horses with or without chronic obstructive pulmonary disease, *Am J Vet Res* 57(5):705-709, 1996.

96. Lavoie JP, Pascoe JR, Kurpershoek CJ: Effect of head and neck position on respiratory mechanics in horses sedated with xylazine, *Am J Vet Res.* 53(9):1652-1657, 1992.

97. Broadstone RV et al: Effects of xylazine on airway function in ponies with recurrent airway obstruction, *Am J Vet Res* 53(10):1813-1817, 1992.

98. Lindegaard C et al: Sedation with detomidine and acepromazine influences the endoscopic evaluation of laryngeal function in horses, *Equine Vet J* 39(6):553-556, 2007.

99. Gasthuys F et al: A preliminary study on the effects of atropine sulphate on bradycardia and heart blocks during romifidine sedation in the horse, *Vet Res Commun* 14:489-502, 1990.

100. Bueno AC et al: Cardiopulmonary and sedative effects of intravenous administration of low doses of medetomidine and xylazine to adult horses, *Am J Vet Res* 60:1371-1376, 1999.

101. Muir WW, Pipers PS: Effects of xylazine on indices of myocardial contractility in the dog, *Am J Vet Res* 38:931-934, 1977.

102. Figueiredo JP et al: Sedative and analgesic effects of romifidine in horses, *Int J Appl Res Vet Med* 3(3):249-258, 2005.

103. Klein LV, Sherman J: Effects of preanesthetic medication, anesthesia, and position of recumbency on central venous pressure in horses, *J Am Vet Med Assoc* 170:216-219, 1977.

104. Roger T, Ruckebusch Y: Colonic α_2-adrenoceptor-mediated responses in the pony, *J Vet Pharmacol Ther* 10:310-318, 1987.

105. Stick JA et al: Effects of xylazine on equine intestinal vascular resistance, motility, compliance, and oxygen consumption, *Am J Vet Res* 48:198-203, 1987.

106. Rutkowski JA, Ross MW, Cullen K: Effects of xylazine and/or butorphanol or neostigmine on myoelectric activity of the cecum and right ventral colon in female ponies, *Am J Vet Res* 50:1096-1101, 1989.

107. Watson TD, Sullivan M: Effects of detomidine on equine oesophageal function as studied by contrast radiography, *Vet Rec* 129 (4):67-69, 1991.

108. Singh S et al: Modification of cardiopulmonary and intestinal motility effects of xylazine with glycopyrrolate in horses, *Can J Vet Res* 61(2):99-107, 1997.

109. Grubb TL et al: Use of yohimibine to reverse prolonged effects of xylazine hydrochloride in a horse being treated with chloramphenicol, *J Am Vet Med Assoc* 210:1771-1773, 1997.

110. Lester GD et al: Effect of α_2-adrenergic, cholinergic, and nonsteriodal anti-inflammatory drugs on myoelectric activity of ileum, cecum, and right ventral colon and on cecal emptying of radiolabeled markers in clinically normal ponies, *Am J Vet Res* 59:320-327, 1998.

111. Merrit AM, Furrow JA, Hartless CS: Effect of xylazine, detomidine, and a combination of xylazine and butorphanol on equine duodenal motility, *Am J Vet Res* 59:619-623, 1998.

112. Sutton DG et al: The effects of xylazine, detomidine, and butorphanol on equine solid phase gastric emptying rate, *Equine Vet J* 34(5):486-492, 2002.

113. Angel I, Bidet S, Langer SZ: Pharmacological characterization of the hyperglycemia induced by α_2-adrenoceptor agonists, *J Pharmacol Exp Ther* 246:1098-1103, 1988.

114. Thurmon JC et al: Xylazine hydrochloride-induced hyperglycemia and hypoinsulinemia in thoroughbred horses, *J Vet Pharmacol Ther* 5:241-245, 1982.

115. Gasthuys F et al: Hyperglycaemia and diuresis during sedation with detomidine in the horse, *J Vet Med* 34:641-648, 1987.

116. Gasthuys F, Vandenhende C, deMoor A: Biochemical changes in blood and urine during halothane anaesthesia with detomidine premedication in the horse, *J Vet Med* 35:655-665, 1988.

117. Latimer FG et al: Cardiopulmonary, blood, and peritoneal fluid alterations associated with abdominal insufflation of carbon dioxide in standing horses, *Equine Vet J* 35(3):283-290, 2003.

118. Trim CM, Hanson RR: Effects of xylazine on renal function and plasma glucose in ponies, *Vet Rec* 118:65-67, 1986.

119. Nunez E et al: Effects of α_2-adrenergic receptor agonists on urine production in horses deprived of food and water, *Am J Vet Res* 65:1342-1346, 2004.

120. Schatzmann U et al: Effects of α_2-agonists on intrauterine pressure and sedation in horses: comparison between detomidine, romifidine, and xylazine, *Zentralbl Veterinarmed A* 41(7):523-529, 1994.

121. Luukkanen L, Katila T, Koskinen E: Some effects of multiple administrations of detomidine during the last trimester of equine pregnancy, *Equine Vet J* 29(5):400-403; 1997.

122. Oijala M, Katila T: Detomidine (Domosedan) in foals: sedative and analgesic effects, *Equine Vet J* 20:327-330, 1988.

123. Robertson SA et al: Effects of intravenous xylazine hydrochloride on blood glucose, plasma insulin, and rectal temperature in neonatal foals, *Equine Vet J* 22(1):43-47, 1990.

124. Garcia-Villar R et al: The pharmacokinetics of xylazine hydrochloride: an interspecific study, *J Vet Pharmacol Ther* 4:87-92, 1981.

125. Salonen JS: Single-dose pharmacokinetics of detomidine in the horse and cow, *J Vet Pharmacol Ther* 12(1):65-72, 1989.

126. Bettschart-Wolfensberger R et al: Pharmacokinetics of medetomidine in ponies and elaboration of a medetomidine infusion regime which provides a constant level of sedation, *Res Vet Sci* 67(1):41-46; 1999.

127. Bettschart-Wolfensberger R et al: Cardiopulmonary effects and pharmacokinetics of intravenous dexmedetomidine in ponies *Equine Vet J* 37(1):60-64, 2005.

128. Lowe JE, Hilfinger J: Analgesic and sedative effects of detomidine in a colic model: blind studies on efficacy and duration of effects, *Proc Am Assoc Equine Pract* 30:225-234, 1984.

129. Kerr DD et al: Sedative and other effects of xylazine given intravenously to horses, *Am J Vet Res* 33:525-532, 1972.

130. Kerr DD et al: Comparison of the effects of xylazine and acetylpromazine maleate in the horse, *Am J Vet Res* 33:777-784, 1972.

131. Greene SA, Thurmon JC: Xylazine—a review of its pharmacology and use in veterinary medicine, *J Vet Pharmacol Ther* 11:295-313, 1988.

132. Freeman SL, England GC: Comparison of sedative effects of romifidine following intravenous, intramuscular, and sublingual administration to horses, *Am J Vet Res* 60(8):954-959, 1999.

133. Ramsay EC et al: Serum concentrations and effects of detomidine delivered orally to horses in three different mediums, *Vet Anaesth Analg* 29:219-222, 2002.

134. Bryant CE, England GC, Clarke KW: Comparison of the sedative effects of medetomidine and xylazine in horses, *Vet Rec* 29(19):421-423, 1991.

135. Muir WW, Skarda RT, Sheehan WC: Hemodynamic and respiratory effects of xylazine-morphine sulfate in horses, *Am J Vet Res* 40:1417-1420, 1979.

136. Robertson JT, Muir WW: A new analgesic drug combination in the horse, *Am J Vet Res* 44:1667-1669, 1983.

137. Brunson DB, Majors LJ: Comparative analgesia of xylazine, xylazine/morphine, xylazine/butorphanol, and xylazine/nalbuphine in the horse, using dental dolorimetry, *Am J Vet Res* 48:1087-1091, 1987.

138. Virtanen R et al: Characterization of the selectivity, specificity, and potency of medetomidine as an α_2-adrenoceptor agonist, *Eur J Pharmacol* 20:150(1-2):9-14; 1988.

139. Jochle W, Hamm D: Sedation and analgesia with Domosedan (detomidine hydrochloride) in horses: dose-response studies on efficacy and its duration: Domosedan symposium, *Acta Vet Scand* 82(suppl):69-84, 1986.

140. Carter SW et al: Cardiopulmonary effects of xylazine sedation in the foal, *Equine Vet J* 22(6):384-388; 1990.

141. Santos M et al: Effects of α_2-adrenoceptor agonists during recovery from isoflurane anaesthesia in horses, *Equine Vet J* 35(2):170-175, 2003.

142. Yamashita K et al: Antagonistic effects of atipamezole on medetomidine-induced sedation in horses, *J Vet Med Sci* 58(10):1049-1052, 1996.

143. Kollias-Baker CA, Court MH, Williams LL: Influence of yohimbine and tolazoline on the cardiovascular, respiratory, and sedative effects of xylazine in the horse, *J Vet Pharmacol Ther* 16(3):350-358, 1993.

144. Ramseyer B, et al: Antagonism of detomidine sedation with atipamezole in horses, *J Vet Anaesth* 25(1):47-51, 1998.

145. Short CE, Grover CD: The use of doxapram hydrochloride with inhalation anesthetics in horses, part II, *Vet Med (Sm Anim Clin)* 65:260-261, 1970.

146. Katila T, Oijala M. The effect of detomidine (Domosedan) on the maintenance of equine pregnancy and fetal development: ten cases, *Equine Vet J* 20:323-326, 1988.

147. Muir WW, Werner LL, Hamlin RL: Effects of xylazine and acetylpromazine upon induced ventricular fibrillation in dogs anesthetized with thiamylal and halothane, *Am J Vet Res* 36:1299-1303, 1975.

148. Gaynor JS, Bednarski RM, Muir WW: Effect of hypercapnia on the arrhythmogenic dose of epinephrine in horses anesthetized with guaifenesin, thiamylal sodium, and halothane, *Am J Vet Res* 54(2):315-321, 1993.

149. Fuentes VO: Sudden death in a stallion after xylazine medication, *Vet Rec* 102:106, 1978.

150. Taylor PM: Possible potentiated sulphonamide and detomidine interactions, *Vet Rec* 6:122(6):143, 1988.

151. Gerlach AT, Dasta JF: Dexmedetomidine: an updated review, *Ann Pharmacother* 41(2):245-252, 2007.

152. Velez LI et al: Systemic toxicity after an ocular exposure to xylazine hydrochloride, *J Emerg Med* 30(4):407-410, 2006.

153. Carruthers SC et al: Xylazine hydrochloride (Rompun) overdose in man, *Clin Toxicol* 15:281-285, 1979.

154. Singh VK et al: Molecular biology of opioid receptors: recent advances, *Neuroimmunomodulation* 4(5-6):285-297, 1997.

155. Alexander SPH, Mathie A, Peters JA: Guide to receptors and channels (GRAC), (2007 revision), *Br J Pharmacol* 150(suppl 1):S1–S168, 2007.

156. Seal US et al: Chemical immobilization and blood analysis of feral horses (Equus caballus), *J Wildl Dis* 21(4):411-416; 1985.

157. Gutstein HB, Huda A: Opioid analgesics. In Goodman LS, Gilman S editors: *The pharmacological basis of therapeutics*, ed 11, edited by Brunton LL, Lazo JS, Parker KL. New York, 2006, McGraw-Hill, pp 547-590.

158. Herz A: Multiple opiate receptors and their functional significance, *J Neural Transm* 18(suppl):227-233, 1983.

159. Thorpe DH: Opiate structure and activity—a guide to understanding the receptor, *Anesth Analg* 63:143-151, 1984.

160. Ossipov MH, Suarez LJ, Spaulding TC: A comparison of the antinociceptive and behavioral effects of intrathecally administered opiates, α_2-adrenergic agonists, and local anesthetics in mice and rats, *Anesth Analg* 67:616-624, 1988.

161. Lal H: Narcotic dependence, narcotic action and dopamine receptors, *Life Sci* 17:483-496, 1978.

162. Hellyer PW et al: Comparison of opioid and α_2-adrenergic receptor binding in horse and dog brain using radioligand autoradiography, *Vet Anaesth Analg* 30(3):172-182, 2003.

163. Kamerling SG et al: Dose-related effects of ethyl ketazocine on nociception, behaviour, and autonomic responses in the horse, *J Pharm Pharmacol* 38:40-45, 1986.

164. Kamerling S et al: Dose-related effects of the kappa agonist U-50 488H on behaviour, nociception, and autonomic response in the horse, *Equine Vet J* 20:114-118, 1988.

165. DeLuca A, Coupar IM: Insights into opioid action in the intestinal tract, *Pharmacol Ther* 69(2):103-115; 1996.

166. Kurz A, Sessler DI: Opioid-induced bowel dysfunction: pathophysiology and potential new therapies, *Drugs* 63(7):649-671, 2003.

167. Boscan P et al: Evaluation of the effects of the opioid agonist morphine on gastrointestinal tract function in horses, *Am J Vet Res* 67(6):992-997; 2006.

168. Muir WW, Skarda RT, Sheehan WC: Cardiopulmonary effects of narcotic agonists and a partial agonist in horses, *Am J Vet Res* 39:1632-1635, 1978.

169. Combie J et al: The pharmacology of narcotic analgesics in the horse. IV. Dose- and time-response relationships for behavioral responses to morphine, meperidine, pentazocine, anileridine, methadone, and hydromorphine, *J Equine Med Surg* 3:377-385, 1979.

170. Tobin T, Woods WE: Pharmacology review: actions of central stimulant drugs in the horse, *Equine Vet J* 3:60-66, 1979.

171. Tobin T et al: The pharmacology of narcotic analgesics in the horse. III. Characteristics of the locomotor effects of fentanyl and apomorphine, *J Equine Med Surg* 3:284-288, 1979.

172. Kamerling SG et al: Dose-related effects of fentanyl on autonomic and behavioral responses in performance horses, *Gen Pharmacol* 16:253-258, 1985.

173. Kalpravidh M: Effects of butorphanol, flunixin, levorphanol, morphine, and xylazine in ponies, *Am J Vet Res* 45(2):217-223, 1984.

174. Muir WW, Robertson JT: Visceral analgesia: effects of xylazine, butorphanol, meperidine, and pentazocine in horses, *Am J Vet Res* 46:2081-2084, 1985.

175. Roger T, Bardon T, Ruckebusch Y: Comparative effects of mu and kappa opiate agonists on the cecocolic motility in the pony, *Can J Vet Res* 58:163-166, 1994.

176. Skarda RT, Muir WW: Comparison of electroacupuncture and butorphanol on respiratory and cardiovascular effects and rectal pain threshold after controlled rectal distention in mares, *Am J Vet Res* 64(2):137-144, 2003.

177. Sellon DC et al: Effects of continuous-rate infusion of butorphanol on physiologic and outcome variables in horses after celiotomy, *J Vet Intern Med* 18:555-563, 2004.

178. Spadavecchia C et al: Effects of butorphanol on the withdrawal reflex using threshold, suprathreshold, and repeated subthreshold electrical stimuli in conscious horses, *Vet Anaesth Analg* 34(1):48-58, 2007.

179. Matthews NS, Lindsay SL: Effect of low-dose butorphanol on halothane minimum alveolar concentration in ponies, *Equine Vet J* 22:325-327, 1990.

180. Clark L et al: Effects of perioperative morphine administration during halothane anaesthesia in horses, *Vet Anaesth Analg* 32:10-15, 2005.

181. Clark L et al: The effects of morphine on the recovery of horses from halothane anaesthesia, *Vet Anaesth Analg* 35(1):22-29, 2008.

182. Mircica E et al: Problems associated with perioperative morphine in horses: a retrospective study, *Vet Anaesth Analg* 30(3):147-155, 2003.

183. Steffey EP, Eisele JH, Baggot JD: Interactions of morphine and isoflurane in horses, *Am J Vet Res* 64(2):166-175, 2003.

184. Thomasy SM et al: The effects of IV fentanyl administration on the minimum alveolar concentration of isoflurane in horses, *Br J Anaesth* 97(2):232-237, 2006.

185. Sanchez LC et al: Effect of fentanyl on visceral and somatic nociception in conscious horses, *J Vet Intern Med* 21(5):1067-1075, 2007.

186. Nolan AM, Chambers JP, Hale GJ: The cardiorespiratory effects of morphine and butorphanol in horses anaesthetized under clinical conditions, *J Vet Anaesth* 18:19-24, 1991.

187. Weld JM et al: The effects of naloxone on endotoxic and hemorrhagic shock in horses, *Res Commun Chem Pathol Pharmacol* 44(2):227-238, 1984.

188. Liu LM et al: Subclass opioid receptors associated with the cardiovascular depression after traumatic shock and the antishock effects of its specific receptor antagonists, *Shock* 24(5):470-475, 2005.

189. Adams SB, Lamer CH, Masty J: Motility of the distal portion of the jejunum and pelvic flexure in ponies: effects of six drugs, *Am J Vet Res* 45:795-799, 1984.

190. Kohn CW, Muir WW: Selected aspects of the clinical pharmacology of visceral analgesics and gut motility modifying drugs in the horse, *J Vet Intern Med* 2:85-91, 1988.

191. Taguchi A et al: Selective postoperative inhibition of gastrointestinal opioid receptors, *N Engl J Med* 345:935-940, 2001.

192. Senior JM et al: Retrospective study of the risk factors and prevalence of colic in horses after orthopaedic surgery, *Vet Rec* 155(11):321-325, 2004.

193. Andersen MS et al: Risk factors for colic in horses after general anaesthesia for MRI or nonabdominal surgery: absence of evidence of effect from perianaesthetic morphine, *Equine Vet J* 38(4):368-374; 2006.

194. Proudman CJ et al: Preoperative and anaesthesia-related risk factors for mortality in equine colic cases, *Vet J* 171(1):89-97, 2006.

195. Burford JH, Corley KT: Morphine-associated pruritus after single extradural administration in a horse, *Vet Anaesth Analg* 33(3):193-198, 2006.

196. Aurich C, Aurich JE, Parvizi N: Opioidergic inhibition of luteinizing hormone and prolactin release changes during pregnancy in pony mares, *J Endocrinol* 169(3):511-518, 2001.

197. Combie JD, Nugent TE, Tobin T: Pharmacokinetics and protein binding of morphine in horses, *Am J Vet Res* 44:870-874, 1983.

198. Tobin T, Miller JR: The pharmacology of narcotic analgesics in the horse. I: The detection, pharmacokinetics, and urinary "clearance time" of pentazocine, *Equine Vet J* 3:191-199, 1979.

199. Kollias-Baker C, Sams R: Detection of morphine in blood and urine samples from horses administered poppy seeds and morphine sulfate orally, *J Anal Toxicol* 26(2):81-86, 2002.

200. Maxwell LK et al: Pharmacokinetics of fentanyl following intravenous and transdermal administration in horses, *Equine Vet J* 35(5):484-490, 2003.

201. Orsini JA et al: Pharmacokinetics of fentanyl delivered transdermally in healthy adult horses—variability among horses and its clinical implications, *J Vet Pharmacol Ther* 29(6):539-546, 2006.

202. Clarke KW, Paton BS: Combined use of detomidine with opiates in the horse, *Equine Vet J* 20:331-334, 1988.

203. Corletto F, Raisis AA, Brearley JC: Comparison of morphine and butorphanol as pre-aneaesthetic agents in combination with romifidine for field castration in ponies, *Vet Anaesth Analg* 32:16-22, 2005

204. Pascoe PJ et al: The pharmacokinetics and locomotor activity of alfentanil in the horse, *J Vet Pharmacol Ther* 14:317-325, 1991.

205. Carregaro AB et al: Effects of buprenorphine on nociception and spontaneous locomotor activity in horses, *Am J Vet Res* 68(3):246-250, 2007. Erratum in *Am J Vet Res* 68(5):523, 2007.

206. Combie J et al: Pharmacology of narcotic analgesics in the horse: selective blockade of narcotic-induced locomotor activity, *Am J Vet Res* 42(5):716-721, 1981.

207. Stevens DR, Klemm WR: Morphine-naloxone interactions: a role for non-specific morphine excitatory effects in withdrawal, *Science* 205:1379-1380, 1979.

208. Kamerline SB, Harma JG, Bagwell CA: Naloxone-induced abdominal distress in the horse, *Equine Vet J* 22(4):241-243, 1990.

209. Dodman NH et al: Investigation into the use of narcotic antagonists in the treatment of a stereotypic behavior pattern (crib-biting) in the horse, *Am J Vet Res* 48:311-319, 1987.

210. Dodman NH et al: Use of narcotic antagonist (nalmefene) to suppress self-mutilative behavior in a stallion, *J Am Vet Med Assoc* 192(11):1585-1586, 1988.

211. Kiley-Worthington M: Stereotypes in horses, *Equine Pract* 5:34-40, 1983.

212. Boscan P et al: Pharmacokinetics of the opioid antagonist N-methyl naltrexone and evaluation of its effects on gastrointestinal tract function in horses treated or not treated with morphine, *Am J Vet Res* 67(6):998-1004, 2006.

213. Jones RS: A review of tranquillisation and sedation in large animals, *Vet Rec* 90(22):613-717, 1972.

11

Local Anesthetic Drugs and Techniques

Roman T. Skarda

William W. Muir

John A.E. Hubbell

KEY POINTS

1. Local anesthetic drugs block sensory and motor nerve activity, producing analgesia and loss of function.
2. Local anesthetics with greater lipid solubility are more potent. Those that are more diffusible produce a faster onset of effect, whereas those that are more protein bound have a longer duration of action.
3. Local anesthetics can be administered at specific sites (local block), near nerves (regional block), topically, and by infusion.
4. Local anesthetics produce analgesic, antiarrhythmic, antishock, central nervous system depressant, anesthetic sparring, mild antiinflammatory, and gastrointestinal promotility effects.
5. Local anesthetics are metabolized in the liver, and metabolites are excreted in the urine. Metabolism and elimination are affected minimally by anesthesia.
6. Local anesthetic overdose can produce bradycardia, heart block, hypotension, delirium, seizures, and respiratory and cardiac arrest. These effects are exaggerated in hypoxemic and acidotic horses.
7. Optimal production of local anesthetic effects depends on the accurate anatomical deposition of the recommended dose of the appropriate drug: meticulous technique.

Local anesthetic drugs are designed to penetrate peripheral nerve barriers and interrupt nerve conduction, thereby producing reversible anesthesia (analgesia) for a predictable duration.[1] Infiltration (local anesthesia), topical application, and peripheral nerve blocks (regional anesthesia), including caudal epidural anesthesia, are the most common local anesthetic techniques used in horses.[2] Major infiltrations of local anesthetic (cervicothoracic ganglion block, sympathetic ganglion block) and central neural blockade techniques (caudal subarachnoid anesthesia, segmental lumbar subarachnoid anesthesia) are used occasionally in special situations. The local anesthetic drug selected and the technical proficiency of the individual performing the procedure (e.g., infiltration, regional) are major determinants of the rate of onset, the duration of drug effect, and the potential for complications (Box 11-1). Most complications are related to inadvertent drug overdose and technique failures, although occasional idiosyncratic and allergic drug reactions occur.

PHYSIOLOGY OF NERVE TRANSMISSION

The conduction of electrical impulses in excitable membranes requires the flow of sodium ions through ion selective channels in response to depolarization of the nerve cell membrane.[3] At rest the concentration of sodium ions is higher outside than inside the nerve, and a transmembrane potential known as the *resting membrane potential* (–70 mV) exists. The permeability of the membrane to sodium ions increases transiently when the nerve is stimulated (depolarized), allowing sodium ions to pass through the membrane by way of sodium selective ion channels that first open and then close in response to depolarization of the membrane.[4] Membrane depolarization also increases membrane permeability to potassium ion, which is at a much higher concentration inside than outside the nerve cell membrane, resulting in potassium efflux and membrane repolarization. The depolarization-repolarization process generates an electrical potential known as an *action potential* that is completed in approximately 1 to 2 msec. The potential difference generated by the action potential between the depolarized nerve membrane and the adjacent segment causes current to flow into the adjacent segment. Sodium channels in the adjacent segment are activated, the membrane depolarizes, and the aforementioned process repeats itself, resulting in the propagation of the action potential along the nerve membrane (Figure 11-1).

Nerve Fiber Types

Peripheral nerve fibers are classified according to their fiber size, physiological function, and rate of impulse transmission (Table 11-1). Myelin is a phospholipid layer that surrounds and insulates the axons of many neurons. The main consequence of a myelin layer (or sheath) is an increase in the speed of impulse propagation along the myelinated nerve fiber. Impulses move more slowly as continuous waves along unmyelinated fibers, but in myelinated fibers they jump or propagate by saltation (saltatory conduction). Myelin increases the fiber diameter and serves as a nonspecific binding site for local anesthetic molecules. The myelin

---

Box 11-1 Factors Determining Local Anesthetic Effect

- Operative site
- Knowledge of local anatomy
- Medical procedure
- Duration of procedure
- The local anesthetic selected
- The technique used
- Technical proficiency
- Temperament of the horse

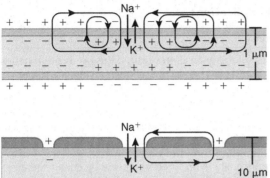

Figure 11–1. Membrane action potential (depolarization-repolarization). Membrane depolarization depends on sodium ions traversing the sodium channels into the axoplasm, whereas repolarization depends on potassium ions leaving the axoplasm. The sodium-potassium pump (sodium-out; potassium-in) helps to restore normal ion concentrations.

sheath is relatively impermeable to local anesthetics. The sodium channel receptors within the plasma membrane become less numerous as the internodal distances increase, with axon diameter contributing to a delay in the onset of motor nerve block by local anesthetics. Therefore the rate of local anesthetic blockade is faster in unmyelinated C fibers than in A fibers because there are fewer diffusion barriers around C fibers than around A fibers, not because of a higher sensitivity of the C fibers to local anesthetic.[5]

Temperature. Cooling of mammalian nerves in vitro slows conduction velocity and increases susceptibility to local anesthetic inhibition of transmission.[6] Moreover, cooling of lidocaine increases its pKa and the relative amount of the protonated (active) form, thereby potentiating anesthetic effect.[7] On the other hand, direct measurement of the lidocaine content of mammalian sciatic nerve shows a 45% reduction in total anesthetic uptake when temperature is decreased from 37° C to 20° C (70° F). However, it is unlikely that cooling of local anesthetics (5° C) before injection of small volumes (5 ml) enhances clinical regional anesthesia because the local anesthetic is rapidly warmed by the surrounding tissue temperature, preventing the nerve from becoming cold.[8]

Electrolytes. There are important interactions among stimulus frequency, tissue electrolyte concentration, and local anesthetics. First, local anesthesia is enhanced by repetitive stimulation (frequency-dependent blockade) because the number of available sodium channels is increased during activation.[9] Only 60% of sodium channels are open during the resting state.[10] This number increases during repetitive stimulation.

Calcium and magnesium ions have an important role in nerve excitability but do not interfere directly with local anesthetic activity.[4] Increasing or decreasing the extracellular calcium ion concentration in nerves causes an increased excitability in myelinated fibers without greatly affecting the resting membrane potential. However, the exact role of calcium on nerve conduction in nerves that have been blocked by local anesthetics remains controversial. One study demonstrated that low calcium concentrations enhance frequency-independent and frequency-dependent lidocaine block, but other studies have ruled out calcium as a regulating mechanism.[4,11] Similarly, alterations in serum magnesium concentrations within the clinically relevant range are unlikely to interfere with nerve conduction, but both ions are known to influence acetylcholine release and the function of the neuromuscular junction (see Chapter 19).

PHARMACOLOGY OF LOCAL ANESTHETICS

Mechanisms of Action

Local anesthetic drugs diffuse through the nerve cell membrane, enter sodium channels, and inhibit the influx of sodium ions, thereby interrupting nerve conduction.[4,12]

General Properties

The chemical properties that determine local anesthetic effect include lipid solubility, dissociation constant, chemical linkage, and protein binding (Table 11-2).[13] Local

Table 11–1.	Classification of nerve fibers and order of blockade				
Nerve characteristics	**Fiber type**				
Nerve group	Aα	Aβ	Aγ	Aδ	B	C
Function	Somatic motor	Touch, pressure	Proprioception	Pain, temperature	Vasoconstriction, preganglionic sympathetic	Pain, postganglionic sympathetic
Myelin	Heavy	Moderate	Moderate	Light	Light	None
Diameter (μM)	12-20	5-12	3-6	2-5	1-3	0.13-1.3
Priority of blockade	5	4	3	2	1	2
Signs of blockade	Loss of motor function	Loss of sensation to touch and pressure	Loss of proprioception	Pain relief, loss of temperature and sensation	Increased skin temperature	Pain relief, loss of temperature and sensation

Table 11–2.   Local anesthetic characteristics and their clinical implications

Characteristic	Correlate	Explanation
Lipid solubility	Potency	Greater lipid solubility facilitates drug diffusion through neural coverings and cell membrane, allowing a lower milligram dose.
Dissociation constant	Time to onset	Determines the portion of an administered dose that exists in the lipid-soluble (uncharged; unionized), tertiary molecular state at a given pH. Local anesthetics with a lower pKa have a greater proportion in the tertiary, diffusible (lipid-soluble) state. This hastens onset to drug effect.
Chemical linkage	Metabolism	Esters are principally hydrolyzed in plasma by cholinesterases; amides are primarily biotransformed in the liver (longer duration).
Protein binding	Duration	Affinity for plasma proteins also corresponds to affinity for protein at the receptor site within sodium channels, prolonging the presence of anesthetic at the site of action and the duration of drug effect.

anesthetic drugs are bases that consist of three essential components: a lipophilic aromatic ring, an intermediate ester or amide chain, and a terminal amine (Figure 11-2 and Table 11-3). Their classification is determined by the nature of the intermediate linkage (ester versus amide), which has a notable effect on their chemical stability and metabolism. Most esters are metabolized rapidly by plasma cholinesterase and have short half-lives when stored in solution without preservatives. The amides are stable for longer periods of time, cannot be hydrolyzed by cholinesterase, and are enzymatically biotransformed in the liver. Local anesthetic bases are formulated as hydrochloride (HCL) salts and exist in a quaternary, or positively charged, water-soluble state when injected. The quaternary form does not penetrate the nerve cell membrane very well, making the time to onset of drug effect highly dependent on the proportion of molecules that convert to a tertiary lipid-soluble or free base (uncharged) form. Lipid solubility is also enhanced by substitution of the aromatic ring (see Figure 11-2). The ionization constant (pKa) of the local anesthetic determines the proportion of molecules that exist in charged (water-soluble) and uncharged (lipid-soluble) form and is greater than 7.4 for all local anesthetics, suggesting that the quaternary (water-soluble) form predominates at physiologic pH (7.4; Table 11-4). Both quaternary or hydrophilic and tertiary or lipid-soluble forms reach the receptor primarily through open sodium channels and bind more strongly to the

closed than the open channel.[1] The free base or uncharged form is able to diffuse through the lipid cell membrane into the axoplasm, where a portion ionizes again. The ionized form of the local anesthetic then diffuses into the sodium channel from the inside of the axon (Figure 11-3). Clinical application of these concepts suggest that local anesthetics with greater lipid solubility are more potent than those with a lower pKa and are more likely to have a faster onset of effect and be effective in inflamed (lower pH) tissues. Finally, affinity of the local anesthetics for plasma proteins (α_1- acid glycoprotein) correlates with their ability to bind to sodium channels and the duration of neural blockade (see Table 11-4).

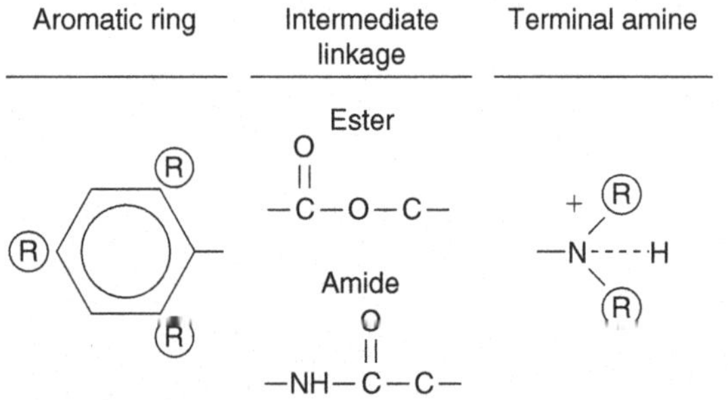

Local Anesthetic Drugs

Potency

A positive correlation exists between the degree of lipid solubility (partition coefficient) and inherent anesthetic potency (see Table 11-2). Relatively insoluble drugs (e.g., procaine) with a high pKa penetrate lipid membranes of large myelinated nerve fibers slowly, so that little conduction block develops. Drugs with the reverse characteristics—high lipid solubility and lower pKa (e.g., mepivacaine)—penetrate diffusion barriers around A-α-nerves relatively easily and thus produce good motor blockade.

Duration of Action

Duration of local anesthetic drug effect is primarily a function of the extent of protein binding and vasoactivity of the local anesthetic. Increasing the side chain of the local anesthetic molecule increases protein binding and prolongs the duration of action of the drug. On the other hand, lidocaine-induced vasodilator causes local anesthetics to be removed from the site of injection faster. This makes lidocaine a shorter-acting anesthetic than prilocaine, even though lidocaine is more protein bound.

Differential Block

Small nerve fibers are considered to be more susceptible than large fibers to conduction block. Studies of differential sensations of desheathed nerves demonstrate various

Figure 11–2. Local anesthetics consist of three principle components: an aromatic ring, intermediate ester or amide linkage, and a terminal amine. *R*, Substitution sites.

Table 11–3.   Name, chemical structure, and clinical use of select local anesthetic drugs

Agent	Trade name	Chemical structure	Main clinical use
Esters			
Cocaine			Topical
Benzocaine	Americaine		Topical
Procaine	Novocain		Infiltration, nerve blocks, epidural
Tetracaine	Pontocaine Amethocaine		Topical, subarachnoid
Amides			
Lidocaine	Xylocaine Lignocaine		Infiltration, nerve blocks, intraarticular, epidural
Mepivacaine	Carbocaine		Infiltration, nerve blocks, intraarticular, epidural
Bupivacaine	Marcaine		Infiltration, nerve blocks, epidural, subarachnoid
Ropivacaine	Naropin		Infiltration, nerve blocks, epidural, subarachnoid

differential rates of block after application of various local anesthetics (e.g., cocaine, procaine, chloroprocaine, tetracaine, lidocaine, bupivacaine, etidocaine, tetrodotoxin, saxitoxin), with C-fibers being blocked before A-α-fibers (see Table 11-1).[14] However, when equilibrium is established between the nerve and local anesthetic solution, the A-α-fibers are blocked at the lowest drug concentration; the intermediate B-fibers are blocked at a higher concentration; and the smallest, slowest conducting C-fibers require the highest drug concentration for conduction blockade.[15,16]

Toxicity

Local anesthetic drugs produce dose-dependent central nervous system (CNS) depression proportional to their inherent local anesthetic potency (Figure 11-4). Therapeutic concentrations are clinically useful for treatment of cardiac arrhythmias, lowering injectable and inhalant anesthetic drug requirements, producing promotility gastrointestinal effects, and treating shock. Local anesthetic drugs may potentiate the CNS depressant effects of sedatives and opioids and can cause vasodilation that contributes to or causes hypotension. Hypotension is treated by stopping the local anesthetic infusion and initiating a dobutamine infusion, if necessary. Higher concentrations can induce seizure activity, presumably as a result of the inhibition of CNS inhibitory tracts (Figure 11-5). Central nervous system signs in horses are rare, self-limiting, and generally easily treated with low dosages of diazepam (0.05 mg/kg intravenously [IV]).

Table 11–4.   Physical, chemical, and biologic properties of commonly used local anesthetic drugs

Drug	Lipid solubility (partition coefficient)	Relative anesthetic potency*	pKa	Onset of action	Plasma protein binding (%)	Duration of action (min)
Low potency, short duration						
Procaine	0.5	1	8.9	Slow	6	60-90
Chloroprocaine	1	1	9.1	Fast	?	30-60
Intermediate potency and duration						
Lidocaine	3	2	7.7	Fast	65	90-180
Mepivacaine	2	2	7.6	Fast	75	120-180
Prilocaine	1	2	7.7	Fast	55	120-240
Intermediate potency, long duration						
Ropivacaine	15	6	8.1	Fast	95	180-360
High potency, long duration						
Tetracaine	80	8	8.6	Slow	80	180-360
Bupivacaine	28	8	8.1	Intermediate	95	180-500

*The potency given is relative to procaine.

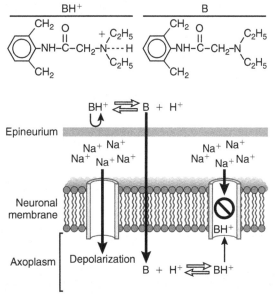

Figure 11–3. Once injected, local anesthetics exist in equilibrium as water soluble quaternary salts *(BH+)* and lipid-soluble tertiary bases *(B)*. The proportion of each is determined by the local anesthetics pKa (see Table 11-2). The lipid-soluble base *(B)* penetrates the neuronal membrane and is transformed to the quaternary state *(BH+)*, which enters and blocks the sodium channel.

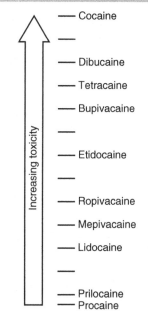

Figure 11–4. Spectrum of local anesthetic drugs according to toxicity.

Local Anesthetic Drug Pharmacology

Procaine

Pharmacology. Procaine HCL (Novocain) was the first synthetic local anesthetic successfully used to produce regional anesthesia. Procaine is an aminobenzoic acid ester, a relatively weak local anesthetic, and has a similar onset of action but short duration compared to other local anesthetic drugs. It is considered the prototype local anesthetic for comparing the potency and toxicity of local anesthetic drugs. Procaine in 2% to 4% aqueous solution is nonirritant, promptly effective after subcutaneous injection, and considerably less toxic than other commonly used local anesthetics.

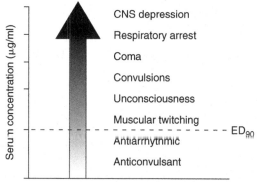

Figure 11–5. Plasma concentration of lidocaine with therapeutic and toxic effects.

Procaine is metabolized in the serum of horses to para-aminobenzoic acid (PABA) and diethylaminoethanol (DEAE) through the action of plasma esterases.[17] Equine synovial fluid has approximately 20% of the procaine esterase activity of plasma.[17] Excretion of procaine and its major metabolite PABA occurs through urinary pathways. Less than 1% of the dose in horses is excreted in urine as parent drug; and this amount varies, depending on the pH of the urine.[18]

The biological half-life for procaine in horses varies according to the route of administration. After intravenous, intramuscular (IM), subcutaneous, and intraarticular administrations of procaine, the elimination half-lives are 50, 125, 65, and 95 min, respectively (Table 11-5).[19] The half-life of procaine administered IM as procaine penicillin is 10 hours. The biological half-life of procaine in synovial fluid after intraarticular injection is 48 minutes, similar to the half-life of procaine after intravenous administration.[20]

The pharmacology, pharmacokinetics, and behavioral effects of procaine have been studied extensively in the horse because its local anesthetic and central stimulant actions could mask lameness and potentially improve performance.[21] Procaine is combined and used therapeutically as a complex with penicillin. Each milliliter of procaine penicillin G (300,000 U/ml) contains 123 mg of procaine. Horses administered procaine penicillin are exposed to relatively large amounts of procaine.[19] Most racing authorities do not allow the presence of procaine or its metabolites in the blood and urine of racing horses.

Clinical pharmacology. Procaine is used for infiltration anesthesia and regional anesthesia and to block pain perception in joints, tendon sheaths, and other structures.[20] A 5-ml amount of 2% procaine solution, injected subcutaneously (SQ) to the palmar and metacarpal nerves and dorsal to the withers in Thoroughbreds and Standardbreds, produces analgesia within 10 minutes that lasts for 90 minutes.[22]

If procaine HCL is used in horses for treatment of spasmodic colic, it relieves pain 5 to 10 minutes after slow intravenous injection of 30 to 40 mg of procaine per 45.5 kg (using a 5% solution) without adverse side effects.[23]

Clinical toxicology. Horses demonstrate signs of CNS excitation after rapid intravenous injection of 2.5 mg of procaine per kilogram of body weight. The signs include deep, rapid, and forced exhalations (blowing); fine muscle tremors on the back and haunches; pawing at the ground; and marked pacing activity. Excitation occurs at high plasma procaine concentrations >800 ng/ml within 30 to 40 seconds and lasts for 4 minutes.[19]

Hypersensitivity. Horses are at least 20 times more sensitive to the central stimulation action of procaine than humans.[19] PABA is responsible for allergic reactions associated with the repeated use of this drug in humans.[24] Localized and generalized reactions to intradermal skin testing have not been reported in horses, although they have been reported in other species.[25]

Lidocaine

Pharmacology. Lidocaine HCL was the first aminoamide-type local anesthetic drug and is derived from xylidine. Lidocaine is probably the most commonly used local anesthetic in clinical practice because of its potency, rapid onset, moderate duration of action, and topical anesthetic activity (see Table 11-4).[13] It is effective at about one half the concentration of procaine. Lidocaine is highly metabolized in the liver; diethylamino acetic acid is the major metabolite.[26] The clearance of lidocaine depends on hepatic blood flow rates and is decreased during general inhalant anesthesia.[27] There is evidence to suggest that lung tissue takes up a considerable amount of lidocaine, thus reducing the concentration in arterial blood and the amount of drug reaching the brain.[28]

Clinical pharmacology. Both 1% to 2% solutions of lidocaine are used for infiltration anesthesia in horses. A 2% solution is commonly used for peripheral nerve blocks and epidural anesthesia. In addition, lidocaine can be administered IV to decrease both injectable and inhalant anesthetic requirements (anesthetic sparing effect) and has been demonstrated to produce promotility effects when administered into the region of celiac ganglia or as an infusion during colic surgery.[29-31] Lidocaine ointments, liposomal creams, jellies, patches, and aerosol preparations are available for topical anesthetic procedures to produce surface anesthesia before intravenous catheter placement, surgery of the larynx

Table 11–5. Pharmacokinetics of procaine in horses

Route of administration	Number of horses tested	Dose of procaine (mg/kg)	Peak concentration (ng/ml)	Time to peak concentration (min)	Half-life for drug elimination (t½β) (min)	Number of horses with CNS excitation
Intravenous	5	2.5	1.2	1	50	5
Intramuscular						
Procaine HCl	9	10	600	20	125	3
Procaine penicillin	20	33,000 IU/kg	280	—	600	1
Subcutaneous	4	3.3	400	20	65	—
Intraarticular	4	0.33	24	60	95	—

Plasma procaine concentration spans Peak concentration, Time to peak concentration, Half-life for drug elimination columns.

CNS, Central nervous system.

and throat, and endotracheal and nasotracheal intubation. Lidocaine patches have been used to protect and desensitize superficial wounds and as a therapy for laminitis, although their efficacy in horses requires validation.[32]

Lidocaine is detected in plasma, urine, and saliva of horses 48 hours after infiltration of the plantar nerves of both pelvic digits with 3.5 ml of 2% lidocaine HCl solution (140 mg; total dosage 0.3 mg/kg), with maximum venous plasma lidocaine concentrations reported to be 0.2 µg/ml 1 hr after injection and with traces of lidocaine detectable 12 and 24 hours after injection.[26,33] Urinary elimination occurs 7 to 48 hours after injection.

Lidocaine administered to horses in doses ranging from 1 to 4 mg/kg causes no significant changes in cardiac output or renal blood flow and is cleared principally by the liver.[27] Negligible quantities of lidocaine are detected in urine of horses (1.7% to 2.5% of injected dose). Plasma clearance of lidocaine in horses (52 ± 11.7 mg/kg) is more than two times greater than estimated hepatic blood flow (22.4 ml/min/kg).[34] Three-day fasting reduces the plasma clearance of IV injected lidocaine (0.42 mg/kg) in horses by 16%, with reductions most likely resulting from a decrease in the intrinsic ability of the liver to remove lidocaine from blood.[34] Apparent distribution volumes of lidocaine in horses are 798 ± 176 ml/kg and remain unaffected by fasting. Lidocaine does not undergo intravascular degradation in horses. Serum lidocaine concentrations are increased in anesthetized compared to awake horses, most likely as a result of anesthetic-associated decreases in liver blood flow.[27] Lidocaine is detectable in arterial and venous plasmas of conscious horses after infiltration of the cervicothoracic (stellate) ganglion with 100 ml of 1% lidocaine HCL solution. Maximum plasma lidocaine concentrations are 1.28 µg/ml and 1.42 µg/ml at 15 to 45 minutes after unilateral and bilateral injections, indicating fast absorption.[29] The maximum venous plasma concentration of lidocaine in horses does not correlate with the total dosage of lidocaine administered, probably because of the difference in the factors that compete with vascular absorption of the drug (e.g., vascularity of the injection site, neural uptake, sequestration of local anesthetic in adipose and fibrous tissues) and interanimal differences in the pharmacokinetics of the drug.

Clinical toxicology. Lidocaine toxicity is most likely to occur immediately after or during intravenous administration. Inadvertent rapid intravenous infusions produce the most dramatic and rapid onset of symptoms (see Figure 11-5). The severity of CNS symptoms and signs depends on the rapidity of administration and exposure of brain cells to local anesthetic rather than a defined concentration in blood.[35] The cardiovascular system is considerably more resistant than the CNS to the toxic effects of intravenous lidocaine.[36] The difference between the intravenous and infusion convulsant doses of lidocaine is probably caused by a high first-pass hepatic extraction and greater tissue distribution of drug after infusion. Acute intravenous toxicity studies in dogs with lidocaine, bupivacaine, and ropivacaine suggest that lidocaine has the least CNS toxic and arrhythmogenic effects and the highest margin of safety between the convulsant dose and lethal dose of the three agents studied.[37] Deaths occur as a result of respiratory arrest after

administration of three times the convulsant dose. Adult horses safely tolerate 250 ml of a 2% lidocaine HCL solution for infiltration of the paralumbar fossa for abdominal surgery. Rapid intravenous bolus administration (>2 mg of lidocaine per kilogram) can induce convulsions in horses.

Hypersensitivity. Allergic reactions to amino-amides are extremely rare, although several cases have been reported.[24] Lidocaine, mepivacaine, and prilocaine solutions that contain the preservative methylparaben, the chemical structure of which is similar to that of PABA, have produced allergic skin reactions.

Mepivacaine

Pharmacology. The local anesthetic profile of mepivacaine is similar to that of lidocaine. Mepivacaine HCL produces profound nerve block with a relatively rapid onset and moderate duration (see Table 10-4). Several differences between mepivacaine and lidocaine exist. Mepivacaine has less vasodilator activity than lidocaine, providing a slightly longer duration of action. Its metabolism in the fetus and newborn may be prolonged.[13] Mepivacaine is less effective as a topical anesthetic than lidocaine, although it has been used for topical anesthesia of the larynx.

Clinical pharmacology. A 2% solution of mepivacaine is useful for infiltration, intraarticular anesthesia, nerve block, and epidural and subarachnoid anesthesia in horses. Postinjection edema after nerve blocks is minimal. Mepivacaine prolongs the time between exposure of a noxious heat stimulus to the metacarpophalangeal joint or dorsal coronary band and also prolongs withdrawal of the limb (latency time) after its local administration to the palmar and metacarpal nerves.[22] Mepivacaine analgesia is achieved earlier (<10 minutes) and lasts approximately twice as long (180 minutes) as procaine. Mepivacaine is detectable in venous plasma during caudal epidural and subarachnoid anesthesia and in cerebrospinal fluid (CSF) during segmental subarachnoid anesthesia in adult horses in concentrations that do not produce measurable direct systemic effects on the cardiovascular system (Table 11-6).[38-40]

Other Local Anesthetics and Drugs Producing Local Anesthetic Effects

Bupivacaine. Bupivacaine HCL (Marcaine) is an amide-linked local anesthetic. Compared with lidocaine and mepivacaine, it is two to four times more potent. It has a slow onset and prolonged duration.[13] Bupivacaine is used in concentrations of 0.124%, 0.25%, 0.5%, and 0.75% for various regional anesthetic procedures, including infiltration, peripheral nerve blocks, and epidural and subarachnoid anesthesia.[41] Bupivacaine is more cardiotoxic than lidocaine, and this toxicity seems to be aggravated by hypoxia and acidemia.[42]

Ropivacaine. Ropivacaine HCL is a long-acting amino-amide local anesthetic that combines the anesthetic potency and long duration of bupivacaine with a lower toxicity profile. It is a congener to mepivacaine and bupivacaine. A 1% ropivacaine solution has an anesthetic profile similar to a 0.75% bupivacaine solution and is considered

Table 11–6. Response to injection of mepivacaine HCl solution (20 mg/ml) in adult horses*

Injection site	Number of horses	Dose of mepivacaine injected (ml)	Onset of analgesia (min)	Maximum dermatomes analgesic	Duration of analgesia (min)	Venous plasma concentration		
						Maximum concentration (μg/ml)	Concentration at cessation of analgesia (μg/ml)	Concentration 120 min after injection (μg/ml)
Caudal epidural (S-3 to S-5)	7	4.6	21.0	S1 to coccyx	102 ± 13	0.05	0.035	0.020
	7	4.1	21.4	S1 to coccyx	81			
Caudal subarachnoid (S2-3)	7	1.3	8.3	SI to coccyx	83 ± 9	0.05	0.02	0.004
	7	1.3	8.2	S1 to coccyx	70			
						Cerebrospinal fluid concentration		
Thoracolumbar subarachnoid (T18-L1)	10	1.5	7.5	T13-L3	47 ± 19	—	204 ± 160	16.8 × 15

*Data are expressed as mean data adjusted to one decimal number.

to be slightly less potent. Its time of onset is short, and it is less cardiotoxic than any other presently available long-acting local anesthetic.[43] Ropivacaine is less lipid soluble; has a lower volume of distribution, greater clearance, and shorter elimination half-life than bupicaine; and undergoes comparatively more rapid hepatic biotransformation and renal clearance. Ropivacaine can be used as a safer alternative to bupivacaine and has been demonstrated to produce long duration of effect (>3 hours) when administered for regional anesthesia (infiltration, epidural, subarachnoid) in horses.[44,45]

Proparacaine. Proparacaine HCL has been approved by the Food and Drug Administration for use as a topical anesthetic in animals. It is the topical agent of choice for corneal anesthesia in horses. The drug is available in aqueous solution containing 0.5% proparacaine HCL (Ophthaine, Ophthetic). Installation of one to three drops on the cornea produces surface anesthesia within 1 minute that lasts for approximately 15 minutes with minimum irritation.[46] It also can be used for analgesia of the ear canal and nose; for minor surgery, including suture removal and foreign body removal; and before tonometry and lacrimal duct catheterization.

Alcohol. Alcohol (ethyl alcohol) is a nonspecific, irritating, hypobaric neurolytic agent.[47] It has local anesthetic properties that appear 10 to 20 minutes after injection, except in the subarachnoid space, where the injection of alcohol in humans is associated with a burning dermatomal pain 5 to 10 minutes after injection.[48] Although its use is discouraged, alcohol has been injected perineurally in horses to produce axonal degeneration distal to the site of injection (e.g., distal limb, tail) as an alternate for performing a neurectomy.[49] Alcohol-induced denervation of coccygeal nerves in horses lasts several months to 1 year, but some return of function occurs after 8 weeks if neurolysis has been incomplete. Efficacy and safety of neurolysis in horses, using epidural ethyl alcohol blocks, have not been reported. Of concern are inaccuracies of the technique, resulting in painful paresthesias; neuritis; and paralysis of bladder, rectum, and pelvic limbs after injection of excessive volumes of alcohol into the caudal epidural space.

Opioids, α₂ agonists, ketamine, tramadol, and their combinations. Various opioids (morphine, methadone, meperidine, hydromorphone, butorphanol), α₂-agonists (xylazine, detomidine, romifidine), dissociative anesthetics (ketamine, tiletamine/zolazepam), tramadol, and their combinations have been administered epidurally or subarachnoidally to horses as analgesics to facilitate surgery of the tail, anus, rectum, vulva, vagina, urethra, and bladder (Table 11-7).[50-55] A major advantage of most of these alternative drugs, especially opioids, is the relative absence of motor blockade (ataxia, recumbency) compared to local anesthetics. In addition, both α₂-agonists and opioids can be antagonized if necessary. The aforementioned drugs or their combinations have been administered to provide pain relief to perform surgical correction of rectovaginal fistula, prolapsed rectum, ovariectomy, and cryptorhidectomy in conscious and anesthetized horses and to facilitate fetotomy, correction of uterine torsion, and a variety of laparoscopic procedures in

anesthetized horses. The pharmacology and pharmacokinetics are described elsewhere in this text (see Chapters 9 and 10), but their doses as local anesthetics are included for comparative purposes.

POTENTIATION AND INHIBITION OF LOCAL ANESTHESIA

Vasoconstrictors

Vasopressors are combined with local anesthetics to produce local vasoconstriction, thereby providing local hemostasis and delaying the absorption of the local anesthetic. Local anesthetics with short duration (e.g., procaine) and those with intermediate duration (e.g., lidocaine, mepivacaine) benefit greatly from the addition of epinephrine to prolong the duration of infiltration anesthesia, peripheral nerve blocks, and epidural anesthesia. The action of long-duration local anesthetics (e.g., prilocaine, bupivacaine, etidocaine, ropivacaine) is also prolonged by the addition of epinephrine, but to a lesser extent. The minimum vasodilator action of prilocaine and the high lipid solubility of bupivacaine and etidocaine are responsible for the diminished effect of epinephrine.[13] The mechanism by which epinephrine prolongs epidural and subarachnoid anesthesia is unclear. It is assumed that the addition of epinephrine to epidural and subarachnoid lidocaine and bupivacaine decreases local blood flow, thereby slowing the absorption and reducing the potential for systemic toxicity.[1,56] However, the improvement of the quality of analgesia with epinephrine is not explained by the classic vasoconstriction effect delaying the absorption of the drug. Improvement might result from epinephrine suppressing noxiously evoked activity of the wide dynamic neurons of the dorsal horns of the spinal cord.[57] The use of epinephrine in obstetric epidural and subarachnoid anesthesia in humans remains controversial. Additional studies are required in horses to determine any potential benefit of adding epinephrine to local anesthetics.[56,58,59] Most local anesthetics are marketed as mildly acidic HCL salts. Adding epinephrine to these solutions decreases the pH of the solutions and the amount of the free protonated anesthetic base available for diffusion through the axonal membrane, thereby potentially slowing the onset of action. Although it is usually desirable to prolong anesthetic activity, the slow onset of action is a disadvantage. Commercially prepared local anesthetic solutions that contain epinephrine have a lower pH than solutions freshly prepared with epinephrine and are less effective for vasoconstriction. Adding epinephrine 1:80,000 to 2% lidocaine HCL solution (pH 5.25) increases the potency of the anesthetic over the commercially available 2% lidocaine solution containing epinephrine 1:800,000 and antioxidant (pH 3.23). A 1:200,000 epinephrine concentration may be prepared by adding 0.1 ml of 1:1000 (0.1 mg) epinephrine to 20 ml of local anesthetic solution. Alternatively, 1:1000 epinephrine may be diluted with preservative-free normal saline.

Raising the pH of the solution immediately before injection shortens time to onset of effect. It should be noted that epinephrine in a solution of pH >7.0 has a markedly reduced life and effectiveness. Any solution prepared by pH adjustment should be used immediately, especially if epinephrine is added.

Table 11–7. Dosages, durations, and adverse effects of local anesthetic drugs used for epidural analgesia in horses*

Drug or combination	Dosages	Onset of action	Duration of anesthesia or analgesia	Adverse effects[†]
Lidocaine	0.22–0.35 mg/kg	5–15 minutes	60–90 minutes	Ataxia or recumbency at higher doses
Lidocaine (2%)	5–8 ml/450 kg			
Mepivacaine (2%)	5–7 ml/450 kg	10–30 minutes	90–120 minutes	
Ropivacaine (0.2%)	5 ml/450 kg	5–10 minutes	3–4 hours	Mild ataxia
Bupivacaine (0.5%)	0.06 mg/kg	10–15 minutes	5–6 hours	Sedation, ataxia
Xylazine	0.17 mg/kg	10–30 minutes	2.5–4 hours	Perineal edema and sweating
Xylazine	0.25–0.35 mg/kg	10–20 minutes	3–5 hours	Mild ataxia
Detomidine	30–60 µg/kg	10–15 minutes	2–3 hours	Sedation, ataxia, cardiovascular depression, second-degree atrioventricular block, diuresis
Romifidine	80 µg/kg	10–20 minutes	?	Inadequate perineal analgesia, bradycardia
Lidocaine and xylazine	0.22 mg/kg and 0.17 mg/kg	5–15 minutes	5.5 hours	Ataxia or recumbency, perineal sweating
Morphine	0.1 mg/kg	4–6 hours	8–18 hours	Skin wheals, sedation
Morphine and detomidine	0.1 mg/kg and 10 µg/kg	20–30 minutes	20–24 hours	Sedation, ataxia
Methadone	0.1 mg/kg	15–20 minutes	5–6 hours	Minimal
Meperidine	0.8 mg/kg	5–15 minutes	4–5 hours	Mild sedation and ataxia
Hydromorphone	0.04 mg/kg	15–20 minutes	3–4 hours	Minimal
Butorphanol	0.05–0.08 mg/kg	NE	NE	
Butorphanol and lidocaine	0.04 mg/kg and 0.25 mg/kg	?	2.5 hours	Change in hind limb gait
Tramadol[‡]	1 mg/kg	30 minutes	8–12 hours	
Tramadol and fentanyl[§]	1 mg/kg and 5 µg/kg	30–60 minutes		
Ketamine	0.5–2.0 mg/kg	5–10 minutes	30–90 minutes	Sedation, mild ataxia with higher doses
Ketamine and morphine[§]	1 mg/kg and 0.1 mg/kg	10–30 minutes	12–18 hours	Sedation, mild ataxia
Ketamine and xylazine	1 mg/kg and 0.5 mg/kg	5–9 minutes	>2 hours	Mild sedation, bradycardia
Tiletamine/zolazepam	0.5–1.0 mg/kg	NE or mild analgesia	NE or mild analgesia	Moderate ataxia, central nervous system excitation muscle fasiculations

*Dose used in clinical practice may be lower to avoid potential complications.
[†]Potential complications, rarely observed.
[‡]Injectable form not available in the United States.
[§]C.C. Natalini, personal communication, 2001.
NE, No analgesic effects reported.

Hyaluronidase

Hyaluronidase depolymerizes hyaluronic acid, the tissue cement or ground substance of the mesenchyme, aiding the local spread of the anesthetic agent.

Addition of hyaluronidase to lidocaine or bupivacaine, 15 U/ml, is reported to hasten onset and provide more effective orbicularis and extraocular muscle akinesia after retrobulbar injections.[60] The addition of 5 U of hyaluronidase/ml of 1% lidocaine with 1:200,000 epinephrine solution in a standard dose and technique for ophthalmic surgery (2 ml as a retrobulbar injection for intraocular anesthesia, 2 ml for upper eyelid anesthesia, and 4 ml for extraorbital facial nerve blockade) does not increase the systemic absorption and CSF concentration of lidocaine in dogs.[61]However, hyaluronidase does not improve the efficacy of local anesthetics administered in other types of nerve blocks.[62,63] The necessity for its use has been questioned since the development of newer local anesthetic agents with improved spreading power.

pH Adjustment

Most local anesthetics are marketed as mildly acidic HCL salts to improve solubility. Raising the pH of lidocaine, mepivacaine, and bupivacaine from 4.5 to 7.2 by adding 1 mEq of sodium bicarbonate per 10 ml of local anesthetic before injection has been shown to accelerate the onset of epidural analgesia and anesthesia.[45,46] Adjustment of local anesthetic pH toward the physiological range is believed to increase the amount of anesthetic base available for diffusion through axonal membranes. Adjusting the pH of 1% lidocaine or 0.25% bupivacaine HCL solution to 5.0 with hydrochloric acid or to pH 7.4 with sodium hydroxide has little or no effect on duration of anesthesia after injection into the infraorbital area or abdominal musculature in humans.[64]

Carbonization of the base preparations of lidocaine does not demonstrate the theoretical expectations of increased diffusion and the effect of the drug in caudal epidural anesthesia in horses.[65]

Inflammation and Local pH Changes

Less than the expected effect or failure to achieve satisfactory anesthesia after injection of local anesthetic agents in acutely inflamed tissues is a recognized clinical phenomenon attributed to tissue acidity. The pH at the site of injection depends on the buffer demand of the injectate and the buffer capacity of the tissue. The buffer capacity of tissues may be influenced by tissue blood flow and factors that influence tissue blood flow (e.g., tissue compression by the injectate, presence of vasoconstrictor in the injectate). The tissue pH changes minimally by the injection of solutions at pH 7.4 but decreases appreciably with injections of solutions at pH 5.0.[64] Solutions that contain epinephrine produce the greatest and most prolonged decreases in pH_t. Decreases in tissue pH after injection of acidic epinephrine-containing solutions can be associated with tissue hypoxia and tissue necrosis along wound edges.[66,67] Clinical and experimental studies in horses and ponies demonstrate complications after diagnostic analgesia of the coffin joint with a lidocaine-penicillin-epinephrine mixture. Irreversible lameness resulting from chronic arthritis and ossifying arthrosis of the coffin joint have developed after intraarticular injection of 2% lidocaine HCl solution with epinephrine (0.012 mg/ml) and sodium penicillin (80,000 U) (pH = 5.9) or ampicillin (0.5 g) (pH 8.1).[68] Epinephrine might act as a catalyst for intraarticular precipitation of lidocaine-penicillin mixtures. Further studies in horses are required to evaluate the role of concurrent drug (e.g., epinephrine, hyaluronidase) administration on local anesthetic absorption and effect in inflamed tissues.

INDICATIONS AND CHOICE OF LOCAL ANESTHETIC

Local anesthetic requirements in horses depend on the operative site, nature and expected duration of surgery, size, temperament and health of the patient, technical skill of the veterinarian, and economics of time and materials (see Box 11-1). Although it is unlikely that any single local anesthetic can provide sufficient versatility for all clinical conditions, 2% lidocaine and mepivacaine HCL solutions produce effective short-term analgesia (see Table 11-4). Local and regional anesthesia using these drugs in equine patients lasts 1 to 2 hours. In general, onset of anesthesia occurs rapidly (within 3 to 5 minutes) during infiltration techniques and subarachnoid administration, followed in order of increasing onset time by minor nerve blocks (5 to 10 minutes), major nerve blocks, and epidural anesthesia (10 to 20 minutes). Epinephrine, 5 µg/ml (1:200,000), occasionally is added to the local anesthetic solution to enhance the onset, prolong the duration, and improve the quality of epidural anesthesia.

EQUIPMENT FOR PERFORMING LOCAL ANESTHESIA

The analgesic technique used varies with each procedure and personal preference. The administration of acepromazine, xylazine, or detomidine alone or in combination with morphine or butorphanol facilitates calming of horses that cannot be controlled by conventional means.[69] Some clinicians prefer stocks for further restraint; however, they can be dangerous to some horses. Sharp and sterile needles, sterile syringes in good working condition, sterile catheters and stylets, and sterile anesthetic solution should always be used. The injection sites, especially puncture sites into joints and epidural and subarachnoid spaces, should be surgically prepared to prevent infection. Avoidance of inflamed areas, aspiration before injection to avoid placing drug into the vascular system instead of the desired tissue, and proper technique are precautions that result in desired effects without complications.

A pneumatic tourniquet can be used in equine orthopedic surgical operations to decrease bleeding, thus providing a clear surgical field, and to facilitate intravenous regional anesthesia of the digit.[70]

Finally, self-evacuating elastomeric pumps, balloons, and computer-operated syringe infusion devices can be used to provide a continuous infusion of local anesthetic into desired locations for extended periods of time (Figure 11-6). These devices help to maintain constant (steady-state) therapeutic blood or tissue concentrations of drug for extended periods of time and help to avoid drug overdose (see Chapter 20).

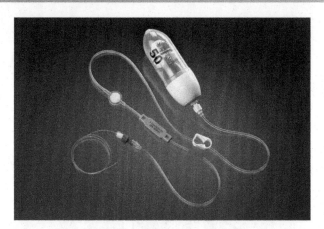

Figure 11–6. An elastomeric balloon reservoir (Surefuser pump system; ReCathCo LLC) infusion line equipped with filter and flow rate (milliliters per hour) casing attached to a fenestrated perineural catheter can be used to deliver local anesthetic to specific sites (peripherally, epidurally) for extended periods of time.

NERVE BLOCKS

Regional Anesthesia of the Head

Ophthalmic Nerve Blocks

Sensory denervation of the eyelids requires anesthesia of four individual nerves: the supraorbital (or frontal), lacrimal, zygomatic, and infratrochlear. The nerves are branches of the trigeminal (fifth) cranial nerve. Palpebral akinesia is achieved by desensitizing the dorsal and ventral branches of the palpebral nerve. A 1.5- to 2.5-cm, 22- to 25-gauge needle is used to inject local anesthetic without epinephrine to each of the listed nerves.

Anesthesia of the upper eyelid. The supraorbital (or frontal) nerve is the nerve most commonly desensitized.[71,72] Blockade of the supraorbital nerve is sufficient to permit a thorough ophthalmic examination. The nerve emerges through the supraorbital foramen. The foramen can be palpated easily with the index finger about 5 to 7 cm dorsal to the medial canthus and in the center of an imaginary triangle formed by grasping the supraorbital process of the frontal bone with the thumb and middle finger and sliding medially. Then 2 ml of local anesthetic is injected into the foramen, 1 ml as the needle is slowly withdrawn, and 2 ml SQ over the foramen. This procedure desensitizes the forehead, including the middle two thirds of the upper eyelid and palpebral motor supply from the medial portion of the palpebral branch of the auriculopalpebral nerve (Figure 11-7, *A*). Other regional nerve blocks may be necessary to suture lacerations or to perform biopsies.[73]

Anesthesia of the lateral canthus and lateral aspect of the upper eyelid is achieved by blocking the lacrimal nerve.[72,73] The needle is inserted percutaneously at the lacrimal canthus and directed mediad along the dorsal rim of the orbit (Figure 11-7, *B*). Then 2 to 3 ml of local anesthetic is injected at this site; and anesthesia of the lacrimal gland, local connective tissue, and temporal angle of the orbit is attained.

Medial canthal anesthesia results after successful placement of 2 to 3 ml of local anesthetic around the infratrochlear nerve.[72,73] This nerve passes through the bony notch or irregularity on the dorsal rim of the orbit near the medial canthus (Figure 11-7, *C*). A deep injection of the anesthetic at this site also desensitizes the nictitans, lacrimal organs, and connective tissues.

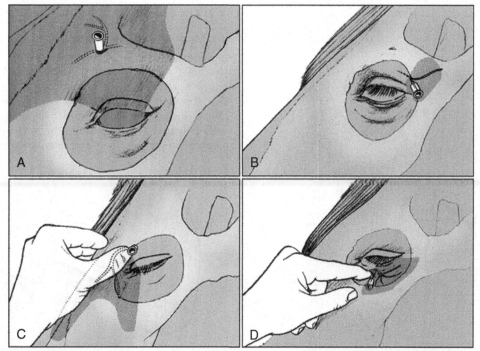

Figure 11–7. A, Needle placement for supraorbital (frontal) nerve block. *Stipple:* Desensitized subcutaneous area after blockade. **B,** Needle placement for lacrimal nerve block. *Stipple:* Desensitized subcutaneous area after blockade. **C,** Needle placement for infratrochlear nerve block. *Stipple:* Desensitized subcutaneous area after blockade. **D,** Needle placement for zygomatic nerve block. *Stipple:* Desensitized subcutaneous area after blockade.

Anesthesia of the lower eyelid.   Anesthesia of the middle two thirds of the lower lid, skin, and connective tissue is produced by successful blockade of the zygomatic nerve.[72,73] The technique is best performed by placing the index finger on the lateral aspect of the bony orbit and supraorbital portion of the zygomatic arch (the site where the rim begins to rise). The needle is inserted medial to the finger and is directed ventrally along the bony orbit, where 3 to 5 ml of the anesthetic is infiltrated SQ (Figure 11-7, D).

Motor paralysis of the orbicularis oculi muscles.   One of the terminal branches of the facial division of the trigeminal nerve is the auriculopalpebral nerve. It carries motor fibers to the orbicularis oculi muscles. Blockade of the auriculopalpebral nerve prevents voluntary closure of the eyelids (akinesia) but does not desensitize the eyelids. Desensitization of this nerve allows examination and treatment of the eye and temporary relief of eyelid spasms and, in conjunction with topical anesthesia, allows removal of foreign bodies from the cornea and other minor ocular surgery. Two principal locations have been suggested to paralyze the palpebral musculature: either depression caudal to the mandible at the ventral edge of the temporal portion of the zygomatic arch or the most dorsal point of the zygomatic arch (Figure 11-8).[73-75] The needle is placed subfascially in each location, and 5 ml of the local anesthetic is injected in a fan-shaped manner.

Anesthesia of the Upper Lip and Nose

Anesthesia of the upper lip and nose is induced by successful blockade of the infraorbital nerve as it emerges from the infraorbital canal.[71,75] The infraorbital foramen is located about one half the distance and 2.5 cm dorsal to a line connecting the nasomaxillary notch and the rostral end of the facial crest. A 2.5-cm, 20-gauge needle is used to make a perineural injection at the bony lip of the infraorbital foramen after displacing the flat levator labii superioris muscle dorsad (Figure 11-9). Injection of 5 ml of the local anes-

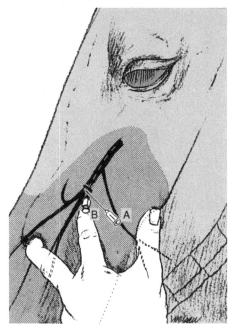

Figure 11–9. Needle placement for infraorbital nerve block at the infraorbital foramen *(A)* and within the infraorbital canal *(B)*. *Stipple:* Desensitized subcutaneous area after blockade.

thetic induces anesthesia of the entire anterior half of the face from the foramen rostrad.

Anesthesia of the Upper Teeth and Maxilla

Local anesthesia is provided for extraction of teeth (as far as the first molar), trephination of the maxillary sinus, and operation on the roof of the nasal cavity and the skin almost to the medial canthus of the eye after a 5-cm, 20-gauge needle is inserted up to 3.5 cm into the infraorbital foramen and 5 ml of local anesthetic is injected (see Figure 11-9).[76,77]

Anesthesia of the Lower Lip

Anesthesia of the lower lip requires deposition of 5 ml of local anesthetic with a 2.5-cm, 22-gauge needle over the mental nerve, rostrad to the mental foramen (Figure 11-10).[75] After displacing the tendon of the pressor labii inferioris muscle dorsad, the lateral border of the mental foramen is easily palpated as a ridge along the horizontal ramus of the mandible in the middle of the interdental space.

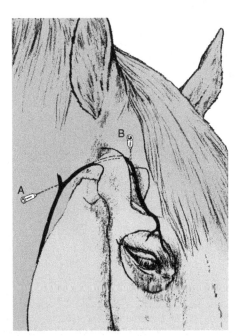

Figure 11–8. Needle placement for auriculopalpebral nerve block (methods *A* and *B*).

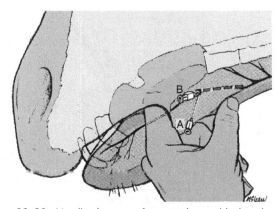

Figure 11–10. Needle placement for mental nerve block at the mental foramen *(A)* and mandibular alveolar nerve block within mandibular canal *(B)*. *Stipple:* Desensitized subcutaneous area after blockade.

Anesthesia of the Lower Incisors and Premolars

If a 7.5-cm, 20-gauge needle is inserted into the mental foramen (see Figure 11-10) and is advanced into the mandibular canal as far as possible in a ventromedial direction, the deposition of 10 ml of anesthetic is adequate to desensitize the mandibular alveolar nerve, thereby extending the area of anesthesia caudal as far as the third premolar.[71,75,78,79]

Other techniques that involve desensitizing the maxillary, mandibular, and ophthalmic nerves are not without dangers and are seldom used.[75,78,80,81]

Anesthesia of the Limbs

Regional anesthesia (peripheral nerve blocks), intraarticular[83] and intrabursal[87] injections, and local infiltration (ring block) are used to provide anesthesia to a surgery site and aid in precise diagnosis, ideal therapy, and accurate prognosis of equine lamenesses.[47,82-90]

There are fewer indications for nerve block in the hind limb when compared with the forelimb, and results are not consistent, probably because of greater technical problems and reduced operator experience.[47,55,82-93] In general, a complete lameness examination, including observation of the horse at rest and in motion, palpation, flexion tests, and the use of hoof testers, is mandatory to define the lameness problem. Pinpointing the involved structures allows a precise clinical and radiographic examination and saves time, effort, and money.

Sterile syringes, needles, and local anesthetic should be used for each injection, along with proper preparation. Aseptic technique should be practiced in all injections to prevent infection. Intraarticular injections require a surgical scrub; clipping the site may or may not be performed. Subcutaneous injections require an alcohol preparation as a minimum preparation.

Nerve blocks and intraarticular injections are performed first on the most distal branches of nerve trunks and joints. The examination should proceed proximally, using a systematic approach to gain as much information as possible in diagnosing the location of the lameness. The needle is best inserted using a distal-to-proximal direction first; it is then attached to the syringe. A local anesthetic should be administered, and adequate time should be given to achieve maximum anesthetic effects. Postblock examination is best accomplished with a combination of deep digital pressure, pressure exerted by hoof testers, manipulation, and testing skin sensation distal to the block. A ballpoint pen can be used for this purpose. The limb should be rubbed down and wrapped to prevent swelling and inflammation after the use of local anesthetics.

Digital Nerves

The palmar (or plantar) digital nerves branch dorsal to the fetlock at the level of the sesamoids, forming the three digital nerves: the dorsal or anterior digital, middle digital, and palmar (or plantar) digital.[86,94-97] The palmar (or plantar) digital nerve and the dorsal branches are important clinically. The palmar (or plantar) digital nerve supplies sensory fibers to the posterior one third of the hoof, including navicular bone and bursa; palmar (plantar) portions of the hoof; laminar corium; and corium of the bars, frog, and sole. The dorsal or anterior digital nerve supplies sensory fibers to the anterior two thirds of the hoof. The middle digital nerve is nonexistent or very small, and it is never blocked.

Palmar (or plantar) digital nerve block. The palmar (or plantar) nerve is palpated on the palmar (or plantar) aspect of the pastern, medially or laterally just palmar to the digital vein and artery. It courses distally over the border of the flexor tendon (Figure 11-11). Approximately 2 ml of local anesthetic is injected SQ over the medial and lateral palmar (plantar) digital nerves midway between the coronary band and fetlock using a 2.5-cm, 20- to 25-gauge needle. The procedure can be done with the leg bearing weight or in an elevated position. Proper nerve blockade desensitizes the posterior one third of the foot, including the navicular bursa, 5 to 10 minutes after completing the injection; and no sensation should be felt when applying the hoof testers over the central third of the frog. Skin desensitization in the bulbs of the heel may be incomplete because of variability of cutaneous nerve branches.

Midpastern ring block. Midpastern ring blocks, although possible, are not commonly used in the clinic. The pastern field block can be achieved by a bilateral palmar (plantar) nerve block and additional subcutaneous and deep injection of 5 to 10 ml of local anesthetic around the pastern proximal to the pastern joint. The structures then anesthetized are the entire digit distal to the injection, including the phalanges P1, P2, P3; proximal and distal interphalangeal joints; entire corium; dorsal branches of the suspensory ligament; and distal extensor tendon. The more commonly used clinical technique is to desensitize the palmar (plantar) digital nerve and the dorsal branch on the lateral and medial aspect of the digit. A 2.5-cm, 22-gauge needle is placed over the palmar (plantar) digital nerve and directed cranially to a depth equal to the length of the needle to inject 3 to 5 ml of local anesthetic.

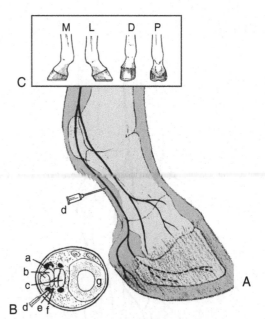

Figure 11-11. Palmar digital nerve blocks of the right forelimb. **A,** Lateral aspect. **B,** Cross-section (*a,* medial palmar digital nerve; *b,* superficial flexor tendon; *c,* deep flexor tendon; *d,* lateral palmar digital nerve; *e,* vein; *f,* artery; *g,* second phalanx). **C,** Desensitized subcutaneous area (*M,* medial aspect; *L,* lateral aspect; *D,* dorsal aspect; *P,* palmar aspect).

Abaxial (basilar) sesamoidean nerve block. The medial and lateral palmar (plantar) nerves are felt by palpating the palmar (plantar) region of the fetlock joint over the abaxial surface of proximal sesamoids, just palmar to the digital artery and vein. A 2.5-cm, 20- to 25-gauge needle is used to inject 3 to 5 ml of local anesthetic SQ at that site (Figure 11-12). Successful injections desensitize the palmar digital nerve and its dorsal branch (i.e., the entire foot, the back of the pastern area, and distal sesamoidean ligaments). Partial numbing of the fetlock area may occur.

Palmar and/or plantar nerve blocks. The palmar or plantar nerves can be desensitized at either a high site (high palmar or high plantar nerve block) or a low site (low palmar or low plantar nerve block). A communicating branch originates from the medial palmar (plantar) nerve proximally. It can be palpated as it crosses distally over the superficial digital tendon to join the lateral palmar (plantar) nerve. Both the lateral and medial palmar (plantar) nerves above or both nerves below the communicating branch must be injected for proper anesthetic effect. Nerve impulses may bypass the blocks if the lateral palmar (plantar) is injected above the origin of the communicating branch and the medial palmar (plantar) nerve is injected below the junction of the communicating branch.

The medial cutaneous antebrachial nerve, a branch of the musculocutaneous nerve (for the dorsal area), and the dorsal branch of the ulnar nerve (for the dorsolateral area) must be desensitized to provide total anesthesia of the metacarpus.[96]

The superficial peroneal nerve (for the dorsal portion) and tibia nerve (for the caudal and caudomedial portion) must also be desensitized for complete anesthesia of the metatarsus.

Low palmar (or plantar) nerve block. This procedure is performed to desensitize almost all the structures distal to the fetlock and fetlock joint except for a small area dorsal to the fetlock joint supplied by sensory fibers of the ulnar and musculocutaneous nerves. While the limb is bearing weight, approximately 2 to 3 ml of local anesthetic is injected at each of the following four points (four-point block) using a 2.5-cm, 20- to 25-gauge needle: the medial and lateral palmar (plantar) nerves and the medial and lateral palmar (plantar) metacarpal nerves. The palmar and plantar nerves (medial/lateral) are desensitized by injecting the local anesthetic between the flexor tendon and suspensory ligament (Figure 11-13). The palmar metacarpal and metatarsal nerves (medial/lateral) are desensitized by injecting the anesthetic between the suspensory ligament and the splint bone (Figure 11-14).[84,85,88-90,95]

High palmar (or plantar) nerve block. The injections for this procedure are performed at the level of the proximal quarter of the metacarpus (or metatarsus) proximal to the communicating branch of the medial and lateral palmar (or plantar) nerves while the limb is elevated or bearing weight (Figure 11-15). A 3.75-cm, 22-gauge needle is placed subfascially into the groove between the suspensory ligament and deep flexor tendon on both the medial and lateral sides. The needle must be inserted perpendicular to the skin surface, more than 4.5 cm distal to the carpometacarpal joint, to avoid penetration of the distopalmar outpouchings of the carpometacarpal joints and infiltration of the distal carpal joints.[95] Injection of 5 ml of anesthetic at these sites desensitizes the palmar metacarpal (or metatarsal) region and all the digits distal to the fetlock. The dorsal metacarpal (or metatarsal) region still has sensation.

Three additional nerves must be desensitized to gain complete anesthesia of the fetlock joint in the forelimb. These nerves include the medial and lateral palmar metacarpal nerves as they emerge from under the splint bones and the medial cutaneous antebrachial nerve as it courses along the medial aspect of the common digital extensor tendon proximal to the fetlock. The dorsal surface of the fetlock in the forelimb is readily desensitized by injecting the local anesthetic SQ around the front of the cannon bone (ring block), thereby desensitizing the dorsal metacarpal nerves.

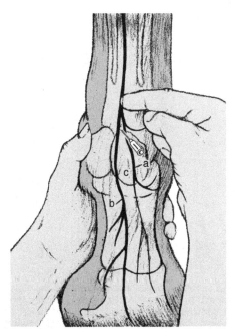

Figure 11-12. Needle placement for right abaxial sesamoidean nerve blocks of the right forelimb, caudolateral aspect (*a*, dorsal digital; *b*, palmar digital nerve; *c*, right sesamoid).

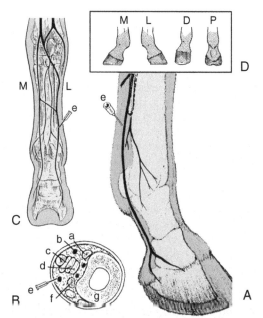

Figure 11-13. Low palmar nerve blocks of the right forelimb. **A,** Lateral aspect. **B,** Cross-section (*a*, second metacarpal bone; *b*, medial palmar nerve; *c*, superficial digital flexor tendon; *d*, deep digital flexor tendon; *e*, lateral palmar nerve; *f*, fourth metacarpal bone; *g*, third metacarpal bone). **C,** Palmar aspect. **D,** Desensitized subcutaneous area (*M*, medial aspect; *L*, lateral aspect; *D*, dorsal aspect; *P*, palmar aspect).

Four additional nerves must be desensitized to completely anesthetize the fetlock joint of the hind limb: the medial and lateral plantar metatarsal nerves and the medial and lateral dorsal metatarsal nerves.[97] The dorsal surface of the fetlock in the hind limb is readily desensitized by subcutaneous deposition of local anesthetic around the front of the cannon bone (ring block), thereby desensitizing the dorsal metatarsal nerves.

High suspensory block. High suspensory block can be produced by inserting a 3.75-cm, 22-gauge needle under the heavy fascia between the superficial digital flexor tendon and suspensory ligament deep to the proximal palmar (plantar) aspect of the metacarpus or metatarsus while the limb is elevated (Figure 11-16). After deposition of 5 ml of local anesthetic solution around the medial and lateral palmar metacarpal or metatarsal nerves, anesthesia of the interosseous muscle (suspensory ligament) and inferior checkligament can be expected in addition to anesthesia of the caudal aspect of the metacarpus (metatarsus) and adjacent splint bones.[93,95,98] Inadvertent infiltration of the distal carpal joints frequently occurs with injection distances from the carpometacarpal joint of 1.5 to 4.5 cm.[95]

Nerve blocks proximal to the carpus. Three nerves must be desensitized to induce anesthesia of the carpus and distal forelimb: the median, ulnar, and branches of the musculocutaneous nerve.[47,84,90,93] The median nerve is desensitized on the medial aspect of the forelimb 5 cm ventral to the elbow joint by inserting a 3.75-cm, 20- to 22-gauge needle between the posterior border of the radius and the muscular belly of the internal flexor carpi radialis and injecting 10 ml of the anesthetic deep to the posterior superficial pectoral muscle (Figure 11-17).

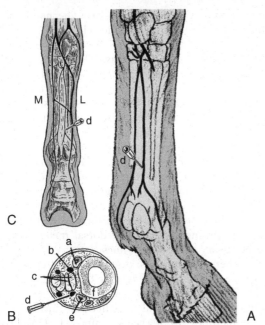

Figure 11-14. Low palmar metacarpal nerve blocks of the right forelimb. Needle placement to lateral palmar metacarpal nerve. **A,** Caudolateral aspect. **B,** Cross-section (*a,* second metacarpal bone; *b,* medial palmar metacarpal nerve; *c,* deep digital flexor tendon; *d,* lateral palmar metacarpal nerve; *e,* fourth metacarpal bone; *f,* third metacarpal bone). **C,** Palmar aspect.

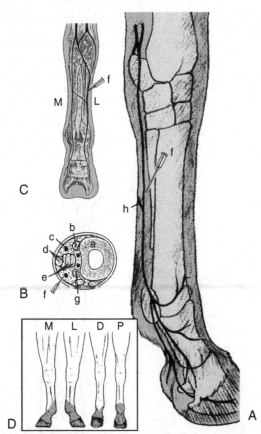

Figure 11-15. High palmar nerve blocks of the right forelimb. Needle placement to lateral palmar nerve. **A,** Caudolateral aspect. **B,** Cross-section (*a,* third metacarpal bone; *b,* second metacarpal bone; *c,* medial palmar nerve; *d,* superficial digital flexor tendon; *e,* deep digital flexor tendon; *f,* lateral palmar nerve; *g,* fourth metacarpal bone; *h,* communicating branch). **C,** Palmar aspect. **D,** Desensitized subcutaneous area (*M,* medial aspect; *L,* lateral aspect; *D,* dorsal aspect; *P,* palmar aspect).

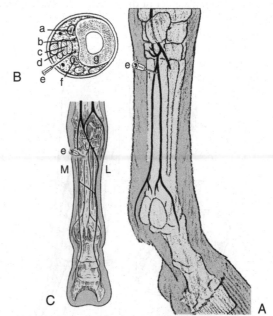

Figure 11-16. Proximal metacarpal nerve blocks of the right forelimb. Needle placement to lateral metacarpal nerve. **A,** Caudolateral aspect. **B,** Cross-section (*a,* second metacarpal bone; *b,* medial palmar metacarpal nerve; *c,* suspensory ligament; *d,* accessory ligament; *e,* medial palmar metacarpal nerve; *f,* fourth metacarpal bone; *g,* third metacarpal bone). **C,** Palmar aspect.

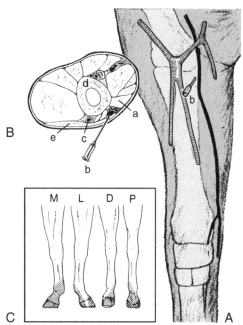

Figure 11–17. Median nerve blocks of the right forelimb. **A,** Craniomedial aspect. **B,** Cross-section (*a,* flexor carpi radialis muscle; *b,* median nerve; *c,* cephalic vein; *d,* radius; *e,* superficial pectoral muscle). **C,** Desensitized cutaneous area (*M,* medial aspect; *L,* lateral aspect; *D,* dorsal aspect; *P,* palmar aspect).

The ulnar nerve is desensitized by inserting a 2.5-cm, 22-gauge needle and placing 5 ml of anesthetic solution 1.5 cm deep beneath the fascia, 10 cm proximal to the accessory carpal bone between the flexor carpi ulnaris and ulnaris lateralis muscles (Figure 11-18).

The medial cutaneous antebrachial nerve, a branch of the musculocutaneous nerve, is desensitized by using a 2.5-cm, 22-gauge needle to deposit 10 ml of anesthetic solution SQ on the anteromedial aspect of the forelimb halfway between the elbow and carpus (Figure 11-19). The nerve is easily palpated just cranial to the cephalic vein.

Nerve blocks proximal to the tarsus. The tibial, saphenous, superficial peroneal (superficial fibular), and deep peroneal (deep fibular) nerves must be desensitized to complete anesthesia of the hind limb from the tarsus distally.[84,90]

The tibial nerve is desensitized by using a 2.5-cm, 22-gauge needle and injecting 20 ml of local anesthetic subfascially between the combined tendons of the gastrocnemius muscle and superficial digital flexor tendon on the medial aspect of the limb, approximately 10 cm proximal to the point of the tarsus while the limb is partially flexed (Figure 11-20). Anesthesia of the posterior metatarsal region and most of the foot, except for the anterolateral region, can be expected. A ring block of the dorsal metatarsal region may be necessary for complete anesthesia.

The saphenous nerve is desensitized after a 2.5-cm, 22-gauge needle is placed SQ on the cranial aspect of the medial saphenous vein proximal to the tibiotarsal joint, and 5 ml of the local anesthetic is injected (Figure 11-21). Sometimes the nerve is composed of two trunks, one extending on the cranial aspect, and one extending on the caudal aspect of the medial saphenous vein. In this case it is best to inject the anesthetic on either side of the vein. The medial aspect of the thigh and part of the metatarsal region will be anesthetized.

The superficial and deep peroneal nerves can be desensitized simultaneously by inserting a 3.75-cm, 22-gauge needle between the long and lateral digital extensor muscles at a site 10 cm proximal to the lateral malleolus of the tibia (Figure 11-22). First, 10 ml of the local anesthetic is deposited SQ around the superficial branch of the nerve. Then the needle is advanced an additional 2 to 3 cm to penetrate the deep fascia and to deposit 15 ml of the anesthetic around the deep branch. The anteriolateral tarsal and metatarsal regions and the joint capsule of the tarsus should be desensitized.[90]

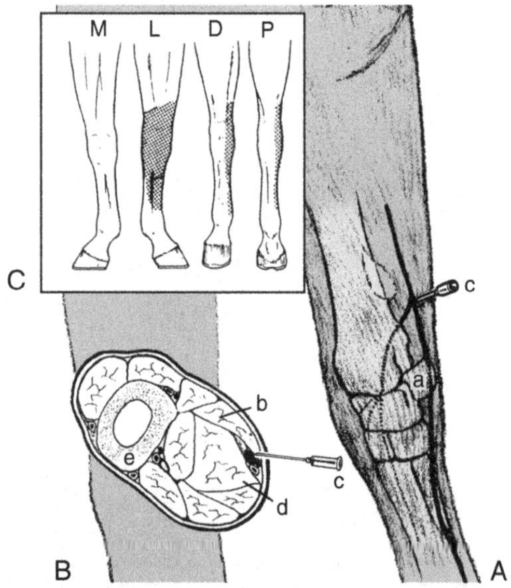

Figure 11–18. Ulnar nerve block of the right forelimb. **A,** Medial aspect. **B,** Cross-section (*a,* accessory carpal bone; *b,* ulnaris lateralis muscle; *c,* ulnar nerve; *d,* flexor carpi ulnaris muscle; *e,* radius). **C,** Desensitized cutaneous area (*M,* medial aspect; *L,* lateral aspect; *D,* dorsal aspect; *P,* palmar aspect).

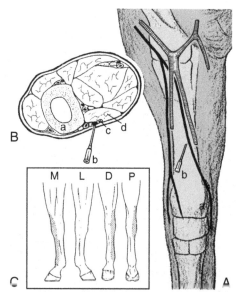

Figure 11–19. Medial cutaneous antebrachial nerve blocks of the right forelimb. **A,** Anteriomedial aspect. **B,** Cross-section (*a,* radius; *b,* medial cutaneous antebrachial nerve (branch of musculocutaneous nerve); *c,* cephalic vein; *d,* medial flexor carpi radialis muscle). **C,** Desensitized cutaneous area (*M,* medial aspect; *L,* lateral aspect; *D,* dorsal aspect; *P,* palmar aspect).

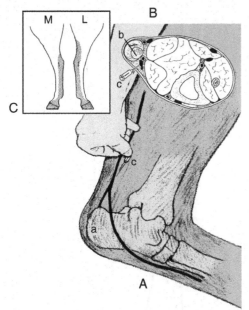

Figure 11-20. Tibial nerve block of the left rear limb. **A,** Medial aspect. **B,** Cross-section (*a,* tarsus; *b,* combined tendons of gastrocnemius and superficial digital flexor tendon; *c,* tibial nerve). **C,** Desensitized cutaneous area (*M,* medial aspect; *L,* lateral aspect).

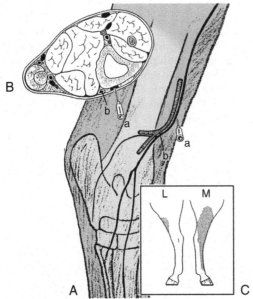

Figure 11-21. Saphenous nerve block of the left rear limb. **A,** Poster aspect. **B,** Cross-section (*a,* saphenous nerve; *b,* medial saphenous vein). **C,** Desensitized cutaneous area (*L,* lateral aspect; *M,* medial aspect).

Intraarticular Injections

Intraarticular coffin block. Intraarticular coffin block is produced by inserting a 5-cm, 20-gauge needle 1.5 cm proximal to the coronet, approximately 2 cm lateral to the vertical center of the pastern and directed obliquely ventral to the tendon toward the extensor process (Figure 11-23). Depth of penetration into the dorsal pouch of the coffin joint capsule is approximately 2.5 cm. Successful injection of 5 to 10 ml of local anesthetic desensitizes the coffin joint (P2-P3) and eventually the navicular bursa. Because the coffin joint and navicular bursa do not communicate, anes-

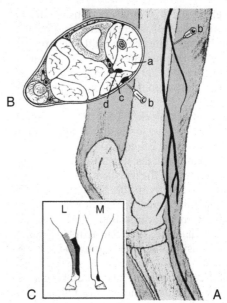

Figure 11-22. Superficial and deep peroneal nerve blockades of the right rear limb. **A,** Posterolateral aspect. **B,** Cross-section (*a,* long digital extensor muscle; *b,* superficial peroneal nerve; *c,* lateral digital extensor muscle; *d,* deep peroneal nerve). **C,** Desensitized cutaneous area. *Stipple:* After superficial peroneal nerve blockade; *solid,* after deep peroneal nerve blockade (*L,* Lateral; *M,* medial).

thesia of the navicular bursa depends on the diffusion of the local anesthetic through the suspensory ligament to the navicular bursa. The procedure is best performed while the limb is bearing weight.

Intraarticular pastern block. The pastern joint (P1-P2) can be entered with ease by inserting a 2.5-cm to 3.75-cm, 20-gauge needle medially or laterally to the midline on the

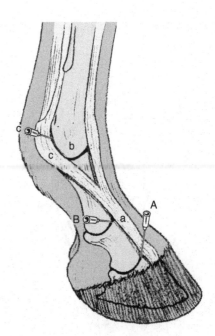

Figure 11-23. Needle placement into (*A*) coffin joint, (*B*) pastern joint, and (*C*) lateral palmar pouch of the fetlock joint capsule. *a,* Common digital extensor tendon; *b,* distal end of third metacarpal bone; *c,* annular ligament.

distal aspect of the first phalanx. The medial and lateral eminences on the distal aspect of the first phalanx are easily palpated at this site. The needle is directed from the point of insertion toward the midline and is inserted approximately 2.5 cm (see Figure 11-23). An injection of 5 to 8 ml of local anesthetic is adequate to desensitize the pastern joint.

Intraarticular fetlock block.   The fetlock is one of the commonly and easily injected joints. Intraarticular fetlock block is induced by inserting a 2.5-cm, 20-gauge needle to penetrate the lateral palmar pouch distal to the splint bone and dorsal to the annular ligament of the fetlock at a depth of approximately 0.5 to 1.5 cm (see Figure 11-23). The joint capsule can be distended by applying digital pressure to the area between the cannon bone (third metacarpal bone) and the suspensory ligament on the medial side. Then 5 to 10 ml of local anesthetic is injected to desensitize the fetlock joint and sesamoids.

Intraarticular carpal blocks.   The radiocarpal and intercarpal are the two most commonly injected carpal joints. The carpometacarpal joint communicates with the intercarpal joint and therefore does not require separate entry. Indentation of the joints can be felt medial or lateral to the palpable extensor carpi radialis tendon when the carpus is flexed. A 2.5-cm, 22-gauge needle is used to deposit 5 to 10 ml of local anesthetic into each joint (Figure 11-24).

Intraarticular elbow block.   The elbow joint is rarely desensitized because it is not usually a source of lameness. A 5-cm, 18-gauge needle is inserted into the depression between the lateral humeral condyle and the radius at the anterior edge of the lateral collateral ligament of the elbow joint (Figure 11-25). Repeated flexion of the elbow joint greatly facilitates the identification of the palpable landmarks. The needle is directed slightly caudomedially to reach the elbow joint at a depth of 3 to 4 cm; up to 20 ml of anesthetic is required.

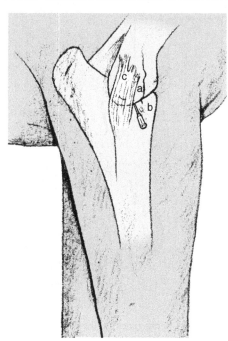

Figure 11–25. Needle placement into elbow joint of the right forelimb. *a,* Lateral humeral condyle; *b,* tuberosity of radius; *c,* lateral ligament.

Bicipital bursa block.   Bicipital bursa block is induced by inserting a 5-cm, 18-gauge needle under the brachial biceps tendon from below. Skin puncture is 4 cm ventral and 1.5 cm posterior to the palpable anterior prominence of the lateral tuberosity of the humerus. The needle is then advanced up to 5 cm in a dorsomedial direction along the humerus to penetrate the bursa (Figure 11-26).

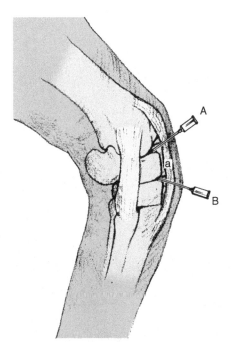

Figure 11–24. Needle placement into *(A)* radiocarpal joint and *(B)* intercarpal joint. *a,* Extensor carpi radialis tendon.

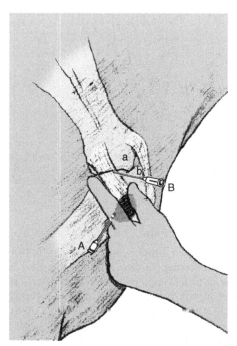

Figure 11–26. Needle placement into *(A)* bicipital bursa and *(B)* shoulder joint of the right forelimb. *a,* Brachial biceps tendon; *b,* anterior portion of lateral tuberosity of humerus.

Intraarticular shoulder block. The shoulder joint can be difficult to enter because of its relative depth. Limb motion or muscle contraction must be prevented to avoid bending a positioned needle. The scapulohumeral joint is entered between the palpable prominent projections of the anterior and posterior portions of the lateral tuberosity of the humerus (see Figure 11-26). Intraarticular shoulder block is induced by inserting a 7.5-cm to 12.5-cm, 18-gauge spinal needle approximately 2.5 cm anterior to this notch and directing it on a horizontal plane in a posteromedial direction toward the opposite elbow. Depth of penetration is up to 10 cm for free flow or aspiration of synovial fluid. A volume of 15 to 30 ml or more of the anesthetic (lidocaine) is frequently required. The shoulder joint may communicate with the bicipital bursa in some horses; therefore injections of local anesthetic into the shoulder joint may also improve a lameness associated with the bicipital bursa in these horses.[91]

Cunean bursa block. The cunean bursa is punctured with a 2.5-cm, 22-gauge needle between the cunean tendon (tendon of the medial branch of the tibialis anterior muscle) and the tarsal bones on the medial aspect of the tarsus (Figure 11-27). At least 10 ml of local anesthetic is injected, and 20 minutes are required for maximum effect.

Intraarticular tarsal blocks. Desensitizing the distal intertarsal and tarsometatarsal joints with local anesthetic improves lameness associated with early bone spavin. If radiographic osteoarthritis has not developed, an intraarticular tarsal block is particularly helpful in diagnosing the lameness. The tarsometatarsal joint is entered most easily on the posterior lateral aspect of the hock over the lateral head of the splint (metatarsal IV; Figure 11-28). Intraarticular tarsal block is induced by inserting a 2.5-cm, 18-gauge needle and injecting 5 ml of anesthetic with minimum pressure.

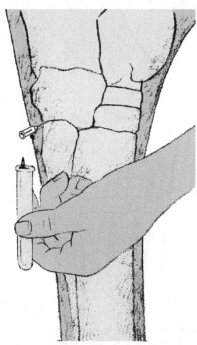

Figure 11–28. Needle placement into the tarsometatarsal joint of the right rear limb, posterolateral aspect.

High-pressure injections of an additional 3 to 4 ml of anesthetic are required to ensure communication to the distal intertarsal joint space.[88]

Alternatively, the intertarsal joint is entered by a 2.5-cm, 22-gauge needle at a right angle to the skin ventral to the cunean tendon on the medial aspect of the tarsus. Approximately 6 ml of local anesthetic solution is injected into the joint space with pressure. Communication between the distal intertarsal and tarsometatarsal joints is variable. Communication can be demonstrated by placing one needle in each of the two joints and observing the local anesthetic flow from one needle after the anesthetic is injected into the other needle.[97] However, both joints should be injected with local anesthetic at separate sites to ensure that both become desensitized.

Intraarticular tibiotarsal block. The tibiotarsal joint is the easiest of all the equine joints to inject. Intraarticular tibiotarsal block is induced by inserting a 2.5-cm, 20-gauge needle 2 to 3 cm ventral to the medial malleolus at the distal end of the tibia on either the medial or lateral side of the saphenous vein (Figure 11-29). The capsule is thin, superficial, and easily observed. The needle is inserted in slight ventral direction toward the anterior medial aspect of the hock to a depth of less than 2 cm. The volume of local anesthetic is 10 to 20 ml.

Intraarticular stifle blocks. The stifle joint is the largest joint in the hind limb. It consists of the femoropatellar pouch enclosing the femoropatellar joint and communicates with the medial femorotibial pouch of the femorotibial joint in most horses. The communicating opening can be obstructed in an inflamed stifle joint, necessitating the injection of local anesthetic or medication into each individual compartment.[90] The femoropatellar pouch is most easily entered

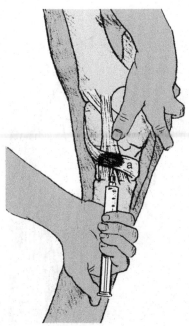

Figure 11–27. Needle placement into cunean bursa of the right rear limb, medial aspect. *a*, Cunean tendon.

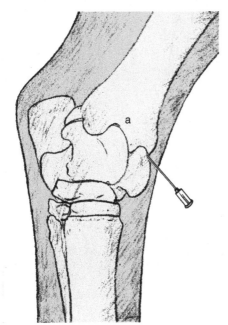

Figure 11–29. Needle placement into the tibiotarsal joint of the left rear limb, medial aspect. *a,* Medial malleolus.

dorsal to the palpable tibial crest between the middle and medial patellar ligaments (Figure 11-30). The lateral femorotibial pouch can be entered between the lateral patellar ligament and the lateral collateral ligament (see Figure 11-30). The medial femorotibial pouch is chosen by some clinicians as an injection site. This pouch is between the medial patellar ligament and the femorotibial ligament dorsal to the proximal medial edge of the tibia (see Figure 11-30). A 5-cm, 18-gauge needle is satisfactory for penetrating the joint capsule and injecting local anesthetic into each pouch.

Trochanteric bursa block. The trochanteric bursa is located on the lateral aspect of the hip between the anterior crest of the great trochanter of the femur and the middle gluteal muscle. Trochanteric bursa block is induced by inserting a 7.5-cm, 18-gauge needle 3 to 5 cm ventral to the anterior crest of the great trochanter and directing it dorsally and medially (Figure 11-31). The bursa should be penetrated to a depth of 3 to 6 cm. A syringe is attached to the needle, and continuous suction is applied. Approximately 10 to 15 ml of local anesthetic is injected after synovial fluid is recovered.

Intraarticular coxofemoral block. The hip joint is the most difficult joint to enter. Several variations of intraarticular coxofemoral block have been described.[83,85,90] The hip joint is blocked by inserting a 15-cm, 14- to 16-gauge spinal needle with stylet between the anterior and posterior eminences of the great trochanter of the femur and advancing it in an anteromedial direction along the femoral neck until the joint capsule is penetrated (see Figure 11-31). Considerable force must be applied to insert the needle while the shaft of the needle is held close to the site of skin penetration. Alternatively, the skin can first be penetrated by a wider-bore needle (3.75-cm, 14-gauge) through which a thinner (15-cm, 18 gauge) and more flexible needle is inserted. Approximately 30 to 50 ml of local anesthetic is injected after synovial fluid is recovered on aspiration. A minimum of 30 minutes is required to reach maximum anesthetic effect and before improvement of the lameness can be assessed.

Laparotomy

At least four techniques for inducing anesthesia of the paralumbar fossa and abdominal wall in the standing horse have been described: (1) infiltration anesthesia, (2) paravertebral thoracolumbar anesthesia, (3) segmental dorsolumbar epidural anesthesia, and (4) thoracolumbar subarachnoid anesthesia (Table 11-8). Any of these techniques may be

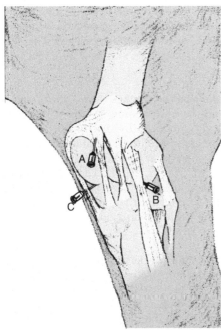

Figure 11–30. Needle placement into *(A)* femoropatellar pouches, *(B)* lateral femorotibial pouch, and *(C)* medial femorotibial pouch of the stifle joint.

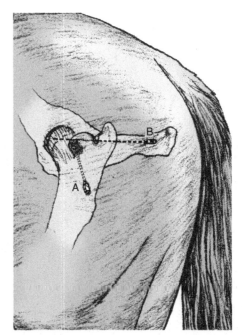

Figure 11–31. Needle placement into *(A)* trochanteric bursa and *(B)* coxofemoral joint.

Table 11–8.	**Techniques for thoracocaudal analgesia in horses**
Technique	**Area blocked**
Paravertebral thoracolumbar	T18-L2
Segmental thoracolumbar subarachnoid	T12-L3
Segmental thoracolumbar epidural	T12-L3
Caudal epidural	S2-coccyx
Continuous caudal epidural	S2-coccyx
Continuous caudal subarachnoid	S2-coccyx

used for surgeries such as exploratory laparotomy, intestinal biopsy, ovariectomy, surgical management of uterine torsion, cesarean section, embryo transfer, castration of stallions with abdominal cryptorchidism, and thoracotomy.

Infiltration Anesthesia

Simple infiltration of the incision line (line block) is the easiest and probably the most commonly used technique for producing anesthesia of the flank in horses. Multiple subcutaneous injections of 1 ml of local anesthetic, 1 to 2 cm apart, are administered using a 2.5-cm, 20-gauge or smaller needle. Successive injections are made slowly and continuously as the needle is inserted at the edge of the desensitized skin. Approximately 10 to 15 ml of anesthetic is adequate for the skin and subcutaneous line block. This is followed by deep infiltration of the muscle layers and parietal peritoneum using a 7.5-cm to 10-cm, 18-gauge needle and 50 to 150 ml of the anesthetic, depending on the area to be desensitized. Adult horses (500 kg) safely tolerate 250-ml 2% lidocaine HCL solution for the line block, which is equivalent to 5 g.[99] Ten to 15 minutes are required for onset of anesthesia. When compared with any other technique, the advantages of the line block are ease of administration and no need for special equipment. Disadvantages of local infiltration anesthesia include distortion of normal tissue architecture, incomplete anesthesia (particularly of the peritoneum), incomplete muscle relaxation of the deeper layers of the abdominal wall, toxicity after injecting significant amounts of anesthetic solution into the peritoneal cavity, and increased cost because of larger doses of anesthetic and time required.

Paravertebral Thoracolumbar Anesthesia

The dorsal and ventral branches of the last thoracic (T18) and first and second lumbar (L1 and L2) spinal nerves are desensitized to induce anesthesia of the skin, musculature, and flank of the midflank region as an alternative to the line block. The T18 to L2 spinal nerves ramify laterally at the intervertebral foramina to form dorsal and ventral branches. The dorsal branches ramify into a medial branch that innervates the lumbar muscles and a lateral branch that innervates the skin of the upper paralumbar fossa.

The lateral cutaneous branches of dorsal spinal nerves T18, L1, and L2 are desensitized by injecting 10 ml of local anesthetic SQ at three sites: between the caudal border of the last rib and distal end of the first lumbar transverse process (for T18), between the first and second transverse processes (for L1), and between the second and third lumbar transverse processes (for L2), respec-

tively. These subcutaneous deposits are made approximately 10 cm from the midline (Figure 11-32). The distance between the injection sites ranges from 3 to 6 cm. A 7.5-cm, 18-gauge needle is used to reach the ventral branches of T18, L1, and L2. The needle is inserted through the desensitized skin at each site until the peritoneum is punctured. Loss of resistance to needle insertion and a slight sucking as air enters the needle are signs that the peritoneum has been entered. The point of the needle should be withdrawn to a retroperitoneal position, where a second deposit of 15 ml of local anesthetic is placed (see Figure 11-32). An additional 5 ml of anesthetic is injected as the needle is withdrawn. Selective ipsilateral anesthesia of the flank (dermatome T18), caudal flank to the lateral surface of the thigh (dermatome L1), and cranial aspect of the thigh to the lateral surface of the stifle (dermatome L2) is a common finding after successful paravertebral blockade.

When compared with infiltration anesthesia, paravertebral anesthesia offers the advantages of small doses of anesthetic; a wide and uniform area of anesthesia and muscle relaxation; and absence of local anesthetic from the operative wound margins, minimizing edema, hematoma, and possible interference with healing. The disadvantages of paravertebral block include difficulty in performing the technique, especially where the landmarks for injection are not identified or when spinal nerves follow a variable course, and loss of motor control of the pelvic limbs resulting from inadvertent desensitization of the third lumbar spinal nerve, which carries motor fibers to the femoral and ischial nerves.

Segmental Dorsolumbar Epidural Anesthesia

Segmental dorsolumbar epidural anesthesia is technically difficult and requires the use of a unidirectional pointed spinal needle and stiff catheter-stylet unit to catheterize the

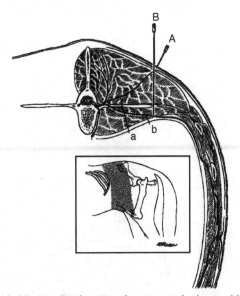

Figure 11–32. Needle placement for paravertebral nerve blockades. **A,** Cranial view of a transsection of the first lumbar vertebra at the location of the intervertebral foramen; *(A)* subcutaneous infiltration; *(B)* retroperitoneal infusion; *a,* dorsal branch; *b,* ventral branch of L1 vertebral nerve. **B,** Desensitized subcutaneous area after blockade of T18, L1, and L2 vertebral nerves.

T18-L1 epidural space from the lumbosacral space. The administration of 4 ml of local anesthetic into the properly placed catheter is sufficient to desensitize the adjacent spinal nerves T18 to L2; and anesthesia of the entire flank region results 10 to 20 minutes after injection and lasts for 50 to 100 minutes.[40] The technique is not practical or readily applicable for use in the field because of frequent kinking and curling of the catheter at the lumbar site with subsequent injection of local anesthetic to the femoral and ischial nerves, thereby producing loss of pelvic limb function.

Thoracolumbar Subarachnoid Anesthesia

Thoracolumbar subarachnoid anesthesia produces the fastest and best controlled surgical anesthesia in horses. However, special equipment and aseptic technique are required.[100] A 17.5-cm, 17-gauge Huber point Tuohy needle with stylet and with the bevel directed cranially is inserted aseptically into the subarachnoid space at the lumbosacral (L6-S1) intervertebral space. This interspace is located 1 to 2 cm caudal of a line drawn between the cranial edge of each tuber sacrale and the dorsal midline. A depression between the dorsal spinous processes of the sixth lumbar (L6) and second sacral (S2) vertebrae can be palpated by applying digital pressure to the skin at the highest point of the gluteal region. Rectal palpation of the ventral lumbosacral eminence may be used to locate the L6-S1 intervertebral space.[100] The skin and thoracolumbar fascia adjacent to the interspinous (L6-S1) ligaments are injected with 5 ml of local anesthetic to help minimize pain during the puncture procedure. The point of the needle is advanced along the median plane perpendicular to the spinal cord until it enters the subarachnoid space. The stylet is removed, and 2 to 3 ml of CSF is aspirated (Figure 11-33). An 80- to 100-cm long (ReCathCo, Allison Park, PA; www.recathco.com) reinforced catheter with a stainless steel spring guide is passed through the needle and advanced approximately 60 cm to the midthoracic area. The needle is withdrawn over the catheter, the spring guide is removed, and a 23-gauge needle and three-way stopcock are attached to the catheter. The catheter is withdrawn a calculated distance to place its tip at T18-L1 (see Figure 11-33). The T18-L1 intervertebral space is located by palpating the depressions between the lumbar spinous processes (L6-L1) and by gradually moving the fingers cranial to the caudal edge of the eighteenth (T18) thoracic spine. A small dose (1.5 to 2 ml) of local anesthetic is injected through the catheter at a rate of approximately 0.5 ml/min. CSF is used to remove the remaining local anesthetic from the catheter. Bilateral segmental anesthesia, extending from spinal cord segment T14 to L3 is maximum 5 to 10 minutes after injection of a 2% solution of mepivacaine HCL solution and lasts for 30 to 60 minutes. Surgical anesthesia is easily maintained by fractional bolus administration of 0.5 ml of the anesthetic at 30-minute intervals or as needed. The duration of anesthesia is determined by the decline of the subarachnoid anesthetic concentration (e.g., mepivacaine) resulting from absorption of drug into the systemic circulation and not hydrolysis in CSF.[39]

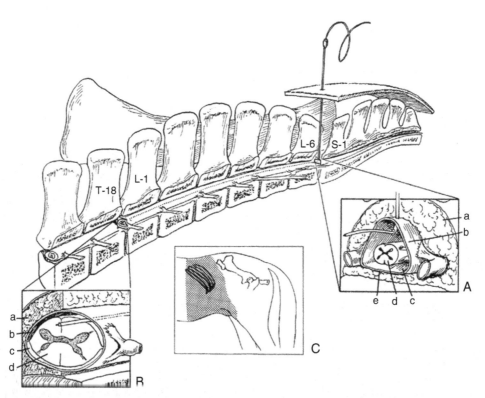

Figure 11–33. Needle and catheter placement for thoracolumbar subarachnoid analgesia. Cranial and left lateral aspect of the thoracolumbar and sacral vertebrae. **A,** Needle tip placement at the lumbosacral subarachnoid space. **B,** Catheter tip placement at the thoracolumbar subarachnoid space. **C,** Desensitized subcutaneous area after segmental blockade. *a,* Epidural space with fat and connective tissue; *b,* dura mater; *c,* arachnoid membrane; *d,* spinal cord; *e,* subarachnoid space with cerebrospinal fluid.

The advantages of thoracolumbar subarachnoid anesthesia compared to dorsolumbar epidural anesthesia include simplicity, deposition of the anesthetic at nerve roots, rapid onset of anesthesia, minimum physiological disturbance, and small doses for maintenance of anesthesia. The disadvantages are the potential for traumatizing the conus medullaris, kinking and curling of the catheter in the subarachnoid space if the wire guide is recessed from the catheter tip, loss of motor control of the pelvic limbs, or hemodynamic disturbances after overdose or injecting the proper dose in a misplaced catheter, and meningitis after septic technique.[100]

Caudal Anesthesia

Caudal epidural anesthesia, continuous caudal epidural anesthesia, and caudal subarachnoid anesthesia are techniques to induce regional anesthesia of the pelvic viscera and genitalia in horses without loss of hind limb motor function. Proper technique should desensitize the caudal and last three pairs of sacral nerves as they emerge from the meninges. The nerves involved are the caudal (for the tail), caudal rectal (for the anal folds, base of the tail, and coccygeal and levator ani muscles), middle rectal (for the perineum, scrotum, and vulva), pudendal (for the penis and vulva), and cranial and caudal gluteal (for the lateral and caudal surface of hip and thigh; Figure 11-34). Blockade of sensory fibers results in loss of sensation to the skin of the tail and croup to the midsacral region, the anus, perineum, vulva, and caudal aspect of the thigh (see Figure 11-34). Blockade of parasympathetic nerve fibers originating from the second, third, and fourth sacral segments of the spinal cord results in relaxation and dilation of the rectum, distal colon, bladder, and reproductive organs. Blockade of motor fibers causes flaccidity of the tail and abolishment of abdominal contractions and may cause weakness of the hind limbs (Table 11-9). The techniques of caudal epidural anesthesia and caudal subarachnoid anesthesia are advocated to control pain and rectal tenesmus associated with irritation of the perineum, anus, rectum, and vagina during difficult labor, and correction of uterine torsion, fetotomy, and various obstetric manipulations. These techniques are commonly used to facilitate surgical procedures such as rectovaginal fistula repairs; prolapsed rectum; Caslick's closure; urethrostomy; tail amputation; or anal, perineal, vulvar, and bladder procedures.

Proper restraint should be used, particularly in fractious horses. The use of a sedative and tranquilizer combination before epidural and subarachnoid injections is often desirable.[69] α_2-Agonists increase urine output in horses, which often results in urination during the surgical procedure.[101]

Caudal Epidural Anesthesia

Caudal epidural anesthesia is used routinely in the horse because it is simple and inexpensive and requires no sophisticated equipment. The technique in horses was first described in 1925; subsequently many have reported its use.[50,51,102-105]

The injection site for caudal epidural anesthesia is the first coccygeal interspace (C_o1-C_o2), identified as the first obvious midline depression caudal to the sacrum (see Table 11-6). The C_o1-C_o2 interspace generally can be palpated as the first movable joint caudal to the sacrum when the tail is raised and lowered. The first coccygeal vertebra usually is fused with the sacrum, and the second is freely movable; thus, C_o1-C_o2 is the site for needle placement (see Figure 11-34). The C_o1-C_o2 interspace may be more difficult to palpate in obese or well-conditioned horses, but it generally lies at the most angular portion of the bend of the tail, 5 to 7 cm cranial to the origin of the first tail hairs and the caudal folds of the tail. Proper restraint should be used, and the horse should be allowed to stand squarely with the croup symmetric.

A 5-cm to 7.5-cm, 18-gauge spinal needle with fitted stylet is inserted in the center of the intercoccygeal space at an angle of about 30 degrees to the horizontal plane until it strikes the floor of the vertebral canal in the standard technique (see Figure 11-34). The needle hub may be filled with isotonic saline solution or anesthetic solution and is slightly withdrawn until the solution is aspirated from the needle hub by epidural subatmospheric pressure. A sucking sound is often heard as the point of the needle enters the epidural

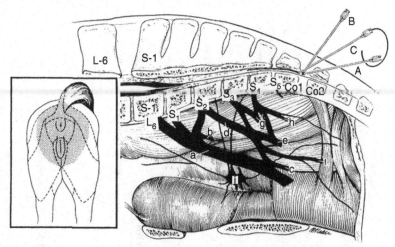

Figure 11-34. *Right,* Needle placement (*A* and *B*) for caudal epidural analgesia. Catheter placement (*C*) for continuous caudal epidural analgesia. The ventral branches of the sixth lumbar (L6) and sacral spinal nerves 1 (S1) to 5 (S5) are shown. Nerve supply to the pelvic viscera of the mare: *a,* sciatic, *b,* caudal gluteal; *c,* caudal cutaneous femoral; *d,* pudendal; *e,* perineal; *f,* distal pudendal; *g,* caudal rectal nerve; *h,* cutaneous nerves; *i,* pelvic plexus. *Left,* Desensitized subcutaneous area after caudal blockade is stippled.

Table 11-9 **Neuroanatomy and effects of caudal epidural analgesia**

Spinal cord segment	Nerves	Branches	Sensory	Motor	Structures supplied		Action
					Parasympathetic	Sympathetic	
Coccygeal	Caudal	—	Most of the tail and skin between anus and tailroot	Coccygeal muscle	—	—	
S5	Caudal rectal (hemorrhoidal)	—	Anal region, tail folds, tail base	Coccygeus and levator and externus muscle	Fibers in caudal rectal nerve	—	Straining in anorectal region resulting from excessive sympathetic stimulation
S4 and 5	Middle rectal	Perineal nerve, caudal scrotal nerves, labial nerves	Perineum, posterior croup, scrotum along its caudal aspects, vulva without clitoris		Pelvic nerves, hypogastric plexus	—	Relaxation of bladder without sphincter, distal colon, rectum, sexual organs
S4, 3, and 2	Pudendal	Dorsal nerve of penis, deep perineal nerve	Penis (corpus cavernosum and spongiosum), clitoris, and vulva	Perineal muscles, fascia of ischiorectal fossa, constrictor vulvae muscle	—	Retractor penis muscle	Prolapse of penis, relaxation of vulva and vagina
Lumbosacral plexus							
S2 and 1	Caudal gluteal	Caudal cutaneous femoral nerve	Lateral and posterior surface of hip and thigh	Extension of hip	—	—	Relaxation of bladder and sphincter of bladder, distal colon, rectum, sexual organs
Sl, L6 and 5	Cranial gluteal	—	Lateral aspect of thigh	Flexor and abductors of hip	—	Splanchnic lumbar nerves (in part)	
Sl, L6 and 5	Ischial	—	Middle to tibial region of foot	Flexor and abductors of hip, flexor of stifle (in part), and extensors of hock and digit	—	—	Ataxia, knuckling of hind fetlock

space. Depth from the skin surface to the neural canal varies between 3 and 7 cm, depending on size and condition of the horse. Correct placement of the needle is further ensured by lack of resistance to the injection of 3 to 5 ml of air into the epidural space and no aspiration of blood.

Alternatively, the spinal needle can be inserted in the center of the C_o1-C_o2 space at a right angle to the general contour of the croup (see Figure 11-34). The needle is first directed ventral in a median plane to the floor of the vertebral canal and is then withdrawn approximately 0.5 cm to avoid injection into the intervertebral disk or ligamentous floor of the canal.

The amount of anesthetic injected is determined by the type of local anesthetic, the size and conformation of the horse, and the extent of regional anesthesia required. A total of 6 to 8 ml of 2% lidocaine HCL solution or its equivalent may be required in a mature 450-kg mare (0.26 to 0.35 mg/kg) to anesthetize the anus, perineum, rectum, vulva, vagina, urethra, and bladder. Other acceptable doses to achieve anesthesia extending from spinal cord segments S1 to coccyx, and thereby producing analgesia of pelvic viscera and genitalia without ataxia of adult horses, are 10 to 12 ml of 2% procaine HCl solution, 5 to 7 ml of 5% procaine HCl solution, 5 to 7 ml of 2% mepivacaine HCl solution, 3 to 5 ml of 5% hexylcaine HCl solution, and 0.17 mg of xylazine/kg diluted in 10 ml of 0.9% sodium chloride (NaCl) solution.[51] Maximum effect should be manifest in 10 to 30 minutes. It is not advisable to redose during this time. Additional quantities of anesthetic can be administered if the needle is left in place and an injection cap is attached. The duration of anesthesia is dose related and lasts from 60 to 90 minutes for 5% procaine and 2% lidocaine, 90 to 120 minutes for 5% hexylcaine and 2% mepivacaine, and 180 to 240 minutes for xylazine. Improper injection technique, anatomical abnormalities, or adhesions resulting from previous epidural injections are some of the most important causes of failed caudal epidural anesthesia.[105] Overdosing can induce serious side effects resulting from rear limb ataxia or motor

blockade, recumbency, and excitement in conscious horses. A horse with hind limb weakness should be supported by a tail-tie for 60 to 90 minutes or until full hind limb control is regained. Infection of the neural canal, another serious potential complication, can be avoided by proper aseptic technique. Trauma to the spinal cord and meninges is nearly impossible because these structures end craniad to the site of injection. Only the coccygeal nerves and the thin phylum terminale remain in the spinal canal at the site of needle penetration, and these structures are not easily damaged.

Continuous Caudal Epidural Anesthesia

Continuous caudal epidural anesthesia in horses can be achieved by aseptically placing a catheter into the epidural space using one of two methods described. A 10.2-cm, 18-gauge thin-walled Tuohy needle with stylet is inserted on the midline into the C_o1-C_o2 interspace while being directed cranially and ventrally at an angle of approximately 45 degrees to the croup in the more simple method (see Figure 11-34).[106] The needle is advanced until an abrupt reduction in resistance to needle passage is noted, indicating piercing through the interarcuate ligament and entry into the vertebral canal. Injection of 10 ml of air should not encounter resistance. Commercially available 91.8-cm, 20-gauge epidural catheters with graduated markings and stylet (Allison Park, PA; www.recathco.com) or medical-grade sterile tubing is introduced into the needle and advanced cranially 2.5 to 4 cm beyond the tip of the needle. The needle is removed from the catheter while the catheter is left in position. A catheter adapter (provided in many kits) is placed into the distal end of the catheter for an injection port. The desired amount of anesthetic solution (4 to 8 ml) is then administered over a period of 1 minute. The syringe should be replaced by a catheter cap to prevent inadvertent dosing between injections.

Alternatively (the more difficult method) a 19.5-cm, 17-gauge Huber-point Tuohy needle with stylet and with the bevel directed caudally is aseptically inserted into the epidural space at the lumbosacral (L6-S1) intervertebral space (Figure 11-35).[50,51,105] Depth of needle penetration ranges

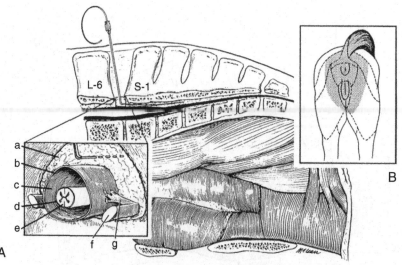

Figure 11–35. Needle placement into the lumbosacral epidural space and catheterization of the sacral epidural space. **A,** Craniolateral view of a transsection of the fifth sacral vertebra at the location of the intervertebral foramen, showing the relation of structures inside the spinal canal: *a,* epidural space with fat and connective tissue; *b,* dura mater; *c,* arachnoid membrane; *d,* pia mater; *e,* spinal cord; *f,* first sacral (S1); *g,* second sacral (S2) spinal nerve. **B,** Desensitized subcutaneous area after caudal blockade is stippled.

from 11 to 14 cm in the adult horse. A catheter reinforced with a stainless steel spring guide is threaded into the needle for 10 to 20 cm. This places the catheter tip at the caudal portion of the sacral (S3-S5) epidural space. Then 4 to 5 ml of local anesthetic is injected after the Huber point needle and wire guide have been removed.

Compared with the needle technique, the advantages of the catheter technique are that the catheter tip is placed at the nerve roots of the pudendal and pelvic nerves, thus minimizing the doses of anesthetic required to produce caudal anesthesia. The catheter also provides a route for repeated administration of small fractional doses of the anesthetic during surgery while the tail is dorsally reflected for immobilization and surgical exposure. The necessity of only one puncture might diminish fibrosis of the extradural space resulting from repeated standard epidural blocks. Disadvantages of the catheter technique include greater potential for infection and greater cost of equipment. Complications with catheters include kinking, curling, and occlusion of the tip with fibrin. Newer catheter designs avoid these problems. Radiographs of the catheter are mandatory if the position of the tubing must be known. The future use of epidural catheters for extending the postoperative analgesia or relieving tenesmus will be less popular with the availability of newer long-acting local anesthetic drugs, narcotics, and α_2-adrenoceptor agonists.

Continuous Caudal Subarachnoid Anesthesia

Lumbosacral subarachnoid anesthesia and anesthesia of the cranial portion of the caudal subarachnoid space in horses was first described in 1901. Injection of local anesthetic into a needle placed into the lumbosacral subarachnoid space is not practical or readily available to use in the field because it produces anesthesia of the pelvic limbs, flank, and lower aspect of the abdomen.[40,50,51] A catheter technique for continuous caudal subarachnoid anesthesia in horses while maintaining pelvic limb function overcomes the problem associated with the needle technique.[38,40,107] First, a 19.5-cm, 17-gauge Huber-point directional needle with stylet and with the bevel directed caudally is inserted aseptically into the subarachnoid space at the lumbosacral (C6-S1) intervertebral space (Figure 11-36). This space is located by palpation of bony landmarks as previously described and is identified by free flow of spinal fluid from the needle hub or by aspiration. A 30-cm Formocath polyethylene catheter (0.625 mm outside diameter), reinforced with a stainless steel spring guide, is then passed through the needle and advanced approximately 15 to 25 cm to the midsacral region.

The catheter tip cannot be advanced beyond the end of the subarachnoid space, which usually is the third sacral (S3) space. The distance between the skin surface and subarachnoid puncture site ranges from 10 to 15 cm, and the distance from the lumbosacral to the caudal subarachnoid space ranges from 8 to 12 cm in adult horses. After removal of 1 to 2 ml of CSF, 1.5 to 2 ml of 2% mepivacaine HCL solution or its equivalent is injected at a rate of approximately 0.5 ml/min (3 minutes). Bilateral caudal anesthesia, extending from spinal cord segments S2 to coccyx, is maximum 5 to 12 minutes after injection and lasts for 20 to 80 minutes.[50,51,107] Surgical anesthesia is easily maintained by fractional bolus administration of 0.5 ml of the anesthetic at 30-minute intervals or as needed.

Subarachnoid administration of local anesthetic when compared with epidural administration requires approximately three times less drug for a similar degree of caudal anesthesia. The onset of anesthesia is twice as fast, and the duration of action is half as long as after epidural injection. Also, asymmetric or incomplete anesthesia resulting from septa within the epidural space or inadequate dispersal of the anesthetic because of epidural fat is avoided. The roots of the spinal nerves within the subarachnoid space are not covered by protective dural sheets and are more readily desensitized. The use of subarachnoid caudal anesthesia in practice is limited because of technical difficulty, potential trauma to the conus medullaris and nerve fibers by the needle or catheter, and the relatively high frequency of postanesthetic myositis.

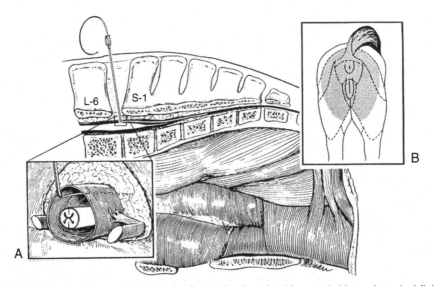

Figure 11–36. Needle placement into the lumbosacral subarachnoid space (with cerebrospinal fluid) and catheterization of the sacral subarachnoid space. **A,** Craniolateral view of a transsection of the first sacral vertebra. **B,** Desensitized subcutaneous area after caudal blockade is stippled. **A** and **B** structures are similar to those in Figure 10-35, *A* and *B*.

Castration

Castration is one of the most commonly performed surgical procedures in general equine practice. Regional anesthesia for castration may be accomplished by injecting local anesthetic drug into the spermatic cord or testis of horses in a standing or laterally recumbent position.[108]

Percutaneous anesthesia of the spermatic cord is accomplished by inserting a 2.5-cm, 20-gauge needle into the cord as close to the external inguinal ring as possible. Approximately 20 to 30 ml of 2% lidocaine HCL solution is injected in a fan-shaped manner without perforating the spermatic artery and vein. The incision sites of the scrotal skin are also desensitized by infiltrating SQ with 5 to 10 ml of local anesthetic. For intratesticular injection, a 6.25-cm, 18-gauge needle is quickly inserted perpendicularly through the tensed skin of the scrotum, and 20 to 30 ml of 2% lidocaine HCL solution is injected into the center of the testis (Figure 11-37). The scrotal tissues along the incision site must also be infiltrated with 5 to 10 ml of the anesthetic. The procedures are repeated to desensitize the opposite testis and scrotum. Ten minutes are allowed for maximum effect, although the anesthetic diffuses quickly (within 90 seconds) from the testis up to the spermatic cord by way of lymph vessels. General anesthesia is often used for recumbent castration.[109]

Therapeutic Local Anesthesia

Infiltration of sympathetic nerves by local anesthetics is effective for relief of vasoconstriction and pain. The two sites where the equine sympathetic nervous system can be desensitized without affecting somatosensory function are the cervicothoracic (stellate) ganglion and paravertebral lumbar sympathetic ganglia.

Cervicothoracic (Stellate) Ganglion Block

Infiltration of the cervicothoracic ganglion (CTG) in horses with local anesthetic effectively interrupts reflex spasm of the local vasculature and pain in the head, neck, and thoracic limb. CTG blockade in horses has been demonstrated as a therapeutic measure for idiopathic shoulder lameness; radial nerve paralysis; eczema of the head and neck; and a variety of diseases of muscle, joints, and tendon sheaths of the front leg. Acute disorders are responsive to a single blockade, whereas chronic conditions require two to three blockades for good results. Infiltration of the CTG in the horse with local anesthetic is a relatively safe procedure when performed from a cranial and paratracheal site.[110] The horse should be confined with both thoracic limbs bearing equal weight. The skin puncture site is 12 to 17 cm dorsal to the intermediate tubercle of the humerus in the jugular furrow dorsal to the jugular vein and carotid artery. This area is surgically scrubbed and infiltrated with 2 to 3 ml of local anesthetic solution. A 25-cm, 16-gauge needle is inserted through the desensitized skin and pushed horizontally or 5 degrees dorsomedially until it impinges on the transverse process or body of the seventh cervical vertebra and 2 to 3 ml of the anesthetic are injected (Figure 11-38). The depth of needle penetration ranges from 11 to 15 cm, depending on the thickness and elasticity of the musculus longus colli. The needle is first withdrawn 5 to 10 cm; its tip is redirected more lateral and ventral, thereby bypassing the seventh cervical vertebra and reaching the articulations of the first and second ribs (see Figure 11-38). The needle will be 15 to 20 cm from the surface of the skin.[110] The needle is correctly placed if there is no air, blood, or spinal fluid on needle aspiration; if there is no resistance to the injection of local anesthetic; and if the block works. Approximately 50 ml of 1% lidocaine HCl in aqueous solution (lidocaine) is injected at this site. An additional 50 ml of lidocaine is injected during withdrawal of the needle for 6 to 10 cm. CTG blockade results in ipsilateral, increased subcutaneous temperature (up to 3° C); profuse sweating of the head, neck, and thoracic limb; ipsilateral Horner's syndrome (e.g., ptosis, mio-

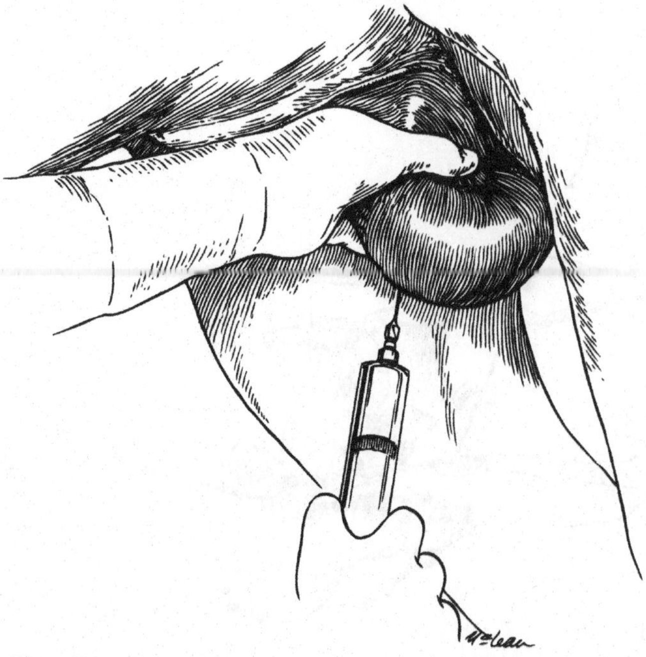

Figure 11-37. Needle placement for right intratesticular injection in a standing horse.

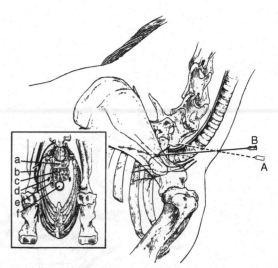

Figure 11-38. Needle placement to the seventh cervical vertebra *(A)* and cervicothoracic (stellate) ganglion *(right side)*. *Inset:* cranial view of a transsection: *a,* seventh cervical vertebra; *b,* ventral branch of the eighth cervical spinal nerve; *c,* longus colli muscle; *d,* right cervicothoracic ganglion; *e,* esophagus; *f,* trachea.

sis, and enophthalmos); and ipsilateral laryngeal paresis (see Chapter 22). These signs are present 10 to 15 minutes after injection and last for more than 75 minutes. Increased skin temperature is related to increased blood flow (vasodilation) to muscle and cutaneous vascular beds. Increased sweating is caused by increased blood supply and thus increased heat in the area, higher metabolism in sweat glands, and central stimulation caused by excitement of the horse. Horner's syndrome is caused by interruption of the oculosympathetic pathway at the site of the CTG or at the site of the ventral sympathetic roots between the eighth cervical and second thoracic spinal nerves.[111,112] Hemodynamic and respiratory alterations induced by unilateral CTG blockade in horses are usually minor. Heart rate, cardiac output, aortic blood pressure, and total peripheral resistance in horses are well maintained; and maximum plasma concentrations of lidocaine are minimal (0.4 to 1.3 µg/ml) after unilateral CTG blockade.[29] Vagal inhibition results in decreased respiratory rates and increased arterial CO_2 tensions. However, hypoventilation in horses is not severe enough to induce significant respiratory acidosis or hypoxemia.[29] Transitory brachial plexus and recurrent laryngeal nerve paralysis and thoracentesis resulting in pneumothorax are potential important complications contraindicating bilateral CTG blockade in horses.

Paravertebral lumbar sympathetic ganglion block

Infiltration of the lumbar sympathetic ganglia in horses with local anesthetic solution is indicated and therapeutically recommended for myositis, periostitis, coxitis, and paralysis of the fibular and penile nerves. The lumbar sympathetic trunk is located between the transverse process of the second and third lumbar (L2 and L3) vertebrae about 15 cm lateral to their spinous processes.[113] Other possible puncture sites are between the eighteenth thoracic and first lumbar vertebrae and between the first and second

and third and fourth lumbar vertebrae, but not between the fourth and fifth lumbar vertebrae, which have a very narrow interspace. The puncture site (between L2 and L3) is aseptically prepared and infiltrated with 2 to 3 ml of local anesthetic. A 25-cm, 16-gauge needle with a marker on the needle shaft is inserted through the desensitized skin and advanced until its tip contacts the transverse process of L2 or L3. The marker is used to note the 15- to 20-cm depth of needle penetration (Figure 11-39, A). The needle is partially withdrawn and then reinserted to walk its tip off the transverse process and locate the intertransverse ligament (angle α). The needle is withdrawn to the subcutaneous area and inserted at angle α and approximately 45 degrees from vertical for the calculated distance, which equals the distance between the marker (skin puncture) and the needle point plus an additional 5 to 8 cm (Figure 11-39, B). Approximately 100 ml of 1% lidocaine HCL solution is slowly injected after aspirating to ensure that the needle tip has not entered the peritoneum or a blood vessel. This amount of anesthetic diffuses throughout the tissues surrounding the sympathetic trunk and two segments rostrally and caudally. Adequate sympathetic blockade is indicated by elevation of the skin and subcutaneous temperature and profuse sweating of the ipsilateral pelvic limb within 10 minutes. Lumbar somatic nerves should not be desensitized by using this technique; thus sensory and motor anesthesia does not result. Nonsedated horses tolerate unilateral lumbar sympathetic ganglion blockade (ULSG block) well. The heart rate and pulse pressure of horses during ULSG block are increased to maintain cardiac output and systemic arterial blood pressure. The respiratory rate in horses during ULSG block is decreased, but alveolar ventilation remains adequate, as indicated by normal arterial blood gas tensions (PO_2, $PaCO_2$) and pH (pHa).[113] Potential complications include puncture of blood vessels, resulting in hematoma, intravascular injection, abdominocentesis, and needle breakage.

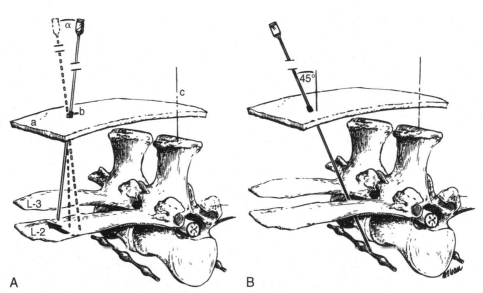

A   B

Figure 11-39. Needle placement to the lumbar sympathetic trunk. **A,** Needle tip at the transverse process. **B,** Right ganglionic chain. *a,* Skin; *b,* marker; *c,* midline.

COMPLICATIONS

Complications associated with use of local and regional anesthesia may be related to the drug administered, poor preparation of the patient, poor equipment, and poor technique (Box 11-2).[51,114-118] Ataxia and recumbency can occur following caudal epidural administration of local anesthetics. Severe pruritus has occurred after the epidural administration of morphine and detomidine in a horse.[116] The ideal practice is to complement local and regional anesthesia with supplementary sedatives or narcotic-tranquilizer combinations during surgery (see Chapter 10). The likelihood of postinjection reaction and breaking needles is low, and the risk can be further reduced by properly restraining the horse and using flexible, disposable needles, and spinal needles with stylet. Nondisposable needles and syringes provide the best equipment for the performance of aseptic regional anesthesia. The owner and trainer should follow medication rules for competition horses because many of the drugs are detectable in plasma and urine.

Systemic Toxicity

Systemic toxicity may occur when excessive amounts of local anesthetic enter the bloodstream resulting from either overdose or inadvertent intravascular injection. The risk in foals is much higher than in adult horses (see Figure 11-5).[119] Strict observance of safe doses and frequent aspiration tests lessen the chances for intravascular injection.

Benzocaine HCL can produce methemoglobinemia in dogs, but benzocaine-induced methemoglobinemia in horses has not been reported.

Local Tissue Toxicity and Nerve Damage

Local anesthetics in conventional concentrations should not produce nerve damage of clinical importance. Experimental studies suggest that both low-potency and high-potency ester local anesthetics (3% 2-chloroprocaine HCl, 10% procaine HCl, 1% tetracaine HCl) and amide local anesthetics (2% mepivacaine HCl, 1.5% etidocaine HCl) can penetrate and break down the perineural sheath and produce nerve injury (e.g., axonal degeneration and demyelination) 48 hours after perineural deposition of drugs.[120] Local anesthetics administered in clinically relevant concentrations can damage skeletal muscle fibers, although the clinical relevance of this finding in horses remains undetermined.[121]

Epinephrine in appropriate doses of 1:200,000 is not neurotoxic. Local anesthetics containing epinephrine must not be injected along wound edges in thin-skinned Thoroughbreds and Arabians because it causes sloughing.[66] Likewise, the combination of lidocaine HCl (20 mg/ml), epinephrine (0.012 mg/ml), and sodium penicillin (800,000 U) must not be injected into the coffin joint of horses. It can cause irreversible lameness based on ossifying arthrosis.[68]

Infection as a complication of regional anesthetic techniques is rarely seen if appropriate sterile technique is used and injection into contaminated areas is avoided. Serious infection in and around the neuraxis is virtually nonexistent, although mild inflammatory reaction occurs at the puncture site. The low incidence of infection in regional anesthesia could be related to the antimicrobial activity of local anesthetic drugs. "Hooked" needles may cause trauma to nerves and nerve trunks.

Tachyphylaxis

Tachyphylaxis or acute tolerance to local anesthetic agents is defined as a decrease in duration, segmental spread, or intensity of regional block after repeated administration of equal doses of the anesthetic. Various local anesthetics, including cocaine, procaine, tetracaine, lidocaine, lidocaine-CO_2, mepivacaine, bupivacaine, etidocaine, and dibucaine, have been used at increasing doses to maintain a given effect during surface anesthesia, conduction block, spinal or epidural anesthesia, and brachial plexus block. The underlying mechanisms of tachyphylaxis are not well understood. Local alterations of disposition and absorption of local anesthetic drugs might play a role in the development of tachyphylaxis.[1] Structural (ester versus amide), pharmacological properties of local anesthetics (short- versus long-acting), technique, mode of administration (intermittent versus continuous), and pharmacodynamic processes (effectiveness at receptor sites) do not appear to be linked to tachyphylaxis.[1,122,123] Time-dependent variations in pain and circadian changes in the duration of local anesthetic action simulate its occurrence (pseudotachyphylaxis).[1,122,123]

REFERENCES

1. Becker DE, Reed KL: Essentials of local anesthetic pharmacology, *Anesth Prog* 53:98-109, 2006.
2. Skarda RT, Tranquilli WJ: Selected anesthetic and analgesic techniques. In Tranquilli WJ, Thurmon JC, Grim KA: *Lumb & Jones veterinary anesthesia and analgesia*, ed 4, 2007, Blackwell Publishing, pp 561-681.
3. Hodgkin AL, Huxley AF: A quantitative description of membrane current and its application to conduction and excitation in nerve, *J Physiol (Lond)* 117:500-544, 1952.
4. Strichartz GR: Molecular mechanisms of nerve block by local anesthetics, *Anesthesiology* 45:421-441, 1976.
5. Wildsmith JA: Peripheral nerve and local anesthetic drugs, *Br J Anesth* 58:692-700, 1986.
6. Rosenberg PH, Heavner JE: Temperature-dependent nerve-blocking action of lidocaine and halothane, *Acta Anesth Scand* 24:314-320, 1980.
7. Sanchez V, Arthur R, Strichartz GR: Fundamental properties of local anesthetics. I. The dependence of lidocaine's ionization and octanol: buffer partitioning on solvent and temperature, *Anesth Analg* 66:159-165, 1987.

Box 11-2 Potential Complications Associated with Local or Regional Analgesic Techniques

- Partial or incomplete analgesic effect
- Nerve toxicity and prolonged nerve blockade
- Allergic skin reactions
- Local infection from contamination
- Accidental intravascular injection and inadvertent overdose
- Muscle fasiculations, ataxia, or recumbency after epidural administration
- Sedation
- Agitation and excitement after larger doses

8. Butterworth JF et al: Cooling lidocaine from room temperature to 5° (neither hastens nor improves median nerve block), *Anesth Analg* 68:S45, 1989.

9. Courtney KR, Kendig JJ, Cohen EN: Frequency dependent conduction block: the role of nerve impulse pattern in local anesthetic potency, *Anesthesiology* 48:111-117, 1978.

10. Fankenhaeuser B: Quantitative description of sodium currents in myelinated nerve fibers of xenopus laevis, *J Physiol* (Lond), 151:491-501, 1960.

11. Saito HS et al: Interactions of lidocaine and calcium in blocking the compound action potential of frog sciatic nerve, *Anesthesiology* 60:205-208, 1984.

12. In Cousins MJ, Brindenbaugh PO, editors: *Neural blockade in clinical anesthesia and pain management*, Philadelphia, 1980, JB Lippincott.

13. Covino BG: Pharmacology of local anaesthetic agents, *Br J Anaesth* 58:701-716, 1986.

14. deJong RH: *Physiology and pharmacology of local anesthesia*, Springfield, Il, 1970, Charles C Thomas.

15. Franz DN, Perry RS: Mechanisms of differential block among single myelinated and non-myelinated axons of procaine, *J Physiol* (Lond) 236:193-210, 1974.

16. Sissen AJ, Covino BG, Gregus J: Differential sensitivities of mammalian nerve fibers to local anesthetic agents, *Anesthesiology* 53:467-474, 1980.

17. Tobin T et al: Pharmacology of procaine in the horse: procaine esterase properties of equine plasma and synovial fluid, *Am J Vet Res* 37:1165-1170, 1976.

18. Evans JA, Lambert MBT: Estimation of procaine in urine of horses, *Vet Rec* 95:316-318, 1974.

19. Tobin T et al: Pharmacology of procaine in the horse: pharmacokinetics and behavioral effects, *Am J Vet Res* 38:637-647, 1977.

20. Wintzer HJ: Pharmacokinetics of procaine injected into the hock joint of the horse, *Equine Vet J* 13:68-69, 1981.

21. Meyer-Jones L: Miscellaneous observations on the clinical effects of injecting solutions and suspensions of procaine hydrochloride into domestic animals, *Vet Med* 45:435-437, 1951.

22. Kamerling SG et al: Differential effects of phenylbutazone and local anesthetics on nociception in the equine, *Eur J Pharmacol* 107:35-41, 1985.

23. Mac Kellar JC: Procaine hydrochloride in the treatment of spasmodic colic in horses, *Vet Rec* 80:44-47, 1967.

24. Brown DT, Beamish D, Wildsmith JAW: Allergic reaction to an amide local anesthetic, *Br J Anaesth* 53:435-437, 1981.

25. Aldrete JA, Johnson DA: Evaluation of intracutaneous testing for investigation of allergy to local anesthetic agents, *Anesth Analg* (Cleve) 49:173-175, 1970.

26. Maes A et al: Determination of lidocaine and its two N-desethylated metabolites in dog and horse plasma by high-performance liquid chromatography combined with electrospray ionization tandem mass spectrometry, *J Chromatogr B Analyt Technol Biomed Life Sci* 852(1-2):180-187, 2007.

27. Feary DJ et al: Influence of general anesthesia on pharmacokinetics of intravenous lidocaine infusion in horses, *Am J Vet Res* 66(4):574-580, 2005.

28. Bertler A et al: In vivo lung uptake of lidocaine in pigs, *Acta Anaesth Scand* 22:530-536, 1978.

29. Skarda RT, Muir WW, Couri D: Plasma lidocaine concentrations in conscious horses after cervicothoracic (stellate) ganglion block with 1% lidocaine HCl solution, *Am J Vet Res* 48:1092-1097, 1987.

30. Malone E et al: Intravenous continuous infusion of lidocaine for treatment of equine ileus, *Vet Surg* 35:60-66, 2006.

31. Doherty TJ, Frazier DL: Effect of intravenous lidocaine on halothane minimum alveolar concentration in ponies, *Equine Vet J* 30(4):300-303, 1998.

32. Bidwell LA, Wilson DV, Caron JP: Lack of systemic absorption of lidocaine from 5% patches placed on horses, *Vet Anaesth Analg* 34(6):443-446, 2007.

33. Courtot D: Elimination of lignocaine in the horse, *Ir Vet J* 33(12):205-208, 215, 1979.

34. Engelking LR et al: Pharmacokinetics of antipyrine, acetaminophen, and lidocaine in fed and fasted horses, *J Vet Pharmacol Ther* 10:73-82, 1985.

35. Scott DB: Toxic effects of local anesthetic agents on the central nervous system, *Br J Anesth* 58:732-735, 1986.

36. Wagman IH, deJong RH, Prince DA: Effects of lidocaine on the central nervous system, *Anesthesiology* 28:155-172, 1967.

37. Arthur GR et al: Acute IV toxicity of LEA-103, a new local anesthetic, compared to lidocaine and bupivacaine in the awake dog, *Anesthesiology* 65:(3A):A182, 1986.

38. Skarda RT, Muir WW, Ibrahim AL: Plasma mepivacaine concentrations after caudal epidural and subarachnoid injection in the horse: comparative study, *Am J Vet Res* 45:1967-1971, 1984.

39. Skarda RT, Muir WW, Ibrahim AL: Spinal fluid concentrations of mepivacaine in horses and procaine in cows after thoracolumbar subarachnoid analgesia, *Am J Vet Res* 46:1020-1024, 1985.

40. Skarda RT, Muir WW: Segmental epidural and subarachnoid analgesia in horses: a comparative study, *Am J Vet Res* 44: 1870-1876, 1983.

41. Derossi R et al: .05% versus racemic 0.5% bupivacaine for caudal epidural analgesia in horses, *J Vet Pharmacol Ther* 28(3): 293-297, 2005.

42. Thomas RD, Behbehani MM, Coyle DE: Cardiovascular toxicity of local anesthetics: an alternative hypothesis, *Anesth Analg* 65:444-450, 1986.

43. Akerman B, Sandberg R, Covino BG: Local anesthetic efficacy of LEA 103—an experimental xylidide agent, *Anesthesiology* 65(3A):A217, 1986.

45. Skarda RT, Muir WW: Analgesic, behavioural, and hemodynamic and respiratory effects of midsacral subarachnoidally administered ropivacaine hydrochloride in mares, *Vet Anaesth Analg* (1):37-50, 2003.

46. Ritchie JM, Cohn PJ, Dripps RD: Cocaine, procaine, and other synthetic local anesthetics. In Goodman LS, Gilman A, editors: *The pharmacological basis of therapeutics*, ed 4, New York, 1970, Macmillan, p 371.

47. Worthman RP: Diagnostic anesthetic injections. In Mansmann RA, McAllister ES, Pratt PW, editors: *Equine medicine and surgery*, ed 3, Santa Barbara, Ca, 1982, American Veterinary Publications, pp 947-952.

48. Hay RC, Yonezawa T, Derrick WS: Control of intractable pain in advanced cancer by subarachnoid alcohol block, *JAMA* 169:1315-1320, 1959.

49. Colter SB: Electromyographic detection and evaluation of tail alterations in show ring horses. In Proceedings of the Sixth Annual Veterinary Medicine Forum, Denver, 1988, ACVIM, pp 421-423.

50. Grosenbaugh DA, Skarda RT, Muir WW: Caudal regional anaesthesia in horses, *Equine Vet Ed* 11(2):98-105, 1999.

51. Robinson EP, Natalini CC: Epidural anesthesia and analgesia in horses, *Vet Clin North Am* (Equine Pract) 18(1):61-82, 2002.

52. Olbrich VH, Mosing M: A comparison of the analgesic effects of caudal epidural methadone and lidocaine in the horse, *Vet Anaesth Analg* 30(3):156-164, 2003.

53. DeRossi R et al: Perineal analgesia and hemodynamic effects of the epidural administration of meperidine or hyperbaric bupivacaine in conscious horses, *Can Vet J* 45(1):42-47, 2004.

54. Ganidagli S et al: Comparison of ropivacaine with a combination of ropivacaine and fentanyl for the caudal epidural anesthesia of mares, *Vet Rec* 154(11):329-332, 2004.

55. Natalini CC, Linardi RL: Analgesic effects of epidural administration of hydromorphone in horses, *Am J Vet Res* 67(1):11-15, 2006.

56. Burm AG et al: Epidural anesthesia with lidocaine and bupivacaine: effects of epinephrine on the plasma concentration profiles, *Anesth Analg* 65:1281-1284, 1986.

57. Collins JG et al: Spinally administered epinephrine suppresses noxiously evoked activity of WDR neurons in the dorsal horn of the spinal cord, *Anesthesiology* 60:269-275, 1984.

58. Brose WG, Cohen SE: Epidural lidocaine for cesarean section: minimum effective epinephrine concentration, *Anesth Analg* 67:S23, 1988.

59. Leicht CH, Carlson JA: Prolongation of lidocaine spinal anesthesia with epinephrine and phenylephrine, *Anesth Analg* 65:365-369, 1986.

60. Nicoll JM et al: Retrobulbar anesthesia: the role of hyaluronidase, *Anesth Analg* 65:1324-1328, 1986.

61. Ludmore I et al: Retrobulbar block: effect of hyaluronidase on lidocaine systemic absorption and CSF diffusion in dogs, *Anesth Analg* 68:S65, 1989.

62. Eckenhoff JE, Kirby CK: The use of hyaluronidase in regional nerve blocks, *Anesthesiology* 12:27-32, 1951.

63. Moore DC: An evaluation of hyaluronidase in local and nerve block analgesia: a review of 519 cases, *Anesthesiology* 11: 470-484, 1950.

64. Buckley FP, Neto GD, Fink BR: Acid and alkaline solutions of local anesthetics: duration of nerve block and tissue pH, *Anesth Analg* 64:477-482, 1985.

65. Schelling CG, Klein LV: Comparison of carbonated lidocaine and lidocaine hydrochloride for caudal epidural analgesia in horses, *Am J Vet Res* 46:1375-1377, 1985.

66. Owen DW: Local nerve blocks. In Proceedings of the Ninth Annual Meeting of the American Association of Equine Practitioners, 1973, pp 152-156.

67. Wennberg E et al: Effects of commercial (pH 3.5) and freshly prepared (pH 6.5) lidocaine adrenaline solutions on tissue pH, *Acta Anaesthesiol Scand* 26:524-527, 1982.

68. Rijkenhuizen ABM: Complications following the diagnostic anesthesia of the coffin joint in horses. In Proceedings of the 15th European Society of Veterinary Surgeons Congress, Bern, Switzerland, Klinik für Nutztiere und Pferde, 1984, pp 7-13.

69. Muir WW: Drugs used to produce standing chemical restraint in horses, *Vet Clin North Am (Large Anim Pract)* 3(1):17-44, 1981.

70. Sandler GA, Scott EA: Vascular responses in equine thoracic limb during and after pneumatic tourniquet application, *Am J Vet Res* 41:648-649, 1980.

71. Bolz W: Ein weiterer Beitrag zur Leitungsanästhesie am Kopf des Pferdes, *Berl Tierärztl Wochenschr* 46:529-530, 1930.

72. Manning JP, St. Clair LE: Palpebral frontal and zygomatic nerve blocks for examination of the equine eye, *Vet Med* 71:187-189, 1976.

73. Merideth RE, Wolf ED: Ophthalmic examination and therapeutic techniques in the horse, *Compend Contin Educ* 3(11): S426-433, 1981.

74. Rubin LF: Auriculopalpebral nerve block as an adjunct to the diagnosis and treatment of ocular inflammation in the horse, *J Am Vet Med Assoc* 144:1387-1388, 1964.

75. Wittman F, Morgenroth H: *Untersuchungen über die Leitungsanästhesie des Nervus infraorbitalis und des Nervus mandibularis bei Zahn-und Kieferoperationen. Festschrift für Eugen Fröhner*, Stuttgart, 1928, Verlag Von Ferdinand Enke, pp 384-399.

76. Edwards JF: Regional anaesthesia of the head of the horse: an up-to-date survey, *Vet Rec* 10:873-975, 1930.

77. Eeckhout AVP: Un procédé pratique pour obtenir l'anesthésie complète des dents molaires supérieures chez le cheval, *Ann Med Vet* 66:10-14, 1921.

78. Bressou C, Cliza S: Contribution a létude de l'anesthésie dentaire chez le cheval et chez le chien, *Rec Med Vet* 107:129-134, 1931.

79. Schönberg F: Anatomische Grundlagen für die Leitungsanästhesie der Zahnnerven beim Pferde, *Berl Tierärztl Wochenschr* 43:1-3, 1927.

79. Hudson R: Local anaesthesia, *Vet Rec* 2:1053-1054, 1930.

80. Lichtenstrn G: Die Verwendung von Tropakokain in der tierärztlichen Chirurgie mit besonderer Berücksichtigung hinsichtlich seiner Verwendbarkeit in der Augapfelinfiltration beim Pferde, *Münch Tierarztl Wochenschr* 55:337-359, 1911.

81. Skarda RT: Practical regional anesthesia. In Mansmann RA, McAllister ES, Pratt PW, editors: *Equine medicine and surgery*, ed 3, vol 1, Santa Barbara, Ca, 1982, American Veterinary Publications, pp 229-238.

82. Adams OR: *Lameness in horses*, ed 3, Philadelphia, 1974, Lea & Febiger, pp 91-112.

83. Brown MP, Valko K: A technique for intraarticular injection of the equine tarso-metatarsal joint, *Vet Med Small Anim Clin* 75:265-270, 1980.

84. Colbern GT: The use of diagnostic nerve block procedures on horses, *Compend Contin Educ* 6(10):611-619, 1984.

85. Van Kruiningen JH: Practical techniques for making injections into joints and bursae of the horse, *J Am Vet Med Assoc* 143:1079-1083, 1963.

86. Gray BW et al: Clinical approach to determine the contribution of the palmar and palmar metacarpal nerves to the innervation of the equine fetlock joint, *Am J Vet Res* 41:940-943, 1980.

87. Lloyd KCK, Stover JM, Pascoe JR: A technique for catheterization of the equine antebrachiocarpal joint, *Am J Vet Res* 49:658-662, 1988.

88. Nyrop KA et al: The role of diagnostic nerve blocks in the equine lameness examination, *Compend Contin Educ* 5(12):669-676, 1983.

89. Stashak TS: Diagnosis of lameness. In Stashak TS, editor: *Adams' lameness in horses*, Philadelphia, 1986, Lea and Febiger, pp 139-142, 659-661.

90. Wheat JD, Jones K: Selected techniques of regional anesthesia, *Vet Clin North Am (Large Anim Pract)* 3(1):223-246, 1981.

90. Lipfert P: Tachyphylaxie von Lokalanaesthetika. Der Anesthesist, *Reg Anaesth* 38:13-20, 1989.

91. Dyson S: Diagnostic technique in the investigation of shoulder lameness, *Equine Vet J* 18:25-28, 1986.

92. Dyson S: Problems associated with the interpretation of results of regional and intraarticular anaesthesia in the horse, *Vet Rec* 12:419-422, 1986.

93. Ordidge RM, Gerring EL: Regional analgesia of the distal limb, *Equine Vet J* 16(2):147-149, 1984.

94. Ford TS, Ross MW, Orsini PG: Communication and boundaries of the middle carpal and carpometacarpal joints in horses, *Am J Vet Res* 49:2161-2164, 1988.

95. Ford TS, Ross MW, Orsini PG: A comparison of methods for proximal palmar metacarpal analgesia in horses, *Vet Surg* 18(2):146-150, 1989.

96. Sack WO: Nerve distribution in the metacarpus and front digit of the horse, *J Am Vet Med Assoc* 167:298-305, 1975.

97. Sack WO: Distal intertarsal and tarsometatarsal joints in the horse: communication and injection sites, *J Am Vet Med Assoc* 179:355-359, 1981.

98. Bramlage LR, Gabel AA, Hackett RA: Avulsion fractures of the origin of the suspensory ligament in the horse, *J Am Vet Med Assoc* 176:1004-1010, 1980.

99. Heavner JE: Local anesthetics, *Vet Clin North Am (Large Anim Pract)* 3(1):209-221, 1981.

100. Skarda RT, Muir WW. Segmental thoracolumbar spinal (subarachnoid) analgesia in conscious horses, *Am J Vet Res* 43:2121-2128, 1982.

101. Nuñez E et al: Effects of alpha$_2$-adrenergic receptor agonists on urine production in horses deprived of food and water, *Am J Vet Res* 65(10):1342-1346, 2004.

102. Fikes LW, Lin HC, Thurmon JC: A preliminary comparison of lidocaine and xylazine as epidural analgesics in ponies, *Vet Surg* 18(1):85-86, 1989.

103. Greene SA, Thurmon JC: Epidural analgesia and sedation for selected equine surgeries, *Equine Pract* 7:14-19, 1985.

104. LeBlanc PH et al: Epidural injection of xylazine for perineal analgesia in horses, *J Am Vet Med Assoc* 193:1405-1408, 1988.

105. Skarda RT: Practical regional anesthesia. In Mansmann RA, McAllister ES, Pratt PW, editors: *Equine medicine*, ed 3, vol 1, Santa Barbara, Ca, 1982, American Veterinary Publications, pp 239-245.

106. Greene EM, Cooper RC: Continuous caudal epidural anesthesia in the horse, *J Am Vet Med Assoc* 184:971-974, 1984.

107. Skarda RT, Muir WW: Continuous caudal epidural and subarachnoid anesthesia in mares: a comparative study, *Am J Vet Res* 44:2290-2298, 1983.

108. Haga HA et al: Effect of intratesticular injection of lidocaine on cardiovascular responses to castration in isoflurane-anesthetized stallions, *Am J Vet Res* 67(3):403-408, 2006.

109. Lowe JE, Dougherty R: Castration of horses and ponies by a primary closure method, *Am Vet Med Assoc* 160:183-185, 1972.

110. Skarda RT et al: Cervicothoracic (stellate) ganglion block in conscious horses, *Am J Vet Res* 47(1):21-26, 1986.

111. Firth EC: Horner's syndrome in the horse: experimental induction and a case report, *Equine Vet J* 10(1):9-13, 1978.

112. Smith JS, Mayhew IG: Horner's syndrome in large animals, *Cornell Vet* 65:529-542, 1977.

113. Skarda RT, Muir WW, Hubbell JA: Paravertebral lumbar sympathetic ganglion block in the horse. In Proceedings of the Second International Congress of Veterinary Anesthesia, Santa Barbara, Ca, 1985, Veterinary Practice Publishing Co, p 160.

114. Burford JH, Corley KT: Morphine-associated pruritus after single extradural administration in a horse, *Vet Anaesth Analg* 55(5):670-680, 1994.

115. Chopin JB, Wright JD: Complication after the use of a combination of lignocaine and xylazine for epidural anaesthesia in a mare, *Aust Vet J* 79(2):354-355, 1995.

116. Haitjema H, Gibson KT: Severe pruritus associated with epidural morphine and detomidine in a horse, *Aust Vet J* 79(4):248-250, 2001.

117. Martin CA et al: Outcome of epidural catheterization for delivery of analgesics in horses: 43 cases (1998-2001), *J Am Vet Med Assoc* 222(10):1394-1398, 2003.

118. Sysel AM et al: Systemic and local effects associated with long-term sepidural catheterization and morphine-detomidine administration in horses, *Vet Surg* 26(2):141-149, 1997.

119. Lansdowne JL et al: Epidural migration of new methylene blue in 0.9% sodium chloride solution or 2% mepivacaine solution following injection into the first intercoccygeal space in foal cadavers and anesthetized foals undergoing laparoscopy, *Am J Vet Res* 66(8):1324-1329, 2005.

120. Kalichman MW, Powell HC, Myers RR: Neurotoxicity of local anesthetics in rat sciatic nerve, *Anesthesiology* 65(3A):A188, 1986.

121. Yagiela JA et al: Comparison of myotoxic effects of lidocaine with epinephrine in rats and humans, *Anesth Analg* 60:471-480, 1981.

122. Liu P, Feldman HS, Covino BG: Acute cardiovascular toxicity of lidocaine, bupivacaine, and etidocaine in anesthetized, ventilated dogs, *Anesthesiology* 53:S231, 1980.

123. Liu P, Feldman HS, Covino BG: Comparative CNS and cardiovascular toxicity of various local anesthetic agents, *Anesthesiology* 55(3):A156, 1981.

Intravenous Anesthetic Drugs

William W. Muir

1. Intravenous anesthetics are administered for induction to and maintenance of anesthesia and as adjuncts to inhalant anesthesia.
2. Total intravenous anesthesia (TIVA) may be safer and produce less stress in horses than inhalant anesthesia.
3. Thiopental and propofol provide rapid onset and offset of anesthetic effects when used as a single dose. Both drugs produce unconsciousness (hypnosis), excellent muscle relaxation, and respiratory depression or apnea. They should not be administered to horses without adequate sedation and relaxation.
4. Ketamine and tiletamine are phencyclidine derivatives that produce a dissociative state of hypnosis and analgesia marked by poor muscle relaxation (catalepsy). They should not be administered to horses without adequate sedation and muscle relaxation.
5. Guaifenesin is an excellent muscle relaxant but a poor anesthetic in horses. It should only be administered to relax horses or coadministered with hypnotics to produce general anesthesia.
6. Chloral hydrate is a longer-acting hypnotic that can be used to produce marked and prolonged sedation in horses.
7. The sole use of succinyl choline for chemical restraint in horses cannot be condoned.
8. Administration of intravenous anesthetic drugs (thiopental, ketamine, guaifenesin) to horses for extended periods of time (>3 hours) may lead to drug accumulation and prolonged recovery times.
9. Poor hemodynamic function, hypoproteinemia, acidemia, and electrolyte disturbances may exaggerate the effects of intravenous anesthetic drugs.

Intravenous anesthetic drugs and intravenous anesthetic techniques are generally administered for shorter-duration surgical procedures or for induction to inhalant anesthesia. The ideal intravenous anesthetic drug or drug combination should provide safe and effective anesthesia without side effects.[1-8] A major advantage would be the ability to reverse or antagonize drug effects should an emergency situation occur. The drug would produce uneventful, excitement-free relaxation and lateral recumbency without cardiorespiratory depression; homeostatic reflexes would remain intact; and hematological and blood chemistry values would remain within normal limits. There would be excellent muscle relaxation and analgesia without excessive central nervous system (CNS) depression during the maintenance phase of anesthesia. Blood flow to vital organs, mus-

cle, and viscera would be optimal. The recovery phase would be highlighted by a rapid return to consciousness but with lingering analgesia and a return of muscle strength without stress or excitement. Horses would be able to stand with minimum or no assistance.

Cardiorespiratory function is compromised by placing horses in lateral or "dorsal" (supine) recumbency (see Chapters 2, 3, and 17). Deleterious cardiorespiratory effects are more pronounced in horses that are large or overweight, have abdominal distention, or are hypovolemic and hypotensive. They are made worse with time and the administration of anesthetic drugs. Most drugs administered as preanesthetic medication also produce cardiorespiratory effects (see Chapter 10). Centrally acting muscle relaxants (benzodiazepines, guaifenesin) administered with opioid agonists (morphine, meperidine), opioid agonist-antagonists (butorphanol, pentazocine), or α_2-adrenoceptor agonists (xylazine, detomidine, romifidine, medetomidine) provide good muscle relaxation and analgesia but can exaggerate cardiorespiratory depression in some horses. The addition of a hypnotic or any drug that increases CNS depression (barbiturate, propofol steroidal anesthetic) or disorganizes brain electrical activity (dissociative anesthetics: ketamine, tiletamine) can further depress or disrupt CNS regulation of cardiorespiratory function, homeostatic reflex responses, and tissue perfusion and oxygenation.

The ideal anesthetic drug of the future will be an injectable anesthetic drug combination capable of being administered for extended periods of time (infused) without ill effects. This drug will have a high safety margin; produce predictable effects; minimize stress (see Chapter 4); and, once reversed, leave the horse normal and comfortable (Box 12-1).

INTRAVENOUS ANESTHETICS

Relatively few intravenous anesthetic drugs are administered to horses. The reasons are related to species, safety, economics, and technical considerations. The greater logistic and technical problems associated with a large and at times frightened and uncooperative horse can be formidable. The use of preanesthetic drugs or drug combinations reduces but does not eliminate many of the problems associated with general anesthesia in horses (see Chapter 10). Barbiturates, dissociative anesthetics, and centrally acting muscle relaxants are used regularly. The coadministration of α_2-adrenoceptor agonists, benzodiazepines, and dissociative anesthetics has become routine for short-term (<10 to 15 minutes) surgical procedures, induction to longer-term intravenous infusion techniques, or inhalant anesthesia (see Chapter 13).

- Highly soluble in water
- Nontissue toxic
- Rapid onset of effect
- Excellent analgesia and muscle relaxation
- Absence of side effects
- Highly predictable
- Dose-dependent duration of action
- Rapid uneventful recovery without ataxia
- Reversible
- Sustained analgesia
- Anxiolytic/reduces stress

The Barbiturates

The administration of barbiturates to produce short-term anesthesia in horses has decreased dramatically. Routinely administered to horses for over 50 years to produce sedation and short-term anesthesia and as anticonvulsants, barbiturates have been largely replaced by centrally acting muscle relaxants (diazepam, midazolam) and dissociative anesthetic (ketamine) drug combinations (see Chapters 13 and 18). Small differences in chemical structure produce marked changes in the onset, duration, and clinical effects of barbiturates (Table 12-1). They are classified on the basis of their duration of action. Only ultrashort-acting barbiturates are administered routinely as single drugs to induce, maintain, or supplement anesthesia in horses. Longer-acting barbiturates (pentobarbital, phenobarbital) were used as sedatives or in combination with other compounds (chloral hydrate, magnesium sulfate) to produce heavy sedation or anesthesia or control seizures.[1,9] Thiamylal and thiopental (thiopentone) are ultrashort-acting thiobarbiturates with similar pharmacological, pharmacokinetic, and pharmacodynamic properties. Only thiopental is used in equine practice today. Pentobarbital (pentobarbitone), considered a short-acting anesthetic, and methohexital (methohexitone), an ultrashort-acting anesthetic, are oxybarbiturates infrequently administered as adjuncts to intravenous or inhalation anesthesia. Bolus intravenous doses of pentobarbital produce significant cardiorespiratory depression and prolonged, uncoordinated, stressful recoveries;

whereas methohexital has the potential to produce muscle fasciculations, pronounced excitatory effects, and seizures, particularly in poorly sedated horses. All barbiturates are weak acids and prepared as sodium (Na^+) salts, which are readily soluble in water but unstable and decompose when exposed to air, heat, or light. For example, pentobarbital is prepared in 20% propylene glycol, 10% alcohol, and 2% benzyl alcohol. Pentobarbital solutions have a pH between 10.5 and 11.5. Thiopental is prepared as a powder and solubilized by adding water or saline sufficient to produce the desired concentration. The maximum safe storage time for thiopental is approximately 2 weeks under ideal conditions, although it is recommended that the drug be prepared immediately before use and administered within 48 hours. Solutions of thiobarbiturates kept for extended periods of time (beyond 48 hours) gradually lose activity, depending on storage conditions. Shelf life can be prolonged by storing dilute solutions (less than 10%) in cool dark places. All barbiturate solutions are alkaline; most have pH values greater than 10. The appearance of small flakes or clouding of a dilute solution of a thiobarbiturate suggests contamination or precipitation resulting from a loss of alkalinity. The addition of 1 to 2 ml of sodium hydroxide helps to restore alkalinity and may cause the solution to become clear.

Barbiturates are hypnotics that produce unconsciousness from which the horse cannot be aroused. They are capable of inducing profound CNS, cardiovascular, and particularly respiratory depression. Barbiturates are frequently incorporated in euthanasia solutions (see Chapter 25). Appropriately administered, they can be used to provide safe and inexpensive short-term anesthesia. Barbiturates are excellent muscle relaxants and excellent adjuncts to other injectable anesthetics or supplements to inhalant anesthesia.

Mechanisms of Action

Barbiturates produce a full range of CNS depressant effects, from mild sedation and sleep to general anesthesia, complete cortical depression, and death. Cerebral metabolic rate and oxygen consumption are decreased. These effects are caused by barbiturate-induced decreases (Na^+, K^+, Ca^{+2}) or increases (Cl^-) in the conductance of various ions across cell membranes, resulting in selective depression of the reticular activating system and polysynaptic responses in all portions of the brain and brainstem. Presynaptic and postsynaptic neurotransmission is inhibited. Barbiturates enhance and mimic the actions of gamma-aminobutyric acid (GABA) at the $GABA_A$ receptor, thereby increasing chloride ion conductance at

Table 12–1. Barbiturates used to produce anesthesia in horses					
Drug	Classification	pH of Solution	Onset of action (sec)	Duration of action (min)	Margin of safety (%)*
Pentobarbital (pentobarbitone)	Short	10-11	30-60	45-90	50-70
Methohexital (methohexitone)	Ultrashort	10-11.5	10-30	3-10	30-50
Thiopental (thiopentone)	Ultrashort	10-11	20-30	3-13	30-50
Thiamylal	Ultrashort	10-11	20-30	5-15	30-50

*Indicates what percent the anesthetic dose is in comparison to the minimum lethal dose.

multiple sites within the CNS, causing membrane hyperpolarization, an increased threshold for excitability, and a reduction in CNS electrical activity. These pharmacological effects are similar to those of the benzodiazepines with which the barbiturates are additive. Extremely elevated serum concentrations of barbiturates activate CNS chloride channels directly, regardless of the influence of GABA, further enhancing their depressant effects. Barbiturates decrease synaptic transmission of excitatory neurotransmitters, including glutamate and acetylcholine at postsynaptic membranes; they produce excellent muscle relaxation and potentiate the peripheral effects of neuromuscular blocking drugs. Barbiturates also depress nervous system transmission in autonomic ganglia and homeostatic reflex mechanisms, which may be partially responsible for their hypotensive effects after bolus administration. Low plasma concentrations of barbiturates can trigger delirium and excitement in horses, leading to stress and hyperalgesia.

Applied Pharmacology

The barbiturates produce dose-dependent depression of all organ system functions. These effects stem directly from their inhibition of membrane ion exchange mechanisms, CNS depression, and reduced cellular metabolic activity. The intensity of these effects depends on the rate of drug administration, the total dosage administered, the horse's physical status, preanesthetic medications, and other concurrent drug administration. For example, the intravenous administration of a seemingly appropriate dose of a thiobarbiturate to an apprehensive horse that is not adequately sedated could result in transient excitement, tachycardia, hyperventilation, hypertension, sweating, muscle fasciculations, involuntary muscle movement, and paddling. Anesthetic dosages of barbiturates decrease CNS impulse transmission, resulting in a decrease in cerebral metabolic rate and oxygen consumption.

Clinically, barbiturates are most noted for producing dose-dependent respiratory depression. Both respiratory rate and tidal volume are decreased after bolus administration of barbiturates. Apnea (1 to 2 minutes) is not uncommon. Barbiturates depress respiratory center response to elevations in arterial concentrations of carbon dioxide (reduce CNS threshold and sensitivity to CO_2) and decreases in oxygenation (PaO_2). Functional residual capacity is reduced secondary to CNS depression and relaxation of the muscles responsible for expanding the chest wall. Laryngospasm and bronchoconstriction are reported to occur in a variety of smaller species but have not been reported in horses. The net result of the respiratory depressant effects is hypoventilation and the development of respiratory acidosis. If respiratory depression is severe (apnea) or prolonged, the partial pressure of oxygen may decrease to values less than 60 mm Hg, resulting in hypoxemia, anaerobic metabolism, and lactic acidosis.

Barbiturates can produce significant dose-dependent cardiovascular depression.[10] In general, the intravenous administration of an ultrashort-acting barbiturate to a properly premedicated, normal healthy horse produces mild hemodynamic changes.[11] However, the bolus administration of thiopental can produce increases in heart rate and decreases in arterial blood pressure, venous return, and the force of cardiac contraction (Figure 12-1).[12] Stroke volume and cardiac output usually decrease, whereas peripheral vascular resistance remains unchanged or increases. These

changes may range from 10% to 25% of baseline values and are exaggerated if the total dosage is administered rapidly. A 50% or greater depression of all hemodynamic variables should be expected if larger doses of thiopental are administered to a horse that is already significantly depressed by the prior administration of preanesthetic medications, other anesthetics, or disease. Blood flow is decreased in proportion to the decrease in cardiac output, but there are no studies describing the effects of barbiturate anesthesia on the distribution of cardiac output in the horse. The thiobarbiturates (thiopental, thiamylal) can produce bradycardia and ventricular arrhythmias and are noted for their ability to sensitize the myocardium of dogs and humans to the arrhythmogenic effects of catecholamines, particularly in the presence of halothane.[13] Experimental or clinical evidence has not confirmed this observation in horses, but bradycardia after intravenous administration of thiopental has occurred.[14,15] The effects of barbiturate anesthesia on the incidence of ventricular arrhythmias, including ventricular fibrillation in horses, is not known.

The pharmacological effects of barbiturates on other organ systems in the horse are not well described, but in general their effects seem to be similar to those produced in other species. Thus barbiturate-induced decreases in cardiac output should result in decreases in cerebral, hepatic, renal, and skeletal muscle blood flows. These changes, in conjunction with barbiturate-induced reductions in cellular metabolism, neuroendocrine function, and myoelectrical activity, usually result in no change or an improved ratio between oxygen consumption and oxygen delivery (organ-sparing effect) and only transient impairment of organ function. The effects of barbiturates on uterine smooth muscle activity in the mare have not been reported, although minimal effects were observed in pregnant mares induced to anesthesia with thiamylal and maintained with halothane or isoflurane.[16] Anesthetic plasma concentrations of barbiturates produce marked fetal respiratory depression and respiratory arrest in the newborn foal.[10] The effects of pentobarbital are theorized to be more prominent than those of the thiopental. Prolonged plasma elimination of barbiturates should be expected in the newborn foal because hepatic microsomal enzyme function is not fully developed.[17] The effect of barbiturates on various hematological and blood chemical values in horses is highly variable but generally associated with minimal changes in packed cell volume, the development of leukopenia, hyperglycemia, respiratory acidemia, and hypoxemia (see Chapter 3; Table 12-2).[18]

Biodisposition

The metabolism and elimination of barbiturates have not been studied extensively in the horse, although there is little reason to believe that important differences exist compared to other species (see Chapter 9).[19-22] Barbiturates are sodium salts of barbituric acid. The substitution of a sulfur atom for oxygen in thiopental markedly enhances its tissue-penetrating (lipid solubility) properties, producing a rapid onset and short duration of action. Once administered intravenously (IV), barbiturate anesthetics rapidly ionize, depending on their ionization constant (pKa; the pH at which 50% of the substance is ionized and 50% is un-ionized), the pH of the blood, and binding to plasma proteins (primarily albumin).

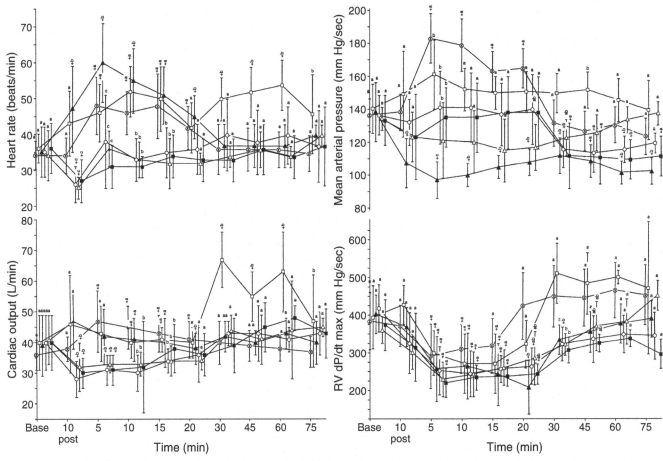

Figure 12–1. Effects of thiamylal (10 mg/kg IV; [X]) and thiamylal preceded by diazepam (0.1 mg/kg IV; [□,]) acepromazine (0.1 mg/kg, IV [▲]), detomidine (10 μg/kg IV [○]), and xylazine (0.5 mg/kg IV [△]; and 1 mg/kg IV [■]) on heart rate, cardiac output, mean arterial pressure, and right ventricular (RV) dP/dt in adult horses; +, $P < 0.05$ difference from baseline; a–d, $P < 0.05$ among groups. (From Muir WW, Mason DE. Effects of diazepam, acepromazine, detomidine and xylazine on thiamylal anesthesia in horses, *Am J Vet Res* 203:1031-1038, 1993.)

Table 12–2.	**Effects of thiopental on hematological and blood chemical values in horses**[27]				
		Minutes after administering anesthesia			
	Preanesthetic value	**5**	**15**	**25**	**Statistical differences**
Leukocyte count (cells/mm³)	9700	7800	7500	6100	!
Packed cell volume (vol %)	32	31	30.5	31	
Blood glucose (mg %)	82.1	85.0	91.2	103.1	!
O₂ content of arterial blood (vol %)	19.2	19.0	18.2	18.4	!!
O₂ content of venous blood (vol %)	14.3	13.5	13.0	12.8	!!
Arterial blood (pH)	7.39	7.31	7.21	35.8	!

!, Statistically significant difference at 1% level before and after administration of thiopental sodium; *!!*, statistically significant difference at the 5% level before and after administration of thiopental sodium (see Chapter 4).

Thiopental is distributed rapidly throughout the horse's plasma volume, with an initial distribution phase half-life of 2 to 4 minutes, a slower redistribution phase of 10 to 20 minutes, and an elimination half-life of approximately 1.5 to 2.5 hours.[22] The terminal half-lives of pentobarbital (3 to 5 hours) and phenobarbital (approx. 10 hours) are much longer. Barbiturates must be in a nonprotein-bound, unionized (nonpolar) state to cross the blood-brain barrier and produce sedative or anesthetic effects. A significant proportion of an injected dose remains in the un-ionized state at physiological pH (7.35 to 7.45). A greater amount of barbiturate remains un-ionized during systemic acidosis, thereby enhancing barbiturate effects. Certain drugs (phenylbutazone, aspirin) or diseases (hepatic, renal) can decrease the plasma protein binding of the thiobarbiturates, further enhancing drug effects. Therefore lipid solubility, plasma pH, and the extent of plasma protein binding have important clinical consequences on the rapidity of action, intensity of effect, and duration of barbiturate activity. Horses that are hypotensive, acidemic, and hypoproteinemic demonstrate a pronounced and prolonged response to the administration of barbiturate drugs. Furthermore, horses that are dehydrated or in shock compensate by centralizing their blood volume, thereby redistributing blood to more vital organs such as the brain, heart, liver, and kidney. This compensatory response decreases the volume of distribution of the drug and lengthens the initial redistribution half-life, leading to an intensification of CNS and cardiorespiratory depressant effects.

Redistribution of ultrashort-acting barbiturates from highly perfused tissues (e.g., brain, heart, lung) to well-perfused lean tissues (e.g., muscle) is responsible for the ultrashort duration of action of the drug.[23] Methohexital is redistributed and is metabolized rapidly in both plasma and liver. Plasma concentrations of thiopental fall rapidly as a result of drug redistribution to lean body tissues (muscle, skin).[22] Clinically, the redistribution of the thiobarbiturate, thiopental, to skeletal muscle is closely related to the clinical duration of action (i.e., the regaining of consciousness and recovery from anesthesia). However, redistribution to fat contributes significantly to the terminal elimination phase and can influence the rate of return to normal consciousness and the rate of recovery from anesthesia. The comparatively prolonged elimination of the barbiturates has important clinical implications in horses because frequent, repeated drug administration can result in drug accumulation and progressive increases in the plasma concentration. The larger the total dosage of thiopental administered, the more dependent the anesthetic and duration of recovery become on hepatic metabolism and renal excretion. Total cumulative dosages of thiobarbiturate thiopental exceeding 15 to 20 mg/kg frequently lead to prolonged and unsatisfactory recoveries. Horses that are hypovolemic or acidotic (dehydration, hemorrhage, shock) should be expected to have a reduced volume of distribution and therefore require a lower total dose of anesthetic. The effects of age, level of fitness, gender, and pregnancy on drug elimination have not been studied in horses.

Acute "tolerance" to the anesthetic effects of thiobarbiturates has been reported in humans and is a potential problem in horses.[24] The initial dose of thiobarbiturate determines the plasma concentration at which the horse regains consciousness. If large bolus injections are administered for induction to anesthesia, larger incremental doses of drug may be required to maintain anesthesia. The mechanism for this phenomenon is unknown but is clinically relevant because

it could lead to the administration of larger doses of thiobarbiturate to maintain anesthesia, producing excessive cardiorespiratory depression and markedly prolonging recovery.

Clinical Use and Antagonism

Pentobarbital and methohexital are rarely used to produce general anesthesia in horses other than for experimental purposes (Table 12-3). Pentobarbital produces a prolonged anesthetic effect and produces hypoventilation, hypotension, and prolonged recovery.[25] Recovery from pentobarbital anesthesia is associated with incoordination, multiple attempts to stand, and stress or excitement. Combinations of pentobarbital, chloral hydrate, and magnesium sulfate historically have been administered to produce sedation and anesthesia in horses and cattle. This drug combination produced good sedation and muscle relaxation but poor hypnosis, analgesia, and recovery. Thiopental (4% to 10% solutions) is administered to horses to produce short-term anesthesia, to induce horses to inhalant anesthesia, and as an adjunct to both injectable or inhalant anesthesia in horses and foals (see Table 12-3).[26,27] Both the induction and recovery from thiopental anesthesia can be associated with excitement, struggling, and incoordination. Appropriate preanesthetic medication should be used; and well-trained, knowledgeable attendants should be available to control or assist the horse's head during induction and recovery from anesthesia.[12]

Properly premedicated horses begin to relax within 10 to 20 seconds after intravenous administration of thiopental. The time of actual relaxation and collapse generally is signaled by the lifting of the horse's head, muscle fasciculations, or a deep breath. Horses that are not adequately tranquilized or sedated may develop generalized muscle tremors or foreleg extensor rigidity. Some horses rear up momentarily and attempt to fall over backward. Skilled technical assistance and the use of hobbles, doors, or gates are useful during this phase (see Chapters 5 and 16). Once recumbent, most horses hypoventilate or develop apnea for periods lasting as short as 15 to 20 seconds. Longer periods of apnea (2 to 3 minutes) can occur and may require physical stimulation to trigger a breath: twisting the base of the ear, pinching the anus, or applying momentary pressure to the chest wall. Anesthesia is short (5 to 10 minutes) and is not associated with a great deal of analgesia. Recovery to a standing position is usually rapid but may be uncoordinated. Recovery may be accompanied by major limb movements, paddling, and rolling from side to side before attempts to stand. Repeated administration of thiopental to maintain anesthesia can lead to cumulative drug effects, resulting in prolonged and

Table 12–3. **Intravenous doses of barbiturates used for induction or maintenance or as adjuncts to anesthesia in horses***

Drug	Induction dose*	Maintenance dose†	Adjunctive dose
Thiopental	5-8 mg/kg	10-15 mg/kg	0.2-0.5 mg/kg
Thiamylal	4-6 mg/kg	10-15 mg/kg	0.2-0.5 mg/kg
Methohexital	2-5 mg/kg	NR	NR
Pentobarbital	NR	15-25 mg/kg	1-3 mg/kg

NR, Not recommended.
*Assumes preanesthetic medication.
†Sole drug used for anesthesia.

awkward recoveries. The horse may initiate multiple attempts to stand and require assistance to do so. The selection and dose of preanesthetic medication can have profound effects on the dose of thiobarbiturate required to induce and maintain anesthesia, the quality of induction and recovery, and the duration of anesthesia.[11] The administration of acepromazine or α_2-adrenoceptor agonists 10 to 20 minutes before induction reduces the dose of anesthetic required for induction, provides additional muscle relaxation and analgesia (xylazine, detomidine, romifidine, medetomidine), prolongs the anesthetic duration, and facilitates uneventful recovery.[13]

Thiopental is used frequently with other intravenous drugs (guaifenesin, ketamine, tiletamine-zolazepam, chloral hydrate) to enhance hypnosis and muscle relaxation or with inhalant anesthesia to provide added hypnosis and muscle relaxation and enhance the maintenance phase of anesthesia (Table 12-4).[4,6,27-29] The CNS depressant effects of barbiturates can persist for extended periods of time in aged, debilitated, dehydrated, diseased (anemic) horses and horses in shock. Metabolic acidosis prolongs the duration of anesthetic effects (see Biodisposition earlier in the chapter). The elimination of barbiturates can be promoted by diuresis and alkalinization of the urine. This can be accomplished by administering 10 to 20 ml/kg of intravenous fluids, furosemide (0.5 to 1.0 mg/kg IV), and sodium bicarbonate (0.5 to 1.0 mg/kg IV). Horses that become apneic after the administration of thiopental should be ventilated manually or mechanically, and pH and blood gases assessed periodically until recovery is complete (see Chapter 17). The administration of 0.2 to 0.5 mg/kg of intravenous doxapram late during the recovery phase increases respiratory rate, tidal volume, and the level of consciousness, which may hasten recovery in some horses.[30] Recovery in pentobarbital-anesthetized ponies can be shortened by administering 0.1 mg/kg of intravenous yohimbine.[31] The latter two techniques for shortening the recovery period are not recommended in clinical situations because of the potential to induce early attempts to stand and associated ataxia.

Complications, Side Effects, and Toxicities

The most frequent complications associated with the intravenous use of barbiturate drugs are unpredictable or inadequate drug effects and apnea. Inadequate or unsatisfactory drug effect can be caused by underdosing, administering dilute solutions of thiopental that have lost activity, improper or inadequate response to sedatives, slow injections, or accidental perivascular injection. Slow injections of methohexital

or thiopental can produce an inadequate effect, particularly in poorly sedated or excited horses. Methohexital is metabolized rapidly, and the thiobarbiturates are redistributed rapidly to muscle in excited horses, resulting in reduced drug concentrations delivered to the CNS. The total time for drug administration should not exceed 20 seconds. Accidental perivascular injection of drug should be suspected if drug effects do not occur within 30 seconds. The rapid or "bolus" injection of methohexital or thiopental is required to obtain the desired effect (see above) but may result in the deposition of a large amount of drug in a perivascular site if an intravenous catheter is not used.[32] This problem can be avoided by using large-bore (14-gauge) intravenous catheters that are fixed securely (see Chapter 7). Large volumes (2 to 4 L) of normal saline or a balanced electrolyte solution should be infused into the perivascular tissues at the site of accidental drug injection to minimize tissue necrosis and prevent abscess formation. Local dilution with fluids and the administration of intravenous nonsteroidal antiinflammatory drugs help to prevent sloughing.

Hypoventilation and apnea are serious and potentially life-threatening side effects. Apnea is usually immediate in onset and transient but can occur after a short period of low tidal volume breaths. The duration of hypoventilation and apnea is directly related to drug concentration, the rate of injection, and the total dosage administered. Rapid injection of concentrated solutions (10%) should be expected to produce apnea, even when low doses are administered. The period of apnea should not be allowed to extend beyond 2 minutes, even if mucous membrane color and pulse pressure are normal. Therapy is directed toward establishing an airway and initiating controlled ventilation (see Chapters 17 and 22).

Prolonged recovery from thiobarbiturate anesthesia should be expected in volume-depleted, hypoproteinemic, or acidemic horses (see previous paragraphs) and foals less than 6 weeks of age. Repeated or large total doses of thiopental (>15 mg/kg IV) can also prolong recovery. This response is the result of delayed metabolism or drug accumulation caused by repeated drug administration. The quality of recovery also decreases with increasing doses of thiopental. Foals less than 6 weeks of age have not fully developed their microsomal enzyme drug-metabolizing capabilities and demonstrate prolonged recovery periods.

Rapid intravenous injections or accidental overdoses of methohexital or thiopental can produce ventricular arrhythmias, cardiovascular collapse, and death. The lethal dose varies

Table 12–4. Thiopental and intravenous anesthetic drug doses in horses

Drug[†]	Dose (mg/kg)	Duration of action (min)	Time to standing (min)
Guaifenesin*	75-150 (10% solution of guaifenesin to effect)	10-20	30-50
Guaifenesin/thiopental	1-2 g thiopental added to 1 L-5% solution guaifenesin	15-30	15-30
Xylazine/ketamine[†]	0.5-1.0/1.7-2.2	10-15	0-35
Chloral hydrate/thiopental[†]	100-150 (to ataxia)	15-25	60-90

*Assume preanesthetic medication.
[†]Thiopental (3-5 mg/kg) can be added with appropriate dose adjustments; thiobarbiturates should not be mixed with ketamine or chloral hydrate.

directly with the concentration of solution and total dosage administered and the rate of drug administration. Acute cardiorespiratory collapse after thiobarbiturate administration is a cardiovascular emergency; cardiopulmonary resuscitative procedures should be instituted immediately (see Chapter 23). Barbiturates can potentiate the CNS depressant effects of all other anesthetic drugs, prolong muscle relaxation, and delay the elimination of drugs that depend on liver metabolism for their elimination. Barbiturates are synergistic with benzodiazepines (see Chapter 10).

Dissociative Anesthetics

Dissociative anesthetics include phencyclidine, ketamine, and tiletamine. The term *dissociative* evolved from their use in humans who reported a feeling of being dissociated from their body and environment after being administered ketamine. Only ketamine has become popular for producing short-term chemical restraint and induction to inhalation anesthesia in horses. Tiletamine is available in combination with the benzodiazepine zolazepam (Telazol). Dissociative anesthetic drugs are noted for their ability to produce catalepsy (plastic or waxy rigidity), poor muscle relaxation, and variable degrees of analgesia. They are administered to horses in combination with sedative-hypnotics, muscle relaxants, and analgesics to produce short-term anesthesia or induce anesthesia before inhalant anesthesia.[33-38] Ketamine and tiletamine are white powders that are highly soluble in water and available commercially as racemic mixtures. Solutions of ketamine are stable for several months. Telazol is stable for at least 10 to 14 days, although color changes can occur and a reduction in solution potency may occur. Neither ketamine nor Telazol is suitable to be administered alone for induction to anesthesia or as the sole anesthetic drug in horses.[10] Intravenous administration in horses is followed by extensor rigidity, a dog-sitting posture, extreme muscle spasm and jerking, purposeless movements, an excited facial expression, profuse sweating, and occasional seizures. Some horses respond violently to normal stimulation, become uncontrollable, and must be restrained with barbiturates or large doses of diazepam.

Mechanism of Action

The mechanism(s) responsible for the effects of ketamine and other dissociative anesthetics is/are complex and incompletely understood.[39] Dissociative anesthetics decrease or alter sensory input without blocking brainstem or spinal pathways. CNS depression does occur in the thalamus and associated pain centers and minimally in the reticular formation, but subcortical areas and the hippocampus undergo activation. Interaction with N-methyl-D-aspartate (NMDA) receptors in the CNS may be responsible for general anesthetic effects and analgesia.[40] Ketamine and tiletamine may also produce analgesia by interaction with opioid receptors in the CNS and inhibit wide-dynamic range neurons in the dorsal horn of the spinal cord.[39] Dissociative anesthetics can induce seizures by producing random electrical discharge in the hippocampus, but, interestingly, they increase the seizure threshold to other known convulsants. The clinical relevance of these findings is uncertain. Ketamine is known to interfere and interact with several centrally acting neurotransmitters, including serotonin, dopamine, and GABA. Increases in brain serotonin and dopamine concentrations produce excitement and increased motor activity in horses and may be partially responsible for the poor muscle relaxant effects of ketamine.[39] Ketamine decreases GABA uptake as well, which increases neuronal membrane chloride conductance, hyperpolarizing nerve cells and decreasing their responsiveness.[41] Finally, ketamine produces complex parasympathetic-sympathetic effects, which lead to varied systemic effects, including tachycardia and reduced gut motility.

Applied Pharmacology

Ketamine and tiletamine/zolazepam should never be administered alone to produce anesthesia in horses but can be used alone to supplement anesthesia. They produce dose-dependent pharmacological effects that are comparatively less depressant than reported for barbiturates or other hypnotics. Clinical doses do not seriously impair ventilation, although there is a tendency for some horses to develop an apneustic (breath-holding) pattern of breathing and reduced minute volume.[10] Arterial $PaCO_2$ remains within normal limits, whereas PaO_2 generally decreases. The influence of position (recumbency) and the development of ventilation-perfusion mismatching on blood gas values are likely of more importance. Pharyngeal and laryngeal reflexes remain active after ketamine administration, and the nasal or oral placement of an endotracheal tube is more difficult than with thiopental anesthesia. Airway resistance is decreased in humans and should be in horses. Assisted or controlled ventilation may be difficult to accomplish in some horses because of poor muscle relaxation and a tendency to "buck" (breathe against) the ventilator during the inspiratory phase. Heart rate, cardiac output, arterial blood pressure, and body temperature may increase after intravenous ketamine or Telazol administration because of increases in CNS sympathetic activation.[42] Circulating concentrations of norepinephrine and epinephrine increase in horses after ketamine administration. Peripheral vascular resistance does not change or increases, which, taken together with increases in heart rate, results in marked increases in myocardial oxygen consumption.

Ketamine can cause direct depression of the myocardium, although clinical doses rarely produce this effect and generally increase heart rate, arterial blood pressure, and cardiac output.[33] Occasionally horses develop sinus heart rates in excess of 60 beats/min, second-degree atrioventricular block, and periodic ventricular depolarizations after intravenous ketamine. Cerebral blood flow, metabolic rate, and intracranial pressure are increased by dissociative anesthetics, contraindicating their use in horses with head trauma or undiagnosed CNS disease. The intravenous use of ketamine in otherwise normal horses requiring a myelogram is uneventful.[10] Lacrimation and ocular and palpebral reflexes are more pronounced in horses administered dissociative anesthetics, although corneal analgesia may be profound, necessitating the use of corneal lubricants to prevent drying. Intraocular pressure may increase but is generally of minimal clinical relevance.[43] Ketamine rapidly crosses the placenta and can produce CNS effects and respiratory depression in the newborn foal.

Biodisposition

The metabolism and elimination of ketamine and its two major metabolites (norketamine, dihydroketamine) have been determined in horses, mules, and mammoth asses.[44-50]

These studies suggest that ketamine is metabolized extensively by the liver and that recovery from anesthesia after a single intravenous dose is almost entirely the result of rapid and extensive redistribution (see Chapter 9).[44-46] Furthermore, ketamine is more than 50% protein bound in the horse. The rapid initial redistribution phase ranges from 2 to 3 minutes, followed by a slower elimination phase ranging from 42 to 70 min.[45] Finally, up to 40% of the initial dose of unmetabolized ketamine remains in the horse after recovery from anesthesia. Norketamine is the main metabolite.[44-46] These findings have important clinical implications in addition to predicting the rapidity of recovery after a single administration. Liver or renal impairment is not expected to significantly affect the duration of action of ketamine after a single dose. Repeated administration or infusions could result in drug accumulation, a prolonged elimination phase, and a correspondingly long duration of recovery.[46] However, the infusion of relatively low doses (0.5 mg/kg/hr) of ketamine for 5 to 6 hours to healthy conscious horses was considered safe and without significant side effects.[50] The predicted duration of action after intravenous administration of 2.2 mg/kg of ketamine is approximately 10 minutes but increases to over 20 minutes when this dose is repeated.[45,51] Repeated doses or hypoproteinemia could prolong anesthesia and predispose to side effects during recovery. The biodisposition of ketamine has not been studied in foals, but based on knowledge of liver-metabolizing capabilities and clinical experience, elimination is believed to be similar to adult horses. The duration of anesthesia after low intravenous doses of xylazine-ketamine to foals ranges from 15 to 30 minutes.[52] The administration of an α_2-adrenoceptor agonist before or simultaneous with ketamine prolongs metabolism and elimination.

Clinical Use and Antagonism

Ketamine and Telazol are used clinically in conjunction with sedative-hypnotics, muscle relaxants, and analgesics to produce short-term intravenous anesthesia or to induce horses to inhalant anesthesia (Table 12-5).[33-38,51-54] They are also administered as adjuncts to general anesthesia to increase anesthetic depth and provide a greater degree of analgesia.[49-50,55] Ketamine and Telazol are not recommended for intramuscular use because of prolonged absorption, unpredictable effects, and poor recovery; although a Telazol-ketamine-detomidine drug combination has been administered intramuscularly to feral horses to produce sedation and immobilization.[10] α_2-Adrenoceptor agonists, guaifenesin, or benzodiazepines (diazepam, midazolam) are administered before or with ketamine to produce short-term intravenous anesthesia (see Chapter 13). The bolus administration or continuous infusion of a xylazine-guaifenesin-ketamine drug combination for surgical procedures lasting 2 hours has been described in ponies (see Chapter 13).[56,57] The drug combination is produced by mixing 250 mg of xylazine and 500 mg of ketamine in 500 ml of solution of 5% dextrose containing 25 g of guaifenesin and administered at a rate of 0.05 ml/kg/min. The key to the successful use of ketamine or Telazol is to administer them to a properly sedated horse and never administer them to inadequately sedated or excitable horses.[58] This means that all horses should receive appropriate tranquilization, sedation, and muscle relaxation before intravenous ketamine or Telazol administration.

Table 12–5.	Intravenous use of ketamine in horses	
Drug	**Dose**	**Duration of action (min)**
Xylazine	1.1 mg/kg	5-15
Ketamine	1.5-2 mg/kg	
Detomidine	5-15 µg/kg	10-25
Ketamine	1.5-2 mg/kg	
Guaifenesin	25-50 mg/kg	15-25
Ketamine	1.5-2 mg/kg	
Xylazine	0.5-1 mg/kg	20-30
Guaifenesin	15-25 mg/kg	
Ketamine	1.5-2 mg/kg	
Diazepam	0.01-0.02 mg/kg	10-20
Xylazine	0.5-1 mg/kg	
Ketamine	1.5-2 mg/kg	
Xylazine	0.3-0.5 mg/kg	15-20
Diazepam	0.1 mg/kg to	
Ketamine*	1.5-2 mg/kg	
Ketamine (as an adjunct to anesthesia)	0.1-0.5 mg/kg	—
Tiletamine/ zolazepam (as an adjunct to anesthesia)	0.1-0.5 mg/kg	—
Xylazine	0.5-1.0 mg/kg	10-20
Tiletamine/ zolazepam	0.5-1.0 mg/kg	

*Diazepam-ketamine administered simultaneously.
Other α_2-agonists are frequently administered as alternatives to xylazine.

Intravenous administration of an α_2-adrenoceptor agonist followed in 2 to 5 minutes by ketamine (1.5 to 2 mg/kg IV) produces quiet, uneventful, excitement-free induction to sternal recumbency followed by lateral recumbency (Figure 12-2; see Table 12-5).[33-38,42,53,54,59,60] α_2-Adrenoceptor agonists produce marked sedation, muscle relaxation, and analgesia. Most horses are somewhat ataxic and assume a sawhorse stance with the neck extended, head lowered, and lower lip relaxed (see Chapter 11). Some horses become markedly ataxic and reluctant to move within 20 to 30 seconds of intravenous ketamine administration and dog-sit before lying on their sternum or become weak in the hind legs and fall to one side or the other. It is extremely important that a knowledgeable person control the horse's head during the induction phase of anesthesia. Horses that recline to a sternal position may be reluctant to roll to lateral recumbency for several seconds but usually can be physically persuaded to do so. Once recumbent, many horses groan during expiration. The pharyngeal and laryngeal reflexes remain active after ketamine or Telazol administration, making the nasal or oral placement of an endotracheal tube more difficult than with thiopental but able to be accomplished. Ocular and palpebral reflexes are active and cannot be used to judge the depth of anesthesia. Intraocular pressure remains unchanged or increases minimally.[43] Lateral nystagmus and

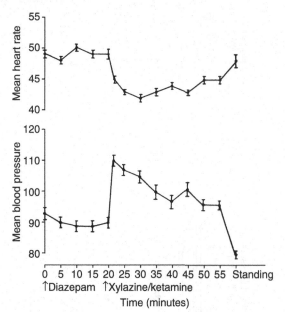

Figure 12-2. Effects of xylazine (1.1 mg/kg IV) and ketamine (2.2 mg/kg IV) on mean heart rate and mean arterial blood pressure in horses and ponies previously administered diazepam (0.22 mg/kg IV). (From Butera ST et al: Diazepam/xylazine/ketamine combination for short-term anesthesia in the horse, *Vet Med (Small Anim Clin)* 73:490, 1978.)

oculogyric movements are frequently present. Respiration may be transiently depressed initially, and hemodynamic variables remain within normal limits or slightly elevated. Blood glucose may increase.[61] Arterial blood pressure may be increased when detomidine is used as preanesthetic medication. The anesthetic period is short, lasting from 5 to 15 minutes, depending on the horse's age, the response to α_2-adrenoceptor agonist, and the severity of the surgical stimulus. Recovery is generally uneventful and begins with the horse rolling to its sternum before attempting to stand. Most horses can stand without assistance within 15 to 25 minutes of α_2-adrenoceptor agonist-ketamine administration. Drug combinations using hypnotics, muscle relaxants, or analgesics and ketamine produce similar effects, although the quality of induction may be improved and recovery prolonged. Repeated doses of ketamine or Telazol administered alone or in combination with tranquilizers or sedatives are occasionally administered to supplement intravenous anesthetic techniques or as adjuncts to inhalant anesthesia (see Chapter 13). Small doses of diazepam or midazolam, α_2-agonists, thiobarbiturates, or thiobarbiturate-guaifenesin drug combinations can be used to enhance or prolong anesthesia, are compatible with ketamine, and do not predispose to awkward or violent recoveries (see Table 12-5).[62] Up to nine supplemental injections of xylazine-ketamine have been administered to horses to prolong anesthesia.[51] Recovery was considered unsatisfactory in five horses.

No specific antagonist reverses the CNS effects of ketamine. The administration of α_2-antagonists (yohimbine, tolazoline, atipamezole) after an α_2-adrenoceptor agonist–ketamine drug combination is contraindicated early after drug administration unless it is an emergency situation. The premature reversal of the α_2-adrenoceptor agonist could lead to excitement, repeated unsuccessful attempts to stand, marked ataxia, hyperresponsiveness to sound and

movement, profuse sweating, tachycardia, hyperventilation, and increases in body temperature. These are all signs of sympathetic activation induced by fear in a semiconscious, uncoordinated horse. However, the administration of an α_2-antagonist 20 to 30 minutes after administering an α_2-adrenoceptor agonist–ketamine drug combination is usually without ill effect and helps to hasten recovery to a standing posture. The administration of the CNS stimulant 4-amino-pyridine has been used to shorten the duration of recovery in xylazine-ketamine anesthetized horses.[63] Intravenous administration of 0.2 mg/kg of 4-amino-pyridine decreases the total recovery time by more than 50% without producing excitement, although ataxia and hyperesthesia persist for a brief period.[63] The respiratory stimulant doxapram can be administered to initiate breathing during an emergency but should not be given to hasten recovery because of the potential excitatory effects. Although not routinely recommended, an α_2-adrenoceptor antagonist (atipamezole, tolazoline) can be administered to horses that remain recumbent for an extended period. The administration of atipamezole (50 to 100 μg/kg) to horses that had spent more than 60 minutes in recovery can result in immediate recovery to standing.

Complications, Side Effects, and Clinical Toxicity

The most common complications associated with the intravenous use of ketamine or tiletamine/zolazepam (Telazol) are failure to induce adequate anesthesia, a short duration of anesthetic effect, and excitement or delirium during the recovery phase.[58] Some horses demonstrate minimal-to-no response after ketamine injection; whereas others become transiently ataxic, dog-sit, or develop a brief period of severe muscle quivering and fasciculation. These responses are unlikely to occur in heavily sedated horses but may be caused by inadvertent perivascular drug administration, a loss of drug activity, or rapid drug redistribution. Shortened anesthesia time is most often the result of inadequate anesthesia, poor analgesia, and surgical stimulation. The primary causes for excitement and delirium and other signs of sympathetic activation during the recovery phase are inadequate sedation or excessive stimulation (loud noises, excessive movement, or bright lights). Additional doses of ketamine generally are ineffective in improving anesthesia but can prolong drug elimination (see Biodisposition earlier in the chapter), resulting in stressful recoveries. Ketamine in combination with an α_2-adrenoceptor agonist at one fourth to one half the original dose should not be administered more than once or twice to prolong anesthetic duration. Horses that become excited can be quieted by administering diazepam or small doses of thiobarbiturate. The combination of guaifenesin and thiopental can be administered as an adjunct to anesthesia to prolong the duration of α_2-adrenoceptor agonist–ketamine anesthesia and quiet the recovery phase.

Ketamine or Telazol can produce marked decreases in ventilation and transient periods of apnea in some horses. Hypercarbia and hypoxemia may result, requiring controlled ventilation or the administration of a respiratory stimulant (see Chapter 17). Large doses of dissociative anesthetics produce direct myocardial depression and can induce myocardial failure, leading to hypotension and the development of pulmonary edema. Hypotension and low cardiac output should be treated with dopamine or dobutamine (see Chapter 22). No other significant complications have been reported to occur in the horse.

Centrally Acting Muscle Relaxants

Centrally acting muscle relaxants (guaifenesin, diazepam, midazolam) are used frequently in conjunction with thiobarbiturates and dissociative anesthetics to enhance intravenous anesthesia in horses. Guaifenesin, a white bacteriostatic-bactericidal powder with a bitter taste, is soluble in sterile water, 0.9% saline, or 5% dextrose. Clinically useful solutions range in concentration from 5% to 15% and frequently have to be heated to prevent precipitation. Once prepared, most solutions are stable at room temperature for up to 1 week. There appears to be no advantage to the choice of diluent other than that related to osmolality.[64] A 10% (100 mg/ml) solution of guaifenesin in sterile water has an osmolality of 242 mOsm/kg, which is similar to that of equine plasma (280 to 310 mOsm/kg). Concentrations of guaifenesin greater than 15% are difficult to keep in solution and may produce hemolysis, hemoglobinuria, and urticaria.[65-67] Accidental perivascular administration produces tissue damage that can result in an inflammatory response, tissue swelling, and thrombophlebitis. Large volumes (800 to 1500 ml) of dilute solutions (5%) of guaifenesin are required to produce recumbency in adult horses, thereby necessitating the use of a large-bore intravenous catheter and method for administering fluids rapidly (pressure bag). Doses of guaifenesin that produce recumbency (100 to 150 mg/kg) are about 20% to 30% of those required to produce cardiopulmonary complications in horses.

Mechanism of Action

Guaifenesin is a centrally acting skeletal muscle relaxant and produces effects similar to the benzodiazepines by binding to specific inhibitory neurotransmitter receptor sites in the brain and spinal cord that are activated by GABA. Guaifenesin is not an anesthetic but selectively blocks polysynaptic reflexes in the spinal cord, reticular formation, and subcortical areas of the brain When used in dosages required to produce recumbency in the horse, it produces sedative-hypnotic effects and variable, although minimal, degrees of analgesia.[68,69] A prominent feature of guaifenesin is the ability to depress impulse transmission in the internuncial neurons of the spinal cord without impairing breathing. Guaifenesin frequently is coadministered with thiopental or ketamine to produce TIVA or induce horses to inhalant anesthesia (see Chapter 13).[56,57,62,70-72]

Applied Pharmacology

Clinically relevant doses of guaifenesin produce comparatively insignificant changes in respiratory rate, heart rate, pulmonary arterial pressure, and cardiac output.[73,74] Arterial blood pressure decreases, and peripheral vascular resistance increases after intravenous guaifenesin administration, but the changes are minimal (Figure 12-3).[74] Cardiac contractility is not depressed and may increase slightly after recumbency. The arterial partial pressure of carbon dioxide is unchanged, and arterial oxygen tension (PaO_2) is transiently decreased (5 minutes) immediately after induction to lateral recumbency. The mechanism responsible for this latter finding is unlikely to result from significant respiratory

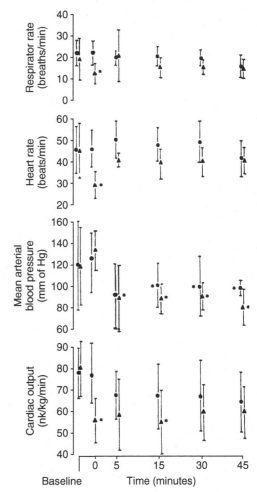

Figure 12–3. The cardiopulmonary effects of guaifenesin (approx. 125 mg/kg IV [●]) and xylazine (1.1 mg/kg IV) guaifenesin (approx. 80 mg/kg IV [▲]) in adult horses. *, P<0.05 from baseline. (From Hubbell JAE, Muir WW, Sams RA: Guaifenesin: cardiopulmonary effects and plasma concentrations in horses, *Am J Vet Res* 41:1751, 1980.)

depression because horses maintained in an upright position after guaifenesin administration demonstrate minimum blood gas alterations (Figure 12-4).[75] Continued infusions of guaifenesin can produce respiratory depression, resulting in respiratory acidosis. The effects of guaifenesin on the distribution of cardiac output to the brain, liver, kidney, and skeletal muscle have not been studied in horses; although it is suspected that they remain relatively normal. Blood chemical values and hematological values are unchanged by guaifenesin if solutions below those that cause hemolysis are used.[76] Guaifenesin is frequently coadministered with various sedative hypnotics (xylazine, detomidine, thiobarbiturates, ketamine) or inhalant anesthetics to produce recumbency and anesthesia. A 33% incidence of apnea has been reported when guaifenesin is infused before the bolus administration of thiamylal sodium for induction to anesthesia.[74] This problem is avoided when ketamine is mixed and administered simultaneously with guaifenesin until recumbency occurs.[56,57,62] Guaifenesin does cross the placental barrier, producing concentrations approximately 30% of that found in the maternal circulation.[74] However, the foals did not show signs of significant depression and responded favorably to physical manipulation.[77] Guaifenesin does not predispose to

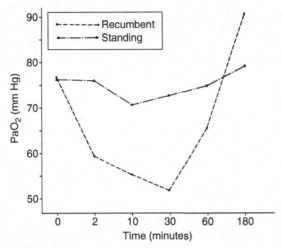

Figure 12–4. The effects of position on arterial oxygen tension (PaO₂ mm Hg) in horses administered guaifenesin (100 mg/kg IV). (From Schatzmann U et al: An investigation of the action and haemolytic effect of glyceryl guaiacolate in the horse, *Equine Vet J* 110:224, 1978.)

premature delivery or abortion in the mare. Studies of its effects on uterine tone in horses have not been reported.

Biodisposition

Guaifenesin is metabolized by the liver, where it is conjugated to a glucuronide and then excreted in the urine (see Chapter 9).[30] Catechol is an intermediate in the metabolic process but does not produce systemic effects. Intravenous guaifenesin undergoes rapid equilibration, requiring approximately 5 to 10 minutes, followed by a longer elimination phase. Studies in ponies and horses suggest a plasma half-life of approximately 60 to 80 minutes.[74,78-80] The half-life is shorter in female than in male ponies and horses and longer in donkeys because of a lower clearance.[81] Some horses and donkeys may require from 4 to 8 hours to stand after 2- to 3-hour infusions (see Chapter 9).

Clinical Use and Antagonism

Guaifenesin can be administered alone but is most frequently administered in conjunction with thiobarbiturates and dissociative anesthetics (ketamine, tiletamine/zolazepam) to produce short-term anesthesia, induce horses to general inhalant anesthesia, and as an adjunct to general anesthesia (Table 12-6; see Chapter 13).[56,57,62,70-72,82] Induction to recumbency is unlike that produced by either the thiobarbiturates or dissociative anesthetics. Large volumes of drug are required to produce recumbency, necessitating a secured intravenous route and continued drug administration until the time of collapse has occurred. The average dosage of guaifenesin required to produce recumbency in ponies and horses ranges from 100 to 150 mg/kg. The administration of this dosage using 5% or 10% solutions may take from 3 to 5 minutes.[83] Most horses become progressively depressed and ataxic during guaifenesin administration and need to be confined and assisted to prevent them from accidentally falling and dislodging the intravenous catheter. Maximum incoordination, ataxia, and buckling of the front legs begin to occur once doses ranging from 75 to 100 mg/kg have been administered. Administering preanesthetic medication or combining guaifenesin with a reduced bolus dose of either thiopental or a dissociative anesthetic minimizes the period of ataxia. Recumbency occurs within 15 to 30 seconds after thiobarbiturate or ketamine administration and may be associated with a transient and short period of hypoventilation. The major advantages of this latter technique are the decrease in the time the horse is ataxic, the removal of intravenous solution apparatus (freeing one assistant), and the ability to predict when the horse will collapse. Transient hypoventilation and apnea are greater concerns in severely debilitated or depressed horses, suggesting that the continuous infusion method to recumbency may be preferred to avoid bolus injections of drug. Horses that are relaxed when they are given guaifenesin retain relatively active palpebral corneal and swallowing reflexes. Tracheal intubation is accomplished easily because the neck and laryngeal muscles are relaxed. The skeletal muscles of the limbs, abdomen,

Table 12–6.	Intravenous anesthetic drug combinations originally developed for field anesthesia in horses	
Drug	**Dose**	**Duration (min)**
Guaifenesin* Thiopental; thiamylal	1-3 g of either thiobarbiturate mixed with guaifenesin to effect	Variable 15-25
2 g Thiamylal in 5% guaifenesin	0.02 ml/kg/min for maintenance	—
Guaifenesin	75-100 mg/kg to ataxia	10-20
Thiopental	4-8 mg/kg 3-6 mg/kg	
Guaifenesin	75-100 mg/kg to ataxia	15-20
Ketamine	1.5-2.2 mg/kg	
250 mg Xylazine; 500 mg ketamine in 5% guaifenesin	1.1 ml/kg for induction 0.05 ml/kg/min for maintenance	—
Guaifenesin	75-100 mg/kg to ataxia	10-20
Tiletamine/zolazepam	0.5-1.0 mg/kg	

*Guaifenesin prepared as a 5% or 10% solution in sterile water.

and neck are relaxed as sedation and analgesia improve with increasing dosages.

Recovery after guaifenesin administration is a gradual process but usually uneventful. Horses that are left in a quiet room with good footing usually roll to a sternal position and stand in one or two attempts. Some horses may become excited or stressed during the recovery process and require additional sedation or assistance to stand. Guaifenesin is compatible with all known preanesthetic and anesthetic drugs used to produce equine anesthesia. Guaifenesin is not an analgesic, and additional analgesics are required to minimize painful surgical stimuli.

Complications, Side Effects, and Toxicity

There are no known antagonists for guaifenesin. There are no reported major complications other than accidental perivascular injection, which can result in thrombophlebitis and hemolysis.[84,85] Occasionally, urticaria is observed in horses administered 10% to 15% guaifenesin concentrations (Figure 12-5).[86] This has occurred after the administration of both freshly made and commercially prepared solutions. The mechanism responsible remains unresolved.

Large intravenous doses of guaifenesin produce an apneustic pattern of breathing or breath holding and hypotension. Irregular breathing patterns and apneustic breathing are signs of drug overdose and occur well before cardiovascular collapse. When hypotension occurs, it generally is caused by bradycardia and decreases in the force of cardiac contraction. Dopamine or dobutamine can be used to increase cardiac contractile force, cardiac output, and arterial blood pressure (see Chapter 22).

OTHER INTRAVENOUS DRUGS

A variety of drugs, including depolarizing neuromuscular blocking drugs, hypnotics, steroidal anesthetics, and neuroleptanalgesics, have been used to produce chemical restraint or short-term anesthesia in the horse. Each drug and drug technique was developed and tested with the goal of producing safe and effective short-term immobilization or anesthesia (see Chapter 13).

Chloral Hydrate

Chloral hydrate is a sedative-hypnotic with a relatively wide therapeutic range. It is no longer available as a veterinary

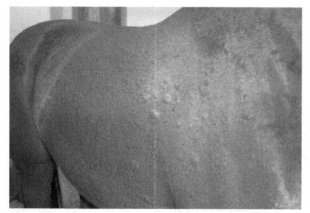

Figure 12–5. Urticaria in an adult Thoroughbred administered a 10% solution of guaifenesin in 5% dextrose.

product in the United States but can be obtained as both oral and intravenous preparations from pharmacies. Chloral hydrate is an excellent sedative with a relatively prolonged duration of effect and is currently used as an inexpensive method of euthanizing horses and cattle[87] (see Chapter 25). It is produced by combining chloral (trichloroacetaldehyde) with water and is available as translucent crystals that are volatile when exposed to air. The drug has a deeply penetrating aromatic odor and a bitter, caustic taste. Chloral hydrate is highly soluble in water (1 g in 0.25 ml of H_2O). Chloral hydrate has been administered as an anticonvulsant, general sedative, and anesthetic to horses.[4,6] The oral route of administration is not recommended (although still frequently used in cattle) because of its irritant effects on the gastric mucosa. Anesthetic doses (125 to 250 mg/kg IV) depress cerebral, respiratory, and vasomotor centers and are approximately 70% to 80% of the minimum lethal dose. These effects, combined with relatively poor analgesic activity, are the primary reasons why chloral hydrate is no longer recommended for intravenous anesthesia in horses.

Mechanism of Action

Chloral hydrate is an excellent sedative-hypnotic but a poor analgesic and anesthetic.[4,6] Increasing sedative doses (50 to 120 mg/kg IV) produce progressive depression of the cerebrum. Anticholinesterase effects are produced at low sedative doses and may potentiate reflex activity. Motor and sensory responses are not noticeably depressed after small-to-large sedative doses, which could have important clinical implications. Anesthetic doses of chloral hydrate produce cerebral and medullary center depression, resulting in muscle relaxation, mild analgesia, and cardiorespiratory depression. The CNS effects can be likened to the consumption of ethanol until stupor and anesthesia are produced. Indeed, horses that recover from chloral hydrate anesthesia appear to be suffering from a "hangover."

Applied Pharmacology

Sedative doses of chloral hydrate produce minimal effects on muscle tone, minute ventilation, arterial blood pressure, or cardiac output in otherwise normal horses.[88-90] Respiratory rate and heart rate may increase, and peripheral vascular resistance decreases during the first 10 to 15 minutes after intravenous administration.[88,89] Anesthetic doses of chloral hydrate reduce both respiratory rate and tidal volume, resulting in hypoventilation (increased $PaCO_2$). Heart rate and arterial blood pressure remain within normal limits, although cardiac output generally is decreased. The effect of recumbency on cardiac output during chloral hydrate anesthesia is unknown. Larger anesthetic doses of chloral hydrate produce decreases in heart rate, the force of cardiac contraction (contractility), and vasodilation, resulting in hypotension and decreases in tissue perfusion. Sudden death during induction to anesthesia after administration of chloral hydrate has been observed.[91] The cause is unknown but hypotension and the development of ventricular arrhythmias are suspected.[91] Both supraventricular and ventricular arrhythmias have been observed in horses after chloral hydrate sedation and anesthesia.[92] The author suggested that chloral hydrate anesthesia predisposes horses to both atrial flutter and fibrillation, proposing the drug as an experimental model to study these arrhythmias.[92]

Chloral hydrate produces anticholinesterase effects, which would be expected to decrease atrial refractoriness, thereby increasing the likelihood of supraventricular arrhythmias. It is not known if chloral hydrate sensitizes the myocardium to catecholamines.

The effects of chloral hydrate on other organ systems (lungs, kidney, gut) are secondary to changes in arterial blood pressure and blood flow. Anesthetic doses produce prolonged decreases in gastrointestinal activity and have resulted in premature delivery and abortion in pregnant mares. Chloral hydrate rapidly crosses the placenta, producing fetal depression.[93]

Biodisposition

Chloral hydrate is metabolized to trichloroethanol and trichloroacetic acid by the liver (see Chapter 9). Unchanged trichloroethanol can be found in the saliva and is excreted as urochloralic acid (trichloroethanol-glucuronic acid) in the urine.[94] Urine urochloralic acid gives a false positive for sugar. Only chloral hydrate and trichloroethanol are known to produce hypnotic effects. The time to peak effect after intravenous administration of chloral hydrate may vary from 5 to 10 minutes. The reason for this delayed onset of effect is unknown but may relate to its conversion to trichloroethanol and relatively slow passage across the blood-brain barrier. Studies conducted in horses suggest a plasma half-life of less than 30 minutes for chloral hydrate and from 1 to 2 hours for trichloroethanol.[94] The relatively long half-life of trichloroethanol may explain the prolonged recoveries from chloral hydrate observed in horses administered large sedative or anesthetic doses.

Clinical Use and Antagonism

Although it is considered extremely safe with a wide therapeutic range, chloral hydrate currently is not marketed for veterinary use in the United States. It can be administered incrementally (to effect) to produce calming and mild sedation without ataxia. More excited horses, stallions, and yearlings require larger doses. Increasing doses produces progressive CNS depression, leading to stupor and ataxia. Chloral hydrate has been administered after promazine or acepromazine and in conjunction with thiobarbiturates, hobbles, or a casting harness to produce short-term anesthesia for castration or minor surgical procedures (Table 12-7).[4,6,88,89] Analgesia using this technique is poor, and this practice is no longer recommended. Past formulations of chloral hydrate were combined with magnesium sulfate (2:1 and 1:1 mixtures) and pentobarbital to increase muscle relaxation and hypnosis, respectively. There is no reported mechanism to reverse the effects of chloral hydrate. Fluid administration and diuresis may promote drug elimination. Chloral hydrate can be solubilized as a 12% solution (120 mg/ml) in water and administered to effect as a euthanasia solution.

Complications, Side Effects, and Toxicity

Chloral hydrate is a safe drug when administered in subanesthetic doses. The chief disadvantage of and principal reason why it is no longer used in general equine practice is its prolonged duration of action; some horses remain stuporous and mildly ataxic for up to 8 hours after a single administration. The word "hangover" has been used to describe prolonged recovery from chloral hydrate

Table 12–7. Intravenous use of chloral hydrate in horses

Drug	Dose (mg/kg)
Chloral hydrate	
Mild sedation-hypnosis	5-10
Moderate sedation-hypnosis	20-50
Profound sedation-hypnosis	50-75
Anesthesia*	150-250
Drug combinations for recumbency†	
Chloral hydrate	100
Thiopental	1.5-2.0
Chloral hydrate	100
Ketamine	1.5-2.0
Promazine	0.6-0.8
7% chloral hydrate	20-40
Thiopental	5-7
Acepromazine	0.04-0.08
7% chloral hydrate	20-40
Thiopental	2-4
Xylazine	0.4-0.6
7% chloral hydrate	20-40
Thiopental	1-2

*Not recommended.
†Requires hobbles or a casting harness and preanesthetic medication.

sedation-hypnosis. Most horses remain quiet and are reluctant to move if left undisturbed. The accidental perivascular or subcutaneous administration of chloral hydrate can produce necrosis, pain, swelling, and sloughing. The occasional development of atrial flutter, fibrillation, and sudden death has been reported after sedative doses of chloral hydrate; but the cause is unknown.[91,92] Chloral hydrate has induced abortion in mares.[95] Anesthetic doses of chloral hydrate can produce marked cardiorespiratory depression, leading to respiratory arrest, profound bradycardia, and electromechanical dissociation resulting in death.[91]

Etorphine/Acepromazine

The drug combination of etorphine, a potent opioid, and acepromazine, a phenothiazine tranquilizer, has been suggested as a convenient neuroleptanalgesic for use in short surgical procedures in horses (Table 12-8).[4,96-102] Etorphine and its antagonist diprenorphine are approved in the United States for immobilization of wild and exotic animals only. The intravenous administration of etorphine alone to adult horses is contraindicated on the basis of severe extensor rigidity and sympathetic discharge that results in profuse sweating, tachycardia, hypertension, hyperthermia, and irregular dyspneic breathing patterns that produce hypercarbia and hypoxemia.[102] A mixture containing 2.25 mg/ml of etorphine (Immobilon) and 10 mg/ml of acepromazine has been available in the United Kingdom since the late 1960s.[4] The advantages of this drug combination are the small doses required to produce immobilization and recumbency, the ability to reverse the "anesthetic" state at any moment with diprenorphine (Revivon), and profound intraoperative analgesia.[101] The intravenous administration of this drug combination to horses produces recumbency within 60 seconds. There may be spastic rigidity, marked muscle fasciculations,

Table 12–8.　Intravenous drugs not commonly used for immobilization or anesthesia in horses

Drug	Dose	Duration	Side effects
Succinylcholine*	0.08 mg/kg	1-3 min	Sympathetic activation, pain, apnea
Etorphine/acepromazine*	100 µg/kg	Until antagonized	Hypoxemia, muscle spasms, lack of effect, anorexia, priapism, reimmobilization, sudden death; deadly to humans
Diprenorphine (antagonist)	30 µg/kg		Muscle spasms, tremors, sweating, excitement, hyperexcitability
Azaperone/metomidate†	0.2 mg/kg/ 3-5 mg/kg	5-10 min	

*No longer acceptable as a field restraint procedure.
†Not yet available in the United States.

coarse muscle tremors, and a state resembling tonic convulsions immediately after immobilization, reminiscent of the use of etorphine alone. Interestingly, inaccurate dosing, particularly a lower dose, is more likely to induce this early response. This is followed by a variable duration of greater relaxation; but rigidity, muscular tremors, sweating, mydriasis, and tachycardia persist throughout the duration of immobilization.[103] Muscle tremors render precise surgical procedures difficult, and male horses may develop engorgement of the penis. The force of cardiac contraction, cardiac output, peripheral vascular resistance, and myocardial oxygen consumption increases. Cardiac arrhythmias are common. The most significant alteration is a decrease in ventilation, often resulting in PaO_2 values less than 45 mm Hg.[100-103] Diprenorphine reverses the immobilization and analgesia within 30 seconds.[104] The horse usually rolls to its sternum and stands shortly thereafter. The disadvantages of etorphine-acepromazine drug combination far outweigh the advantages and include: (1) respiratory depression leading to hypoxemia and cyanosis; (2) hypertension and cardiac arrhythmias; (3) poor muscle relaxation and muscle spasms; (4) enterohepatic cycling of etorphine, resulting in excitement, aimless walking, and reimmobilization for up to 4 hours after drug administration; (5) behavioral changes after reversal or recovery from immobilization; (6) the reversal of analgesia after the administration of diprenorphine; and (7) it is lethal to humans in minute doses, necessitating extreme caution during its use and the availability of naloxone should an accidental injection occur. In addition to these problems, etorphine-acepromazine drug combination has been reported to produce no effect, profuse epistaxis, anorexia (lasting 48 hours), priapism, respiratory arrest, cardiac arrest, and sudden death after intravenous administration to horses.[105-107]

Propofol

Propofol is a popular intravenous anesthetic in humans, dogs, and cats. Although chemically unrelated to the ultra-short-acting hypnotic anesthetics thiopental, methohexital, and etomidate, propofol acts by a similar mechanism of action (i.e., it potentiates the GABA-induced chloride current by binding with the β-subunit of $GABA_A$ receptors at both spinal and supraspinal sites).[108] Propofol is an excellent hypnotic and muscle relaxant, minimizes the stress response during induction to anesthesia, and possesses both antiepileptic and antiemetic properties.[109] Its extensive distribution,

rapid clearance, and limited accumulation are responsible for rapid recovery from anesthesia with minimum hangover.[110] These attributes have led several authors to investigate its use as a single bolus injection, as an intermittent bolus, or as part of a balanced or TIVA infusion technique in horses.[111-116] Respiratory depression and apnea during induction to anesthesia and the potential to produce respiratory depression during the maintenance of inhalant anesthesia have delayed and may prevent approval for general use in equine practice.[10,112,113]

The pharmacokinetic, pharmacodynamic, and clinical effects of propofol in horses are similar to those observed in other species and include a rapid onset of effect, a short duration of anesthesia, and rapid recovery.[111] Induction doses of propofol produce an initial period of hypotension and respiratory depression and can trigger excitement.[111,112,117,118] Recovery from anesthesia is rapid, uneventful, and generally typified by good skeletal muscle strength and minimum ataxia.[111,112] Propofol is unlikely to replace current induction techniques or maintenance practices ($α_2$-adrenoceptor agonist–ketamine, diazepam-ketamine) in horses because of unpredictable behavioral responses during induction to anesthesia and the potential for hypoventilation, apnea, and low PaO_2, particularly in horses in dorsal recumbency; but it may be useful as an adjunct to inhalant anesthesia.[112,113,116,119] Some have suggested that depressant effects of propofol may be related to the choice of induction technique and that appropriate infusions of propofol (approximately 6 mg/kg/hr) in combination with medetomidine (3.5 µg/kg/hr) can be used to provide stable anesthesia and prompt recovery from anesthesia without hypoxemia[116,120-123] (see Chapter 13). Additional studies are needed in horses with naturally occurring disease before propofol can be recommended as an intravenous anesthetic.

Metomidate, Etomidate, Alphaxalone/Alphadolone

Various short-acting, nonbarbiturate, intravenous anesthetics (metomidate, etomidate, alphaxalone/alphadolone) originally developed for use in humans have been administered to horses to produce short-term anesthesia or induction to inhalant anesthesia. The potential advantages of these compounds in horses are their hypnotic effects, relatively short duration of action (approximately 10 to 15 minutes), and the maintenance of near normal cardiorespiratory values. However, their clinical use generally requires that sedatives and muscle relaxants be administered before anesthesia or coadmininstered to enhance the quality of anesthesia, prolong the anesthetic effect, or quiet the recovery period. Metomidate, etomidate. and alphaxalone/alphadolone produce sweating, muscular tremors, and involuntary leg and head movements during induction to anesthesia.[124,125] Excitement and convulsions have occurred during recovery, requiring resedation or anesthesia (thiobarbiturates, ketamine). Horses that recover without becoming excited do so quickly and are hyperresponsive to audible or visual stimulation. Alphaxalone/alphadolone administration produces short-term (5 to 10 minutes) anesthesia characterized by excitement during induction, poor muscle relaxation and muscle spasms after recumbency, and excitement and hyperresponsiveness to audible and visual stimuli during recovery. Although this general response is modified, it still occurs after preanesthetic medication using α_2-adrenoceptor agonists.[10]

Efforts to improve the safety and quality of intravenous anesthetics in horses rely on the combination of reversible, receptor-specific sedative-analgesics; short-acting, noncumulative hypnotics; and mild or short-acting muscle relaxants. The ideal short-term intravenous anesthetic for horses has yet to be developed, but continued clinical research has advanced current practice considerably.

REFERENCES

1. Crispin SM: Methods of equine general anaesthesia in clinical practice, *Equine Vet J* 13:19-26, 1981.
2. McGrath CJ, Easley KJ, Rowe MV: Anesthesia of horses under field conditions, *Vet Med Small Anim Clin* 77:1643-1646, 1982.
3. Geiser DR: Practical equine injectable anesthesia, *J Am Vet Med Assoc* 182:547-577, 1983.
4. Taylor P: Field anaesthesia in the horse, *In Pract 5 Vet Rec* (suppl):112-119, 1983.
5. Klein L: Anesthesia for neonatal foals, *Vet Clin North Am (Equine Pract)* 1(1):77-89, 1985.
6. Benson GJ, Thurmon JC: Intravenous anesthesia, *Vet Clin North Am (Equine Pract)* 6(3):513-528, 1990.
7. Taylor PM: Equine stress responses to anaesthesia, *Br J Anaesth* 63(6):702-709, 1989.
8. Luna SP, Taylor PM, Wheeler MJ: Cardiorespiratory, endocrine, and metabolic changes in ponies undergoing intravenous or inhalation anaesthesia, *J Vet Pharmacol Ther* 19(4):251-258, 1996.
9. Král E: Anesthesia using a mixture of chloral hydrate, magnesium sulfate, and pentobarbital in horses, *Vet Med (Praha)* 19(2):157-164, 1974.
10. Muir WW: Unpublished observations.
11. Muir WW, Mason DE: Effects of diazepam, acepromazine, detomidine, and xylazine on thiamylal anesthesia in horses, *J Am Vet Med Assoc* 203(7):1031-1038, 1993.
12. Butera ST et al: Xylazine/sodium thiopental combination for short-term anesthesia in the horse, *Vet Med (Small Anim Clin)* 5:765-769, 1980.
13. Muir WW: Thiobarbiturate-induced dysrhythmias: the role of heart rate and autonomic imbalance, *Am J Vet Res* 38(9):1377-1381, 1977.
14. Gaynor JS, Bednarski RM, Muir WW: Effect of xylazine on the arrhythmogenic dose of epinephrine in thiamylal/halothane-anesthetized horses, *Am J Vet Res* 53(12):2350-2354, 1992.
15. Gaynor JS, Bednarski RM, Muir WW: Effect of hypercapnia on the arrhythmogenic dose of epinephrine in horses anesthetized with guaifenesin, thiamylal sodium, and halothane, *Am J Vet Res* 54(2):315-321, 1993.
16. Daunt DA: Actions of isoflurane and halothane in pregnant mares, *J Am Vet Med Assoc* 201(9):1367-1374, 1992.
17. Spehar AM et al: Preliminary study on the pharmacokinetics of phenobarbital in the neonatal foal, *Equine Vet J* 16(4):368-371, 1984.
18. Taylor PM: The stress response to anaesthesia in ponies: barbiturate anaesthesia, *Equine Vet J* 22(5):307-312, 1990.
19. Alexander F, Nicholson JD: The blood and saliva clearances of phenobarbitone and pentobarbitone in the horse, *Biochem Pharmacol* 17:203-210, 1968.
20. Spehar AM et al: Preliminary study on the pharmacokinetics of phenobarbital in the neonatal foal, *Equine Vet J* 16:368-371, 1984.
21. Reimer JM, Sweeney RW: Pharmacokinetics of phenobarbital after repeated oral administration in normal horses, *J Vet Pharmacol Ther* 15(3):301-304, 1992.
22. Abass BT et al: Pharmacokinetics of thiopentone in the horse, *J Vet Pharmacol Ther* 17(5):331-338, 1994.
23. Saidman LJ: Uptake, distribution, and elimination of barbiturates. In Eger EI, editor: *Anesthetic uptake and action*, Baltimore, 1974, Williams & Wilkins, p 272
24. Dundee JW, Price HL, Dripps RD: Acute tolerance to thiopentone in man, *Br J Anaesth* 28:344-352, 1956.
25. O'Scanaill T: Pentobarbitone sodium as an anaesthetic in the horse, *Vet Rec* 109:125, 1981.
26. Jones EW, Johnson L, Heinze CD: Thiopental sodium anesthesia in the horse: a rapid induction technique, *J Am Vet Med Assoc* 137:119-122, Jul 15, 1960.
27. Tyagi RPS et al: Effects of thiopental sodium (pentothal sodium) anesthesia on the horse, *Cornell Vet* 54:584-602, 1964.
28. Tavernor WD, Lees P: The influence of thiopentone and suxamethonium on cardiovascular and respiratory function in the horse, *Res Vet Sci* 2:45-53, 1970.
29. Taylor PF: Thiopentone anaesthesia in horses, *Aust Vet J* 39:122-125, 1963.
30. Wernette KM et al: Doxapram: cardiopulmonary effects in the horse, *Am J Vet Res* 47(6):1360-1362, 1986.
31. McGruder JP, Hsu WH: Antagonism of xylazine-pentobarbital anesthesia by yohimbine in ponies, *Am J Vet Res* 46:1276-1281, 1985.
32. Jones RS: The effects of the extravascular injection of thiopentone in the horse, *Br Vet J* 124:72-77, 1968.
33. Muir WW, Skarda RT, Milne DW: Evaluation of xylazine and ketamine hydrochloride for anesthesia in horses, *Am J Vet Res* 38:195-201, 1977.
34. Ellis RG et al: Intravenously administered xylazine and ketamine HCl for anesthesia in horses, *J Equine Med Surg* 1:259-265, 1977.
35. Butera ST et al: Diazepam/xylazine/ketamine combination for short-term anesthesia in the horse, *Vet Med (Small Anim Clin)* 73:490-499, 1978.
36. Fisher RJ: A field trial of ketamine anaesthesia in the horse, *Equine Vet J* 16:176-179, 1984.
37. Luna SP, Taylor PM, Massone F: Midazolam and ketamine induction before halothane anaesthesia in ponies: cardiorespiratory, endocrine and metabolic changes, *J Vet Pharmacol Ther* 20(2):153-159, 1997.
38. Bennett RC et al: Comparison of detomidine/ketamine and guaiphenesin/thiopentone for induction of anaesthesia in horses maintained with halothane, *Vet Rec* 142:541-545, 1998.
39. Reves JG et al: Intravenous nonopioid anesthetics. In Ronald D, editor: *Goodman and Gilman's the pharmacological basis of therapeutics*, ed 6, New York, 2005, Macmillan, pp 346-347.
40. Visser E, Schug SA: The role of ketamine in pain management, *Biomed Pharmacother* 60(7):341-348, 2006.
41. Mori K et al: A neurophysiologic study of ketamine anesthesia in the cat, *Anesthesiology* 35:373-383, 1971.

42. Muir WW, Gadawski JE, Grosenbaugh DA: Cardiorespiratory effects of a tiletamine/zolazepam-ketamine-detomidine combination in horses, *Am J Vet Res* 60(6):770-774, 1999.

43. Trim CM, Colbern GT, Martin CL: Effect of xylazine and ketamine on intraocular pressure in horses, *Vet Rec* 117:442-443, 1985.

44. Kaka JS, Klavano PA, Hayton WL: Pharmacokinetics of ketamine in the horse, *Am J Vet Res* 40(7):978-981, 1979.

45. Waterman AE, Robertson SA, Lane JG: Pharmacokinetics of intravenously administered ketamine in the horse, *Res Vet Sci* 42(2):162-166, 1987.

46. Muir WW, Sams R: Effects of ketamine infusion on halothane minimal alveolar concentration in horses, *Am J Vet Res* 53(10):1802-1806, 1992.

47. Matthews NS et al: Pharmacokinetics of ketamine in mules and mammoth asses premedicated with xylazine, *Equine Vet J* 26(3):241-243, 1994.

48. Fielding CL et al: Pharmacokinetics and clinical effects of a subanesthetic continuous rate infusion of ketamine in awake horses, *Am J Vet Res* 67(9):1484-1490, 2006.

49. Knobloch M et al: Antinociceptive effects, metabolism, and disposition of ketamine in ponies under target-controlled drug infusion, *Toxicol Appl Pharmacol* 216(3):373-386, 2006.

50. Lankveld DP et al: Pharmacodynamic effects and pharmacokinetic profile of a long-term continuous rate infusion of racemic ketamine in healthy conscious horses, *J Vet Pharmacol Ther* 29(6):477-488, 2006.

51. McCarty JE, Trim CM, Ferguson D: Prolongation of anesthesia with xylazine, ketamine, and guaifenesin in horses: 64 cases (1986-1989), *J Am Vet Med Assoc* 197:1646-1650, 1990.

52. Schmidt-Oechtering GU: Anesthesia of horses with xylazine and ketamine: anesthesia of foals, *Tierarztl Prax* 17(4):388-393, 1989.

53. Hubbell JAE, Bednarski RM, Muir WW: Xylazine and tiletamine-zolazepam anesthesia in horses, *Am J Vet Res* 50(5):737-742, 1989.

54. Short CE, Tracy CH, Sanders E: Investigating xylazine's utility when used with Telazol in equine anesthesia, *Vet Med* 84:228-233, 1989.

55. Kushiro T et al: Anesthetic and cardiovascular effects of balanced anesthesia using constant rate infusion of midazolam-ketamine-medetomidine with inhalation of oxygen-sevoflurane (MKM-OS anesthesia) in horses, *J Vet Med Sci* 67(4):379-384, 2005.

56. Muir WW, Skarda RT, Sheehan W: Evaluation of xylazine, guaifenesin, and ketamine hydrochloride for restraint in horses, *Am J Vet Res* 39:1274-1278, 1978.

57. Greene SA et al: Cardiopulmonary effects of continuous intravenous infusion of guaifenesin, ketamine, and xylazine in ponies, *Am J Vet Res* 47:2364-2367, 1986.

58. Trim CM, Adams JG, Hovda LR: Failure of ketamine to induce anesthesia in two horses, *J Am Vet Med Assoc* 190:201-202, 1987.

59. Clarke KW, Taylor PM, Watkins SB: Detomidine/ketamine anaesthesia in the horse, *Acta Vet Scand* 82:167-179, 1986.

60. Hall LW, Taylor PM: Clinical trial of xylazine with ketamine in equine anaesthesia, *Vet Rec* 108:489-493, 1981.

61. Tranquilli WJ et al: Hyperglycemia and hypoinsulinemia during xylazine-ketamine anesthesia in Thoroughbred Horses, *Am J Vet Res* 45:11-14, 1984.

62. Muir WW et al: Evaluation of thiamylal, guaifenesin, and ketamine hydrochloride combinations administered prior to halothane anesthesia in horses, *J Equine Med Surg* 3:178-184, 1979.

63. Kitzman JV et al: Antagonism of xylazine and ketamine anesthesia by 4-aminopyridine and yohimbine in geldings, *Am J Vet Res* 45:875-879, 1984.

64. Grandy JL, McDonell WN: Evaluation of concentrated solutions of guaifenesin for equine anesthesia, *J Am Vet Med Assoc* 176:619-622, 1980.

65. Berger FM, Hubbard CV, Ludwig BJ: Hemolytic action of water soluble compounds related to mephenesin, *Proc Soc Exp Biol Med* 82:232-235, 1953.

66. Truitt EB, Patterson RB: Comparative haemolytic activity of mephenesin, guaiacol glycerol ether, and methocarbamol in vitro and in vivo, *Proc Soc Exp Biol Med* 95:422-428, 1957.

67. Mostert JW, Metz J: Observations on the hemolytic activity of guaiacol glycerol ether, *Br J Anaesth* 35:461-464, 1963.

68. Funk KA: Glyceryl guaiacolate: a centrally acting muscle relaxant, *Equine Vet J* 2:173-178, 1970.

69. Funk KA: Glyceryl guaiacolate: some effects and indications in horses, *Equine Vet J* 5:15-19, 1973.

70. Taylor PM et al: Cardiovascular effects of surgical castration during anaesthesia maintained with halothane or infusion of detomidine, ketamine, and guaifenesin in ponies, *Equine Vet J* 30(4):304-309, 1998.

71. Bennett RC et al: Comparison of detomidine/ketamine and guaiphenesin/thiopentone for induction of anaesthesia in horses maintained with halothane, *Vet Rec* 142(20):541-545, 1998.

72. Gangl M et al: Comparison of thiopentone/guaifenesin, ketamine/guaifenesin, and ketamine/midazolam for the induction of horses to be anaesthetised with isoflurane, *Vet Rec* 149(5):147-151, 2001.

73. Tavernor WD: The influence of guaiacol glycerol ether on cardiovascular and respiratory function in the horse, *Res Vet Sci* 11(1):91-93, 1970.

74. Hubbell JA, Muir WW, Sams RA: Guaifenesin: cardiopulmonary effects and plasma concentrations in horses, *Am J Vet Res* 41(11):1751-1755, 1980.

75. Schatzmann U et al: An investigation of the action and haemolytic effect of glyceryl guaiacolate in the horse, *Equine Vet J* 10:224-228, 1978.

76. Garner HE, Rosborough JP, Amend JF: Effects of glyceryl guaiacolate on certain serum, plasma, and cellular parameters in ponies, *Vet Med Small Anim Clin* 67(4):408-412, 1972.

77. Silva R et al: Clinical inquiries: is guaifenesin safe during pregnancy?, *J Fam Pract* 56(8):669-670, 2007.

78. Davis LE, Wolff WA: Pharmacokinetics and metabolism of glyceryl guaiacolate in ponies, *Am J Vet Res* 31(3):469-473, 1970.

79. Ketelaars HC, van Dieten JS, Lagerweij E: Guaiacol glyceryl ether study in horses and ponies. 1. The pharmacokinetics after a single IV injection, *Berl Munch Tierarztl Wochenschr* 92(11):211-214, 1979.

80. Taylor PM et al: Total intravenous anaesthesia in ponies using detomidine, ketamine, and guaiphenesin: pharmacokinetics, cardiopulmonary and endocrine effects, *Res Vet Sci* 59(1):17-23, 1995.

81. Matthews NS et al: Pharmacokinetics and cardiopulmonary effects of guaifenesin in donkeys, *J Vet Pharmacol Ther* 20(6):442-446, 1997.

82. Schatzman U: The induction of general anaesthesia in the horse with glyceryl guaiacolate: comparison when used alone and with sodium thiamylal (Surital), *Equine Vet J* 6(4):164-169; 1974.

83. Grandy JL, McDonell WN: Evaluation of concentrated solutions of guaifenesin for equine anesthesia, *J Am Vet Med Assoc* 176(7):619-622, 1980.

84. Dickson LR et al: Jugular thrombophlebitis resulting from an anaesthetic induction technique in the horse, *Equine Vet J* 22(3):177-179, 1990.

85. Herschl MA, Trim CM, Mahaffey EA: Effects of 5% and 10% guaifenesin infusion on equine vascular endothelium, *Vet Surg* 21(6):494-497, 1992.

86. Matthews NS et al: Urticarial response during anesthesia in a horse, *Equine Vet J* 25(6):555-556; 1993.

87. Jones RS et al: Euthanasia of horses, *Vet Rec* 13:130(24):544, 1992.

88. Gabel AA, Hamlin R, Smith CR: Effects of promazine and chloral hydrate on the cardiovascular system of the horse, *Am J Vet Res* 25:1151-1158, 1964.

89. Gabel AA: Promazine, chloral hydrate, and ultra-short-acting barbiturate anesthesia in horses, *J Am Vet Med Assoc* 15(140):564-571, 1962.

90. Schneider J, Stief E: The behavior of specific parameters of acid-base balance, heart rate, and depth of anesthesia during chloral hydrate anesthesia and chloral hydrate-My 301 anesthesia in horses, *Arch Exp Veterinarmed* 41(2):276-284, 1987.

91. Turner DM, Davis PE: Cardiac failure in a horse during chloral hydrate-chloroform anaesthesia, *Aust Vet J* 45:423-426, 1969.

92. DetweilerDK: *Experimental and clinical observations on auricular fibrillation in horses.* In Proceedings of the Annual Meeting of the American Veterinary Medical Association, Atlantic City, NJ, 1952, pp 119-129.

93. Allen WE: Equine abortion and chloral hydrate, *Vet Rec* 118(14):407, 1986.

94. Alexander F, Horner MW, Moss MS: The salivary secretion and clearance in the horse of chloral hydrate and its metabolites, *Biochem Pharmacol* 16:1305-1311, 1967.

95. Akpokodje JU, Akusu MO, Osuagwu AIA: Abortion of twins following chloral hydrate anaesthesia in a mare, *Vet Rec* 118:306, 1986.

96. Hillidge CJ: The use of immobilon, *Vet Rec* 87:669, 1970.

97. Hillidge CJ, Lees P: Fatality after revivon, *Vet Rec* 84:476, 1974.

98. Lakin CNS: Anaesthesia and revivon, *Vet Rec* 94:555-556, 1974.

99. Mitchell RJ: The use of immobilon, *Vet Rec* 87:600, 1970.

100. Jenkins JT et al: The use of etorphine-acepromazine (analgesic-tranquilizer) mixtures in horses, *Vet Rec* 90:207-210, 1972.

101. Stockman MJR: The use of immobilon, *Vet Rec* 87:518-519, 1970.

102. Schlarmann B et al: Clinical pharmacology of an etorphine-acepromazine preparation: experiments in dogs and horses, *Am J Vet Res* 34:411-415, 1973.

103. Hillidge CJ et al: Influence of acepromazine/etorphine and azaperone/metomidate on serum enzyme activities in the horse, *Res Vet Sci* 17:395-397, 1974.

104. Evans DJ: Anaesthesia and revivon, *Vet Rec* 95:70-71, 1974.

105. Brook D: Fatality after revivon, *Vet Rec* 84:476-477, 1974.

106. Clayton-Jones DG: Fatality after revivon, Vet Rec 84:477, 1974.

107. Sampson JH: Fatality after revivon, *Vet Rec* 84:477, 1974.

108. Jurd R, Arras M, Lambert S, Drexster B: General anesthetic actions in vivo strongly attenuate by a point mutation in the $GABA_A$ receptor beta3 subunit, *FASEB J* 17:250-252, 2003.

109. Smith I et al: Propofol: an update on its clinical use, *Anesthesiology* 81(4):1005-1043, 1994.

110. Nolan A et al: Simultaneous infusions of propofol and ketamine in ponies premedicated with detomidine: a pharmacokinetic study, *Res Vet Sci* 60(3):262-266, 1996.

111. Nolan AM, Hall LW: Total intravenous anaesthesia in the horse with propofol, *Equine Vet J* 17(5):394-398, 1985.

112. Mama KR, Steffey EP, Pascoe PJ: Evaluation of propofol as a general anesthetic for horses, *Vet Surg* 24(2):188-194, 1995.

113. Mama KR, Steffey EP, Pascoe PJ: Evaluation of propofol for general anesthesia in premedicated horses, *Am J Vet Res* 57(4):512-516, 1996.

114. Frias AF et al: Evaluation of different doses of propofol in xylazine pre-medicated horses, *Vet Anaesth Analg* 30(4):193-201, 2003.

115. Oku K et al: Cardiovascular effects of continuous propofol infusion in horses, *J Vet Med Sci* 68(8):773-778, 2006.

116. Umar MA et al: Evaluation of total intravenous anesthesia with propofol or ketamine-medetomidine-propofol combination in horses, *J Am Vet Med Assoc* 228(8):1221-1227, 2006.

117. Nolan A et al: Simultaneous infusions of propofol and ketamine in ponies premedicated with detomidine: a pharmacokinetic study, *Res Vet Sci* 60(3):262-266, 1996.

118. Flaherty D et al: A pharmacodynamic study of propofol or propofol and ketamine infusions in ponies undergoing surgery, *Res Vet Sci* 62(2):179-184, 1997.

119. Matthews NS et al: Detomidine-propofol anesthesia for abdominal surgery in horses, *Vet Surg* 28(3):196-201, 1999.

120. Bettschart-Wolfensberger R et al: Cardiopulmonary effects of prolonged anesthesia via propofol-medetomidine infusion in ponies, *Am J Vet Res* 62(9):1428-1435, 2001.

121. Bettschart-Wolfensberger R et al: Infusion of a combination of propofol and medetomidine for long-term anesthesia in ponies, *Am J Vet Res* 62(4):500-507, 2001.

122. Ohta M et al: Propofol-ketamine anesthesia for internal fixation of fractures in Racehorses, *J Vet Med Sci* 66(11):1433-1436, 2004.

123. Bettschart-Wolfensberger R et al: Total intravenous anaesthesia in horses using medetomidine and propofol, *Vet Anaesth Analg* 32(6):348-354, 2005.

124. Hillidge CJ, Lees P, Serrano L: Investigations of azaperone/metomidate anaesthesia in the horse, *Vet Rec* 93:307-311, 1973.

125. Eales FA: Effects of saffan administered intravenously in the horse, *Vet Rec* 99:270-272, 1976.

Intravenous Anesthetic and Analgesic Adjuncts to Inhalation Anesthesia

Kazuto Yamashita

William W. Muir

KEY POINTS

1. Combinations of intravenous anesthetic drugs can be administered to produce excellent short- or long-term anesthesia and as adjuncts to inhalant anesthesia.
2. Total intravenous anesthesia may be safer and less stressful than inhalant anesthesia. Safety is further enhanced by oxygen supplementation.
3. Intravenous analgesic adjuncts reduce the dose requirement for inhalant anesthetics (anesthetic-sparing effects).
4. Total intravenous anesthesia and intravenous analgesic adjuncts generally produce less cardiovascular depression than inhalant anesthetics.
5. Prolonged administration of multiple intravenous anesthetic drugs may lead to drug accumulation, drug interactions, and prolonged recovery times.

Intravenous anesthetic drugs and techniques are the primary means for producing general anesthesia in equine practice. For the equine surgeon, induction and maintenance of general anesthesia with intravenous drugs (i.e., total intravenous anesthesia [TIVA]) has many potential advantages over inhalation anesthesia. The use of TIVA reduces the cost of equipment, the requirement for an oxygen source (facilities), and the potential hazard from high-pressure tanks (see Chapter 16). In addition, TIVA eliminates any possible hazards to humans associated with exposure to trace concentrations of volatile and gaseous anesthetics drugs. The administration of a mixture of detomidine, ketamine, and guaifenesin (DKG) as TIVA in horses provided much better cardiovascular function and suppression of the endocrine stress response during anesthesia than inhalation anesthesia with halothane (Figures 13-1 to 13-3).[1-4] The administration of propofol and sufentanil as TIVA in humans reduced the production of proinflammatory cytokines (such as interleukin [IL]-2, IL-6, IL-8, IL-12, tumor necrosis factor-α [TNF-α], interferon-γ) and antiinflammatory cytokines (such as IL-10, IL-1 receptor agonist, transforming growth factor-β), compared with inhalation anesthesia with sevoflurane.[5,6] It has also been demonstrated that ketamine inhibits lipopolysaccharide-induced TNF-α and IL-6 in an equine macrophage cell line.[7] Together these studies suggest that TIVA produces favorable effects on endocrine and inflammatory responses triggered by anesthesia and surgery.

A major concern regarding the use of TIVA in horses is that the long-acting and cumulative effects of many intravenous anesthetic drugs may prolong or result in a poor quality of recovery. Inhalation anesthesia is more controllable than TIVA and preferred for prolonged periods of anesthesia (>60 to 90 minutes), regardless of the potential for vasodilation, hypotension, and lower cardiac output values (see Chapter 15).[8-10] However, intravenous analgesics or anesthetic adjuncts can be administered to horses during inhalant anesthesia to minimize inhalant anesthetic requirements and ensure adequate pain relief during the operative and postoperative period. Several intravenous analgesic adjuncts (IVAAs), including but not limited to lidocaine, ketamine, and medetomidine coadministered with inhalation anesthesia, provided better transition and maintenance of anesthesia, reduced inhalant requirements, and improved cardiovascular function in horses.[11-16] Both TIVA and IVAA coadministered with inhalant anesthetics provide safer and more effective general anesthesia in horses than the use of inhalant anesthesia alone.

PHARMACOKINETICS AND PHARMACODYNAMICS OF INTRAVENOUS AGENTS

The production of analgesia and anesthesia following the administration of intravenous drugs is related to the plasma concentration (Cp) of the drug, which can be predicted based on knowledge of the pharmacokinetic parameters of the drug: clearance, volume of distribution, and half-life (see Chapter 9; Table 13-1).

Rapid (15 to 60 seconds) intravenous ("bolus") administration of drugs produces high Cp values, a rapid onset of anesthetic drug and analgesic effects, and the greatest drug response. The slower drug administration rates used to maintain TIVA or IVAAs require a longer time (minutes; hours) to attain and maintain a constant Cp and are frequently preceded by intravenous bolus ("loading") doses. The onset of anesthetic and analgesic effects is delayed because of the slower delivery of infused drugs (Figure 13-4). The time required to reach a steady-state Cp during infusion can be estimated by the elimination half-life of the drug. The Cp of intravenous drugs is equal to 90% of its final steady-state value after 3.3 half-lives (see Chapter 9 and Figure 13-4).

The continuous variable rate infusion of intravenous anesthetic drugs to produce a desired effect provides a practical and highly controllable method for producing or supplementing inhalant anesthesia and is the logical extension of the more traditional incremental intravenous bolus dose method, which inevitably leads to cyclical fluctuations in

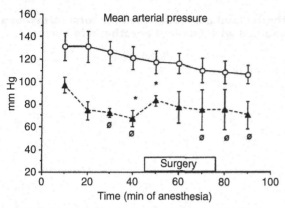

Figure 13–1. Arterial blood pressure (mean ± SD) during anesthesia and surgery with detomidine/ketamine/guaiphenesin (DKG) *(O)* or halothane (▲) (HAL) in 16 ponies. There was no significant change with time in DKG. °Significant decrease from 10-minute value in the HAL group. All DKG points were significantly higher than HAL. *Significant increase between 40 and 50 minutes in HAL group only. (From Taylor PM et al: Cardiovascular effects of surgical castration during anaesthesia maintained with halothane or infusion of detomidine, ketamine, and guaifenesin in ponies, *Equine Vet J* 30:304-309, 1998.)

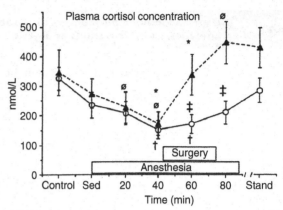

Figure 13–3. Plasma cortisol concentration (mean ± SD) during anesthesia and surgery with detomidine/ketamine/guaiphenesin (DKG) *(O)* or halothane (▲) (HAL) in 16 ponies. °Significant change from control value in HAL group. *Significant increase between 40 and 60 min in HAL group only. †Significant change from control value in GKD group. ‡Significant difference between DKG and HAL. (From Taylor PM et al: Cardiovascular effects of surgical castration during anaesthesia maintained with halothane or infusion of detomidine, ketamine, and guaifenesin in ponies, *Equine Vet J* 30:304-309, 1998.)

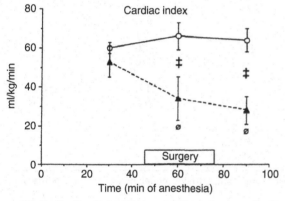

Figure 13–2. Cardiac index (mean ± SD) during anesthesia and surgery with detomidine/ketamine/guaiphenesin (DKG) *(O)* or halothane (▲) (HAL) in 16 ponies. There was no significant change with time in DKG. °Significant decrease from 30-minute value in the HAL group. ‡Significant difference between DKG and HAL. *BW,* Body weight. (From Taylor PM et al: Cardiovascular effects of surgical castration during anaesthesia maintained with halothane or infusion of detomidine, ketamine, and guaifenesin in ponies, *Equine Vet J* 30: 304-309, 1998.)

Cp, anesthetic depth, and cardiorespiratory function that follow each bolus dose (see Figure 13-4). Initial bolus doses, "loading doses," and infusions are established from pharmacokinetic data and modified as needed to attain the desired goals (hypnosis, analgesia, muscle relaxation). A loading dose can be administered to achieve an effective Cp rapidly. This approach is similar to administering a high inspired concentration (over pressure) of inhalant anesthetic during the initial phase of anesthesia to speed the onset of an inhalant anesthetic central nervous system (CNS) depressant effect. Smaller loading doses generally require greater initial maintenance infusion rates to attain and maintain anesthesia. Subsequent drug administration is reduced to maintain the Cp within the "therapeutic window" (minimum effective

concentration to toxicity) and avoid drug-related side effects (see Figure 13-4). The rate of administration of TIVA is titrated on an empirical basis, depending on the horse's cardiorespiratory status and physical response to surgical stimulation. With time, the infusion rate required to maintain any Cp becomes solely dependent on the elimination rate (clearance) of the drug. Thus the infusion rate needed to maintain a given Cp decreases as a function of the infusion duration and should be balanced (titrated) to attain optimum anesthetic and cardiopulmonary effects.

TOTAL INTRAVENOUS ANESTHESIA TECHNIQUES IN HORSES

The routine use of TIVA for prolonged periods of anesthesia in horses is hampered by cumulative drug effects, prolonged time for drug elimination, and expense. Many drugs are long acting and cumulative. Therefore extending the length of anesthesia by administering an intravenous drug for a longer period may result in a prolonged and poor-quality recovery. The ideal drugs for TIVA have pharmacokinetic properties that indicate that neither they nor their active metabolites are cumulative when infused into horses for prolonged periods. Current TIVA techniques can be grouped into three categories: (1) those that are suitable for short-term procedures such as castration (<30 minutes) and that result in a very rapid recovery, (2) those suitable for intermediate-duration procedures (medium-term; <90 minutes), and (3) those that could be extended indefinitely (hours).

Total Intravenous Anesthesia for Short-Duration (<30 Minutes) Procedures

Adequate anesthesia for procedures lasting 10 to 15 minutes can be produced and extended with incremental intermittent boluses of intravenous drugs. The most popular combinations of drugs selected for short-term anesthesia are combinations of α₂-adrenoceptor agonists (xylazine,

Table 13–1. **Pharmacokinetic parameters of sedatives, anesthetics, and analgesics used for total intravenous anesthesia or intravenous analgesic adjuncts combined with inhalant anesthesia in horses**

Drugs	Compartment model	Elimination half-life (minutes)	Volume of distribution (L/kg)	Total systemic clearance (ml/kg/min)	References
Acepromazine	2-comp.	185	6.6	49.2	86
	2-comp.	52-149	2.87-6.57	19.6-170.8	87
Guaifenesin	1-comp.	88-128	0.77-0.82	4.3-6.4	88
Diazepam	2-comp.	450-792	1.98-2.25	1.9-3.4	89
Xylazine	2-comp.	50	2.46	21.0	90
Detomidine	2-comp.	71	0.74	7.1	91
Medetomidine	2-comp.	51	1.10	66.7	92 (ponies)
Ketamine					
After xylazine	2-comp.	42	1.63	26.6	93
After xylazine	2-comp.	66	2.72	31.1	94
With propofol	2-comp.	90	1.43	23.9	63 (ponies)
Constant rate infusion	2-comp.				95
Thiopental					
With halothane	3-comp.	147	0.74	3.53	96
With isoflurane	3-comp.	222	1.13	3.64	96 (ponies)
Thiamylal	2-comp.	312	3.14	5.9	97 (ponies)
Propofol					
With ketamine	3-comp.	69	0.89	33.1	63 (ponies)
Morphine	3-comp.	3,377	7.95*	0.79*	98
Fentanyl	3-comp.	130	0.68	5.9	99
Awake	3-comp.	60	0.37	9.2	70
With isoflurane	3-comp.	68	0.26	6.3	70
Alfentanil					
Awake	2-comp.	22	0.45	14.1	69
With halothane	2-comp.	56	1.20	14.0	69
With isoflurane	2-comp.	68	1.37	13.6	69
Butorphanol					
Bolus IV	2-comp.	44	1.25	21.0	100
Constant rate infusion	non-comp.	34	1.10	18.5	100
Lidocaine infusion					
Awake	non-comp.	79	0.79	29	76
With sevoflurane	non-comp.	54	0.40	15	76
In surgical cases	non-comp.	65	0.70	25	75

1-comp., One-compartment model; *2-comp.*, two-compartment model; *3-comp.*, three-compartment model; *non-comp.*, noncompartmental analysis was performed.
*A rough estimate from original data.

detomidine, medetomidine, romifidine) administered with dissociative anesthetics (ketamine, Telazol) or barbiturates (thiopental).[17,18] Centrally acting muscle relaxants (guaifenesin, benzodiazepines [diazepam, midazolam]) are frequently administered in conjunction with ketamine and thiopental to ensure smooth induction to anesthesia.[19] Tiletamine-zolazepam, a 1:1 combination of tiletamine, a dissociative anesthetic, and zolazepam, a benzodiazepine tranquilizer, can also be used for induction (see Chapter 10).[20,21] Butorphanol, an opioid agonist-antagonist, is frequently coadministered with α2-adrenoceptor agonists to enhance analgesia during surgery.[22]

Drug combinations that are infused to produce short-term anesthesia in horses generally incorporate analgesic drugs (α2-adrenoceptor agonists, opioids, dissociative anesthetics), muscle relaxants (guaifenesin, diazepam, midazolam), and hypnotics (thiopental; Table 13-2). Reduced doses of thiopental (0.5 to 1 mg/kg intravenously [IV]) can be administered to extend anesthesia that has been induced

with either thiopental or an α2-agonist–ketamine drug combination. Larger total doses of thiopental (>10 mg/kg), even when administered incrementally, may be safe but prolong recovery. Anesthesia induced with an α2-adrenoceptor agonist and ketamine may be extended by the administration of ketamine (0.5 to 1 mg/kg IV); but muscle relaxation may be poor; and there is the potential for undesirable CNS excitatory effects unless sedation is still adequate.

Xylazine-Ketamine

The intravenous administration of xylazine (1.1 mg/kg) followed in 3 to 5 minutes by ketamine (2.2 mg/kg IV) produces quiet, uneventful, and excitement-free induction to recumbency in most horses.[18,23,24] Xylazine produces marked sedation, muscle relaxation, and analgesia. Most horses become ataxic and assume a sawhorse stance with the neck and head lowered and lower lip relaxed (see Chapter 10). Ataxia and usually dog-sitting, if their head is raised as they weaken before lying on their sternum, are apparent within 20 to 30

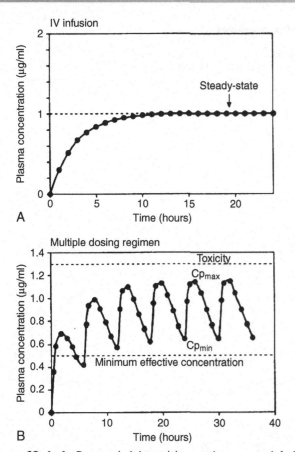

Figure 13–4. A, Drugs administered by continuous-rate infusion reach a steady-state value that can be predicted by their half-lives (i.e., 90% of steady-state in 3.3 half-lives). **B,** The Cp varies between Cp_{max} and Cp_{min} when drugs are administered at regular intervals (hours). Fluctuations between Cp_{max} and Cp_{min} at steady state increase as the dosing interval increases and can be predicted by the half-life of the drug. The Cp_{max} is equal to two times the Cp_{min} when the dosing interval is equal to the half-life of the drug. (Revised from Muir WW, Sams RA: Pharmacologic principles and pain: pharmacokinetics and pharmacodynamics. In Gaynor JS, Muir WW, editors: *Handbook of veterinary pain management,* ed 2, St Louis, 2009, Mosby.)

seconds after intravenous ketamine administration. Some horses become weak in the hind legs and fall to one side or the other. Induction (time from intravenous drug administration to recumbency) is relatively short, 30 to 45 seconds, but longer than the time required following intravenous thiopental administration, most likely because of a difference in uptake of drug by the brain (thiobarbiturates are highly lipid soluble).[25] It is extremely important that an experienced person control the horse's head during the induction phase of anesthesia. Horses that recline to a sternal position may be reluctant to roll to lateral recumbency for several seconds but usually can be physically persuaded to do so. Once recumbent, many horses groan during expiration. The pharyngeal and laryngeal reflexes remain active, making the nasal or oral placement of an endotracheal tube more difficult but able to be accomplished. Skeletal muscle relaxation can be improved by coadministration of a benzodiazepine (diazepam 0.01 to 0.05 mg/kg IV) with ketamine for induction (instead of ketamine alone), although respiratory depression may occur. Ocular and palpebral reflexes are active and cannot be used

to judge the depth of anesthesia. Intraocular pressure remains unchanged or increases minimally.[26] Lateral nystagmus and oculogyric movements are frequently present. Respiration may be depressed transiently ($PaCO_2$ 40 to 50 mm Hg), and the arterial partial pressure of oxygen (PaO_2) may decrease to 60 mm Hg during recumbency in spontaneously breathing horses.[27] Hemodynamic variables remain normal but may become slightly elevated, and blood glucose may increase.[18, 28] The anesthetic period is short, lasting 5 to 15 minutes, depending on the horse's age, the response to xylazine (or another α_2-agonist), and the severity of the surgical stimulus. Recovery is generally uneventful and begins with the horse rolling to its sternum before attempting to stand. Most horses stand without assistance within 15 to 25 minutes after ketamine administration.

When necessary, repeated reduced doses of ketamine and xylazine have been administered to prolong the duration of anesthesia in horses.[27] One study in adult horses reported that the duration of anesthesia could be extended by one to seven supplemental intravenous injections of xylazine (0.31 ± 0.07 mg/kg)-ketamine (0.68 ± 0.20 mg/kg).[27] The time from induction of anesthesia to the first supplemental xylazine-ketamine injection was 13 ± 4 minutes, and the time between supplemental injections was 12 ± 4 minutes. The time to standing from the last injection of xylazine-ketamine was prolonged (>50 minutes) in horses administered two or more supplemental doses compared to horses that did not receive supplemental doses (approximately 30 minutes).

Xylazine-Butorphanol-Ketamine[24]

The intravenous coadministration of xylazine (1.1 mg/kg) and butorphanol (0.04 mg/kg) followed in 3 to 5 minutes by ketamine (2.2 mg/kg IV) usually produces rapid and smooth induction to anesthesia. The anesthetic period is short, lasting 5 to 15 minutes. Respiratory rate may decrease briefly during the early phase of anesthesia. The $PaCO_2$ is maintained between 40 and 50 mm Hg, but the PaO_2 decreases to 60 mm Hg during recumbency and spontaneous breathing, similar to xylazine-ketamine drug combination. Hemodynamic variables remain within normal limits. Recovery from anesthesia is generally good to excellent, and most horses stand without assistance within 30 minutes after ketamine administration.

Xylazine-Diazepam-Ketamine[29]

The intravenous administration of xylazine (1.1 mg/kg) followed in 3 to 5 minutes by ketamine (2.2 mg/kg IV) coadministered with diazepam (0.04 mg/kg IV) enhances muscle relaxation, resulting in quiet, uneventful, and excitement-free induction. Muscle relaxation is improved compared to xylazine-ketamine, and anesthesia time is slightly increased (approximately 15 minutes). Hemodynamic variables remain within normal limits (Figures 13-5 and 13-6). The PaO_2 decreases to 60 mm Hg during spontaneous breathing (Figure 13-7) similar to xylazine-ketamine drug combination. Most horses stand with minimum-to-mild ataxia on their first attempt within 35 minutes of drug administration.

Xylazine-Guaifenesin-Ketamine[19]

Sedation is produced by intravenous administration of xylazine (1.1 mg/kg). Three to five minutes later, a 5% or 10%

Table 13–2.   Total intravenous anesthesia for short-duration procedures

Drug combinations	Intravenous dose	Mean duration of anesthesia or lateral recumbency (min)	Mean time to stand (min)	References
Xylazine Ketamine	1.1 mg/kg 2.2 mg/kg	30, 15, 20, <15, 23	31, 18, 33, 23, 26	35, 30, 23, 24, 16

Xylazine
  Butorphanol
  Ketamine
	1.1 mg/kg
	0.04 mg/kg
	2.2 mg/kg
		15<	24	24

Xylazine
  Guaifenesin
  Ketamine
	1.1 mg/kg
	35-50 mg/kg (to ataxia),
	2.2 mg/kg
		23	40	19

Xylazine
  Diazepam
  Ketamine
	1.1 mg/kg
	0.04 mg/kg
	2.2 mg/kg
		16	32	29

Xylazine Tiletamine-zolazepam	1.1 mg/kg 1.1 mg/kg	<20, 15	32, 31	20, 24
Detomidine Ketamine	20 μg/kg 2.2 mg/kg	15	27	24

Detomidine
  Butorphanol
  Ketamine
	20 μg/kg
	0.04 mg/kg
	2.2 mg/kg
		15	36	24

Romifidine
  Diazepam
  Ketamine
	100 μg/kg
	0.04 mg/kg
	2.2 mg/kg
		21	44	29

Xylazine Thiopental	1.1 mg/kg 5.5 mg/kg	46, 25	47, 31	35, 16
Xylazine Thiamylal	1.0 mg/kg 6.0 mg/kg	38	50	17
Xylazine Methohexital	1.1 mg/kg 2.8 mg/kg	33, 25	34, 28	35,16

Xylazine
  Guaifenesin
  Thiopental
	1.1 mg/kg
	to ataxia
	5 mg/kg
			30 to 40	

Xylazine Propofol	1 mg/kg 4 mg/kg	30	33	38

Xylazine
  Midazolam
  Propofol
	1 mg/kg
	0.02 mg/kg
	3 mg/kg
		26	35	40

Detomidine Propofol	15 μg/kg 4 mg/kg	33	41	38

solution of guaifenesin is infused into the jugular vein until the horse demonstrates signs of marked ataxia (35 to 50 mg/kg). A bolus intravenous dose of ketamine (2.2 mg/kg) produces quiet, uneventful, and excitement-free induction. Cardiorespiratory depression is minimal during anesthesia.[19] Recovery is quiet and uneventful, with full-standing recovery occurring in approximately 40 to 60 minutes. This technique is similar to the administration of xylazine-diazepam-ketamine but ensures adequate muscle relaxation since guaifenesin can be administered to effect before administering ketamine. Alternatively, 1 to 2 g of ketamine can be added to 1000 ml of a 10% solution of guaifenesin and administered until recumbency is produced. The latter technique requires a longer time to induce anesthesia than the bolus administration of diazepam-ketamine but avoids the potential negative consequences of bolus drug administration on cardiorespiratory function in high-risk patients.

Xylazine-Tiletamine-Zolazepam[20,24,30]

Sedation is produced by intravenous xylazine (1.1 mg/kg) followed in 3 to 5 minutes by tiletamine-zolazepam (1.1 mg/

kg IV). Induction to anesthesia is similar to xylazine-ketamine, but the duration of anesthesia is longer (15 to 20 minutes). Larger doses of tiletamine-zolazepam (1.65 mg/kg IV) prolong the duration of anesthesia. The PaO_2 decreases to 60 mm Hg, and the $PaCO_2$ is maintained between 40 and 50 mm Hg in spontaneously breathing recumbent horses, similar to other ketamine drug combinations. Hemodynamic variables remain within normal limits. Recovery is usually satisfactory but can be unsatisfactory. Most horses can stand without assistance within 35 minutes of tiletamine-zolazepam administration. However, some horses may require several attempts to stand and may fall minutes after standing successfully.

Detomidine-Ketamine[24,31]

The intravenous administration of detomidine (20 μg/kg) followed in 3 to 5 minutes by ketamine (2.2 mg/kg IV) produces rapid and smooth induction to sternal and lateral recumbency.[31,32] Induction to anesthesia is rarely unsatisfactory but occasionally requires the administration of thiopental in some horses. The anesthetic period is short, lasting

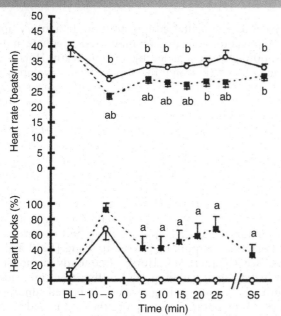

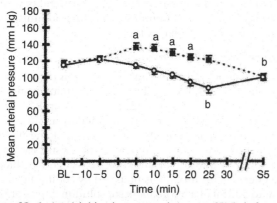

Figure 13–5. Heart rate (mean ± SEM) and percent of horses with 2-degree atrioventricular heart blocks before premedication (baseline, *BL*), 5 minutes after premedication with xylazine or romifidine (−5 minutes), following diazepam/ketamine (5 to 25 minutes), and 5 minutes after standing (*S5*). Difference (P<0.05) between the romifidine (■) and xylazine (O) treatment groups are illustrated by *a*, and differences relative to baseline values within a treatment group are illustrated by *b*. (From Kerr CL, McDonell WN, Young SS: A comparison of romifidine and xylazine when used with diazepam/ketamine for short duration anesthesia in the horse, *Can Vet J* 37:601-609, 1996.)

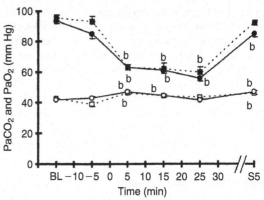

Figure 13–7. $PaCO_2$ (open symbols) and PaO_2 (closed symbols) concentrations (mean ± SEM) before premedication (baseline, *BL*), 5 minutes after premedication with romifidine (*squares*) or xylazine (*circles*) followed by diazepam/ketamine (5 to 25), and 5 minutes after standing (*S5*) from romifidine/diazepam/ketamine (■, □) and xylazine/diazepam/ketamine (●, O) anesthesia. Differences (P<0.05) relative to baseline within a treatment group are illustrated by *b*; difference between treatment groups were not significant. (From Kerr CL, McDonell WN, Young SS: A comparison of romifidine and xylazine when used with diazepam/ketamine for short duration anesthesia in the horse, *Can Vet J* 37: 601-609, 1996.)

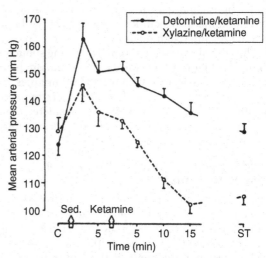

Figure 13–8. Comparison of xylazine (*O*; 1.1 mg/kg IV)-ketamine (2.2 mg/kg IV), and detomidine (●; 20 µg/kg IV)-ketamine (2.2 mg/kg IV) on mean arterial blood pressure in horses and ponies. (From Clarke KW, Taylor PM, Watkins SB: Detomidine/ketamine anaesthesia in the horse, *Acta Vet Scand* 82:167, 1986.)

Figure 13–6. Arterial blood pressure (mean ± SEM) before premedication (baseline, *BL*), 5 min after premedication with xylazine or romifidine (−5), following diazepam/ketamine (5 25), and 5 minutes after standing (*S5*). Differences between romifidine/diazepam/ketamine (■) and xylazine/diazepam/ketamine (*O*) groups are illustrated by *a* and differences relative to baseline within a treatment group are illustrated by *b*. (From Kerr CL, McDonell WN, Young SS: A comparison of romifidine and xylazine when used with diazepam/ketamine for short duration anesthesia in the horse, *Can Vet J* 37:601-609, 1996.)

5 to 15 minutes. Higher arterial blood pressure has been observed with detomidine-ketamine than with xylazine-ketamine (Figure 13-8). Respiratory depression is similar to that of xylazine-ketamine.[31] The PaO_2 decreases to 60 mm Hg during recumbency, although $PaCO_2$ is maintained between 40 and 50 mm Hg during spontaneous breathing. Recovery from anesthesia after administration of detomidine-ketamine

is not as good as that produced by xylazine-ketamine. Some horses demonstrate incoordination or excitement during recovery. Most horses can stand within 30 to 35 minutes following ketamine administration. The higher arterial blood pressure and poor recovery may be caused by lingering vasoconstriction and lingering sedation, ataxia, and muscle weakness resulting from the prolonged cardiopulmonary depression associated with detomidine.[32-34]

Detomidine-Butorphanol-Ketamine[24]

The intravenous administration of detomidine (20 µg/kg) and butorphanol (0.04 mg/kg) followed in 3 to 5 minutes by ketamine (2.2 mg/kg IV) generally produces smooth induction, but significant ataxia may occur in some horses before induction to anesthesia. The anesthetic period is short, lasting 15 minutes. The $PaCO_2$ is maintained between 40 and 50 mm Hg during spontaneous breathing, although the PaO_2 decreases to 60 mm Hg during recumbency. Hemodynamic variables remain within normal limits. Recovery is satisfactory but generally not as uneventful as that produced with xylazine-butorphanol-ketamine. Horses may show some ataxia during recovery. Most horses can stand within 40 to 60 minutes of ketamine administration.

Romifidine-Diazepam-Ketamine[29]

The intravenous administration of romifidine (100 μg/kg) followed in 3 to 5 minutes by ketamine (2.2 mg/kg IV)-diazepam (0.04 mg/kg IV) drug combination produces quiet, uneventful, and excitement-free induction. The romifidine-diazepam-ketamine drug combination produces a longer duration (15 to 20 minutes) of anesthesia than the xylazine-diazepam-ketamine drug combination. The duration of anesthesia can be extended safely to 30 minutes with supplemental doses of ketamine alone with no adverse effects on recovery.[29] Higher arterial blood pressure is produced in horses anesthetized with romifidine-diazepam-ketamine than with xylazine-diazepam-ketamine. There is a greater incidence of second-degree atrioventricular heart block during romifidine-diazepam-ketamine anesthesia than with xylazine-diazepam-ketamine drug combination (see Figure 18-6). The PaO_2 decreases to 60 mm Hg during spontaneous breathing (see Figure 13-7). Most horses stand on their first attempt without assistance within 50 to 60 minutes. There is mild ataxia once standing. The administration of diazepam with ketamine after romifidine is considered essential to avoid muscle rigidity or muscle tremors during induction and recovery from anesthesia.

Xylazine-Thiopental, Xylazine-Thiamylal, or Xylazine-Methohexital[17,25,35,36]

The intravenous administration of 4% to 10% solutions of thiopental (5 to 8 mg/kg) produces short-term (5- to 15-minute) general anesthesia in horses. The choice of barbiturates (thiopental, thiamylal, methohexital) is based on preference, although thiopental is thought to be associated with fewer side effects and adverse events. These ultrashort-acting barbiturates are administered by rapid intravenous injection (bolus injection) to hasten the onset of anesthesia, avoid struggling, and minimize involuntary muscle activity and movement during induction. Induction is rapid (10 to 20 seconds), and recovery is relatively uneventful. Both the induction and recovery phases of anesthesia can be associated with excitement, struggling, and incoordination. Appropriate preanesthetic medication is essential in all horses induced to anesthesia with ultrashort-acting barbiturates. The administration of supplemental doses of thiobarbiturates is not required in most horses. A well-trained, experienced person is required to control the horse's head during induction and recovery from anesthesia.

The intravenous administration of xylazine (1.1 mg/kg) followed in 3 to 5 minutes by thiopental (5 to 8 mg/kg IV) or thiamylal (4 to 6 mg/kg IV) produces rapid and smooth induction to anesthesia in most horses. Properly premedicated horses begin to relax within 15 to 20 seconds of intravenous thiopental administration. Temporary apnea and hypoventilation are common, and adequate muscle relaxation is often signaled by a deep breath. Horses that are not adequately tranquilized or sedated develop generalized muscle fasciculations and foreleg extensor rigidity or may rear up momentarily, attempt to fall over backward, or run in place (paddle) after recumbency. Skilled, experienced assistance is important when this occurs. The duration of apnea generally lasts for 15 to 20 seconds but can be as long as 3 minutes and may require physical stimulation (twisting the base of ear, pinching the anus, applying momentary pressure to the chest wall) to initiate breathing. Anesthesia is short (5 to 10 minutes) and not associated with significant analgesia. Recovery to a standing position is usually rapid but may be uncoordinated. The horse may require assistance to stand (head and tail ropes; see Chapter 21). Horses frequently demonstrate limb movements, paddling, and rolling from one side to the other before attempting to stand. Repeated administration of thiopental to maintain anesthesia can lead to drug accumulation and result in prolonged and uncoordinated recoveries. The horse may require multiple attempts to stand and require assistance.

The intravenous administration of xylazine (1.1 mg/kg) followed in 3 to 5 minutes by methohexital (2 to 5 mg/kg IV) generally produces rapid and smooth induction. The quality of induction depends on the preanesthetic sedative effect. Induction to anesthesia and lateral recumbency is similar to that of thiopental. The breathing rhythm is often abnormal, and Biot's breathing (deep breaths interposed with apnea) frequently occurs. Anesthesia lasts for about 5 minutes, and the horse usually begins attempts to stand within about 20 to 30 minutes from drug administration. Recovery is usually quiet and uneventful.

Xylazine-Guaifenesin-Thiopental[37]

The intravenous administration of xylazine (1.1 mg/kg), followed in 3 to 5 minutes by the intravenous administration of a 5% or 10% guaifenesin solution until the horse shows marked ataxia (to effect) and then by an intravenous bolus of thiopental (5 mg/kg), produces rapid and uneventful induction to anesthesia. Induction to anesthesia can also be achieved by infusion of a mixture of guaifenesin-thiopental to effect.[37] This mixture is prepared by adding 1 g of thiopental to 500 ml of a 5% guaifenesin solution. Stress or panic has occurred in horses that are not adequately sedated and do not succumb to the relaxant effects of the guaifenesin-thiopental drug combination. A small bolus dose of thiopental (0.5 to 1 mg/kg IV) may be required to hasten induction to anesthesia during these circumstances. Recovery occurs within 30 to 40 minutes, and residual muscle weakness is common if high doses of guaifenesin are used.

Xylazine-Propofol, Detomidine-Propofol, or Xylazine-Midazolam-Propofol

The administration of propofol (4 mg/kg IV) for short-term anesthesia[38-40] without premedication produces short-term anesthesia and very rapid and smooth recovery.[38] However, transition to lateral recumbency is slow, and leg paddling is common.[38] Tachycardia (heart rate 60 to 80 beats/min) is common during anesthesia. The intravenous administration of xylazine (1 mg/kg) or detomidine (15 μg/kg) prevents tachycardia and enhances the quality of induction but fails to prevent all of the undesirable characteristics of propofol, including hypoventilation and apnea.[39] The intravenous administration of xylazine (1 mg/kg) and midazolam (0.04 mg/kg) minimizes paddling, but excessive muscle fasciculations and tremors still remain undesirable characteristics of propofol induction to anesthesia.[40] The $PaCO_2$ generally is maintained between 40 and 50 mm Hg during spontaneous breathing, but the PaO_2 decreases to 60 mm Hg during recumbency.[39,40] Hemodynamic variables remain within normal limits.[39,40]

Total Intravenous Anesthesia for Intermediate-Duration (30 to 90 Minutes) Procedures

Surgical procedures requiring anesthesia for more than 30 minutes can be achieved with various combinations of α_2-adrenoceptor agonists, dissociative anesthetics, and centrally acting muscle relaxants (Table 13-3). These drug combinations can be administered as intermittent intravenous boluses or by infusion.[3,37,41-44] The use of guaifenesin, ketamine, and xylazine to induce and maintain anesthesia in horses (triple drip) was first reported in 1978 and

Table 13–3. Total intravenous anesthesia for intermediate-duration procedures

Protocols	Premedication	Induction	Maintenance	References
KD/KX	Xylazine 1.1 mg/kg Butorphanol 0.04 mg/kg IV	Ketamine 2.2 mg/kg Diazepam 0.06 mg/kg IV	Bolus IV of ketamine 0.25 mg/kg Xylazine 0.25 mg/kg (repeat as needed to maintain anesthesia)	37
TZKD	Xylazine 1.1 mg/kg Butorphanol 0.04 mg/kg IV	TZKD mixture 0.007 ml/kg IV	Bolus IV of TZKD mixture 0.002 ml/kg (repeat as needed to maintain anesthesia) TZKD mixture is prepared by adding 4 ml of ketamine (100 mg/ml) and 1 ml of detomidine (10 mg/ml) to an unreconstituted 5-ml bottle of tiletamine-zolazepam.	37, 21
GKX infusion (triple drip)	Xylazine 1.1 mg/kg IV alone or combined with Butorphanol 0.04 mg/kg IV	Ketamine 2.2 mg/kg IV or GKX mixture is infused to effect (1.1 ml/kg)	GKX mixture 1.5 ml/kg/hr CRI (temporary increases in the infusion rate until movement ceases) GKX mixture is prepared by adding 2.5 ml of xylazine (100 mg/ml) and 5 ml of ketamine (100 mg/ml) to 500 ml of 5% guaifenesin	37, 42
GKD infusion	Detomidine 20 μg/kg IV	Ketamine 2 mg/kg IV	GKD mixture 0.6-0.8 ml/kg/hr CRI GKD mixture consists of guaifenesin (100 mg/ml), ketamine (4 mg/ml), and detomidine (40 μg/ml)	3
CK infusion	Acepromazine 0.03 mg/kg Xylazine 1 mg/kg IV	Ketamine 2 mg/kg IV	CK infusion rate: climazolam 0.4 mg/kg/hr ketamine 6 mg/kg/hr Antagonized by sarmazenil 0.04 mg/kg IV at 20 minutes after the cessation of CK infusion	44
GKR infusion	Romifidine 100 μg/kg IV	Ketamine 2.2 mg/kg IV	GKR infusion rate: Guaifenesin 100 mg/kg/hr ketamine 6.6 mg/kg/hr Romifidine (82.5 μg/ml)	46
MKM infusion	Medetomidine 5 μg/kg IV	Ketamine 2.5 mg/kg Midazolam 0.04 mg/kg IV	MKM mixture 0.1 ml/kg/hr constant rate infusion MKM mixture is prepared by mixing 8 ml of midazolam (5 mg/ml), 20 ml of ketamine (100 mg/ml), and 5 ml of medetomidine (1 mg/ml) and adjusted final volume to 50 ml by saline	41

CK, Climazolam-ketamine; *GKD*, guaifenesin-ketamine-diazepam; *GKR*, guaifenesin-ketamine-romifidine; *GKX*, guaifenesin-ketamine-xylazine; *KD*, ketamine-diazepam; *KX*, ketamine-xylazine; *MKM*, midazolam-ketamine-medetomidine.

popularized in 1986.[19, 30] This technique and modifications using different α_2-adrenoceptor agonists or water-soluble benzodiazepines can be safely administered to horses for procedures lasting for 90 minutes.[3,27,37,41,42,44]

The combinations of α_2-adrenoceptor agonists, dissociative anesthetics, and centrally acting muscle relaxants in horses produce minimum cardiovascular depression and moderate hypoventilation ($PaCO_2$ 50 to 60 mm Hg; Figures 13-9 to 13-11).[43] Hypoxia during anesthesia may occur in horses spontaneously breathing room air.[41] Supplemental oxygen is recommended to prevent hypoxia during triple-drip TIVA for intermediate-duration procedures.

Ketamine-Diazepam/Ketamine-Xylazine[37]

Anesthesia can be produced in horses by the intravenous administration of xylazine (1.1 mg/kg) with or without butorphanol (0.02 mg/kg IV), followed 10 to 15 minutes later by ketamine (2.2 mg/kg IV) and diazepam (KD) (0.06 mg/kg IV). Anesthesia can be maintained by repeated intravenous administration of ketamine (0.25 mg/kg) and xylazine (KX) (0.25 mg/kg) as needed. The administration of xylazine-butorphanol produces good sedation and analgesia and minimizes the need for physical restraint. The intravenous administration of KD following the xylazine-butorphanol

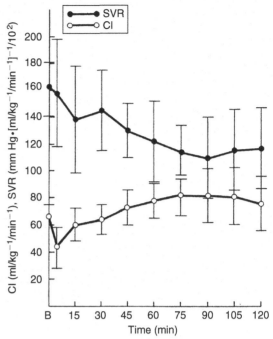

Figure 13–10. Cardiac index *(CI)* and systemic vascular resistance *(SVR;* mean ± SD) of ponies anesthetized with guaifenesin, ketamine, and xylazine (50, 1, and 0.5 mg/ml, respectively, in 5% dextrose in water) administered IV at 1.1 ml/kg followed by continuous intravenous infusion at a rate of 2.75 ml/kg/hr and spontaneously breathing oxygen. B, baseline. (From Greene SA et al: Cardiopulmonary effects of continuous intravenous infusion of guaifenesin, ketamine, and xylazine in ponies, *Am J Vet Res* 47:2364-2367, 1986.)

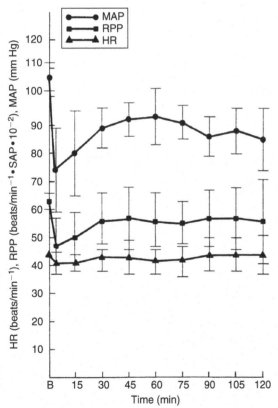

Figure 13–9. Heart rate *(HR)*, mean arterial blood pressure *(MAP)*, and rate-pressure product *(RPP;* mean ± SD) of ponies anesthetized with guaifenesin, ketamine, and xylazine (50, 1.0, and 0.5 mg/ml, respectively, in 5% dextrose in water) administered IV at 1.1 ml/kg followed by continuous intravenous infusion at a rate of 2.75 ml/kg/hr and spontaneously breathing oxygen. *SAP,* Systolic arterial blood pressure; *B,* baseline. (From Greene SA et al: Cardiopulmonary effects of continuous intravenous infusion of guaifenesin, ketamine, and xylazine in ponies, *Am J Vet Res* 47:2364-2367, 1986.)

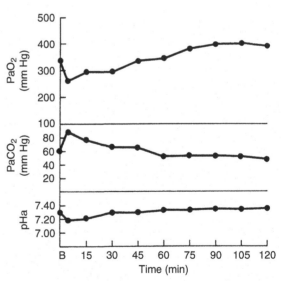

Figure 13–11. Blood gas values and pH of ponies anesthetized with guaifenesin, ketamine, and xylazine (50, 1, and 0.5 mg/ml, respectively, in 5% dextrose in water) administered IV at 1.1 ml/kg followed by continuous intravenous infusion at a rate of 2.75 ml/kg/hr and spontaneously breathing oxygen. B, Baseline. (From Greene SA et al: Cardiopulmonary effects of continuous intravenous infusion of guaifenesin, ketamine, and xylazine in ponies, *Am J Vet Res* 47:2364-2367, 1986.)

premedication produces quiet, uneventful, and excitement-free induction in most horses.

Horses may require three to five doses of KX to maintain anesthesia (38 ± 10 minutes) for cryptorchid castration (surgery time 21 ± 4 minutes).[37] Additional analgesia (local anesthetic; see Chapter 11) or inhalation anesthesia may be required in some horses because of movement in response to surgical stimulation. Hypoxia and hypoventilation are within clinically acceptable limits in horses breathing 100% oxygen spontaneously. Hemodynamic variables remain within normal limits. Recovery is uneventful, and horses usually stand (1.2 ± 0.4 attempts) within 18 ± 6 minutes from the end of the last anesthetic drug administration.

Tiletamine-Zolazepam-Ketamine-Detomidine[37]

Anesthesia can be produced in horses by the intravenous administration of xylazine (1.1 mg/kg) and butorphanol (0.02 mg/kg) followed in 10 to 15 minutes by tiletamine-zolazepam (0.67 mg/kg IV), ketamine (0.53 mg/kg IV), and detomidine (13 μg/kg IV) (TZKD). Anesthesia is maintained by repeated intravenous doses of tiletamine-zolazepam (0.22 mg/kg IV), ketamine (0.18 mg/kg IV), and detomidine (4 μg/kg IV) as needed. The TZKD drug combination is prepared by adding 4 ml of ketamine (100 mg/ml) and 1 ml of detomidine (10 mg/ml) to an un-reconstituted 5-ml bottle of tiletamine-zolazepam. This combination is administered at a dose of 0.007 ml/kg for induction of anesthesia and 0.002 ml/kg as a bolus dose for maintenance. The intravenous administration of TZKD following xylazine-butorphanol premedication produces quiet, uneventful, and excitement-free induction in most horses. Horses may require three to four additional bolus doses to maintain anesthesia (41 ± 9 minutes) for cryptorchid castration (surgery time 20 ± 5 minutes).[37] Arterial blood pressure remains within normal values during anesthesia. Hypoxia and hypoventilation are not common in horses allowed to spontaneously breathe 100% oxygen. However, recovery is poor, and horses require 3.7 ± 5.5 attempts to stand at 15 ± 8 minutes from the end of anesthetic drug administration. This drug combination (TZKD) has also been administered intramuscularly to sedate and anesthetize wild or feral horses.

Ketamine-Xylazine Infusion[39]

Xylazine and ketamine (KX) can be administered to produce TIVA in horses. Anesthesia was produced and safely maintained for approximately 1 hour by infusion of xylazine (35 μg/kg/min) and ketamine (90 to 150 μg/kg/min) with 100% inspired oxygen or xylazine (35 to 70 μg/kg/min) and ketamine (120 to 150 μg/kg/min) in 100% inspired oxygen.[39] Anesthesia was maintained satisfactorily with various infusions of xylazine and ketamine, although the combination of xylazine (70 μg/kg/min) and ketamine (90 to 150 μg/kg/min) produced the best results. Ketamine alone (150 μg/kg/min) produced the best cardiovascular function, but the quality of surgical anesthesia was poor. All horses that received supplemental oxygen hypoventilated, but $PaCO_2$ remained within acceptable limits. The degree of hypoxemia during KX anesthesia was similar to that observed with inhalation anesthesia, emphasizing the importance of oxygen supplementation. Recovery was good to excellent with all drug combinations. Most horses stood 45 to 90 minutes after KX infusion.

Climazolam-Ketamine Infusion[44]

The intravenous administration of ketamine (2 mg/kg) followed by climazolam (CK) (0.2 mg/kg IV) produces smooth and calm induction to anesthesia in ponies premedicated with acepromazine (0.03 mg/kg IV) and xylazine (1 mg/kg IV). Anesthesia can be maintained for up to 120 minutes by infusion of climazolam (0.4 mg/kg/hr) and ketamine (6 mg/kg/hr). Moderate hypoventilation and mild hypoxia may occur during anesthesia in spontaneously breathing horses supplemented with oxygen. Hemodynamic variables remain within normal limits. The intravenous administration of sarmazenil (0.04 mg/kg), a benzodiazepine antagonist, 20 minutes after the infusion was stopped, shortened and enhanced recovery from anesthesia. The ponies stood 7.2 ± 6 minutes after the injection of sarmazenil; however, recovery was not ideal in two of six ponies.

Guaifenesin-Ketamine-Xylazine Infusion (Triple Drip)[19,37,42,43]

Anesthesia can be induced and maintained in sedated horses by an infusion of triple drip.[37] A mixture of guaifenesin (50 mg/ml), ketamine (1 mg/ml), and xylazine (GKX) (0.5 mg/ml) is administered to effect (recumbency), and anesthesia is maintained by an infusion of the same drug combination (1 to 1.5 ml/kg/hr). The infusion rate is increased or decreased as needed to maintain anesthesia. The mixture is prepared by adding 2.5 ml of xylazine (100 mg/ml) and 5 ml of ketamine (100 mg/ml) to 500 ml of 5% guaifenesin (50 mg/ml). The intravenous administration of GKX drug combination after sedation with xylazine (1.1 mg/kg IV)-butorphanol (0.04 mg/kg IV) produces quiet, uneventful, and excitement-free induction in most horses.[37] Hemodynamic variables remain within normal limits. Hypoxia and hypoventilation do not occur in horses allowed to spontaneously breathe 100% oxygen. Recovery is judged to be good, and horses usually stand on their first attempt in 12 ± 5 minutes from the end of anesthetic drug administration. Recovery from prolonged infusion (>60 minutes) of triple drip may take more than 1 hour.

The intravenous administration of xylazine (1.1 mg/kg) followed by ketamine (2.2 mg/kg IV) for anesthetic induction, followed by an intravenous infusion of a GKX drug combination (50 mg/ml of guaifenesin, 1 mg/ml of ketamine, and 0.5 mg/ml of xylazine; triple drip) at a rate of 2.75 ml/kg/hr (guaifenesin 137.5 mg/kg/hr, ketamine 2.75 mg/kg/hr, xylazine 1.375 mg/kg/hr) produces good-to-excellent TIVA for 60 to 90 minutes. Cardiopulmonary depression is minimal (see Figures 13-9 to 13-11).

The clinical efficacy of triple drip has been evaluated in horses induced to anesthesia with xylazine (1 mg/kg IV) and ketamine (2 mg/kg IV), with detomidine (20 μg/kg IV) and ketamine (1 mg/kg), with xylazine (1 mg/kg IV) and thiopental (5.5 mg/kg IV), or with detomidine (20 μg/kg IV) and thiopental (5.5 mg/kg IV). Anesthesia is maintained by an infusion of guaifenesin (100 mg/ml)-ketamine (2 mg/ml)-xylazine (1 mg/ml) drug combination. The median duration of infusion in one study was 65 minutes (ranging from 51 to 95 minutes), and median infusion rate was 1.1 ml/kg/hr (ranging from 1 to 1.4 ml/kg/hr).[43] Anesthesia was satisfactory in 36 horses, although laryngeal reflex interfered with laryngeal surgery in two horses, and the diuretic effect (α_2-agonist–mediated; see Chapter 10) of the infusion was considered inconvenient during urogenital surgery. Hypoxia and hypoventilation did not occur in horses spontaneously breathing oxygen-enriched air, and hemodynamic variables remained within normal limits. Recovery was judged to be good in most horses, and the median time to standing was 38 minutes (ranging from 30.5 to 46.5 minutes) from the cessation of infusion.

Guaifenesin-Ketamine-Detomidine Infusion[2,3,45]

A GKD drug combination can be administered to produce anesthesia in horses and has been compared to halothane. Cardiovascular and respiratory function are better maintained during GKD TIVA than inhalation anesthesia (see Figures 13-1 to 13-3).[3]

Surgical anesthesia can be maintained for 90 minutes with an infusion of guaifenesin (100 mg/ml)-ketamine (4 mg/ml)-detomidine (40 μg/ml) using an infusion rate of 0.8 ml/kg/hr for the first 60 minutes and then 0.6 ml/kg/hr for the remaining 30 minutes. Horses were administered detomidine (20 μg/kg IV) and ketamine (2 mg/kg IV) for induction to anesthesia and breathed room air supplemented with oxygen.[1] The GKD drug combination provided better cardiorespiratory function than halothane for surgical castration without compromising clinical conditions for surgery. Recovery was acceptable, and horses stood in 46 ± 30 minutes from the end of anesthetic drug administration.

Guaifenesin-Ketamine-Romifidine Infusion[46]

A guaifenesin-ketamine-romifidine (GKR) drug combination has been compared with halothane anesthesia in horses. Horses were premedicated with intravenous romifidine (100 μg/kg) and anesthetized with ketamine (2.2 mg/kg IV). Guaifenesin (50 mg/kg IV) was administered immediately after induction of anesthesia, followed by a constant-rate infusion of romifidine (82.5 μg/kg/hr), ketamine (6.6 mg/kg/hr), and guaifenesin (100 mg/kg/hr) for the first 30 minutes after the induction. The infusion rates of romifidine and ketamine remained constant, but the rate of guaifenesin administration was reduced to 50 mg/kg/hr for the remaining 45 minutes. The horses breathed 100% oxygen. TIVA with the mixture of GKR provided better cardiorespiratory function during anesthesia than halothane.

Midazolam-Ketamine-Medetomidine Infusion[41]

The intravenous administration of ketamine (2 mg/kg) and the short-acting, water-soluble benzodiazepine midazolam (0.04 mg/kg) produces smooth and calm induction to anesthesia in horses premedicated with medetomidine (5 μg/kg IV).[41] Horses can be castrated using a mixture of midazolam (0.8 mg/ml)-ketamine (40 mg/ml)-medetomidine (MKM) (0.1 mg/ml) as TIVA. The mixture is prepared by mixing 8 ml of midazolam (5 mg/ml), 20 ml of ketamine (100 mg/ml), and 5 ml of medetomidine (1 mg/ml) and then adjusting to a final volume of 50 ml with saline. The MKM drug combination is infused at a rate of 0.091 ± 0.021 ml/kg/hr for surgical anesthesia. Recovery from anesthesia is good, and horses stand 33 ± 13 minutes from the end of anesthetic drug administration.

The administration of MKM (0.1 ml/kg/hr) to spontaneously breathing horses for 60 minutes produced a $PaCO_2$ of approximately 50 mm Hg and a PaO_2 of 60 mm Hg. Hemodynamic variables remained within normal limits.

Recovery was good to acceptable, and the horses stood in 59 ± 22 minutes after stopping drug administration. Inspired air should be supplemented with oxygen to prevent hypoxemia in spontaneously breathing horses.

Total Intravenous Anesthesia for Prolonged Procedures (120 Minutes and More)

Propofol is the only intravenous anesthetic that has been evaluated and is sufficiently noncumulative to be used for prolonged TIVA in horses.[47-50] Following premedication with xylazine (0.5 mg/kg IV), horses can be anesthetized satisfactorily by an infusion of propofol administered at a rate of 0.2 mg/kg/min after induction to anesthesia with propofol (2 mg/kg IV). However, propofol is a poor analgesic and causes substantial respiratory depression and moderate cardiovascular depression at doses required to produce surgical anesthesia (see Chapter 12; Figures 13-12 to 13-15).[50-53]

Propofol is prepared commercially as 10 mg/ml in a lipid (Intralipid) formulation without preservative. Large volumes of propofol (150 to 300 ml) are required for induction and maintenance of anesthesia in sedated horses, making expense an issue. The quality of anesthetic induction is unpredictable[54] (see TIVA for Short-Term Procedures: Xylazine-Propofol, Detomidine-Propofol, or Xylazine-Midazolam-Propofol earlier in the chapter). The anesthetic effects of a new micellar microemulsion preparation of propofol have been compared to commercially available lipid propofol formulation in horses.[55] The micellar microemulsion preparation has similar anesthetic effects to those of the lipid propofol formulation. In addition, the micellar microemulsion preparation is anticipated to have comparatively low production costs and can be manufactured in higher concentrations. Propofol is unsatisfactory as the sole anesthetic for horses because of its poor analgesia, the large volumes required, cost, and significant respiratory depression produced.

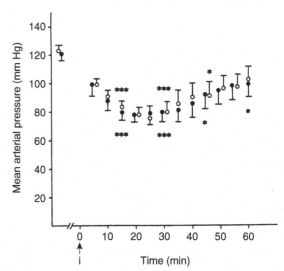

Figure 13–12. Effect of two infusion rates of propofol on mean arterial blood pressure (mm Hg; mean ± SEM; n=6). Control values are shown preinduction. ○, 0.15 mg per kilogram of body weight per minute; ●, 0.2 mg per kilogram of body weight per minute; *i*, induction. *$P<0.05$; ***$P<0.001$. (From Nolan AM, Hall LW: Total intravenous anaesthesia in the horse with propofol, *Equine Vet J* 17:394, 1985.)

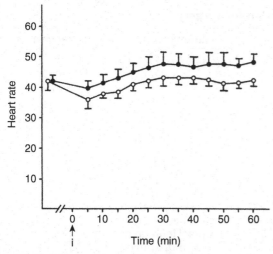

Figure 13–13. Effects of two infusion rates of propofol on heart rate (mean ± SEM; n=6). Control values are shown before induction. ○, 0.15 mg per kilogram of body weight per minute; ●, 0.2 mg per kilogram of body weight per minute; i, induction. (From Nolan AM, Hall LW: Total intravenous anaesthesia in the horse with propofol, *Equine Vet J* 17:394, 1985.)

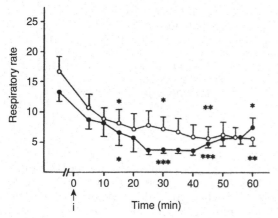

Figure 13–14. Effect of two infusion rates of propofol on respiratory rate (mean ± SEM; n=6). Control values are shown before induction. ○, 0.15 mg per kilogram of body weight per minute; ●, 0.2 mg per kilogram of body weight per minute. *P<0.05; **P<0.01; ***P<0.001. (From Nolan AM, Hall LW: Total intravenous anaesthesia in the horse with propofol, *Equine Vet J* 17:394, 1985.)

The minimum infusion rate (MIR) is the median effective dose (ED_{50}) of an intravenous anesthetic required to prevent movement in response to a surgical stimulus.[56] The MIR concept is not considered as useful as MAC for inhalation anesthetics because the pharmacokinetics of intravenous anesthetics vary considerably among horses. Furthermore, unlike MAC, MIR may be more of a time-dependent variable. The approach currently used to determine MIR in human medicine is to determine the target Cp required to prevent a positive response to a surgical stimulus in 50% of the patients (Cp_{50}). The MIR of propofol in horses ranges from 0.14 to 0.20 mg/kg/min.[56,57] Since there is no practical method for estimating the plasma drug concentration in real time during routine equine surgery, adjusting the rate of drug administration to prevent a response to surgical

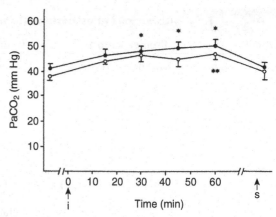

Figure 13–15. Effects of two infusion rates of propofol on PCO_2 (mm Hg). Results are (mean ± SEM; n=6). Control values are shown before induction. ○, 0.15 mg per kilogram of body weight per minute; ● 0.2 per kilogram of body weight per minute; i, induction; S, standing. *P<0.05; **P<0.01. (From Nolan AM, Hall LW: Total intravenous anaesthesia in the horse with propofol, *Equine Vet J* 17:394, 1985.)

stimulus in 95% of the horses (ED_{95}) would be more meaningful. The dose of propofol required to prevent a response to surgical stimulation in 95% (ED_{95}) of ponies and horses may be greater than 0.28 mg/kg/min and may impose clinically significant cardiorespiratory effects.[52] A number of studies have looked at methods to reduce the dose of propofol by providing analgesia and further sedation (Table 13-4).[51,58-62] Several studies have suggested that the MIR of propofol in horses can be effectively reduced to values ranging from 0.10 ± 0.02 to 0.18 ± 0.04 mg/kg/min by premedication with xylazine (1 mg/kg IV) or detomidine (15 μg/kg IV), respectively.[56,57]

Additional studies are necessary to determine if the hypnotic effects of propofol are adequate to provide safe and effective surgical anesthesia in horses that have been administered supplemental sedative or analgesic therapies.

Ketamine-Propofol Infusion[51,60,63]

Ketamine significantly reduces propofol requirements for surgery in ponies.[51] Anesthesia in ponies can be produced by administering detomidine (20 μg/kg IV) followed by ketamine (2.2 mg/kg IV) and maintained with propofol, 0.33 ± 0.05 mg/kg/min alone or 12 ± 0.01 mg/kg/min when administered with ketamine (2.4 mg/kg/hr).

Seven Thoroughbred Horses were anesthetized with propofol (3 mg/kg IV) after sedation with xylazine (1 mg/kg IV) and midazolam (0.05 mg/kg IV).[60] Anesthesia was maintained for 124 ± 11 minutes (ranging from 112 to 140 minutes) with ketamine (3 mg/kg/hr) and propofol (0.16 ± 0.02 mg/kg/min) for repair of a simple longitudinal fracture of the proximal phalanx or third metacarpus. Cardiovascular function was adequate; however, positive-pressure ventilation was required in all horses. Recovery was good in five horses and fair in two horses. The horses stood in 70 ± 23 minutes after the cessation of propofol infusion.

Medetomidine-Propofol Infusion[47-49,58]

The simultaneous infusion of medetomidine (3.5 μg/kg/hr) and propofol significantly reduces the MIR of propofol (0.06 to 0.1 mg/kg/min) in ponies.[49] The cardiopulmonary effects

Table 13–4. **Total intravenous anesthesia with propofol infusion for surgery**

Protocols	Premedication	Induction	Maintenance	References
Propofol infusion alone	Xylazine 0.5 mg/kg	Propofol 2 mg/kg IV	Propofol infusion rate: 0.28 mg/kg/min in one pony	52
	Detomidine 15 µg/kg IV	Propofol 2 mg/kg IV	Propofol infusion rate: 0.18 mg/kg/min in 12 horses	59
	Detomidine 20 µg/kg IV	Ketamine 2 mg/kg IV	Propofol infusion rate: 0.33 mg/kg/min in four ponies	51
	Medetomidine 5 µg/kg IV	Midazolam 0.04 mg/kg IV Ketamine 2.5 mg/kg IV	Propofol infusion rate: 0.22 mg/kg/min in six horses	61
Ketamine-propofol infusion	Detomidine 20 µg/kg IV	Ketamine 2 mg/kg IV	Ketamine 2.4 mg/kg/hr Propofol infusion rate: 0.12 mg/kg/min in four ponies	51
	Xylazine 1 mg/kg IV Midazolam 0.05 mg/kg IV	Propofol 3 mg/kg IV	Ketamine 3 mg/kg/hr Propofol infusion rate: 0.16 mg/kg/min in seven horses	60
Medetomidine-propofol infusion	Medetomidine 7 µg/kg IV	Ketamine 2 mg/kg IV	Medetomidine 3.5 µg/kg/hr Propofol infusion rate: 0.10-0.11 mg/kg/min in 50 horses	58
Ketamine-medetomidine-propofol infusion	Medetomidine 5 µg/kg IV	Ketamine 2.5 mg/kg Midazolam 0.04 mg/kg IV	Ketamine 1 mg/kg/hr Medetomidine 1.25 µg/kg/hr Propofol infusion rate: 0.14 mg/kg/min in six horses	61

and the quality of anesthesia produced by medetomidine (7 µg/kg IV)-ketamine (2 mg/kg) induction to anesthesia, followed by 4 hours of medetomidine (3.5 µg/kg/min)-propofol (0.89 to 1 mg/kg/hr) anesthesia, has also been evaluated.[48] Induction to anesthesia is considered excellent, and the response to painful stimuli is minimal. Cardiopulmonary variables remain within acceptable limits. Recovery to standing averages 31 ± 10 minutes, and the ponies stand within one or two attempts.

Anesthesia in horses produced by the administration of intravenous ketamine (2 mg/kg) after sedation with medetomidine (7 µg/kg IV) was maintained with medetomidine (3.5 µg/kg/hr) and propofol (0.1 to 0.11 mg/kg/min).[58] A variety of surgical procedures (orthopedic, integumentary, elective abdominal) have been performed (total time: 46 to 225 minutes) using this drug combination. Cardiovascular function is acceptable, and blood pressure support generally is not required. Positive-pressure ventilation is required in the majority of horses, however. Recovery is uneventful, and horses stand in 42 ± 20 minutes (12 to 98 minutes) from the end of anesthetic drug administration.

Ketamine-Medetomidine-Propofol Infusion[50,61]

The simultaneous infusion of ketamine and medetomidine significantly reduces the propofol requirement for surgery in horses. Anesthesia produced by medetomidine (5 µg/kg IV), followed in 3 to 5 minutes by midazolam (0.04 mg/kg IV) and ketamine (2.5 mg/kg IV), can be maintained for 1.5 to 4 hours with propofol infusion with or without ketamine (1 mg/kg/hr) and medetomidine (1.25 µg/kg/hr). The mean infusion rate of propofol is 0.22 ± 0.03 mg/kg/min in horses anesthetized with propofol alone and 0.14 ± 0.02 mg/kg/min in horses anesthetized with ketamine-medetomidine-propofol. Heart rate and arterial blood pressure remain within acceptable limits during both infusions. Respiratory depression and apnea resulting in hypoventilation and hypoxia are common during the early stages of anesthesia. Positive pressure ventilation is required in most horses. Ketamine-medetomidine-propofol infusion provides satisfactory anesthesia and better recovery than propofol infusion alone. Recovery is satisfactory in horses anesthetized with propofol alone, and horses stand in 87 ± 36 to 132 ± 31 minutes after the cessation of drug administration, depending on the duration of anesthesia (1.5 versus 4 hours). Recovery generally is good in horses anesthetized with ketamine-medetomidine-propofol, and horses stand in 62 ± 10 to 92 ± 21 minutes after the cessation of drug administration, depending on the duration of anesthesia (1.5 versus 4 hours).

INTRAVENOUS ANALGESIC ADJUNCTS IN COMBINATION WITH INHALATION ANESTHESIA IN HORSES

Horses are commonly anesthetized with volatile inhalant anesthetic drugs for prolonged surgical procedures. Inhaled anesthetics cause dose-related cardiopulmonary depression, which contributes to the high mortality rate associated with equine anesthesia (see Chapter 22).[8-10,64] The coadministration of analgesic drugs has the potential to reduce the amount of inhalation anesthetic required to maintain anesthesia by providing analgesia or altering consciousness. The intravenous administration (i.e., IVAA) of opioids;[65-71] ketamine;[13] α_2-adrenoceptor agonists;[72] lidocaine;[11,73-77] or α_2-adrenoceptor agonists, ketamine, and centrally acting muscle relaxants[12,14-16] has been investigated in horses during inhalation anesthesia.

Opioid Infusion

The administration of opioids provides perioperative analgesia, improves hemodynamics, and minimizes the requirement for inhalation anesthesia. However, several studies have demonstrated that morphine and alfentanil do not consistently decrease the MAC of inhalant anesthetics in horses.[78,79] No statistically significant positive effects of perioperative morphine (0.15 mg/kg IV followed by 0.1 mg/kg/hr) administration have been identified in horses anesthetized with halothane for elective surgical procedures, although a better quality of anesthesia and reduced requirements for additional anesthetic drugs without significant hemodynamic or ventilatory changes were reported.[65] Fentanyl reduces MAC in horses, but this decrease is small compared to other species. For example, fentanyl infusion producing a Cp of 13 ng/ml reduces isoflurane MAC by 18% in horses (see Chapter 10).[71] Fentanyl Cp values of 6 to 14 ng/ml decrease isoflurane MAC by 82%, 53%, and 25% in humans, dogs, and pigs, respectively.[50,61,77] Further studies are required to determine the effects and relative resistance of horses to the MAC-lowering effects of opioids is required.

Ketamine Infusion

Ketamine is used frequently as an adjunct to inhalant anesthesia in horses.[18,19,27,36,42,43,51,60,61] Ketamine Cp values greater than 1 µg/ml reduce halothane MAC and produce beneficial hemodynamic effects.[13] The degree of MAC reduction is directly correlated with the square root of the Cp of ketamine, reaching a maximum of 37% at a Cp of 10.8 ± 2.7 µg/ml (Figure 13-16). Cardiac output increases sig-

nificantly during ketamine infusions and halothane MAC reduction (Figure 13-17). A Cp of ketamine of approximately 1 µg/ml is an appropriate minimum target value for initiating an anesthetic effect in horses.

Medetomidine Infusion

The MAC of desflurane is reduced in ponies administered medetomidine (3.5 µg/kg/hr) and induced to anesthesia with medetomidine (7 µg/kg IV) and ketamine (2 mg/kg IV).[72] Medetomidine infusion reduces desflurane MAC from values ranging from 7% to 7.6% to 5.3%.[80,81] Cardiopulmonary values remain stable throughout anesthesia. The time taken for the ponies to stand after discontinuing desflurane ranges from 5.8 to 26 minutes, and the quality of recovery is good to excellent.

Lidocaine Infusion

Lidocaine can be administered to horses to improve analgesia, reduce inhalant anesthetic requirements (anesthetic sparing) and improve gastrointestinal motility.[73,74,82-84] Infusion of lidocaine produces dose-dependent reduction in the MAC of inhalation anesthetics in ponies and may also decrease the incidence of postoperative ileus through analgesic and antiinflammatory effects (Figure 13-18).[74,82,85] A lidocaine bolus (2 mg/kg) followed by an infusion (3 mg/kg/hr) until the end of anesthesia may increase ataxia and prolong recovery time in horses. Discontinuing the lidocaine infusion 30 minutes before the end of surgery reduces Cp concentrations and any untoward effects that lidocaine may have on recovery.[77]

Various drug combinations incorporating opioids, local anesthetics, and dissociative anesthetics are being investigated as IVAAs in horses. The principal goals of these studies are to improve analgesia both during and after surgery and to provide a safer anesthetic experience by reducing the inhaled or injectable anesthetic requirement. Several popular drug combinations in small animals have been administered to adult horses to supplement inhalant anesthesia for soft tissue or orthopedic surgical procedures. The administration of morphine (0.1 mg/kg/hr)-lidocaine (3 mg/kg/hr)-ketamine (MLK) (1.5 mg/kg/hr)

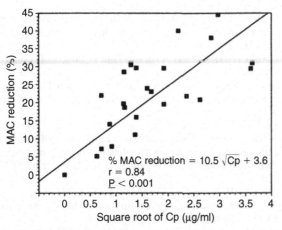

Figure 13-16. Halothane MAC reduction in horses versus the square root of the Cp (■) concentration. (From Muir WW, Sams R: Effects of ketamine infusion on halothane minimal alveolar concentration in horses, *Am J Vet Res* 53:1802, 1992.)

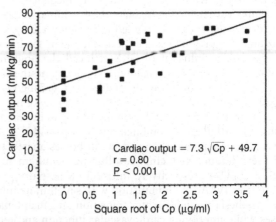

Figure 13-17. Cardiac output in horses versus the square root of the Cp (■) concentration. (From Muir WW, Sams R: Effects of ketamine infusion on halothane minimal alveolar concentration in horses, *Am J Vet Res* 53:1802, 1992.)

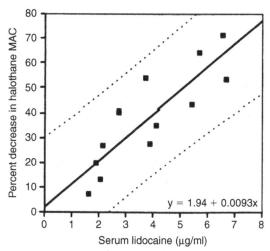

Figure 13–18. Correlation between serum lidocaine concentration and percent decrease in halothane MAC (r = 0.86, P<0.0003). Data for all ponies fall within 95% confidence interval (dashed line) for the equation describing the linear relationship between the two variables. (From Doherty TJ, Frazier DL: Effect of intravenous lidocaine on halothane MAC in ponies, *Equine Vet J* 30:340-343, 1998.)

with or without medetomidine (20 µg/kg/hr; M²LK) has been demonstrated to reduce inhalant anesthetic requirements by 50% in some horses while simultaneously improving hemodynamics. Recovery from anesthesia has been uneventful. Additional studies are required to determine the range of pharmacological effects and practicality of these formulations for improving general anesthesia in horses.

Simultaneous Infusion of Guaifenesin-Ketamine-Xylazine, Guaifenesin-Ketamine-Medetomidine, or Midazolam-Ketamine-Medetomidine During Inhalant Anesthesia

Anesthesia for surgical procedures can be produced by α_2-agonists, ketamine, and centrally acting muscle relaxants such as triple drip (see TIVA for Intermediate-Duration Procedures earlier in the chapter). Lower infusion rates of triple drip (guaifenesin 30 mg/kg/hr, ketamine 1.2 mg/kg/hr, xylazine 0.3 mg/kg/hr) reduce the requirement for inhalant anesthesia. The infusion of GKX reduced the amount of sevoflurane required to maintain surgical anesthesia by 62%.[16] Low-dose infusion of guaifenesin (25 mg/kg/hr)-ketamine (1 mg/kg/hr)-medetomidine (1.25 µg/kg/hr) and midazolam (0.02 mg/kg/hr)-ketamine (1 mg/kg/hr)-medetomidine (1.25 µg/kg/hr) combinations also provided significant analgesic and anesthetic effects in horses anesthetized with sevoflurane, reducing sevoflurane requirement by 50%[15] and 60%,[12] respectively. Infusion of these drug combinations as IVAAs in combination with sevoflurane inhalation anesthesia provides better transition and maintenance phases while improving cardiovascular function and reducing the number of attempts needed to stand after completion of anesthesia, compared with inhalation of sevoflurane alone.[12,14-16]

CONCLUSION

The administration of anesthetic drugs to horses should be individualized and tailored to the horse's physiology, size, and physical status. The development and use of one or two predetermined anesthetic protocols for all horses is practical and reduces the chance for error; however, they must be designed to provide adequate hypnosis and analgesia throughout and after anesthesia. Anesthetic protocols must be designed to optimize cardiorespiratory function while providing adequate intraoperative and operative analgesia in sick or severely compromised horses. The administration of TIVA and IVAAs in conjunction with reduced concentrations of inhalant anesthesia provides the opportunity to improve anesthetic safety and efficacy in horses.

REFERENCES

1. Luna SP, Taylor PM, Bloomfield M: Endocrine changes in cerebrospinal fluid, pituitary effluent, and peripheral plasma of anesthetized ponies, *Am J Vet Res* 58:765-770, 1997.
2. Luna SP, Taylor PM, Wheeler MJ: Cardiorespiratory, endocrine, and metabolic changes in ponies undergoing intravenous or inhalation anaesthesia, *J Vet Pharmacol Ther* 19:251-258, 1996.
3. Taylor PM et al: Cardiovascular effects of surgical castration during anaesthesia maintained with halothane or infusion of detomidine, ketamine, and guaifenesin in ponies, *Equine Vet J* 30:304-309, 1998.
4. Taylor PM et al: Total intravenous anaesthesia in ponies using detomidine, ketamine, and guaiphenesin: pharmacokinetics, cardiopulmonary and endocrine effects, *Res Vet Sci* 59:17-23, 1995.
5. El Azab SR et al: Effect of VIMA with sevoflurane versus TIVA with propofol or midazolam-sufentanil on the cytokine response during CABG surgery, *Eur J Anaesthesiol* 19:276-282, 2002.
6. Schneemlich CE, Bank U: Release of pro- and antiinflammatory cytokines during different anesthesia procedures, *Anaesthesiol Reanim* 26:4-10, 2001.
7. Lankveld DP et al: Ketamine inhibits LPS-induced tumor necrosis factor-α and interleukin-6 in an equine macrophage cell line, *Vet Res* 36:257-262, 2005.
8. Grosenbaugh DA, Muir WW: Cardiorespiratory effects of sevoflurane, isoflurane, and halothane anesthesia in horses, *Am J Vet Res* 59:101-106, 1998.
9. Steffey EP, Howland D: Cardiovascular effects of halothane in the horses, *Am J Vet Res* 39:611-615, 1978.
10. Steffey EP, Howland D: Comparison of circulatory and respiratory effects of isoflurane and halothane anesthesia in horses, *Am J Vet Res* 41:821-825, 1980.
11. Dzitiki TB, Hellebrekers LJ, van Dijk P: Effects of intravenous lidocaine on isoflurane concentration, physiological parameters, metabolic parameters, and stress-related hormones in horses undergoing surgery, *J Vet Med A Physiol Pathol Clin Med* 50:190-195, 2003.
12. Kushiro T et al: Anesthetic and cardiovascular effects of balanced anesthesia using constant rate infusion of midazolam-ketamine-medetomidine with inhalation of oxygen-sevoflurane (MKM-OS anesthesia) in horses, *J Vet Med Sci* 67:379-384, 2005.
13. Muir WW, Sams R: Effects of ketamine infusion on halothane minimal alveolar concentration in horses, *Am J Vet Res* 53:1802-1806, 1992.
14. Yamashita K et al: Infusion of guaifenesin, ketamine, and medetomidine in combination with inhalation of sevoflurane versus inhalation of sevoflurane alone for anesthesia of horses, *J Am Vet Med Assoc* 221:1150-1155, 2002.

15. Yamashita K et al: Combination of continuous infusion using a mixture of guaifenesin-ketamine-medetomidine and sevoflurane anesthesia in horses, *J Vet Med Sci* 62:229-235, 2000.

16. Yamashita K et al: Combination of continuous intravenous infusion anesthesia of guaifenesin-ketamine-xylazine and sevoflurane anesthesia in horses, *J Jpn Vet Med Assoc* 50:645-648, 1997.

17. Muir WW, Mason DE: Effects of diazepam, acepromazine, detomidine, and xylazine on thiamylal anesthesia in horses, *J Am Vet Med Assoc* 203:1031-1038, 1993.

18. Muir WW, Skarda RT, Milne DW: Evaluation of xylazine and ketamine hydrochloride for anesthesia in horses, *Am J Vet Res* 38:195-201, 1977.

19. Muir WW, Skarda RT, Sheehan W: Evaluation of xylazine, guaifenesin, and ketamine hydrochloride for restraint in horses, *Am J Vet Res* 39:1274-1278, 1978.

20. Hubbell JA, Bednarski RM, Muir WW: Xylazine and tiletamine-zolazepam anesthesia in horses, *Am J Vet Res* 50:737-742, 1989.

21. Muir WW, Gadawski JE, Grosenbaugh DA: Cardiorespiratory effects of a tiletamine/zolazepam-ketamine-detomidine combination in horses, *Am J Vet Res* 60:770-774, 1999.

22. Muir WW, Sams RA: Pharmacologic principles and pain: pharmacokinetics and pharmacodynamics. In Gaynor JS, Muir WW, editors: *Handbook of veterinary pain management*, St Louis, 2002, Mosby, p. 111-141.

23. Hall LW, Taylor PM: Clinical trial of xylazine with ketamine in equine anaesthesia, *Vet Rec* 108:489-493, 1981.

24. Matthews NS et al: A comparison of injectable anesthetic combinations in horses, *Vet Surg* 20:268-273, 1991.

25. Butera ST et al: Xylazine/sodium thiopental combination for short-term anesthesia in the horse, *Vet Med Small Anim Clin* 75:765-770, 1980.

26. Trim CM, Colbern GT, Martin CL: Effect of xylazine and ketamine on intraocular pressure in horses, *Vet Rec* 117:442-443, 1985.

27. McCarty JE, Trim CM, Ferguson D: Prolongation of anesthesia with xylazine, ketamine, and guaifenesin in horses: 64 cases (1986-1989), *J Am Vet Med Assoc* 197:1646-1650, 1990.

28. Tranquilli WJ et al: Hyperglycemia and hypoinsulinemia during xylazine-ketamine anesthesia in Thoroughbred Horses, *Am J Vet Res* 45:11-14, 1984.

29. Kerr CL, McDonell WN, Young SS: A comparison of romifidine and xylazine when used with diazepam/ketamine for short-duration anesthesia in the horse, *Can Vet J* 37:601-609, 1996.

30. Cuvelliez S et al: Intravenous anesthesia in the horse: comparison of xylazine-ketamine and xylazine-tiletamine-zolazepam combinations, *Can Vet J* 36:613-618, 1995.

31. Clarke KW, Taylor PM, Watkins SB: Detomidine/ketamine anaesthesia in the horse, *Acta Vet Scand* 82(suppl):167-179, 1986.

32. Jochle W, Hamm D: Sedation and analgesia with Dormosedan (detomidine hydrochloride) in horses: dose response studies on efficacy and its duration, *Acta Vet Scand* 82(suppl):69-84, 1986.

33. Wagner AE, Muir WW, Hinchcliff KW: Cardiovascular effects of xylazine and detomidine in horses, *Am J Vet Res* 52:651-657, 1991.

34. Yamashita K et al: Cardiovascular effects of medetomidine, detomidine, and xylazine in horses, *J Vet Med Sci* 62:1025-1032, 2000.

35. Brouwer GJ, Hall LW, Kuchel TR: Intravenous anaesthesia in horses after xylazine premedication, *Vet Rec* 107:241-245, 1980.

36. Watkins SB et al: A clinical trial of three anaesthetic regimens for the castration of ponies, *Vet Rec* 120:274-276, 1987.

37. Muir WW et al: Comparison of four drug combinations for total intravenous anesthesia of horses undergoing surgical removal of an abdominal testis, *J Am Vet Med Assoc* 217:869-873, 2000.

38. Mama KR, Steffey EP, Pascoe PJ: Evaluation of propofol for general anesthesia in premedicated horses, *Am J Vet Res* 57:512-516, 1996.

39. Mama KR et al: Evaluation of xylazine and ketamine for total intravenous anesthesia in horses, *Am J Vet Res* 66:1002-1007, 2005.

40. Oku K et al: Clinical observations during induction and recovery of xylazine-midazolam-propofol anesthesia in horses, *J Vet Med Sci* 65:805-808, 2003.

41. Yamashita K et al: Anesthetic and cardiopulmonary effects of total intravenous anesthesia using a midazolam, ketamine, and medetomidine drug combination in horses, *J Vet Med Sci* 69:7-13, 2007.

42. Young LE et al: Clinical evaluation of an infusion of xylazine, guaifenesin, and ketamine for maintenance of anaesthesia in horses, *Equine Vet J* 25:115-119, 1993.

43. Greene SA et al: Cardiopulmonary effects of continuous intravenous infusion of guaifenesin, ketamine, and xylazine in ponies, *Am J Vet Res* 47:2364-2367, 1986.

44. Bettschart-Wolfensberger R et al: Physiologic effects of anesthesia induced and maintained by intravenous administration of a climazolam-ketamine combination in ponies premedicated with acepromazine and xylazine, *Am J Vet Res* 57:1472-1477, 1996.

45. Taylor PM et al: Physiological effects of total intravenous surgical anesthesia using guaifenesin-ketamine-detomidine in horses, *J Vet Anaesth* 19:24-31, 1992.

46. McMurphy RM et al: Comparison of the cardiopulmonary effects of anesthesia maintained by continuous infusion of romifidine, guaifenesin, and ketamine with anesthesia maintained by inhalation of halothane in horses, *Am J Vet Res* 63:1655-1661, 2002.

47. Bettschart-Wolfensberger R et al: Cardiopulmonary effects of prolonged anesthesia via propofol-medetomidine infusion in ponies, *Am J Vet Res* 62:1428-1435, 2001.

48. Bettschart-Wolfensberger R et al: Medetomidine-ketamine anaesthesia induction followed by medetomidine-propofol in ponies: infusion rates and cardiopulmonary side effects, *Equine Vet J* 35:308-313, 2003.

49. Bettschart-Wolfensberger R et al: Infusion of a combination of propofol and medetomidine for long-term anesthesia in ponies, *Am J Vet Res* 62:500-507, 2001.

50. Umar MA et al: Evaluation of cardiovascular effects of total intravenous anesthesia with propofol or a combination of ketamine-medetomidine-propofol in horses, *Am J Vet Res* 68:121-127, 2007.

51. Flaherty D et al: A pharmacodynamic study of propofol or propofol and ketamine infusions in ponies undergoing surgery, *Res Vet Sci* 62:179-184, 1997.

52. Nolan AM, Hall LW: Total intravenous anaesthesia in the horse with propofol, *Equine Vet J* 17:394-398, 1985.

53. Oku K et al: Cardiovascular effects of continuous propofol infusion in horses, *J Vet Med Sci* 68:773-778, 2006.

54. Mama KR, Steffey EP, Pascoe PJ: Evaluation of propofol as a general anesthetic for horses, *Vet Surg* 24:188-194, 1995.

55. Boscan P et al: Comparison of high (5%) and low (1%) concentrations of micellar microemulsion propofol formulations with a standard (1%) lipid emulsion in horses, *Am J Vet Res* 67:1476-1483, 2006.

56. Oku K et al: The minimum infusion rate (MIR) of propofol for total intravenous anesthesia after premedication with xylazine in horses, *J Vet Med Sci* 67:569-575, 2005.

57. Katayama Y et al: Minimum infusion rate of propofol in horses, *Jpn J Vet Anesth Surg* 38(suppl 1):in press, 2007.

58. Bettschart-Wolfensberger R et al: Total intravenous anaesthesia in horses using medetomidine and propofol, *Vet Anaesth Analg* 32:348-354, 2005.

59. Matthews NS et al: Detomidine-propofol anesthesia for abdominal surgery in horses, *Vet Surg* 28:196-201, 1999.

60. Ohta M et al: Propofol-ketamine anesthesia for internal fixation of fractures in Racehorses, *J Vet Med Sci* 66:1433-1436, 2004.

61. Umar MA et al: Evaluation of total intravenous anesthesia with propofol or ketamine-medetomidine-propofol combination in horses, *J Am Vet Med Assoc* 228:1221-1227, 2006.

62. Frias AF et al: Evaluation of different doses of propofol in xylazine pre-medicated horses, *Vet Anaesth Analg* 30:193-201, 2003.

63. Nolan A et al: Simultaneous infusions of propofol and ketamine in ponies premedicated with detomidine: a pharmacokinetic study, *Res Vet Sci* 60:262-266, 1996.

64. Johnston GM et al: Confidential enquiry into perioperative equine fatalities (CEPEF-1): preliminary results, *Equine Vet J* 27:193-200, 1995.

65. Clark L et al: Effects of perioperative morphine administration during halothane anaesthesia in horses, *Vet Anaesth Analg* 32:10-15, 2005.

66. Hellyer PW et al: Effects of diazepam and flumazenil on minimum alveolar concentration for dogs anesthetized with isoflurane or a combination of isoflurane and fentanyl, *Am J Vet Res* 62:555-560, 2001.

67. McEwan AI et al: Isoflurane minimum alveolar concentration reduction by fentanyl, *Anesthesiology* 78:864-869, 1993.

68. Moon PF et al: Effect of fentanyl on the minimum alveolar concentration of isoflurane in swine, *Anesthesiology* 83:535-542, 1995.

69. Pascoe PJ et al: The pharmacokinetics and locomotor activity of alfentanil in the horse, *J Vet Pharmacol Ther* 14:317-325, 1991.

70. Thomasy SM et al: Influence of general anaesthesia on the pharmacokinetics of intravenous fentanyl and its primary metabolite in horses, *Equine Vet J* 39:54-58, 2007.

71. Thomasy SM et al: The effects of intravenous fentanyl administration on the minimum alveolar concentration of isoflurane in horses, *Br J Anaesth* 97:232-237, 2006.

72. Bettschart-Wolfensberger R et al: Minimal alveolar concentration of desflurane in combination with an infusion of medetomidine for the anaesthesia of ponies, *Vet Rec* 148:264-267, 2001.

73. Dizitiki TB, Hellebrekers LJ, van Dijik P: Effects of intravenous lidocaine on isoflurane concentration, physiological parameters, metabolic parameters, and stress-related hormones in horses undergoing surgery, *J Vet Med A Physiol Pathol Clin Med* 50:190-195, 2003.

74. Doherty TJ, Frazier DL: Effect of intravenous lidocaine on halothane MAC in ponies, *Equine Vet J* 30:340-343, 1998.

75. Feary DJ et al: Influence of gastrointestinal tract disease on pharmacokinetics of lidocaine after intravenous infusion in anesthetized horses, *Am J Vet Res* 66:574-580, 2005.

76. Feary DJ et al: Influence of general anesthesia on pharmacokinetics of intravenous lidocaine infusion in horses, *Am J Vet Res* 66:574-580, 2005.

77. Valverde A et al: Effect of a constant rate infusion of lidocaine on the quality of recovery from sevoflurane or isoflurane general anaesthesia in horses, *Equine Vet J* 37:559-564, 2005.

78. Pascoe PJ et al: Evaluation of the effect of alfentanil on the minimum alveolar concentration of halothane in horses, *Am J Vet Res* 54:1327-1332, 1993.

79. Steffey EP, Eisele JH, Baggot JD: Interactions of morphine and isoflurane in horses, *Am J Vet Res* 64:166-175, 2003.

80. Clarke KW et al: Desflurane anaesthesia in the horse: minimum alveolar concentration following induction of anaesthesia with xylazine and ketamine, *J Vet Anaesth* 23:56-59, 1996.

81. Tendillo FJ et al: Anesthetic potency of desflurane in the horse: determination of the minimum alveolar concentration, *Vet Surg* 26:354-357, 1997.

82. Nellgard P et al: Small-bowel obstruction and the effects of lidocaine, atropine, and hexamethonium on inflammation and fluid losses, *Acta Anaesthesiol Scand* 40:287-292, 1996.

83. Murrell JC et al: Investigation of the EEG effects of intravenous lidocaine during halothane anesthesia in ponies, *Vet Anaesth Analg* 32:212-221, 2005.

84. Robertson SA et al: Effect of systemic lidocaine on visceral and somatic nociception in conscious horses, *Equine Vet J* 37:122-127, 2005.

85. Brianceau P et al: Intravenous lidocaine and small-intestine size, abdominal fluid and outcome after colic surgery in horse, *J Vet Intern Med* 16:736-741, 2002.

86. Ballard S et al: The pharmacokinetics, pharmacological responses, and behavioral effects of acepromazine in the horse, *J Vet Pharmacol Ther* 5:21-31, 1982.

87. Marroum PJ et al: Pharmacokinetics and pharmacodynamics of acepromazine in horses, *Am J Vet Res* 55:1428-1433, 1994.

88. Matthews NS et al: Pharmacokinetics and cardiopulmonary effects of guaifenesin in donkeys, *J Vet Pharmacol Ther* 20:442-446, 1997.

89. Shini S, Klaus AM, Hapke HJ: Kinetics of elimination of diazepam after intravenous injection in horses, *Dtsch Tierartztl Wochenschr* 104:22-25, 1997.

90. Garcia-Villar R et al: The pharmacokinetics of xylazine hydrochloride: an interspecific study, *J Vet Pharmacol Ther* 4:87-92, 1981.

91. Salonen JS et al: Single-dose pharmacokinetics of detomidine in the horse and cow, *J Vet Pharmacol Ther* 12:65-72, 1989.

92. Bettschart-Wolfensberger R et al: Pharmacokinetics of medetomidine in ponies and elaboration of a medetomidine infusion regime which provides a constant level of sedation, *Res Vet Sci* 67:41-46, 1999.

93. Kaka JS, Klavano PA, Hayton WL: Pharmacokinetics of ketamine in the horse, *Am J Vet Res* 40:978-981, 1979.

94. Waterman AE, Robertson SA, Lane JG: Pharmacokinetics of intravenously administered ketamine in the horse, *Res Vet Sci* 42:162-166, 1987.

95. Fielding CL et al: Pharmacokinetics and clinical effects of a subanesthetic continuous rate infusion of ketamine in awake horses, *Am J Vet Res* 67:1484-1490, 2006.

96. Abass BT et al: Pharmacokinetics of thiopentone in horses, *J Vet Pharmacol Ther* 17:331-338, 1994.

97. Young DB et al: Effects of phenylbutazone on thiamylal disposition and anesthesia in ponies, *J Vet Pharmacol Ther* 17:389-393, 1994.

98. Combie JD, Nugent TE, Tobin T: Pharmacokinetics and protein binding of morphine in horses, *Am J Vet Res* 44:870-874, 1983.

99. Maxwell LK et al: Pharmacokinetics of fentanyl following intravenous and transdermal administration in horses, *Equine Vet J* 35:484-490, 2003.

100. Sellon DC et al: Pharmacokinetics and adverse effects of butorphanol administered by single intravenous injection or continuous intravenous infusion in horses, *Am J Vet Res* 62:183-189, 2001.

14

Tracheal and Nasal Intubation

Richard M. Bednarski

KEY POINTS

1. Horses are obligate nose breathers. If the nasal passages are occluded, a tracheostomy must be performed.
2. The maintenance of a patent airway is the principal goal of anesthesia.
3. Tracheal intubation is the surest method of maintaining a patent airway and minimizing aspiration.
4. Endotracheal tubes are easily placed "blindly" per os.
5. Endotracheal tubes should be composed of nonreactive materials.
6. Great care must be taken when cleaning endotracheal tubes to avoid irritation or damage to the upper respiratory system or trachea mucosa from cleaning procedures or subsequent use.
7. Some horses may require the placement of a nasotracheal tube or an endotracheal tube during recovery to minimize or avoid upper airway obstruction during the recovery period.
8. Upper airway obstruction during recovery is an emergency and requires nasotracheal intubation or a tracheotomy and the placement of a breathing tube.

Horses are obligate nasal breathers. The placement of a tracheal tube (orotracheal intubation) is essential for the maintenance of an unobstructed airway, the efficient delivery of oxygen and inhalant anesthetics, and assisted or controlled ventilation. Tracheal intubation is the passage of a tube through the nose or mouth or a tracheotomy into the trachea to secure a patent airway.[1] Tracheal intubation was first described by the Scottish physician Sir William Macewen in 1880.[2] However, tracheal intubation in the horse was not performed routinely until the 1950s, coinciding with the development of large-animal inhalation anesthetic delivery equipment and the introduction of halothane anesthesia.[3] Inhalation anesthesia before 1950 was routinely performed using a mask or inhaler (diethyl ether, chloroform) for delivery of chloroform.

ANATOMY

The nasal cavity begins at the external nares and communicates caudally with the pharynx. The external nares are oval in outline; each is divided into dorsal and ventral compartments by the alar fold. The alar folds are retracted by the caninus, dilatator naris, and levator nasolabialis muscles, which are relaxed by sedatives, particularly α_2-agonists, predisposing some horses to upper airway obstruction. The dorsal compartment extends caudally as a blind pouch, which terminates at the junction of the nasal bone and nasal process of the premaxilla.[4] The ventral compartment communicates with the nasal cavity. The nasal cavity is divided into three meatus by two turbinates (Figure 14-1). The ventral meatus provides the most direct communication of the nasal cavity with the pharynx. The turbinates are highly vascular, and the meatus are small. This predisposes the turbinates to hemorrhage from poorly performed nasotracheal intubation and the meatus to obstruction from edema (supine position, head down) after prolonged intubation.

More than half of the larynx is located cranial to the ramus of the mandible when the head and neck are in the normal, slightly flexed position. The long axis of the larynx is horizontal with the head in this position. More of the larynx is proportionally located behind the posterior border of the rami of the mandible with the head and neck extended.[4] The larynx is bordered dorsally by the pharynx and the origin of the esophagus. Laterally it is bordered by the cavity of the pharynx. It is attached ventrally indirectly to the base of the tongue by the hyoid bone.

Five cartilages comprise the framework of the larynx. The cricoid, thyroid, and epiglottic cartilages are unpaired; and the arytenoid cartilage is paired. The most lateral cartilage is the thyroid. Cranially the thyroid cartilage has a prominence that can be palpated externally. It articulates posteriorly with the cricoid. Ventrally the cricothyroid ligament stabilizes and connects the two thyroid and cricoid cartilages. This is the ligament that is incised during a laryngotomy. The paired arytenoid cartilages lie medially to the thyroid and cranially to the cricoid cartilages. The caudal portion of the arytenoids articulates with the cricoid cartilage. The vocal ligaments are attached dorsally to the vocal processes of the arytenoids and ventrally to the thyroid. These ligaments, covered by the vocal folds, form the framework for the glottis (Figure 14-2). The epiglottic cartilage is thin and flexible at its apex. It is attached at its base to the thyroid cartilage. The tip of the epiglottic cartilage usually is situated dorsal to the posterior border of the soft palate, which is the reason the horse typically does not mouth breathe. However, the epiglottis can become displaced during recovery from anesthesia, resulting in upper airway obstruction and a typical expiratory noise.

The extrinsic muscles of the larynx serve to abduct, adduct, or tense the vocal folds, thereby regulating the diameter of the glottis. The paired cricoarytenoid muscle is the only abductor of the vocal folds. It attaches cranially to the muscular process of the arytenoid; and, when it contracts, it rotates the arytenoid outward and dilates the glottis.

The mucosa of the larynx is stratified squamous cell epithelium caudally to the vocal folds, where it continues as pseudostratified columnar epithelium. The mucosa presents a fold (the ventricular folds) located cranially to the glottis. Just caudal to the ventricular folds are the openings

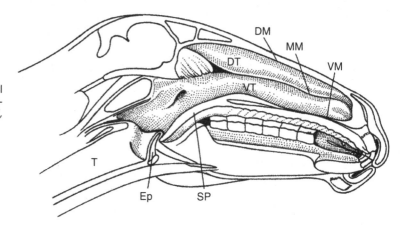

Figure 14–1. Sagittal section of the head. *DM,* Dorsal meatus; *DT,* dorsal nasal turbinate; *Ep,* epiglottis; *VT,* ventral nasal turbinate; *MM,* middle meatus; *SP,* soft palate; *VM,* ventral meatus; *T,* tracheal lumen.

to the laryngeal saccules (see Figure 14-2). The vocal folds are caudal to these openings, and the space between these folds is termed the *rima glottis*. The vocal folds appear whitish because there is no submucosa overlying the vocal ligaments. The glottis is the area of the larynx with the narrowest diameter. Disease of the larynx can distort the normal anatomy and result in difficult intubation (Figures 14-3 to 14-7).

The paired vagus nerves supply sensory and motor innervation to the larynx. Sensory innervation is through the cranial laryngeal nerves, and motor innervation is through the recurrent laryngeal nerves, with the exception of the cricothyroid muscle, which is innervated by the cranial laryngeal nerve. The nerves within the larynx may be damaged from tracheal intubation, resulting in laryngeal motor dysfunction after extubation (paresis, paralysis) that can be life threatening unless the endotracheal tube is replaced or a tracheotomy is performed.

PURPOSES OF INTUBATION

Tracheal intubation serves many useful functions (Box 14-1). It ensures a patent airway. The normal protective laryngeal closing reflex is obtunded during inhalant or injectable anesthesia.[5] Proper tracheal intubation prevents aspiration of oral cavity fluids, blood, and surgical flush solutions. Regurgitation rarely occurs in normal horses. An anesthetized horse with an indwelling nasogastric tube can regurgitate, particularly during surgical manipulation of the stomach during colic surgery. Surgery of the nasal cavity, sinuses, guttural pouches, pharynx, and larynx can result in considerable hemorrhage. Furthermore, lavage solutions instilled into these surgical fields increases the volume of fluid accumulating in the larynx. Inflation of the endotracheal tube cuff helps to prevent aspiration of foreign material.

Tracheal intubation maintains airway patency in horses with airway pathology such as laryngeal hemiplegia or chondritis, nasal trauma, and airway space-occupying lesions (see Figures 14-4 through 14-7). Respiratory depression imposed by anesthesia reduces the horse's ability to overcome increases in airway resistance caused by the above abnormalities. Tracheal intubation minimizes increased airway resistance.[6]

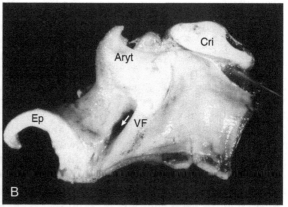

Figure 14–2. Larynx and related structures. **A,** Viewed from the front. **B,** Sagittal section. *Aryt,* = left arytenoid; *Cri,* cricoid; *Ep,* epiglottis; *G,* glottis; *SP,* soft palate; *VF,* left vocal fold. *Arrow* indicates opening to right laryngeal saccule.

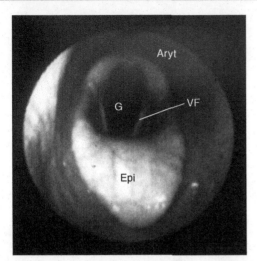

Figure 14–3. Endoscopic view of a normal larynx with arytenoids in abduction. Endoscope has been inserted into the pharynx through the ventral nasal meatus. The soft palate is in the normal position ventral to the epiglottis. *Aryt,* Arytenoid; *Epi,* epiglottis; *G,* glottis; *VF,* vocal fold.

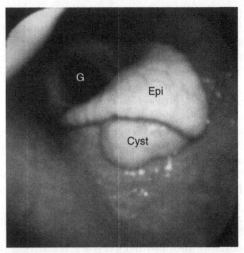

Figure 14–6. Subepiglottic cyst. *Epi,* Epiglottis; *G,* glottis.

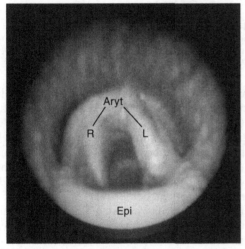

Figure 14–4. Larynx exhibiting left laryngeal hemiplegia. Note the right arytenoid is in abduction and the left arytenoid is not. *Aryt,* Right *(R)* and left *(L)* arytenoids; *Epi,* epiglottis.

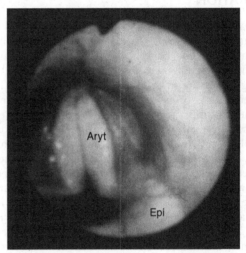

Figure 14–7. Normal larynx with the arytenoids in adduction. Occasionally the arytenoid cartilages adduct when touched by the endotracheal tube. This prohibits insertion of the endotracheal tube. *Aryt,* arytenoids; *Epi,* epiglottis.

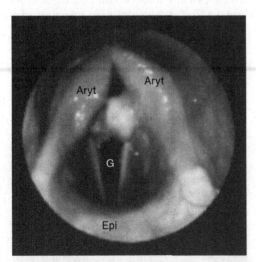

Figure 14–5. Chrondritis of right and left arytenoid cartilages. *Aryt,* Arytenoid; *Epi,* epiglottis; *G,* glottis.

Box 14–1	**Reasons for Tracheal Intubation**

1. Ensure a patent airway
2. Prevent aspiration
3. Minimize airway resistance
4. Facilitate administration of inhalant anesthetics
5. Facilitate assisted or controlled ventilation
6. Facilitate tracheal toilet
7. Control or scavenge waste gases
8. Maintain airway control during airway or oral cavity laser procedures

Tracheal intubation facilitates administration of inhalation anesthetics. Effective delivery of inhalation anesthesia requires a leak-free delivery apparatus. Leak-free masks are difficult to position and maintain. Entrainment of room air around a loose-fitting mask can result in the unpredictable delivery of inhaled anesthetics.

A leak-free tracheal tube prevents escape of anesthetic vapors into the environment. Exposure of personnel to trace amounts of anesthetic gas is considered a health hazard, and it may have legal ramifications.[7,8] Waste gas concentrations are significantly greater when an uncuffed tracheal tube is used compared to a cuffed tracheal tube.[9]

Tracheal intubation facilitates assisted and controlled ventilation. Assisted or controlled ventilation through a mask can result in gas accumulation in the esophagus and stomach. Upper airway pressures greater than 25 cm of H_2O, which develop from positive-pressure ventilation through a mask, can force air through a relaxed cricopharyngeal sphincter, resulting in gas accumulation in the stomach.

COMPLICATIONS OF TRACHEAL INTUBATION

Tracheal intubation is an invasive procedure and is not without risk, although the advantages far outweigh the disadvantages. The complications of tracheal intubation have been documented extensively in humans;[10] and, although there are few reports of complications in horses, the incidence is probably likely to be high.[11-15] One study documented upper airway lesions in 38 of 38 horses after "routine" intubation.[13] Most reported complications are referable to mucosal damage of the mouth, nasal meatus, larynx, and trachea (Box 14-2). Damage to the tracheal and laryngeal mucosa is the most frequently reported complication and occurs wherever the tube contacts the mucosa (Figure 14-8).[13] Lesions include edema, ecchymotic hemorrhage, and epithelial desquamation.[13] They usually resolve within 7 days after extubation and are not associated with permanent damage.[13] Similar lesions are reported after nasotracheal intubation.[14] Interestingly there is no correlation between the number of unsuccessful attempts to intubate and laryngeal trauma.[13]

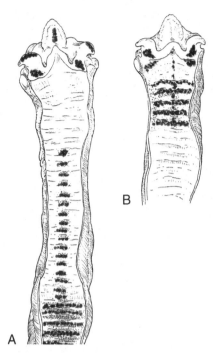

Figure 14–8. Pattern of contact zone and injury. **A,** with cuffed. **B,** Cole tracheal tubes. (From Heath RB et al: Laryngotracheal lesions following routine orotracheal intubation in the horse, *Equine Vet J* 21:434, 1989.)

Ischemic tracheal damage can occur if the tracheal tube cuff pressure on the tracheal wall exceeds capillary perfusion pressure (20 to 30 mm Hg).[15] Pressures greater than 50 mm Hg for approximately 15 minutes destroy the epithelium, leaving the basement membrane visible.[15] Unfortunately, intracuff pressure is not always an accurate reflection of cuff pressure against the mucosa of the trachea because of differences in endotracheal cuff compliance.[16] The intracuff pressure needed to seal the airway using a commonly available equine tracheal tube has been shown to be between 59 and 73 mm Hg.[17]

Other complications associated with tracheal intubation include obstruction of the tube caused by blood or mucus and inward compression of the wall of the endotracheal tube by an excessively inflated cuff or excessive neck flexion (Figure 14-9).[18] Accidental disconnection of the tube

---

Box 14–2   Reported Complications of Tracheal Intubation in the Horse

Summary of Lesions

1. Laryngeal hematomas on epiglottis and arytenoids (1 horse)[15]

2. Swollen tongue (1 horse)[15]

3. Pharyngeal perforation (1 case)[11]

4. Trauma and retroversion of epiglottis (3 of 9 horses).[12]

5. Nasotracheal intubation–mucosal damage (5 of 7 horses). Nasal meatus; arytenoids; trachea; dorsal pharyngeal recess; vocal folds; entrance to guttural pouch; Right laryngeal hemiplegia[14]

6. Laryngeal and tracheal mucosal damage (38 of 38 horses)[13]

7. Laryngeal paresis or paralysis

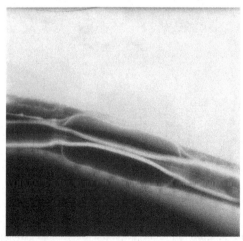

Figure 14–9. Radiograph of an excessively inflated cuff.

from the Y piece can occur, particularly when the connection is covered by surgical drapes. Endobronchial intubation can occur in young horses and ponies. For this reason the distance of tube insertion should be assessed before intubation in relatively short-necked horses or foals to avoid this eventuality. Ventral flexion of the neck can cause the distal end of the tracheal tube to migrate caudally[19] and potentially endobronchially. This could become important during procedures requiring extreme head flexion such as cervical radiography.

PREOPERATIVE EVALUATION

Preanesthetic evaluation should consider the anatomical, pathological, and surgical issues that will influence the route (nasal versus oral) of intubation. The external nares should be evaluated for discharge, particularly if nasotracheal intubation is to be performed. Airflow through each nostril can be confirmed by occluding the opposite nostril. Palpation and observation of the nasal bones for distortion can suggest fractures, tumors, or sinusitis. The larynx and trachea should be palpated to detect any obvious anatomical defects such as atrophied laryngeal musculature or collapsed or damaged tracheal rings. Any suspicion of abnormality should be followed by endoscopic evaluation.

Certain surgical procedures are facilitated using nasal rather than oral intubation. These include mandibular fracture repair, some cheek-teeth repulsions, laser procedures of the oral cavity, and other oral surgeries. Horses with a history of arytenoid paralysis or chondritis caused by trauma may be difficult to intubate (see Figures 14-4 through 14-6). Smaller tracheal tubes should be available because of the potential for reduced laryngeal diameter. Somewhat smaller-diameter but adequate tracheal tubes facilitate ventricular sacculectomy without extubation.

EQUIPMENT

Tracheal Tubes

Tracheal tubes used for horses are relatively long and of large diameter. The tracheal tubes used in foals weighing less than 40 to 50 kg usually are longer than those of similar diameter used in dogs (Figures 14-10 and 14-11).

Tracheal tubes are made from rubber, polyvinyl chloride plastic, or silicone (Table 14-1). Rubber tubes have poor resistance to kinking, cause tissue reactions, and break down with heat sterilization. Medical-grade silicone is very nonreactive and can be heat sterilized without deteriorating. However, silicone tubes kink easily when bent. Polyvinyl chloride is fairly rigid and conforms well to the

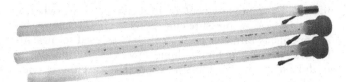

Figure 14–10. Tracheal tubes used in adult horses (22-30 mm). Note the different adapters for connection to the Y piece. (Smith Medical/Surgivet, Waukesha, WI.)

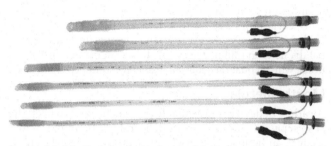

Figure 14–11. Foal-size tracheal tubes (10-22 mm). (Smith Medical/Surgivet, Waukesha, WI.)

anatomical shape of the upper airway at body temperature. Most polyvinyl chloride is relatively nonreactive. Heat sterilization is not recommended because polyvinyl chloride is thermolabile. Tubes bearing the designation *I.T., F-29,* or *Z-79* have been tested and found free of tissue toxicity.[10] Tracheal tubes currently used in horses do not bear this designation; therefore the reactivity of the tube material is unknown.

The tracheal tube cuff seals the space between the tracheal tube and the tracheal wall, helping to minimize or prevent aspiration of fluid and leakage of air and anesthetic gases around the tube. Cuff inflation also centers the tube in the trachea, thereby preventing the tube tip from traumatizing the tracheal mucosa. Tracheal tube cuffs are designated as either low residual volume (high pressure) or high residual volume (low pressure). High–residual volume cuffs generally induce less tracheal damage because they seal the airway at lower intracuff pressures. However, evidence is lacking that short-term (several hours) intubation with a properly inflated high-pressure cuff causes more damage than short-term intubation with a low-pressure cuff.[10] Proper cuff inflation implies inflation until the cuff just seals the trachea against air leak at peak positive inspiratory pressure (20 to 30 mm Hg). Low-volume–high-pressure cuffed tracheal tubes such as those commonly used for equine orotracheal intubation exert less pressure on the tracheal wall than

Table 14–1. Tracheal tubes available for use in horses			
Source	Tube material	Cuff	Sizes (internal diameter, mm)
Smith Medical/Surgivet Inc. Waukesha, WI	Silicone	Low volume	14-30
Smith Medical/Surgivet Inc Waukesha, WI	Silicone	Low volume	Foal Series nasotracheal tubes: 7-14
Jorvet, Loveland, CO	Rubber	Low volume	Up to 16

indicated by measurement of intracuff pressure; whereas high-volume–low-pressure cuffs exert tracheal pressure that approximates intracuff pressure.[17] Devices used to measure intracuff pressure in high-volume–low-pressure cuffs are not useful for estimating pressure exerted against the tracheal wall by equine tracheal tubes (Figure 14-12). A cuff-tracheal wall contact pressure of between 20 and 30 cm of H_2O is adequate to seal the airway and prevent mucosal damage.[18] Cuff inflation should be readjusted frequently during anesthesia if nitrous oxide is used in the anesthetic gas mixture to prevent excessive intracuff pressure from developing as a result of diffusion of nitrous oxide into the cuff.[19]

Tracheal tubes are available in a variety of diameters (see Table 14-1). Tube size is indicated by either the internal or external diameter in millimeters. Some tubes are marked in French units, which equal the external diameter multiplied by 3.

Mouth Specula

A variety of devices are available that can be used to keep the jaws separated for examination or oral intubation. A dental wedge can be inserted between the upper and lower cheek teeth. A more economical and easier-to-use device is a 5-cm

Table 14–2.	Tracheal tube lubricants and cleaning and disinfecting agents
Lubricants	**Remarks**
Water	Effective lubricant for oral tracheal intubation
Sterile water-soluble gel	Suitable for oral or nasal tracheal intubation
Water-soluble gel with lidocaine	Facilitates nasal tracheal intubation in awake animals
Cleaning and disinfecting agents	
Agent	**Spectrum of activity**
Soaps and detergents	Useful for removing gross contaminants
Chlorhexidine	Gram (+), gram (–); virucidal; nonsporicidal
Glutaraldehyde	Gram (+), gram (–), virucidal; sporicidal
Alcohols	Gram (+), gram (–); virucidal; nonsporicidal

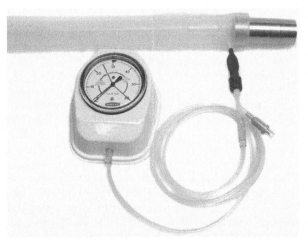

Figure 14–12. Device for measuring intracuff pressure.

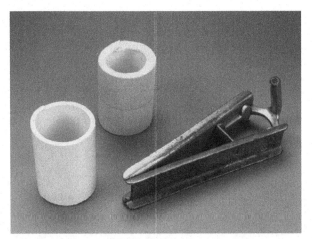

Figure 14–13. Devices for holding the mouth open during intubation. From *left* to *right*: 5-cm diameter PVC pipe; PVC pipe wrapped with tape to intcrease the friction of the pipe between the incisors; Bayer mouth wedge (Jorvet, Loveland, CO).

diameter, 10-cm length of PVC pipe wrapped with elastic bandage to prevent slippage. The pipe is inserted between the upper and lower incisors. The tracheal tube is inserted through the hole in the pipe (Figure 14-13). A smaller 3-cm diameter pipe can be used in smaller horses and foals.

Lubricants

Various lubricants can be applied to the tracheal tube to facilitate passage (Table 14-2). Water or a water-soluble gel is adequate. Gels containing local anesthetics offer no advantage and may increase the incidence of postintubation irritation.[20] A gel containing local anesthetic (lidocaine) can be applied to the first few centimeters of the nasal passage to facilitate nasotracheal intubation in awake horses.

CLEANING, STERILIZATION, AND REPAIR OF TRACHEAL TUBES

Tracheal tubes for horses are expensive and not disposable. They should be cleaned and disinfected to prevent nosocomial infection. Silicone is the only tracheal tube material that can withstand steam autoclaving; manufacturer recommendations for temperature and contact time should be followed. Disinfection is usually most easily accomplished using soaps and chemical disinfectants (see Table 14-2).

Tubes should be rinsed of exudate and secretions immediately or, if this is not possible, soaked in a solution of water and detergent to prevent drying of organic material. The presence of organic material impedes chemical disinfection; thus the tube should be cleaned thoroughly inside and out and rinsed with water. After being cleaned of gross contamination, tracheal tubes can be soaked in a disinfectant solution such as glutaraldehyde to further reduce the chance for nosocomial infection. The endotracheal tubes should then be rinsed thoroughly and allowed to dry. Tracheal tubes that are not adequately rinsed of chemical disinfectants can induce tissue reactions. Glutaraldehyde is the only cold disinfectant that is bactericidal, sporicidal, fungicidal, and virucidal. The tracheal tube should remain in the disinfectant solution for at least 10 minutes.

Ethylene oxide gas can be used to sterilize equipment that cannot be steam autoclaved but is recommended only as a last resort. Ethylene oxide penetrates into crevices and effectively kills all organisms. It is hazardous to personnel unless expensive equipment is installed to vent the gas properly.[18] Acute effects include respiratory and ocular irritation, cramps, and convulsions.[18] Known chronic effects of ethylene oxide include respiratory infections, anemia, and behavior changes.[18] Tracheal tubes should be aerated for at least 7 days before use after exposure to ethylene oxide unless commercial aerators are used. Improper aeration results in severe laryngotracheitis caused by ethylene glycol residue formed by the reaction of ethylene oxide and water.[21]

Equine tracheal tube cuffs are fragile and predisposed to laceration from sharp cheek teeth. A kit to replace damaged equine endotracheal tube cuffs on silicone tubes is available commercially (Surgivet, Waukesha WI). The replacement process is described by the manufacturer and is relatively simple to perform.

INTUBATION TECHNIQUE

A physical examination and evaluation of the horse's upper airway and mouth should be performed before anesthesia. The horse's mouth should be thoroughly rinsed with water before anesthetic induction (see Chapter 6). Even horses muzzled for several hours may retain food in the cheek pouch area. A large-dose syringe or a garden hose is inserted lateral to the cheek teeth, and a stream of water is directed into the cheek pouch area (Figure 14-14). Both sides of the mouth are flushed until no food residue is observed in the effluence.

Orotracheal Intubation

The largest-diameter tube that can be inserted without excessive force should be selected (Table 14-3). The cuff is inflated before insertion and observed for leaks; then it is deflated. Anesthetic technique should provide a depth of anesthesia sufficient to relax the masseter muscles and permit insertion of the mouth speculum (Figure 14-15). The head and neck of the horse should be extended to align the oral cavity with the larynx and trachea (Figure 14-16). The

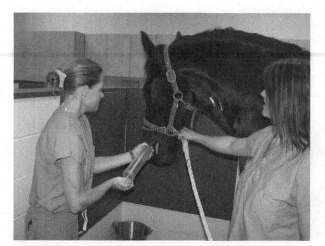

Figure 14–14. Dose syringe filled with water inserted into the cheek pouch to wash food debris from mouth intubation.

Table 14–3.	Suggested sizes for tracheal tubes	
	Cuffed tube, internal diameter (mm)	
Body weight (kg)	Oral	Nasal
450 or greater	26-30	18-22
200-400	22-26	14-16
100-250	16-22	12-14
<100	10-14	7-11

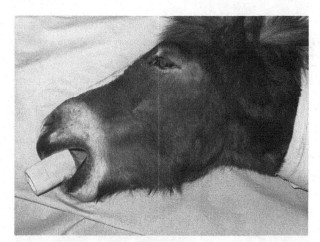

Figure 14–15. PVC pipe inserted between incisors.

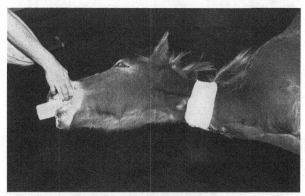

Figure 14–16. Head dorsal flexed to align the oral cavity with the larynx.

horse's tongue is retracted through the interdental space. The lubricated tracheal tube is inserted into the mouth and advanced into the pharynx, carefully avoiding the cheek teeth. It is advanced with the concave surface of the tube directed toward the palate. It is rotated approximately 180 degrees as the tip of the tube enters the pharynx while it continues to be advanced into and through the larynx.

Several attempts may be necessary before the tube enters the larynx (Figure 14-17). Unsuccessful attempts result from reflection of the tube into the pharyngeal wall or esophagus and are evident by a resistance to further tube advancement and vertical movement of the larynx (Figure 14-18). The tracheal tube should be retracted approximately 10 cm when this resistance is felt, rotated approximately 90 to 180

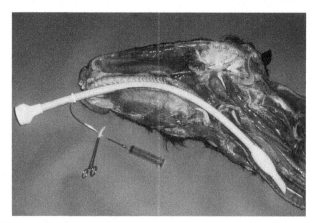

Figure 14–17. Sagittal section of head and neck illustrating correct placement of tube.

degrees, and readvanced until it passes without resistance past the larynx. A small stomach tube or long endoscope can be used as a guide during difficult intubations (Figure 14-19). The stomach tube should be inserted into the larynx and then used as a stylet for insertion of the tracheal tube.

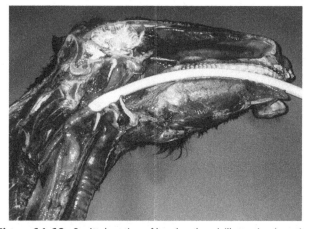

Figure 14–18. Sagittal section of head and neck illustrating insertion of tube into the esophagus.

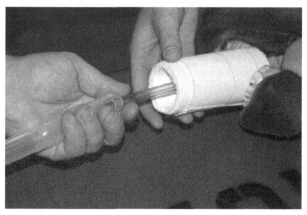

Figure 14–19. A stomach tube inserted into the larynx is used as a stylet to guide the endotracheal tube into the larynx.

If the tracheal tube is inserted properly, airflow can be detected at the end of the tracheal tube during the horse's spontaneous respiration or when the chest is compressed. Water vapor should also be observed condensing on the inner surface of the tube with correct tracheal tube insertion. The cuff is inflated with air to seal the airway when the lung is pressurized to 20 to 30 cm of H_2O. This is accomplished by connecting the patient end of the tube to the Y piece of the breathing circuit and squeezing the rebreathing bag or compressing the ventilator bellows to develop a pressure within the breathing circuit of 20 to 30 cm of H_2O. Leaks can be detected by listening for a rush of air from the nostrils, detecting the odor of the inhalation anesthetic, or the inability to maintain a positive airway pressure.

NASOTRACHEAL INTUBATION

Nasotracheal intubation can be performed in the awake or anesthetized horse (Figure 14-20, *A*). Awake intubation is very useful for inducing anesthesia in foals when using an inhalation anesthetic such as isoflurane or sevoflurane (Figure 14-20, *B*). Struggle-free induction usually occurs within 2 to 3 minutes.[22]

A smaller-diameter tube is used for nasotracheal intubation than that used for orotracheal intubation (see Table 14-3).

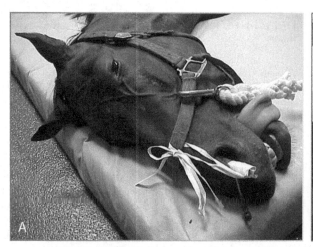

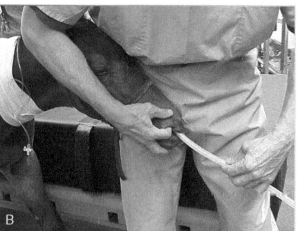

Figure 14–20. A, Endotracheal tube inserted into the larynx through the ventral nasal meatus. **B,** Nasotracheal intubation is easily performed in sedated foals.

The technique is identical to that of passing a stomach tube through the nasal cavity. The tip of the nasotracheal tube should be well lubricated and inserted through the nostril in a ventral-medial direction, directing the tube tip into the ventral nasal meatus. The tracheal tube is slowly and gently advanced into the pharynx. It should be withdrawn if progress within the nasal cavity is stopped. Resistance to the tube advancing within the nasal cavity indicates that too large a diameter tube is being used or that the tube is not being directed into the ventral meatus. Once the tube enters the pharynx, the intubation procedure is similar to that described for orotracheal intubation. The tracheal tube can be diverted into the esophagus during awake intubation if the horse swallows. The tube should be retracted a few centimeters, and the process repeated. If repeated swallowing prevents tracheal intubation, attempts to intubate the horse through the opposite nostril can inexplicably result in success.

The relatively smaller airway produced by nasotracheal intubation increases resistance to breathing. The nasal tube should be exchanged for an orally inserted tube of larger diameter if the increased resistance creates respiratory distress.

TRACHEOSTOMY

Tracheostomy is performed as an emergency procedure for upper respiratory obstruction or as an elective procedure to facilitate some surgical procedures (Figure 14-21). The tracheostomy site should be prepared surgically and infiltrated with 2% lidocaine in a nonemergency situation in an awake horse.

A longitudinal 10- to 12-cm long ventral midline incision is made at the junction between the cranial one third and middle one third of the neck. The musculature overlying the trachea is thin and easily separated, and the tracheal rings are palpable. Muscle and fascia are divided until the tracheal rings are exposed. A transverse incision is made between two tracheal rings using a No. 10 scalpel blade. An incision one third to one half the circumference of the trachea, centered over the ventral trachea, is made. A sucking sound of air denotes entry into the tracheal lumen. The incision between the rings is extended with scissors or forceps, and the tracheal or tracheostomy tube inserted. A standard equine tracheal tube can be used; however, care should be taken to avoid damage to the tracheal mucosa or endobronchial intubation. The tracheostomy tube size should be smaller than that chosen for orotracheal intubation because of the difficulty and potential trauma associated with inserting the tube between tracheal rings (Figure 14-22).

CONSIDERATIONS FOR LASER PROCEDURES OF THE UPPER AIRWAY AND ORAL CAVITY

The use of lasers for upper airway surgery of the soft palate, arytenoid cartilage, epiglottis, and larynx has become increasingly common.[23] Secure orotracheal intubation isolates the lower airway from the surgical site, ensuring continued delivery of oxygen and anesthetic gas while preventing inhalation of laser-induced smog from tissue coagulation.[10,23] Inadvertant laser contact with the tracheal tube can burn a hole through the tracheal tube wall and result in an airway fire as the laser contacts the oxygen-enriched gas within the tube. Currently no laser-safe tracheal tube is available for equine use. The external wall of the tracheal tube proximal to the cuff can be shielded from the laser with aluminum adhesive-backed tape (3M No. 425 1-inch aluminum tape) or moistened roll gauze.[10] Although tubes made of silicone or rubber can ignite in room air, a 40% FiO_2 can be used to minimize the risk of airway fire and maintain adequate oxygenation. The reduction in FiO_2 can be accomplished with nitrogen or helium.[10,24] A 60% He/40% O_2 inspired gas mixture eliminates the need for tracheal tube shielding.[24]

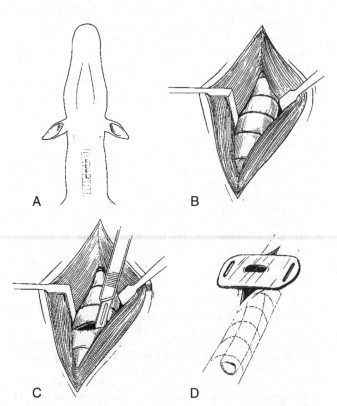

Figure 14–21. A, Longitudinal 10- to 12-cm ventral midline incision. **B,** Exposure of the tracheal rings. **C,** Transverse incision between two tracheal rings. The incision is approximately one third to one half the circumference of the trachea. **D,** Correctly positioned tube.

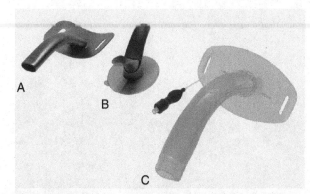

Figure 14–22. Tracheostomy tubes. **A,** Custom manufactured stainless steel J tube (not commercially available). **B,** Self-retaining tube (Jorvet, Loveland, CO). **C,** Silicone J tube (Smith's Medical/Surgivet, Waukesha, WI).

EXTUBATION

Extubation is a relatively simple procedure. The tracheal tube is removed carefully after the horse regains its swallowing reflex by first deflating the tracheal tube cuff. Swallowing indicates the ability to protect the airway from foreign material. Moving the tube slightly while the horse is awakening from anesthesia often stimulates the swallowing reflex. The tracheal tube can be left in place until the horse is standing (Figure 14-23). This is an advantage when there is nasal turbinate edema or some other cause for upper airway obstruction. Nasal airway obstruction is common in supine horses following prolonged anesthesia when the head is below the level of the heart. Alternatively a small tracheal tube can be inserted into the larynx before recovery before the tracheal tube is removed. The tubes should be fastened to the horse's halter with tape or gauze to avoid aspiration of the tube into the airway (Figure 14-24).

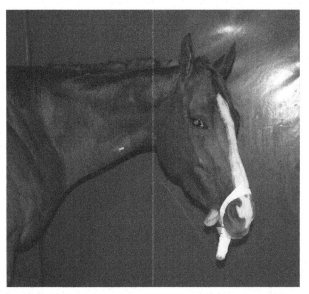

Figure 14–23. Recovery to standing with oral tracheal tube in place.

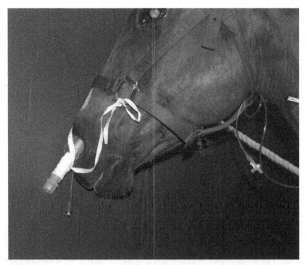

Figure 14–24. Recovery to standing with nasal tube in place.

COMPLICATIONS AFTER EXTUBATION

Nasal edema can develop in anesthetized horses. The amount of edema varies, and most horses develop edema during dorsal recumbency. Nasal congestion can result in significant upper airway obstruction after extubation. Upper airway obstruction can cause loud inspiratory snoring. Edema quickly disappears in most horses after extubation and does not require treatment, but occasionally it may be severe enough to cause a functional obstruction requiring treatment. The horse can be reintubated and allowed to stand with the tube in place (see Figure 14-24). Alternatively 30- to 40-cm lengths of soft plastic tubing, foal-sized tracheal tubes, or specially designed nasal tubes (SurgiVet, Waukesha, WI) can be inserted into one or both nostrils to bypass the edema. Phenylephrine (10 ml, 0.15% solution) divided and deposited along the full length of both ventral meatus may reduce the need for insertion of nasal tubes during recovery.[25] Other less common causes for upper respiratory obstruction after extubation include dorsal displacement of the soft palate above (dorsal to) the epiglottis. A displaced epiglottis results in airway obstruction as the soft palate enters the larynx during inspiration. Soft palate displacement is easily corrected by inducing swallowing. Swallowing can be induced by either gentle manipulation of the larynx or reinsertion of the tracheal tube.[26]

Occasionally horses show signs of respiratory obstruction resulting from arytenoid paralysis.[27] The cause is unknown but may require tracheostomy. Laryngeal paralysis can occur and generally resolves within several hours to days. It is usually accompanied by a loud shrill noise with exaggerated inspiratory efforts (abdominal lift). A small nasotracheal tube should be quickly inserted in the trachea. A tracheotomy should be performed if a nasotracheal tube cannot be placed. Once the horse becomes hypoxic and physically uncontrollable, tracheostomy is not possible until the horse collapses from hypoxia. Hypoxia or negative pressure can produce pulmonary edema.

REFERENCES

1. *Stedman's Medical Dictionary*: ed. 27, Baltimore, 2000, Lippincott Williams & Wilkins, p 918.
2. Macewen W: Clinical observations on the introduction of tracheal tubes by the mouth instead of performing tracheotomy or laryngotomy, *Br Med J* 2:163-165, 1880.
3. Hall LW: Bromochlorotrifluorethane (Fluothane): a new volatile anesthetic agent, *Vet Rec* 69:615-617, 1957.
4. Sisson S, Grossman JD: The respiratory system. In *The anatomy of the domestic animals*, Philadelphia, 1953, Saunders.
5. Robinson E: Radiographic assessment of laryngeal reflexes in ketamine-anesthetized cats, *Am J Vet Res* 47:1569-1572, 1986.
6. Tomasic M, Mann L, Soma L: Effects of sedation, anesthesia, and endotracheal intubation on respiratory mechanics in adult horses, *Am J Vet Res* 58:641-646, 1997.
7. Paddleford RR: Anesthetic waste gases and your health. In Short CE, editor: *Principles and practice of veterinary anesthesia*, Baltimore, 1987, Williams & Wilkins.
0. Whitcher CE, Cohen EN, Trudell JR. Chronic exposure to anesthetic gases in the operating room, *Anesthesiology* 35: 348-353, 1971.
9. Trim CM: Complications associated with the use of the cuffless endotracheal tube in the horse, *J Am Vet Med Assoc* 185: 541-542, 1984.

10. Lewis FR, Schlobohm RM, Thomas AN: Prevention of complications from prolonged tracheal intubation, *Am J Surg* 135:452-457, 1978.
11. Brock KA: Pharyngeal trauma from endotracheal intubation in a colt, *J Am Vet Med Assoc* 187:944-946, 1985.
12. Dodman NH, Koblik PD, Court MH: Retroversion of the epiglottis as a complication of endotracheal intubation in the horse: a pilot study, *Vet Surg* 15:275-278, 1986.
13. Heath RB et al: Laryngotracheal lesions following routine orotracheal intubation in the horse, *Equine Vet J* 21:434-437, 1989.
14. Holland M et al: Laryngotracheal injury associated with nasotracheal intubation in the horse, *J Am Vet Med Assoc* 189:1447-1450, 1986.
15. Nordin U: The trachea and cuff-induced tracheal injury, *Acta Otolaryngol (Stockh)* 7(suppl 345):7-69, 1977.
16. Bernhard WN et al: Adjustment of intracuff pressure to prevent aspiration, *Anesthesiology* 50:363-366, 1979.
17. Touzot-Jourde G, Stedman N, Trim CM: The effects of two endotracheal tube cuff inflation pressures on liquid aspiration and tracheal wall damage in horses, *Vet Anaesth Analg* 32: 23-29, 2005.
18. Dorsch JA, Dorsch SE: *Understanding anesthesia equipment*, ed 4, Baltimore, 1999, Williams & Wilkins.
19. Raeder JC, Borchgrevink PC, Sellevold OM: Tracheal tube cuff pressures: the effects of different gas mixtures, *Anaesthesia* 40:444-447, 1985.
20. Loeser EA et al: The influence of endotracheal tube cuff design and cuff lubrication on postoperative sore throat, *Anesthesiology* 58:376-379, 1983.
21. Belani KG, Preidkalns J: An epidemic of pseudomembranous laryngotracheitis: complications following extubation, *Anesthesiology* 47:530-531, 1977.
22. Webb AI: Nasal intubation in the foal, *J Am Vet Med Assoc* 185:48-51, 1984.
23. Driessen B et al: Hazards associated with laser surgery in the airway of the horse: implications for the anesthetic management. In Steffey EP, editor: *Recent advances in anesthetic management of large domestic animals: International Veterinary Information Service,* www.ivis.org, Ithaca, NY, 2003.
24. Driessen B, Nann L, Klein L: Use of a helium/oxygen carrier gas mixture for inhalation anesthesia during laser surgery in the airway of the horse, In Steffey EP, editor: *Recent advances in anesthetic management of large domestic animals: International Veterinary Information Service,* www.ivis.org, Ithaca, NY, 2003.
25. Lukasik VM et al: Intranasal phenylephrine reduces postanesthetic upper airway obstruction in horses, *Equine Vet J* 29: 236-238, 1997.
26. Riebold TW, Goble DO, Geiser DR: *Large animal anesthesia, principles and techniques*, Ames, 1982, Iowa State Press.
27. Abrahamsen EJ et al: Bilateral arytenoid cartilage paralysis after inhalation anesthesia in a horse, *J Am Vet Med Assoc* 197:1363-1365, 1990.

15

Inhalation Anesthetics and Gases

Eugene P. Steffey

1. The drug delivery system for inhalant anesthetics is the lung. Ventilation produces rapid changes in the concentration of inhaled gases or vapors in the lungs.
2. Uptake of inhaled anesthetics depends primarily on ventilation, the blood solubility of the inhaled drug, cardiac output, and the partial pressure difference of the inhalant between the venous blood and alveoli (blood gas partition coefficient).
3. Tissues serve as depots for anesthetic drugs. Tissue uptake depends on tissue solubility and tissue blood flow. Changes in distribution of blood flow to vessel-rich group (e.g., brain, heart, liver), muscle group (e.g., skeletal muscle), and fat group tissues influence the uptake of inhalant anesthetics.
4. Inhalant anesthetics produce dose-related cardiorespiratory depression, resulting in decreases in cardiac output, arterial blood pressure, tissue perfusion, and tissue oxygenation.
5. Inhalant anesthetics depress compensatory responses, especially baroreceptor reflex control of arterial blood pressure in horses.
6. The gas nitrous oxide is of limited value in horses because of low potency, the potential for hypoxemia, and the development of bloat and ileus.
7. Metabolism of inhalant anesthetics is minimal for isoflurane, sevoflurane, and desflurane.
8. Scavenging methods for the elimination of trace inhalant anesthetic gases should be used to limit personnel exposure.

FUNDAMENTALS OF INHALATION ANESTHESIA

General anesthesia produced largely or exclusively by the controlled administration of gaseous or volatile drugs is commonly known as *inhalation anesthesia*. Inhalation (or inhaled) anesthetics are a group of drugs that, either by themselves or in combination with other types of drugs, produce general anesthesia by an unknown mechanism. Inhalation anesthetics are grouped into three categories for the purpose of this chapter. The first grouping and the focus of this chapter is composed of (listed according to historical introduction to clinical practice in North America) halothane, isoflurane, desflurane, and sevoflurane. Isoflurane is now the most commonly used equine inhalation anesthetic; and halothane is the agent of longest use, having been introduced to clinical practice in 1957. Sevoflurane recently has gained a notable share of the commercial market in North America and has replaced halothane as the second most commonly used inhalation anesthetic for animal patients, including horses. The second group includes only N_2O, a gas stored under pressure

in cylinders (see Chapter 16). Because of its limited anesthetic potency in horses and some relatively unique physical properties, its clinical use requires careful evaluation of its advantages and disadvantages. A third group includes volatile liquids such as chloroform, diethyl ether, methoxyflurane, and enflurane (a chemical isomer of isoflurane). These drugs are no longer used to anesthetize horses, especially in North America; thus they are only of historical interest and receive only occasional brief mention (mostly for comparison) in this chapter. Readers with greater interest in the development and clinical use of these drugs are referred to an earlier edition of this text or other early editions of veterinary anesthesia texts of broader species coverage.[1-4]

Inhalation anesthetics have justifiably played an important role in the anesthetic management of horses for more than five decades. They are broadly credited with reducing morbidity and mortality, especially under clinical circumstances, which include physiologically compromised patients and procedures requiring prolonged or complicated anesthetic management.

Contemporary inhalation anesthetics are popular because they are the most controllable method for producing general anesthesia in horses. The magnitude of depression of the central nervous system (CNS) (i.e., anesthetic depth) and the function of other vital organs are easily regulated by altering the partial pressure or concentration of anesthetic in the inspired gas. Recent technology also permits accurate breath-to-breath monitoring of both inspired and expired anesthetic concentration (partial pressure), thereby ensuring accurate inhalant anesthetic concentrations. Antidotes are not required, and the incidence of direct toxicity or other adverse reactions is minimal.

Administration of inhalation anesthetics usually necessitates use of special-delivery equipment or machines, which, although adding to the cost and complexity of anesthetic management, provide additional health-related benefits to equine patients (see Chapter 16). For example, the equipment includes a fresh gas reservoir bag or bellows and a source of oxygen. The respiratory rate and tidal breath (volume in milliliters) of the patient can be quantitated more easily by watching the tidal excursions of the gas reservoir bag of the anesthetic machine (see Chapter 16). Positive-pressure ventilation is facilitated by manual or mechanically controlled compression of the same reservoir. Because general anesthesia and recumbency reduce the horse's ability to oxygenate its arterial blood,[5] the supplementation of the horse's inspired gas with oxygen is a particular advantage provided by the use of an anesthetic machine.

Despite their general excellence, all contemporary inhaled anesthetics produce side effects. For example, they all depress circulatory and respiratory system function. They are degraded, and some resultant products are toxic. Accordingly, the search for an ideal inhalant anesthetic continues (Box 15-1).

<table>
<tr><td colspan="2">

Box 15–1 Characteristics of the Ideal Inhalation Anesthetic for Horses

- Stable shelf life without preservatives
- Nonflammable
- Compatible with existing delivery equipment
- Easily vaporized under ambient conditions
- Low blood solubility to foster rapid changes in anesthetic depth
- Potent anesthetic (i.e., anesthesia at low inspired concentrations)
- Not irritating to airways
- Absence of cardiopulmonary depression
- Compatible with catecholamines and other vasoactive drugs
- Not metabolized
- Skeletal muscle relaxation
- Lingering analgesic effects
- Absence of hepatic and renal toxicity
- Rapid, controlled, coordinated recovery
- Inexpensive (both agent and agent delivery)

</td></tr>
</table>

and maintain an optimum partial pressure of anesthetic in the CNS (brain and spinal cord). The molecular nature of inhalation anesthetics and their physicochemical properties are important determinants of their actions and the safety of their administration.

Chemical and Physical Properties

The physicochemical properties of inhalant anesthetics determine how drugs are supplied by the manufacturer, govern the method of anesthetic administration, and influence their uptake and elimination by patients (Table 15-1). A brief review of some of these properties may be helpful, especially considering each in light of the ideal anesthetic (see Box 15-1). For example, early inhalation anesthetics were flammable and liable to cause explosions. Development of nonflammable anesthetics became mandatory as the use of electronic equipment in the operating room increased. Advances in halogen (especially fluorine) chemistry permitted the synthesis of halogenated ethers and hydrocarbons, which were both potent and nonflammable. Unfortunately, the halogen ion, especially fluoride, is also toxic to some tissues (e.g., kidneys) and of substantial concern if the parent compound is not resistant to in vitro or in vivo (or both) degradation.

An ideal inhalation anesthetic would be easily vaporized at ambient temperatures. That is, the vapor pressure of a volatile drug must be sufficient to provide enough molecules in the vapor phase to produce anesthesia under ambient conditions. Other things being equal, the higher the vapor pressure, the higher the concentration of drug deliverable to the patient. The contemporary volatile liquids demonstrate this desirable characteristic. Nitrous oxide (N_2O) can be delivered at even higher concentrations; however, it is stored as a gas under pressure, which, compared to the volatile liquids, complicates storage practices.

GENERAL CHARACTERISTICS OF INHALATION ANESTHETICS

The fundamental goal of inhalation anesthesia is to immobilize the horse, obtund pain, and help provide optimum conditions for surgery or other health improvement-related procedures. To accomplish this it is necessary to achieve

Table 15–1. Some chemical and physical properties of modern inhalation anesthetics

Property	Desflurane	Halothane	Isoflurane	Sevoflurane	Nitrous oxide
Trade name	Suprane	Fluothane	Forane Aerrane, Isoflo	Ultane	N_2O
Formula	$CHF_2-O_2-CHFCF_3$	$CF_3CHClBr$	$CHF_2-O-CHClCF_3$	$CH_2F-O-CH(CF_3)_2$	N_2O
Molecular weight	168	197	185	200	44
Boiling point (° C)	23.5	50	49	59	
Vapor pressure (mm Hg at 20° C)	664	244	240	160	
Vapor concentration (% saturated at 20° C)	87	32	32	21	100
Milliliters of vapor per milliliter of liquid @ 20° C	210	227	195	183	
Preservative	No	Yes	No	No	No
Stability in moist soda lime	Stable	Stable	Stable	Unstable	Stable
Solubility*					
Blood:gas	0.5	2.4	1.4	0.7	0.5
Oil:gas	19	224	98	47	1.4
Rubber:gas	16	120	62	31	1.2

Data from references 55,204,216,259-262.
*Partition coefficients for human blood and olive oil at 37° C and rubber at room temperature.

Present-day inhalation anesthetics have a prolonged shelf life, and most are uncontaminated by preservatives or breakdown. Excepting halothane, contemporary inhalant anesthetics do not require additives to the liquid anesthetic to promote shelf life. However, isoflurane, desflurane, and sevoflurane react with CO_2 absorbents of the anesthetic delivery apparatus (notably Baralime [as a result no longer commercially available in the United States] and soda lime) and degrade to toxic products to varying degrees. Such degradation produces heat and breakdown products, including compound A in the case of sevoflurane, and carbon monoxide (CO) in the case of desflurane and isoflurane. More recent CO_2 absorbents (Amsorb, Sodasorb LF) have been specifically formulated to inhibit the degradation on anesthetic gases (CO; compound A) while retaining their CO_2 absorption efficiency.

The solubility of inhalation anesthetics (see Table 15-1) is generally expressed in terms of a partition coefficient (PC). The PC describes the relative capacity per unit volume of two solvents (e.g., blood and gas) for a specified anesthetic (i.e., it is a ratio of the concentration of the anesthetic between two phases after equilibration). Because solubility is temperature sensitive, it is important to compare PCs at similar temperatures, preferably body temperature (commonly 37° C). As background it should be remembered that anesthetic vapors and gases such as respiratory gases, O_2 and CO_2, equilibrate between two phases according to pressure gradients. At equilibrium the partial pressure of anesthetic in the two phases is the same, but the concentration in the two phases may differ markedly. Thus the PC describes the magnitude of difference of the volume of anesthetic in the two phases when the partial pressure in the two phases is equal. For example, consider an anesthetic X with a blood:gas (air) PC of 2.5. In this case the PC indicates that at equilibrium the concentration of this anesthetic is two and a half times greater in blood than in the gaseous phase, whereas the partial pressure of the anesthetic is the same in both phases. Alternatively, consider an anesthetic Y with a PC of 0.5. The magnitude of the PC of anesthetic Y indicates that the anesthetic is only half as soluble in blood as it is in air. Comparing the PC of anesthetic X and anesthetic Y, it is apparent that anesthetic X is much more soluble in blood than anesthetic Y (about five times more soluble). The clinical relevance in this example is that, other things being equal, induction of anesthesia will proceed faster with anesthetic Y because a higher PC is related to a slower anesthetic induction. As noted in Table 15-1, anesthetic X is halothane, and anesthetic Y is desflurane (or N_2O). At least two other PCs are commonly used in evaluating the clinical use of inhaled anesthetics: the oil:gas and rubber:gas PCs (see Table 15-1). The oil:gas PC (blood:gas PC) correlates inversely with anesthetic potency and describes the capacity of lipids for the anesthetic. The rubber:gas PC is useful because it describes the magnitude of absorption of anesthetic by rubber. Loss of anesthetic into rubber (or other materials of the anesthetic delivery apparatus) retards the delivery of anesthetic to the patient. Tissue solubility is also important but for simplicity is not listed in Table 15-1 or discussed here. Specific tissue solubilities of inhalation anesthetics in horses are available.[6-10]

Minimum Alveolar Concentration

The relationship of an administered dose of anesthetic to the magnitude of effect it causes is an expression of the potency of the anesthetic. Attempts to assess anesthetic potency are long-standing, and an appropriate expression of CNS depression (insensibility) is necessary because there are obvious needs to compare effects on vital organ function by equipotent doses of different anesthetics. In 1963 Markel and Eger[11] described what has become the major index of anesthetic potency for inhalation anesthetics: minimum alveolar concentration (MAC).

MAC is the *minimum alveolar concentration* of an inhaled anesthetic, at 1 atmosphere, that prevents gross purposeful skeletal muscle movement in response to a noxious stimulus (Box 15-2).[9,11] MAC corresponds to the ED_{50} (i.e., the median anesthetic concentration), the dose at which half of the animals are anesthetized and half are not. The dose corresponding to 95% anesthesia (i.e., ED_{95}), at least in humans, may be as much as 40% greater than MAC.[12] It must be stressed that MAC is the *alveolar* anesthetic concentration, not the inspired anesthetic concentration or the concentration represented by a specific vaporizer dial setting.

Also important is that MAC is defined in terms of a percent of 1 atmosphere and therefore represents an alveolar anesthetic partial pressure. The concentration of anesthetic in air or oxygen is proportional to its partial pressure:

$$\frac{\text{Partial Pressure}}{\text{Total Pressure}} \times 100 = \text{concentration in vol\%}$$
$$\text{(e.g., atmosphere)}$$

The concentration of anesthetic in media other than gas (i.e., blood or tissue) is the product of its solubility and partial pressure in that media. Therefore, unlike reference to the gas phase, the terms *partial pressure* and *concentration of anesthetics in blood or tissues* should not be used interchangeably. The term *tension* is sometimes used synonymously with partial pressure. Presuming, after sufficient time, that there is equilibrium between the alveolar gas and arterial blood anesthetic partial pressure and the arterial blood and brain anesthetic partial pressure, MAC should represent the partial pressure of anesthetic at its site of action: the CNS. An appreciation of the latter point (i.e., a focus on anesthetic partial pressure) is necessary because a given partial pressure of anesthetic may result in different concentrations of anesthetic in different body phases (e.g., gas, blood, lipid). Furthermore, although the partial pressure of an anesthetic at MAC should not vary, the alveolar concentration changes with changes in ambient pressure (e.g., altitude). The alveolar concentration at altitude is higher than that at sea level for the same anesthetic conditions.[9,13]

Finally, it is important to remember that MAC is determined in healthy animals under laboratory conditions in the absence of other drugs and circumstances common to the clinical use of inhaled anesthetics, which may alter the requirement for anesthesia.

Box 15–2   Minimum Alveolar Concentration (MAC)

- The end-alveolar concentration of an inhalation anesthetic that prevents gross purposeful movement in response to a painful stimulus in 50% of patients

- An index of relative potency of inhalation anesthetics

MAC values determined in healthy adult horses differ among inhalation anesthetics (Table 15-2). As noted, halothane is the most potent of the contemporary inhalation drugs (i.e., has the lowest MAC, 0.9%), and N_2O is the least potent (i.e., general anesthesia of healthy horses is not possible with N_2O alone under ambient conditions).[14] Notice also that 0.9% halothane provides a similar or equivalent level of anesthesia as 1.3% isoflurane.

Equipotent doses (e.g., equivalent concentrations at MAC) are useful for comparing effects of inhalation anesthetics on vital organ function. This concept is discussed later in this chapter when effects of drugs are compared and contrasted. In this regard anesthetic dose is defined in multiples of MAC (e.g., 1.0, 1.5, 2.0 times the MAC).

Remember that greater than a 1.0 MAC level of anesthesia is necessary to produce immobility in *all* surgical patients. Although a 1.0 MAC is helpful for comparing anesthetic effects, it represents on average a light level of anesthesia and does not provide adequate anesthesia in about 50% of patients. On the other hand, 2.0 MAC is a deep level of anesthesia and may represent an anesthetic overdose in many patients. As a guideline, most patients require 1.2 to 1.4 MAC or less for an adequate level of surgical anesthesia, especially considering that during clinical anesthesia multiple anesthetic adjuvant drugs are commonly coadministered.

The variability of MAC in a single species is generally small and is not influenced substantially by gender, duration of anesthesia, variation in $PaCO_2$ (from 10 to 90 mm Hg), metabolic alkalosis or acidosis, variation in PaO_2 between 40 and 500 mm Hg, moderate anemia, or hypotension.[9,13] However, a number of physiological drug-related factors impact MAC; some increasing and some decreasing the anesthetic requirement (i.e., MAC). A variety of effects described largely from studies of dogs and humans are known to affect MAC (Box 15-3). There is no reason to doubt that these same factors similarly influence MAC in horses.

Monitoring the Response to Anesthetics

The horse's response to anesthesia must be monitored to minimize the likelihood of arousal during surgery and to avoid anesthetic overdose and death. There are two basic approaches to providing an appropriate anesthetic depth. First, a dose of

Box 15–3	Factors Influencing Inhalation Anesthetic Requirement (Minimum Alveolar Concentration)[48,170]
Increase	Hyperthermia (to 42° C)
	Hypernatremia
	Drugs causing central nervous system stimulation (e.g., amphetamines, ephedrine)
No change	Duration of anesthesia
	Hyperkalemia, hypokalemia
	Gender
	$PaCO_2$ (15 to 95 mm Hg)
	PaO_2 >40 mm Hg
	$\overline{AP}$ >50 mm Hg
	Metabolic acid-base changes
Decrease	Hypothermia
	Hyponatremia
	Pregnancy
	PaO_2 <40 mm Hg
	$PaCO_2$ >95 mm Hg
	$\overline{AP}$ <50 mm Hg
	Increasing adult age
	Drugs causing central nervous system depression (e.g., preanesthetic medication, injectable anesthetics, other inhaled anesthetics; see Chapters 11 and 12)

anesthetic that should produce a desired effect can be administered (i.e., a multiple of MAC).[12] The accompanying disadvantage of this technique is that some horses are exposed to an excessive amount of anesthetic over the course of their anesthetic management, and the incidence of undesirable side effects, including death, increases. This results because horses differ in their sensitivities to anesthetics and noxious stimulation. In addition, the magnitude of depression at a given dose of anesthetic varies considerably because the intensity and duration of noxious (surgical) stimulation vary during an operation. Alternatively, the anesthetist perfects his or her clinical skills and titrates the anesthetic dose against the horse's response to noxious stimulation.

Both techniques referred to in the previous paragraph are used to attain and maintain proper anesthetic "depth" in usual clinical practice. First, a predetermined anesthetic dose (vaporizer dial setting or inspired or end-expired concentration) is administered on the basis of the drug used and patient circumstances. This is followed by a fine adjustment of that dose based on repeated observations of the horse's response to surgical stimulation. It is desirable to seek the least amount of anesthetic compatible with the surgical procedure. It is usually in the horse's best interest for the anesthetist to err on the side of insufficient anesthesia rather than excessive depression. Inhalant anesthetic dose can be reduced, and effects augmented by coadministering analgesic adjuncts (α_2-agonists, ketamine; see Chapter 18).

The transition from consciousness to complete surgical anesthesia was originally described by Guedel.[15] He defined four stages of anesthesia (awake, delirium, surgical, medullary depression) and described pupillary alteration, eye movements, and respiratory changes that were used for many years to estimate depth of diethyl ether anesthesia in unpre-

Table 15–2.	Minimum alveolar concentration* compared with other useful anesthetic concentrations in healthy adult horses		
		Useful delivered concentrations (vol %)[†]	
Drug	MAC*	Induction	Maintenance
Halothane	0.9[104] – 1.05[263]	3-5	1-3
Isoflurane	1.31[104] – 1.64[89]	3-5	1-3.5
Sevoflurane	2.31[241] – 2.84[200]	4-6	2.5-5
Desflurane	7.02[264] – 8.06[201]	9-12	7-9
Nitrous oxide	205[14]	60	≤50

*Vol % determined in horses.
[†]Actual concentration differs widely, depending on clinical conditions and accompanying additional anesthetic and/or adjuvant drugs.

medicated human patients. Stage 3, surgical anesthesia, was divided into four planes and characterized by depression of respiration, circulation protective reflexes, and muscle tone. These stages and planes of anesthesia in relation to animals are described elsewhere.[16,17] The variability among species, contemporary anesthetics, and anesthetic practices is so great that no similar uniform system applies today. Nevertheless, evaluation of the patient's physiological responses is important to anesthetic dose requirement and is applicable to the horse (Box 15-4). In using various stages as a guide to determining anesthetic dose, it is important to recognize that the moment-to-moment patient outcome is a balance between anesthetic-induced CNS depression and arousal by noxious stimulation. The intensity of stimulation is variable and arbitrarily graded strong or weak. Skin incision and intestinal, nerve, and ovarian traction represent strong stimuli; whereas intestinal suturing and arthroscopic surgery are often weak stimuli.

For practical purposes, three planes of surgical anesthesia are recognized in the horse: too light, adequate, and too deep. Although individual circumstances may vary and depend on numerous factors, the characteristics of premedicated horses anesthetized with a regimen of a ketamine-based anesthetic induction and inhalation anesthetic maintenance are definable (Table 15-3).

PHARMACOKINETICS OF INHALED ANESTHETICS

The precise mechanism of action of inhaled drugs is not known; however, it is clear that sites of action are within the brain and more recently recognized in the spinal cord.[18-24] The pharmacokinetics of inhalation anesthetics include, but are not limited to, anesthetic delivery to the lungs, uptake into the systemic circulation, distribution to the brain (and other tissues), and elimination.[9,25] Inhalation anesthetics, like respiratory gases (e.g., oxygen [O_2] and carbon dioxide [CO_2]), "move" down partial pressure gradients from regions of higher pressure to those of lower pressure (Figure 15-1). It is necessary to achieve a critical partial pressure of anesthetic in the CNS to achieve a desired anesthetic effect.

Box 15–4   Useful Variables to Consider in Clinical Assessment of Anesthetic Depth

Cardiovascular System
Heart rate and rhythm*
Arterial blood pressure†
Mucous membrane color
Capillary refill time

Respiratory System
Breathing frequency†
Ventilatory volume (tidal and minute ventilation)*
Character of breathing†
Arterial or end-tidal CO_2 partial pressure†

Muscle
Presence or absence of gross purposeful movement†
Shivering or trembling*
Muscle tone

Eye
Eye position or movement of eye†
Pupil size
Pupil response to light
Palpebral reflex
Corneal reflex
Lacrimation*

Miscellaneous
Body temperature
Laryngeal reflex*
Swallowing†
Sweating*
Urine flow*
Anal sphincter tone

Specificity in assessment of anesthetic depth of horses: *moderate; †high.

Table 15–3.   Some general characteristics of horses at three levels of general anesthesia*

Variable	Anesthetic plane		
	Too light	Adequate	Too deep
Heart rate	28-60	28-36	<28
Arterial blood pressure (systolic)	>100	90-120	<90
Breathing rate	>8	4-8	<4
Character of breathing	Irregular	Regular	Regular or irregular
Arterial CO_2 partial pressure	<50	50-70	>70
Eye position	Nystagmus	"Wandering"	Central fix
Palpebral reflex	+	±	−
Corneal reflex	+	+	±
Lacrimation	+	±	−
Purposeful muscle movement	+	−	−
Swallowing			
Sweating	+	−	−

*Spontaneously breathing adult horses are presumed premedicated with an α_2-agonist; anesthesia is induced with benzodiazepine and ketamine, perhaps including guaifenesin; and anesthesia is maintained with an inhaled, volatile anesthetic delivered in oxygen.

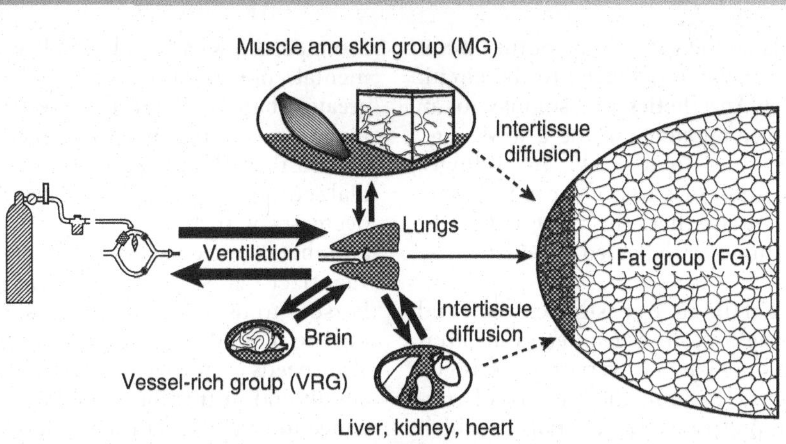

Figure 15–1. The drug delivery system for inhalant anesthetics is the lung. Adequate ventilation and cardiac output determine anesthetic delivery to the three major tissue groups: the muscle group (MG); the fat group (FG); and the vessel-rich group (VRG), which has the highest blood flow per gram of tissue and includes the heart, liver, kidney, and brain. The thicker arrows (e.g., *VRG*) represent greater blood flow and greater drug delivery. The FG has the lowest blood flow per gram of tissue (*thin arrows*) but is represented by a large circle because it can function as an anesthetic depot because of a much higher affinity (tissue/blood partition coefficient) for inhalant anesthetics than the other tissues (*VRG, MG*). More and more inhalant anesthetic is taken up by the FG (*shaded area in FG*) during longer anesthetic episodes. In addition, inhalant anesthetic is transferred (intertissue diffusion) to the FG (interrupted lines) during longer anesthetic episodes. Very little inhalant anesthetic is lost as a result of metabolism. Less inhalant anesthetic is taken up by the MG or FG during short-duration anesthesia (< 60 minutes), leading to more rapid recovery from anesthesia and fewer lingering inhalant anesthetic-related drug effects (disorientation, depression, weakness, ataxia).

By controlling the partial pressure of anesthetic delivered to the anesthetic machine, a gradient is established between the anesthetic machine and the CNS. In time the CNS partial pressure of anesthetic equilibrates with that in arterial blood, and arterial blood anesthetic partial pressure equilibrates with the alveolar partial pressure. Thus the alveolar anesthetic tension is of pivotal importance in attaining and maintaining a level of anesthesia; it also determines the magnitude of drug elsewhere in the body. The measurement of alveolar anesthetic tension becomes a reliable method of monitoring anesthetic dose (e.g., MAC). The inspired anesthetic is reduced to zero during anesthetic recovery so that a reversal in gradients occurs, and the anesthetic moves down the gradient from CNS to blood to alveoli to atmosphere when the anesthetic partial pressure is essentially zero.

Anesthetic Uptake: Factors That Determine the Alveolar Partial Pressure of Anesthetic

The alveolar anesthetic tension is a balance between anesthetic input (i.e., delivery to alveoli) and uptake (by blood) from the lungs (Box 15-5).

Box 15–5 Factors Affecting Alveolar Uptake/Elimination[9]

- Inspired concentration
- Ventilation
- Solubility
- Cardiac output
- Alveolar to mixed venous partial pressure difference
- Tissue uptake
- Tissue capacity and tissue blood flow

Delivery to Alveoli

The magnitude and rate of anesthetic delivery to the alveoli depend on the inspired concentration and alveolar ventilation. Increasing the inspired concentration (e.g., increasing the vaporizer dial setting) and supplementing alveolar ventilation (e.g., controlled mechanical ventilation) increase delivery of anesthetic and cause the alveolar anesthetic tension to rise. This in turn results in a more rapid induction of anesthesia. Conversely, a decreased inspired partial pressure or decreased ventilation decreases the alveolar anesthetic partial pressure and slows induction of anesthesia.

Characteristics of the equipment used to deliver inhalation anesthetics to adult horses significantly influence the development of, and changes in, inspired concentration and in turn the magnitude and rate of rise of anesthetic (and O_2) in the lungs (see Chapter 16).[26,27]

Anesthetic Delivery Apparatus

Both the horse's large size and its accompanying large minute ventilatory volume and gas flow rate impose some unique requirements for anesthetic delivery equipment (see Chapter 16). For example, unlike smaller animals, a to-and-fro or, most commonly, a circle breathing circuit is all but mandatory for safely managing inhalation anesthesia in adult horses under clinical conditions. A large-animal anesthetic machine (LAAM) usually includes a circle patient breathing circuit. Breathing circuits consist of large-bore tubing and include a rebreathing or reservoir bag with a capacity of at least 20 L and a CO_2 absorber of about 6-L capacity. This is in contrast to a comparable system for anesthetic management of humans or dogs and cats that has a smaller *total* internal gas volume of about 5 to 7 L. The large internal gas volume of a LAAM dilutes inflowing (delivered; i.e., the concentration from the vaporizer) anesthetic gases and delays the time for equilibration between delivered and inspired anesthetic partial pressure. Consequently, the equilibration time depends on the gas volume of the circuit and the rate at which anesthetic is delivered to the circuit (i.e., fresh gas inflow).[9,27] Anesthetics are soluble to an important degree in some components of the LAAM (e.g., rubber, soda lime, plastics; see Table 15-1). Accordingly, depending on the composition of parts of the LAAM and the magnitude of uptake of anesthetic by these materials, the "apparent" dilution volume for delivered anesthetic may be further influenced.

To minimize the impact of the large anesthetic circuit and potential delays in reaching a desired inspired concentration, the anesthetist should: (1) avoid oversized anesthetic delivery and CO_2 absorbers; (2) limit the amount of rubber goods in the circuit in preference to materials in which anesthetics are less soluble; and (3) when possible, limit the volume of the rebreathing bag and the length of "elephant" hoses that compose the breathing circuitry.

Alternatively, a large fresh gas inflow rate may be used to decrease the delay in the rate of rise of the inspired oxygen and the alveolar partial pressure of anesthetic (Figure 15-2). However, there are limits to this tactic. First, high gas inflow wastes carrier gas and anesthetic drug, making this technique more costly, especially with the two newest anesthetic agents desflurane and sevoflurane. Second, in the absence of waste gas scavenging equipment, operating room personnel are undesirably exposed to greater environmental concentrations of anesthetic. Finally, at flow rates greater than 10 L/min, the anesthetic output of many normally functioning precision, agent-specific vaporizers may be less than the dialed concentration (especially at higher dial settings; e.g., 3% or more); and vaporizer output further decreases with time.[28-31] The consequence is that inspired anesthetic concentration may actually decrease (for a given vaporizer dial setting). A clinical compromise for an adult horse is to use fresh gas inflows totaling 8 to 10 L/min during the first 10 to 15 minutes of anesthesia (this maneuver also speeds denitrogenation [80% N_2 in air] of the breathing circuit and in turn hastens the increase of inspired oxygen concentration)[26] and then reduce inflow to about 3 to 6 L/min, depending on clinical conditions.

Physical Consequences of Uptake

Before proceeding to examine the impact of factors influencing removal of anesthetic from the alveolus, it is important to highlight briefly two physical consequences of anesthetic uptake that influence the inspired concentration: the concentration effect and the second gas effect. These two factors influence the rate of rise of the inspired concentration as opposed to the upper limit or absolute magnitude of the inspired concentration.

Concentration effect.[9,32] Increasing the inspired concentration accelerates the rate of rise of the alveolar concentration. This phenomenon is commonly known as the concentration effect[32] and is caused by augmentation of alveolar ventilation, which concentrates anesthetic molecules in the alveoli.

Second gas effect.[9,33,34] The second gas effect occurs when two anesthetics are administered concurrently.[9,35] It is especially related to circumstances in which one of these two gases (i.e., the first gas) is given in a high concentration. Because of the high concentration (i.e., large pressure gradient for escape from the lung), the large volume uptake of the first gas from the lung by blood accelerates the rate of rise of the concurrently administered second gas. This phenomenon results from the same two factors that produce the concentration effect: a concentrating action caused by anesthetic uptake and an augmentation of alveolar ventilation. The second gas, the inhalant anesthetic, is clinically most important when considered in association with the use of N_2O.

The consequences of these two effects are, at best, of questionable importance to the anesthetic management of horses. The influence of the LAAM likely blunts or prevents any practical impact in the anesthetic management of adult horses. These effects may have marginal clinical importance in the anesthetic management of foals because smaller breathing circuits are used and the uptake of N_2O by the foal during the first 5 to 10 minutes of anesthesia is probably sufficiently large to produce a detectable second gas effect. But even this explanation does not provide strong evidence of clinical relevance.[36]

Uptake by Blood

Anesthetic uptake from the lung by blood is the product of three factors: anesthetic solubility (i.e., blood/gas

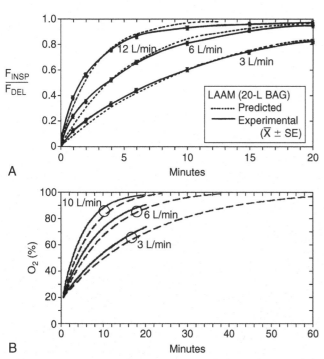

Figure 15–2. A, Rate of increase of inspired halothane concentration toward a constant delivered concentration (F_{insp}/F_{Del}) in a 32-L large-animal anesthetic machine *(LAAM)* at fresh gas inflow rates of 3, 6, and 12 L/min. **B,** Measured *(solid line)* and predicted *(dotted line)* rate of increase of oxygen (O_2) concentration for a large-animal circle-anesthetic system with a 40-L breathing bag and inflow of fresh O_2 at rates of 3, 6, and 10 L/min. Time 0 = start of inflow of fresh O_2. **(A** From Steffey EP, Howland D: Rate of change of halothane concentration in a large-animal anesthetic circle system, *Am J Vet Res* 48:1993, 1977.) **(B** From Solano AM, Brosnan RJ, Steffey EP: Rate of change of oxygen concentration for a large-animal circle anesthetic system, *Am J Vet Res* 66:1675, 2005.)

PC of the drug), cardiac output, and the difference in anesthetic partial pressure in alveolar gas and venous blood (i.e., the intercompartment gradient for anesthetic molecule movement).

It is perhaps helpful at this point to refocus on the primary objective, which is to achieve an optimal partial pressure of anesthetic in the brain. It is also valuable to remember that the brain (and other body tissues) tends to equilibrate with the partial pressure of anesthetic drug brought to it by arterial blood and that the partial pressure in arterial blood equilibrates with the alveolar anesthetic partial pressure (i.e., alveolar partial pressure > arterial partial pressure > brain [CNS] partial pressure). Therefore maintaining an optimal alveolar anesthetic partial pressure is a reliable method for controlling and mirroring the anesthetic partial pressure in the brain.

An unimpeded transfer of anesthetic from the lungs to the blood is necessary for anesthetic induction. Efficient transfer of anesthetic may be influenced by impediments to diffusion or improper matching of ventilation and lung blood flow. Normally the alveolar capillary membrane is no barrier to diffusion of inhaled anesthetics. However, maldistribution of ventilation and blood flow frequently exists, even in normal horses during inhalation anesthesia. Intrapulmonary shunts or shuntlike effects (e.g., perfusion of unventilated alveoli) tend to slow anesthetic induction because shunted blood contains no anesthetic and dilutes the partial pressure of anesthetic in blood from ventilated alveoli properly matched with blood flow (see Chapter 2).

A high pressure gradient between the alveoli and venous blood enhances removal of anesthetic from the lungs and thereby decreases the alveolar anesthetic partial pressure. Other things being equal (including a similar and constant inspired anesthetic partial pressure), an anesthetic with a relatively high blood/gas PC (i.e., highly blood soluble) fosters a large pressure gradient between blood and alveoli and thereby tends to maintain a lower alveolar partial pressure of anesthetic and retard the rise of the anesthetic partial pressure of the brain. Similarly, cardiac output influences anesthetic uptake. An elevated cardiac output (e.g., an excited patient or a patient responding to heightened intensity of surgical stimulation) increases the amount of blood matched with alveoli per unit time and results in a more rapid uptake. Consequently, the rate of rise of the alveolar anesthetic partial pressure and anesthetic induction is slowed. A low cardiac output (e.g., as occurs in shock) decreases the uptake from the lung and alveolar partial pressure increases more rapidly. Because a greater proportion of drug taken up by blood is distributed to the CNS (vessel-rich group tissue), induction of anesthesia is more rapid. Finally, maintaining a low venous blood partial pressure of anesthetic prolongs the development of an anesthetic state. For a given alveolar anesthetic partial pressure, the magnitude of venous partial pressure is a reflection of tissue uptake. Tissue uptake in turn is governed by factors similar to those that govern uptake from the lung: anesthetic solubility in tissues (i.e., the tissue/blood PC), tissue (i.e., regional) blood flow, and the anesthetic partial pressure difference between arterial blood and the tissue (i.e., the intercompartment transfer gradient). For example, conditions that tend to cause blood flow to muscle to increase (e.g., excitement, exercise, stress) may produce delays in attaining adequate alveolar anesthetic partial pressure because of the large tissue

reservoir for anesthetic, which delays adequate brain anesthetic levels.

Three factors can further influence the magnitude of arterial-to-venous anesthetic partial pressure gradient: loss across the skin,[37] loss into closed gas spaces, and metabolism. None of these is a major factor in anesthetic uptake or the rate of rise of alveolar anesthetic partial pressure during clinical anesthesia. Transcutaneous movement of anesthetic occurs, but in small quantity. However, the other two factors play a role in anesthetic uptake and management and are addressed in later sections.

Summary

Understanding the factors that determine a rapid rise in alveolar anesthetic partial pressure is important to skillful, effective control of inhalation anesthesia. Factors that promote an increase in alveolar anesthetic tension foster improved control of general anesthesia and are related to increased alveolar delivery and decreased removal of anesthetic from alveoli. Increased delivery is accomplished by factors increasing the inspired tension of anesthetic and an increased ventilatory (alveolar) minute volume. Decreased removal from the alveoli is related to a decreased anesthetic solubility, cardiac output, or alveolar-venous anesthetic partial pressure gradient.

Anesthetic Elimination

Many of the factors that regulate the rate of fall of the alveolar anesthetic partial pressure (i.e., recovery from anesthesia) are identical to those governing the previously discussed rate of rise (i.e., anesthetic induction) and include alveolar ventilation, anesthetic solubility, and cardiac output (see Box 15-5).

The alveolar anesthetic partial pressure rapidly declines after anesthetic is removed from the inspired breath. The initial decrease (first few moments) is very rapid and related to washout of the functional residual capacity by ventilation. In general, large minute alveolar ventilation speeds this decrease, whereas a low alveolar ventilatory volume (hypoventilation) delays anesthetic removal from the body and the rate of recovery. At this point it must be stressed that *minute alveolar ventilation* is the operant term and that both frequency of breathing and the effective breath size (i.e., tidal volume minus dead space volume) determine the magnitude of minute alveolar ventilation. An increase or decrease in frequency of breathing does not in itself signify elevated or depressed alveolar ventilation (see Chapter 2).

Washout

As ventilation removes anesthetic from the alveoli, a gradient in anesthetic partial pressure develops between the pulmonary arterial blood (i.e., venous blood returning from tissues) and the alveoli. This gradient fosters anesthetic movement from blood to the alveoli, and this intercompartmental exchange in turn opposes the effect of ventilation to lower the amount of alveolar anesthetic. The magnitude of impact is related again to anesthetic solubility (i.e., its blood gas PC). The slowing effect (i.e., delayed recovery) is greater with a higher blood-soluble drug such as halothane, less with sevoflurane, and least with low blood-soluble drugs such as N_2O and desflurane. This is because for soluble drugs there is far more anesthetic in blood (i.e., more anesthetic molecules) for a given partial pressure and the blood serves as a larger reservoir of anesthetic. Accordingly, all other factors being equal, the alveolar partial pressure of anesthetic decreases more slowly with more soluble drugs.

Although the speed of recovery from inhalation anesthesia depends largely on drug solubility in blood, anesthetic washout from the blood is also related to anesthetic concentration and duration.[38] Anesthetic recovery differs from induction in this regard. The accumulation and storage of anesthetic in tissues differs with anesthetic dose and time. Consequently, tissues are variably equilibrated with anesthetic at the end of anesthesia. If large quantities of inhaled anesthetic are dissolved in blood and other tissues (i.e., soluble anesthetics), they serve as a reservoir that maintains the alveolar partial pressure (when the partial pressure gradients are reversed to foster anesthetic removal at the conclusion of anesthesia); the result is a slower recovery. Consequently, it is expected that, other variables being constant, recovery will be longer after halothane than isoflurane. Incomplete equilibration of anesthetic between tissues and blood allows the alveolar anesthetic partial pressure to fall most rapidly. Thus recovery time after a short exposure to an inhalant anesthetic is less than after a longer exposure (greater tissue accumulation) to a similar alveolar concentration (see Figure 15-1).

The patient breathing circuit may further limit the rate of recovery. Here, as during anesthetic induction, the volume of the circuit commonly used in the anesthetic management of adult horses is of special and substantial concern. If the patient is not disconnected from the circuit at the end of anesthesia, recovery is delayed by the large volume of anesthetic resident in the existing circuit gas, rebreathing of previously exhaled anesthetic, and reentry of anesthetic from rubber and other components of the circuit (see Table 15-1). If there are specific reasons the equine patient must continue to breathe from the circuit at the end of anesthetic delivery (an important safety consideration for patient and staff) and recovery time is of some concern, maneu-

vers that hasten drug loss from the anesthetic circuit (i.e., flush ["flush valve"] the system a few times with pure oxygen, maintain a small but adequate rebreathing bag size for tidal breathing, and increase the fresh gas [anesthetic-free] inflow) can be instituted.

Diffusion Hypoxia

During recovery from anesthesia that includes N_2O, the movement of large volumes of N_2O into the lungs may cause a condition termed *diffusion hypoxia*.[9,14,25,39] It deserves particular emphasis when discussing the anesthetic management of horses (see The Gaseous Anesthetic—Nitrous Oxide later in the chapter).

Biotransformation

The illusion that inhalation anesthetics are chemically inert and resistant to biotransformation (metabolism) in the body has been shattered,[40] and it is now recognized that inhalation drugs undergo varying degrees of metabolism (Table 15-4).[41-44] Biotransformation occurs primarily in the liver but also to lesser degrees in the lung, kidney, and intestinal tract.[45]

Metabolism is low enough that it does not influence the rate of anesthetic induction; however, it may minimally influence (shorten) anesthetic recovery from the more soluble anesthetic drugs such as halothane. Metabolism of sevoflurane, but especially isoflurane and desflurane, is too small (see Table 15-4) to have an important impact in this regard.[46,47] However, of greater practical and clinical significance is the relationship of biodegradation and production of metabolites that may be systemically toxic.[48,49] This is discussed in greater depth later in this chapter.

PHARMACODYNAMICS: THE ACTIONS AND TOXICITY OF INHALATION ANESTHETICS

The actions of inhaled anesthetics on organ systems are in reality side effects that accompany general anesthesia

Table 15–4.   Biotransformation of inhalation anesthetics in humans*

Anesthetic	Anesthetic recovered as metabolites (%)	Principal metabolites[265]
Halothane[43,144]	20-25	Trifluoroacetic acid Cl Br (chlorotrifluoroethane, chlorodifluoroethene, Fl)†
Sevoflurane[220]	3	Hexafluoroisopropanolol Fl
Isoflurane[189]	0.17	Trifluoroacetic acid Trifluoroacetaldehyde Trifluoroacetylchloride
Desflurane[220]	0.02	Trifluoroacetic acid Fl CO_2 Water
Nitrous oxide[45]	0.004	N_2 Inactivated methionine synthase Reduced cobalamin (vitamin B_{12})

*Similar patterns of metabolism in horses.
†Reductive metabolism.

Table 15–5. **Comparative summary of characteristics of halothane, isoflurane, sevoflurane, and desflurane**

Characteristic							
Chemical stability	[D]*	>	I	>	S	>	H
Blood solubility	H	>	I	>	S	>	[D]
MAC	D	>	S	>	I	>	[H]
Circulatory depression†	H	>	I	≥	S	>	[D]
Dysrhythmia with catecholamines	H	>	[I]	=	[S]	=	[D]
Respiratory depression	D	≥	S	≥	I	>	[H]
Apneic dose of inhalant	D (11%)‡	>	[H] (2.6%)	>	I (2.3%)	=	S (2.3%)
Muscle relaxation	[D]	≥	[S]	≥	[I]	>	H
Metabolism	H	>	S	>	I	>	[D]
Seizure activity	S	>	[D]	=	[I]	=	[H]

D, Desflurane; H, halothane; I, isoflurane; S, sevoflurane.
*Brackets indicate desired superiority.
†During conditions of controlled ventilation.
‡Requires further investigation.

(Table 15-5). Knowledge of these properties is required for the safe conduct of general anesthesia in horses. The influence of inhaled drugs on the circulatory, respiratory, and other life-support systems may be general (i.e., common to most or all drugs), or it may be a more specific or prominent influence of one drug.

The properties of the volatile agents (noted in historical order) halothane, isoflurane, desflurane, and sevoflurane are discussed because they are in present use for anesthetic management of horses and specific data derived from controlled laboratory and clinical studies are available. When possible, data from healthy, young adult horses exposed to known alveolar concentrations of inhalation drugs are emphasized. Results of measurements from spontaneously breathing horses form the basis for comparing actions of inhalation anesthetics because this condition more commonly mimics general clinical practice. The response of surgical patients may be different from data derived under laboratory circumstances because other variables (e.g., surgery, blood loss, pain) confound interpretation in the clinical setting. The impact of coexisting factors such as disease, surgical stimulation, adjuvant drug therapy, extremes of age, anesthetic duration, intermittent positive-pressure ventilation (IPPV), and altered intravascular fluid volume must be considered and are mentioned when specific information from studies of horses is known.

The Volatile Anesthetics

Halothane

Effects on cardiovascular function. Halothane causes a dose-related depression of cardiovascular function in horses, ponies,[50-54] and other species.[55,56]

Cardiac output. Halothane causes a decrease in cardiac output compared to values in awake, unsedated, or lightly tranquilized horses;[5] the magnitude of this decrease is related to the alveolar inhalant anesthetic concentration of halothane (Figure 15-3).[53,54] The cardiac output usually decreases because the stroke volume of the heart decreases.[54] In vitro[57] and in vivo[58] studies of heart muscle show that contractility is reduced by halothane.

The horse's heart rate usually changes minimally (perhaps an increase) or not at all during inhalant anesthesia (see

Figure 15-3).[5,53,54] There may be an inconsistent increase or decrease at the extremes of an anesthetic dose.

Halothane may increase the automaticity of the heart muscle. Spontaneous dysrhythmias have been reported in horses anesthetized with halothane,[54,59,60] but clinical and laboratory experience suggests that their overall incidence is low.[61] Impulses from ectopic sites within the atria and especially the ventricles are possible responses to endogenous or injected catecholamines, but halothane sensitization of the myocardium to catecholamines may not be clinically relevant in horses.[62] Increased secretion of catecholamines may occur as a result of surgical stimulation and insufficient anesthesia or from an elevation in arterial CO_2 tension ($PaCO_2$) secondary to hypoventilation.[63] Epinephrine is sometimes injected during surgery to aid in the control of local tissue bleeding or as part of resuscitative therapy. Although dysrhythmias in horses are usually infrequent and benign, they may be important in the presence of other factors such as cardiac disease, hypotension, and electrolyte abnormalities.

Dysrhythmias during halothane anesthesia are also increased by hypercapnia[62] or sympathomimetic drugs (e.g., ephedrine, norepinephrine, phenylephrine, dopamine, and dobutamine) commonly administered to increase blood pressure and improve circulatory system function.[50,61,64-66] The incidence of ventricular dysrhythmias is low with clinical doses of ephedrine and phenylephrine but increased in horses with colic, endotoxemia, or shock.[66]

The baroreceptor reflex is a short-term central mechanism for systemic arterial blood pressure homeostasis. An acute decrease or increase in arterial blood pressure is detected by the baroreceptors and tends to cause a reflex increase or decrease, respectively, in heart rate. The sensitivity of the baroreceptor reflex in adult horses is particularly sensitive to inhalant anesthesia and markedly depressed in the horse by halothane.[64]

Systemic arterial blood pressure. Halothane decreases arterial blood pressure. The magnitude of this reduction is directly related to the alveolar anesthetic concentration (see Figure 15-3).[14,50-54]

The decrease in arterial blood pressure that accompanies an increase in alveolar halothane concentration is related to the decrease in cardiac output because total vascular resistance does not change greatly or may increase.[53]

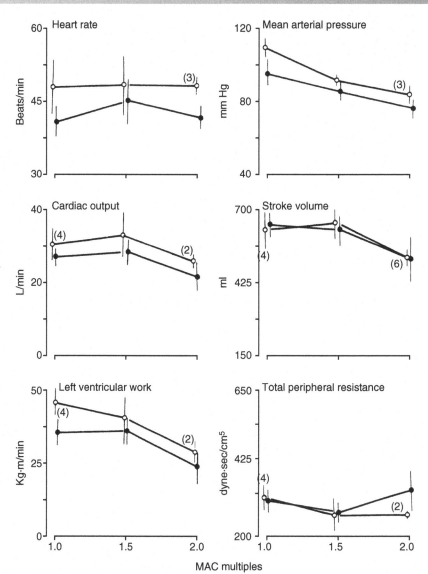

Figure 15–3. Effects of isoflurane (○) and halothane (●) in five horses during spontaneous ventilation. There are no significant differences between isoflurane and halothane at equipotent doses (i.e. equal MAC multiples). (), number of horses if less than 5. (From Steffey EP, Howland D: Comparison of circulatory and respiratory effects of isoflurane and halothane anesthesia in horses, *Am J Vet Res* 41:821, 1980.)

Modifiers of circulatory effects

Controlled ventilation. Controlled mechanical IPPV is commonly used in the anesthetic management of horses to maintain or normalize $PaCO_2$. Equipotent alveolar doses of halothane are more depressing to equine circulatory system function (especially cardiac output) when ventilation is mechanically controlled and $PaCO_2$ is normal compared with conditions of spontaneous ventilation (Figure 15-4).[53,54,67] The magnitude of the effect of IPPV on hemodynamics may be influenced further by body position (i.e., more depressing in dorsally recumbent [supine] horses compared to similar conditions in a lateral posture).[68]

The influence of IPPV is probably related to at least two factors. First, an elevated intrathoracic pressure caused by mechanical ventilation depresses return of blood (venous return) to the heart and thereby limits the stroke volume of the heart. Second, halothane depresses ventilation and causes $PaCO_2$ to increase in a dose-related fashion (see Effects on Respiratory Function and Chapter 17). The net effect of hypercapnia in anesthetized normal animals is usually to heighten sympathetic nervous system activity as evidenced by increased plasma epinephrine and norepinephrine concentrations.[63,69] This condition in turn causes an increase in

cardiac output and systemic arterial blood pressure[56,63,69,70] but may be associated with increased risk of developing ventricular arrhythmias (especially in association with halothane).[62]

Hypoxemia. Compared to normoxic halothane-anesthetized horses, heart rate and cardiac output are increased during hypoxemia.[71]

Surgery and noxious stimulation. Surgery and other forms of noxious stimulation modify the circulatory effects of halothane in horses[14,54,72,73] and other species,[55,56,74] presumably by causing pain or stress that stimulates the sympathetic nervous system (see Chapter 4).

Noxious stimulation may increase arterial blood pressure at light levels of halothane anesthesia (i.e., 1.2 to 1.5 MAC). Hypertension may occur in conjunction with pain.[75] The magnitude of rise in blood pressure accompanying noxious stimulation varies with degree and duration of stimulation, increasing anesthetic depth and/or accompanying adjuvant drugs (*infra-vida*).[56,73,74,76] Paradoxically, at very light levels (i.e., around 1.0 MAC or less) a small decrease rather than an increase in blood pressure occasionally may occur.

Severe blood loss. Arterial blood pressure decreases as blood loss increases. The horse's heart rate does not change dramatically during halothane anesthesia and severe hemorrhage.[77]

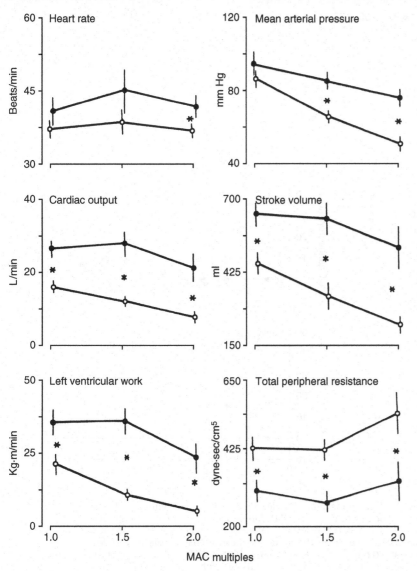

Figure 15–4. Effects of halothane during spontaneous (●) and controlled (○) ventilation in five horses. The mean ± SE is indicated. *MAC,* Minimum alveolar concentration for horses. *Indicates significance P<0.05. Note the lower peripheral vascular resistance and greater cardiac output and stroke volume during spontaneous ventilation. (Data adapted from studies of Steffey and Howland.[53] (From Steffey EP, Howland D: Comparison of circulatory and respiratory effects of isoflurane and halothane anesthesia in horses, *Am J Vet Res* 41:821, 1980.)

Duration of anesthesia. The cardiovascular effects of halothane change with the duration of anesthesia. Halothane anesthesia lasting 5 to 6 hours in humans is associated with an increase in cardiac output and heart rate.[55,78,79] These time-related changes are prevented if humans are administered propranolol before anesthesia, suggesting the mechanism relates to increased sympathetic nervous system activity.[80]

Time-related increases in arterial blood pressure, stroke volume, and cardiac output are noted consistently in studies of laterally recumbent horses (Figure 15-5).[54,71,81,82] Time-related adjustments are noted, regardless of the mode of ventilation,[82,83] but may be modified by body posture.[81,84-86] Although these changes in cardiovascular function are probably of little clinical relevance (anesthetic durations of 2 hours or less), they must be considered when interpreting results of data from halothane studies in horses.

Coexisting drugs. Prior or concurrent drug therapy may influence cardiovascular function by altering anesthetic requirement (i.e., MAC) or by the specific cardiovascular actions of the drug. For example, drugs such as acepromazine and xylazine are popularly administered before the induction of anesthesia to produce calming and sedation (see Chapter 10). They likely decrease MAC to varying degrees,[87-89] but they also have direct cardiovascular effects.[90] Accordingly, they may decrease arterial blood pressure beyond what might be expected by halothane alone.[91] The mechanism for this action differs between these two injectable drugs and includes a decrease in cardiac output (xylazine) versus a decrease in total peripheral vascular resistance (i.e., vasodilation with acepromazine). The administration of analgesic anesthetic adjuncts may help to decrease the amount of inhalant drug required to maintain anesthetic, thereby improving hemodynamics while improving analgesia.[92]

Anesthetic induction drugs such as thiobarbiturates and guaifenesin also confound the primary effects of halothane and may accentuate cardiovascular depression (see Chapter 12).[93-95] In contrast, the presence of sympathomimetic drugs such as ephedrine,[50] dopamine, dobutamine,[65,96,97] and phenylephrine[97,98] lessen the depressive aspects of halothane-induced circulatory system depression and are frequently administered clinically to counteract arterial hypotension (see Chapters 22 and 23). Concurrent use of opioids such as morphine (and possibly fentanyl) increase heart rate and or systemic arterial blood pressure.[99,100]

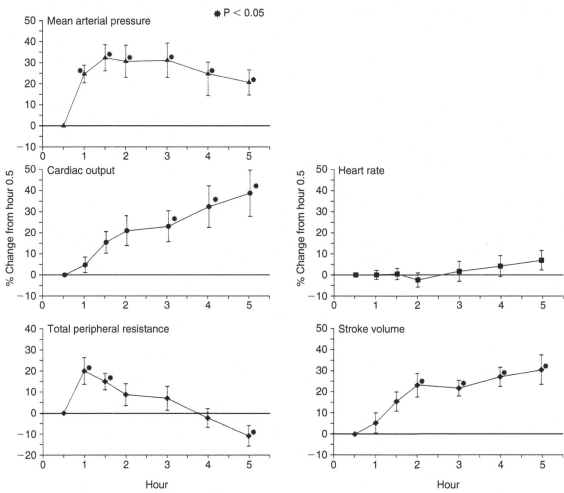

Figure 15–5. Time-related changes (mean ± SE) in mean arterial blood pressure, cardiac output, and total peripheral resistance *(left);* and heart rate and stroke volume *(right)* during 5 hours of a constant alveolar concentration (1.06%) of halothane in 10 spontaneously breathing, laterally recumbent horses. * Indicates significant difference (P<0.05) from the 0.5-hour value. Note the increase in mean arterial pressure and cardiac output with little or no change in heart rate. (From Steffey EP, Kelly AB, Woliner MJ: Time-related responses of spontaneously breathing, laterally recumbent horses to prolonged anesthesia with halothane, *Am J Vet Res* 48:952, 1987.)

Effects on respiratory function

Anesthetic dose. Halothane and other inhaled anesthetics cause a dose-related depression in respiratory system function that is characterized by an increase in the partial pressure of CO_2 in arterial blood (Figure 15-6) and a decreased ability to oxygenate arterial blood. This latter effect is manifested as an increased difference between the partial pressure of oxygen in alveolar gas and arterial blood and perhaps hypoxemia.[5,53,54,101-105] The magnitude of this depression for a given dose of halothane is substantially greater in horses than other commonly studied species, including humans (Figure 15-7), despite similar blood gas values in these species when the individuals are awake and unmedicated.[78,101,104-108]

Compared with awake conditions, light halothane anesthesia is associated with a decrease in breathing frequency. The magnitude of respiratory rate depression does not change appreciably or may increase slightly as anesthetic dose is increased from 1.0 MAC to 2.0 MAC (see Figure 15-6).[53,104] Tidal volume tends to decrease over the same range.[109] Respiratory rate decreases at very deep levels (i.e.,

greater than 2.0 MAC) of anesthesia. The average alveolar concentration of halothane at which the horse's spontaneous respiratory effort ceases for at least 1 minute (i.e., the apneic concentration) is 2.4% or 2.6% MAC (see Table 15-5).[104]

Modifiers of ventilatory responses

Mode of ventilation. To compensate for halothane-induced respiratory depression, ventilation is frequently assisted or controlled by mechanical means (see Chapter 17). The horse regulates its own rate of breathing, and the anesthetist determines the horse's tidal volume during assisted ventilation. Accordingly, assisted ventilation may improve the efficiency of oxygenating blood (and thereby the arterial oxygen partial pressure [$PaCO_2$]) and minimize the work of breathing, but it is not especially effective in lowering the $PaCO_2$.[67,110] Controlled ventilation of the lungs (i.e., controlled tidal volume and respiratory rate) is necessary to predictably decrease and maintain a normal $PaCO_2$ during inhalation anesthesia.

Surgery and noxious stimulation. Like cardiovascular function, noxious stimulation accompanying surgery may result in CNS arousal sufficient to increase ventilation.[76,111,112]

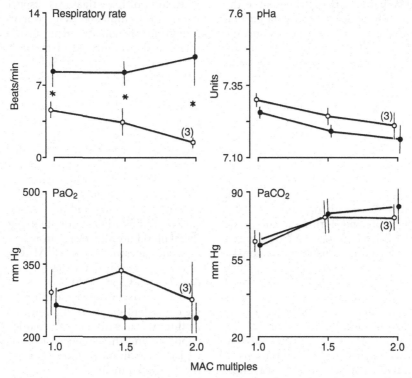

Figure 15–6. Respiratory effects of halothane (●) and isoflurane (○) in five horses during spontaneous ventilation.[53] The mean ± SE is indicated; and the number of observations, if fewer than 5, is indicated in parentheses. Significant differences (P< 0.05) between observations during halothane and isoflurane anesthesia are indicated by*. (From Steffey EP, Howland D: Comparison of circulatory and respiratory effects of isoflurane and halothane anesthesia in horses, *Am J Vet Res* 41:821, 1980.)

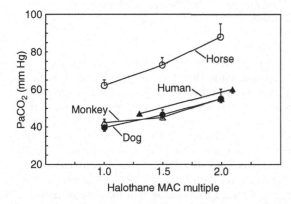

Figure 15–7. Arterial PCO₂ (mean ± SE) in spontaneously breathing, healthy dogs, horses, humans, and monkeys during halothane-oxygen anesthesia. The anesthetic level is expressed as a MAC multiple for each species. Data are from Steffey et al. (dog, n = 8),[106] Steffey et al. (horse, n = 7),[104] Bahlman et al. (human, n = 8),[78] and Steffey et al. (monkey, n = 6).[107]

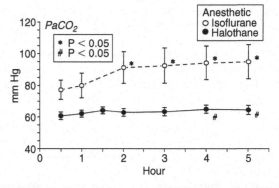

Figure 15–8. Time-related changes in PaCO₂ in spontaneously breathing horses anesthetized for 5 hours with a constant, equipotent end-tidal concentration (1.2 MAC) of halothane (n = 10)[82] or isoflurane (n = 10).[161]

The increase in ventilation may be sufficient to decrease PaCO₂ by 5 to 10 mm Hg.

Duration of anesthesia. The duration of a constant dose of halothane may also affect PaCO₂ (Figure 15-8). Results of studies in horses anesthetized for more than 5 hours at 1.2 MAC halothane suggest that PaCO₂ may rise a few millimeters of Mercury over time.[81,82] Because horses are rarely anesthetized for such long periods in clinical practice and the change in PaCO₂ found in reported horse studies was relatively small, this finding is probably of little clinical relevance.

Of greater clinical importance is the variability in arterial oxygen tension accompanying long-duration anesthesia and body posture.[81-86] Impaired arterial oxygenation is probably more likely related to events common to general anesthesia and body posture than uniquely related to halothane anesthesia (see Chapter 2).

Effects on the central nervous system. Administration of halothane increases cerebral blood flow (CBF) in humans and dogs.[113,114] Studies of ponies show similar results.[51] Since halothane can increase CBF in horses, it should also increase cerebral blood volume and in turn cerebrospinal fluid pressure (intracranial pressure or ICP) in this species as in others.[70] This could be particularly detrimental to the horse, given the extremes in head position during general anesthesia relative to normal awake circumstances and the associated large hydrostatic gradients between head and heart.[115] An increase in $PaCO_2$ increases ICP in halothane-anesthetized horses.[70]

There is considerable investigative activity related to neurological monitoring of anesthetized human patients, and it is understandable that applications used for this purpose in humans be considered during anesthetic management of horses. The electroencephalographic responses to halothane anesthesia (and other anesthetics) in horses varies. All anesthetic drugs do not produce the same changes in electroencephalogram (EEG) (raw or processed) pattern with changes in anesthetic dose. Anesthetic adjuvant drugs administered immediately before and during the anesthetic period further confound EEG recordings and thus interpretation. However, some general EEG patterns are consistent. In general, inhalation anesthetic drugs affect frequency (expressed in cycles/sec [Hz]) and amplitude (expressed in microvolts [μV]) of EEG waveforms. The brain waves become larger and slower in frequency compared to the awake condition in halothane-anesthetized horses,[116-119] similar to results in humans.[120] There is a further slowing of the EEG wave pattern with increasing concentrations of halothane. The EEG wave flattens (isoelectric EEG) at clinically excessive, cardiovascularly toxic doses. Surgical stimulation alters EEG pattern responses.[121]

Effects on the liver and its function. Like most inhaled anesthetics, halothane causes depression of hepatic function, which is likely dose related. Such depression may be exaggerated by decreased organ blood flow.

A study in dogs suggests that halothane markedly inhibits the drug-metabolizing capacity by the liver.[122] A reduction in intrinsic hepatic clearance of drugs fosters delayed drug removal or increases in plasma drug concentration during (e.g., fentanyl) anesthesia.[100,123] Prolonged or heightened plasma concentrations of some drugs have important toxic implications, especially if the physical status of the patient is already markedly compromised. Hepatic function usually returns to normal shortly after the termination of anesthesia unless conditions are severe enough to cause direct toxicity.

All of the contemporary inhaled anesthetics are capable of causing hepatotoxicity in laboratory animals. Evidence of injury may vary from slight-to-moderate increases in plasma levels of hepatic enzymes to the rare case, especially in humans, of fulminant hepatic failure. The liver damage most commonly described is centrilobular necrosis, and the incidence is greatest with halothane.[42]

Halothane-induced hepatotoxicity has rarely been reported in horses.[124-126] Laboratory and clinical studies using horses and ponies indicate that there are alterations in hepatic function and hepatic cell integrity associated with halothane anesthesia.[17,127-132] Horses anesthetized for more than 3 hours with halothane anesthesia are more likely to develop clinically important elevations in serum levels of hepatic-derived enzymes (e.g., transaminase, sorbitol dehydrogenase) than multiple short exposures.[128,133,134] Minimum or no increase in serum level would be expected following a single short (i.e., less than 1.5 hours) period of halothane anesthesia.

Results of investigations, especially in rats but including ponies, indicate that concurrent hypoxia or prior induction of hepatic drug-metabolizing enzymes may increase the likelihood of clinical signs of liver dysfunction after anesthesia.[42,129] Subsequent studies suggest that prolonged arterial hypotension[130,134] or hypoxemia[71,133] further increases the magnitude and duration of serum hepatic-derived enzyme concentrations after halothane anesthesia.

Effects on the kidney and its function. Inhalation anesthetics depress renal blood flow, glomerular filtration rate, and urinary flow in humans.[55] The effects reverse rapidly when anesthesia is discontinued. Results of studies of halothane-anesthetized ponies and horses under laboratory and clinical conditions indicate qualitatively similar responses.[51,131] Renal blood flow decreases from awake values by about 36% in ponies anesthetized at 1.0 MAC halothane.[51] Renal blood flow progressively decreases further with increasing alveolar dose (e.g., 73% at 2.0 MAC).

Serum urea nitrogen, creatinine, and inorganic phosphate are consistently increased immediately after halothane (and isoflurane) anesthesia.[131,132] Reduced anesthetic dose time exposure and the concurrent use of polyionic intravenous replacement fluids or both decrease the extent of the anesthesia-related insult.

Anesthetic-induced reductions in renal (and/or hepatic) function prolong or heighten plasma concentrations of some drugs. Although there is evidence of such concerns in horses anesthetized with halothane,[135] such effects are more broadly related to conditions associated with general anesthesia rather than the specific inhalation drug administered.[123,136]

Other effects

Malignant hyperthermia. Malignant hyperthermia (MH) is a potentially life-threatening pharmacogenetic myopathy most commonly reported in susceptible swine and human patients. Its occurrence has been reported in the horse.[137-141] MH is characterized by a rapid rise in body temperature in individuals anesthetized with a variety of drugs and techniques that frequently include halothane (see Chapter 22). Halothane is considered the most potent triggering drug among the contemporary inhaled anesthetics. The syndrome is referred to as malignant because of its rapid progression to irreversibility. The etiology in the horse was discussed recently.[142]

Changes in blood components. Results from several studies[130-132] using horses anesthetized with halothane indicate no clinically important changes in perianesthetic or postanesthetic serum electrolyte concentrations or quantitative evaluations of red and white blood cells (i.e., complete blood counts). Glucose frequently is transiently elevated immediately after anesthesia (see Chapter 4). There is also a mild leukocytosis (i.e., increased numbers of bands and mature neutrophils) noted for up to 1 to 2 days after halothane anesthesia. These transient changes are judged to be of no clinical relevance.

Halothane anesthesia is associated with a temporary, mild (but statistically significant) decrease in platelet number and function.[143] Platelet numbers declined during 8.0 MAC hours of halothane, but the platelet count returned to normal within 24 hours of anesthetic recovery. Platelet aggregation was reduced significantly during the anesthetic period and for up to 4 days after anesthesia. These findings are judged to be of little clinical consequence in healthy horses.

Biotransformation. About 20% to 25% of the administered halothane undergoes biotransformation (see Table 15-4), largely in the liver; and the rest is eliminated unchanged by way of the respiratory system (mostly) and other routes.[43,144] The major metabolite is trifluoroacetic acid, which is eliminated in the urine. Chloride, bromide, and only a very small amount of fluoride ions are also eliminated.[44] Increased plasma bromide concentration after halothane has been reported for both foals and horses.[145,146]

Isoflurane

Effects on cardiovascular function.
Isoflurane depresses cardiovascular function in horses in a dose-related manner.[53,104,147,148] The effects of isoflurane are qualitatively similar to those of halothane but less pronounced at surgical phases of anesthesia. Studies in a variety of species, including horses, indicate that, compared to halothane, a greater margin of cardiovascular safety is associated with isoflurane.[55,127,149-153]

Studies of unmedicated, spontaneously breathing horses suggest that a dose of 1.2 MAC isoflurane does not significantly alter cardiac output from awake values because a reduction in stroke volume is counterbalanced by a tendency for heart rate to increase.[154] Furthermore, isoflurane reduces afterload (time-dependent decrease in peripheral vascular resistance; see Figure 15-3; Figure 15-9).[9,154] Increases in heart rate are a characteristic of isoflurane and have also been noted in studies of foals.[149,155,156]

Mechanical ventilation in isoflurane-anesthetized horses impairs cardiovascular function compared to horses breathing spontaneously.[53,157] Similar studies in isoflurane-anesthetized horses indicate less depressed cardiac output during mechanical ventilation than in similarly managed halothane-anesthetized horses (Figure 15-10).[53,83,157] The magnitude of this sparing effect on cardiac output is greater with isoflurane as anesthetic dose is increased.

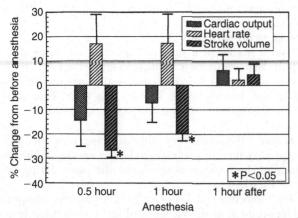

Figure 15–9. Changes (mean ± SE) in cardiac output and its determinants associated with 1.2 MAC isoflurane in O_2 anesthesia in seven horses. (From Steffey EP et al: Cardiovascular and respiratory measurements in awake and isoflurane-anesthetized horses, *Am J Vet Res* 48:7, 1987.)

Isoflurane decreases arterial blood pressure (Figure 15-11). The magnitude of the decrease in arterial blood pressure is anesthetic dose related and similar with equipotent doses of isoflurane versus halothane in adult horses[53,104,154] and foals.[149,156,158] However, studies of mechanically ventilated ponies suggest a greater reduction in arterial blood pressure by isoflurane.[51,147] The incidence of cardiac dysrhythmias after injection of vasoactive substances (catecholamines) is reduced substantially during isoflurane anesthesia.[55,66,151,159,160]

The duration of isoflurane anesthesia influences the magnitude of cardiovascular changes produced in horses.[83,161] Arterial blood pressure and cardiac output increase with time during prolonged constant-dose anesthesia compared with baseline values (Figure 15-12).[161,162] However, associated surgery and anesthetic adjuvant drugs may modify this temporal response.[92,127,152]

Postanesthetic myopathy is a potential complication of general anesthesia and has been attributed, at least in part, to ischemic muscle damage secondary to inadequate blood pressure and blood flow during anesthesia and recumbency.[130,163-166] Accordingly, techniques that preserve the adequacy of blood flow to muscles are of substantial interest. Muscle perfusion is increased during isoflurane anesthesia in humans.[55,167] Studies of muscle blood flow in horses are limited and conflicting, but results to date generally support the view that isoflurane, like halothane, reduces skeletal muscle blood flow (compared with that of awake conditions) and that any differences between isoflurane and halothane in their effect on skeletal muscle blood flow are small at best.[148,168-171] However, more recently reported studies show that microvascular and global muscle blood flow is higher during isoflurane anesthesia compared to halothane.[98,172,173]

Effects on respiratory system function.
Isoflurane, like halothane, depresses respiratory system function and causes hypercapnia (see Figure 15-6).[54,55,101,104,109,161,174] The magnitude of depression is dose and time related and at least equal to or greater than that produced by halothane (see Figures 15-6 and Figure 15-8). Controlled mechanical ventilation may be used to avoid excessive hypercapnia.

Breathing during isoflurane anesthesia is usually characterized by a low breathing rate, large tidal volume, and high inspiratory flow rate.[109,154,161,174,175] Coughing and breath holding, frequently noted in humans with acute exposure to isoflurane, is not usually observed in horses.[33,101,134,175]

The average concentration of isoflurane causing apnea of at least a 60-second duration in horses was earlier found to be 3.2% or about 2.3 MAC.[104] This value ranks isoflurane as a more potent respiratory depressant than halothane.

Effects on the central nervous system.
Isoflurane anesthesia is associated with an increase in CBF and ICP similar to that in humans and like halothane anesthesia in ponies and horses.[147,176,177] Increases are further related to dose, mode of ventilation, and body posture.[178-180]

The frequency and voltage of EEG activity increase in humans at subanesthetic levels of isoflurane. The frequency of electrical activity slows with increasing doses, and periods of EEG suppression begin at 1.5 MAC. At 2.0 MAC, electrical

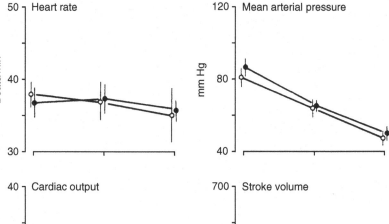

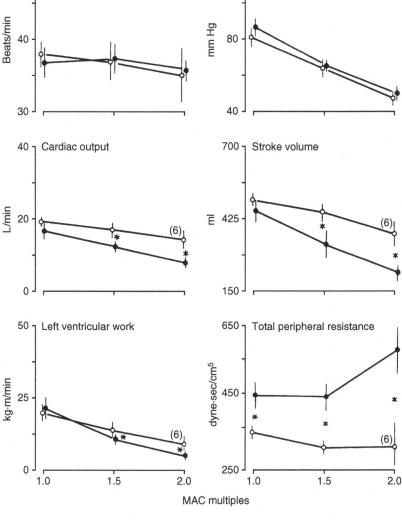

Figure 15–10. Effects of halothane (●) and isoflurane (○) in seven horses during controlled ventilation and a constant $PaCO_2$. The mean ± SE is indicated; and the number of observations, if not seven, is indicated in parentheses. MAC is the minimum alveolarconcentration for each drug in the horse. Significant differences (P< 0.05) in observations at equipotent concentrations (i.e., equal MAC multiples) of halothane and isoflurane are indicated by *. (Data adapted from studies of Steffey et al.[53] (From Steffey EP: Inhalation anesthesia. In White NA, Moore JN, editors: *Current practices in equine surgery,* Philadelphia, 1990, JB Lippincott, p 77.)

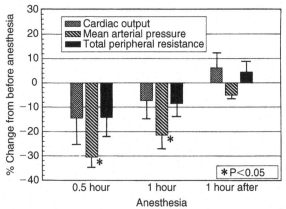

Figure 15–11. Changes (mean ± SE) in mean arterial blood pressure and its determinants associated with 1.2 MAC isoflurane in O_2 anesthesia in seven horses. (From Steffey EP et al: Cardiovascular and respiratory measurements in awake and isoflurane-anesthetized horses, *Am J Vet Res* 48:7, 1987.)

silence predominates.[181,182] The EEG effects of isoflurane in horses are similar to those reported in humans.[118] Like isoflurane-anesthetized humans but unlike conditions with halothane in either horses or humans, EEG burst suppression is seen at higher anesthetic doses than might occur clinically (1.5 MAC in humans; electrical silence occurs at about 2.0 MAC).[182] Burst suppression is not seen at clinically relevant halothane doses (i.e., 2.0 MAC or less). Surgical stimulation may or may not alter the depressed EEG pattern.[183,184]

Effects on other organs

Liver. Studies in a variety of animals, including horses, indicate that isoflurane is unlikely to injure the liver.[55,127,185,186] Hypoxemia during anesthesia may cause increases in serum markers of hepatic insult but are less than those associated with similar conditions during halothane anesthesia in horses.[133]

Kidney. Isoflurane reversibly decreases renal blood flow and urinary flow in ponies[170] and other species.[55] The magnitude of these effects is similar to that seen during halothane anesthesia.

The molecular stability of isoflurane minimizes the potential for production of toxic metabolites (such as fluoride ion), which might cause kidney damage (see Table 15-4).[42,146] The quantity of fluoride released by biodegradation is insufficient to cause renal cellular damage.[55,146]

Blood. Total leukocyte and immature and mature neutrophil numbers are increased for 24 hours after prolonged

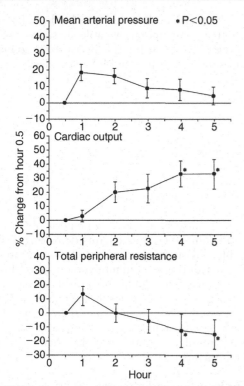

Figure 15–12. Time-related changes in mean arterial blood pressure and its determinants during constant 1.2 MAC (1.57% end-tidal) isoflurane in O_2 anesthesia in spontaneously breathing horses. *Indicates P<0.05 versus 0.5-hour observation. (From Steffey EP et al: Cardiopulmonary function during 5 hours of constant-dose isoflurane in laterally recumbent, spontaneously breathing horses, *J Vet Pharmacol Ther* 10:290, 1987.)

isoflurane anesthesia in horses.[186] These changes are similar to those that occur after halothane anesthesia and are compatible with signs of generalized physiological stress.

Like halothane, isoflurane anesthesia temporarily reduces circulating platelet number and function in horses, but these effects are small and transient.[187,188]

Biotransformation. The biotransformation of isoflurane is substantially less than that of the other volatile anesthetics (see Table 15-4).[42,55,189] The resistance to biodegradation is evidenced by a small rise in serum fluoride levels during and after isoflurane anesthesia in humans and rats.[55] Adult horses also metabolize isoflurane to fluoride ion at rates similar to those in humans.[146] On the other hand, the serum fluoride levels in foals are not changed after clinical exposure to isoflurane

Anesthetic induction and recovery. The lower blood solubility of isoflurane compared to halothane facilitates a more rapid anesthetic induction and recovery.[9,127,156,190-192] The quality of isoflurane induction and recovery in foals and ponies is at least comparable and frequently more rapid than that for halothane.[156,190] Foals are usually alert earlier in the recovery period, and recovery is generally considered "crisper."

The quality of recovery from isoflurane by adult horses is judged clinically to be more variable than with foals. Reports of overall better recovery with halothane[150,191,193] and a greater incidence of rough recovery after isoflurane

(compared with halothane)[194] blemish an otherwise very good appraisal of the clinical actions of isoflurane. The administration of α_2-agonists during the recovery period may improve the quality, but prolong the duration, of recovery.[195] Although there are no guarantees for an uneventful recovery from anesthesia with any anesthetic technique, careful consideration of the effects of isoflurane on recovery in potentially complicated recovery situations or after certain surgical procedures (e.g., long bone fractures) in horses is prudent.

Desflurane

Desflurane was first synthesized in the 1960s but only released for clinical use in human patients in 1992. Despite more than 10 years of availability, information describing the effects of desflurane is limited. It is structurally related to isoflurane (see Table 15-1) but differs from isoflurane in some notable and clinically important ways. First, the vapor pressure curve for desflurane is steep, and it boils at room temperature (22.8° C). These characteristics preclude delivery of desflurane from commonly used vaporizers. Variation in ambient temperature causes clinically unacceptable fluctuations in delivered desflurane concentrations. Second, it is the least soluble in blood of the contemporary volatile anesthetics, similar to that of N_2O, thus providing the most rapid anesthetic uptake and recovery of all the currently available volatile anesthetics. Third, its anesthetic potency in horses is only about one sixth that of isoflurane, thereby limiting inspired O_2 concentration considerably; a consideration for horses that is not trivial, even at sea level.

Effects on cardiovascular function. Laboratory studies of human volunteers and animals indicate that the cardiovascular effects of desflurane are qualitatively similar to those of isoflurane, which in turn is less depressing than halothane.[196,197] In the absence of the confounding effects of associated drugs, available information from horses indicates that desflurane depresses blood pressure and cardiac output in a dose-related manner. However, when the effects of desflurane are compared to those of sevoflurane and isoflurane, desflurane is less depressing within the dosage range of 1.0 to 1.5 MAC (Figure 15-13).[53,195,198-201] Indeed, the magnitude of cardiac output per kilogram in spontaneously breathing horses was near values reported for that in awake horses.[195,199,201] Heart rate tends to be greater during desflurane (and sevoflurane) anesthesia in otherwise unmedicated horses and tends to increase with dose. Desflurane is less arrhythmogenic than halothane and similar to isoflurane.[202] As previously noted with halothane and isoflurane, IPPV increases the depressant effect of desflurane; however, the combined depressant effect of dose and IPPV is less with desflurane than with other inhaled anesthetics, including sevoflurane at least at doses less than 1.5 MAC.[199,201] Above 1.5 MAC, desflurane appears to lose its hemodynamic advantage and becomes a cardiovascular depressant equal to or possibly greater than the other volatile anesthetics.[197,203]

Effects on respiratory system function. Desflurane is a potent respiratory depressant in horses[195,201] and ponies.[199] Respiratory depression during desflurane anesthesia is greater than that typical of responses to other volatile agents in humans under similar conditions as judged by the

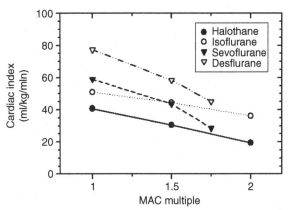

Figure 15–13. The effects of alveolar dose (expressed as multiples of MAC) of four contemporary inhalation anesthetics on the cardiac output (indexed to body mass) of adult horses during controlled ventilation. Plotted data sets are from reported, similarly conducted studies in my laboratory.[53,200,201] Note the effects of halothane versus-desflurane and the similarity of isoflurane and sevoflurane at clinically relevant anesthetic concentrations (<1.5 MAC).

magnitude of rise in $PaCO_2$ from normal.[204,205] Respiratory depression in horses is as great or greater than that caused by halothane or isoflurane.[53,104,150,201] Respiratory rate in horses is especially depressed by desflurane compared to halothane but similar to that with isoflurane and sevoflurane.[201] A breathing rate of four or less per minute is common. Desflurane is a mild respiratory irritant in humans and provokes coughing or breath holding during anesthetic induction by mask. Experience to date suggest this is not of concern in foals (author's experience) or adult horses.[201]

Effects on other organs

Liver. The low level of biodegradation of desflurane, the favorable hemodynamics (especially the sustained cardiac output at clinical levels of anesthesia), and the rapid elimination from the body following anesthesia predict hepatic safety (see Table 15-4). This is supported by studies of humans[206] and animals,[207,208] including horses.[201]

Desflurane causes an increase in hepatic arterial blood flow in dogs compared to awake conditions.[209] Total hepatic blood flow decreased slightly, but only at the deepest levels of anesthesia (1.75 and 2.0 MAC) because hepatic portal blood flow decreased.[209] The same dogs were similarly studied during isoflurane anesthesia, and no differences in hepatic arterial or total hepatic blood flow were noted. Presuming that blood flow results in dogs apply to horses, desflurane, like isoflurane, would be less likely than halothane to be associated with hepatic injury during hypoxemic conditions;[207] this circumstance is not unusual during anesthetic management of horses.

Kidney. The molecular stability of desflurane, like that of isoflurane, minimizes the potential for production of renal toxic metabolites such as fluoride ion.[201] At least in dogs, renal blood flow is not decreased by desflurane.[209]

Biotransformation. Desflurane is expected to be metabolized in a manner similar to that of isoflurane because of its structural similarity to isoflurane.[42] Although biotransformation of these two anesthetics is qualitatively similar, the magnitude of breakdown of desflurane is quantitatively less; from studies of humans, less than one tenth of that of iso-

flurane.[189,210] Indeed, desflurane resists biodegradation more than any other contemporary volatile anesthetic (see Table 15-4). Levels of inorganic fluoride measured in serum taken from horses before, during, and following desflurane anesthesia are comparable to results of studies of humans.[201]

Although minimally degraded in the body, desflurane (and to lesser degrees isoflurane, sevoflurane, and halothane [the latter two nearly negligible])[211] degrade in the presence of desiccated CO_2 absorbents (e.g., soda lime) to form carbon monoxide (CO). Reported injury is rare, but abnormal levels of CO have been reported in anesthetized humans; the highest level was associated with desflurane anesthesia.[212] The production of CO by desflurane is inconsequential when newly formulated CO_2 absorbents (Sodasorb LF, Amsorb) are used. No reports of CO concentrations in equine anesthetic circuits delivering desflurane are available, although increases in CO concentration have been reported during the administration of isoflurane to horses.[213] Carboxyhemoglobin does not change (in my experience) during clinical use of desflurane in horses. However, fresh gas flow rates have been greater than 4 L/min in these circumstances with adult horses. Reduced fresh gas flow rate during prolonged anesthetic management may produce a different outcome.

Anesthetic induction and recovery. The low blood solubility of desflurane predicts that it should provide the most rapid and complete recovery from a comparable depth and duration of anesthesia compared to other volatile anesthetics. Results of studies of rats and humans support[38,214] this conclusion, as does limited data from studies of horses and ponies.[199,201,215]

Sevoflurane

Sevoflurane was synthesized in the early 1970s, and its characteristics were first described in 1975;[216] but it was not introduced clinically for human patients until the 1980s in Japan and in 1995 in the United States. The blood solubility of sevoflurane is less than that of isoflurane but greater than that of desflurane (see Table 15-1), and it is able to be degraded to compound A (a nephrotoxin in rats) in the presence of commonly used CO_2 absorbents (e.g., soda lime and Baralyme [no longer available]) in anesthetic breathing circuits (see Table 15-2). Studies in horses have not demonstrated significant anesthetic circuit concentrations of compound A, and the presence of low amounts is considered clinically irrelevant.[200,217] Furthermore, the production of compound A is likely to be inconsequential if Sodasorb LF and Amsorb are used as CO_2 absorbents.

Effects on cardiovascular function. The cardiovascular effects of sevoflurane are qualitatively and quantitatively similar to those of isoflurane,[218-221] including foals[222] and adult horses.[150,198,200] Sevoflurane may be of greater insult to cardiovascular performance than similar conditions with isoflurane at a dose greater than 1.5 MAC (see Figure 15-13), although one clinical investigation suggests that sevoflurane anesthesia in horses requires less hemodynamic support than does isoflurane.[200] The impact of IPPV on reducing hemodynamics compared to conditions of spontaneous ventilation in sevoflurane-anesthetized horses is also similar to that of isoflurane at least in doses of 1 to 1.5 MAC (see Figure 15-13). Like other inhalation anesthetics, the duration of sevoflurane anesthesia modifies some of its cardiovascular effects.[162] Sevoflurane does not increase the arrhythmogenicity of the heart,[216] and the arrhythmogenic dose of epinephrine is similar at least in dogs[223] and cats[224] similarly anesthetized with isoflurane and sevoflurane. Results of comparable studies have not been reported for horses.

Effects on respiratory system function. Horses anesthetized with sevoflurane breathe at low frequency and are hypercapnic. The magnitude of respiratory depression is dose dependent and similar to effects from isoflurane in adult horses anesthetized at or below 1.5 MAC[150,198,225] and in foals.[222] At greater doses, the potency of sevoflurane as a respiratory depressant relative to other volatile agents remains unresolved in the horse but is at least equivalent to similar conditions with isoflurane.

Effects on other organs

Liver. The impact of volatile anesthetics on hepatic blood flow had been evaluated in a variety of species.[226] Most anesthetics decrease portal blood flow because cardiac output decreases. Hepatic blood flow may increase slightly but is usually not sufficient to prevent a reduction in total flow to the liver.[227] Hepatic blood flow is usually the lowest during halothane and only modestly decreased by sevoflurane or isoflurane.[228] Similar studies of the impact of inhalant anesthetics on hepatic blood flow in horses has not been reported.

Administration of sevoflurane to horses not undergoing surgery and studied under laboratory conditions produced no important anesthetic-specific changes in blood biochemical analytes indicative of liver cell injury.[198,200,229] Similarly, blood tests and histopathological analysis of liver from horses anesthetized for an unusually prolonged time (18 hours) showed no remarkable evidence of hepatocellular damage.[217]

Kidney. The inhaled anesthetics differentially alter normal renal physiology. Like other agents, sevoflurane may decrease renal blood flow and glomerular filtration rate, which in turn decreases urine production.

Nephrotoxicity from inorganic fluoride released after metabolism of fluorinated volatile anesthetics is possible. Most notable in this regard is the nephrotoxicity produced in humans following the administration and metabolism of a no-longer-administered inhaled anesthetic, methoxyflurane. The nephrotoxic threshold of serum fluoride in humans is commonly considered to be 50 μmol/L.[48]

Sevoflurane is broken down in the liver, and inorganic fluoride is released in this process (see Table 15-4). However, there has been no evidence of gross changes in renal histology or function in humans following sevoflurane anesthesia.[230] Similarly, serum inorganic fluoride concentrations approaching or exceeding nephrotoxic levels (in rats and humans) have been measured during and following prolonged anesthesia in horses,[200] but no injury has been reported. Current opinion on why fluoride ion produced by methoxyflurane, but not sevoflurane, damaged human kidneys relates to two issues: (1) the greater blood solubility of methoxyflurane versus sevoflurane and therefore greater duration of exposure to fluoride ion increase; and (2) unlike sevoflurane, degradation of methoxyflurane

occurs in the kidney, and it is speculated that high intrarenal fluoride production contributes to local toxicity.[42,231] From newly reported data, an additional hypothesis has been proposed: along with fluoride, a cotoxic metabolite (dichloroacetic acid) is produced during methoxyflurane degradation but not during sevoflurane anesthesia (or other anesthetics). This by-product is responsible for the renal toxicity of methoxyflurane. Therefore this circumstance could account for the difference in toxic outcomes between anesthetics despite their similarities in serum fluoride level.[232,233]

Caution regarding the renal effects of sevoflurane in horses with renal disease or associated with co-contributors to renal toxicity seems warranted since the degradation of sevoflurane by CO_2 (especially desiccated) absorbents produces another renal toxic substance, compound A.[234] The concentration threshold of compound A for renal toxicity in rats is reached in clinical practice.[235,236] In recognition of possible renal damage from compound A, the package labeling for sevoflurane warns physicians to adjust inspired concentrations and fresh gas flow rate to minimize exposure (i.e., a human patient's exposure should not exceed 2.0 MAC hours at flow rates of 1 to <2 L/min fresh gas inflow). Fresh gas inflow rates of <1 L/min are not recommended. However, it is questionable whether the production of compound A during sevoflurane anesthesia is clinically relevant in horses; and, as stated earlier, newer CO_2 absorbents have made this issue academic.[237]

There has been no significant clinical renal toxicity reported for human or animal patients anesthetized with sevoflurane. In cases in which kidney-associated changes have occurred, they have been transient and associated with prolonged exposure, implying total exposure (i.e., time and concentration, not just concentration, are important). Regardless, it has been recommended that sevoflurane not be used in human patients with impaired renal function.[42,238]

Biotransformation. Like all fluorinated volatile anesthetics, sevoflurane is defluorinated in the liver (see Table 15-4).[239] Sevoflurane defluorination is increased by prior induction of microsomal enzymes with drugs such as phenobarbital.[240] Serum Fl⁻ concentrations from horses anesthetized with sevoflurane are similar to those in humans under comparable conditions and with prolonged exposure can exceed 50 μmol/L.[198,200,217]

Anesthetic induction and recovery. Horses anesthetized with sevoflurane do not show signs of airway irritation such as coughing.[200,222,241] Following anesthetic induction with injectable drugs administered intravenously, transition to sevoflurane anesthesia is qualitatively unremarkable. Despite a low blood solubility favoring a more rapid anesthetic induction with sevoflurane compared to isoflurane, times to anesthetic induction for these two agents in the absence of other drugs are similar.[222] The volume of components of the anesthetic breathing circuit, vaporizer setting, and fresh gas inflow to the breathing circuit are important modifiers of anesthetic induction time beyond the agent's physical characteristics.[26,242]

Rapid recovery from general anesthesia is commonly regarded as a principal goal in the management of horses to facilitate safe return to a wakeful, standing state and cardiopulmonary stability. Results from studies in rats indicate that a low blood solubility facilitates more rapid recovery from anesthesia than an inhalant anesthetic with a higher solubility.[38] Thus recovery from sevoflurane is faster than from isoflurane but slower than from desflurane.[150,199,201] Anesthetic dose and duration are also important modifiers of the speed of anesthetic recovery in rats and humans (i.e., other conditions equal, the shorter the anesthesia time or lower the anesthetic dose or both, the shorter the recovery time).[38,243] Comparisons of results of different but similarly conducted studies in horses anesthetized without adjuvant drugs provide indirect evidence that these same outcomes apply also to horses.[192,200,201] However, in a study of six foals anesthetized for about 2 hours, there was no difference in recovery characteristics between isoflurane and sevoflurane.[222] Conversely, in a clinical trial of 60 Draft Horses, sevoflurane produced the most rapid, controlled, and uneventful recovery from anesthesia compared to halothane and isoflurane (W Muir, unpublished data, 2003).

Most studies (laboratory and clinical) reporting recovery events of horses following inhalation anesthesia used a management plan that included adjuvant drugs administered for anesthetic induction, to supplement anesthetic maintenance, and/or just before or during the anesthetic recovery period in an attempt to pharmacologically facilitate a smooth, atraumatic transition from recumbency to standing. Some report experiences with sevoflurane and adjuvant drugs.[92,225,229,244-246] Other studies were designed to compare equine recovery from a sevoflurane-based anesthetic plan with an isoflurane-based management scheme.[150,247,248] In total, these studies reported widely varying clinical or quasi-clinical circumstances in which horses recovering from sevoflurane anesthesia generally experience a smooth, safe recovery. Seemingly, recovery times from sevoflurane anesthesia are comparable to those of isoflurane and often faster.

The Gaseous Anesthetic—Nitrous Oxide

N_2O is frequently used as a vehicle for potent volatile anesthetics or as a supplement to drugs injected intravenously.[35] Its beneficial effects in humans are rapid anesthetic induction and recovery, minimum circulatory system depression, and a reduction of the amount of concurrently administered more potent anesthetics (resulting in less overall cardiovascular and other organ system depression). Recent evidence suggests that the analgesic effects of N_2O are opioid in nature and may involve blockade of N-methyl-D-aspartate (NMDA) receptors (see Chapter 20).[249,250]

N_2O is of less value in the anesthetic management of horses than in humans because it has only about half of the anesthetic potency in horses as in humans (see Table 15-2).[13,14,50] The limited potency in horses necessitates the use of high concentrations, ideally 50% to 75% N_2O to provide at least minimum anesthetic effects. Therefore the concurrently inspired O_2 concentration is in the range of 50% to 25%. As a result, its use is associated with an increased risk of hypoxemia in horses when compared with the more common practice of using only O_2 as a vehicle for volatile anesthetics. Hypoxia is an additional concern at the termination of anesthesia if the patient is abruptly permitted to breathe air following N_2O breathing. The elimination of a large volume of N_2O (because of its relatively low solubility in blood), especially within the first few moments, dilutes the alveolar O_2 concentration, which may in turn cause hypoxemia (i.e., diffusion hypoxia).[251]

Finally, the high partial pressure of N_2O in blood and its low blood:gas PC (see Table 15-2) causes it to diffuse readily into air containing gas spaces. The volume of these spaces thereby increases because of the lesser solubility of nitrogen and greater transfer of N_2O. A common consequence is expansion of gastrointestinal gas, ileus, and abdominal bloat.[14,154,206,252]

The clinical use of N_2O in the anesthetic management of horses is less obvious than for human or small animal patients. On the basis of present information, with the possible exception of its use in foals (and even in this case theoretical advantages are equivocal), the overall disadvantages of N_2O use in horses generally outweigh any minor advantages it may provide. There may be some advantage to facilitating anesthetic induction by inhalation anesthetics in foals. There is a large volume uptake of N_2O from the lungs during the early moments of anesthetic induction with N_2O and the administration of a second potent inhaled anesthetic (e.g., isoflurane), which in turn increases the rate of rise of the alveolar concentration of the second anesthetic (second gas effect). This may speed anesthetic induction slightly.[9]

TRACE CONCENTRATIONS OF INHALATION ANESTHETICS: OCCUPATIONAL EXPOSURE

Inhalation anesthetics are usually administered to horses in a surgical facility operating room. Some of these gases enter the operating room atmosphere, exposing operating room personnel to risk from chronic exposure to low inhalant anesthetic gas concentrations. This is of concern because epidemiological studies of humans and laboratory studies of animals have suggested that chronic exposure to trace levels of anesthetics may constitute a health hazard. Concerns relate to fetal death, spontaneous abortion, birth defects, or cancer.[253] The data remain equivocal; even today a firm cause-and-effect relationship between chronic exposure to trace levels of anesthetics and human health problems does not exist. Although controversy remains, personnel exposure should be minimized. Concentrations of anesthetics delivered to patients are usually reported on a volume-per-volume basis as % of 1 atmosphere (e.g., MAC for isoflurane in the horse is 1.3%. On the other hand, waste anesthetic gases are usually reported on a volume-per-volume basis in parts per million [ppm]). In this case 1.3% isoflurane is equivalent to 13,000 ppm. Maximum decreased levels of exposure have been suggested by the National Institute of Occupational Safety and Health (NIOSH) as 25 ppm for N_2O and 2 ppm for halogenated anesthetic drugs.[254,255] These levels are very low but are readily achievable in operating room settings of a contemporary equine hospital that is properly ventilated. Equine operating rooms are by necessity relatively large with large entrances and good ventilation supporting large room air change over. In addition, anesthetic practices for horses are less conducive to operating room contamination than the management of small animal or human patients; for example, inhalation anesthetic induction by mask, high fresh gas delivery to small patient anesthetic delivery circuit, and use of N_2O are standards of care for small animals and humans.

Methods for reduction and control of anesthetic exposure levels below NIOSH-recommended standards include clean up of sources of gas/vapor spillage, adequate ventilation of anesthetizing areas, and use of waste anesthetic gas scavenging and disposal systems (see Chapter 16).[255,256] Frequent monitoring of anesthetic gas/vapor concentrations is of obvious value, especially in areas of high use since recommended exposure thresholds are lower than concentrations most humans can recognize.[257] Finally, educating personnel exposed to inhalation anesthetics is of value because it makes them aware of potential problems and methods for controlling exposure levels.[258]

REFERENCES

1. Hall LW: *Wright's veterinary anaesthesia and analgesia*, ed 7, London, 1971, Baillière Tindall.
2. Lumb WV, Jones EW: *Veterinary anesthesia*, Philadelphia, 1973, Lea & Febiger.
3. Short CE: *Principles and practice of veterinary anesthesia*, Baltimore, 1987, Williams & Wilkins.
4. Soma LR: *Textbook of veterinary anesthesia*, Baltimore, 1971, Williams & Wilkins.
5. Hall LW, Gillespie JR, Tyler WS: Alveolar-arterial oxygen tension differences in anesthetized horses, *Br J Anaesth* 40:560-568, 1968.
6. Pearson MRB, Weaver BMQ, Staddon GE: The influence of tissue solubility on the perfusion distribution of inhaled anesthetics. In Grandy J et al, editors: *Proceedings of the Second International Congress of Veterinary Anesthesia*, Santa Barbara, 1985, Veterinary Practice Publishing, Co.; pp 101-102.
7. Weaver BMQ, Webb AI: Tissue composition and halothane solubility in the horse, *Br J Anaesth* 53:487-493, 1981.
8. Webb AI, Weaver BMQ: Solubility of halothane in equine tissues at 37° C, *Br J Anaesth* 53:479-486, 1981.
9. Eger EI II: *Anesthetic uptake and action*, Baltimore, 1974, Williams & Wilkins.
10. Webb AI: The effect of species differences in the uptake and distribution of inhalant anesthetic agents. In Grandy J et al, editors: *Proceedings of the Second International Congress of Veterinary Anesthesia*, Santa Barbara, 1985, Veterinary Practice Publishing Co; pp. 27-32.
11. Merkel G, Eger EI II: A comparative study of halothane and halopropane anesthesia: including method for determining equipotency, *Anesthesiology* 24:346-357, 1963.
12. deJong RH, Eger EI II: MAC expanded: AD50 and AD95 values of common inhalation anesthetics in man, *Anesthesiology* 42:408-419, 1975.
13. Quasha AL, Eger EI II, Tinker JH: Determination and applications of MAC, *Anesthesiology* 53:315-334, 1980.
14. Steffey EP, Howland D Jr: Potency of halothane-N2O in the horse, *Am J Vet Res* 39:1141-1146, 1978.
15. Guedel AE: Stages of anesthesia and reclassification of the signs of anesthesia, *Anesth Analg* 6:157-162, 1927.
16. Hall LW, Clarke KW: *Veterinary anaesthesia*, ed 8, London, 1983, Baillière Tindall.
17. Lumb WV, Jones EW: *Veterinary anesthesia*, ed 2, Philadelphia, 1984, Lea & Febiger.
18. Antognini JF, Schwartz K: Exaggerated anesthetic requirements in the preferentially anesthetized brain, *Anesthesiology* 79:1244-1249, 1993.
19. Rampil IJ: Anesthetic potency is not altered after hypothermic spinal cord transection in rats, *Anesthesiology* 80:606-610, 1994.
20. Rampil IJ, Mason P, Singh H: Anesthetic potency (MAC) is independent of forebrain structures in the rat, *Anesthesiology* 78:707-712, 1993.
21. Antognini JF, Carstens E, Raines DE: *Neural mechanisms of anesthesia*, Totowa, NJ, 2003, Humana Press.
22. Eger EI, II, Eisenkraft JB, Weiskopf RB: *The pharmacology of inhaled anesthetics*, ed 2, San Francisco, 2003, Dannemiller Memorial Educational Foundation.
23. Koblin DD: Mechanisms of action. In Miller RD, editor: *Miller's anesthesia*, ed 6, Philadelphia, 2005, Elsevier Churchill Livingstone, pp 105-130.
24. Rubin E, Miller KW, Roth SH: *Molecular and cellular mechanisms of alcohol and anesthetics*, New York, 2006, The New York Academy of Sciences.
25. Eger EI, II: Uptake and distribution. In Miller RD, editor: *Miller's anesthesia*, ed 6, Philadelphia, 2005, Elsevier, Churchill Livingstone, pp 131-153.
26. Solano AM, Brosnan RJ, Steffey EP: Rate of change of oxygen concentration for a large animal circle anesthetic system, *Am J Vet Res* 66:1675-1678, 2005.
27. Steffey EP, Berry JD: Flow rates for an intermittent positive pressure breathing-anesthetic delivery apparatus for horses, *Am J Vet Res* 38:685-687, 1977.
28. Dorsch JA, Dorsch SE: *Understanding anesthesia equipment*, ed 4, Baltimore, 1999, Williams & Wilkins.
29. Paterson GM, Hulands GH, Nunn JF: Evolution of a new halothane vaporizer: the Cyprane Fluotec Mark 3, *Br J Anaesth* 41:109-119, 1969.
30. Steffey EP, Woliner M, Howland D: Evaluation of an isoflurane vaporizer: the Cyprane Fortec, *Anesth Analg* 61:457-464, 1982.
31. Steffey EP, Woliner MJ, Howland D: Accuracy of isoflurane delivery by halothane-specific vaporizers, *Am J Vet Res* 44:1071-1078, 1983.
32. Eger EI II: Effect of inspired anesthetic concentration on the rate of rise of alveolar concentration, *Anesthesiology* 24:153-157, 1963.
33. Epstein RM et al: Influence of the concentration effect on the uptake of anesthetic mixtures: the second gas effect, *Anesthesiology* 25:364-371, 1964.
34. Stoelting RK, Eger EI II: An additional explanation for the second gas effect: a concentrating effort, *Anesthesiology* 30:273-277, 1969.
35. Eger EI II: *Nitrous oxide/N₂O*, ed 1, New York, 1985, Elsevier.
36. Mapleson WW, Korman B: The second gas effect is a valid concept, *Anesth Analg* 89:1326, 1999.
37. Stoelting RK, Eger EI II: Percutaneous loss of nitrous oxide, cyclopropane, ether, and halothane in man, *Anesthesiology* 30:278-283, 1969.
38. Eger EI, II, Johnson BH: Rates of awakening from anesthesia with I-653, halothane, isoflurane, and sevoflurane: a test of the effect of anesthetic concentration and duration in rats, *Anesth Analg* 66:977-983, 1987.
39. Fink BR: Diffusion anoxia, *Anesthesiology* 16:511-519, 1955.
40. Van Dyke RA, Chenoweth MB, Van Poznak A: Metabolism of volatile anesthetics. I. Conversion in vivo of several anesthetics to $14CO_2$ and chloride, *Biochem Pharmacol* 13:1239-1247, 1964.
41. Holaday DA, Rudofsky S, Treuhaft PS: The metabolic degradation of methoxyflurane in man, *Anesthesiology* 33:579-593, 1970.
42. Martin JL Jr, Njoku DB: Metabolism and toxicity of modern inhaled anesthetics. In Miller RD, editor: *Miller's anesthesia*, ed 6, Philadelphia, 2005, Elsevier Churchill Livingstone, pp 231-272.
43. Rehder K et al: Halothane biotransformation in man: a quantitative study, *Anesthesiology* 28:711-715, 1967.

44. Stier A et al: Urinary excretion of bromide in halothane anesthesia, *Anesth Analg* 43:723-728, 1964.

45. Hong K et al: Metabolism of nitrous oxide by human and rat intestinal contents, *Anesthesiology* 52:16-19, 1980.

46. Carpenter RL et al: Does the duration of anesthetic administration affect the pharmacokinetics or metabolism of inhaled anesthetics in humans?, *Anesth Analg* 66:1-8, 1987.

47. Carpenter RL et al: The extent of metabolism of inhaled anesthetics in humans, *Anesthesiology* 65:201-206, 1986.

48. Mazze RI, Trudell JR, Cousins MJ: Methoxyflurane metabolism and renal dysfunction: clinical correlation in man, *Anesthesiology* 35:247-252, 1971.

49. Van Dyke R: Biotransformation of volatile anaesthetics with special emphasis on the role of metabolism in the toxicity of anaesthetics, *Can Anaesth Soc J* 20:21-33, 1973.

50. Grandy JL et al: Cardiopulmonary effects of ephedrine in halothane-anesthetized horses, *J Vet Pharmacol Ther* 12:389-396, 1989.

51. Manohar M, Goetz TE: Cerebral, renal, adrenal, intestinal, and pancreatic circulation in conscious ponies and during 1.0, 1.5, and 2.0 minimal alveolar concentrations of halothane-O$_2$ anesthesia, *Am J Vet Res* 46:2492-2498, 1985.

52. Steffey EP: Circulatory effects of inhalation anaesthetics in dogs and horses, *Proc Assoc Vet Anaesth Gr Britain Ireland* 10:S82-S98, 1982.

53. Steffey EP, Howland D, Jr: Comparison of circulatory and respiratory effects of isoflurane and halothane anesthesia in horses, *Am J Vet Res* 41:821-825, 1980.

54. Steffey EP, Howland DJ: Cardiovascular effects of halothane in the horse, *Am J Vet Res* 39:611-615, 1978.

55. Eger EI II: *Isoflurane (Forane): a compendium and reference*, ed 2, Madison, 1985, Anaquest.

56. Pagel PS et al: Cardiovascular pharmacology. In Miller RD, editor: *Miller's anesthesia*, ed 6, Philadelphia, 2005, Elsevier Churchill Livingstone, pp 191-229.

57. Sugai N, Shimosato S, Estsen BE: Effect of halothane on force-velocity relations and dynamic stiffness of isolated heart muscle, *Anesthesiology* 29:267-274, 1968.

58. Sonntag H et al: Left ventricular function in conscious man during halothane anesthesia, *Anesthesiology* 48:320-324, 1978.

59. Eberly VE et al: Cardiovascular values in the horse during halothane anesthesia, *Am J Vet Res* 29:305-314, 1968.

60. Vasko KA: Preliminary report on the effects of halothane on cardiac action and blood pressure in the horse, *Am J Vet Res* 23:248-250, 1962.

61. Lees P, Tavernor WD: Influence of halothane and catecholamines on heart rate and rhythm in the horse, *Br J Pharmacol* 39:149-159, 1970.

62. Gaynor JS, Bednarski RM, Muir WW III: Effect of hypercapnia on the arrhythmogenic dose of epinephrine in horses anesthetized with guaifenesin, thiamylal sodium, and halothane, *Am J Vet Res* 54:315-321, 1993.

63. Wagner AE, Bednarski RM, Muir WW III: Hemodynamic effects of carbon dioxide during intermittent positive-pressure ventilation in horses, *Am J Vet Res* 51:1922-1929, 1990.

64. Hellyer PW et al: The effects of halothane and isoflurane on baroreflex sensitivity in the horse, *Am J Vet Res* 50:2127-2134, 1989.

65. Swanson CR et al: Hemodynamic responses in halothane-anesthetized horses given infusions of dopamine or dobutamine, *Am J Vet Res* 46:365-371, 1985.

66. Tucker WK, Rackstein AD, Munson ES: Comparison of arrhythmic doses of adrenaline, metaraminol, ephedrine, and phenylephrine, during isoflurane and halothane anesthesia in dogs, *Br J Anaesth* 46:392-396, 1974.

67. Hodgson DS et al: Effects of spontaneous, assisted, and controlled ventilation in halothane-anesthetized geldings, *Am J Vet Res* 47:992-996, 1986.

68. McMurphy RM, Blissitt KJ: Effects of controlled ventilation on indices of ventricular function in halothane-anesthetized horses, *Vet Surg* 28:130, 1999.

69. Khanna AK et al: Cardiopulmonary effects of hypercapnia during controlled intermittent positive-pressure ventilation in the horse, *Can J Vet Res* 59:213-221, 1995.

70. Cullen LK et al: Effect of high PaCO$_2$ and time on cerebrospinal fluid and intraocular pressure in halothane-anesthetized horses, *Am J Vet Res* 51:300-304, 1990.

71. Steffey EP, Willits N, Woliner M: Hemodynamic and respiratory responses to variable arterial partial pressure of oxygen in halothane-anesthetized horses during spontaneous and controlled ventilation, *Am J Vet Res* 53:1850-1858, 1992.

72. Donaldson LL, Trostle SS, White NA: Cardiopulmonary changes associated with abdominal insufflation of carbon dioxide in mechanically ventilated, dorsally recumbent, halothane-anaesthetised horses, *Equine Vet J* 30:144-151, 1998.

73. Wagner AE et al: Hemodynamic function during neurectomy in halothane-anesthetized horses with or without constant dose detomidine infusion, *Vet Surg* 21:248-256, 1992.

74. Roizen MF, Horrigan RW, Frazer BM: Anesthetic doses blocking adrenergic (stress) and cardiovascular responses to incision—MAC BAR, *Anesthesiology* 54:390-398, 1981.

75. Abrahamsen E et al: Tourniquet-induced hypotension in horses, *J Am Vet Med Assoc* 194:386-388, 1989.

76. Steffey EP, Pascoe PJ: Xylazine blunts the cardiovascular but not the respiratory response induced by noxious stimulation in isoflurane-anesthetized horses. In *Proceedings of the Seventh International Congress of Veterinary Anesthesia*, Bern, Switzerland, 2000, p 55.

77. Wilson DV, Rondenay Y, Shance PU: The cardiopulmonary effects of severe blood loss in anesthetized horses, *Vet Anaesth Analg* 30:81-87, 2003.

78. Bahlman SH et al: The cardiovascular effects of halothane in man during spontaneous ventilation, *Anesthesiology* 36:494-502, 1972.

79. Eger EI II et al: Cardiovascular effects of halothane in man, *Anesthesiology* 32:396-409, 1970.

80. Price HL et al: Evidence for b-receptor activation produced by halothane in man, *Anesthesiology* 32:389-395, 1970.

81. Steffey EP et al: Effect of body posture on cardiopulmonary function in horses during 5 hours of constant-dose halothane anesthesia, *Am J Vet Res* 51:11-16, 1990.

82. Steffey EP, Kelly AB, Woliner MJ: Time-related responses of spontaneously breathing, laterally recumbent horses to prolonged anesthesia with halothane, *Am J Vet Res* 48:952-957, 1987.

83. Dunlop CI et al: Temporal effects of halothane and isoflurane in laterally recumbent ventilated male horses, *Am J Vet Res* 48:1250-1255, 1987.

84. Nyman G, Funkquist B, Kvart C: Postural effects on blood gas tension, blood pressure, heart rate, ECG, and respiratory rate during prolonged anaesthesia in the horse, *J Vet Med* 35:54-62, 1988.

85. Steffey EP, Woliner MJ, Dunlop C: Effects of 5 hours of constant 1.2 MAC halothane in sternally recumbent, spontaneously breathing horses, *Equine Vet J* 22:433-436, 1990.

86. Stegmann GF, Littlejohn A: The effect of lateral and dorsal recumbency on cardiopulmonary function in the anaesthetised horse, *J S Afr Vet Assoc* 58:21-29, 1987.

87. Doherty TJ, Geiser DR, Rohrbach BW: Effect of acepromazine and butorphanol on halothane minimum alveolar concentration in ponies, *Equine Vet J* 29:374-376, 1997.

88. Muir WW III, Wagner AE, Hinchcliff KW: Cardiorespiratory and MAC reducing effects of α$_1$ adrenoreceptor agonists in horses. In Short CE, Vanpoznak A, editors: *Animal pain*, New York, 1992, Churchill Livingstone, pp 201-212.

89. Steffey EP, Pascoe PJ, Woliner MJ, et al: Effects of xylazine hydrochloride during isoflurane-induced anesthesia in horses, *Am J Vet Res* 61:1225-1231, 2000.

90. Muir WW III, Skarda RT, Sheehan W: Hemodynamics and respiratory effects of a xylazine-acetylpromazine drug combination in horses, *Am J Vet Res* 40:1518-1522, 1979.
91. Steffey EP et al: Cardiovascular and respiratory effects of acetylpromazine and xylazine on halothane-anesthetized horses, *J Vet Pharmacol Ther* 8:290-302, 1985.
92. Kushiro T et al: Anesthetic and cardiovascular effects of balanced anesthesia using constant rate infusion of midazolam-ketamine-medetomidine with inhalation of oxygen-sevoflurane (MKM-OS anesthesia) in horses, *J Vet Med Sci* 67:379-384, 2005.
93. Hubbell JAE, Muir WW III, Sams RA: Guaifenesin: cardiopulmonary effects and plasma concentrations in horses, *Am J Vet Res* 41:1751-1755, 1980.
94. Muir WW et al: Evaluation of thiamylal, guaifenesin, and ketamine hydrochloride combinations administered prior to halothane anesthesia in horses, *J Equine Med Surg* 3:178-184, 1979.
95. Pascoe PJ, McDonell WN, Fox AE: Hypotensive potential of supplemental guaiphenesin doses during halothane anesthesia in the horse. In Grandy J et al, editors: *Proceedings of the Second International Congress of Veterinary Anesthesia,* Santa Barbara, 1985, Veterinary Practice Publishing Co.; pp. 61-62.
96. Dyson DH, Pascoe PJ: Influence of preinduction methoxamine, lactated Ringer solution, hypertonic saline solution infusion, or postinduction dobutamine infusion on anesthetic-induced hypotension in horses, *Am J Vet Res* 51:17-21, 1990.
97. Linton RA et al: Cardiac output measured by lithium dilution, thermodilution, and transesophageal Doppler echocardiography in anesthetized horses, *Am J Vet Res* 61:731-737, 2000.
98. Raisis AL et al: Measurements of hind limb blood flow recorded using Doppler ultrasound during administration of vasoactive agents in halothane-anesthetized horses, *Vet Radiol Ultrasound* 41:64-72, 2000.
99. Steffey EP, Eisele JH, Baggot JD: Interactions of morphine and isoflurane in horses, *Am J Vet Res* 64:166-175, 2003.
100. Thomasy SM et al: The effects of intravenous fentanyl administration on the minimum alveolar concentration of isoflurane in horses, *Br J Anaesth* 97:232-237, 2006.
101. Farber NE, Pagel PS, Warltier DC: Pulmonary pharmacology. In Miller RD, editor: *Miller's anesthesia,* ed 6, Philadelphia, 2005, Elsevier Churchill Livingstone, pp 155-189.
102. Gillespie JR, Tyler WS, Hall LW: Cardiopulmonary dysfunction in anesthetized, laterally recumbent horses, *Am J Vet Res* 30:61-72, 1969.
103. Hall LW: Disturbances of cardiopulmonary function in anesthetized horses, *Equine Vet J* 3:95-98, 1971.
104. Steffey EP et al: Enflurane, halothane, and isoflurane potency in horses, *Am J Vet Res* 38:1037-1039, 1977.
105. Wilson WC, Benumof JL: Respiratory physiology and respiratory function during anesthesia. In Miller RD, editor: *Miller's anesthesia,* ed 6, Philadelphia, 2005, Elsevier Churchill Livingstone, pp 679-722.
106. Steffey EP, Farver TB, Woliner MJ: Circulatory and respiratory effects of methoxyflurane in dogs: comparison of halothane, *Am J Vet Res* 45:2574-2579, 1984.
107. Steffey EP et al: Cardiovascular effect of halothane in the stump-tailed macaque during spontaneous and controlled ventilation, *Am J Vet Res* 35:1315-1319, 1974.
108. Steffey EP et al: Circulatory effects of halothane and halothane-nitrous oxide anesthesia in the dog: spontaneous ventilation, *Am J Vet Res* 36:197-200, 1975.
109. Hodgson DS et al: Ventilatory effects of isoflurane anesthesia in horses, *Vet Surg* 14:74, 1985.
110. Steffey EP et al: Body position and mode of ventilation influences arterial pH, oxygen, and carbon dioxide tensions in halothane-anesthetized horses, *Am J Vet Res* 38:379-382, 2977.
111. Eger EI II et al: Surgical stimulation antagonizes the respiratory depression produced by Forane, *Anesthesiology* 36:544-549, 1972.
112. France CJ et al: Ventilatory effects of isoflurane (Forane) or halothane when combined with morphine, nitrous oxide, and surgery, *Br J Anaesth* 46:117-120, 1974.
113. Artru AA: Relationship between cerebral blood volume and CSF pressure during anesthesia with halothane or enflurane in dogs, *Anesthesiology* 58:533-539, 1983.
114. Wollman H et al: Cerebral circulation of man during halothane anesthesia: effects of hypocarbia and *d*-tubocurarine, *Anesthesiology* 25:180-184, 1964.
115. Brosnan RJ et al: Direct measurement of intracranial pressure in adult horses, *Am J Vet Res* 63:1252-1256, 2002.
116. Auer JA, Amend JF, Granier HE, et al: Electroencephalographic response during volatile anesthesia in domestic ponies: a comparative study of isoflurane, enflurane, methoxyflurane, and halothane, *J Equine Med Surg* 3:130-134, 1979.
117. Grabow J, Anslow RO, Spalatin J: Electroencephalographic recordings with multicontact depth probes in a horse, *Am J Vet Res* 30:1239-1243, 1969.
118. Johnson CB, Taylor PM: Comparison of the effects of halothane, isoflurane, and methoxyflurane on the electroencephalogram of the horse, *Br J Anaesth* 81:748-753, 1998.
119. Johnson CB, Young SS, Taylor PM: Analysis of the frequency spectrum of the equine electroencephalogram during halothane anaesthesia, *Res Vet Sci* 56:373-378, 1994.
120. Mahla ME, Black S, Cucchiara RF: Neurologic monitoring. In Miller RD, editor: *Miller's anesthesia,* ed 6, Philadelphia, 2005, Elsevier Churchill Livingstone, pp 1511-1550.
121. Murrell JC et al: Changes in the EEG during castration in horses and ponies anaesthetized with halothane, *Vet Anaesth Analg* 30:138-146, 2003.
122. Reilly CS et al: The effect of halothane on drug disposition: contribution of changes in intrinsic drug metabolizing capacity and hepatic blood flow, *Anesthesiology* 63:70-76, 1985.
123. Thomasy SM et al: Influence of general anesthesia on the pharmacokinetics of intravenous fentanyl and its primary metabolite in horses, *Equine Vet J* 39:54-58, 2007.
124. Gopinath C, Jones RS, Ford EJH: The effect of repeated administration of halothane on the liver of the horse, *J Pathol* 102:107-114, 1970.
125. Lees P, Mullen PA, Tavernor WD: Influence of anaesthesia with volatile agents on the equine liver, *Br J Anaesth* 45:570-578, 1973.
126. Wolff WA, Lumb WV, Ramsay MK: Effects of halothane and chloroform anesthesia on the equine liver, *Am J Vet Res* 28:1363-1372, 1967.
127. Durongphongtorn S et al: Comparison of hemodynamic, clinicopathologic, and gastrointestinal motility effects and recovery characteristics of anesthesia with isoflurane and halothane in horses undergoing arthroscopic surgery, *Am J Vet Res* 67:32-42, 2006.
128. Engelking LR et al: Effects of halothane anesthesia on equine liver function, *Am J Vet Res* 45:607-615, 1984.
129. Gopinath C, Ford EJ: The influence of hepatic microsomal aminopyrine demethylase activity on halothane hepatotoxicity in the horse, *J Pathol* 119:105-112, 1976.
130. Grandy JL et al: Arterial hypotension and the development of postanesthetic myopathy in halothane-anesthetized horses, *Am J Vet Res* 48:192-197, 1987.
131. Steffey EP et al: Alterations in horse blood cell count and biochemical values after halothane anesthesia, *Am J Vet Res* 41:934-939, 1980.
132. Stover SM et al: Hematologic and biochemical values associated with multiple halothane anesthesias and minor surgical trauma of horses, *Am J Vet Res* 49:236-241, 1988.

133. Whitehair KJ et al: Effects of inhalation anesthetic agents on response of horses to 3 hours of hypoxemia, *Am J Vet Res* 57:351-360, 1996.

134. Lindsay WA et al: Induction of equine postanesthetic myositis after halothane-induced hypotension, *Am J Vet Res* 50: 404-410, 1989.

135. Smith CM et al: Effects of halothane anesthesia on the clearance of gentamicin sulfate in horses, *Am J Vet Res* 49:19-22, 1988.

136. Feary DJ et al: Influence of general anesthesia on pharmacokinetics of intravenous lidocaine infusion in horses, *Am J Vet Res* 66:574-580, 2005.

137. Aleman M et al: Malignant hyperthermia in a horse anesthetized with halothane, *J Vet Intern Med* 19:363-367, 2005.

138. Klein L et al: Postanesthetic equine myopathy suggestive of malignant hyperthermia: a case report, *Vet Surg* 18:479-482, 1989.

139. Klein LV: Case report: a hot horse, *Vet Anesth* 2:41-42, 1975.

140. Manley SV, Kelly AB, Hodgson D: Malignant hyperthermia-like reactions in three anesthetized horses, *J Am Vet Med Assoc* 183:85-89, 1983.

141. Waldron-Mease E et al: Malignant hyperthermia in a halothane-anesthetized horse, *J Am Vet Med Assoc* 179:896-898, 1981.

142. Aleman M et al: Association of a mutation in the ryanodine receptor 1 gene with equine malignant hyperthermia, *Muscle Nerve* 30:356-365, 2004.

143. Kelly AB et al: Immediate and long-term effects of halothane anesthesia on equine platelet function, *J Vet Pharmacol Ther* 8:284-289, 1985.

144. Cascorbi HF, Blake DA, Helrich M: Differences in the biotransformation of halothane in man, *Anesthesiology* 32: 119-123, 1970.

145. de Moor A et al: Increased plasma bromide concentration in the horse after halothane anesthesia, *Am J Vet Res* 39: 1624-1626, 1978.

146. Rice SA, Steffey EP: Metabolism of halothane and isoflurane in horses, *Vet Surg* 14:76, 1985.

147. Manohar M et al: Systemic distribution of blood flow in ponies during 1.45%, 1.96%, and 2.39% end-tidal isoflurane O₂ anesthesia, *Am J Vet Res* 48:1504-1511, 1987.

148. Serteyn D et al: Measurements of muscular microcirculation by laser Doppler flowmetry in isoflurane and halothane anaesthetised horses, *Vet Rec* 121:324-326, 1987.

149. Dunlop CI et al: Cardiopulmonary effects of isoflurane and halothane in spontaneously ventilating foals, *Vet Surg* 19:315, 1990.

150. Grosenbaugh DA, Muir WW III: Cardiorespiratory effects of sevoflurane, isoflurane, and halothane anesthesia in horses, *Am J Vet Res* 59:101-106, 1998.

151. Johnston GM et al: Is isoflurane safer than halothane in equine anaesthesia? Results from a prospective multicentre randomised controlled trial, *Equine Vet J* 36:64-71, 2004.

152. Raisis AL et al: The effects of halothane and isoflurane on cardiovascular function in laterally recumbent horses, *Br J Anaesth* 95:317-325, 2005.

153. Roberts SL, Gilbert M, Tinker JH: Isoflurane has a greater margin of safety than halothane in swine with and without major surgery or critical coronary stenosis, *Anesth Analg* 66:485-492, 1987.

154. Steffey EP et al: Cardiovascular and respiratory measurements in awake and isoflurane-anesthetized horses, *Am J Vet Res* 48:7-12, 1987.

155. Dunlop CI et al: Comparative cardiopulmonary effects of halothane and isoflurane between adult horses and foals. In *Proceedings of the Fourth International Congress of Veterinary Anesthesia*, Utrecht, Netherlands, 1991, p 128.

156. Steffey EP et al: Clinical investigations of halothane and isoflurane for induction and maintenance of foal anesthesia, *J Vet Pharmacol Ther* 14:300-309, 1991.

157. Edner A, Nyman G, Essen-Gustavsson B: The effects of spontaneous and mechanical ventilation on central cardiovascular function and peripheral perfusion during isoflurane anaesthesia in horses, *Vet Anaesth Analg* 32:136-146, 2005.

158. Hodgson DS et al: Cardiopulmonary effects of isoflurane in foals, *Vet Surg* 19:316, 1990.

159. Joas TA, Stevens WC: Comparison of the arrhythmic doses of epinephrine during Forane, halothane, and fluroxene anesthesia in dogs, *Anesthesiology* 35:48-53, 1971.

160. Johnston RR, Eger EI, II, Wilson C: A comparative interaction of epinephrine with enflurane, isoflurane, and halothane in man, *Anesth Analg* 55:709-712, 1976.

161. Steffey EP et al: Cardiopulmonary function during 5 hours of constant-dose isoflurane in laterally recumbent, spontaneously breathing horses, *J Vet Pharmacol Ther* 10:290-297, 1987.

162. Yamanaka T et al: Time-related changes of the cardiovascular system during maintenance anesthesia with sevoflurane and isoflurane in horses, *J Vet Med Sci* 63:527-532, 2001.

163. Duke T et al: Clinical observations surrounding an increased incidence of postanesthetic myopathy in halothane-anesthetized horses, *Vet Anaesth Analg* 33:122-127, 2006.

164. Klein L: A review of 50 cases of postoperative myopathy in the horse—intrinsic and management factors affecting risk, In *Proceedings of the American Association of Equine Practitioners*, Miami Beach, Florida, 1979, pp 89-94.

165. Lindsay WA, McDonell W, Bignell W: Equine postanesthetic forelimb lameness: intracompartmental muscle pressure changes and biochemical pattern, *Am J Vet Res* 41:1919-1924, 1980.

166. Trim CM, Mason J: Post-anaesthetic forelimb lameness in horses, *Equine Vet J* 5:71-76, 1973.

167. Stevens WC et al: The cardiovascular effects of a new inhalation anesthetic, Forane, in human volunteers at constant arterial carbon dioxide tension, *Anesthesiology* 35:8-16, 1971.

168. Goetz TE et al: Isoflurane anesthesia at 1.1, 1.5, or 1.8 MAC does not increase equine skeletal muscle perfusion. In *Third Equine Colic Research Symposium*, Athens, Greece, 1988, p 48.

169. Goetz TE et al: A study of the effect of isoflurane anaesthesia on equine skeletal muscle perfusion, *Equine Vet J* 7: S133-S137, 1989.

170. Manohar M, Gustafson R, Nganwa D: Skeletal muscle perfusion during prolonged 2.03% end-tidal isoflurane-O₂ anesthesia in isocapnic ponies, *Am J Vet Res* 48:946-951, 1987.

171. Weaver BMQ et al: Muscle perfusion during isoflurane anesthesia. In *Proceedings of the International Congress of Veterinary Anesthesia*, Brisbane, Australia, 1988, p 3.

172. Lee YHL, Clarke KW, Alibhai HIK: effects of the intramuscular blood flow and cardiopulmonary function of anesthetised ponies of changing from halothane to isoflurane maintenance and vice versa, *Vet Rec* 143:629-633, 1998.

173. Raisis AL: Skeletal muscle blood flow in anaesthetized horses. Part II: effects of anaesthetics and vasoactive agents, *Vet Anaesth Analg* 32:331-337, 2005.

174. Brosnan RJ, Imai A, Steffey EP: Quantification of dose-dependent respiratory depression in isoflurane-anesthetized horses, *Vet Anaesth Analg* 29:104, 2001.

175. Hodgson DS et al: Alteration in breathing patterns of horses during halothane and isoflurane anesthetic induction. In Grandy J et al, editors: *Proceedings of the Second International Congress of Veterinary Anesthesia*, Santa Barbara, Ca, 1985, Veterinary Practice Publishing Co.: pp 195-196.

176. Brosnan RJ et al: Intracranial and cerebral perfusion pressures in awake versus isoflurane-anesthetized horses. In *Proceedings of the American College of Veterinary Anesthesia*, New Orleans, 2001, p 36.

177. Patel PM, Drummond JC: Cerebral physiology and the effects of anesthetics and techniques. In Miller RD, editor: *Miller's anesthesia,* ed 6, Philadelphia, 2005, Elsevier Churchill Livingstone, pp 813-857.

178. Brosnan RJ et al: Effects of duration of isoflurane anesthesia and mode of ventilation on intracranial and cerebral perfusion pressures in horses, *Am J Vet Res* 64:1444-1448, 2003.

179. Brosnan RJ et al: Effects of body position on intracranial and cerebral perfusion pressures in isoflurane-anesthetized horses, *J Appl Physiol* 92:2542-2546, 2002.

180. Brosnan RJ et al: Effects of ventilation and isoflurane end-tidal concentration on intracranial and cerebral perfusion pressures in horses, *Am J Vet Res* 64:21-25, 2003.

181. Clark DL, Hosick EC, Neigh JL: Neural effects of isoflurane (Forane) in man, *Anesthesiology* 39:261-270, 1973.

182. Eger EI II, Stevens WC, Cromwell TH: The electroencephalogram in man anesthetized with Forane, *Anesthesiology* 35:504-508, 1971.

183. Haga HA, Dolvik NI: Electroencephalographic and cardiovascular variables as nociceptive indicators in isoflurane-anaesthetized horses, *Vet Anaesth Analg* 32:128-135, 2005.

184. Otto KA et al: Differences in quantitated electroencephalographic variables during surgical stimulation of horses anesthetized with isoflurane, *Vet Surg* 25:249-255, 1996.

185. Engelking LR et al: Effects of isoflurane anesthesia on equine liver function, *Am J Vet Res* 45:616, 1984.

186. Steffey EP, Zinkl J, Howland DJ: Minimal changes in blood cell counts and biochemical values associated with prolonged isoflurane anesthesia of horses, *Am J Vet Res* 40:1646-1648, 1979.

187. Kelly AB, Steffey EP, McNeal D: Isoflurane anesthesia effects equine platelets, *Proc Fed Am Soc Exp Biol* 44:1644, 1985.

188. Kelly AB et al: Comparative hemostatic effects of halothane and isoflurane anesthesia in the horse. In Grandy J et al, editors: *Proceedings of the Second International Congress of Veterinary Anesthesia,* Santa Barbara, 1985, Veterinary Practice Publishing Co.; pp 65-66.

189. Holaday DA et al: Resistance of isoflurane to biotransformation in man, *Anesthesiology* 43:325-332, 1975.

190. Auer JA et al: Recovery from anaesthesia in ponies: a comparative study of the effects of isoflurane, enflurane, methoxyflurane, and halothane, *Equine Vet J* 10:18-23, 1978.

191. Donaldson LL et al: The recovery of horses from inhalant anesthesia: a comparison of halothane and isoflurane, *Vet Surg* 29:92-101, 2000.

192. Whitehair KJ et al: Recovery of horses from inhalation anesthesia, *Am J Vet Res* 54:1693-1702, 1993.

193. Taylor PM, Watkins SB: Isoflurane in the horse, *J Assoc Vet Anaesth Gr Britain Ireland* 12:191-195, 1984.

194. Rose JA, Rose EM, Peterson PR: Clinical experience with isoflurane anesthesia in foals and adult horses, *Proc Am AssocEquine Pract* 34:555-561, 1988.

195. Santos M et al: Cardiovascular effects of desflurane in horses, *Vet Anaesth Analg* 32:355-359, 2005.

196. Weiskopf RB et al: Cardiovascular actions of desflurane in normocarbic volunteers, *Anesth Analg* 73:143-156, 1991.

197. Weiskopf RB et al: Cardiovascular effects of I-653 in swine, *Anesthesiology* 69:303-309, 1988.

198. Aida H et al: Cardiovascular and pulmonary effects of sevoflurane anesthesia in horses, *Vet Surg* 25:164-170, 1996.

199. Clarke KW et al: Cardiopulmonary effects of desflurane in ponies, after induction of anaesthesia with xylazine and ketamine, *Vet Rec* 139:180-185, 1996.

200. Driessen B et al: Differences in need for hemodynamic support in horses anesthetized with sevoflurane as compared to isoflurane, *Vet Anaesth Analg* 33:356-367, 2006.

201. Steffey EP et al: Effects of desflurane and mode of ventilation on cardiovascular and respiratory functions and clinicopathologic variables in horses, *Am J Vet Res* 66:669-677, 2005.

202. Weiskopf RB et al: Epinephrine-induced premature ventricular contractions and changes in arterial blood pressure and heart rate during I-653, isoflurane, and halothane anesthesia in swine, *Anesthesiology* 70:293-298, 1989.

203. Weiskopf RB et al: Cardiovascular safety and actions of high concentrations of I-653 and isoflurane in swine, *Anesthesiology* 70:793-799, 1989.

204. Eger EI II: *Desflurane (Suprane): a compendium and reference,* Rutherford Healthpress Publishing Group.

205. Warltier DC, Pagel PS: Cardiovascular and respiratory actions of desflurane: is desflurane different from isoflurane? *Anesth Analg* 75:S17-S31, 1992.

206. Jones RM et al: Biotransformation and hepato-renal function in volunteers after exposure to desflurane (I-653), *Br J Anaesth* 64:482-487, 1990.

207. Eger EI II et al: Studies of the toxicity of I-653, halothane, and isoflurane in enzyme-induced, hypoxic rats, *Anesth Analg* 66:1227-1230, 1987.

208. Holmes MA et al: Hepatocellular integrity in swine after prolonged desflurane (I- 653) and isoflurane anesthesia: evaluation of plasma alanine aminotransferase activity, *Anesth Analg* 71:249-253, 1990.

209. Merin RG et al: Comparison of the effects of isoflurane and desflurane on cardiovascular dynamics and regional blood flow in the chronically instrumented dog, *Anesthesiology* 74:568-574, 1991.

210. Sutton TS et al: Fluoride metabolites after prolonged exposure of volunteers and patients to desflurane, *Anesth Analg* 73:180-185, 1991.

211. Fang ZX et al: Carbon monoxide production from degradation of desflurane, enflurane, isoflurane, halothane, and sevoflurane by soda lime and baralyme, *Anesth Analg* 80:1187-1193, 1995.

212. Berry PD, Sessler DI, Larson MD: Severe carbon monoxide poisoning during desflurane anesthesia, *Anesthesiology* 90:613-616, 1999.

213. Dodam JR et al: Inhaled carbon monoxide concentration during halothane or isoflurane anesthesia in horses, *Vet Surg* 28:506-512, 1999.

214. Ghouri AF, Bodner M, White PF: Recovery profile after desflurane nitrous oxide versus isoflurane nitrous oxide in outpatients, *Anesthesiology* 74:419-424, 1991.

215. Steffey EP et al: A laboratory study of horses recovering from desflurane and isoflurane anaesthesia, *Vet Anaesth Analg* 29:90, 2002.

216. Wallin RF et al: Sevoflurane: a new inhalational anesthetic agent, *Anesth Analg* 54:758-766, 1975.

217. Driessen B et al: Serum fluoride concentrations, biochemical and histopathological changes associated with prolonged sevoflurane anaesthesia in horses, *J Vet Med Assoc* 49:337-347, 2002.

218. Bernard JM et al: Effects of sevoflurane and isoflurane on cardiac and coronary dynamics in chronically instrumented dogs, *Anesthesiology* 72:659-662, 1990.

219. Ebert TJ, Harkin CP, Muzi M: Cardiovascular responses to sevoflurane: a review, *Anesth Analg* 81:S11-S22, 1995.

220. Eger EI II: New inhaled anesthetics, *Anesthesiology* 80:906-922, 1994.

221. Manohar M, Parks CM: Porcine systemic and regional organ blood flow during 1.0 and 1.5 minimum alveolar concentrations of sevoflurane anesthesia without and with 50% nitrous oxide, *J Pharmacol Exp Ther* 231:640-648, 1984.

222. Read MR et al: Cardiopulmonary effects and induction and recovery characteristics of isoflurane and sevoflurane in foals, *J Am Vet Med Assoc* 221:393-398, 2002.

223. Hayashi Y et al: Arrhythmogenic threshold of epinephrine during sevoflurane, enflurane, and isoflurane anesthesia in dogs, *Anesthesiology* 69:145-147, 1988.

224. Hikasa Y et al: Ventricular arrhythmogenic dose of adrenaline during sevoflurane, isoflurane, and halothane anaesthesia either with or without ketamine or thiopentone in cats, *Res Vet Sci* 60:134-137, 1996.

225. Aida H et al: Use of sevoflurane for anesthetic management of horses during thoracotomy, *Am J Vet Res* 61:1430-1437, 2000.

226. O'Connor CJ, Rothenberg DM, Tuman KJ: Anesthesia and the hepatobiliary system. In Miller RD, editor: *Miller's anesthesia,* ed 6, Philadelphia, 2005, Elsevier Churchill Livingstone, pp 2209-2229.

227. Gelman S: General anesthesia and hepatic circulation, *Can J Physiol Pharmacol* 65:1762-1779, 1987.

228. Frink EJ Jr et al: The effects of sevoflurane, halothane, enflurane, and isoflurane on hepatic blood flow and oxygenation in chronically instrumented greyhound dogs, *Anesthesiology* 76:85-90, 1992.

229. Hikasa Y, Takase K, Ogasawara S: Sevoflurane and oxygen anaesthesia following administration of atropine-xylazine-guaifenesin-thiopental in spontaneously breathing horses, *J Vet Med Assoc* 41:700-708, 1994.

230. Holaday DA, Smith FR: Clinical characteristics and biotransformation of sevoflurane in healthy human volunteers, *Anesthesiology* 54:100-106, 1981.

231. Kharasch ED, Hankins DC, Thummel KE: Human kidney methoxyflurane and sevoflurane metabolism-intrarenal fluoride production as a possible mechanism of methoxyflurane nephrotoxicity, *Anesthesiology* 82:689-699, 1995.

232. Kharasch ED et al: New insights into the mechanism of methoxyflurane nephrotoxicity and implications for anesthetic development (Part 1), *Anesthesiology* 105:726-736, 2006.

233. Kharasch ED et al: New insights into the mechanism of methoxyflurane nephrotoxicity and implications for anesthetic development (Part 2), *Anesthesiology* 105:737-745, 2006.

234. Mazze RI: The safety of sevoflurane in humans, *Anesthesiology* 77:1062-1063, 1992.

235. Gonsowski CT et al: Toxicity of compound A in rats: effect of a 3-hour administration, *Anesthesiology* 80:556-565, 1994.

236. Gonsowski CT et al: Toxicity of compound A in rats: effect of increasing duration of administration, *Anesthesiology* 80:566-573, 1994.

237. Croinin DF, Shorten GD: Anesthesia and renal disease, *Curr Opin Anaesth* 15:359-363, 2002.

238. Mazze RI, Jamison R: Renal effects of sevoflurane, *Anesthesiology* 83:443-445, 1995.

239. Kharasch ED: Biotransformation of sevoflurane, *Anesth Analg* 81:S27-S38, 1995.

240. Cook TL et al: A comparison of renal effects and metabolism of sevoflurane and methoxyflurane in enzyme-induced rats, *Anesth Analg* 54:829-835, 1975.

241. Aida H et al: Determination of the minimum alveolar concentration (MAC) and physical response to sevoflurane inhalation in horses, *J Vet Med Sci* 56:1161-1165, 1994.

242. Steffey EP, Howland DJ: The rate of change of halothane concentration in a large animal circle anesthetic system, *Am J Vet Res* 38:1993-1996, 1977.

243. Eger EI et al: The effect of anesthetic duration on kinetic and recovery characteristics of desflurane versus sevoflurane, and on the kinetic characteristics of compound A, in volunteers, *Anesth Analg* 86:414-421, 1998.

244. Matthews NS et al: Sevoflurane anaesthesia in clinical equine cases: maintenance and recovery, *J Vet Anaesth* 26:13-17, 1999.

245. Ohta M et al: Anesthetic management with sevoflurane and oxygen for orthopedic surgeries in Racehorses, *J Vet Med Sci* 62:1017-1020, 2000.

246. Yamashita K et al: Combination of continuous intravenous infusion using a mixture of guaifenesin-ketamine-medetomidine and sevoflurane anesthesia in horses, *J Vet Med Sci* 62:229-235, 2000.

247. Matthews NS et al: Recovery from sevoflurane anesthesia in horses: comparison to isoflurane and effect of postmedication with xylazine, *Vet Surg* 27:480-485, 1998.

248. Valverde A et al: Effect of a constant rate infusion of lidocaine on the quality of recovery from sevoflurane or isoflurane general anaesthesia in horses, *Equine Vet J* 37:559-564, 2005.

249. Eger EI et al: Contrasting roles of the N-methyl-D-aspartate receptor in production of immobilization by conventional and aromatic anesthetics, *Anesth Analg* 102:1397-1406, 2006.

250. Emmanouil DE, Quock RM: Advances in understanding the actions of nitrous oxide, *Anesth Prog* 54:9-18, 2007.

251. Moens Y, de Moor A: Diffusion of nitrous oxide into the intestinal lumen of ponies during halothane-nitrous oxide anesthesia, *Am J Vet Res* 42:1750-1753, 1981.

252. Steffey EP et al: Nitrous oxide increases the accumulation rate and decreases the uptake of bowel gases, *Anesth Analg* 58:405-408, 1979.

253. Cohen EN et al: Occupational disease among operating room personnel: a national study, *Anesthesiology* 41:321-340, 1974.

254. National Institute for Occupational Safety and Health: *Criteria for a recommended standard: occupational exposure to waste anesthetic gases and vapors,* Washington, DC, 1977, DHEW (NIOSH), Report No 77-140.

255. Whitcher C: *Development and evaluation of methods for the elimination of waste anesthetic gases and vapors in hospitals,* Washington, DC, 1975, DHEW Publications, Report No 75-137.

256. Manley SV, McDonell WF: Recommendations for reduction of anesthetic gas pollution, *J Am Vet Med Assoc* 176:519-524, 1980.

257. Flemming DC, Johnstone RE: Recognition thresholds for diethyl ether and halothane, *Anesthesiology* 46:68-69, 1977.

258. Lecky JH: Anesthetic pollution in the operating room: a notice to operating room personnel, *Anesthesiology* 52:157-159, 1980.

259. Jones RM: Desflurane and sevoflurane: inhalation anaesthetics for this decade?, *Br J Anaesth* 65:527-536, 1990.

260. Lowe HJ, Ernst EA: *The quantitative practice of anesthesia: use of closed circuit,* ed 1, Baltimore, 1981, Williams & Wilkins.

261. Miller EDJ, Greene NM: Waking up to desflurane: the anesthetic for the 90s?, *Anesth Analg* 70:1-2, 1990.

262. Targ AG, Yasuda N, Eger EI II: Solubility of I-653, sevoflurane, isoflurane, and halothane in plastics and rubber composing a conventional anesthetic circuit, *Anesth Analg* 69:218-225, 1989.

263. Bennett RC et al: Influence of morphine sulfate on the halothane sparing effect of xylazine hydrochloride in horses, *Am J Vet Res* 65:519-526, 2004.

264. Tendillo FJ et al: Anesthetic potency of desflurane in the horse: determination of the minimum alveolar concentration, *Vet Surg* 26:354-357, 1997.

265. Kronen PW: Anesthetic management of the horse: inhalation anesthesia. In Steffey EP, editor: *Recent advances in anesthetic management of large domestic animals* (International Veterinary Information Services Website). January 31, 2003. Accessed September 13, 2005, from http://www.ivis.org/advances/Steffey_Anesthesia/kronen/chapter_frm.asp?LA=1.

16

Anesthetic Equipment

Richard M. Bednarski

KEY POINTS

1. Short-duration equine anesthesia can be performed with minimum equipment, but a means to support breathing and hemodynamics should be available.
2. Infusion pumps and anesthetic machines provide the ability to administer a controlled amount of injectable or inhalant anesthetic, respectively.
3. Most inhalant anesthetic vaporizers are temperature- and flow-compensated and deliver accurate concentrations of inhalant anesthetic over a wide flow range.
4. Many equine anesthetic machines are equipped with a ventilator. Anesthesia ventilators are equipped with either ascending bellows (ascends during expiration) or descending bellows (descends during expiration) (see Chapter 17).
5. Horses less than 200 kg of body weight can be anesthetized using standard small animal anesthetic machines. Larger horses require larger breathing circuits to minimize resistance to breathing and provide a large breathing reservoir.
6. All personnel should be trained on the safe use of flow meters, compressed gas cylinders, and gas supply pressure systems.
7. The duration of use of carbon dioxide absorbent material should be monitored and is approximately 6 to 8 hours in adult horses.
8. Anesthetic machines should be tested for leaks before each use (pressurized to 30 cm H_2O).

All equipment, breathing hoses, and Y pieces should be cleaned and dried after every use.

Equipment requirements for equine anesthesia are determined by the anesthetic technique performed. Syringes, needles, and solution administration sets are the only equipment required for field anesthetic techniques limited to the use of injectable drugs. However, endotracheal tubes and oxygen delivery equipment may be needed in the event of complications. Most long-term anesthetic procedures (longer than 1 hour) are performed using inhalation anesthesia. The delivery of inhalation anesthetics requires familiarity with various relatively complex pieces of equipment. Intravenous catheters, syringe infusion pumps, ventilators, and patient monitoring devices are discussed elsewhere (see Chapters 7, 8, and 17).[1]

SYSTEMS FOR DELIVERY OF MEDICAL GASES

Oxygen, nitrous oxide, or air can be delivered directly to the anesthetic apparatus from compressed gas cylinders, compressors (air, O_2), or remote gas source through a pipeline system.

Compressed Gas Cylinders and Connections

Compressed gas cylinders are most commonly used for medical gas storage. All of the commonly used gases are available in cylinders (Table 16-1). Gas cylinders are relatively inexpensive, portable, and available in various sizes. Popular color-coded cylinder sizes used with anesthetic equipment include E, G, or H (see Table 16-1). The E cylinders are pin indexed (see following paragraphs) to ensure proper connection to the regulator or hanger yoke of the anesthetic apparatus. The large G and H cylinders have specific screw threads and valve stem sizes to ensure appropriate connection. Compressed gas cylinders are potentially dangerous if they are handled inappropriately; there are reports of serious accidents associated with improper storage and handling.[1,2] Large cylinders should always be secured to a wall or set into a stable base; they should be transported only after they are secured to mobile carts specifically designed for this purpose. Small cylinders should be carried in the vertical position with the hand securely around the valve body. Publications are available that detail safe handling and storage of compressed gases.[3,4]

Cylinders filled solely with gas (e.g., oxygen) undergo a pressure drop when gas is used. The pressure drop is proportional to the amount of gas remaining within the tank. Knowing the pressure in the tank, the number of liters in a full cylinder (see Table 16-1), and the flow rate of gas (i.e., oxygen) being used permits calculation of the amount of time the flow of gas will continue. For example, a G cylinder with 500 psi (approximately 25% of a full tank) contains approximately 1300 L and will provide a continuous flow of oxygen at a rate of 5 L/min for 260 minutes. Nitrous oxide cylinders are part liquid and part gas. They do not undergo a pressure drop until all the liquid has volatized. The only way to determine how much nitrous oxide remains in a tank is to weigh the cylinder and compare this with the weight of the cylinder when full. Full E cylinders of nitrous oxide contain 1590 L of gas at standard temperature and pressure ($0°$ C, 1 atm = 14.7 psi). Most small animal anesthetic machines are equipped with hanger yokes for attachment of small E cylinders to the anesthetic machine. These hanger yokes have a pin index system with the pins located in specific positions for specific gases (Figure 16-1). Large G or H cylinders can be connected individually to the anesthetic apparatus through high-pressure conductive tubing, using a diameter index safety system gas-specific connector (Figure 16-2) or a yoke block connector, which fits into the pin-indexed hanger yoke (Figure 16-3).

G or H cylinders used for central hospital gas supply systems are connected to a manifold that connects multiple cylinders to a hospital supply line (Figure 16-4). Most manifolds have a provision to trigger an alarm and automatically

Table 16–1.   Compressed gases

		Cylinder specifications (liters, STP)			
		E	**G**	**H**	
Agent	**Color**	**(10 cm × 75 cm)**	**(20 cm × 138 cm)**	**(23 cm × 138 cm)**	**Filling pressure (psi)**
Oxygen	Green (United States) Black with white top (United Kingdom)	655	5290	6910	2200
Nitrous oxide	Blue	1590	12,110	14,520	750

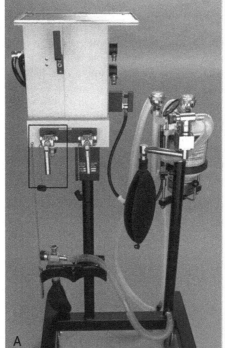
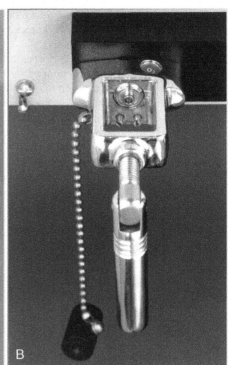

Figure 16–1. A, Hanger yoke for attachment of an oxygen cylinder. Note the pin index system. **B**, Close-up of boxed area in **A**.

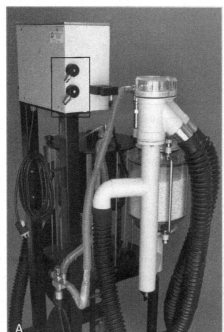
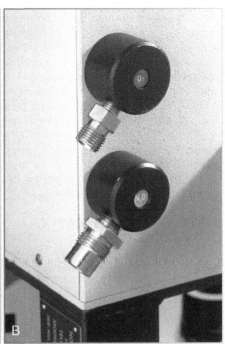

Figure 16–2. A, Diameter index safety system for attachment of oxygen and nitrous oxide high-pressure hoses. Note the different configuration of the two connections. **B**, Close-up of boxed area in **A**.

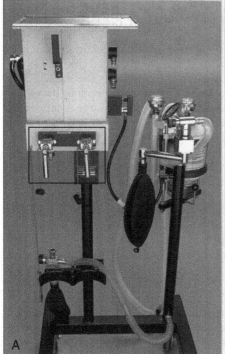
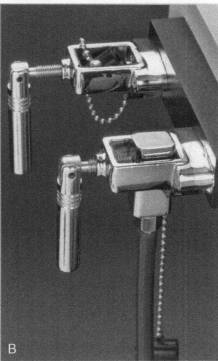

Figure 16–3. A, Yoke block connector for attachment of high-pressure oxygen delivery hose to an anesthetic machine not equipped with a diameter index safety system fitting. **B,** Close-up of boxed area in **A.**

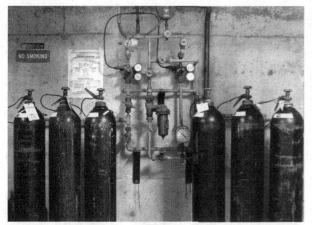

Figure 16–4. Manifold for connection of several compressed gas cylinders to a pressure regulator and common gas line. This is a system for delivery of nitrogen.

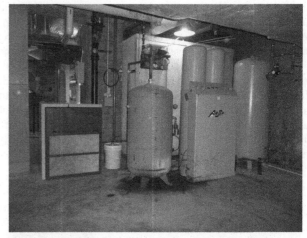

Figure 16–5. This oxygen generator is capable of producing 22 L/min of oxygen. (Air Sep Corp, Buffalo, NY.)

switch to an auxiliary bank of cylinders when the pressure in the primary cylinder bank reaches a predetermined low pressure (generally below 50 psi). Central hospital gas supply systems should have a shut-off valve in the pipeline supplying each area of the hospital. This permits isolation of leaks and repair without shutting off supply to the entire hospital.[1,5]

Oxygen-Generating Systems

Oxygen-generating systems can be installed in veterinary hospitals as alternatives to oxygen cylinders (Figure 16-5). Oxygen is generated continually but requires electrical power. Oxygen-concentrating devices are available in a variety of sizes, with delivery capabilities sufficient for equine anesthesia. These units use a series of molecular sieves (zeolite) to adsorb nitrogen. The sieves continually regenerate their oxygen-concentrating capability and can produce 90% to 95% oxygen; however, the output may be as low as 73%, and frequent checks of the system with an oxygen analyzer are recommended.[6]

Liquid Oxygen

Oxygen can be liquefied and stored in insulated cylinders at –148° C (Figure 16-6).[1] One cubic foot of liquid oxygen yields 860 cubic feet (24,000 L) of gaseous oxygen at 20° C (70° F). This type of oxygen storage is more economical than gas-containing cylinders but is not economical if use is infrequent because of evaporative loss from the cylinder. Liquid oxygen tanks of suitable size can be refilled by the supplier and transported to the hospital.

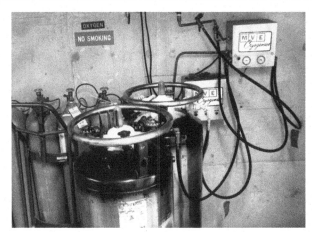

Figure 16–6. Liquid oxygen cylinder delivery system. Note the reserve supply of oxygen cylinders connected to a manifold for a back-up system.

Pressure Regulators

Pressure regulators decrease cylinder pressure to a predetermined constant level, usually between 50 and 60 psi (340 to 400 kPa), thereby maintaining a constant flow of gas in the face of a changing pressure supply. Regulators are built into many small animal anesthetic machines. They are generally an integral component of the hospital supply manifold or can be attached to individual cylinders. Regulators have specific fittings that match the valve outlet threads and stems of specific cylinders. Some regulators have a fixed delivered pressure, whereas others allow adjustment of the delivered pressure. Stand-alone pressure regulators are equipped with a gauge that indicates the cylinder pressure and a separate gauge that reflects delivery pressure, whereas regulators that are built into the anesthetic machine typically indicate only the pressure within the attached cylinder.

COMPONENTS OF THE ANESTHETIC MACHINE AND BREATHING CIRCUIT

The anesthetic machine and breathing circuit are designed to facilitate controlled delivery of oxygen and anesthetic gases and remove carbon dioxide from the exhaled gas. Anesthetic machines and circuits differ widely in appearance; however, most machines have the same components, albeit configured differently.

Oxygen Fail-Safe

Most commercially manufactured anesthetic machines have a valve or alarm intended to prevent air or nitrous oxide (if used) from being delivered through the anesthetic machine if the oxygen supply fails. This does not prevent the delivery of a hypoxic gas mixture, even if an adequate supply of oxygen is connected to the machine. For example, the nitrous oxide flowmeter can still be adjusted to deliver nitrous oxide to the breathing circuit even if the oxygen flowmeter is in the off position, as long as the hospital oxygen supply is connected to the machine or the oxygen cylinder is turned on. Nitrous oxide is not commonly used in horses; however, the oxygen flow setting should be monitored during the anesthetic procedure to prevent inadvertent delivery of a hypoxic mixture.

Flowmeters

A flowmeter is present for each type of gas (Figure 16-7). The flowmeter controls and displays the rate (L/min) of gas flow. The type of flowmeter used on most anesthetic machines consists of a valve adjusted by a color- and tactile-coded control knob; a tapered glass tube inscribed with numbers that correspond to gas flow rates; and a float, which rises within the tapered glass tube to indicate the flow rate of gas. As the valve is opened, gas flows into the tapered tube, and the float rises within the tube until the gravitational force acting on the float is balanced by the force of gas entering the bottom of the tube. The more gas that is allowed to

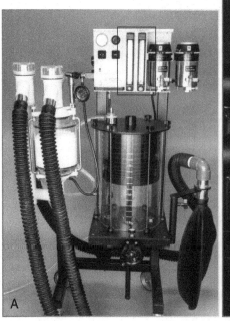
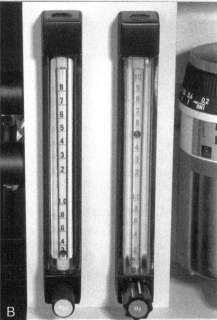

Figure 16–7. A, Oxygen and nitrous oxide flowmeters. The flow corresponds to the numbers opposite the widest portion of the float (in this instance, the center of the ball). **B,** Close-up of boxed area in **A.**

enter the tube, the higher the float rises within the tube. Gas passes between the float and the walls of the tube, exits from the top of the flowmeter, and is delivered to the vaporizer or fresh gas outlet.

Flowmeters are gas specific and should only be used for the type of gas for which they were designed. Because the physical properties of the different gases vary, the viscosity and density of gas affect the flow rate. Gas density also varies with altitude. Therefore at high altitude when high flow rates are used, flowmeters deliver relatively more gas than indicated by the calibration scale.[1] The owner's manual should be consulted for correction factors when using flowmeters at high altitude.

Oxygen Flush Valve

The oxygen flush valve delivers oxygen directly into the breathing circuit at relatively high flow rates. The oxygen bypasses the anesthetic vaporizer. Most oxygen flush valves deliver oxygen between 35 and 75 L/min.[1] Activation of the oxygen flush valve is activated and will fill the anesthetic circuit with 100% oxygen and dilute the anesthetic gas concentration.

Vaporizers

The anesthetic vaporizer converts the volatile liquid inhalation anesthetic from a liquid to vapor. Modern vaporizers (precision type) provide precisely determined vapor concentrations, regardless of the temperature and incoming gas flow rate perfusing the vaporizer (Figures 16-8 and 16-9).[6] Molecules of anesthetic liquid continually leave the surface of the liquid to enter a vapor phase. Equilibrium is reached when the number of molecules leaving the liquid equals the number reentering the liquid from the vapor. The pressure exerted by the vapor at equilibrium is termed the *saturated vapor pressure* and is the highest partial pressure the vapor can achieve at a given temperature.[1] The saturated vapor pressure of an inhalation anesthetic within an anesthetic vaporizer determines the maximum concentra-

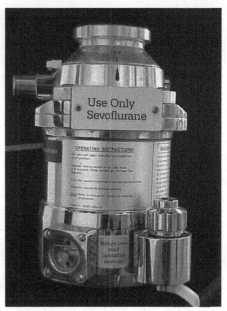

Figure 16–9. Sevoflurane vaporizer.

tion of anesthetic gas achievable at a given temperature. The saturated vapor pressure for the commonly used inhalation anesthetics is reached rapidly within a closed container such as an anesthetic vaporizer. Vapor pressure changes only in response to changes in temperature. Heating the anesthetic increases the vapor pressure because more molecules are likely to leave the liquid phase. Cooling the anesthetic liquid lowers the vapor pressure. If the saturated vapor pressure (partial pressure) at a given temperature is divided by the barometric pressure, the maximum concentration of the inhalation anesthetic (saturated inhalant anesthetic vapor concentration) can be calculated and expressed in terms of *volume percent*. For example, if the saturated vapor pressure of drug X is 240 mm Hg at 20° C, at a barometric pressure equal to 760 mm Hg (1 atm) the saturated vapor concentration of drug X is 240/760 = 32%. To achieve an appropriate safe delivered concentration, modern vaporizers split the carrier gas (oxygen or an oxygen blend from the flowmeters) within the vaporizer such that a portion is diverted into the vaporization chamber to combine with saturated anesthetic vapor. This saturated vapor leaving the vaporization chamber is diluted by the portion of the carrier gas that bypasses the vaporization chamber. The result is a final concentration (e.g., 1% to 5% for isoflurane) exiting the vaporizer that matches the operator's dialed setting (Figure 16-10).

As vaporization continues, the anesthetic within the vaporizer cools (*heat of vaporization*). Heat is extracted from the environment to offset the cooling. Vaporizers are usually designed to minimize the decrease in temperature of the anesthetic brought about by vaporization. The *specific heat* is the quantity of heat required to raise the temperature of 1 g of substance 1° C.[1] Anesthetic vaporizers are constructed of materials with a high specific heat so that they change temperature slowly. The *thermal conductivity* of the material from which the vaporizer is constructed must be high so that heat can be conducted rapidly from the environment to the liquid. Vaporizers are usually constructed

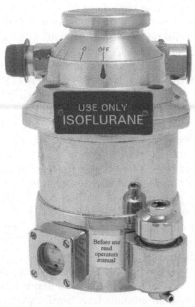

Figure 16–8. Isoflurane vaporizer.

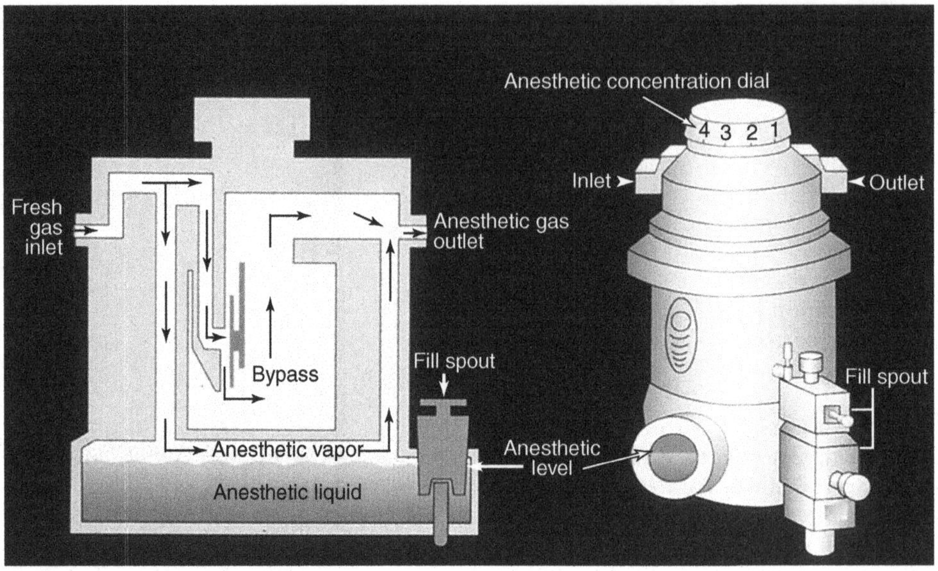

Figure 16–10. Schematic diagram illustrating the method used by a "precision" vaporizer to control the delivered concentration.

of copper or brass, two materials with high specific heat and thermal conductivity to minimize temperature elevations. Temperature drops from vaporization and changes in ambient temperature affect anesthetic liquid temperature and influence vaporizer output unless the vaporizer is temperature compensated. Most vaporizers have an internal mechanism that automatically adjusts flow by a thermostatic mechanism, allowing more or less vapor to exit the vaporization or bypass chamber. Modern vaporizers deliver a constant known concentration of vapor independent of fluctuations in temperature. The specific methods that different vaporizers use to accomplish precise delivery of vapor are proprietary.

A variety of vaporizers are used for equine anesthesia. Most are agent-specific and flow rate and temperature "compensated" and should only be used with one specific inhalation anesthetic. Anesthetic concentration output generally is constant when oxygen flow rates are between 300 ml and 10 L/min. The owner's manual should be consulted before use to determine the limits of both temperature and flow compensation.

Vaporizers should be removed from machines, cleaned, and recalibrated every 1 to 3 years or whenever the anesthetic concentration delivered by the vaporizer becomes questionable. Most vaporizers should not be tilted or laid on their side. This causes liquid anesthetic to spill into the vaporizer bypass outlet, potentially resulting in dangerously high anesthetic concentrations being delivered into the breathing circuit. The vaporizer should be emptied, and a high flow of oxygen allowed to flow through it until no anesthetic vapor is detected at the vaporizer outlet.

Common Gas Outlet

The common gas outlet delivers gas from the flowmeters and vaporizers to the anesthetic breathing circuit. This outlet is generally fitted with a standard 15-mm female opening (Figure 16-11) into which a connector and length of tubing are attached. This tubing is connected to the anesthetic breathing circuit and delivers the fresh carrier gas (i.e., oxygen) and anesthetic vapor.

Anesthetic Breathing Circuits

The breathing circuit conducts oxygen and anesthetic gases from the common gas outlet to the patient and removes exhaled gases from the patient (Box 16-1).[7] Breathing circuits have been classified in a number of ways, and the terminology can be confusing.[1] Breathing circuits in which the exhaled gases are partially rebreathed (exhaled gas minus carbon dioxide) use one-way valves to unidirectionally route gases through carbon dioxide–absorbent material and back to the horse (Figure 16-12). Alternatively, a valveless to-and-fro system is used, and gases are exhaled through the carbon dioxide–absorbent material into a reservoir bag and drawn back through the absorbent material during inhalation (Figure 16-13). Most classification systems refer to these circuits as "semiclosed" or "closed." The distinction between the two circuits refers to exposure to atmospheric air and the position of the pressure release or pop-off valve. Closed systems use fresh gas flow rates just equal to the horse's minute oxygen consumption; thus these circuits can be completely "closed" to the atmosphere (closed pop-off valve). Semiclosed systems use fresh gas flow rates that are greater than the horse's minute oxygen consumption; therefore the pressure relief (pop-off) valve remains open to vent the excess gas. Both circle and to-and-fro systems can be used as closed or semiclosed systems, depending on the fresh gas flow rate. These systems have similar components: carbon dioxide absorption canister, pressure relief (pop-off) valve, and reservoir bag. In addition, the circle system uses one-way valves, a Y piece, and corrugated breathing hoses. The advantages and disadvantages of the circle and to-and-fro breathing circuits are different (Table 16-2).

These features are present on most modern equine inhalation anesthetic machines. Machines manufactured for use in humans or small animals have similar components and can be used for horses that weigh less than 200 kg.[8]

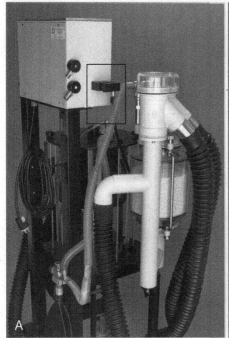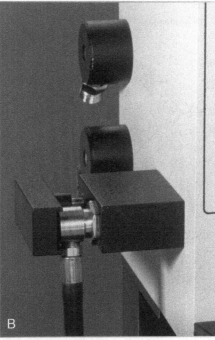

Figure 16–11. A, This 15-mm common gas outlet carries gas from the flowmeter and vaporizer to the breathing circuit. Note the protective cover that eliminates inadvertent disconnection. **B,** Close-up of boxed area in **A**.

Carbon Dioxide Absorption Canister

Carbon dioxide is absorbed by chemical reaction. Sodium, potassium, barium, and calcium hydroxides react with carbon dioxide and water to generate carbonates of these alkaline earth metals. The absorbent material producing this reaction is contained within a plastic or metal canister. Most absorption materials contain at least 75% calcium hydroxide; 14% to 19% water; and, depending on the manufacturer, small amounts of sodium or potassium hydroxides as activators.[1] The activators have been incriminated in the production of compound A (sevoflurane), carbon monoxide (desflurane > isoflurane > sevoflurane), and other breakdown compounds, particularly in desiccated

---

Box 16–1   Required Features of Anesthetic Apparatus Suitable for Delivery of Inhalation Anesthesia to Horses[7]

- Oxygen supply and oxygen flowmeter capable of delivering at least a 10 L/min

- Oxygen supply line (O_2 flush valve) that bypasses the vaporizer

- Vaporizer capable of delivering a known concentration of anesthetic vapor

- Wide-bore breathing tubing at least equal to the tracheal diameter; circle anesthetic circuits should contain one-way valves

- Pressure relief (pop-off) valve

- Carbon dioxide absorber

- Breathing bag large enough to assist or control breathing

- Appropriate low dead space endotracheal tube connection

---

absorbent.[9,10] Production of hydrogen gas from sevoflurane degradation has been incriminated. Absorbents that do not contain activators (sodium and potassium hydroxides) do not produce this phenomenon. To date no evidence of morbidity in horses related to any of these breakdown products exists.[10] Regardless, carbon dioxide absorbents that do not contain these activators (e.g., Amsorb, Sodasorb LF) are available.

The absorbent material removes carbon dioxide from the exhaled gas and in the process generates heat and moisture.[11] Approximately 13,700 calories of heat are generated per mole of CO_2 absorbed. However, absorbent temperatures greater than 200° C have been documented when desiccated absorbent containing barium reacts with sevoflurane. Absorbent material containing barium hydroxide has been withdrawn. Heat production is a crude method of checking absorbent activity. An active canister feels warm to the touch and can remain warm for an extended period of time after carbon dioxide consumption capability has been exhausted. The canister in a to-and-fro apparatus minimizes heat loss through the lungs because of its location and proximity to the patient's airway. Relatively high fresh gas flow rates and the construction of the canister with a material of high thermal conductivity such as steel or brass help prevent temperature rise. One study in horses failed to demonstrate an increase in body temperature during 90-minute use of a to-and-fro system. Absorbent material can desiccate when the oxygen flowmeter is inadvertently left on or when bulk absorbent supplies are left uncovered and exposed to dry room air. These high circuit temperatures can predispose to explosion and fire within the breathing circuit.

The contents of the CO_2 canister become less alkaline as absorption proceeds, and a pH-sensitive color indicator within the absorption granules indicates the degree of absorbent exhaustion. Color change (and thus exhaustion)

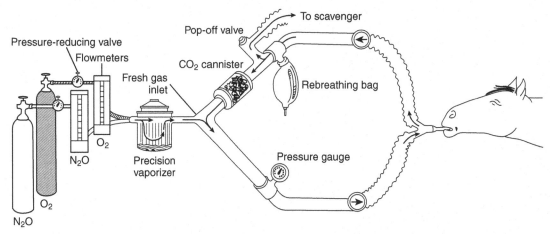

Figure 16–12. Schematic diagram of the components of a circle rebreathing circuit.

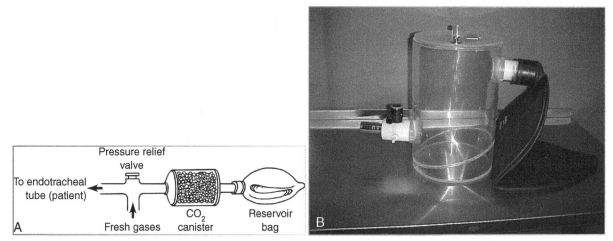

Figure 16–13. A, Schematic diagram of a to-and-fro rebreathing apparatus. **B,** To-and-fro rebreathing apparatus. (**B,** Courtesy Tom Riebold, Oregon State University)

Table 16–2. **Comparison of to-and-fro and circle breathing circuits**	
To-and-fro	**Circle**
Relatively simple with rugged construction	Relatively complex and expensive
Easily disassembled for cleaning	Relatively difficult to disassemble
Easily transportable	Not easily transported
Relatively rapid change in anesthetic concentration for a given fresh gas flow	Relatively slow change in anesthetic concentration for a given fresh gas flow
Excessive heat produced near endotracheal tube attachment	Temperature relatively uniform throughout circuit
Alkaline dust may be inhaled	Minimum chance of inhaling alkaline dust
Relatively awkward to use	Long hoses make connection to endotracheal tube easy
Dead space increases relatively rapidly	Dead space remains constant

is greatest at the canister inlet and spreads parabolically from the center of the canister to the walls, where resistance to gas flow is the least.[1] The greater the color change, the more complete the exhaustion. There is some degree of regeneration of the absorbent material within approximately 30 minutes of nonuse; the color change indicator returns to the original color. However, the color change is minimal,

and the color change indicator quickly returns if the absorbent material is put back into use.[1]

Absorbents are available that will not "regenerate" (e.g., Sodasorb LF); therefore the color change of the expired granules is permanent. The duration that absorbent material is effective before it must be changed varies with the size of the horse, the individual CO_2 production (metabolic rate) of the horse, the fresh gas flow rate, the size of the canister, and the location of the canister in relation to the patient's airway and other components of the breathing circuit. The single best method of deciding when to change the CO_2 absorbent material is to monitor inspired gas for CO_2. A progressively increasing inspired CO_2 concentration generally indicates CO_2 absorbent exhaustion or channeling. In the absence of a capnometer, color change and time of use should be noted. A canister containing 5 kg of absorbent material typically remains active for 6 to 8 hours of anesthesia (assuming a 450-kg horse and a 5-L/min O_2 flow rate). Ideally the canister size should be large enough when packed with absorbent granules that the air space within the canister is equal to the patient's tidal volume (approximately 10 ml/kg).[12] The air space (volume of air within the filled canister) when filled with 4- to 8-mesh size granules should be approximately 48% to 55% of the canister volume.[12,13] Therefore, for optimum efficiency the canister volume for a 450-kg horse should be approximately 10 L. Most commercially available large animal (LA) machine canisters have a 5-L volume. Canisters sized for use in small animals or humans are sufficient for use in horses or ponies weighing up to 200 kg because these canisters usually have a 1500- to 3000-ml capacity. Canister size is most critical in the to-and-fro system[13] because the CO_2 content of the system progressively increases with time as a result of progressively increasing dead space breathing (CO_2 absorbent exhaustion).[14] Too large a canister in to-and-fro systems causes exhaled gases to concentrate in the area near the patient, resulting in rapid exhaustion and increase in apparatus dead space. Too small a canister results in some of the tidal volume passing through the canister on exhalation. This gas is not in contact with the absorbent during the expiratory pause. During inhalation, when the gas is drawn back through the canister, absorption may not be complete, and some CO_2 can be rebreathed.

Canisters should be filled uniformly by gently tapping or agitating the canister during filling to prevent channeling of exhaled gas through the absorbent material. Channeling results in preferential passage of gas through discrete areas of the absorbent canister and can result in rebreathing of CO_2. The CO_2 canisters should not be packed too tightly because this crushes the granules and increases the amount of caustic dust within the canister. A small air space should be left at the entrance to the CO_2 canister to ensure an even flow of gas through the absorber surface.

Reservoir Bag

The reservoir bag (rebreathing bag) provides a buffer for changing volumes within the breathing system and a means to assist or control breathing. It also provides a visual indication of spontaneous ventilation. Ideally the maximum volume of the reservoir bag should be 5 to 10 times the tidal volume (450 kg × 10 ml/kg = 4500 × 5 = 22500 [22.5L]). Reserve bags available for adult horses are usually 15 or 30 L. A 5-L bag attached to a small animal machine is suitable for animals weighing less than 200 kg.

Pressure Relief (Pop-Off) Valve

The pressure relief valve is intended to vent gas from the breathing circuit and control the pressure within. The greater the fresh gas flow rate, the more gas escapes through the pop-off valve. The valve is left in the open position at all times when fresh gas flow rates exceed the horse's oxygen consumption, except during periods of assisted or mechanical ventilation (large animal machines equipped with ventilators). A pressure relief valve is integrated into the air. This valve automatically "opens" (expiration) and "closes" (inspiration) during the mechanical respiratory cycle (see Chapter 17). Excess gas within the breathing system is vented to the atmosphere through a waste gas scavenger system. Most pop-off valves can be adjusted manually to vary the pressure within the system at which gas is expelled. Circuit gas is expelled from the circuit when pressure reaches between 0.5 and 1.5 cm H_2O and the pressure relief valve is in the fully open position. Pressure relief valves frequently are fitted with a collection device that directs waste gas to a gas scavenging system through a flexible corrugated hose (Figure 16-14).

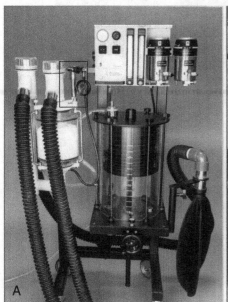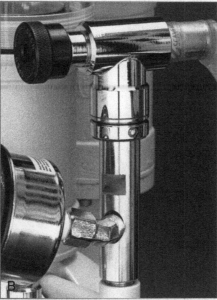

Figure 16–14. A, Adjustable pressure relief (pop-off) valve configured for attachment to a waste gas scavenging system. **B,** Close-up of boxed area in **A.**

The pressure relief valve is located near the endotracheal tube connection in a to-and-fro system. This is an awkward location, particularly when the horse's head is covered with surgical drapes. The pressure relief valve can be located at several sites in a circle system. When located at the Y piece, CO_2-absorbent is maximally conserved during spontaneous respiration because some alveolar gas, which has a relatively high CO_2 content, exits the pressure relief valve. As with the to-and-fro system, this is an awkward location. Most pressure relief (pop-off) valves in circle anesthetic circuits are located between the patient and the CO_2 canister (see Figure 16-14). This location is readily accessible and conserves absorbent by venting some alveolar gas.

Unidirectional Valves

Two unidirectional valves are located within the circle system and are responsible for maintenance of one-way gas flow. These valves direct flow to the horse through one breathing hose and away from the horse through the other breathing hose. Properly functioning valves, particularly the exhalation valve, minimize rebreathing of exhaled gases that have not yet reached the absorbent canister. Unidirectional valves should be relatively lightweight and constructed so they do not stick when coated with moisture from exhaled gas. They are usually covered with a clear plastic dome so proper valve operation can be viewed.

Breathing Hoses

Breathing hoses constructed of lightweight plastic or rubber are corrugated to prevent kinking and turbulent flow.[1] Resistance to flow is inversely proportional to the radius raised to the fourth power; therefore larger-diameter tubes offer less resistance than smaller-diameter tubes. Breathing hoses that are equal in diameter or larger than the horse's trachea should be used for anesthetic periods greater than 1 hour. Resistance measurements of four different equine anesthetic circuits reveal that resistance is higher in circuits with a tubing diameter of 37 mm than those with a tubing diameter of 50 mm.[14] Interestingly, normal arterial carbon dioxide concentrations were observed in adult horses (mean weight = 454 kg) during spontaneous ventilation, when 22 mm-diameter (adult human) hoses were used for 1 hour of inhalation anesthesia.[15] The increase in resistance from these small-diameter tubes was overcome by an increased work of breathing.[16] Most large animal circle breathing circuit hoses have an internal diameter of approximately 50 mm. This is greater than the diameter of the majority of equine tracheas.[7]

Hoses can expand (are compliant) during positive-pressure ventilation, reducing the delivered volume to the lung. This is referred to as *wasted ventilation*.[1] This wasted ventilation has not been quantified for equine breathing circuits, but for rubber 22-mm hoses it is approximately 1 to 4 ml/cm H_2O.[17] This value approaches 50 to 70 ml/cm H_2O for 50-mm diameter hoses and is likely inconsequential in adult horses.

Y Piece Connector

The Y piece connects the inspiratory and expiratory hoses of the circle anesthetic circuit to a mask or endotracheal tube. Some Y pieces contain a pressure relief valve (see preceding paragraphs) and the unidirectional valves and are not recommended because of the frequency of mechanical failures. The endotracheal tube is attached to the Y piece using a plastic or metal sleeve adapter (Figure 16-15). Alternatively, some endotracheal tubes have a flexible adapter that slides over the Y piece (Figure 16-16).

Fresh Gas Flow Rates

Both circle and to-and-fro systems can be operated using relatively low fresh gas flow rates, which results in conservation of anesthetic gases. An oxygen flow rate that

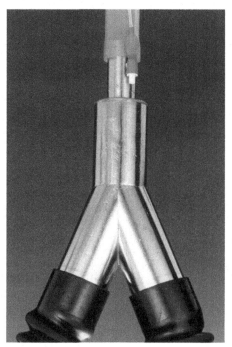

Figure 16–15. A plastic or metal sleeve connects the endotracheal tube to the Y piece.

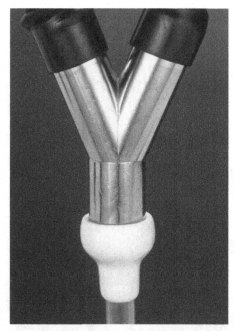

Figure 16–16. A flexible end of the tube slides over the Y piece.

just equals the horse's minute oxygen consumption (10 × body weight (kg)$^{3/4}$), or approximately 2.2 ml/kg of body weight, minimizes the amount of anesthetic gas used and the amount eliminated as waste. Using this fresh gas flow is considered a low-flow system. Use of such a system in horses has been described.[18] The disadvantage of low-flow oxygen is that the relatively low fresh gas flow rates and a conventional vaporizer can delay or prevent the attainment of a sufficient anesthetic concentration within the system to induce anesthesia. In addition, the anesthetic concentration within the anesthetic circuit cannot be changed rapidly. These disadvantages are in part related to the relatively large volume of the equine anesthetic circuit and the relatively large lung volume of horses. Flow rates equal to the horse's minute oxygen consumption are perhaps better suited for use in a to-and-fro system, which has a smaller volume than a circle system. The time necessary to achieve a 63% change in inspired halothane concentration in a typical 32-L large animal circle system using oxygen flow rates of 3, 6, and 12 L/min is 10.7, 5.3, and 2.7 minutes, respectively[19] (see Chapter 15 and Figure 15-2). The connection of an adult horse to the breathing circuit significantly slows the increase in anesthetic concentration (longer time constant).[19] Similar time constants have been demonstrated for the rate of change in the concentration of oxygen within the breathing circuit.[20] Uptake of anesthetic gas by system components (rubber hoses, reservoir bags) also slows the anesthetic concentration rate of rise.[20] Therefore oxygen flow rates for an equine circle system should be adjusted to 8 to 12 L/min for the first 10 to 15 minutes after induction to anesthesia. The flow can then be reduced to anything greater than or equal to a closed system flow rate during the maintenance phase of anesthesia. The recommended oxygen flow rate for equine to-and-fro breathing systems is similar to that of the circle systems.[21]

EQUINE ANESTHETIC MACHINES

A variety of anesthetic delivery systems are available for delivery of inhalation anesthetic drugs to horses (Table 16-3 and Figures 16-17 to 16-21; see Chapter 17). Most machines incorporate a circle system with an out-of-circle vaporizer. Some machines are equipped with a mechanical ventilator. One commonly used equine anesthetic machine (e.g., North American Drager large animal anesthetic machine) is no longer manufactured. However, used machines periodically are available. A qualified anesthesia service representative should inspect used machines before use.

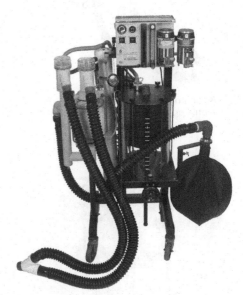

Figure 16–17. NA Dragar anesthetic machine with ventilator. (NA Dragar, Telford, PA.)

Table 16–3. **Commercially available equine anesthetic machines**	
Manufacturer	**Features**
NA Dragar, Telford, PA	Narkovet E2: Circle system mounted on frame with wheels. No longer manufactured.
	Large Animal Control Center: Circle system with ventilator. No longer manufactured.
JD Medical Distributing, Phoenix, AZ	LAVC 2000 CM: Circle system with ventilator. Many variations exist and can be custom ordered.
Matrx Medical, Inc. Mid County Dr. Orchard Park, NY 14127 800 847-1000 Matrxmedical.com	VML: Circle system on frame with wheels; no ventilator attached.
Smiths Medical PM Inc./Surgivet Waukesha, WI	LDS 3000 Anesthesia machine: circle system with optional cart and ventilator.
Mallard Medical Inc. 20268 Skypark Dr. Redding, CA 96002 Phone: (530) 226-0727 Fax: (530) 226-0713	Model 2800C: Large animal circle and integrated microprocessor controlled ventilator with ascending bellows.
	Model 2800CP: Large and small animal circle and integrated microprocessor controlled ventilators with ascending bellows.
Vetland Medical Sales & Services LLC 2601 Holloway Rd. Louisville, KY 40299	Vetland LAS 4000: Dragar-like circle with reconditioned NA Dragar ventilator.

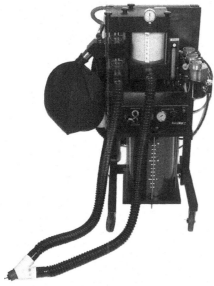

Figure 16–18. Smith Medical/Surgivet large animal anesthetic machine with ventilator. (Smith Medical/Surgivet, Waukesha, WI.)

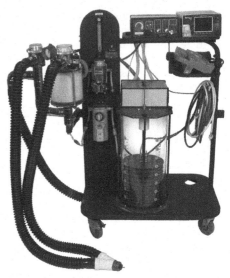

Figure 16–20. Mallard Medical large animal anesthetic machine with ventilator. (Model 2800, Mallard Medical Inc, Redding, CA.)

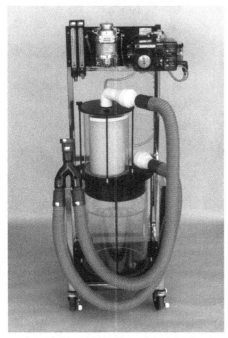

Figure 16–19. JD Medical anesthetic machine and ventilator. This machine is adapted for use in foals. Note the smaller absorption canister and plate within bellows chamber. (JD Medical Corp., Phoenix, AZ.)

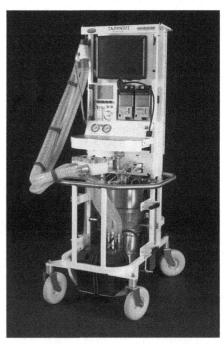

Figure 16–21. Tafonius ventilator and anesthetic machine with integral monitoring capabilities.

MACHINE AND BREATHING CIRCUIT CHECK

Every new anesthetic machine should be assembled by the manufacturer's representative and verified and tested for correct function. Ideally the machine should be serviced at least once per year by a manufacturer-trained representative. Such things as worn gaskets, leaky hoses, and improperly functioning pressure relief valves can be repaired or replaced.

Proper function of the anesthetic machine should be verified daily to reduce unanticipated intraoperative problems. Specific machine-check procedures should be performed daily; others should be performed before each anesthetic episode (Box 16-2). The user's manual should be consulted for a complete check procedure because no universal checklist is appropriate for all anesthetic machines.

Cylinders should be shut off at the end of the day to prevent depletion of gases through leaks within the piping system. Before each day's surgery, the hospital gas supply should be checked to verify that it contains enough gas for completion of the day's surgeries. Gas cylinders should be opened, and the pressure within the piping system should

- Inspect machine components
  - Turn flowmeters off
  - Turn vaporizer(s) off, fill, close filler caps
  - Fill CO_2 absorbent canister properly[†]
  - Ensure presence of one-way valves[†]
- Affirm adequate oxygen supply
  - Check cylinder pressure or turn on oxygen generator
  - Connect machine to hospital supply or to individual cylinders
  - Close cylinders and check for high pressure leaks by observing pressure gauge[†]
  - Reopen O_2 supply
- Test flowmeter
  - Be certain float drops completely to zero and rises smoothly[†]
  - Turn off flowmeter
- Check breathing circuit
  - Verify proper, tight connections
  - Occlude Y piece, close pressure relief valve, pressurize circuit to 30 cm H_2O, check for leaks (rate of <250 ml/min)
  - Open pressure relief valve and verify proper relief valve function
- Check ventilator
  - Connect to electric supply if necessary
  - Connect ventilator bellows to breathing circuit
  - Turn ventilator to on position, close pressure relief valve, occlude Y piece, interrupt just before peak ascent, bellows will not descend if leak-free
- Check waste gas scavenging system
  - Confirm transfer tubing properly connected to pressure relief valve[†]
  - Turn on vacuum pump *or*
  - Assume active charcoal canister is not exhausted

*This generic machine check should be modified according to the particular equipment used.
[†]If machine is to be used repeatedly during the day, these procedures need be performed only before the first case of the day.

be between 50 and 65 psi. The quantity of gas needed varies with the length of surgery, fresh gas flow rates, and type of equipment used. For example, an NA Drager large animal anesthetic machine with ventilator on and adjusted for a 450-kg horse will consume all the oxygen in one G cylinder (5300 L) in 1 to 2 hours. An oxygen cylinder backup system should be tested if an oxygen-generating device is used.

The flowmeter(s) should be turned on and off to check that the float rises smoothly within the flowmeter tube. Proper function of the oxygen fail-safe system should be verified. All gases to the machine and all flowmeters should be turned on. The oxygen supply source is then shut off (disconnected), and the oxygen pressure is allowed to drop to zero. If the flowmeters of the other gases fall to zero, the fail-safe is functioning properly. The flowmeters should return to their original setting when the oxygen source is turned on.

Leaks can occur at any connection and can be detected by following the user's manual.[1] A generic check involves connecting a pressure manometer (gauge from a standard sphygmomanometer) to the common gas outlet. The oxygen flowmeter is turned on slowly (with the vaporizer on) until a pressure of 30 cm H_2O is registered on the gauge. The flow is turned off, and the time it takes for the pressure to drop to 20 cm H_2O should be noted. This should be at least 10 seconds.[1]

The vaporizer should be filled, taking care to fully tighten the filler cap after filling. Vaporizers should always be filled with the vaporizer and flowmeters in the off position.

Breathing Circuit

A "leak test" should be performed on every anesthetic machine before use. The hoses and reservoir bag should be attached to the machine, and the pressure relief valve closed. The opening of the Y piece should be occluded, and the oxygen flush valve activated. The pressure within the system should rise to 30 cm H_2O. It should not decrease if the system is leak free. Leaks are present within the system if the pressure drops. The leak can be quantified by turning the oxygen flowmeter on and observing the flow rate at which the pressure no longer drops. A leak rate of less than 250 ml/min is acceptable. The relatively large volume of an equine breathing circuit may require a substantial time interval with the Y piece occluded to detect relatively small leaks. The most common sources of leaks are at connections, from cracks in old rubber articles (hoses, reservoir bags), loose one-way valve dome fittings, or an improperly sealed CO_2 absorbent canister resulting from worn gaskets or pieces of absorbent material between the gasket and canister.

The integrity of the anesthetic ventilator bellows (if available) should be verified. The outlet from a descending bellows ventilator should be occluded after the bellows is allowed to rise to its fully compressed configuration. The bellows should not fall if it is leak free. Holes in the bellows allow gas to enter the breathing system from the surrounding cylinder, causing higher than expected airway pressures.[22] The ascending bellows ventilators should be filled by rotating the oxygen flush valve and then occluding the hose connecting the ventilator to the breathing circuit. A gradual descent of the bellows indicates a leak. Manufacturer's instructions should be followed because not all ventilators can be leak checked as described.

Unidirectional valves should be inspected visually, and function verified. Inspiratory valve malfunction can result in rebreathing of exhaled gas and severe hypercarbia.[23] The exhalation valve should rise when someone blows through the Y piece. Integrity of the inspiratory valve is not easily verified without observing its correct motion during the patient's respiratory cycle. The carbon dioxide absorbent should be changed as necessary. Criteria for changing absorbent material were discussed previously.

COMPLICATIONS RELATED TO THE ANESTHETIC MACHINE AND BREATHING CIRCUITS

Verification of machine function before anesthesia (see Box 16-2) helps to prevent intraoperative complications related to machine and breathing circuit malfunction. However, operator error can still occur (see Chapter 1; Table 16-4). Systematic vigilance helps to identify problems related to the anesthetic machine and breathing circuit.

WASTE GAS DISPOSAL (SCAVENGER) SYSTEMS

Exposure of operating room personnel to trace gas concentrations is a concern.[1] Exposure to trace inhalant anesthetic gas has been linked to headaches, increased irritability, impaired cognitive and motor function, carcinogenesis, abortion, congenital anomalies, hepatic and renal dysfunction, and infertility in humans. Although evidence fails to confirm a link between chronic exposure to trace amounts of inhaled anesthetic gas and toxicity,[24,25] all practical precautions

Table 16–4.	Common complications related to the anesthetic machine and breathing circuit
Clinical sign	**Possible cause**
Improper anesthetic depth	Vaporizer* 1. Vaporizer empty 2. Vaporizer off 3. Vaporizer not calibrated 4. Vaporizer filled with wrong drug *Breathing circuit†* 1. Leaks in breathing hoses 2. Leaks in reservoir bag 3. Leaks at endotracheal tube connector or cuff 4. Leaks around CO_2 absorbent canister
Inadequate pressure in breathing circuit	1. Leaks as listed previously 2. Waste gas scavenging system applying too much vacuum to pressure relief (pop-off) valve 3. Flowmeter off 4. Exhausted gas supply
Excessive pressure in breathing circuit	1. Vacuum of waste gas scavenging system too low 2. Pressure relief valve (pop-off) closed or improperly adjusted
Abnormal breathing patterns or excessive $PaCO_2$	1. Exhausted or channeled CO_2 absorbent 2. Absorbent canister too small or inadequately filled (especially to-and-fro) 3. Unidirectional valves stuck open or absent 4. Same factors listed under inadequate breathing circuit pressure

*With these, the patient can appear either too light or too deep.
†With these, the patient will appear too light.

should be taken to reduce exposure to trace anesthetic gas. Exposure to inhalant anesthetic gas can occur before and during anesthesia and particularly during the recovery period once the horse is disconnected from the anesthetic machine. Only a comprehensive effort directed at limiting trace gas concentrations during all phases of anesthesia can ensure limited exposure.

Anesthetic vaporizers should be filled carefully in a well-ventilated room. Vaporizers should be filled before anesthetic induction, not during surgery, to avoid exposure of operating room personnel. Special filling devices are available that reduce pollution while the vaporizer is being filled. The anesthetic system should be tested for leaks, and recovery from anesthesia should occur in well-ventilated recovery stalls. The personnel recovering the horse should not be near the endotracheal tube. Trace concentrations of inhaled anesthetic gas are significant in recovery rooms; concentrations are greatest within 1 m of the endotracheal tube.[24]

Anesthetic machines should be equipped with a waste gas disposal system that transfers gas escaping from the pressure relief valve to a remote site. Gas scavenging devices attach to the pressure relief valve through a specially configured collection device (see Figure 16-14). Most scavenging devices (Figure 16-22) incorporate: (1) transfer tubing, which conducts gas from the specially configured pressure relief valve; (2) an interface, which prevents excessive negative or positive pressure from developing within the scavenging and breathing system; (3) a disposal system, which is either active (vacuum) or passive (Chapter 16). Gas scavenging systems that include all of these components are available commercially. Most commercially available units are equipped with a vacuum pump for generation of negative pressure. Various home-made devices can be used. Homemade scavenger systems generally use the passive methods for gas removal and direct gas by way of a hose connected to the pressure relief valve: (1) through a wall to the outdoors;

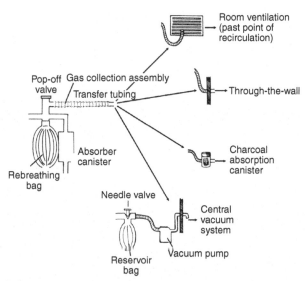

Figure 16–22. Schematic diagram illustrating various gas scavenging techniques. (From Muir WW et al: *Handbook of veterinary anesthesia*, ed 4, St Louis, 2007, Mosby Elsevier.)

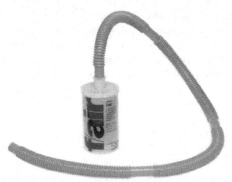

Figure 16–23. Charcoal canister for passive collection of waste gas from the pressure relief valve. The free end of the hose connects to the pressure relief valve.

(2) to the air intake of a portable wall air conditioner; (3) to a room ventilation intake duct, which must enter the ventilation system past any point of recirculation; or (4) to an activated charcoal canister. Activated charcoal canisters (Figure 16-23), although effective with relatively low fresh gas flow rates, become ineffective at high fresh gas flow rates typically used for adult horses. They are exhausted rapidly and do not remove nitrous oxide.

CLEANING AND DISINFECTION OF ANESTHETIC MACHINES AND BREATHING CIRCUITS

Microbial contamination of anesthetic breathing circuits and subsequent infection of horses using that same breathing circuit is rare.[1] Some studies document failure of the anesthetic machine and breathing circuit to transmit microbes; however, there are reports of transmission of organisms through the breathing circuit.[26,27] Equine anesthesia equipment is physically difficult to disinfect and sterilize because of its large size. Portions of the breathing circuit that are removed easily such as the reservoir bag, corrugated hoses, Y piece, and ventilator hoses can be removed, cleaned (by hand, dishwasher, or autoclave), and allowed to dry after each use. Having more than one set of these plastic or rubber goods available if multiple daily surgeries are performed is helpful. Plastic or rubber goods and the endotracheal tube should be washed in a mild detergent solution and rinsed well to remove dirt, mucus, blood, and other particulate material. These items

can be soaked in a cold disinfectant solution such as glutaraldehyde (after washing and rinsing), rinsed again with water, and allowed to dry. Glutaraldehyde is the only cold disinfectant that is bactericidal, sporicidal, fungicidal, and virucidal.[6] Manufacturer's directions for correct dilution and use must be followed.

The absorbent canister should be wiped dry when the absorbent is changed; and the one-way valves should be disassembled, wiped, and allowed to air dry at the end of the day. The dome valve covers can be left off the machine overnight to facilitate evaporative drying of the circuit. If contamination of the breathing circuit is suspected, the stationary portions of the breathing circuit, including the absorbent canister, one-way valves, and pressure relief valve, should be cleaned and disinfected.

The exterior of the machine should be wiped clean with a cloth and mild detergent solution or proprietary spray cleaner. The user's manual should be consulted to determine which cleaners will not harm the finish.

Gas sterilization of anesthesia equipment, particularly endotracheal tubes, should be avoided. Severe burns of the respiratory tract can result from improper aeration of endotracheal tubes sterilized with ethylene oxide. Aeration by exposure to room air should be for a minimum of 7 days, although actual aeration time depends on the composition of the sterilized article.[1]

SURGICAL TABLES AND PROTECTIVE PADDING

Most modern surgery tables use electrically operated hydraulic systems to position the horse in the correct plane and at the correct height (Table 16-5; Figures 16-24 and 16-25). Tables should be constructed of materials that are durable, easily cleaned, corrosion resistant, and mobile. Most surgery tables typically are set on wheels or casters to transport the horse to and from the surgical suite. Sometimes an overhead hoist is used to lift the horse onto the surgery table (Figure 16-26). Tables can be custom made to accommodate a variety of induction techniques and facility specifications. Transportable tables are available that can be used for remote or field surgeries. Inflatable tables have been developed that lift the horse to a suitable height and can be deflated to return the horse to the ground. Tables should be equipped to provide head and leg support (see Figures 16-24 and 16-25). These supports allow relatively easy positioning of the horse in dorsal or

Table 16–5. **Surgical tables**	
Manufacturer	**Features**
Shanks Veterinary Equipment, Milledgeville, IL	*Equine surgery table:* Hydraulic scissors lift action; heavy gauge metal with vinyl-coated surface; head and leg supports *Hydraulic tilt table:* Removable wheels; tilts from vertical to horizontal
Kimzey Welding Works, Woodland, CA	Hydraulic scissors lift; stainless steel construction; head and leg supports
Snell 2000 Ltd. Castle Cary, Somerset, United Kingdom BA7 7DW	Pneumatic lift; polyurethane-coated fabric; portable and suitable for field use

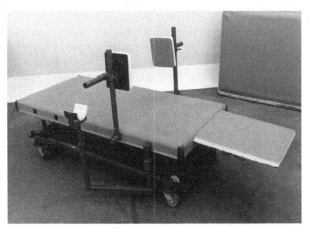

Figure 16–24. Portable hydraulically operated table with removable head and leg supports. (Shanks Veterinary Equipment, Milledgeville, IL.)

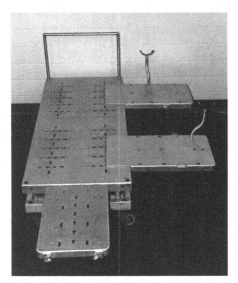

Figure 16–25. Portable hydraulically operated table with removable adjustable head and leg supports. (Kimzey Welding Works, Woodland, CA.)

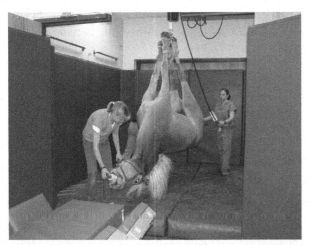

Figure 16–26. Horse being lifted onto surgical table using overhead hoist and leg shackles. (New England Equine MSC, Dover, NH.)

lateral recumbency and help prevent excessive pressure on large muscle groups, bony prominences, and nerves. Padding should always be used to protect the horse from direct contact with hard surfaces. A variety of protective padding devices are available (Box 16-3). Foam, air, and water have been used for the padding material. The least expensive padding involves inserting partially inflated automobile tire inner tubes under pressure points (hips and shoulders). Ideally the horse's weight should be distributed evenly, and padding should cover the entire table contact surface. Pads should be lightweight, portable, and covered with a washable surface so they can be removed from the surgical table for cleaning and storage. Various-size pads should be available to provide additional padding or assist in positioning the horse.

Slings

Slings that attach to an overhead hoist or counterbalance frame can be used to assist recovery from anesthesia (see Chapter 21). They help to support the horse in the standing position during recovery from general anesthesia.[28] Personnel must be trained and experienced with the use and techniques required for a sling recovery.

Pools

Orthopedic injuries are a leading cause for euthanasia in horses recovering from anesthesia (see Chapter 21). The rationale for using a pool is to reduce stressful forces on the horse's limbs during its attempts to stand. Pools can be used to facilitate recovery from anesthesia.[29,30] The horse is transported to the pool in a sling and suspended in the pool by the sling or a specially designed raftlike flotation device until recovery is complete. Horses must be heavily sedated or anesthetized during transport to the pool. The horse's head must be controlled. Personnel must be trained and experienced, and at least one person must stay with the horse at all times. A pool 2.6 m deep, 1.2 m wide, and 3.7 m long with a hydraulically operated floor has been designed and proven to be safe and practical for recovering horses from anesthesia. The pool can be equipped with a jet ski to provide a whirlpool effect.

Box 16–3	**Protective Padding Manufacturers**

Dandy Products, Inc.
   3314 State Route 131
   Goshen, OH 45122
A & A Pad Co
   Maryville TN 37803
   865-970-7400
Shanks Veterinary Equipment
   Milledgeville, IL

REFERENCES

1. Dorsch JA, Dorsch SE: *Understanding anesthesia equipment*, ed 4, Baltimore, 1999, Williams and Wilkins.
2. Webb AI, Warren RG: Hazards and precautions associated with the use of compressed gases, *J Am Vet Med Assoc* 181: 1491-1495, 1982.

3. Compressed Gas Association: *Safe handling of compressed gases in containers*, CGA Pamphlet P-1, ed 10, New York, 2006, Compressed Gas Association.

4. Compressed Gas Association: *Characteristics and safe handling of medical gases*, CGA Pamphlet P-2, ed 9, New York, 2006, Compressed Gas Association.

5. Compressed Gas Association: *Oxygen CGA G-4*, ed 9, New York, 2002, Compressed Gas Association.

6. Steffey EP, Hodgson DS, Kupershoek C: Monitoring oxygen concentrating devices (letter to the editor), *J Am Vet Med Assoc* 184:626-638, 1984.

7. Rex MAE: Apparatus available for equine anaesthesia, *Aust Vet* 148:283-287, 1972.

8. Hartsfield SM: Machines and breathing systems for administration of inhalation anesthetics. In Short CE, editor: *Principles and practice of veterinary anesthesia*, Baltimore, 1987, Williams & Wilkins, pp 395-418.

9. Fang Z et al: Carbon monoxide production from degradation of desflurane, enflurane, isoflurane, halothane, and sevoflurane by soda lime and Baralyme, *Anesth Analg* 80:1187-1193, 1995.

10. Dodam JR et al: Inhaled carbon monoxide concentration during halothane or isoflurane anesthesia in horses, *Vet Surg* 28:506-511, 1999.

11. Riebold TW, Coble DO, Geiser DR. In Riebold TW, Geiser DR, Goble DO, editors, *Large animal anesthesia: principles and technique*, Ames, 1995, Iowa State University Press, p 69.

12. Elam JO: The design of circle absorbers, *Anesthesiology* 19: 99-100, 1958.

13. Ten Pas RH, Brown ES, Elam JO: Carbon dioxide absorption, *Anesthesiology* 19:231-239, 1958.

14. Purchase IFH: Function tests on four large animal anaesthetic circuits, *Vet Rec* 77:913-919, 1965.

15. Short CE: Evaluation of closed, semiclosed, and nonrebreathing inhalation anesthesia systems in the horse, *J Am Vet Med Assoc* 157:1500-1503, 1970.

16. Nunn JF, Ezi-Ashi TI: The respiratory effects of resistance to breathing in anesthetized man, *Anesthesiology* 22:174-185, 1961.

17. Mushin WW et al: *Automatic ventilation of the lungs*, ed 3, Oxford, 1980, Blackwell Scientific Publications.

18. Olson KN et al: Closed circuit liquid injection isoflurane anesthesia in the horse, *Vet Surg* 22:73-78, 1993.

19. Steffey EP, Howland D: Rate of change of halothane concentration in a large animal circle anesthetic system, *Am J Vet Res* 38:1993-1996, 1977.

20. Solano AM, Brosnan RJ, Steffey DP: Rate of change of oxygen concentration for a large animal circle anesthetic system, *Am J Vet Res* 66:10, 2005.

21. Thurmon JC, Benson GJ: Inhalation anesthetic delivery equipment and its maintenance, *Vet Clin North Am (Large Anim Pract)* 3(1):73-96, 1981.

22. Klein LV: An unusual cause of increasing airway pressure during anesthesia, *Vet Surg* 3:239-242, 1989.

23. Baxter GM, Adams JE, Johnson JJ: Severe hypercarbia resulting from inspiratory valve malfunction in two anesthetized horses, *J Am Vet Med Assoc* 198:123, 1991.

24. Milligan JE: Waste anesthetic gas concentrations in a veterinary recovery room, *J Am Vet Med Assoc* 181:1540-1542, 1982.

25. Shuhaiber S et al: A prospective-controlled study of pregnant veterinary staff exposed to inhaled anesthetics and x-rays, *Int J Occup Med Environ Health* 15:363-373, 2002.

26. du Moulin GC, Saubermann AJ: The anesthesia machine and circle system are not likely to be sources of bacterial contamination, *Anesthesiology* 47:353-358, 1977.

27. Langevin PB, Rand KH, Layon JA: The potential for dissemination of mycobacterium tuberculosis through the anesthesia breathing circuit, *Chest* 115:4; 1107-1114, 1999.

28. Taylor EL et al: Use of the Anderson sling suspension system for recovery of horses from general anesthesia, *Vet Surg* 34: 559-564, 2005.

29. Sullivan EK et al: Use of a pool-raft system for recovery of horses from general anesthesia: 393 horses (1984-2000), *J Am Vet Med Assoc* 221(7):1014-1018, 2002.

30. Richter MC et al: Cardiopulmonary function in horse during anesthetic recovery in a hydropool, *Am J Vet Res* 62(12): 1903-1910, 2001.

Oxygen Supplementation and Ventilatory Support

Carolyn L. Kerr

Wayne N. McDonell

Dramatic physiological alterations occur in horses during general anesthesia and recumbency. Typical changes include a decrease in both arterial oxygen partial pressure (PaO_2) and cardiac output. Therefore tissue oxygen delivery is reduced, and in some cases it may not meet tissue requirements. Hypoventilation and a subsequent increase in arterial carbon dioxide partial pressure ($PaCO_2$) are common consequences of most anesthetic regimens. Unfortunately, information on the incidence and impact of specific types of respiratory dysfunctions on morbidity or mortality in anesthetized horses is not available. Despite the lack of statistics, most would agree that under certain circumstances oxygen supplementation and ventilatory support are indicated in horses to improve oxygen delivery and carbon dioxide removal from the body. For example, oxygen supplementation and ventilatory support may be required to achieve and maintain acceptable PaO_2 levels in anesthetized horses positioned in dorsal recumbency. Ventilatory support is commonly used to control $PaCO_2$ levels, achieve a constant end-tidal inhalant concentration, and produce a stable plane of anesthesia in horses subjected to procedures undertaken with inhalant anesthetic drugs. Considerable controversy exists regarding the appropriate goals for ventilatory support and the optimum methods to achieve them

in the horse. Specifically the optimum inspired oxygen concentration (FiO_2), the significance of ventilation-perfusion mismatching and atelectasis, and the best method for recruiting atelectic regions of lung are a few of the current issues requiring clarification.

HISTORICAL CONSIDERATIONS

The desire to improve outcomes associated with intrathoracic surgery combined with epidemics of poliomyelitis inspired the development of ventilators for human patients. Although intrathoracic surgery is performed only rarely in the horse, the respiratory dysfunction associated with anesthesia, recumbency, and positioning has been recognized since the late 1960s. Interest in mechanical ventilators followed the identification of hypoxemia, hypoventilation, and ventilation-perfusion inequalities in the anesthetized horse. Equipment designed for use in humans was modified for horses in the 1960s and 1970s.[1-3] These initial ventilators were a bag-in-a-barrel design, whereby a Bird ventilator controlled the flow of gas into a barrel and compressed a rebreathing bag located within the barrel. The compression of the bag forced the gas within the bag into the horses lungs. This basic design concept of a mechanized method of squeezing the rebreathing bag is still used in all anesthesia ventilators currently in use for the horse.

SPECIAL CONSIDERATIONS REGARDING EQUINE ANATOMY AND PHYSIOLOGY

Conducting Airways

Horses, unlike dogs and cats, are obligate nose breathers. Fortunately, they possess large nasal passages that are not usually prone to airway obstruction during induction and maintenance of anesthesia or for the short period of time when they are positioned in lateral recumbency. However, when anesthetized and placed in dorsal recumbency for prolonged periods (>1 hour), venous congestion and edema can lead to partial or complete obstruction of the nasal passages, particularly when the head is lower than the body. Therefore placement of an endotracheal tube is recommended to maintain airway patency and facilitate the delivery of oxygen and/or the institution of ventilatory support. Nasotracheal or orotracheal intubation is performed easily in the horse, even at light planes of anesthesia.

The tidal volume (VT), or the volume of gas breathed in and out with inspiration and expiration, is approximately 10 to 13 ml/kg in the awake horse. The physiological dead space, which includes anatomical and alveolar dead space, has been measured to be approximately 5 ml/kg in the horse, making the dead space-to-VT ratio approximately 50%.[4] Compared to other species (e.g., the dog and human), the ratio of the physiological dead space to VT is large. The relatively large dead space volume is of particular importance when providing ventilatory support to anesthetized horses since low VT ventilation (5 to 6 ml/kg), which is recommended in some species, requires a far greater minute ventilation to achieve a similar degree of alveolar ventilation (Figure 17-1). Physiological dead space increases immediately after anesthesia and recumbency and may increase over time during anesthesia in spontaneously breathing horses, particularly when they are placed in dorsal recumbency.[5,6] This increase in dead space observed with anesthesia and recumbency in the horse is a result of an increase in ventilation-perfusion mismatching and right-to-left vascular shunting through the lung.[7] Reductions in cardiac output and lung volume, an alteration in lung/thoracic wall mechanics, and gravitational forces on pulmonary blood flow contribute to these changes. The impact of mechanical ventilation on dead space in the horse is likely similar to that of other species in which the method of ventilation has been shown to impact the relative amount of dead space. For example, alveolar dead space has been shown to increase or decrease with the institution of mechanical ventilation in a spontaneously breathing horse.[6,8] In general, strategies that use a low VT or require large airway pressures are more likely to result in either a relatively greater percent of the inspired gas ventilating dead space or an actual increase in alveolar dead space.

Pulmonary Mechanics

During spontaneous breathing the lungs are expanded because of the negative pressure generated in the pleural space as a result of inspiratory muscle activity. Typical maximum transpulmonary pressure in the spontaneously breathing horse is approximately 5 cm H_2O (see Chapter 2). All ventilators currently used use positive pressure to expand the lungs. The peak inspiratory pressure (PIP) between the airway and the atmosphere (e.g., the transpulmonary pressure) required to deliver a VT of 10 to 15 ml/kg in the anesthetized healthy horse is approximately 20 to

35 cm H_2O. The major difference between the transpulmonary pressures in the recumbent anesthetized horse versus the standing, spontaneously breathing horse results from the impact of the thoracic wall and diaphragm. Specifically, when positive-pressure ventilation (PPV) is used, the pressure applied to the lungs must also expand the chest wall and diaphragm. Typical PIP values required in horses are also markedly different from those required in other species such as the dog or cat. For example, PIP values of approximately 12 to 15 cm H_2O are required to deliver a VT of 10 to 15 ml/kg in the latter species. Variations in the force required to enlarge the thoracic cavity by expanding the chest wall and diaphragm are responsible for these differences.

Gas Exchange Units

Overall, anesthesia and the assumption of recumbency in the horse produce physiological changes relatively similar to those that occur in other species; however, some marked differences exist. For example, the degree of respiratory depression and the resulting increase in $PaCO_2$ are relatively higher in the spontaneously breathing horse than in the dog at equipotent inhalant concentrations.[9] Similarly in the horse $PaCO_2$ often increases over time during spontaneous breathing when inhalant anesthetics are delivered at a constant end-tidal concentration,[10] whereas in the dog $PaCO_2$ levels generally remain constant. For these reasons ventilatory support is used frequently in the horse when the duration of inhalant anesthesia is expected to exceed 60 minutes.

One of the most notable differences between the horse and smaller animals when placed under anesthesia is the much greater decrease in PaO_2 and increase in the alveolar-arterial oxygen gradient. Under normal conditions an animal's PaO_2 should be approximately five times the inspired oxygen concentration (%), based on the predicted alveolar gas equation. For example, in a standing awake horse breathing room air (21% oxygen), the measured PaO_2 is approximately 90 to 100 mm Hg ($5 \times 20\%$). The PaO_2 values should be near or exceed 500 mm Hg based on the alveolar gas content when breathing 100% oxygen ($5 \times 100\%$). In contrast, under general anesthesia typical oxygen levels in horses breathing room air are 55 to 70 mm Hg,[11] markedly lower than in other species anesthetized using similar regimens. PaO_2 values in the horse can be as low as 50 to 60 mm Hg during inhalant anesthesia even when inspired oxygen concentrations are near 100%, although they are generally in the 200- to 300–mm Hg range.[12] Gross ventilation-perfusion mismatching with lung collapse, alveolar atelectasis, and intrapulmonary vascular shunting are the main causes responsible for the lower than predicted PaO_2 in the anesthetized horse.[13-15] To address the reduction in PaO_2, therapy has focused on two approaches. First, the inspired oxygen fraction is increased; and second, ventilatory strategies aimed at decreasing atelectasis and therefore intrapulmonary shunt have been attempted. The latter so-called recruitment maneuvers are not without consequence.

The presence of communicating passages in the distal airways and alveoli (pores of Kohn) helps provide collateral ventilation within the lung despite the numerous factors tending to decrease the efficiency of gas exchange in the horse lung. Pores of Kohn may not play a large role in efficient gas exchange in the healthy horse but may help

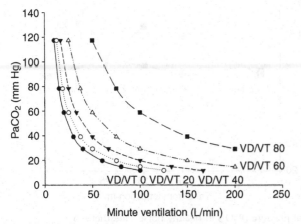

Figure 17–1. Relationship between $PaCO_2$ (mm Hg) and minute ventilation (L/min) when dead space to VT ratio *(VD/VT)* increases from 0 to 80%. The VD/VT is approximately 50% in the conscious horse. A larger VT generally produces lower VD/VT ratios, thereby decreasing the minute ventilation required to achieve the desired $PaCO_2$ level.

maintain lung inflation, albeit with a prolonged inflation time (increased time constant; see Chapter 2).

INDICATIONS FOR OXYGEN SUPPLEMENTATION

Oxygen supplementation or, more specifically, increasing the oxygen fraction (FiO_2) of the patient's inspired gas, is indicated in the spontaneously breathing horse or foal with acceptable $PaCO_2$ levels but PaO_2 values below 60 mm Hg (Box 17-1). Clinically, unless blood gas analysis is available, it is hard to determine the oxygen status of a horse unless it is very severe and cyanosis is present. The inspired O_2 content should be supplemented whenever possible, and the horse's ventilatory effort closely monitored. The PaO_2 tension usually falls to 55 to 70 mm Hg; whereas $PaCO_2$ tension remains

within the normal range of 35 to 45 mm Hg in horses breathing room air (21% O_2) anesthetized with a combination of an α_2-agonist, muscle relaxant (benzodiazepine or guaifenesin), and dissociative anesthetics (ketamine; Figure 17-2, *A*). A PaO_2 of 60 mm Hg, while low, still saturates 90% of the hemoglobin; therefore oxygen delivery should be adequate (see Chapter 2). However, if the horse hypoventilates (f <4, VT <10 ml/kg) while breathing room air, arterial and alveolar carbon dioxide concentrations increase, PaO_2 falls even further, and hypoxemia may develop. In short the ventilation-perfusion mismatch and lower PaO_2 erode most of the anesthetized horse's safety reserve in regard to oxygen supply. The impact of hypoventilation on the alveolar oxygen content is decreased with oxygen supplementation, and arterial oxygenation improves (Figure 17-2, *B*). The impact of hypoventilation (carbon dioxide concentration) on alveolar oxygen tensions with varying inspired oxygen concentrations is significant in anesthetized spontaneously breathing horses (Figure 17-3). The degree of improvement in arterial oxygen concentration with increased inspired oxygen depends on the degree of ventilation-perfusion mismatching and vascular shunting through the lung (Table 17-1). The degree of vascular shunt in healthy horses anesthetized and placed in lateral or dorsal recumbency varies from 15% to 25%, respectively. The benefit of oxygen supplementation on PaO_2 with this degree of shunt can be observed, even at inspired oxygen concentrations as low as 40%. Unfortunately, certain pathological situations can produce a large enough right-to-left shunt (e.g., 50%) that the benefit of low and even high oxygen supplementation is minimal.

The exact PaO_2 value at which oxygen delivery is impaired and leads to adverse consequences depends on several factors, including the animal's size, cardiac output, hemoglobin content, and duration of impaired oxygenation. In general however, if the PaO_2 is below 60 mm Hg, oxygen supplementation is recommended. A PaO_2 value of 60 mm Hg, which corresponds to an SaO_2 of approximately 93% in the horse, is generally the limit considered acceptable since small decreases in PaO_2 below this level can result in large changes in hemoglobin saturation and therefore the oxygen content of arterial blood.

Box 17-1 Indications for Oxygen Supplementation and Ventilation

Oxygen Supplementation
- Hypoxemia
  - PaO_2 <60 mm Hg
- Hb <5 g/dl

Ventilation
- Apnea (hypoxemia)
  - PaO_2 <60 mm Hg
- Hypoventilation (hypercapnia)
  - $PaCO_2$ >70 mm Hg
- Decrease the work of breathing
- Stabilize inhalant anesthesia
- Facilitate surgery (thoracotomy, thoracoscopy)
- Use unique positioning for special surgical procedures (laparoscopy, fetotomy)
- Administration of neuromuscular blocking drugs

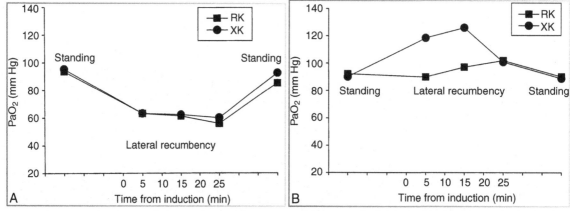

Figure 17-2. A, Typical changes in arterial oxygen partial pressure (PaO_2) in healthy horses anesthetized with intravenous anesthetics and breathing room air.[11] Note the similarity between the two anesthetic regimens (romifidine/diazepam/ketamine [RK] versus xylazine/diazepam/ketamine [XK]). Also note the persistently low PaO_2 values (approximately 60 mm Hg) during the entire period of lateral recumbency and a return to near normal PaO_2 values shortly after the horses stand. **B,** Maintenance of PaO_2 values (>90 mm Hg) during intravenous anesthesia and lateral recumbency during insufflation of 15 L/min of oxygen into a nasotracheal tube inserted to the midtrachea region.[12]

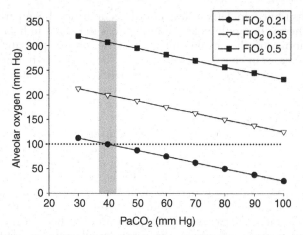

Figure 17–3. The relationship between fraction of alveolar oxygen partial pressure (mm Hg) and the $PaCO_2$ (mm Hg) with different fractional concentrations of inspired oxygen (FiO_2) (FiO_2 0.21=21%). The alveolar PaO_2 increases from 100 mm Hg to over 300 mm Hg (■) at a eucapneic level ($PaCO_2$ = 40 mm Hg; shaded area) as FiO_2 increases from 0.21 (room air; λ) to 0.35 (∇) and finally to 0.50 (■).

Table 17–1.	The predicted PaO_2 (mm Hg) with increasing amounts of intrapulmonary shunt and different fractions of inspired oxygen (FiO_2)			
		% Shunt			
		5%	10%	20%	50%
FiO_2	21%	110	100	90	45
	50%	240	180	100	50
	100%	600	500	290	55

INDICATIONS FOR VENTILATORY SUPPORT

The respiratory indications for instituting ventilatory support in a patient include the presence of apnea, moderate-to-severe-hypercapnia, hypoxemia in the presence of increased inspired oxygen content, and/or an excessive work of breathing (see Box 17-1). The primary objectives of ventilatory support are to optimize a patient's carbon dioxide removal from the lung (ventilation) and to deliver oxygen to the alveoli. In addition to improving ventilation and potentially oxygenation, the institution of ventilatory support can speed the rate of change in alveolar inhalant anesthetic concentration by increasing alveolar ventilation. This latter consequence facilitates changing the depth of anesthesia when maintaining anesthesia with an inhalant anesthetic. It is also easier to maintain a stable plane of anesthesia with inhalant anesthetics when ventilatory support is used: the drug delivery system for an inhalant anesthetic is the lung. Ventilatory support is essential whenever neuromuscular blocking agents are used or when surgical interventions of the thorax (diaphragmatic hernia repair, thoracotomy, and thoracoscopy) are performed.

Tissue oxygenation and ventilation are not isolated events and must be considered together when instituting mechanical ventilation with the goal of improving arterial oxygen or carbon dioxide concentrations. For example, the horse's cardiac output and intrapulmonary shunt fraction

can dramatically alter the impact of oxygen supplementation and/or mechanical ventilation on subsequent arterial blood gas partial pressures. The initiation of PPV can influence a patient's cardiac output, pulmonary vascular resistance, and intrapulmonary vascular shunt to varying degrees. The interrelationship between mechanical ventilation and hemodynamic status highlights the importance of assessing the impact of ventilation and should be considered before initiating ventilatory support in severely ill horses (Figure 17-4). For example, the initiation of intermittent positive-pressure ventilation (IPPV) in horses with intestinal obstruction (colic) and severely distended abdomens (tympany) may reduce cardiac output and arterial blood pressure to unacceptably low values. IPPV should not be initiated until the horse's bowel is decompressed or the abdomen has been opened surgically, thereby decreasing pressure in the abdominal cavity and on the diaphragm and facilitating venous return.

Although the clinical incidence of apnea in the anesthetized horse has not been reported, numerous research investigations have clearly shown dose-dependent respiratory depression with both injectable and inhalant anesthetics.[9,16] As previously mentioned, the impact of hypoventilation and apnea on a patient's oxygenation depends on the inspired oxygen fraction (FiO_2). Hypoventilation and apnea quickly lead to a low alveolar oxygen partial pressure and, as a result, hypoxemia within 1 to 2 minutes. In contrast, the PaO_2 generally remains in an acceptable range for at least 5 minutes during apnea when a horse has high alveolar oxygen partial pressures caused by exposure to high levels of inspired oxygen (apneic oxygenation; Figure 17-5).[17] Furthermore, the $PaCO_2$ concentration rises at approximately 3 to 6 mm Hg per minute during apnea, assuming normal metabolic rate, irrespective of the FiO_2. Therefore, when apnea does occur, positive-pressure ventilatory support is required within minutes to prevent rapid increases in $PaCO_2$ levels.

A horse's $PaCO_2$ levels can be adjusted easily to achieve a target level by adjusting the delivered VT and respiratory

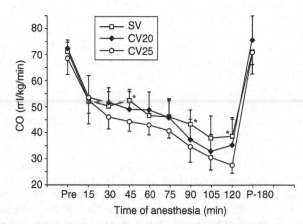

Figure 17–4. Sequential changes in cardiac output (CO) in seven Thoroughbred mares after anesthesia with xylazine-midazolam-ketamine followed halothane in oxygen. Cardiac output was determined before anesthesia and during spontaneous ventilation *(SV)* (□), controlled ventilation *(CV)* with a peak inspired of 20 (♦), and 25 (○) cm H_2O. *$P<0.05$ SV versus CV25. (From Mizuno Y et al: Cardiovascular effects of intermittent positive-pressure ventilation in the anesthetized horse, *J Vet Med Sci* 56:39, 1994.)

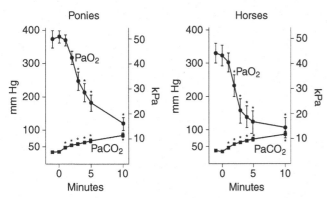

Figure 17–5. Changes in arterial oxygen and carbon dioxide tensions in six ponies (145 to 186 kg) and six horses (409 to 586 kg) during 10 minutes of apneic oxygenation (tracheal insufflations at the thoracic inlet) with 15 L/min O_2. Note the rapid decrease in PaO_2 during the first 3 minutes of insufflation. (From Blaze CA, Robinson NE: Apneic oxygenation in anesthetized ponies and horses, *Vet Res Commun* 11:281, 1987.)

rate with a ventilator or ventilatory assist device. However, although instituting ventilatory support in the apneic patient is clearly indicated, both the optimum and acceptable ranges of $PaCO_2$ levels in the anesthetized horse remain controversial. Typical $PaCO_2$ levels reported in spontaneously breathing healthy horses range from 60 to 80 mm Hg during surgical planes of anesthesia maintained with halothane, isoflurane, sevoflurane, or desflurane.[9,10,16,18] The degree of hypercapnia generally is greater in horses positioned in dorsal recumbency than in those positioned in lateral recumbency and tends to increase with the duration of anesthesia.[10,18,19] The degree of respiratory depression in horses maintained on intravenous infusions of injectable anesthetic drug is variable, with some authors reporting $PaCO_2$ levels similar to those of inhalant anesthetics; whereas others report less marked respiratory depression with injectable anesthetics.[20]

Hypercapnia in horses under general anesthesia is primarily a result of the depressant effects of anesthetics on the central respiratory centers. This depression is manifested in the horse by a decrease in respiratory rate and/or VT. The relative change in respiratory rate and VT may vary with the anesthetic protocol used. For example, horses maintained on isoflurane may have a greater decrease in respiratory rate but $PaCO_2$ levels similar to those of horses maintained with equipotent doses of halothane. An increased work of breathing resulting from the positional changes associated with general anesthesia likely contributes to hypoventilation and ventilation-perfusion mismatch. Horses positioned on their back with their forelimbs pulled back along their sides to facilitate surgical correction of vertebral instability generally hypoventilate and may have markedly elevated $PaCO_2$ and low (<100 mm Hg) PaO_2 even when breathing 100% oxygen. The effects of general anesthetics on the respiratory center are primarily responsible for the increase in $PaCO_2$ levels observed in horses during general anesthesia and prevent or minimize the normal compensatory changes in breathing rate or VT necessary to maintain normocapnia with positional changes. This conclusion is supported by the observation that the $PaCO_2$ is normal in awake ponies/horses

positioned in lateral and dorsal recumbency.[21] Similarly, whereas intrapulmonary shunting does not result in hypercapnia in the awake horse because of compensatory increases in alveolar ventilation, no compensatory increase in ventilation occurs in the anesthetized horse because of central respiratory depression. Intrapulmonary shunting contributes slightly to the hypercapnia observed in anesthetized horses.

Ventilatory support should be considered when $PaCO_2$ levels exceed 70 mm Hg (pH <7.25 to 7.20). Blood gas analysis is frequently not available under field or even general practice situations. In general, if a horse's respiratory rate decreases below 4 breaths/min, $PaCO_2$ levels generally increase to above 75 to 80 mm Hg, assuming normal metabolic rates. Increases in $PaCO_2$ can produce both positive and negative effects on the cardiovascular system. Mild increases in $PaCO_2$ ($PaCO_2$ = 40 to 70 mm Hg) during anesthesia result in vasodilation, decreased vascular resistance, and a potential increase in cardiac output. Large increases in $PaCO_2$ ($PaCO_2$ >70 mm Hg) during anesthesia produce myocardial depression, an impairment of cellular homeostasis and enzymatic function as a result of the decrease in arterial pH (pH <7.20), and an increased risk of cardiac arrhythmias as a result of sympathetic activation and increased levels of circulating catecholamines (Box 17-2).[22,23] Whereas increases in $PaCO_2$ have a direct myocardial depressant effect as determined in isolated heart preparations, mild-to-moderate hypercapnia has indirect cardiovascular stimulating and vasodilating effects in intact animals.[22,24] Therefore hypercapnia may help offset some of the negative cardiovascular effects of agents used to maintain general anesthesia.

Box 17–2 Effects of Increases in PaCO$_2$

Mild-to-Moderate (40 to 70 mm Hg)
- Increased cardiac output
- Decreased systemic vascular resistance
- Increased tissue blood flow (perfusion)
- Modulates cerebral blood flow
  - Hypercapnia: Cerebral vasodilation
  - Hypocapnia: Cerebral vasoconstriction
- Right shift in the oxyhemoglobin dissociation curve
- Increased tissue oxygenation and oxygen availability

Moderate-to-Severe (>70 mm Hg)
- Decrease in blood pH
  - Increase serum potassium (K^+)
- Myocardial depression
- Sympathetic activation and catecholamine release
  - Sinus tachycardia
  - Cardiac arrhythmias
- Impairment of cellular homeostasis and enzymatic function
- Central nervous system depression

Once the decision to ventilate mechanically has been made, setting the ventilator with the goal of achieving eucapnia in the patient is not recommended, at least in the healthy horse. The rationale for permitting an above-normal $PaCO_2$ is to minimize the direct cardiovascular depressant effects of PPV and maintain the indirect stimulatory effects of moderate increases in $PaCO_2$ on the cardiovascular system. In support of this approach are results of investigations evaluating the hemodynamic effects of PPV and studies evaluating the effects of increased $PaCO_2$ levels on hemodynamic variables in the anesthetized mechanically ventilated horse.[22, 24] For example, horses anesthetized using a PPV strategy that resulted in $PaCO_2$ values of 35 to 45 mm Hg had greater decreases in mean arterial blood pressure and cardiac output than horses ventilated with a lower minute ventilation and therefore higher $PaCO_2$.[25] Furthermore, under experimental conditions in which horses were ventilated with a constant minute ventilation and $PaCO_2$ was adjusted by altering the inspired carbon dioxide concentration, moderate levels of hypercapnia ($PaCO_2 \approx 80$ mm Hg) were shown to increase systemic arterial blood pressure and cardiac output while heart rate remained at baseline levels (Figure 17-6).[24] It is also easier and faster to reestablish spontaneous respiration at the end of the anesthetic period when $PaCO_2$ is elevated versus eucapnia or below-normal $PaCO_2$ levels.

Spontaneously breathing horses receiving oxygen supplementation with PaO_2 values below 80 mm Hg will likely benefit from ventilatory support. Unlike $PaCO_2$ values, achieving specific PaO_2 values is not easily accomplished. If ventilation is controlled soon after induction of anesthesia, PaO_2 generally is maintained at higher levels than in horses that are permitted to spontaneously ventilate for a period of time (>30 minutes) following induction.[19] Several authors have reported improvements in PaO_2 in horses transferred from spontaneous to mechanical ventilation; but others have reported inconsistent responses, with some horses showing no improvement and some actually showing a decrease in PaO_2.[18,26-28] Most important, once hypoxemia is present, oxygenation is not improved consistently with mechanical ventilation.[19] For example, in a prospective clinical trial PaO_2 improved in only 50% of spontaneously breathing dorsally recumbent hypoxemic horses with the initiation of mechanical ventilation. It is likely that, once a critical amount of atelectasis is present in the equine lung, it is difficult to recruit that portion of the lung using traditional ventilation strategies. The use of a ventilatory strategy that includes both positive end-expiratory pressure (PEEP) and inotropic support has been shown to improve oxygen levels.[29,30] However, it is unknown whether this strategy improves oxygenation status in a horse that is hypoxemic. Similarly a recent investigation in ponies showed improvement in oxygenation with a recruitment maneuver that used stepwise increases in PEEP. The recruitment maneuver was performed by increasing the PIP to 45, 50, and 55 cm H_2O while maintaining PEEP at 20 cm H_2O.[31] The authors suggested that this recruitment maneuver produced acceptable adverse cardiovascular effects, although the technique has yet to be tested in hypoxemic horses. Others have suggested that recruitment maneuvers need to be performed early (<30 minutes) during anesthesia since oxygenation may not improve with mechanical ventilation in horses once hypoxemia is present.[19] Mechanical ventilation from the onset of general anesthesia and recumbency results in a greater PaO_2 and a lower incidence of hypoxemia, particularly when a prolonged duration of anesthesia is anticipated.[19] It is not known at this time whether this recommendation should be modified based on the type of anesthetic protocol used (i.e., inhalant versus injectable anesthesia or a combination of injectable and inhalant).

Although rarely measured clinically, one can assume that the work of breathing is increased during anesthesia in horses. For example, when a small endotracheal tube must be used because of airway diameter or is used electively to facilitate surgical access to the pharynx or larynx, the work of breathing is increased and may add to the risk of clinically significant hypoventilation. Similarly the horse's conformation, positioning, including limb positioning, or an increase in intraabdominal pressure as occurs with some types of colic (tympany) laparoscopy or abdominal accidents can also increase the work of breathing by reducing thoracic and diaphragmatic compliance (Figure 17-7).[31a] It is recommended that mechanical ventilation be considered early in the anesthetic period and that hemodynamic status (arterial blood pressure) be monitored closely and supported when necessary.

EQUIPMENT

Methods of Increasing the Fraction of Inspired Oxygen (FiO_2)

A source of oxygen and a method of delivering oxygen are required to increase the FiO_2. Bulk tanks or large cylinders of liquid or pressurized oxygen are used most commonly in hospital environments, whereas small portable cylinders of pressurized oxygen are suitable in the field. To safely and efficiently deliver the oxygen from a tank or cylinder,

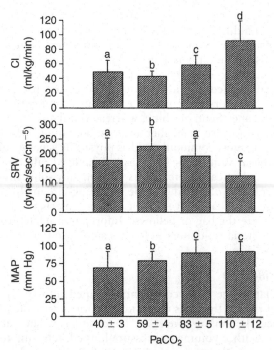

Figure 17–6. The effects of increases in $PaCO_2$ on cardiac index *(CI)*, systemic vascular resistance *(SVR)*, and mean arterial blood pressure *(MAP)* in eight mature horses weighing 425 to 550 kg. Groups with same letter *(a-d)* are not different; $p<0.05$.[24]

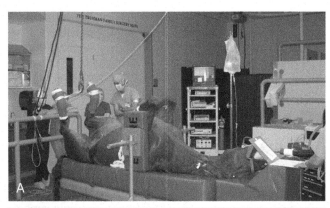

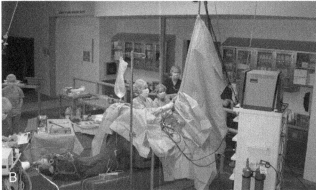

Figure 17–7. A and **B,** The horse's position can have a significant effect on pulmonary gas exchange. Supine horses that have their hindquarters elevated for laparoscopic procedures (**B**) in which the abdomen is insufflated with carbon dioxide are particularly susceptible to ventilation-perfusion mismatch, hypoxemia, and hypercarbia if not ventilated.

a regulator that attaches to the oxygen source and reduces the pressure of the oxygen leaving the tank is required (see Chapter 16).

Several different options exist that permit the delivery of oxygen from the oxygen source to the animal. The most efficient system for maximizing the inspired oxygen content is to place an orotracheal or nasotracheal tube into the patient and connect this to an anesthetic machine with a regulated oxygen supply and a functional carbon dioxide removal system. If the airway is sealed, oxygen concentrations greater than 90% can be achieved in a standard large animal anesthetic breathing circuit within 10 to 15 minutes by using high oxygen flow rates (see Chapter 15). If tracheal intubation is not possible or desired, the anesthetic breathing circuit can be attached to a mask that can be placed over the horse's or foal's muzzle. Unfortunately, this results in large equipment-associated dead space and is not well tolerated in most adult horses. For the most part, oxygen delivery via mask is limited to use in the foal for the purposes of preoxygenation before induction of anesthesia with injectable anesthetics or during the coadministration of inhalant anesthetic agents.

The oxygen source can originate from a flexible oxygen line and a demand valve.[32] The demand valve in turn is designed to fit to an orotracheal or nasotracheal tube. A demand valve results in the delivery of an increased FiO_2 with spontaneous ventilation but is primarily used to provide assisted or controlled breaths.[33] The demand valve increases airway resistance and should not be left in place during spontaneous breathing. It is most commonly used to provide IPPV when weaning horses from mechanical to spontaneous ventilation at the termination of anesthesia.

Nasal, pharyngeal, intratracheal, or transtracheal insufflation can also be used to increase the FiO_2, with the oxygen being delivered via various lengths of soft flexible tubing connected to a flowmeter, regulator, and a source of oxygen.[17,34] The animal breathes a combination of room air and supplemental oxygen, resulting in an alveolar oxygen content ranging from approximately 30% to 70%. In general, the further distal in the airway the oxygen is delivered, the greater the increase in FiO_2 for a particular oxygen flow rate. Tracheal oxygen inflation (15 L/min) in spontaneously breathing horses under injectable anesthesia placed in lateral recumbency results in PaO_2 values similar to or above those observed in standing horses breathing room air. Controlled studies in which horses receive a variety of FiO_2 values delivered at the distal end of the endotracheal tube have not been performed. Insufflation with this latter method using oxygen flow rates of 15 L/min is still routinely performed because of the potential benefit on PaO_2 in the patient with impaired ventilation.

Mechanical Ventilators

Ventilators can be designed as self-contained stand-alone units or as components designed to integrate with an anesthetic machine. The latter design is marketed either as part of the anesthetic machine or as a physically separate unit that connects to the anesthetic breathing circuit. Critical care ventilators (including high-frequency ventilators) that are designed for the long-term support of ventilation are usually marketed as stand-alone ventilators that provide humidification of the inspired gases and control of the inspired O_2 concentration (%). Anesthesia ventilators are most commonly designed to be compatible with inhalant anesthetic delivery systems that are integral or easily incorporated into anesthetic circuits (see Chapter 16). Most ventilators designed for equine use are incorporated into the anesthetic machine, whereas ventilators currently marketed for use in smaller animals, including foals up to 80 kg, are most commonly sold as physically separate units. Anesthesia ventilators serve as mechanized, although at times sophisticated, substitutes for manually squeezing the reservoir bag of the anesthetic breathing circuit. In other words, a mechanical ventilator acts as a mechanical hand to squeeze the bag or bellows.[1] Information related to use of anesthesia ventilators in foals is similar to that for adult horses.[35]

Classification

Ventilators are most commonly grouped into two major categories on the basis of the major control variable, often termed the *limiting, preset,* or *target variable.* The categories are either volume or pressure limited, referring to the VT delivered to the patient or the PIP generated by the ventilator within the patient breathing circuit (Box 17-3). Other variables that may be controlled and that can impact the target volume or pressure value include the inspiratory

---

Box 17-3 Common Modes of Mechanical Ventilation Used for Horses

Pressure-Limited

- Pressure-**controlled** ventilation (rate and volume controlled)
  - Set to a predetermined pressure; time-triggered, time-cycled, pressure-limited; also referred to as intermittent positive-pressure ventilation
- Pressure-**support** (assisted) ventilation
  - Set to a predetermined pressure; patient-triggered, pressure-limited

Volume-Limited

- Controlled mechanical ventilation (rate and volume controlled)
  - Predetermined rate and volume
- Assist-controlled mechanical ventilation
  - Patient-triggered, predetermined tidal volume
- Intermittent mandatory ventilation
  - Spontaneous breathing; mandatory timed breathes delivered at a predetermined tidal volume

NOTE: Several equine ventilators can be operated in a volume-controlled pressure-limited mode

---

flow rate (flow-limited) and the duration of inspiration and expiration (time-limited). Additional characteristics that may be used to describe ventilators include their power source, drive mechanism, cycling mechanism, and bellows type.

Major control (limiting, preset or target) variable. As stated previously, most anesthesia ventilators are described as volume- or pressure-controlled ventilators and are operated as limited, preset, or targeted ventilators, since it is one of these latter variables that the operator controls and it is this variable that determines the maximum volume or pressure obtained during a delivered breath. Specifically with a volume-targeted ventilator, the VT to be delivered to the patient is preset, whereas in the pressure-targeted ventilator the operator sets the PIP. As previously mentioned, the inspiratory flow rate, duration of inspiration, inspiratory:expiratory ratio (I:E ratio), and/or the respiratory time may impact the achievement of the VT or PIP goal with both types of ventilators. The inspiratory flow rate and the duration of inspiration indirectly control the VT with many volume-targeted ventilators. In addition, in volume-preset ventilators the apparent VT set on the ventilator may differ from that actually delivered to the patient because of variations in the compliance of the breathing circuit, the rate of fresh gas entry into the breathing circuit (flowmeter settings), or the presence of leaks. The volume delivered when using a pressure-targeted ventilator may vary, depending on the preset PIP, the compliance and resistance of the patient's respiratory system and breathing circuit, and the location of the pressure sensor.

Power source. Sources of power to drive mechanical ventilators include electricity or compressed gas. Most ventilators used for ventilating horses use a combination of electricity and compressed gas; however, two early generation ventilators (North American Drager large animal anesthetic machine and the JD Medical [see Chapter 16]) use only compressed gas and therefore may be preferred when electricity is not available.

Driving mechanism. The drive mechanism refers to the mechanism by which the bellows is compressed during inspiration. For most anesthesia ventilators ventilation is pneumatically driven, and a double circuit exists whereby the gas driving the ventilator is separate from the gases (O_2 and inhalant anesthetic) delivered to the anesthetic circuit. Most commonly, a compressed gas is responsible for applying pressure to a bag or bellows, which contains the gas (O_2 and inhalant anesthetic) delivered to the patient. Therefore the bellows physically separates the gas in the patient circuit from the driving gas.[1] The content of the compressed or driving gas may vary, depending on the ventilator type; however, most ventilators use 100% oxygen as the driving gas as a matter of convenience. Although oxygen is potentially more expensive than using air or air mixture to compress the bellows, compression of the bellows with oxygen may protect against hypoxemia, particularly if there is a leak in the bellows.

Cycling mechanism. Most equine anesthesia ventilators are used in the control mode (rate and volume/pressure predetermined) and therefore are cycled based on time. In other words, the ventilator is set to a preset number of breaths per minute and VT; inspiration is initiated to deliver a predetermined volume or pressure, regardless of the phase of the horse's own respiratory efforts (see Box 17-3).

Bellows type. Bellows are described by the direction of bellows movement during the expiratory phase of the ventilatory cycle (Figure 17-8). When the bellows descends during inspiration and ascends during expiration, the bellows is termed *standing* or *ascending*. Generally there is a certain degree of PEEP with ascending bellows caused by the weight of the bellows, unless the ventilator has a system to adjust the pressure within the bellows housing during expiration. The bellows ascends during inspiration and descends during expiration with descending, or hanging, bellows. Most new ventilators generally incorporate an ascending bellows. Ascending bellows do not fully ascend in the presence of a significant leak in the circuit and therefore are considered safer. By contrast, the ventilator continues to ascend during inspiration and descend during exhalation with the descending or hanging bellows, despite the presence of a leak in the circuit.

Operating principles of ascending bellow ventilators. As mentioned, ventilators basically are a mechanical substitute for manually squeezing the reservoir bag on the anesthetic breathing circuit. Most of the currently available equine ventilators connect to the breathing circuit at the rebreathing bag connector (i.e., their connecting hose replaces the breathing bag). The pressure relief (pop-off) valve on the

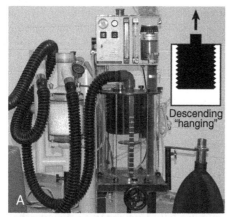

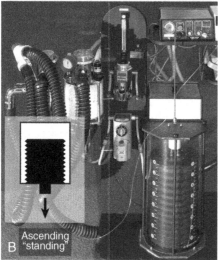

Figure 17–8. Bellows type. **A,** Descending (hanging) bellows descends during expiration. **B,** Ascending (standing) bellows ascends during expiration.

anesthetic breathing circuit must be closed before initiating a positive-pressure breath. Accumulation of excess gas (volume) in the circuit is controlled by a pressure relief valve built into the ventilator. Driving gas enters the space surrounding the bellows with the initiation of a breath, exerting pressure on the outside of the bellows in the case of classic pneumatically driven, double-circuit volume, or pressure-preset ventilators. The ventilator pressure relief valve closes as the pressure within the bellows increases; and the bellows compresses, forcing a preset volume of gas within the bellows into the anesthetic machine breathing circuit and the horse. The pressure within the bellows chamber is reduced to zero at the termination of the breath; the gas exhaled by the patient refills the bellows; and the relief valve opens, eliminating any excess gas within the patient breathing circuit. A scavenging hose should be connected to the pressure-relief valve (most ventilators incorporate this) on the ventilator if inhalant anesthetics are used. A pressure-measuring device (e.g., positive-negative manometer) positioned in the anesthetic rebreathing circuit or connected to the bellows helps to ensure that the PIP delivered to the animal is not excessive, the pressure in the bellows returns to zero, and the desired level of PEEP (e.g., 0 to 15 cm H_2O) on exhalation is not excessive.[29]

Modes of Mechanical Ventilation

All methods currently used for providing ventilatory support in adult horses use positive pressure to expand the lung and promote gas exchange. As a result, the modes of ventilation described in the following paragraphs are all considered positive-pressure ventilatory modes.

Intermittent positive-pressure ventilation.   Periodic delivery of a positive-pressure breath to a spontaneously breathing patient is termed *IPPV*. IPPV can be accomplished by manually applying pressure to the rebreathing bag of the anesthetic machine while the pressure relief valve (pop-off valve) is closed or by intermittently delivering a positive-pressure breath using a mechanical ventilator or demand valve. It is generally not regarded as a suitable method of maintaining a patient's minute ventilation for a prolonged period of time. Occasionally IPPV is used to "sigh," or maximally inflate the lungs during anesthesia, with the goal of recruiting atelectatic regions of lung.[31] The value of this technique in the horse is not known. IPPV is also used to wean a patient off controlled ventilation at the end of an anesthetic period.

Assisted ventilation.   The ventilator delivers a preset volume or pressure in response to an initiated breath. The horse determines respiratory rate but not VT. Assisted ventilation is used infrequently in horses during general anesthesia since mechanical ventilation is most commonly used to prevent inadequate ventilation and assisted ventilation does not guarantee the delivery of a set minute ventilation, nor does it lower $PaCO_2$ levels to the desired level.

Controlled mechanical ventilation (continuous or conventional mandatory ventilation).   The ventilator is set to deliver a volume of gas (e.g., the VT) at a preset frequency (respiratory rate) during mechanical ventilation (continuous or conventional mandatory ventilation [CMV]), independent of the patient's ventilatory efforts. This is the most common type of ventilatory support used during anesthesia in horses. The ventilator is set to deliver a target VT (ml) or PIP (mm Hg or cm H_2O), depending on the design of the specific ventilator used (see Chapter 16). The ventilatory settings are generally adjusted to achieve target $PaCO_2$ (50 to 70 mm Hg). Either manual ventilation (physically squeezing the breathing bag) or the use of a demand valve can also be used to provide controlled ventilation. However, these latter techniques are cumbersome and not as reliable or consistent in providing appropriate minute ventilation. It is rare for a horse to initiate ventilatory efforts during surgical planes of anesthesia with delivery of adequate minute ventilation when a controlled ventilatory mode is employed. Exceptions would be when PaO_2 values fall below 60 to 80 mm Hg or if a machine malfunction leads to increases in the horse's $PaCO_2$ despite use of a ventilator.

Ventilator Settings

Several different ventilators are manufactured for equine use, and many old models that are no longer marketed remain in use. Considerable variation exists in their design and the specific features that the operator can adjust, although the basic principles remain consistent among designs.

Tidal volume.   The VT is the amount of gas breathed in or exhaled during a single breath. Adjustment of the volume of the bellows determines the maximum volume of gas, or VT, that can be delivered into the breathing circuit during a given respiratory cycle by a volume-targeted ventilator (see Chapter 16). The operator must also adjust the inspiratory flow rate and/or inspiratory time to optimize the gas delivery during inspiration. The PIP determines the VT delivered when using a pressure-targeted ventilator (see Chapter 16). Achieving peak pressure depends on the operator setting an adequate inspiratory flow rate and inspiratory time. The actual volume of gas that leaves a mechanical ventilator and participates in gas exchange is influenced by the compliance of the ventilatory circuit, the mechanical dead space, and the horse's physiological dead space. In general it is preferable to use lower respiratory frequencies and larger VTs during anesthesia in horses. The recommended VT for adult horses ranges from 12 to 16 ml/kg (Table 17-2).

Frequency or respiratory rate.   The frequency or respiratory rate adjustment determines the number of respiratory cycles per minute. A rate of 6 to 8 breaths per minute, with a 12- to 16-ml/kg VT, generally produces a $PaCO_2$ within the range of 45 to 60 mm Hg.

Inspiratory flow rate.   The inspiratory flow rate adjusts the volume of gas per unit time that enters the chamber containing the bag or bellows and therefore determines the rate (ml/sec) that gas leaves the bag and enters the horse. The minimum required inspiratory flow rate for most ventilators is 0.5 to 1 L/kg/min, mandating that large animal ventilators be able to deliver 400 to 600 L/min.[2] Generally the inspiratory flow rate is set at a high enough value, which permits the operator to adjust only the inspiratory time.

Inspiratory time.   The inspiratory time is the period between the beginning and end of the flow of inspiratory gases. The inspiratory time in the spontaneously breathing horse is generally 2 to 3 seconds, and positive-pressure ventilators are adjusted to deliver the VT during the same 2- to 3-second period (see Table 17-2). The inspiratory flow rate can influence and limit the inspiratory time, particularly when ventilating larger horses. For example, a ventilator adjusted to deliver an inspiratory flow rate of 200 L/min (approximately 3.3 L/sec) would not be able to deliver a VT of 12 L to an 800-kg horse (15 ml/kg) in less than 3 sec-

onds (3.3 L/sec × 3 sec = 9.9 L). The inspiratory flow rate can be adjusted on most ventilators and would need to be increased to greater than 250 L/min (approximately 4 L/sec) to deliver the required VT (12 L) in less than 3 seconds.

Inspiratory:expiratory ratio.   Most currently available ventilators permit the operator to control the relative time of inspiration and expiration, also known as the I:E ratio. The operator can set the I:E ratio on some ventilators or indirectly set the I:E ratio by adjusting the inspiratory flow rate, the inspiratory time, and the respiratory rate. The traditional "rule" for ventilator use across species is that the expiratory phase should be twice as long as the inspiratory phase (I:E ratio of at least 1:2) to permit time for adequate lung deflation and venous return to the heart during the expiratory phase. A relatively longer inspiratory time (e.g., an I:E ratio of 1:1 to 1:1.5) results in a greater time for recruitment of atelectatic areas of lung or lung regions with low compliance or slow time constants (see Chapter 2). However, the longer inspiratory time results in a longer time during which there is increased intrathoracic pressure and therefore a greater possibility of hemodynamic compromise. The I:E ratio should initially be set at 1:2 to 1:3 in horses, with subsequent adjustments based on monitoring of gas exchange (PaO_2 and $PaCO_2$) and hemodynamics (arterial blood pressure, cardiac output; see Table 17-2).

Positive end-expiratory pressure.   PEEP is the positive pressure that the ventilator maintains within the breathing circuit at the end of expiration. PEEP can be applied during both controlled and assisted ventilation. Ascending (standing; see Figure 17-8) bellows ventilators typically result in an inherent PEEP because the weight of the bellows impedes the patient's exhalation. However, some ventilators have mechanisms incorporated into the ventilator that reduce the end-expiratory pressure to zero. PEEP is used to recruit atelectatic regions of lung and improve oxygenation (Box 17-4). The amount of PEEP typically is adjusted and displayed in units of centimeters of H_2O on some critical care ventilators. Typical values of PEEP range from 5 to 15 cm H_2O, but in horses higher PEEP values may be needed to achieve the desired pulmonary changes.[29,30] These higher PEEP values may improve arterial oxygenation but can reduce venous return and cardiac output unless appropriate fluid therapy

Table 17–2.	**Recommended ventilatory settings for adult horses and foals**	
	Adult horse	**Foal (< 3 months)**
VT (ml/kg)	12-15	10-12
Respiratory rate (breaths/min)	6-8	8-10
Inspiratory:expiratory ratio	1:2 or 1:3	1:3
Inspiratory time (seconds)	2-3	2
Peak inspiratory pressure (cm H_2O)	20-30	12-15

Box 17–4	**Effects of Positive End-Expiratory Pressure (PEEP)**

- Preserves, stabilizes, and recruits lung units
- Increases functional lung capacity
- Reduces shunt fraction
- Improves arterial oxygenation (PaO_2)
- Increases central venous pressure
- Decreases venous return, cardiac output, and arterial blood pressure
- Increases intracranial pressure
- May contribute to pulmonary barotraumas when improperly applied

and inotropes are used (Figure 17-9).[36] Accurate control of PEEP is not typically a feature of equine mechanical ventilators at the present time, and PEEP is usually estimated from a pressure manometer that records the pressure within the circuit throughout the respiratory cycle.

Peak inspiratory pressure. The peak pressure within the breathing circuit at the end of inspiration (PIP) is directly related to the delivered VT. The PIP required to deliver a VT of 12 to16 ml/kg is highly variable in the horse and depends on the horse's position, body condition, degree of abdominal distention, and lung compliance. Typically PIP values of 20 cm H_2O are appropriate in laterally recumbent horses, and PIP values of 25 to 35 cm H_2O are adequate in dorsally recumbent horses. The required PIP may exceed 55 cm H_2O in a horse with abdominal distention. Generally PIP values should not exceed 30 cm H_2O. Values greater than 40 cm H_2O may be harmful to the normal horse lung and should not be sustained.

Expiratory time. The time from the end of inspiration to the initiation of inspiration is referred to as the expiratory time. On some ventilators this variable is used to set the respiratory rate (time between breaths). Adequate expiratory time (I:E ≥ 1:2) is required to permit complete exhalation and avoid the trapping of gas within the lung.

Inspiratory sensitivity. The threshold negative pressure generated by a patient during inspiration can trigger the ventilator to initiate a positive-pressure breath and is referred to as the *inspiratory sensitivity*. Pressure-targeted ventilators that are capable of being used in assist mode may have this feature. Inspired sensitivity or effort is not used with CMV.

Ventilators for Equine Use
Volume-Targeted Ventilators

Mallard large animal ventilator. Several different models of the Mallard large animal ventilator exist (e.g., 2800, 2800B, 2800C); however, they are all similar in design (i.e., they are all volume-targeted, double-circuit ventilators). The operator adjusts the inspiratory flow (10 to 600 L /min) and inspiratory time to achieve the desired VT

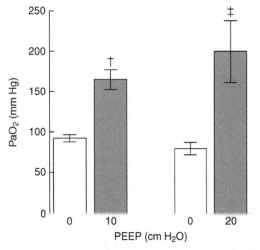

Figure 17-9. Effects of three levels of positive end-expiratory pressure *(PEEP)* (0, 10, 20 cm H_2O) on PaO_2 in horses undergoing colic surgery.[29]

within 2 to 3 seconds, which is estimated by visualizing the liter gradations on the outside of the bellows assembly. Mallard ventilators are electronically controlled and electronically and pneumatically powered with a pneumatic driving system; they are designed to provide ventilation only in the controlled mode. The pneumatic driving mechanism requires a driving pressure of 40 to 60 pounds per square inch (psi) of either oxygen or, with adjustment, air as the driving gas. They are time-cycled ventilators with an ascending (standing) bellows (see Figure 17-8). Because of the bellows design, a horse can breathe spontaneously while the ventilator is in the standby or off mode with only a minimal increase in the work of breathing when the ventilator is connected to the anesthetic system. The 2800 and 2800B models have a 21-L capacity bellows, whereas the 2800C model has an 18-L bellows. The adjustable settings include the off/standby/on knob, respiratory frequency, inspiratory flow rate, and inspiratory time knob. Inspiratory pressure can be obtained from a positive-negative pressure gauge positioned on the top of the bellows. The ventilator can be set in the standby mode during setting up and leak testing before use. The respiratory frequency can be adjusted from 2 to 15 breaths/min. The inspiratory flow rate can be dialed into the low, medium, or high range; but these settings do not provide more detail regarding specific flow rates. The inspiratory flow rate should be adjusted to the medium or high range for adult horses, and the inspiratory time should be adjusted to achieve the desired VT. The I:E ratio is calculated based on the respiratory rate and inspiratory time and is not directly adjusted, but it is calculated and digitally displayed. A PEEP adjustment knob exists; however, it is not designed to set a predetermined PEEP. Instead this control adjusts the PEEP settings from the naturally occurring PEEP level of approximately 5 cm H_2O (because of the ascending bellows design) to atmospheric pressure (zero PEEP) by adjusting a pneumatic vacuum pump that creates a negative pressure within the bellows chamber during expiration. A manual button on the ventilator also permits the delivery of a breath irrespective of the ventilatory settings. This control can be used to provide ventilation if there is an interruption in electrical power. The interface hose, which exits at the bottom of the bellows, attaches to the circle system rebreathing bag mount. The hosing is designed to disconnect at the base of the bellows assembly, thereby optimizing the drainage of fluid and drying of the interior of the bellows. A "releasing" fixture at the top of the bellows is used to maintain the bellows in the fully inflated position when not in use to facilitate drying of the inside of the bellows assembly. The "release" fixture is released when the ventilator is hooked up to the circle system with an occluded Y piece on the breathing circuit and a closed pressure relief (pop-off) valve to test for leaks in the circuit and ventilator. The Mallard ventilator is quieter than other equine ventilators. An MRI-compatible model is available.

Surgivet DHV 1000 LA ventilator. The DHV 1000 LA ventilator is a volume-targeted, double-circuit ventilator. It is electrically controlled, electronically and pneumatically powered, and time cycled with a descending (hanging) bellows. The maximum volume delivered is adjusted manually by adjusting the size of the bellows. The operator adjusts the inspiratory flow rate and inspiratory time to control the VT. The DHV 1000 LA ventilator is designed for controlled ventilation only. The control settings include an on/off switch, breaths per minute, inspiratory time, and inspiratory flow. The PIP is also displayed on the ventilator housing. An MRI-compatible model is available.

Drager large animal ventilator.   The Drager AV ventilator marketed with the Narkovet E large animal system was the first available Drager large animal ventilator. The subsequent model, the Drager AV-E ventilator, was marketed with the Narkovet E-2 large animal system. Although neither ventilator is currently being manufactured, they are still in use. Both ventilators are volume-targeted, double-circuit ventilators designed for use in the controlled ventilatory mode. They are electronically controlled, and the power source is both electronic and pneumatic. The bellows are pneumatically driven, and they are time cycled with a descending (hanging) bellows. The maximum volume delivered is adjusted by manually altering the size of the bellows (4 to 15 L) through adjustment of the degree to which the bellows descends (see Chapter 16). This is done using a rotary device located on the front housing of the bellows, which in turn adjusts the bellows stop plate. Additional settings include an on/off switch, frequency, and inspiratory flow rate. In the Drager AV ventilator the I:E ratio is set at 1:2, whereas in the Drager AV-E ventilator the I:E ratio can be adjusted from 1:1 to 1:4.5. The ventilator connects to the circuit at the top of the bellows assembly via a corrugated hose that detaches from the rebreathing bag mounting system. To dry the inside of the bellows, the top of the bellows housing must be removed and dried manually.

Alpha 400.   The Alpha 400 (France) is a circle system anesthetic machine and electrically controlled volume-cycled ventilator designed specifically for horses. The anesthetic machine and ventilator can be powered by compressed air or O_2. The ventilator can be operated in controlled or assist modes and during spontaneous ventilation. The operator, independent of respiratory efforts, determines the tidal volume, ventilatory frequency, and minute volume. The negative pressure necessary to trigger inspiration (assist mode) is determined by the operator. The peak inspiratory airway pressure (1 to 60 cm H_2O) and inspiratory trigger pressure (–1 to –20 cm H_2O). Minute volume (15 to 78 L) and respiratory rate (3 to 20) are adjustable. These settings can be changed easily during the course of anesthesia. Inspiratory, expiratory, and mean airway pressures; minute volume; and respiratory rate are digitally displayed. PEEP can be applied by means of an adjustable PEEP valve. The Alpha 400 is mobile and adjustable in height (100 to 140 cm). The bellows (10 L or 25 L size) is situated in a graduated plexiglas chamber. A water vapor collector and a manual pop-off relief valve are on the left side of the bellows. Four absorbent canisters (1 kg each) are positioned at the four corners of the rebreathing circuit.

Pressure-Cycled Ventilators

JD Medical LAV-3000 and LAV-2000.   The LAV-3000 is a stand-alone ventilator, and the LAV-2000 is a ventilator integrated with a large animal anesthetic circuit. Both are pressure-preset ventilators with a double-circuit design. Therefore, setting the inspiratory pressure on the ventilator controls the delivered VT. The descending (hanging) bellows is pneumatically driven with a modified mark 7 Bird ventilator (see Chapter 16). The Bird ventilator, which was originally manufactured for human applications, is modified to supply the gas to the bellows housing during inspiration, forcing the bellows upward. The interface hosing connects to the top of the bellows assembly; and, as with the Drager and Surgivet machines, disassembly is required for drying and cleaning. These ventilators can be used in assist, control, or assist-control modes. The control settings include the inspiratory pressure (5 to 65 cm H_2O), the inspiratory flow rate (0 to 450 L/min), the expiratory time (5 to 15 seconds), and the inspiratory sensitivity (–0.5 to –5 cm H_2O). Unlike the original homemade Bird "bag-in-a-box" ventilators that were historically used, the LAV-3000 and LAV-2000 ventilators are designed to permit a visual estimate of the VT based on the bellows movement against a scale.[1] They are also designed to permit automatic release of excess gas volumes in the bellows on exhalation. Most homemade systems do not have this feature, and it is easy to develop excessive exhalation pressures (PEEP).

Volume- or Pressure-Cycled Ventilator

Smith respirator LA 2100.   The Smith Respirator LA 2100 (Netherlands) is a volume-cycled pressure-limited version of the older "Smith" mechanical ventilator. PIP can be controlled by a manual valve for expiratory gases at the bottom of the bellows. It is operated by compressed gas and designed as a stand-alone unit that is easy to move because of its large wheels. The Smith respirator LA 2100 can be connected to any existing circle anesthetic system and provides controlled or assisted ventilation. A front panel permits touch control of ventilatory parameters, including minute volume, VT, and respiratory frequency in either assist or control modes. The I:E ratio is adjustable from 1:2 to 1:5 by increasing resistance of air insufflation. There is also an option to apply a breath hold to maintain a positive pressure in the lung at the end of insufflation. The anesthetist controls the time and pressure of this function. The bellows is situated beside a big plastic front cover; thus turning the machine on requires a check of VT and appropriate machine operation. Anesthetic waste gases are removed from the machine by 19-mm tubes.

The entire panel system must be opened for cleaning, which is not very easy in practice.

Tafonius (wind god).   Tafonius (Hollowell EMC) is a fully computerized large animal anesthesia machine with integral monitoring and a volume- or pressure-cycled ventilator. The electronics have direct control over the movement of the breathing gases. The layer of pneumatic driving force and all driving gas consumption has been eliminated. Tafonius uses a linear actuator to move a piston in response to operator settings and a pressure feedback signal. A linear actuator is similar in appearance to a hydraulic piston; however, a servomotor controls it with great precision. The linear actuator is capable of moving the piston a distance that translates to VTs up to 20 L with a resolution of 50 ml. The piston moves at any velocity and changes velocity translating to inspiratory flow. The current design can deliver 1200 L/min to a peak pressure of 80 cm H_2O. This control over volume and flow with feedback from the airway pressure measured at the patient Y piece makes the machine capable of generating inspiratory and expiratory waveforms desired for any size horse.

Ventilatory Assist Devices

Demand Valve

A demand valve consists of a specialized valve that is designed to connect to a pressurized source of oxygen via an oxygen supply hose and to the proximal end of an endotracheal tube.[32] Most demand valves are supplied with different-size adapters to permit use with a range of endotracheal tube sizes; however, the valve can be attached to a stomach tube (used as an endotracheal tube) in an emergency. It permits the controlled delivery of oxygen at a flow rate of 160 to 280 L/min. The actual flow achieved depends on both the supply gas pressure and the specific valve design. Demand valves require an oxygen source with a supply pressure of 50 to 80 psi, with the greater pressures resulting in higher flow rates. Flow of oxygen is initiated by the operator manually depressing a triggering button or by a sensor that detects negative airway pressure that is generated during inspiratory efforts. Flow of oxygen ends when the horse terminates its inspiratory efforts or when the operator releases the triggering button. The demand valve can be used for either IPPV or for CMV. In either situation the horse's $PaCO_2$ and PaO_2 can be improved. The delivered VT is estimated when using the demand valve to deliver a positive-pressure breath based on the degree of chest wall movement and the duration of the inspired breath. Exhalation is passive with this system; however, the resistance to exhalation is markedly increased through the demand valve. Therefore it is recommended that the valve be disconnected from the endotracheal tube at the end of inspiration to permit unobstructed exhalation. The resistance to breathing also limits the use of the demand valve in spontaneously ventilating horses since the increased work of breathing generally results in an increased $PaCO_2$. Modifications to the valve have been attempted to reduce the work of breathing; however, a model that creates adequate inspiratory flow without a decrease in the inspired oxygen fraction while minimizing the resistance to breathing is not currently available.[33]

BASICS OF VENTILATOR SETUP

Regardless of design, the same general principles are applied when preparing ventilators for use (Box 17-5). Both the anesthetic circuit and the mechanical ventilator should be

---

Box 17-5 Preparing Ventilators for Use

- Connect the power source of the ventilator.
- Connect the pneumatic driving gas.
- Connect the interface hose to the anesthetic machine.
- Close the pressure release valve on the anesthetic machine.
- Connect the scavenging hose to the ventilatory-scavenging outlet.
- Set the ventilator control dials for the individual patient.
- "Leak test" the anesthetic machine and ventilator.

---

tested for leaks before anesthetizing the horse. The anesthetic system should be connected to the supply gases and electrical source. The anesthetic delivery system should be assembled with a breathing circuit and rebreathing bag, and a pressure test performed. In brief this involves sealing the breathing circuit at the patient end (at the Y piece adaptor), closing the pressure relief (pop-off) valve, and using either the oxygen flush valve or the oxygen flowmeter to pressurize the circuit to 20 cm H_2O (see Box 17-5). Ideally this pressure should be maintained for at least 30 seconds without additional oxygen entering the circuit via either the flush or the flowmeter. If the pressure within the circuit decreases, the fresh gas flow should be turned on to determine the minimum flow required to maintain the circuit pressure at 20 cm H_2O. If the fresh gas flow is less than 200 ml/min, it is considered acceptable. Following the pressure test of the anesthetic system, the pressure relief valve should remain closed, and the scavenging hoses should be transferred from this valve to the ventilator-scavenging outlet on the ventilator. The rebreathing bag can be removed, interface hosing from the ventilator can be connected to the anesthetic machine on the bag mount, and the ventilator can be tested for leaks. A leak in either system prevents the ventilator from delivering a PIP breath of appropriate volume, in the appropriate time, and potentially leads to room contamination with inhaled anesthetics if they are in use. The breathing circuit can be sealed at the Y piece (site of connection of the endotracheal tube adaptor), and the bellows filled using the oxygen flush valve when setting up a ventilator with an ascending (standing) bellows. The bellows should remain fully inflated when the bellows is filled and the oxygen inflow stopped. Ventilators with descending (hanging) bellows can be pressure tested by attaching an anesthesia rebreathing bag to the Y piece, partially filling the bag using the oxygen flush valve, and then triggering the ventilator (see Figure 17-8). Sufficient VT should be delivered to the bag at the Y piece to create a circuit pressure at end-inspiration of at least 10 to 20 cm H_2O. The peak pressure should remain constant with repeated delivery of the positive-pressure breath if no leaks are present in the system. A similar system can be set up to test a pressure-targeted ventilator.

Following attachment of the power sources (electrical and pneumatic), driving gases, and scavenging systems and after pressure testing the ventilator, the controlled variables should be adjusted before starting the ventilator. Inappropriate settings could lead to lung injury and/or excessive hemodynamic depression. Recommended settings for mechanical ventilation are made on the basis of the horse's size (VT), observation of the respiratory rate and degree of thoracic expansion, or the use of capnography or arterial blood gas analysis (see Table 17-2).

Horses can be ventilated mechanically immediately after induction to anesthesia and connection to the anesthetic system. The anesthetic breathing circuit can be connected after securing and sealing the airway with an orotracheal or nasotracheal tube; and the mechanical ventilator started, assuming that the systems have been leak tested and set up as described previously. Alternatively, the horse can be connected to the anesthetic machine and allowed to breathe spontaneously before initiating mechanical ventilation. The gas and electrical supply to the ventilator should be checked. The rebreathing bag on the patient's breathing circuit should be emptied into the scavenge system, and the interface hosing from the ventilator bellows should replace the rebreathing bag. The pressure-relief valve should be closed, and the scavenge hose transferred to the ventilator. Generally it is not necessary to use neuromuscular paralyzing drugs to prevent patient-ventilator interaction (the patient fighting or bucking the ventilator) when initiating mechanical ventilation because of the respiratory depressant effects of the general anesthetics in the horse. It is rare for a horse to initiate spontaneous breaths, assuming adequate oxygenation if the horse's $PaCO_2$ is maintained below 60 mm Hg.

The horse can be weaned from the ventilator (resume spontaneous ventilation) by reducing the ventilatory settings for VT and/or rate, thereby increasing $PaCO_2$. The elevation in $PaCO_2$ stimulates the horse to initiate spontaneous breathing before disconnection from the anesthetic machine. In general, the return of spontaneous ventilation is easily accomplished once the delivery of anesthetic drugs and therefore the degree of respiratory depression are reduced. Alternatively the ventilator can be turned off abruptly, the rebreathing bag reattached to the anesthetic circuit, and intermittent positive-pressure breaths delivered manually at a reduced frequency (2 to 3 breaths/min) until ventilation resumes. Horses in which ventilation was abruptly discontinued (producing a brief period of apnea) had higher $PaCO_2$ levels compared to horses that were weaned off ventilation and were spontaneously breathing before removal from the anesthetic machine. Arterial blood gas levels were similar in both groups of horses within 5 minutes.[37] Horses in which ventilation was not reduced before abrupt discontinuation of support began breathing in approximately 5 minutes.[37] If the latter approach to removing a horse from controlled ventilation is taken, the anesthetist should be prepared to reinstitute PPV if the horse does not resume breathing within 5 to 6 minutes. Use of a pulse oximeter is recommended to monitor for hypoxemia.

RESPIRATORY EFFECTS OF OXYGEN SUPPLEMENTATION AND MECHANICAL VENTILATION

Recumbency in anesthetized adult horses consistently results in a decrease in PaO_2 values as a result of a reduction in lung volume, ventilation-perfusion inequalities, and an increase in the intrapulmonary shunting of blood.[13,15] Supplementation of the inspired gases with oxygen (increased FiO_2) in spontaneously breathing or mechanically ventilated anesthetized horses consistently increases PaO_2 and the oxygen content of arterial blood (CaO_2).[18,26,38,39] The $PaCO_2$ also increases slightly during oxygen supplementation in spontaneously breathing horses because of the removal of the stimulation of the respiratory center by low PaO_2.[38,39] The PaO_2 does not increase in direct proportion to FiO_2 as a result of ventilation-perfusion inequalities and intrapulmonary shunt. Nonetheless, PaO_2 generally increases to values that result in a saturation of oxygen (SpO_2) of greater than 95%. Temporal changes in the response to oxygen supplementation on PaO_2 have been reported in the spontaneously breathing horses administered an inhalant anesthetic and breathing >90% oxygen.[10] Specifically PaO_2 values remain stable over time or may

decrease in laterally recumbent anesthetized horses spontaneously breathing >90% oxygen, whereas the PaO_2 decreases with time in horses placed in dorsal recumbency.[10,13,19,26,38] Atelectasis and the increase in ventilation-perfusion inequalities are responsible for the progressive time-related decrease in PaO_2 and increase in pulmonary shunt fraction during elevated FiO_2. Increased FiO_2 values administered with inhalant anesthesia "wash out" alveolar nitrogen (80% of room air); and the replacement of nitrogen with an easily absorbed gas (oxygen) is likely responsible for time-related increases in shunt fraction. Nitrogen in the alveoli normally has somewhat of a protective ("splinting") effect since it is not readily absorbed by the blood. Experimentally, oxygen supplementation resulting in an FiO_2 >85% in anesthetized spontaneously breathing horses increases the degree of intrapulmonary shunt.[38,39] Once atelectasis develops in the spontaneously breathing horse, it will likely persist even after return to a lower FiO_2 unless some method of alveolar recruitment is used (Box 17-6).[31,39] Mechanical ventilation, when instituted early in the anesthetic period, results in a lower shunt fraction than in spontaneously breathing horses by minimizing the development of airway closure and atelectasis.[13,19] Unlike the spontaneously breathing horse, oxygenation and the degree of shunt remain constant over time in horses that are mechanically ventilated unless abdominal tympany develops.[19]

The optimum FiO_2 in adult spontaneously breathing or ventilated horses that provides optimum oxygenation (PaO_2) while minimizing the development of atelectasis has not been determined. Unfortunately, without blood gas analysis it is difficult to accurately assess an individual horse's oxygen status. Providing room air (e.g., 0.21 FiO_2) results in low arterial oxygen levels that could impair oxygen delivery to tissues in some horses; therefore an FiO_2 of at least 30% to 50% is recommended for prolonged inhalant or intravenous general anesthesia. Most horses in which anesthesia is maintained with inhalant anesthetics receive over 90% oxygen from the anesthetic machine. Interestingly, the administration of acepromazine (0.035 mg/kg IM)

Box 17–6 Recruitment of Atelectic Lung Areas in Horses

- Recruitment maneuvers should be instituted early when PaO_2 is <60 mm Hg during inhalant anesthesia in 100% oxygen
- Monitor arterial blood pressure and systolic arterial blood pressure variation
- Administer fluids and support arterial blood pressure when necessary
- Specific recruitment maneuvers include:
  - Incremental PEEP in 5 cm H_2O steps every 30 seconds to 25 cm H_2O
  - PIP of 30-45 cm H_2O held for 15 to 30 seconds
  - PIP of 30-45 cm H_2O held for 15 to 30 seconds while maintaining 10-20 cm H_2O PEEP
  - Stepwise increase in PIP from 45, 50, and 55 cm H_2O while maintaining PEEP at 10 to 20 cm H_2O

approximately 30 minutes before dissociative anesthesia improved hemodynamics and arterial oxygenation in laterally recumbent spontaneously breathing horses.[399]

CARDIOVASCULAR EFFECTS OF OXYGEN SUPPLEMENTATION AND MECHANICAL VENTILATION

Controlled positive-pressure ventilation can result in a decrease in cardiac output, systemic arterial blood pressure, and oxygen delivery.[18,25,40,41] The magnitude of these changes depends on the health status of the horse, the ventilatory strategy used, and the horse's blood volume (Box 17-7). Some studies in healthy horses have shown no significant effect of CMV on cardiac output, stroke volume, or oxygen delivery for up to 90 minutes.[25,28] The negative cardiovascular effects of mechanical ventilation that occur are partly indirect through lowering carbon dioxide levels.[22,24] Mechanical ventilation directly affects cardiovascular function by changing intrathoracic pressure. The positive pressure during inspiration reduces venous return and alters lung volume and the distribution of pulmonary blood flow and autonomic tone (Figure 17-10). To date the relative significance of the direct versus indirect effects on cardiovascular performance has not been determined. The effect of changes in intrathoracic pressure on right ventricular performance during PPV is likely the predominant factor influencing cardiovascular function. Irrespective of cause, the potential for a decrease in cardiac output, arterial blood pressure, and oxygen delivery should be anticipated whenever PPV (IPPV or CMV) is instituted in horses; and it is recommended that blood pressure be monitored in ventilated horses and inotropic support be available if needed.

Effect of Changes in Intrathoracic Pressure on Venous Return and Right Heart Function

Intrathoracic pressure normally decreases during inspiration and spontaneous ventilation. Systemic venous return depends on the pressure gradient between the peripheral systemic

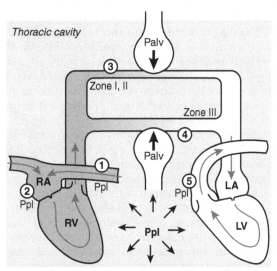

Figure 17–10. Effects of mechanical ventilation and increases in *l*, pleural pressure *(Ppl)* on venous return; *2*, right atrial pressure; *3*, pulmonary capillaries (right ventricular afterload); *4*, capillary blood volume; and *5*, aortic blood volume (left ventricular afterload). Mechanical ventilation increases right arterial pressure and right ventricular afterload, squeezes blood out of pulmonary capillaries toward the left ventricle, and reduces left ventricular afterload. The decrease in venous return and right ventricular output during the inspiratory phase of mechanical ventilation causes a decrease in left ventricular filling and output during the expiratory period, leading to mild variations (ups and downs) in the systolic arterial blood pressure in normovolemic horses over a single mechanical breath. Systolic pressure variation (SPV) correlates with blood volume status and becomes pronounced in hypovolemic horses. Adequate fluid therapy helps to minimize SPV.

veins (e.g., extrathoracic) and right atrium (e.g., intrathoracic). Blood flow into the thorax and right atrium (venous return) increases during spontaneous inspiration. Right ventricular preload and stroke volume increase, assuming normal contractile function (Starling effect) of the heart. In contrast, intrathoracic pressure increases during inspiration and PPV, thereby decreasing venous return to the right atrium. Right ventricular preload and right ventricular stroke volume decrease, potentially resulting in a decrease in cardiac output and arterial blood pressure (see Figure 17-10). The mean airway pressure and therefore mean intrathoracic pressure are key factors determining the impact of PPV on right ventricular preload and cardiac output.[41] Ventilation strategies that minimize PIP, PEEP, and the duration of inspiration reduce the impact of ventilation on right ventricular performance.

Most mechanical ventilatory strategies used in horses have been shown to impact cardiovascular performance.[25] A pressure-targeted ventilatory mode in which the PIP was adjusted to 20 cm H_2O resulted in less depressant cardiovascular changes than a PIP of 25 cm H_2O. The horses with the latter changes had a significantly lower $PaCO_2$, which may have contributed to the differences in hemodynamic outcome. PEEP values ranging from 5 to 30 cm H_2O produced a negative effect on cardiac output, systemic arterial pressures, and oxygen delivery.[36] These later findings suggest that impaired venous return produced by the increase in mean intrathoracic pressure was responsible for the reduced cardiac output in anesthetized horses.

The blood volume status of the horse affects the response to mechanical ventilation. Specifically, the negative effects of PPV with or without PEEP are greater in hypovolemic

---

Box 17–7 Deleterious Consequences of Mechanical Ventilation

- Decreased cardiac output (decreased venous return, compression of the heart)
- Decreased arterial blood pressure (MAP = CO × SVR)
- Inactivation of pulmonary surfactant (stiff lung)
- Barotrauma: lung injury caused by elevated transpulmonary pressure leading to large increases in regional lung distention and causing interstitial emphysema, air embolism
- Volutrauma: increased alveolar-capillary permeability; edema caused by ventilation at high lung volumes
- Atelectrauma: lung injury caused by repetitive opening/closing of lung units following ventilation at low tidal volumes
- Biotrauma: activation of inflammatory cells and release of cytokines caused by ventilation of injured or diseased lung

or vasodilated (endotoxic or septic) horses than in normal normovolemic horses. Venous return and right ventricular preload increase during inspiration because of the increase in intrathoracic pressure compresses the vena cava and the right atrium. Right ventricular afterload increases because pulmonary capillaries are compressed by the pressure generated in the alveoli during inspiration, leading to a decrease in right ventricular ejection. The inspiratory decrease in right ventricular output produces a decrease in left ventricular filling and output a few heartbeats later during expiration. Stabilization and replacement of the intravascular volume should be attempted before anesthesia and minimizes the effects of PPV on right ventricular function. Alternatively, if the horse is anesthetized and the cardiovascular effects of PPV are profound (large cyclical variation in arterial pressure values during IPPV), fluids should be administered, and inotropic support instituted (Figure 17-11).

Effect of Changes in Intrathoracic Pressure on the Left Ventricle

Changes in intrathoracic pressure affect the left ventricle via alterations in left ventricular afterload, which is proportional to the transmural pressure of the intrathoracic aorta. During spontaneous ventilation, when the intrathoracic pressure decreases on inspiration, the transmural aortic pressure and therefore left ventricular afterload increases. During PPV, intrathoracic pressure increases, and transmural aortic pressure and therefore afterload decrease. Stroke volume increases during inspiration as a result of the decrease in left ventricular afterload and the increase in left ventricular preload produced by blood being squeezed out of the pulmonary capillaries during PPV. Large cyclical variations (Δup; Δdown) in systolic pressure (SP) during a single mechanical breath compared to that measured during a long expiratory pause or apnea (SPref) suggest hypovolemia or poor ventricular function and the need for fluid or inotropic support (see Figures 17-10 and 17-11). The magnitude of the changes in right and left ventricular afterload and systolic pressure variation (SPV) associated with PPV are relatively inconsequential (SPV <10 to 15 mm Hg) in horses with normal myocardial contractility and blood volume, resulting in minimal changes in stroke volume and cardiac output.[42]

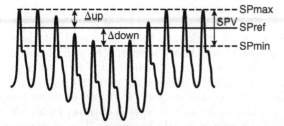

Figure 17–11. Arterial systolic pressure *(SP)* and systolic pressure variation *(SPV)* during mechanical ventilation. The maximum *(SPmax)* and minimum *(SPmin)* systolic pressure measured during mechanical inspiration and expiration. The increase (Δup) and decrease (Δdown) in systolic arterial blood pressure compared to systolic blood pressure at end-expiration *(SPref)* should be less than 10 mm Hg. A large SPV and, more important, large Δdown (>10 mm Hg) indicate hypovolemia even if systolic arterial blood pressure and heart rate are relatively normal.

Effects of Changing Lung Volume

Pulmonary vascular resistance is the major determinant of right ventricular afterload. Pulmonary vascular resistance is determined by the tone of both the alveolar and extra-alveolar vessels, which change as lung volume changes. The total pulmonary vascular resistance is at its lowest at functional residual capacity (FRC) and increases when FRC increases or decreases (see Chapter 2). Reducing lung volume below the normal FRC increases pulmonary vascular resistance. Similarly, if lung volume is well above FRC, which could occur with a ventilatory strategy that uses both high PEEP and large VTs, pulmonary vascular resistance increases. The impact of pulmonary vascular resistance on right ventricular output is not likely to be clinically significant in healthy horses if positive-pressure ventilation is performed at close-to-normal lung volumes.

Heart Rate Changes with Ventilation

Heart rate increases during inspiration and spontaneous ventilation because of a withdrawal of vagal tone. Cyclical fluctuation in vagal tone during respiration may be responsible for sinus arrhythmia (see Chapter 3). When the lungs are hyperinflated or excessive VTs are used, vagal tone increases, and heart rate tends to decrease. It is unlikely that a decrease in heart rate with inspiration will occur when using a normal VT in horses; however, a very large breath or sigh may trigger this reflex.

EFFECTS OF MECHANICAL VENTILATION ON CEREBRAL PERFUSION

General anesthesia substantially alters intracranial hemostasis by changing cerebral perfusion pressure (CPP) and/or intracranial pressure (ICP). The consequences of these changes have not been shown to have any detectable clinical significance in healthy horses. Improper anesthetic management could adversely affect outcome in horses with intracranial pathology by reducing cerebral perfusion to the point that cerebral ischemia occurs or cerebral herniation occurs secondary to raised ICP. CPP is a function of both mean arterial pressure (MAP) and ICP: CPP = MAP − ICP. ICP in turn is determined by intracranial volume, which is composed of intracranial tissue, cerebrospinal fluid, and blood. Anesthesia can alter CPP and ICP by changing MAP and/or ICP through changes in cerebral blood flow. Cerebral blood flow also depends on $PaCO_2$, PaO_2, and ICP. The correlation of these variables with cerebral blood flow is complex and may change over time.[43] Positive-pressure ventilation influences CPP and ICP indirectly via its effects on $PaCO_2$, MAP, and venous return. Specifically, by maintaining $PaCO_2$ within a normal range, the vasodilator effect of carbon dioxide on the cerebral vasculature is reduced, and increases in cerebral blood flow and ICP are minimized.[43] CPP may decrease during PPV as a result of a decrease in MAP secondary to anesthetic- and ventilation-induced decreases in cardiac output. Ventilatory strategies that result in high mean airway pressure such as modes that use a high PEEP or prolonged inspiratory time have a greater negative impact on CPP and therefore should be avoided in a patient with decreased CPP. Alternatively, prolonged expiratory times may improve venous return from the brain, thereby increasing CPP.

MONITORING VENTILATORY SUPPORT

Monitoring horses during the institution and maintenance of PPV should include an assessment of the patient's ventilation ($PaCO_2$), oxygenation (PaO_2), peak airway pressure (PIP), and hemodynamic variables such as heart rate and arterial blood pressure. The depth of anesthesia should be assessed frequently (see Chapter 8).

Observation of the degree of chest wall expansion and respiratory rate may be the sole indicator of the adequacy of alveolar ventilation when performing IPPV with a demand valve. Use of the recommended respiratory rates and VTs or PIPs (see Table 17-2) generally produces adequate alveolar ventilation in recumbent healthy horses. Nevertheless, considerable variability exists, and some horses may be underventilated or overventilated. The adequacy of alveolar ventilation is most accurately assessed by the determination of $PaCO_2$. The measurement of end-tidal carbon dioxide ($ETCO_2$) is a viable alternative if blood gas analysis is not available. The $ETCO_2$ tends to be lower than $PaCO_2$ levels by 5 to 12 mm Hg in adult horses during general anesthesia. Larger differences occur in horses with ventilation-perfusion inequalities and intrapulmonary shunt.[5,44] The $ETCO_2$ can be used to follow trends in alveolar ventilation in healthy horses and foals, although the accuracy may decrease with time. The $ETCO_2$ is a relatively inaccurate indicator of $PaCO_2$ during spontaneous ventilation in adult horses because of the impact of anatomical dead space ventilation and should not be relied on, particularly in the compromised animal.[6,8,44]

Oxygenation in the adult horse is assessed most accurately by determining the PaO_2 (see Chapter 8). Unfortunately, this may not always be possible. Visual assessment of mucous membrane color or a pulse oximeter (SpO_2) helps to assess hemoglobin saturation with oxygen. Most standard human lingual probes applied to the tongue in adult horses tend to underestimate SpO_2.[44,45] Small differences between SpO_2 and SaO_2 can lead to important therapeutic decisions because of the small numerical range over which hemoglobin is saturated with oxygen (see Chapter 2). Therefore caution should be used when interpreting SpO_2 readings, particularly in anemic horses and when the pulse oximeter does not accurately assess the heart rate.[44] Considerable variation in the accuracy and reliability of individual monitors exists, and failure to obtain accurate readings can occur.[45]

Monitoring airway pressures with currently available anesthetic machines and ventilators typically involves observing the PIP and the PEEP on a manometer placed within the breathing circuit. Typical PIP values in normal horses range from 20 to 25 cm H_2O when PEEP is zero; however, tremendous variations exist, depending on the horse's position and the degree of abdominal distention. For example, abdominal distention may require that PIP values exceed 50 cm H_2O to deliver a VT of 10 ml/kg. The PIP and PEEP should remain relatively constant throughout the anesthetic period in healthy horses unless ventilatory variables are changed.

Monitoring heart rate and rhythm, arterial blood pressure, and capillary perfusion is extremely important when mechanical ventilation is first instituted.

COMPLICATIONS OF VENTILATORY SUPPORT

The most common side effect associated with IPPV of healthy horses or foals is related to the cardiovascular consequences of using a positive pressure to inflate the lungs. Decreases in blood pressure and cardiac output should be anticipated if PIP is elevated, inspiratory or expiratory time are prolonged, and the depth of anesthesia is maintained constant.[40] A marked reduction in blood pressure may be observed in hypovolemic or vasodilated horses when inspiratory time is prolonged or excessive VTs are delivered (see Figure 17-11).

Lung injury resulting from positive-pressure ventilation is rare in the healthy horse; it is more likely in horses with preexisting lung injury if extreme VTs are used (>30 to 40 ml/kg). Lung injury resulting from excessive volume expansion of the lung is referred to as volutrauma. Lung injury resulting from excessive inspiratory pressure is referred to as *pulmonary barotrauma*. Regardless of cause (volume or pressure), injury to the airways or lungs is of greater concern in horses with preexisting lung injury or disease because of regional differences in lung compliance or atelectasis. A small portion of the lung that is compliant or aerated may receive all or the majority of the delivered VT as a result of the heterogeneous pattern of lung injury. Volutrauma or barotrauma occurs as a result of overstretching the lung and the shear forces that are created at the junction of the collapsed and aerated portions of lung. The use of standard VT ventilation (12 to 15 ml/kg) has not been shown to result in lung injury in normal horses that do not have preexisting lung injury, despite the presence of ventilation-perfusion mismatch or atelectasis. This is true even in horses with chronic obstructive lung disease or heaves. One study suggested that IPPV increased the percent of neutrophils and protein content in bronchoalveolar lavage fluid taken from dependent lung regions in anesthetized spontaneously breathing horses; however the study lacked controls, and the changes reported were transient.[46] Further investigation regarding differences in the inflammation response in horses subjected to different ventilatory strategies (PIP, FiO_2) is warranted.

Prolonged exposure to oxygen can result in lung injury. However, this is unlikely to occur when O_2 exposure is less than 8 to 12 hours even when FiO_2 is >90%. If the FiO_2 is kept below 60%, oxygen toxicity is unlikely to contribute to the progression of lung injury, even when prolonged oxygen therapy is required (e.g., in the foal with respiratory failure). Ventilator-associated pneumonia is one of the most common complications of prolonged ventilatory support in humans, and it is likely to be a risk factor for foals requiring prolonged ventilatory support. The risk of pneumonia is very low with routine PPV in healthy horses if appropriate maintenance and hygiene of equipment is practiced (see Chapter 16). Anesthesia and PPV could facilitate progression of lung injury and the spread of pneumonia in horses with preexisting bacterial pneumonia. The advantages and disadvantages of PPV must be considered on an individual basis. It is also imperative that the ventilator bellows and anesthetic tubing be thoroughly cleaned and disinfected after use in a diseased horse (see Chapter 16).

Although complications related to orotracheal intubation are rare, they have been reported in the horse and include tracheal mucosal damage, arytenoid cartilage paralysis, pharyngeal perforation, and retrograde inversion of the epiglottis (see Chapter 22).[47-49] Some mucosal damage to the arytenoid cartilages may occur during tracheal intubation; however, the clinical significance of this mucosal damage has yet to be determined (see Chapter 14). Tracheal mucosal injury can be minimized by monitoring and maintaining intracuff inflation pressure (approximately 80 cm H_2O).[49] Appropriate patient positioning, tube size selection, and intubation technique should be practiced in all cases to minimize laryngeal trauma and ventilator-associated complications (see Chapter 14).

Ventilator malfunction can occur as a result of operator-related errors or mechanical failure of the equipment. Although relatively simple in design and principle, the effective use of a ventilator and CMV requires a basic knowledge of respiration and practical experience in the application of PPV to horses. Ventilation of horses by inexperienced personnel is likely to produce volume or pressure trauma, hypoventilation or hyperventilation, and cardiovascular compromise. Typical ventilator malfunctions include but are not limited to leaks, bellows malfunction, and stuck breathing valves (Tables 17-3 and 17-4).

Table 17–3. Problem solving with a volume-targeted ventilator

Malfunction	Potential causes	Action
Ascending bellows not filling	Disconnection from endotracheal tube Leak in bellows or anesthetic machine Inadequate oxygen flow (<3 ml/kg/min) Patient "bucking" the ventilator	Check all connections Verify that pressure relief valve (pop-off valve) is closed Check endotracheal tube cuff inflation Check oxygen flow meter and increase if necessary Assess patient for ventilatory efforts; if "bucking". ventilator, see Patient "bucking" the ventilator later in the table Check and close water drain (spit) valve if necessary
Long inspiratory time	Incorrect ventilatory flow rate settings; low inspiratory flow rate, long inspiratory time; inadequate pressure in the gas source driving the bellows	Verify adequacy of inspiratory flow rate Shorten inspiratory time if required Verify I:E settings Verify respiratory rate setting Check pressure in gas source driving the bellows
Short inspiratory time	Incorrect ventilatory settings (inadequate inspiratory time caused by high I:E ratio with rapid inspiratory flow rates)	Verify I:E settings Increase (prolong) inspiratory time Verify respiratory rate settings Verify adequate VT Verify inspiratory flow rate
Long end-inspiratory hold	Ventilator setting (low rate with I:E ratio of 1:1-1:4)	Verify I:E ratio Increase respiratory rate
Patient "bucking" the ventilator	Inappropriate ventilator settings resulting in hypercapnia Exhausted soda lime or malfunction of anesthetic system one-way valves Inadequate depth of anesthesia (pain) Hypoxemia	Check ventilator settings Assess adequacy of ventilation; if inadequate, readjust VT or rate Assess patient's depth of anesthesia; if inadequate, deepen plane of anesthesia Treat pain Assess patient's oxygenation; if hypoxemic, adjust ventilator settings or reposition patient Check soda lime and one-way valve function
Failure to deliver adequate VT	Incorrect ventilatory settings	Verify adequate inspiratory flow rate Verify adequate inspiratory time (rate and I:E ratio) Verify adequate preset volume
Excessive airway pressure	Incorrect ventilator setting Low compliance (i.e., stiff) respiratory system (lung, chest wall, and/or diaphragm) Airway or endotracheal tube obstructions (kink, clot, mucus)	Verify VT setting (e.g., not excessive) Consider intraabdominal pressure; deflate if possible Consider pneumothorax and treat accordingly Consider primary lung disease and adjust respiratory rate and VT Verify no obstructions or partial obstructions within the airway or breathing circuit

Table 17–4. Problem solving with a pressure-targeted ventilator

Malfunction	Potential causes	Action
Long inspiratory time	Leak in bellows or anesthetic machine Incorrect ventilator settings: inadequate inspiratory flow rate, I:E ratio, and respiratory rate Inadequate pressure in the gas source driving the bellows	Check all connections, airway seal, and pressure relief valve Verify inspiratory flow rate Verify I:E ratio setting Verify respiratory rate Verify pressure of gases driving the bellows
Short inspiratory time	Obstruction Decreased compliance of respiratory system Incorrect ventilatory settings	Check all hoses for kinks Check endotracheal tube for obstruction Consider intraabdominal pressure: deflate if possible Consider pneumothorax and treat accordingly Verify peak inspiratory pressure settings
Patient "bucking" the ventilator	Inappropriate ventilator settings resulting in hypercapnia Exhausted soda lime or malfunction of anesthetic system one-way valves Inadequate depth of anesthesia (pain) Hypoxemia	Check ventilator settings Assess adequacy of ventilation; if inadequate, increase VT or rate Assess patient's depth of anesthesia; if inadequate, deepen plane of anesthesia Treat pain Assess patient's oxygenation; if hypoxemic, adjust ventilator settings or reposition patient Check soda lime and one-way valve function

SPECIAL SITUATIONS

Mechanical ventilation helps to maintain normal blood gases and the delivery of inhalant anesthetic drugs, thereby helping to stabilize the maintenance phase of anesthesia. Mechanical ventilation also facilitates the use of neuromuscular blocking drugs during ophthalmologic and orthopedic surgical procedures (see Chapter 19).

Abdominal Exploratory in the Adult Horse

Horses requiring anesthesia for abdominal surgery (colic, cesarean section) can vary tremendously in their respiratory and hemodynamic status. Increases in the work of breathing and obvious respiratory compromise may be evident in some horses before anesthesia, secondary to extreme abdominal distention. The duration of anesthesia may be prolonged (>90 minutes), and horses are generally positioned on their backs. These factors warrant the use of oxygen supplementation and ventilatory support after producing anesthesia and securing an airway with an orotracheal tube. Many horses benefit from oxygen supplementation before induction of anesthesia; however, this may be technically difficult to achieve, and studies that document the beneficial effect of preoxygenation on PaO_2 values after the onset of recumbency in the horse are limited. Abdominal distention and bloat can impair ventilation and markedly decrease venous return in recumbent horses. PIP values of 50 to 60 cm H_2O may be required to deliver a 10-ml/kg VT in the horse with abdominal distention caused by the low compliance of the thoracic cage as a result of the cranial movement of the diaphragm. Horses with excessive abdominal distention (bloat, tympany) should be allowed to breathe spontaneously and be trocharized or anesthetized, and the abdomen should be opened before initiating PPV to avoid the combined negative effects of increased abdominal and intrathoracic pressure on cardiac output and arterial blood pressure. Ventilation can be initiated once abdominal distention (pressure) is reduced or the abdomen is surgically opened, thereby removing intraabdominal pressure. When using a volume-targeted ventilator, an initial VT of 10 to 12 ml/kg with an I:E ratio of 1:3 should be delivered to minimize the potential negative impact of PPV, particularly in hypovolemic horses (see Figure 17-11). The goal of this strategy is to minimize mean airway and intrathoracic pressures and hemodynamic depression while providing adequate ventilation with increased inspired oxygen and a hemoglobin saturation of 100%. The PIP that results from PPV depends on the VT and the inspiratory flow rates; airway resistance; and, most important, pulmonary compliance. Inotropic support (e.g., dobutamine 1 to 2 μg/kg/min) may be required during inhalational anesthesia and PPV, even before blood pressure measurements are obtained. Ventilatory settings can be adjusted once hemodynamic and arterial blood gas variables are available. The optimum $PaCO_2$ is generally between 50 and 60 mm Hg unless marked metabolic (nonrespiratory) acidosis is present. Moderate-to-severe hypoxemia is not uncommon in horses with abdominal crises. Fortunately, abdominal decompression often results in an immediate improvement in oxygenation without adjusting ventilator settings. Although "sighing" the horse with intermittent large VT breaths (25 to 30 ml/kg) has not been shown to improve oxygenation in the normal horse, this strategy and other recruitment techniques may recruit atelectic lung units following an enterotomy or decompression of the viscera (see Box 17-6). This is usually accomplished by decreasing the respiratory rate to 2 to 3 breaths/min for a couple of minutes while increasing the VT to 25 to 30 ml/kg and adjusting the I:E ratio to 1:3 or 1:4. After the "sighing," VTs, rates, and I:E ratios are returned to the previous settings.

The use of PEEP in horses requiring surgery for colic is reported to significantly improve PaO_2 values; however, overall tissue oxygen delivery was not assessed (Figure 17-9).[29] Nevertheless, the use of PEEP or a recruitment maneuver may be a viable therapeutic option in hemodynamically stable hypoxemic horses that remain hypoxemic following abdominal decompression. The change in position from dorsal to lateral recumbency during recovery can help to minimize ventilation-perfusion mismatching and intrapulmonary shunt. Horses that are in lateral recumbency should be recovered with the same side down as during the surgery. Rolling the horses to the other side to facilitate recovery may further compromise lung function.[34] Oxygen supplementation should follow PPV support when spontaneous ventilation resumes.

Foals

Foals with hypoxemia and/or respiratory failure may require oxygen supplementation and/or ventilatory support. Fortunately, critical care ventilators designed for humans can be used in foals that require long-term ventilatory support for neurological disorders, septicemia, or primary respiratory problems.[50]

Emergency surgery may necessitate general anesthesia in the first few weeks of life to repair a ruptured bladder or resect an infected umbilicus. The foal may or may not have primary respiratory disease. The foal's respiratory systems should be examined for secondary or concurrent respiratory disease or infections before anesthesia. Foals have a very compliant chest wall, which predisposes them to a decrease in FRC during general anesthesia and recumbency. Their oxygen consumption and work of breathing are also greater than those of the adult horse, and their cardiovascular homeostatic protective mechanisms are less developed. The work of breathing may be increased further as a result of abdominal distention. Foals may be more prone to respiratory muscle fatigue and/or the respiratory depressant effects of anesthetic drugs. Oxygen supplementation and/or ventilatory support are often required. Oxygen supplementation should be instituted before induction of anesthesia if the development of hypoxemia is a concern. The goals for PPV are similar to those in adult horses, although the initial recommended respiratory rates and VTs are different (see Table 17-2). The increased chest wall compliance results in a lower PIP. Foals often have a patent ductus arteriosus with mild left-to-right shunting of blood in the first few days of life. Hypoxemia, atelectasis, and high mean airway pressures increase pulmonary vascular resistance that can produce right-to-left shunting of blood and reduce oxygenation. An unexpected decrease in oxygenation in a foal with high PIP values may indicate right-to-left shunting of blood through the patent ductus arteriosus. A strategy that minimizes PIP and higher respiratory rates should be used if this occurs.

SUMMARY

Mechanical ventilation of horses improves gas (PaO_2, $PaCO_2$) exchange, ensures inhalant anesthetic delivery, provides a more stable level of inhalant anesthesia, facilitates the use of unique surgical positions and neuromuscular blocking drugs, and serves as an indirect method for monitoring blood volume (hypovolemia). When properly applied, the hemodynamic consequences of mechanical ventilation are inconsequential and easily managed by fluid therapy and pharmacological support.

REFERENCES

1. Thurmon JC, Menhusen MJ, Hartsfield SM: A multivolume ventilator-bellows and air compressor for use with a Bird Mark IX respirator in large animal inhalation anesthesia, *Vet Anesthesiol* 2:34-39, 1975.
2. Steffey EP, Berry JD: Flow rates from an intermittent positive-pressure breathing-anesthetic delivery apparatus for horses, *Am J Vet Res* 38:685-687, 1977.
3. Thurmon JC, Benson GJ: Inhalation anesthetic delivery equipment and its maintenance, *Vet Clin North Am (Large Anim Pract)* 3:73-96, 1981.
4. Gallivan GJ, McDonell WN, Forrest JB: Comparative ventilation and gas exchange in the horse and the cow, *Res Vet Sci* 46:331-336, 1989.
5. Geiser DR, Rohrbach BW: Use of end-tidal CO_2 tension to predict arterial CO_2 values in isoflurane-anesthetized equine neonates, *Am J Vet Res* 53:1617-1621, 1992.
6. Neto FJT et al: The effect of changing the mode of ventilation on the arterial-to-end-tidal CO_2 difference and physiological dead space in laterally and dorsally recumbent horses during halothane anesthesia, *Vet Surg* 29:200-205, 2000.
7. Nyman G, Henenstierna G: Ventilation-perfusion relationship in the anaesthetised horse, *Equine Vet J* 21:274-281, 1989.
8. Moens Y: Arterial-alveolar carbon dioxide tension difference and alveolar dead space in halothane-anaesthetised horses, *Equine Vet J* 21:282-284, 1989.
9. Steffey EP et al: Effects of sevoflurane dose and mode of ventilation on cardiopulmonary function and blood biochemical variables in horses, *Am J Vet Res* 66:606-614, 2005.
10. Steffey EP et al: Cardiopulmonary function during 5 hours of constant-dose isoflurane in laterally recumbent, spontaneously breathing horses, *J Vet Pharmacol Ther* 10:290-297, 1987.
11. Kerr CL, McDonell WN, Young SS: A comparison of romifidine and xylazine when used with diazepam/ketamine for short-duration anesthesia in the horse, *Can Vet J* 37:601-609, 1996.
12. Kerr CL, McDonell WN, Young SS: Cardiopulmonary effects of romifidine/ketamine or xylazine/ketamine when used for short-duration anesthesia in the horse, *Can J Vet Res* 68:274-282, 2004.
13. Hall LW: Disturbances of cardiopulmonary function in anesthetized horses, *Equine Vet J* 3:95-98, 1971.
14. Dobson A et al: Changes in blood flow distribution in equine lungs induced by anaesthesia, *Q J Exp Physiol* 70:283-297, 1985.
15. Nyman G et al: Atelectasis causes gas exchange impairment in the anaesthetised horse, *Equine Vet J* 22:317-324, 1990.
16. Steffey EP et al: Effects of desflurane and mode of ventilation on cardiovascular and respiratory functions and clinicopathologic variables in horses, *Am J Vet Res* 66:669-677, 2005.
17. Blaze CA, Robinson NE: Apneic oxygenation in anesthetized ponies and horses, *Vet Res Commun* 11:281-291, 1987.
18. Steffey EP et al: Body position and mode of ventilation influences arterial pH, oxygen, and carbon dioxide tensions in halothane-anesthetized horses, *Am J Vet Res* 38:379-382, 1977.
19. Day TK et al: Blood gas values during intermittent positive-pressure ventilation and spontaneous ventilation in 160 anesthetized horses positioned in lateral or dorsal recumbency, *Vet Surg* 24:266-276, 1995.
20. Taylor PM et al: Total intravenous anaesthesia in ponies using detomidine, ketamine, and guaiphenesin: pharmacokinetics, cardiopulmonary and endocrine effects, *Res Vet Sci* 59:17-23, 1995.

21. Hall LW: Cardiovascular and pulmonary effects of recumbency in two conscious ponies, *Equine Vet J* 16:89-92, 1984.
22. Wagner AE, Bednarski RM, Muir III WM: Hemodynamic effects of carbon dioxide during intermittent positive-pressure ventilation in horses, *Am J Vet Res* 51:1922-1929, 1990.
23. Akca O: Optimizing the intraoperative management of carbon dioxide concentration, *Curr Opin Anaesthesiol* 19:19-25, 2006.
24. Khanna AK et al: Cardiopulmonary effects of hypercapnia during controlled intermittent positive-pressure ventilation in the horse, *Can J Vet Res* 59:213-221, 1995.
25. Mizuno Y et al: Cardiovascular effects of intermittent positive-pressure ventilation in the anesthetized horse, *J Vet Med Sci* 56:39-44, 1994.
26. Gleed RD, Dobson A: Improvement in arterial oxygen tension with change in posture in anaesthetised horses, *Res Vet Sci* 44:255-259, 1988.
27. Nyman C et al: Selective mechanical ventilation of dependent lung regions in the anaesthetized horse in dorsal recumbency, *Br J Anaesth* 59:1027-1034, 1987.
28. Edner A, Nyman G, Essen-Gustavesson B: The effects of spontaneous and mechanical ventilation on central cardiovascular function and peripheral perfusion during isoflurane anaesthesia in horses, *Vet Anaesth Analg* 32:136-146, 2005.
29. Wilson DV, McFeely AM: Positive end-expiratory pressure during colic surgery in horses: 74 cases (1986-1988), *J Am Vet Med Assoc* 199:917-921, 1991.
30. Swanson CR, Muir WW: Hemodynamic and respiratory responses in halothane-anesthetized horses exposed to positive end-expiratory pressure alone and with dobutamine, *Am J Vet Res* 49:539-542, 1988.
31. Wettstein D et al: Effects of an alveolar recruitment maneuver on cardiovascular and respiratory parameters during total intravenous anesthesia in ponies, *Am J Vet Res* 67:152-159, 2006.
31a. Moens Y et al: Distribution of inspired gas to each lung in the anaesthetized horse and influence of body shape, *Equine Vet J:* 27:110-116, 1995.
32. Watney GCG, Watkins SB, Hall LW: Effects of a demand valve on pulmonary ventilation in spontaneously breathing, anaesthetised horses, *Vet Rec* 117:358-362, 1985.
33. Johnson CB, Adma EN, Taylor PM: Evaluation of a modification of the Hudson demand valve in ventilation and spontaneously breathing horses, *Vet Rec* 135:569-572, 1994.
34. Mason DE, Muir WW, Wade A: Arterial blood gas tensions in the horse during recovery from anesthesia, *J Am Vet Med Assoc* 190:989-994, 1987.
35. Hartsfield SM: Airway management and ventilation. In Thurman JC, Tranquilli WJ, Benson GJ, editors: *Lumb and Jones' veterinary anesthesia*, Baltimore, 1996, Williams & Wilkins.
36. Wilson DV, Soma LR: Cardiopulmonary effects of positive end-expiratory pressure in anesthetized, mechanically ventilated ponies, *Am J Vet Res* 51:734-739, 1990.
37. Wright BD, Hildebrand SV: An evaluation of apnea or spontaneous ventilation in early recovery following mechanical ventilation in the anesthetized horse, *J Vet Anaesth Analg* 28:26-33, 2001.
38. Cuvelliez SG et al: Cardiovascular and respiratory effects of inspired oxygen fraction in halothane-anesthetized horses, *Am J Vet Res* 51:1226-1231, 1990.
39. Marntell S, Nyman G, Hedenstierna G: High inspired oxygen concentrations increase intrapulmonary shunt in anaesthetized horses, *Vet Anaesth Analg* 32:338-347, 2005.
39a. Marntell S et al: Effects of acepromazine on pulmonary gas exchange and circulation during sedation and dissociative anaesthesia in horses, *Anesth Analg* 32:83-93, 2005.
40. Hodgson DS et al: Effects of spontaneous, assisted, and controlled modes in halothane-anesthetized geldings, *Am J Vet Res* 47:992-996, 1986.
41. Slutsky AS: Lung injury caused by mechanical ventilation, *Chest* 116:9S-15S, 1999.
42. Michard F: Changes in arterial pressure during mechanical ventilation, *Anesthesiology* 103:419-428, 2005.
43. Brosnan RJ et al: Effects of duration of isoflurane anesthesia and mode of ventilation on intracranial and cerebral perfusion pressures in horses, *Am J Vet Res* 64:1444-1448, 2003.
44. Koenig J, McDonnell W, Valverde A: Accuracy of pulse oximetry and capnography in healthy and compromised horses during spontaneous and controlled ventilation, *Can J Vet Res* 67:169-174, 2003.
45. Matthews NS, Hartke S, Allen JC Jr: An evaluation of pulse oximeters in dogs, cats, and horses, *Vet Anaesth Analg* 30:3-14, 2003.
46. Ito S, Hobo S, Kasashima Y: Bronchoalveolar lavage fluid findings in the atelectatic regions of anesthetized horses, *J Vet Med Sci* 65:1011-1013, 2003.
47. Heath RB et al.: Laryngotracheal lesions following routine orotracheal intubation in the horse, *Equine Vet J* 21:434-437, 1989.
48. Abrahamsen EJ et al: Bilateral arytenoid cartilage paralysis after inhalation anesthesia in a horse, *J Am Vet Med Assoc* 197:1363-1365, 1990.
49. Touozot-Jouorde G, Stedman NL, Trim CM: The effects of two endotracheal tube cuff inflation pressures on liquid aspiration and tracheal wall damage in horses, *Vet Anaesth Analg* 32:23-29, 2005.
50. Palmer JE: Ventilatory support of the critically ill foal, *Vet Clin North Am (Equine Pract)* 21:457-486, 2005.

18

Anesthesia and Analgesia for Donkeys and Mules

Nora S. Matthews

KEY POINTS

1. Donkeys and mules have unique anatomical, physiological, and behavioral characteristics that are different from those of horses and that can affect anesthetic management.
2. Many donkeys and mules are stubborn and reluctant to move, especially after sedation.
3. Donkeys tend to be stoic and mask pain until it is severe.
4. Donkeys metabolize many anesthetic and analgesic drugs at different rates than horses. Doses or dosing intervals need to be adjusted accordingly.
5. Monitoring donkeys and mules under anesthesia is different than monitoring horses; more reliance on blood pressure and close observation of respiratory patterns are indicated.

Donkeys and mules present unique differences from horses. Mules are more variable in behavior, and their body type depends on the dam (e.g., Arab mares produce different foals than Draft Mares). *Donkeys* (burros) are of the species *Equus asinus*. Donkeys are registered on the basis of size in the United States. *Miniature* donkeys are less than 34 inches at the withers. *Standard* donkeys range in size from 34 to 54 inches at the withers, whereas *mammoth* donkeys are greater than 54 inches at the withers. *Mules* are produced from breeding a jackass (male donkey) to a mare (female horse). A hinny is produced by breeding a stallion to a jenny (female donkey), but mules and hinnies may be indistinguishable (Figure 18-1). Although both donkeys and mules have long ears, mules show horse characteristics (e.g., a more refined head, characteristic of the breed of horse used) and have a tail similar to that of a horse. The donkey has a tail similar to that of a cow, with only a switch of hair at the end.[1]

Agricultural use of donkeys and mules in North America has declined markedly since the early 1900s. Donkeys are used to guard sheep, goats, and calves from wild predators; whereas mules are used for logging and farm work. Both are primarily used for recreation (riding, driving, and packing) and as pets. Mule and donkey owners are frequently in touch with other owners through local and national clubs and organizations (Box 18-1). The United States is the largest producer of mules in the world. Both donkeys and mules are exported for use for transporting goods, agricultural products, water, and fuel; plowing; weeding; pulling carts; and recreational packing. It is estimated that over 50 million donkeys and mules are being used for these activities throughout the world (Global Livestock Production and Health Atlas, Food and Agriculture Organization, United Nations, NY, NY). A list of charitable organizations that provide veterinary care for these animals and who have collected useful information about their care is contained in Box 18-1.

PREOPERATIVE EVALUATION

Behavioral Differences

Behavioral differences are most evident in donkeys that have had little handling or training. Donkeys do not respond like horses when confronted with something new. They usually become immobile until acclimated (hence their reputation for stubbornness). Patience is required when trying to get them to perform tasks such as entering a stock or trailer. They are not easily "bullied" into movement. A nose twitch is frequently ineffective in restraining donkeys (in part because it slides off the nose easily). Donkeys may be adequately restrained by snubbing the head rope securely to a stout fixed object. Mules can be more difficult to work with than donkeys (unless well trained) and are considerably more dangerous because of their larger size. It is strongly recommended to have an experienced mule handler available when working with untrained mules. Both mules and donkeys may strike without warning.

Donkeys and mules are stoic, making it difficult to assess pain or illness; it is likely that they are sicker or have more pain than casual observation and physical examination suggest. There is a myth that says that donkeys and mules don't colic. This is not true, but mild bouts of colic are rarely observed because of their stoic nature. Since donkeys and mules may be quite ill before being presented for treatment or surgery, they present a significant anesthesia risk (see Chapter 22).

Physiological Differences

There are numerous physiological differences between donkeys and horses.[2] Donkeys are adapted to the desert; increases in hematocrit, commonly seen with dehydration in horses, do not occur until donkeys are approximately 30% dehydrated. Therefore assessing moderate dehydration by packed cell volume or hematocrit is inaccurate. Although generally resistant to disease, donkeys are susceptible to hyperlipidemia when anorexic.[3] Any donkey that is "off feed" should have triglyceride levels checked. In addition, mule foals are more likely to have neonatal isoerythrolysis than horse foals.[4] Hyperkalemic periodic paralysis has not been reported in mules; anecdotal reports suggest that a mare positive for this defect does not produce a mule with the defect.

Anatomical Differences

Anatomical differences that are relevant to anesthesia include: (1) the anatomy of the branches of the facial artery (i.e., the artery that is located under the temporal crest) makes it difficult to place an arterial catheter in that location; and (2) the jugular vein is located in the same position in the donkey as in the horse, but the cutaneous colli muscle

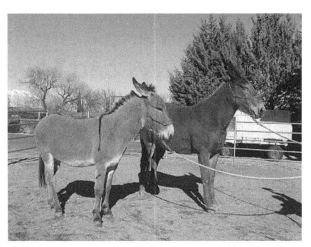

Figure 18–1. Donkeys are of the species *Equus asinus*. A mule is produced by breeding a male donkey to a mare. Mules (background) are larger than donkeys (foreground), have characteristics similar to those of horses, and are frequently used as pack animals. (Courtesy Dr. Craig London, Rock Creek Pack Station, Bishop, CA, www.rock creekpackstation.co).

| Box 18–1 | **Organizations Devoted to Donkeys and Mules** |

American Donkey and Mule Society (ADMS)
P.O. Box 1210
Lewisville, TX 75667

Canadian Donkey and Mule Association
Canadian Livestock Records Corporation
2417 Holly Lane
Ottawa, Ontario, CANADA K1V OM7

The Donkey Sanctuary
Sidmouth
Devon, EX10 ONU
UNITED KINGDOM

is a sheet of fascia and the skin is thicker; thus needles should be angled more perpendicular to the skin, similar to performing an intravenous injection in cattle when placing a jugular catheter.[5] A neck rope may make the jugular vein more visible.

Normal Values

Normal values for body temperature, respiration, and heart rate are slightly different than for horses. The donkey is thermolabile. Body temperature may increase to a greater degree than expected in donkeys in a hot climate or following exercise. Heart rate responses appear to be similar to those in horses and are a good indicator of stress or pain when other indicators (such as appearance) do not indicate stress. Normal resting respiratory rates for donkeys are higher than in horses; 20 to 30 breaths/min is normal.

Normal baseline values for most hematological and biochemical indices have been published for donkeys and mules, and slight differences from horses are normal.[6-8] Normal values from horses should not be extrapolated to

either donkeys or mules. Some normal values have not been documented; normal plasma protein levels and adrenocorticotropic hormone values have not been established for young donkeys and mules, making it difficult to diagnose some conditions (e.g., failure of passive immunity or cushingoid syndrome) with certainty.

Preoperative Analgesia in Donkeys and Mules

Preoperative analgesia is particularly important in donkeys and mules and should have the primary emphasis, especially for painful (e.g., orthopedic) conditions. Inadequate pain management can occur easily in donkeys because pain is not easily recognized and differences in drug metabolism have not been investigated adequately. Failure to provide adequate preoperative analgesia may result in inadvertent anesthetic overdose, resulting in cardiovascular collapse soon after induction. This situation is similar to but more common than that in horses in severe pain or those with chronic painful conditions (e.g., chronic laminitis); but, since it is easier to recognize severe pain in horses, it is less likely to occur. Donkeys require higher doses of nonsteroidal antiinflammatory drugs or shorter dosing intervals to achieve a degree of analgesia similar to that produced in horses since they metabolize many drugs more rapidly than horses (Table 18-1). This is especially true of miniature donkeys since they metabolize flunixin more rapidly than standard donkeys.

PREMEDICATION AND SEDATION FOR STANDING PROCEDURES

Most sedatives and preanesthetic medications used in horses can be administered to donkeys and mules with good results (see Chapters 10, 12, and 13). Generally mules require 50% more drug than donkeys or horses to achieve adequate sedation. Standing procedures can be accomplished with the same drugs or their combinations (e.g., acepromazine with xylazine; xylazine with butorphanol) used in horses. Larger doses (two to three times larger) and combination drug therapies are required for untrained, excited, or feral horses, donkeys, and mules (see Table 18-1).[9] The route of administration affects the dose required; generally the

Table 18–1.	**Suggested analgesics, dose, and dosing intervals for donkeys and mules**		
	Dose (mg/	Dosing interval	
Drug	kg), Route	Donkeys	Mules
Phenylbutazone	4.4, IV, PO	bid-tid	bid
Vedaprofen	1.0, PO	bid	NA*
Flunixin	1.1, IV	tid	NA
Carprofen	0.7, IV, PO	q24h	NA
Meloxicam	0.6, IV	bid-tid	NA
Buprenorphine	0.003-006, IV†	NA	NA
Nalbuphine	0.1, IV	NA	NA

bid, Twice a day; *IV*, intravenously; *NA*, not applicable; *PO*, orally; *tid*, three times a day.
*No pharmacokinetic data available.
†Combined with sedative.

amount of the intravenous dose required is twice that of the intramuscular dose. The same precautions should be observed for sedated mules or donkeys as for untrained or feral horses since they are more likely to bite or kick. It is not uncommon for donkeys to lie down after being administered a preanesthetic dose of xylazine; they do not fall down but deliberately lie down when they become uncoordinated. Anesthetic-induction drugs can be administered with the donkey in sternal recumbency.

INDUCTION AND MAINTENANCE OF GENERAL ANESTHESIA WITH INJECTABLE DRUGS

Smooth induction and maintenance of anesthesia depend on adequate sedation. A variety of injectable drugs are advocated for induction and maintenance of anesthesia (Table 18-2). Ketamine after sedation with an α_2-agonist is generally acceptable but is metabolized more rapidly in donkeys and mules than in horses. Faster metabolism in conjunction with a more rapid distribution phase results in higher doses and more frequent readministration (shorter dosing intervals; see Chapter 9).[10] This is especially important in miniature donkeys in which a surgical plane of anesthesia will not be achieved if horse doses of xylazine and ketamine are administered. If repeat administration of ketamine (by bolus or infusion) is not possible, a local block with lidocaine helps to ensure adequate analgesia during the latter stages of the procedure. The addition of butorphanol to a xylazine-ketamine drug combination enhances analgesia and extends the duration of anesthesia.

Guaifenesin-Ketamine-Xylazine Administration to Donkeys

The drug combination guaifenesin-ketamine-xylazine (GKX) produces smooth induction and maintenance of anesthesia in donkeys. Preanesthetic medication with xylazine (1.1 mg/kg intravenously [IV]) or an equivalent dose of another α_2-adrenoceptor agonist (e.g., romifidine, detomidine) usually produces adequate sedation. Induction to anesthesia is accomplished by rapid infusion (gravity flow) of 1 L of 5% guaifenesin to which 2 g of ketamine and 500 mg of xylazine have been added. Once the donkey is recumbent, the infusion rate is reduced to approximately 1 ml/kg/hr (based on eye signs, respiratory rate and pattern, and heart rate). The increased concentration of ketamine (rapidly metabolized in donkeys) compared to that used in horses (1 g/L) is important because donkeys are more sensitive to the respiratory depressant effects of guaifenesin.[11] Anesthetic induction in mules can be accomplished by administering xylazine (1.6 mg/kg IV) followed by ketamine (2.2 mg/kg IV); then the GKX drug combination is infused to effect.

Thiopental used alone or in combination with guaifenesin produces anesthesia in donkeys and mules with good results; but caution is required if guaifenesin is used since less guaifenesin is required to produce anesthesia in donkeys and the biological half-life is longer (see Table 18-2).[11]

Other drugs that can be administered to donkeys and mules are tiletamine-zolazepam (Telazol). This drug combination provides a slightly longer period of anesthesia and is recommended for miniature donkeys.[12] Propofol can be

Table 18–2. **Preanesthetics and anesthetics for induction or injectable anesthesia in donkeys and mules**		
Drug	**Dose: Donkeys (mg/kg IV)**	**Dose: Mules (mg/kg IV)**
Preanesthetics		
Xylazine	0.6-1.0	1.0-1.6
Detomidine	0.005-0.02	0.01-0.03
Romifidine	0.1	0.15
Butorphanol	0.02-0.04	0.02-0.04
Diazepam	0.03	0.03
Acepromazine	0.05	0.05-0.1
Midazolam	0.06	0.06
Induction		
Ketamine	2.2*	2.2*
Thiopental	5.0	5.0
Tiletamine-zolazepam	1.1	1.1
Guaifenesin	20-35 with ketamine or thiopental	20-35 with ketamine or thiopental
Propofol	2.2	NA†
Maintenance		
Propofol	0.2-0.3 mg/kg/min	NA
G-K-X‡	1.1 ml/kg/hr	1-2 ml/kg/hr
G.G. with thiopental§	"To effect" with careful monitoring of respiration	

*More rapidly metabolized than in the horse; must redose at shorter intervals.
†No information available.
‡50 mg/ml; 2 mg/ml; 0.5 mg/ml.
§50 mg/ml; 3 mg/ml.

used for induction and maintenance in donkeys following sedation with xylazine. Since apnea and desaturation are common problems with propofol, it is not recommended for use unless intubation or oxygen supplementation is available.

MAINTENANCE WITH INHALANT ANESTHETICS

Endotracheal intubation and maintenance with inhalant anesthetics is preferred for longer procedures in donkeys and mules. Endotracheal intubation is easily achieved using the same technique as in horses; on occasion it may be necessary to use a slightly smaller endotracheal tube, especially if the depth of anesthesia is not sufficient to produce adequate relaxation for intubation. Additional injectable anesthetic drugs, preferably thiopental, should be available to deepen anesthesia if required. Miniature donkeys (especially those with dwarflike features) may have hypoplastic tracheas and abnormal airway anatomy similar to that of (dwarflike) miniature horses.

Minimum alveolar concentration (MAC) values for halothane and isoflurane in donkeys are similar to those of horses.[13] The MAC value for sevoflurane has not been determined in donkeys and mules, but clinical experience suggests that the same vaporizer settings should be used. Donkeys and mules are monitored using procedures and techniques identical to those used for horses (see Monitoring Anesthesia).

I have observed several donkeys that experienced severe bradycardia and profound hypotension after induction to general anesthesia with inhalant anesthetics. Anticholinergics and inotropic drugs reversed this process. All of these donkeys had very painful orthopedic conditions (i.e., "three-legged" lame, severe laminitis), which may have produced an exaggerated sympathoadrenal response and may not have been adequately treated with analgesics before surgery because of a failure to recognize pain.

MONITORING ANESTHESIA

Anesthetic monitoring in donkeys and mules is similar to that for horses with some subtle differences. Eye signs (nystagmus, corneal and palpebral reflexes, rotation of the eyeball) are helpful and similar to those in horses, but they are not as reliable in donkeys. Direct or indirect monitoring of arterial blood pressure is strongly recommended; blood pressure increases as the patient gets "light" and is a more reliable indicator of depth of anesthesia than eye signs. When placing an arterial catheter, the (thicker) skin should be perforated with a needle before introducing the catheter to prevent "burring" of the catheter. Branches of the facial artery and the dorsal metatarsal and auricular arteries are good sites for arterial catheter placement.

Treatment of hypotension (defined as a mean arterial pressure less than 60 mm Hg) should be similar to that in horses; the plane of anesthesia should be decreased if possible, intravenous fluids should be increased, and inotrope drugs should be administered until appropriate blood pressure is restored (see Chapter 22). An increase in

hematocrit may not be seen with mild-to-moderate dehydration in donkeys or mules; thus the anesthetist should not rely on packed cell volume as an initial guide for fluid administration.

Respiratory rate and pattern should be observed carefully; normal respiratory rates are greater in donkeys than in horses, but breath holding may occur during a painful procedure. An increase in tidal volume and spontaneous "sighing" are usually suggestive of a very light plane of anesthesia.

Postanesthetic myositis is less likely to occur in donkeys than horses since they have much less muscle mass. Myositis and myopathy can occur in mules, especially Draft Mules. Care should be taken to pad body surfaces and superficial nerves (i.e., facial and radial) appropriately (see Chapter 21).

It is important to ensure that airflow is not compromised in donkeys that are not orotracheally intubated. The head should be positioned to ensure that the airway is not kinked or obstructed by their excessive nasal tissue. Straightening the position of the head relative to the neck or placing a nasal cannula usually relieves inspiratory noise.

RECOVERY FROM ANESTHESIA

Recovery from anesthesia is usually not affected by the occasional hysteria seen in horses because donkeys generally are calmer (see Chapter 21). Analgesia should be provided. Donkeys generally lie quietly until they are able to regain a sternal position and stand; they may make a half attempt to stand and lie back down if not coordinated enough. It is generally not necessary to "hand recover" donkeys. They frequently stand hind-end first (like a cow) or get up on one knee with the hind legs first. Mules are highly variable in their response to recovery and may require assistance with head and tail ropes similar to horses.

ANALGESIA

The analgesics used in horses are appropriate for donkeys and mules; but the dose or dosing interval should be adjusted, and pain should be assessed frequently (see Table 18-1). There are currently no data on the usefulness of transdermal fentanyl (patches) in donkeys or mules. Although fentanyl concentrations are achieved rapidly in horses via the transdermal route, donkeys have thicker skin, which could inhibit fentanyl absorption and produce differences in the rate of absorption from dermal sites (e.g., a thick fascial layer on the neck might prevent absorption). Epidural administration of local anesthetic drugs and other analgesics are very useful in providing anesthesia for procedures of the caudal region or analgesia for postoperative pain (see Chapter 11).[14] No differences between donkeys and mules and horses have been reported using epidural or spinal techniques.

In conclusion, although it is tempting to treat donkeys and mules like horses, there are subtle and at times significant differences in physiology, behavior, and response to anesthetic drugs that must be taken into account to provide successful and minimally stressful anesthesia.

REFERENCES

1. Taylor TS, Matthews NS, Blanchard TL: Introduction to donkeys in the US: elementary assology, *N Engl J Large Anim Health* 1:21-28, 2001.
2. Yousef MR: The burro: a new backyard pet: its physiology and survival, *Calif Vet* 33:31-34, Oct 1979.
3. Watson TDG et al: An investigation of the relationships between body condition and plasma lipid and lipoprotein concentrations in 24 donkeys, *Vet Rec* 127:498-500, 1990.
4. Traub-Dargatz JL : Neonatal isoerythrolysis in mule foals, *J Am Vet Med Assoc* 206:67-70, 1995.
5. Sobti VK, Dhiman N, Singh KI: Ultrasonography of normal palmar metacarpal soft tissues in donkeys, *Indian J Vet Surg* 17:37-38, 1996.
6. Zinkl JG et al: Reference ranges and the influence of age and sex on hematologic and serum biochemical values in donkeys, *Am J Vet Res* 51:408-413, 1990.
7. Mori E et al: Reference values on serum biochemical parameters of Brazilian donkey breed, *J Equine Vet Sci* 23:358-364, 2003.
8. Terkawi A, Tabbaa D, Al-Omari Y: Estimation of normal haematology values of local donkeys in Syria. In *Proceedings of the Fourth Colloquium on Working Equines*, Hama, Syria, 2002, pp 115-118.
9. Hubbell JAE et al: Anesthetic, cardiorespiratory, and metabolic effects of four intravenous anesthetic regimens induced in horses immediately after maximal exercise, *Am J Vet Res* 61:1545-1552, 2000.
10. Matthews NS et al: Pharmacokinetics of ketamine in mules and mammoth asses premedicated with xylazine, *Equine Vet J* 26:241-243, 1994.
11. Matthews NS et al: Pharmacokinetics and pharmacodynamics of guaifenesin in donkeys, *Vet Surg* 25:184, 1996.
12. Matthews NS, Taylor TS, Sullivan JA: A comparison of three combinations of injectable anesthetics in miniature donkeys, *Vet Anaesth Analg* 29:36-42, 2002.
13. Mercer DE, Matthews NS: Minimum alveolar concentrations of halothane and isoflurane in donkeys and MAC-sparing effect of butorphanol. In Proceedings of the Fifteenth PanVet Congress, Campo Grande, Brazil, 1996, p 129.
14. Shoukry M, Seleh M, Fouad K: Epidural anaesthesia in donkeys, *Vet Rec* 97:450-452, 1975.

19

Peripheral Muscle Relaxants

John A.E. Hubbell

William W. Muir

Neuromuscular blocking drugs (NMBDs) are used frequently in human anesthesia to provide laryngeal relaxation for endotracheal intubation and to enhance skeletal muscle relaxation to facilitate surgery. The administration of NMBDs to horses facilitates delicate ophthalmic surgeries (phacoemulsification of cataracts), fracture repair, and ventilation when intraabdominal pressure is high and deep levels of anesthesia are contraindicated because of cardiovascular instability. Relaxation of abdominal muscles is especially useful when a flank incision is used (e.g., for excision of granulosa cell tumors). Neuromuscular blockade also allows better control of horses that are difficult to manage because of unreliable signs of anesthesia. Newer NMBDs with short and predictable durations of action, minimum cumulative effects, and few cardiovascular side effects have been developed. The neuromuscular and cardiovascular responses to several NMBDs have been studied in horses. Inexpensive clinical monitors can be used to adjust dose requirements and ensure that muscle function has recovered before awakening; safety improves when NMBDs are used in conjunction with point-of-care blood gas analyzers.

Regardless of the potential benefits of neuromuscular blockade, the use of NMBDs in horses remains limited to university settings and specialized referral hospitals. The reasons for their limited use are multifactorial. Endotracheal intubation is easily accomplished in the horse even when swallowing reflexes remain intact. Controlled ventilation is accomplished easily in most horses by maintaining the arterial carbon dioxide tension at values below 55 to 60 mm Hg. Monitoring anesthetic depth is more difficult if NMBDs are used: the ability to use eyelid (palpebral) and ocular (corneal) reflex responses is not available because of muscle paralysis. Furthermore, the horse cannot move if it regains consciousness or in response to a noxious stimulus. Of utmost concern is the need for the return of sufficient muscular strength to stand during recovery from anesthesia (see Chapter 21). On balance, the use of NMBDs is likely to remain limited in horses. The barbaric and once widespread use of succinylcholine (depolarizing NMBD) for immobilization and castration of awake horses mercifully has been all but abandoned in favor of safer, more humane methods (see Chapter 12).

PHYSIOLOGY AND PHARMACOLOGY OF THE NEUROMUSCULAR JUNCTION

Normal Neuromuscular Transmission

Motor Nerve Terminal: Acetylcholine Synthesis and Release

The motor nerve terminal is a metabolically active structure containing a high density of mitochondria, membrane ion channels, ionic exchange systems, and cholinergic and adrenergic receptors.[1] An active choline uptake system and the intracellular enzyme choline acetyltransferase provide for acetylcholine synthesis. Some of the synthesized acetylcholine is packaged into small membrane-bound structures referred to as *vesicles*. These vesicles, containing "quanta" of acetylcholine of several thousand molecules each, tend to be concentrated in groups at areas of thickened cell membrane referred to as *active zones* (Figure 19-1). The packages of acetylcholine in the motor nerve terminal represent the *readily releasable fraction*. Calcium ions enter the cell at the peak of the action potential (when the motor end plate is depolarized) either through ion-specific channels or aided by an Na/Ca antiporter system. Calcium entry, which is enhanced by cyclic adenosine monophosphate, results in binding of the acetylcholine-containing vesicles to the cell membrane and acetylcholine release into the synaptic cleft. The release

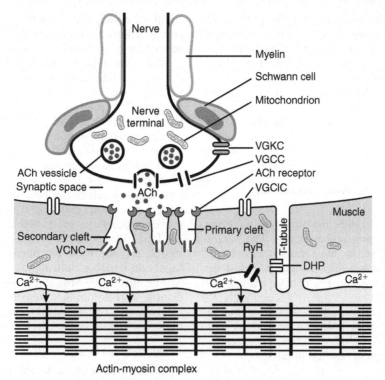

Figure 19–1. Schematic representation of the neuromuscular junction. Aectylcholine *(ACh)* vesicles are shown aggregated near "active zones" in the motor nerve terminal. Across the synaptic cleft, ACh receptors are clustered primarily on crests of synaptic folds in the motor end plate region of the sarcolemma. Voltage-gated *(VG)* potassium (K), sodium (N), chloride (CL), and calcium (C) channels regulate ACh release and transmembrane ionic fluxes. Membrane depolarization initiated by interaction of ACh with ACh receptors opens VGNCs, resulting in membrane depolarization and activation of dihydropyridine *(DHP)* receptors in the T tubules and ryanodine receptors *(RyR)* in the sarcoplasmic reticulum. DHP-RyR receptor activation releases large amounts of calcium, which causes muscle contraction (excitation-contraction coupling). (Modified from Dreyer F: Acetylcholine receptor, *Br J Anaesth* 54:115, 1982.)

mechanism is not entirely understood, but it is sensitive to changes in extracellular calcium ion concentration and also affected by the total amount of calcium ion entering the cell. Calcium entry and the release processes are terminated by potassium efflux from the motor nerve as the membrane repolarizes. During sustained neuromuscular activity the additional acetylcholine required for release is mobilized from stores within the motor nerve terminal. Binding of released acetylcholine to cholinergic receptors on the motor nerve terminal may function as a stimulus for this mobilization.

Motor End Plate: Acetylcholine Receptor, Propagation of Action Potential, Activation of Contractile Process

The acetylcholine receptors on the motor end plate are concentrated along the shoulders of the folds defining secondary clefts in the sarcolemma.[1,2] The receptors are made up of five subunit proteins forming a cylinder with a central pore ion channel. Each receptor unit has two sites for acetylcholine binding. Depolarization of the motor end plate occurs when both receptors bind acetylcholine, causing a conformational change in the channel complex, opening it to the inward flow of positive ions (Figure 19-2). Acetylcholinesterase is also closely associated with the postjunctional membrane, both on the folds and in the clefts.

Cholinergic receptors are concentrated at the motor end-plate region of the sarcolemma in normal skeletal muscle.

When the motor end plate is depolarized, the action potential is propagated to voltage-sensitive sodium channels in the adjacent sarcolemma. The wave of depolarization is carried into the interior of the cell by way of the T tubules to the sarcoplasmic reticulum, triggering the release of intracellular calcium, which activates the contractile machinery (see Figure 19-1). Acetylcholine leaves the postjunctional receptor rapidly and is degraded by acetylcholinesterase. The motor end plate subsequently repolarizes, and the contractile process is inactivated.

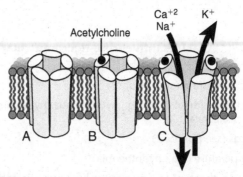

Figure 19–2. Schematic illustration of the relationship of the ACh-receptor complex to the conformational state of the nonspecific cation channel in the motor end-plate membrane. When both acetylcholine receptors bind agonist molecules, the ionophore complex is activated, allowing the flow of positive ions. *A,* Inactive; *B,* binding of one ACh molecule does not activate; *C,* binding of two ACh molecules activates channel. (From Dreyer F: Acetylcholine receptor, *Br J Anaesth* 54:115, 1982.)

Voluntary motion results when brief volleys of nerve action potentials reach the motor nerve terminal and acetylcholine is released in successive bursts, first from the readily releasable fraction and then from the mobilizable store. There is a very large margin of safety in normal animals in both the quantity of acetylcholine available for release and the number of acetylcholine receptors on the motor end plate; the number of receptors is far in excess of that required for depolarization of the end plate. Therefore depolarization of a nerve invariably results in contraction of all of the fibers in the motor unit, with acetylcholine and receptors to spare.

Pathological Alterations to Neuromuscular Transmission

Neuromuscular transmission can be impaired by alterations at a number of steps in the previous processes. The horse's breed, age, sex, nutritional status, liver and renal function, serum potassium concentration, blood glucose, acid-base status, and body temperature and the concurrent administration of NMBD-potentiating drugs (e.g., aminoglycoside antibiotics) must be considered before administering NMBDs (Box 19-1). Several pathological conditions that produce myasthenic syndromes in horses can potentiate the effects and duration of action of NMBDs in horses.

Channelopathies

Various ion cellular membrane channelopathies are responsible for a variety of neuromuscular diseases in humans that can intensify and prolong the effects of NMBDs, including hyperkalemic periodic paralysis (HYPP; voltage-gated Na^+ channel) and malignant hyperthermia (ligand-gated Ca^{+2} channel). Mutant Na^+ channels result in sustained Na^+ currents and prolonged membrane depolarization that can be exaggerated by NMBDs (see preceding paragraph). HYPP is an inherited autosomal-codominant genetic disease of Quarter Horses.[2-4] Potassium efflux from muscle results in a reduction of the transmembrane gradient, lowering the membrane resting potential. When the resting potential is sufficiently lowered, an action potential cannot be propagated, and muscle contraction is not initiated. An episode of HYPP could occur at any point during anesthesia but is most common during induction or recovery from anesthesia. Clinical attacks are precipitated by stress; are recurrent; and are characterized by muscle fasciculation and spasm, drooling, prolapse of

---

Box 19–1 Factors Influencing Neuromuscular Transmission

- Acid-base state (e.g., acidosis)
- Electrolyte imbalance (e.g., hypokalemia, hyperkalemia, hypocalcemia)
- Drugs (see Box 19-2)
- Temperature (e.g., hypothermia)
- Muscle diseases (e.g., myopathy, hyperkalemic periodic paralysis)
- Neurological diseases (e.g., equine protozoal myelitis, cervical vertebral instability)
- Liver/renal function

---

the third eyelid, and respiratory stridor. The cardiovascular complications of HYPP (bradycardia, cardiac arrest) require immediate treatment (see Chapter 22).

Malignant hyperthermia is a myopathy that features acute abnormal cellular calcium cycling. The loss of control leads to hypermetabolism, excessive continual muscle contraction, and the generation of heat. Succinylcholine and halothane anesthesia are well-documented triggering drugs for malignant hyperthermia in humans and swine. There are case reports of malignant hyperthermia-like reactions in anesthetized horses administered succinylcholine.[5-7] Postanesthetic clinical myopathy and/or massive elevation in serum creatinine kinase levels occur. Four of six halothane-anesthetized ponies given succinylcholine became hyperthermic, with muscle rigidity and protracted fasciculations seen in two of the four.[8] The ponies survived and showed no evidence of muscle damage in the postoperative period. Such effects are highly undesirable clinically.

The effects of NMBDs in horses with a history of muscle disorders are not known. Regardless, it would seem prudent to avoid the use of NMBDs, especially succinylcholine, in horses with muscle disorders.

Botulinum Toxicosis

Botulinum toxin binds to the motor nerve terminal, preventing the release of acetylcholine.[9] The toxin can be inactivated by antitoxin in the early stages of botulism. After irreversible binding and entry into the motor nerve terminal are completed, the antitoxin is ineffective. Binding of the toxin is use dependent in that it is accelerated by voluntary neuromuscular activity and by drugs such as neostigmine that normally enhance neuromuscular transmission. These drugs temporarily increase muscle strength but may ultimately worsen the condition.

Organophosphate Toxicosis and Other Toxins

Inhibition of cholinesterase by organophosphates results in accumulation of acetylcholine at the neuromuscular junction, initially causing excessive muscle activity (tremors, fasciculations) and later paralysis resulting from desensitization of cholinergic receptors. The presence of organophosphates would appear to have the potential to potentiate NMBDs, but the administration of trichlorfon does not affect the dose requirement or duration of action of atracurium in anesthetized horses.[10] Tetrodotoxin (puffer fish) and saxitoxin (red tide shellfish) specifically block sodium channels in excitable membranes, preventing spread of the action potential in nerve and muscle. Death is from respiratory paralysis.

CLINICAL PHARMACOLOGY OF NEUROMUSCULAR BLOCKING DRUGS

Actions of Neuromuscular Blocking Drugs

All NMBDs are large hydrophilic molecules containing at least one quaternary ammonium group that mimics the receptor binding site for acetylcholine.[11-13] They are categorized into two groups, depolarizing and nondepolarizing drugs (Table 19-1). Nondepolarizing NMBDs (e.g., atracurium) competitively bind to acetylcholine receptor sites, thereby inhibiting membrane depolarization to produce muscle paralysis. Nondepolarizing NMBD effects can be overcome or intensified by increasing or decreasing,

Table 19–1. Dose requirements for neuromuscular blocking agents and facilitatory drugs in horses

Drug	Dose (µg/kg)	Duration (min)	Side effect
Nondepolarizing blocking agents			
Atracurium	50-100 CRI: 0.1 ± 0.4 mg/kg/hr	28	Minimal cardiovascular effects
Pancuronium	82 ± 7.3	20-35	Tachycardia Ventricular arrhythmias Hypertension
Rocuronium[22]	200	45	Slight increases in heart rate and blood pressure
Depolarizing blocking agents			
Succinylcholine	100 CRI: 2200/hr	4-5 (Infusion)	Hyperkalemia Increased intracranial and intraocular pressure Myalgia Cardiac arrhythmia
Facilitatory drugs			
Neostigmine	30-50 Incremental dosing: 15-30, 5 minutes apart		Muscarinic effects: bradycardia, hypotension, salivation, diarrhea Increased airway secretions Increased gastrointestinal motility
Edrophonium	500-1000 slowly (over 60 seconds) Incremental dosing: 250-500, 3 minutes apart		Minimal side effects Increase in arterial blood pressure Treatment with anticholinergic agent not necessary

CRI, Continuous-rate infusion.

the concentration of acetylcholine at the motor end plate. Depolarizing drugs (e.g., succinylcholine) act like the neurotransmitter acetylcholine and produce depolarization of the motor end plate, resulting in muscle fasciculations (i.e., muscle contraction), complete membrane depolarization, and failure of action potential generation.

Nondepolarizing Drugs

Nondepolarizing NMBDs bind to acetylcholine receptors on the motor end plate, blocking access to acetylcholine. This action competitively inhibits the action of acetylcholine, preventing opening of the nonspecific cation channels and thus muscle contraction. Muscle contraction cannot occur, and muscle tone is reduced. Injection of a large dose of a nondepolarizing NMBD causes a progressive loss of strength (*fade*) as the concentration of the drug in muscle increases. Blockade of 70% to 75% of receptors at an individual motor end plate inactivates the contractile process in that fiber because ion flow through the remaining channels generates insufficient current for depolarization. Muscle strength diminishes as more fibers are inactivated until complete paralysis occurs. The action of nondepolarizing NMBDs is *competitive* with acetylcholine. During partial paralysis, increasing the amount of acetylcholine in the synaptic cleft (by inhibiting acetylcholinesterase or repetitively stimulating the motor nerve) partially restores muscular strength. The additional acetylcholine displaces the nondepolarizing NMBDs from some of the receptors.

Nondepolarizing NMBDs also bind to the motor nerve terminal, where they interfere with the mobilization of acetylcholine. The presynaptic effect of blocking drugs is seen during rapid nerve stimulation or voluntary effort in which initial muscle contraction is strong but muscle strength fades as acetylcholine release fails with time.[12]

Depolarizing Drugs: Phase I Block

The mechanism of action of the depolarizing blocking drugs is more complicated and less understood than that of the nondepolarizing drugs.[11,12] Succinylcholine binds to postsynaptic acetylcholine receptors and acts initially as an agonist, opening ion channels and depolarizing the motor end plate. *Muscle fasciculations* precede skeletal muscle paralysis. They first appear on the neck and shoulders of the horse and then progress to the trunk and hind limbs. Fasciculations are the result of uncoordinated contractions of motor units caused by the release of acetylcholine, which in turn is caused by presynaptic stimulation of motor nerves.

Depolarizing NMBD effects depend on their rate of clearance from the synaptic cleft. Sodium channel activity (gating) in the adjacent sarcolemma is both voltage and time dependent.[2] At rest the voltage-dependent gate is closed, and the time-dependent gate is open. The voltage-dependent gate opens in response to the depolarization of the motor end plate, and ion flow continues until the time-dependent gate closes. The time-dependent gate cannot reopen until the voltage-dependent gate repolarizes. Continued presence of depolarizing current (resulting from the presence of depolarizing blockers) at the motor end plate keeps the voltage-dependent gates from closing; thus the perijunctional muscle zone remains insensitive. Therefore phase I of paralysis with depolarizing drugs is the result of persistent depolarization of the motor end plate with inactivation of the adjacent sarcolemma. Clinical doses of succinylcholine are designed to produce only phase I block. Termination of the block depends on the metabolism of succinylcholine and subsequent repolarization of the motor end plate.

Depolarizing Drugs: Phase II Block

The character of blockade changes with time. A very large single dose of succinylcholine, repeated smaller doses, or an infusion causes depolarizing block to become more like nondepolarizing blockade. Phase II block is not completely understood and may involve multiple factors, including ion channel block, desensitization of receptors, and ionic imbalance across the motor nerve terminals and end-plate membranes.[11] Fade occurs with repetitive nerve stimulation during phase II block. Development of phase II block and its reversibility with cholinesterase inhibitors varies with the dose of succinylcholine, duration of exposure, species, muscle groups, type of anesthetic, and the individual patient.

Other Compounds Affecting Neuromuscular Transmission

A variety of toxins and experimental drugs (Tetrodotoxin) are used as pharmacological tools for studying neuromuscular transmission. α-Bungarotoxin and erabutoxin irreversibly block postjunctional (but not prejunctional) acetylcholine receptors.[14] Trimethaphan, decamethonium, and histrionicotoxin block ion channels; and hemicholinium blocks choline uptake and the synthesis of acetylcholine. Vesamicol blocks loading of acetylcholine into vesicles.[15] 4-Aminopyridine causes prolongation of potassium ion reflux, leading to enhanced calcium entry into the motor nerve terminal and increased acetylcholine release.[16]

Many drugs that are used clinically, including antibiotics, antiepileptics (e.g., barbiturates), diuretics (e.g., furosemide), local anesthetics (e.g., lidocaine), calcium channel blockers (e.g., diltiazem), and anesthetics (e.g., isoflurane, sevoflurane, propofol), can interfere with membrane channels (i.e., sodium, calcium) or intracellular biomolecular mechanisms to intensify neuromuscular blockade and prolong muscle weakness (Box 19-2).[2] Aminoglycoside antibiotics, polymyxin B, lincomycin, and tetracyclines potentiate nondepolarizing neuromuscular block. Aminoglycoside antibiotics (e.g., gentamicin) inhibit the prejunctional release of acetylcholine and also depress postjunctional receptor sensitivity to acetylcholine. Tetracyclines (e.g., oxytetracycline) decrease postjunctional receptor sensitivity to acetylcholine. Cephalosporin and potassium-free penicillins have not been reported to affect neuromuscular function. Inhalant and injectable anesthetic drugs can intensify the effects of NMBDs, although this effect depends more on the horse's health (anesthetic risk; see Chapter 6) than on additive or synergistic drug effects. Halothane-anesthetized horses administered atracurium infusions that reduce twitch strengths to 40% of baseline values experience further reductions in twitch strength within 7 minutes of gentamicin administration.[17] Recovery to 75% of twitch strength was longer when gentamicin was

---

Box 19–2 Examples of Drugs That Could Interfere with Neuromuscular Transmission

Volatile and Injectable Anesthetics
- Isoflurane
- Sevoflurane
- Desflurane
- Barbiturates
- Ketamine
- Propofol

Antibiotics
- Polymyxin B
- Gentamicin
- Oxytetracycline

Intravenous Local Anesthetics
- Lidocaine

Ca^{+2} Channel Blockers
- Diltiazem

Diuretics
- Furosemide

---

present, but the differences were not clinically significant. Acetylcholine esterase inhibitors (e.g., edrophonium) and calcium ion may partially antagonize the effects of the antibiotic at the neuromuscular junction.[17]

Other Effects of Neuromuscular Blocking Drugs

Autonomic Effects of Nondepolarizing Drugs

Most NMBDs have the potential to affect autonomic ganglia when administered in excessive doses. The nature and magnitude of clinical effects are variable, depending on the drug and anesthetic technique used. In general, however, cardiovascular effects are minimal when clinical doses of pancuronium, gallamine, metocurine, atracurium, and rocuronium are administered to anesthetized horses.[18-23]

Autonomic Effects of Succinylcholine

Because of its structural similarity to acetylcholine, succinylcholine depolarizes autonomic ganglia and postganglionic parasympathetic cholinergic receptors. Succinylcholine has a dual effect on the isolated heart as in skeletal muscle. Negative inotropic and chronotropic effects are observed after the administration of low concentrations of succinylcholine (similar to those seen with acetylcholine), whereas positive effects are observed after the administration of high concentrations or after prolonged exposure.[24] The cardiovascular effects of clinical doses of succinylcholine usually produce an increase in blood pressure and transient increases in heart rate in halothane-anesthetized horses.[24,25] Increases in heart rate and arterial blood pressure are less pronounced during controlled ventilation than during spontaneous ventilation. Injection of succinylcholine can result in a period of apnea lasting for 2 to 4 minutes and occasionally is accompanied by bradycardia, wandering pacemaker, and sinus arrest (baroreceptor reflex response to hypertension) in spontaneously breathing anesthetized horses.[25,26]

Marked hypertension (systolic arterial blood pressures over 400 mm Hg) and tachycardia accompanied by ventricular extrasystoles occur after succinylcholine administration in awake or thiopental-anesthetized horses.[26-28] In awake horses these effects are partly the result of the depolarizing action of succinylcholine at sympathetic ganglia, hypoxemia, and hypercarbia; but they are more likely the result of extreme stress associated with muscle paralysis and an inability to remain standing, ventilate, or move. Death has occurred immediately after the administration of succinylcholine and also after recovery from immobilization. Cardiovascular damage has been suggested as a contributing factor.[26]

Histamine Release

d-Tubocurarine and mivacurium can cause histamine release in people. The effect is rarely clinically significant and is clinically irrelevant when atracurium or rocuronium is administered to horses.[2,29] Clinical manifestations of histamine release have not been reported in horses given NMBDs.

Potassium Release

Succinylcholine infusion can result in mild-to-moderate elevations in serum potassium levels in normal horses.[13,24,30] No clinical effects of hyperkalemia were reported. Succinylcholine aggravates potassium release (occasionally leading to cardiovascular arrest) in human patients suffering from burns, crush injuries, spinal cord and peripheral nerve injuries, and some neuromuscular diseases.

Effects on Intraocular Pressure

Extraocular muscles are tonic in nature and multiply innervated. Contractions of the extraocular muscles may be prolonged following succinylcholine administration. A transient increase in intraocular pressure occurs after succinylcholine injection in anesthetized humans and horses.[30] The increase in pressure is generally of minimal clinical relevance in the normal eye but may be dangerous in horses with a corneal laceration or otherwise compromised globe. This potentially devastating complication has not been reported in the horse, but succinylcholine should be avoided in horses with unstable eye injuries. Nondepolarizing blocking drugs do not increase intraocular pressure.

Myalgia and Myoglobinuria

Complaints of muscle pain in humans after succinylcholine administration are common.[2] The relation between the incidence and severity of postoperative myalgia is controversial. It is not known whether horses experience myalgia. Massive myoglobin release has been reported after succinylcholine administration to human patients with clinical or subclinical myopathy. Myoglobinuria did not occur in normal halothane-anesthetized horses given succinylcholine nor were plasma muscle enzyme concentrations increased compared to horses not given succinylcholine.[31]

Central Nervous System Effects and Placental Transfer of Neuromuscular Blocking Drugs

NMBDs are highly hydrophilic; however, small amounts may cross the blood-brain and placenta barriers in low concentrations. Pancuronium administration decreases halothane requirements in humans.[32] The reduction may be the result of reduced central nervous system (CNS) stimulation from muscle spindle afferents during paralysis rather than a direct effect on the CNS. Other studies have shown no effect by nondepolarizing relaxants on the CNS.[33] Halothane-anesthetized dogs given five times the 100% neuromuscular blocking dose of atracurium have shown evidence of arousal on an electroencephalogram, the cause of which was attributed to laudanosine.[33]

Doses of pancuronium, d-tubocurarine, gallamine, and succinylcholine far in excess of those causing 100% blockade in pregnant cats and ferrets produce minimum effect on the fetus.[34] Placental transfer of pancuronium and atracurium can be demonstrated in humans, but blood concentrations are low and not clinically relevant.[35,36] Placental transfer of NMBDs has not been studied in horses. Normal clinical doses of atracurium to pregnant mares do not produce clinical effects in the fetus (authors' experience).

Protein Binding, Metabolism, and Excretion of Neuromuscular Blocking Drugs

Nondepolarizing Drugs

All the nondepolarizing drugs except pancuronium have been shown to bind significantly to plasma proteins.[2] Theoretically, disease conditions altering plasma protein binding (liver and renal dysfunction) would be expected to alter the bioavailability of NMBDs, but the effect is likely to be unpredictable.

Atracurium is the most commonly used nondepolarizing blocking drug in horses.[37-39] It has two proposed pathways for elimination, which do not involve renal or hepatic mechanisms. Thus the elimination of atracurium is unaltered in renal and hepatic failure. It is hydrolyzed by nonspecific plasma esterases, is unstable at physiological pH and temperature, and undergoes spontaneous degradation (Hoffman elimination) on injection.[2] Atracurium produces dose-dependent neuromuscular blockade when administered to anesthetized horses; it is noncumulative; and neuromuscular blockade is not prolonged in horses with impaired pseudocholinesterase activity.

Gallamine and metocurine are excreted almost entirely by the kidneys; thus their effects are longer lasting and unpredictable in patients with renal failure. The effects of gallamine may persist for 2 to 3 hours in healthy halothane-anesthetized horses because of reduced renal blood flow and clearance during anesthesia.[40] The kidney is also the major organ of elimination for pancuronium and its metabolites, and the effects may be prolonged in horses with renal failure.[2,41] d-Tubocurarine and vecuronium are not commonly used to produce neuromuscular blockade in horses.

Depolarizing Drugs

Succinylcholine is a depolarizing NMBD. Its duration of action is highly dependent on the concentration of plasma cholinesterase (pseudocholinesterase) and therefore liver function.[13] Much of the injected dose is hydrolyzed before it reaches the neuromuscular junction. Normal horses administered a single paralyzing dose of succinylcholine fully recover neuromuscular function in 5 to 15 minutes (see Table 19-1). Respiratory paralysis persists for 30 to 120 seconds. Pseudocholinesterase activity is lower for several weeks in horses and ponies administered anthelmintic doses of organophosphate compounds, thereby intensifying and prolonging succinylcholine effects. The prolongation of effect is of clinical significance: death could result if mechanical ventilation is unavailable. The risks of unpredictable, and at times prolonged, paralysis increase in intraocular pressure; the potential for hyperthermia, electrolyte, and acid-based disturbances markedly detracts from the clinical use of succinylcholine as an NMBD in horses.

PHYSIOLOGICAL ALTERATIONS AFFECTING NEUROMUSCULAR BLOCKADE

Exercise, Temperature, and Acid-Base Balance

Most reports of clinically relevant alterations of body temperature and acid-base and electrolyte concentrations on the intensity of neuromuscular blockade are highly variable and inconclusive. Exercise does not alter the responsiveness of horses to the nondepolarizing NMBD metocurine.[20] Hypercarbia (arterial partial pressures of carbon dioxide in excess of 50 mm Hg) may impede reversal of nondepolarizing blockade. Positive-pressure ventilation should be maintained until adequate reversal is achieved.

Electrolyte Disturbances

Magnesium

Excessive plasma magnesium concentrations decrease the release of acetylcholine from the motor nerve terminal and the sensitivity of postjunctional cholinergic receptors to acetylcholine. Muscle contractility is also depressed. Intravenously administered magnesium salts cause clinical muscle relaxation. If exceptionally large doses of magnesium-containing cathartics are administered orally, significant increases in blood levels may occur.

Calcium

Acetylcholine release is impaired during hypocalcemia. Overall muscle weakness may be present, but tremors and tetanic spasms occur because the threshold for nerve and muscle membrane depolarization is lowered. Administration of calcium salts partially antagonizes nondepolarizing blockade and blockade caused by aminoglycoside antibiotics or magnesium.[2]

Potassium

Results of in vitro studies suggest that acute elevations in extracellular potassium can partially antagonize nondepolarizing blockade, whereas acute hypokalemia potentiates blockade. The effect of potassium alterations on neuromuscular blockade in chronic disease states is unpredictable.

REVERSAL OF NONDEPOLARIZING BLOCKADE

The binding of nondepolarizing blocking drugs to the motor end-plate receptor is competitive with acetylcholine. Increasing the concentration of acetylcholine in the synaptic cleft favors its interaction with the receptor, displacing the nondepolarizing NMBD drug and restoring neuromuscular function.[2]

Mechanism of Action of Drugs That Facilitate Neuromuscular Junction Function

The acetylcholine released into the synaptic cleft is rapidly hydrolyzed by acetylcholinesterase and resorbed into the presynaptic nerve terminal; thus its presence at the motor end plate is fleeting. Edrophonium, neostigmine, and pyridostigmine are drugs that inhibit acetylcholinesterase, antagonizing the effects of nondepolarizing blockade.[42] Edrophonium forms only electrostatic and hydrogen bonds to acetylcholinesterase; whereas neostigmine and pyridostigmine are hydrolyzed by the enzyme, leaving a carbamyl group attached. Edrophonium is shorter acting but is as effective as neostigmine and pyridostigmine.

4-Aminopyridine antagonizes nondepolarizing NMBDs.[43] It acts presynaptically to decrease potassium efflux during depolarization of the motor nerve terminal, prolonging the action potential and enhancing calcium entry into the presynaptic nerve terminal. Although 4-aminopyridine has been shown to act synergistically with cholinesterase inhibitors to antagonize nondepolarizing and antibiotic-induced neuromuscular blockade, it has not been marketed for clinical use. 4-Aminopyridine produces significant dose-related peripheral and central nervous excitatory effects when given to awake animals and humans.[43]

Autonomic Effects of the Facilitory Drugs

The cholinesterase inhibitors have effects at autonomic muscarinic cholinergic sites. Vagal effects predominate, and pronounced bradycardia can occur if an anticholinergic drug (e.g., atropine, glycopyrrolate) is not administered before reversal of neuromuscular blockade. Neostigmine administered in incremental doses of 10 to 20 µg/kg 7 minutes apart has little or no effect on heart rate and blood pressure in halothane-anesthetized horses, but airway secretions and gastrointestinal motility are increased unless an anticholinergic drug has been administered.[41,42] Edrophonium administration, 0.5 to 1 mg/kg intravenously, is frequently followed by an increase in arterial blood pressure.[41]

MONITORING NEUROMUSCULAR BLOCKADE

Methods for determining when sufficient neuromuscular blockade has been attained to accomplish the intended surgical procedure, when additional NMBD is required, when sufficient neuromuscular function has returned to support adequate breathing, and when enough muscle strength has returned for the horse to stand are currently based on the use of a nerve stimulator and clinical signs.[2,40,42,44]

Quantitative Techniques

Neuromuscular function can be monitored mechanically or electrically. Both methods involve electrical stimulation of a peripheral nerve and evaluation of the evoked muscle response. Experimentally, mechanical responses are measured with a force displacement transducer or strain gauge. Immobilization of the limb is required for determination of measured isometric tension. Electrical monitoring involves measurement of the evoked muscle compound action potential using electrodes placed over a motor end point. Systems for measuring isometric-evoked hind limb twitch tension in horses have been described, but the equipment is too cumbersome for routine clinical use.[42] A simpler system has been used for monitoring lip twitch response in horses.[44] The advantage of monitoring the compound muscle action potential in the equine is that the cumbersome apparatus for immobilizing the limb and measuring and recording tension are not necessary for obtaining quantitative information. Adhesive skin electrodes are used for stimulation and recording. The electrical response correlates reasonably well with mechanical twitch, although it underestimates the degree of relaxation and thus residual relaxation may be undetected.[44]

Clinical Monitoring: Estimation of Mechanical Responses

Mechanical responses to nerve stimulation are usually estimated in the clinical setting by observation (Figure 19-3). Assessment of the degree of neuromuscular blockade depends on the ability of the technique to demonstrate neuromuscular blockade and the ability of the operator to recognize it.

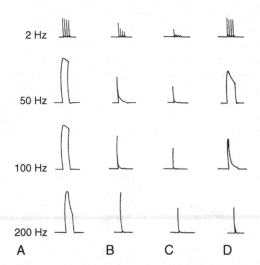

Figure 19–3. Mechanical responses to electrical stimulation of the peroneal nerve at various frequencies in a halothane-anesthetized horse. **A**, Before neuromuscular blockade, tension is well maintained at stimulus frequencies up to 100 Hz. **B**, Partial blockade with pancuronium, twitch tension (first response at 2 Hz) is depressed 25% compared with **A** and fade (decreasing magnitude of the mechanical response) is obvious at 2 Hz. At tetanic frequencies, initial evoked tension is depressed and fade is marked. **C**, An additional dose of pancuronium causes twitch depression of about 60% during 2-Hz stimulation; third and fourth responses are barely visible. **D**, Partial recovery. Twitch tension and 2-Hz responses are normal, but fade is still present during tetanic stimulation. (From Klein L: Neuromuscular blocking agents in equine anesthesia, *Vet Clin North Am (Large Anim Pract)* 3:136, 1981.)

Muscle Sensitivity to Blocking Drugs

Muscles of the trunk generally are more resistant to NMBDs than are limb muscles. The facial muscles in the horse are more resistant to blocking drugs than the limb muscles.[19,42] If the facial nerve is used to monitor neuromuscular blockade, the degree of blockade of the limbs may be underestimated, leading to administration of excessive doses of the NMBD. In addition, residual blockade and resistance to the effects of nondepolarizing NMBDs may be undetected. Residual neuromuscular blockade and resistance to the effects of NMBDs have not been investigated adequately in horses.

Responses to Nerve Stimulation

Absence of a twitch response to a single nerve stimulus obviously indicates 100% blockade of neuromuscular transmission. Maintaining 100% blockade by repeated injections of nondepolarizing blocking drugs may result in prolonged action and incomplete reversal; therefore complete paralysis should be avoided. Seventy-five to 85% neuromuscular blockade is usually sufficient for most surgical procedures, but quantification of the degree of partial blockade by observation or palpation of a single twitch is difficult. A baseline (unblocked) twitch is necessary for comparison, and subtle differences may not be detectable. During recovery and reversal from nondepolarizing blockade, the single twitch response (stimulus delivered at a frequency of 0.1 Hz or less) is normal even when measured quantitatively. Significant clinical impairment of neuromuscular function can exist when no blockade is detectable using single twitch techniques (see Figure 19-3).

The train-of-four (T4) response to electrical stimulation is a sensitive indicator of the adequacy of skeletal muscle function and clinical relaxation. Four electrical pulses are delivered (2 Hz), and the resulting muscle contractions are observed. Four muscle contractions are produced in the absence of blockade. Fade in the T4 response is typical of effects produced by nondepolarizing NMBDs and becomes more pronounced with increasing blockade (Figure 19-4). The disappearance of the fourth and third responses during T4 stimulation correlates reasonably well with 75% to 85%

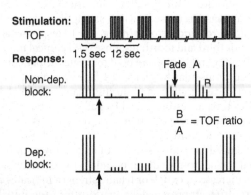

Figure 19–4. Relation between percent twitch depression, train-of-four fade ratio (tension of fourth response divided by first response during 2-Hz stimulation; *B/A = TOF ratio*), and train-of-four count (number of responses visible after four stimuli at 2 Hz) *(top, middle)*. Schematic representation of responses to train-of-four stimulation of 2 Hz during nondepolarizing blockade *(middle)* and during phase I depolarizing blockade *(bottom)*. (Modified from Klein L: Neuromuscular blocking agents. In Short CE, editor: *Principles and practice of veterinary anesthesia*, Baltimore, 1987, Williams & Wilkins.)

twitch depression (see Figure 19-4). The T4 fade increases for all drugs with time.[40]

Restoration of a T4 fade ratio (tension of the fourth response compared to that of the first response) of 70% or greater correlates well with the adequate return of clinical neuromuscular function during recovery in humans. Unfortunately, detection of differences in the strength of contraction can be difficult. Thus T4 responses are useful for maintaining blockade but may be misleading when judging recovery.[42] During phase I block with succinylcholine, T4 response is flat, with fade occurring if phase II block ensues.

Slight degrees of fade during tetanic stimulation, in contrast to T4 stimulation, are easily detected by observation and palpation. The higher the rate of stimulation, the more sensitive is the response to partial blockade (see Figure 19-3). Significant fade may still be present at 100 Hz during antagonism when a sustained response to 50 Hz stimulation has been achieved. Some but not all of this fade can be eliminated by the administration of NMBD antagonists.

Suggestions for monitoring neuromuscular blockade in anesthetized horses

Sites and stimulation rates. Responses to nerve stimulation should be obtained before administering the NMBD to ensure that a nerve can be located, the stimulator is functioning properly, and the response can be observed for later comparison. The peroneal and facial nerves are located superficially in horses and can be found easily by palpation. The peroneal nerve is preferred because it more accurately reflects the function of the trunk muscles. The peroneal nerve can be identified by locating the midpoint of the patellar ligaments and moving laterally along the lateral edge of the tibial plateau until the head of the fibula is felt (Figure 19-5). Moving the fingers distal along the fibula of the adult horse will detect the peroneal nerve approximately 8 to 10 cm from the proximal end. The facial nerve is easily palpated just ventral to the eye (Figure 19-6). A stimulator with 2-, 50-, and 100-Hz capabilities should be available. The negative electrode is placed directly over the nerve, and the positive electrode is placed a few centimeters proximal to the negative electrode. The stimulus strength should be increased beyond the point at which no further increase in muscle twitch strength is detected.

Monitoring criteria: peroneal nerve. The T4 response (absence of fourth or third and fourth response) and clinical impression of the degree of relaxation are used to titrate the patient to adequate neuromuscular blockade. T4 fade does not occur during onset of vecuronium and during phase I succinylcholine blockade; thus an estimate of blockade must be made from twitch or tetanic strength when using these drugs.[40] The reappearance of the third or fourth twitch is used as an indicator of the need for administration of an additional dose of the NMBD if the neuromuscular blockade is to be maintained. An obvious increase in twitch or tetanic strength indicates a need for more drug. Approximately one fourth of the initial dose or an infusion of the NMBD can be administered. An infusion could also be used to maintain succinylcholine block.[24,31]

Pharmacological antagonism of nondepolarizing neuromuscular blockade should not be attempted if 100% paralysis persists. Pharmacological antagonism is most effective if partial spontaneous recovery has occurred, as evidenced by the presence of all four responses to T4. Responses should be

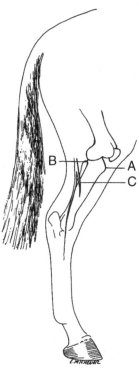

Figure 19–5. Subcutaneous location of the peroneal nerve in the horse. **A**, Tibial tuberosity. **B**, Head of fibula. **C**, Motor branch of peroneal nerve to digital extensor muscles, which can be palpated as it crosses the shaft of the fibula. (From Klein L: Neuromuscular blocking agents in equine anesthesia, *Vet Clin North Am (Large Anim Pract)* 3:136, 1981.)

observed to 5-second tetanic stimulation at 50 Hz repeated at 3- and 5-minute intervals after administration of edrophonium or neostigmine. Fade is estimated at 100 Hz when tetanus is sustained at 50 Hz and additional reversal drugs are given until no further improvement occurs.

Monitoring criteria: facial nerve. Differential monitoring criteria must be used if the facial nerve is stimulated. The facial muscles are resistant to neuromuscular blockade, and fade develops very slowly after drug administration. An obvious decrease in initial tetanic tension usually can be detected

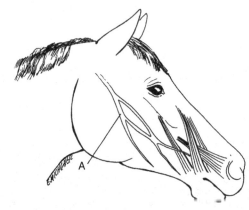

Figure 19–6. Subcutaneous location of the facial nerve in the horse. The active electrode should be placed approximately at the level of the lateral canthus of the eye *(A)* to avoid direct muscle stimulation. (From Klein L: Neuromuscular blocking agents in equine anesthesia, *Vet Clin North Am (Large Anim Pract)* 3:136, 1981.)

during onset of neuromuscular blockade. This parameter, along with clinical criteria (e.g., weakening of spontaneous limb movement, relaxation of abdominal muscles), can be used to detect adequate neuromuscular blockade. Nearly complete elimination of fade during 100-Hz stimulation of the facial nerve is usually possible during reversal.

Clinical Evaluation of Muscle Strength

Inspiratory effort (force) can be estimated by occluding the neck of the rebreathing bag and observing the pressure gauge on the anesthetic breathing circuit during spontaneous respiratory effort. A lightly anesthetized horse should be able to generate at least 15 cm H_2O negative pressure during inspiration. Alternatively, the endotracheal tube can be occluded, and intercostal and diaphragmatic function can be estimated subjectively during a voluntary effort.

The horse is observed in recovery for signs of muscle weakness: inability to keep the eyelids closed tightly, inability to hold the head up, and muscle fasciculations during attempts to stand. Additional facilitory drugs should be administered if weakness is thought to be caused by residual nondepolarizing blockade. The patient's history and condition should be assessed carefully for other causes of weakness when postanesthetic weakness is present despite appropriate doses of antagonists (1 mg/kg of edrophonium or 50 μg/kg of neostigmine). Excessive antagonist dosage can result in depolarizing blockade.[45]

ADMINISTRATION OF NEUROMUSCULAR BLOCKING DRUGS TO ANESTHETIZED HORSES

Positive-pressure ventilation should always be available and initiated before injection of the NMBD (see Chapter 17). Adequate anesthesia (insensibility) should be established because skeletal muscle reflexes are absent. The dose of NMBD should be titrated to effect because there can be marked variation in relaxant requirements among horses. An initial test dose (i.e., approximately 50% of the dose reported to cause 80% to 90% blockade [see Table 19-1]), should be administered, and the response assessed. The effect of each injected dose is nearly maximum at 3 minutes, and the requirements for additional drug can be determined (Figure 19-7). The same technique can be used observing the T4 response to a handheld stimulator, but fade occurs somewhat more slowly than twitch depression. Observations of T4 fade, although not as accurate as tension recordings, are reliable enough for clinical use when nondepolarizing NMBDs are administered.

Atracurium is the most frequently used NMBD in anesthetized horses. It is administered as an intravenous bolus or by infusion.[21,23,37,39] Atracurium (0.05 to 0.1 mg/kg) produces maximum effects within 5 minutes of intravenous administration. Recovery usually occurs within 15 minutes of drug administration. Subsequent doses should be administered at approximately 50% of the original dose. If a longer duration of paralysis is desired, atracurium can be administered by infusion, 0.1 to 0.4 mg/kg/ hour.[37] Muscle strength usually returns within 20 minutes after discontinuation of the infusion. Residual weakness can be antagonized by the administration of neostigmine or edrophonium (see Table 19-1).

ADMINISTRATION OF NEUROMUSCULAR FACILITORY DRUGS TO ANESTHETIZED HORSES

Some degree of spontaneous recovery (i.e., all four twitches present during T4 stimulation or respiratory movements) should be present before pharmacological antagonism is attempted because excessive doses of the antagonists could potentiate neuromuscular blockade (see Table 19-1). Incremental doses of edrophonium (250 to 500 μg/kg) 3 minutes apart or neostigmine (15 to 30 μg/kg) 5 minutes apart can be administered to obtain optimum reversal (see Table 19-1). Atropine (10 to 20 μg/kg intravenously) or glycopyrrolate (5 to 10 μg/kg intravenously) should be given before the first dose of neostigmine if bradycardia, airway secretions, or gastrointestinal hypermotility is a concern. Neuromuscular monitoring should continue until optimum reversal is assured. Although cardiovascular depression from edrophonium and neostigmine given incrementally is rare in the horse, monitoring of the electrocardiogram and arterial blood pressure should be continued during anticholinesterase drug administration (see Chapter 8). Significant bradycardia with hypotension can be treated with atropine or glycopyrrolate. If anticholinergics are not effective, ephedrine (20 to 40 μg/kg), dopamine (1 to 5 μg/kg/min), or epinephrine (6 to 8 μg/kg) should be given intravenously (see Chapter 22).

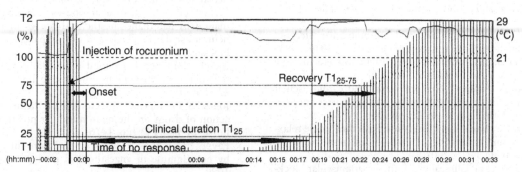

Figure 19–7. Graphic representation of a train-of-four (TOF) stimulation recorded on the memory card of the TOF guard before and after 0.4 mg/kg of rocuronium in a horse illustrating the pharmacodynamic parameters measured. The upper thin line indicates the skin temperature *(scale on left axis)*. The clinical duration of no response and recovery to 25% to 75% of baseline muscle twitch strength are illustrated. (From Auer U, Uray C, Mosing M: Observations on the muscle relaxant rocuronium bromide in the horse—a dose-response study, *Vet Anaesth Analg* 34:75-81, 2007.)

REFERENCES

1. Naguib M et al: Advances in neurobiology of the neuromuscular junction, *Anesthesiology* 96:202-231, 2002.
2. Naguib M, Lien C: Pharmacology of muscle relaxants and their antagonists. In Miller RD, editor: *Miller's anesthesia*, ed 6, Philadelphia, 2005, Elsevier Churchill Livingstone, pp 481-572.
3. Naylor JM: Hyperkalemic periodic paralysis, *Vet Clin North Am (Equine Pract)* 13:129, 1997.
4. Naylor JM et al: Hyperkalemic periodic paralysis in homozygous and heterozygous horses: a co-dominant genetic condition, *Equine Vet J* 31:153-159, 1999.
5. Waldron-Mease E, Klein LV, Rosenberg H: Malignant hyperthermia in a halothane-anesthetized horse, *J Am Vet Med Assoc* 179:896, 1981.
6. Manley SV, Kelly AB, Hodgson D: Malignant hyperthermia-like reactions in three anesthetized horses, *J Am Vet Med Assoc* 183:85, 1983.
7. Riedesel DH, Hildebrand SV: Unusual response following use of succinylcholine in a horse anesthetized with halothane, *J Am Vet Med Assoc* 187:507, 1985.
8. Hildebrand SV, Howitt GA: Succinylcholine infusion associated with hyperthermia in ponies anesthetized with halothane, *Am J Vet Res* 44:2280, 1983.
9. Galey FD: Botulism in the horse, *Vet Clin North Am (Equine Pract)* 17:579, 2001.
10. Hildebrand SV, Hill T, Holland M: The effect of the organophosphate trichlorphon on the neuromuscular blocking activity of atracurium in halothane-anesthetized horses, *J Vet Pharmacol Ther* 12:277, 1989.
11. Bowman WC: *Pharmacology of neuromuscular function*, ed 2, London, 1990, Wright.
12. Bowman WC: Neuromuscular block, *Br J Pharmacol* 147: S277, 2006.
13. Martinez EA: Neuromuscular blocking drugs, *Vet Clin North Am (Equine Pract)* 18:181, 2002.
14. Bowman WC, Marshall IG, Gibb AJ: Is there feedback control of transmitter release at the neuromuscular junction? *Semin Anesth* 3:275, 1984.
15. Prior C, Marshall IG, Parsons SM: The pharmacology of vesamicol: an inhibitor of the vesicular acetylcholine transporter, *Gen Pharmacol* 23:1017, 1992.
16. Saint DA: The effects of 4-aminopyridine and tetraethylammonium on the kinetics of transmitter release at the mammalian neuromuscular synapse, *Can J Physiol Pharmacol* 67:1045, 1989.
17. Hildebrand SV, Hill T: Interaction of gentamycin and atracurium in anaesthetized horse, *Equine Vet J* 26:209, 1994.
18. Klein L et al: Cumulative dose responses to gallamine, pancuronium, and neostigmine in halothane-anesthetized horses: neuromuscular and cardiovascular effects, *Am J Vet Res* 44:786, 1983.
19. Manley SV et al: Cardiovascular and neuromuscular effects of pancuronium bromide in the pony, *Am J Vet Res* 44:1349, 1983.
20. White DA et al: Determination of sensitivity to metocurine in exercised horses, *Am J Vet Res* 53:757, 1992.
21. Hildebrand SV, Arpin D: Neuromuscular and cardiovascular effects of atracurium administered to healthy horses anesthetized with halothane, *Am J Vet Res* 49:1066, 1988.
22. Auer U, Uray C, Mosing M: Observations on the muscle relaxant rocuronium bromide in the horse—a dose-response study, *Vet Anaesth Analg* 34:75, 2007.
23. Hildebrand SV et al: Clinical use of the neuromuscular blocking agents atracurium and pancuronium for equine anesthesia, *J Am Vet Med Assoc* 195:212, 1989.

24. Benson GJ et al: Physiologic effects of succinylcholine chloride in mechanically ventilated horses anesthetized with halothane in oxygen, *Am J Vet Res* 40:1411, 1979.
25. Lees P, Travenor WD: The influence of suxamethonium on cardiovascular and respiratory function in the anesthetized horse, *Br J Pharmacol* 36:116, 1969.
26. Lakskn LH, Loomis LN, Steel JD: Muscular relaxants and cardiovascular damage: with special reference to succinylcholine chloride, *Aust Vet J* 35(6):269-275, 1959.
27. Travenor WD, Lees P: The influence of thiopentone and succinylcholine on cardiovascular and respiratory functions in the horse, *Res Vet Sci* 11:45, 1970.
28. Zinn RS, Gabel AA, Heath RB: Effects of succinylcholine and promazine on the cardiovascular and respiratory systems of horses, *J Am Vet Med Assoc* 157:1495, 1970.
29. Naguib M et al: Histamine-release haemodynamic changes produced by rocuronium, vecuronium, mivacurium, atracurium, and tubocurarine, *Br J Anaesth* 75:588, 1995.
30. Benson GJ et al: Intraocular tension of the horse: effects of succinylcholine and halothane anesthesia, *Am J Vet Res* 42:1831, 1981.
31. Benson GJ et al: Biochemical effects of succinylcholine chloride in mechanically ventilated horses anesthetized with halothane in oxygen, *Am J Vet Res* 41:754, 1980.
32. Forbes AR, Cohen NG, Eger EI: Pancuronium reduces halothane requirement in man, *Anesth Analg* 58:497, 1979.
33. Lanier WL, Milde JH, Michenfelder JD: The cerebral effects of pancuronium and atracurium in halothane-anesthetized dogs, *Anesthesiology* 63:589, 1985.
34. Evans CA, Waud DR: Do maternally administered neuromuscular blocking agents interfere with fetal neuromuscular transmission? *Anesth Analg* 52:548, 1973.
35. Duvaldestin P et al: The placental transfer of pancuronium and its pharmacokinetics during caesarian section, *Acta Anaesth Scand* 22:327, 1978.
36. Flynn PJ, Frank M, Hughes R: Use of atracurium in caesarean section, *Br J Anaesth* 56:599, 1984.
37. Hildebrand SV, Hill T: Effects of atracurium administered by continuous intravenous infusion in halothane-anesthetized horses, *Am J Vet Res* 50:2124, 1989.
38. Aida H et al: Use of sevoflurane for anesthetic management of horses during thoracotomy, *Am J Vet Res* 61:1430, 2000.
39. Senior JM et al: Clinical use of atracurium in horses undergoing ophthalmic surgery, *Vet Anaesth Analg* 28:207, 2001.
40. Klein LV, Hopkins J, Rosenberg H: Different relationship of train-of-four to twitch and tetanus for vecuronium, pancuronium, and gallamine, *Anesthesiology* 59:A275, 1983.
41. Hildebrand SV, Howitt GA: Antagonism of pancuronium neuromuscular blockade in halothane-anesthetized ponies using neostigmine and edrophonium, *Am J Vet Res* 45:2276, 1984.
42. Klein L et al: Mechanical responses to peroneal nerve stimulation in halothane-anesthetized horses in the absence of neuromuscular blockade and during partial nondepolarizing blockage, *Am J Vet Res* 44:783, 1983.
43. Klen L, Hopkins J: Behavioral and cardiorespiratory responses to 4-aminopyridine in healthy awake horses, *Am J Vet Res* 42:1655, 1981.
44. Jones RS, Prentice DE: A technique for the investigation of the action of drugs on the neuromuscular junction in the intact horse, *Br Vet J* 132:226, 1976.
45. Payne JP, Hughes R, Azawi SA: Neuromuscular blockade by neostigmine in anaesthetized man, *Br J Anaesth* 52:69, 1980.

20

Perioperative Pain Management

Phillip Lerche
William W. Muir

The recognition, assessment, and treatment of pain in horses should be an essential goal or objective in every equine practice. Appreciation of the mechanisms responsible for pathological pain in conjunction with focused methods and techniques for recognizing, assessing (subjective, objective) and treating pain continue to evolve, thus improving the horse's quality of life (QOL).[1] Increased education and emphasis on the importance of the negative consequences of pain are reshaping equine veterinarians' attitudes toward the importance of pain to the well-being of horses.[2-4] The primary responsibility of the equine anesthetist has been to produce hypnosis (unconsciousness), muscle relaxation, and analgesia, in the safest way possible. Additional goals are the reduction of stress and the treatment of pain before, during, and after any surgical event (see Chapter 4).

Whether caused by naturally occurring disease (e.g., strain, tissue trauma, infection, gastrointestinal obstruction) or resulting from surgery (e.g., castration, arthroscopy, fracture repair, abdominal surgery), pain can have serious behavioral, physiological, neurohumoral, metabolical, and immunological effects, which are deleterious if left untreated (see Chapter 4). Indeed, if acute pain is not addressed, it may progress to chronic pain, leading to poor performance, weight loss, and increased susceptibility to infection, a disease entity now recognized as "sickness syndrome."[5] Thus it is the obligation of every equine veterinary surgeon to recognize, assess, and alleviate pain throughout anesthesia and in the perioperative period.[2,3]

PHYSIOLOGY OF PAIN

Pain can be defined as "an unpleasant sensory and emotional experience (a perception) that elicits protective motor actions, resulting in learned avoidance, and is capable of modifying species-specific behavior, including social behavior."[3] Thus pain is a complex experience that is different for each animal, which may have evolved as a hierarchal homeostatic system to protect and maintain the integrity of the body.[6] The pain experience comprises detection of tissue injury by the nervous system (*nociception*); conscious perception of pain; behavioral responses or changes; and discomfort, which, if allowed to progress, may ultimately result in extreme suffering.[1,7]

The neurophysiological role of pain is to produce signals that protect the animal from tissue damage. The perception of noxious stimuli is called *nociception*. Nociception consists of five processes: *transduction, transmission, modulation, projection,* and *perception* (Figure 20-1). Noxious stimuli are sensed and transduced into electrical signals by "pain receptors" (nociceptors) and transmitted to the spinal cord by small-diameter, high-threshold A-delta (Aδ) and C sensory nerve fibers.[8] These sensory impulses are modulated (suppressed or amplified) in the dorsal horn of the spinal cord and transmitted (projected) to the brain, where they are perceived and initiate physiological and behavioral responses.

Pain of short duration, in which minimal or no tissue injury occurs, is referred to as *physiological pain*. Acute pain initiates preprogrammed, discrete, and relatively "static" behavioral and neuroendocrine responses characterized by basic stimulus-response patterns. In contrast, *pathological* or *clinical pain* usually results from physical injury to tissues but can be experienced in the absence of a noxious stimulus (*spontaneous pain*), in response to a normally innocuous stimulus (*allodynia*), or as an exaggerated response to a noxious stimulus (*hyperalgesia*). Pathological pain is usually classified on the basis of mechanism, duration (acute [hours], chronic [days, years]), and severity. Unrelenting pain can initiate neurobiological processes that may become dynamic and exaggerate (neuroplasticity) the response of the nervous system (Box 20-1).[9-12]

Inflammation and nerve injury produce similar, tissue-specific activating and sensitizing substances, including but not limited to histamine, serotonin, bradykinin, leukotrienes, prostaglandins, interleukins, neutrophil-chemotactic peptides, nerve growth factors, adenosine triphosphate, substance P (a neuropeptide), H$^+$, and K$^+$.[10] These mediators combine to form a "sensitizing soup," which activates functional and inactive ("silent") nociceptors and lowers the activation threshold of (sensitizes) peripheral nerve endings, leading to *peripheral sensitization* (see Figure 20-1).[1,8,10] *Primary hyperalgesia* is the direct result of peripheral sensitization (see Box 20-1). Furthermore, neurotransmitters and proinflammatory cytokines (tumor necrosis factor, nitrous oxide, interleukin [IL]-1, IL-6, adenosine triphosphate) released by activated peripheral sensory afferents can stimulate glial cells (astrocytes, microglia) in the central nervous system (CNS) (immune-to-brain

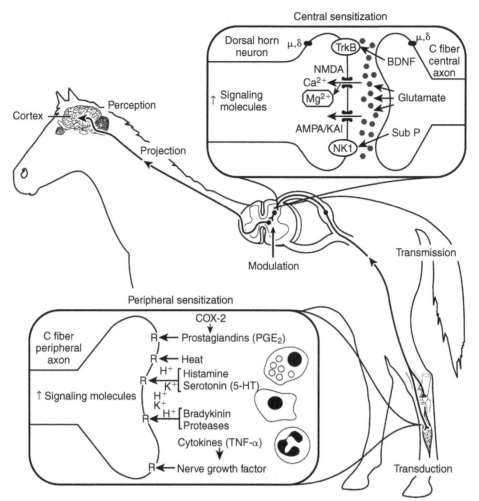

Figure 20–1. Noxious (thermal, mechanical, chemical) stimuli are transduced to electric potentials (action potentials) that are transmitted to the spinal cord, where they are modulated and then projected to the brain (perception). Glutamate is a major excitatory neurotransmitter in the dorsal horn of the spinal cord and normally activates α-amino-3-hydroxy-5-isoxazole propionic acid *(AMPA)* and kainite *(KAI)* receptors. Tissue damage and inflammation lower the threshold of nociceptors and activate "silent" nociceptors, leading to peripheral sensitization and hyperalgesia. Temporal summation of nociceptive input activates *N*-methyl-D-aspartate *(NMDA)* and neurokinin *(NK1)* receptors in the spinal cord, resulting in central sensitization and secondary hyperalgesia. *BDNF*, Brain-derived neurotropic factor; *COX-2*, cyclooxygenase 2; *5-HT*, 5-hydroxy-tryptamine; *Sub P*, substance P; *TNF-α*, tumor necrosis factor α; *TrkB*, tyrosine kinase B. See text for details. (From Muir WW: Pain management. In Reed SM, Bayly WM, Sellon DC, editors: *Equine internal medicine,* ed 3, St Louis, 2010, Saunders.)

Box 20–1	Terms Used to Describe Pain

Pain: Unpleasant sensory or emotional experience associated with actual or potential tissue damage or described in terms of such damage.

1. Noxious stimulus: stimulus (mechanical, chemical, thermal) of sufficient intensity to threaten or overtly cause tissue damage

2. Nociception: the process of pain perception via pain receptors (nociceptors), transmission of noxious (painful) stimuli; includes transduction, transmission, modulation, projection, and perception

3. Peripheral sensitization: increase in the excitability and responsiveness of peripheral nerve terminals

4. Central sensitization: increase in the excitability and responsiveness of neurons in the spinal cord

5. Hyperalgesia: increased response (hypersensitivity) to a noxious stimulus that is normally painful; either at the site of injury (primary) or in surrounding undamaged tissue (secondary)

6. Hyperesthesia: increased sensitivity to stimuli

7. Hyperpathia: a greatly exaggerated pain sensation to painful stimuli

8. Allodynia: pain produced by nonpainful (nonnoxious) stimuli

9. Preemptive analgesia: the prevention or minimization of pain by the administration of analgesics before the production of pain or the introduction of a noxious stimulus (surgery) if pain already exists; the goal of preemptive analgesia is to provide a therapeutic intervention in advance of pain to prevent or minimize the central nervous system response to a noxious stimulus

10. Multimodal therapy: the administration of multiple drugs that act by different mechanisms of action to produce the desired (analgesic) effect

communication), which, in conjunction with repetitive and sustained nociceptive input, are responsible for activation of dorsal horn sensory neurons and temporal summation (*wind up*), respectively.[5,10,11] Wind up involves the activation of dorsal horn N-methyl-D-aspartate (NMDA) and tachykinin receptors and results in *central sensitization* and an exaggerated pain response state that can last for hours to days beyond the initial noxious stimulus (see Figure 20-1). Central sensitization is likely responsible for the hypersensitivity to noxious or harmless stimuli at sites distant from the area of primary injury (*secondary hyperalgesia*).[11]

CONSEQUENCES OF PAIN

Untreated pain causes activation of sympathoneuroadrenal pathways, leading to elevations in cortisol, norepinephrine, and epinephrine and a decrease in insulin (see Chapter 4; Table 20-1). The immediate results are vasoconstriction, increased myocardial work, and increased myocardial oxygen consumption. Blood flow and therefore oxygen delivery to the gut and kidneys decrease, similar to the flight-or-fight response; whereas skeletal muscle blood flow increases. If left unchecked, these sympathoneuroadrenal-hemodynamic changes precipitate a catabolic state, increasing morbidity and mortality. Horses in pain stand at the back of the stall; are uninterested in food; are apprehensive, restless, or unwilling to move; have trouble sleeping or lying down; and are less social. All of these factors and others can be used to suggest an increased level of stress and potentially distress and are indicators of a decrease in QOL.[3] Notably painful or agitated horses generally require higher doses of sedative and anesthetic drugs (see Chapter 21). Increased drug doses put the

horse at risk for increased drug-related side effects and toxicity, leading to higher perioperative morbidity and mortality.

PAIN ASSESSMENT

Pain is a multi-faceted, complex experience that is specific to each animal, although similar and somewhat predictable species-specific indicators and physiological responses are routinely considered when assessing pain in horses (Box 20-2).[13] The owner, trainer, or handler is a useful source of information regarding behavioral changes; and a thorough patient history and physical examination can provide important details that may not be noticed in a hospital environment or stable visit.

There is no single parameter that is considered pathognomonic for pain. The consequences of pain, behavioral and physiological, should be evaluated and used collectively to draw a conclusion (see Box 20-2; Table 20-1).[13] Pain recognition and assessment in horses is challenging and relies on a thorough understanding of normal equine behavior and physiology, with the proviso that a horse may behave differently in the hospital than it does at home.[14-16] Behaviors may be masked in unfamiliar surroundings or in the presence of strangers. Remote cameras or one-way windows (observation or recovery stall) are very useful in assessing equine behavior. Pain responses may be different, depending on breed and age. Draught horses are considered to be more stoic than "hot-blooded" breeds such as Thoroughbreds and Arabians. Young horses and foals generally are more likely to exhibit painful behaviors than mature horses.

Physiological responses may be helpful in detecting pain, although some patients in pain, particularly those with chronic pain, may show little or no change in physiological variables (see Table 20-1).[4,14] For example, increases in heart rate and a reduction in heart rate variability have been associated with acute moderate-to-severe pain (laminitis fracture, colic).[14,17] An experimental study of tarsocrural joint–induced pain in horses demonstrated a positive correlation between a multifactorial composite pain scale (CPS) and noninvasive arterial blood pressure and cortisol.[18]

The assessment for pain-associated behaviors should follow a systematic approach. Distance observation of the horse should be completed first to avoid possible masking of

Table 20–1.	Consequences of untreated pain
Effect	Consequence
Peripheral sensitization	Primary hyperalgesia
Central sensitization	Secondary hyperalgesia Allodynia
Sympathetic stimulation	Tachycardia, tachypnea Peripheral vasoconstriction Increased myocardial work Increased myocardial oxygen consumption Decreased blood flow (oxygen delivery) to abdominal organs
Neuroendocrine	Adrenocorticotropic hormone release ↑ Cortisol ↑ Norepinephrine ↑ Epinephrine ↓ Insulin
Stress	↓ Appetite Insomnia Immunosuppression ↓ Quality of life
Anesthesia	↑ Drug requirement and risk

Box 20–2 Indicators of Pain, Stress, and Well-Being

- Attitude
- Behavior
- Posture
- Activity
- Appearance
- Appetite
- Facial expression
- Interaction with attendants
- Response to handling
- Willingness to perform work

behaviors. Pain-related behaviors include but are not limited to abnormal postures or head movements, decreased locomotion, more time spent at the back of the stall, stomping or pawing the floor, nervousness, apprehension, or depression (Box 20-3).[15,16,18] Indicators of abdominal pain include vocalization, rolling, kicking at the abdomen, and stretching.[16] Distance observation should be followed by silent observation of the horse. The assessment continues with verbal interaction. Horses in pain are unlikely to investigate or interact with a person at the stall and may not respond to the observer's voice.[16,18,19] A common response is for the horse to remain at the back of the stall, ignoring its environment.[15] The final step is to perform a physical examination, which usually begins with a physical stimulus that would not normally initiate a painful response (such as petting or stroking) followed by physical manipulation and more aggressive palpation of the painful area. This may involve manipulation of the head, neck, or limbs in horses. Quantitative sensory testing (QST) using von Frey filaments, hoof testers, and thermal and mechanical stimuli can also help to identify and quantify focal or generalized pain in horses.[20-24]

Pain Assessment Tools

Equine- and disease-specific (orthopedic, colic, laminitis) pain assessment (pain scoring) instruments are developing. A variety of descriptive, categorical, numerical, visual analog, and QST scaling systems have been evaluated and used to quantify pain in horses.[19-26] Most of these instruments require validation and emphasize that observer or evaluator training is essential to obtaining meaningful results.

The simplest types of pain assessment scales are verbal rating and descriptive (Box 20-4). These scales are easy to use, can be completed rapidly, and provide subjective assessment of the horse's pain but are generally not objective (quantitative) enough for assessing subtle changes.[25] The visual analog scale (VAS) provides a semiobjective scoring method for evaluating pain in horses (Figure 20-2). The evaluator places a time-dated mark (typically an X) on a 100-mm line; the extreme left represents no pain, and the extreme right represents the worst pain imaginable. A horse with severe colic that is violently throwing itself down and injuring itself and attendant personnel might be an example at the far right side of a VAS. In addition to its simplicity, the principle advantage of the VAS is its ability to track trends, providing the same evaluator is assessing pain.[25]

Numerical rating scales list parameters in categories with point values associated with each specific criterion for the development of composite pain scales (CPS). No numerical scale can cover every possible pain-associated parameter; thus usually only those criteria with the highest specificity and sensitivity are selected (Table 20-2).[15,16,18] The

Box 20–3	Behavioral Indicators of Pain in Horses

- Restless, agitated, and anxious (acute: moderate/severe)
- Dullness and depression (chronic: moderate)
- Rigid stance and reluctance to move
- Noninteractive; stands at back of stall
- Fixed stare and dilated nostrils
- Aggression towards own foal
- Aggression towards handlers and other horses
- Vocalization (deep groaning, grunting)
- Lowered head carriage
- Rolling
- Kicking at abdomen
- Flank watching
- Stretching
- Weight-shifting between limbs
- Limb guarding
- Abnormal weight distribution
- Pointing, hanging, and rotating limbs
- Abnormal movement
- Arched back
- Headshaking
- Abnormal bit behavior
- Altered eating; anorexia, food pocketing

Box 20–4	Simple Descriptive Pain Scale

- No pain
- Mild pain
- Moderate pain
- Severe pain

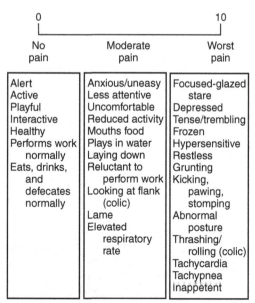

Figure 20–2. The visual analog scale is a simple, practical method for recording and trending the severity of pain and the efficacy of therapy. (From Muir WW: Pain management. In Reed SM, Bayly WM, Sellon DC, editors: *Equine internal medicine*, ed 3, St Louis, 2010, Saunders).

Table 20–2. Multifactorial numerical rating composite pain scale for horses

Parameters	Criteria	Score
Physiological data		
Heart rate	Within 10% of initial value	0
	11%-30% above initial value	1
	31%-50% increase	2
	>50% increase	3
Respiratory rate	Within 10% of initial value	0
	11%-30% above initial value	1
	31%-50% increase	2
	>50% increase	3
Digestive sounds	Normal motility	0
	Decreased motility	1
	Hypomotility	2
	No motility	3
Rectal temperature	Within 0.5° C of initial value	0
	Differs by less than 1° C of initial value	1
	Differs by less than 1.5° C	2
	Differs by less than 2° C	3
Response to observer		
Interaction	Pays attention to humans	0
	Exaggerated response to auditory stimuli	1
	Exaggerated-to-aggressive response to auditory stimuli	2
	Stupor, prostration, no response to auditory stimuli	3
Response to palpation	No reaction	0
	Mild reaction	1
	Resistance to palpation	2
	Violent reaction	3
Behavior		
Demeanor	Bright, lowered head and ears, no reluctance to move	0
	Bright, alert, occasional head movements, no reluctance to move	1
	Restless, pricked-up ears, abnormal facial expression, dilated pupils	2
	Excited, continuous body movement, abnormal facial expression	3
Sweating	None	0
	Damp to the touch	1
	Wet to the touch	2
	Wet to the touch, beads of sweat visible	3
	Excessive sweating, beads of sweat running off the horse	
Kicking at abdomen	Standing quietly, no kicking	0
	Occasional kicking (1-2 times/5 min)	1
	Frequent kicking (3-4 times/5 min)	2
	Excessive kicking (>4 times/5 min), intermittent attempts to lie down and roll	3
Pawing at the floor (limb pointing or hanging)	Quietly standing, no pawing	0
	Occasional pawing (1-2 times/5 min)	1
	Frequent pawing (3-4 times/5 min)	2
	Excessive pawing (>4 times/5 min)	3
Posture (weight distribution, comfort)	Stands quietly, walks normally	0
	Occasional weight shift, slight muscle tremors	1
	Nonweight-bearing, abnormal weight distribution	2
	Prostration, muscle tremors	3
Head movement	No evidence of discomfort, head mostly straight	0
	Intermittent lateral/vertical head movements, occasional flank watching (1-2 times/5 min), lip curling (1-2 times/5 min)	1
	Intermittent and rapid lateral/vertical head movements, frequent flank watching (3-4 times/5 min), lip curling (3-4 times/5 min)	2
	Continuous head movements, excessive flank watching (>4 times/5 min), lip curling (>4 times/5 min)	3
Appetite	Eats hay readily	0
	Hesitates to eat hay	1
	Shows little interest in hay, eats very little or takes hay into mouth but does not chew or swallow	2
	Neither shows interest in nor eats hay	3
Total possible score		39

Adapted from Bussières G et al: Development of a composite orthopaedic pain scale in horses, *Res Vet Sci* 85(2):294-306, 2008.

individual scores are added to provide a total pain score, which is used to direct and evaluate pain therapies. Generally a higher number indicates increased pain and an increased analgesic requirement. Multifactorial numerical rating pain scales for evaluating pain in horses have the potential to provide more sensitive and quantitative methods to evaluate pain, although there is evidence to suggest that pain must be reduced by 25%-50% to be clinically relevant.[27]

Pain scores decrease when analgesic therapy is effective, providing the method of evaluation is sensitive and comprehensive enough to detect change. Use of a CPS that considers the mechanism, origin, and duration of pain helps to evaluate pain and develop treatment plans.[9,28] Pain may be inflammatory, neuropathic, neoplastic, or idiopathic. It can be *somatic* (superficial [e.g., skin] or deep [e.g., bone, tendon, ligament]) or *visceral* (e.g., pleuritis, peritonitis, colic) in origin. It may be acute (minutes, hours) or chronic (days, months). Both somatic and visceral pain may exist at the same time (e.g., chronic osteoarthritis (OA) pain in a horse with acute colic). The location, severity, and duration of pain determine the frequency of evaluation and suggest analgesic therapy. Horses undergoing major surgery (e.g., long bone fracture, colic) may need to be assessed constantly, whereas horses with chronic pain may require much less frequent evaluation. Behaviors that are associated with acute pain generally decrease with effective pain management, and normal behaviors return. These horses generally become more interactive, begin to eat more frequently, rest more comfortably, develop a more normal posture and locomotion, and are more likely to interact with caregivers. It is virtually impossible to remove all pain that an animal is experiencing; the goal is to reduce the pain score and by so doing improve the horse's QOL.[29,30] Improving the horse's QOL is the goal of all pain therapy programs and emphasizes the use of QOL scales in conjunction with CPS to ensure that every horse experiences optimum physical, psychological, and social well-being (Box 20-5).

TREATING PERIOPERATIVE AND OPERATIVE PAIN

Preemptive (preventive) and *multimodal* analgesia are two key therapeutic concepts that have evolved from studies evaluating the efficacy of analgesic therapies (see Box 20-1).[31,32] Multiple mechanisms, receptors, and mediators are involved in the nociceptive process and are responsible for the development of peripheral and central sensitization. Perioperative pain management should begin before surgery. Analgesics can be administered separately (e.g., nonsteroidal antiinflammatory drugs [NSAIDs]) or as a component of premedication (e.g., α_2-adrenoceptor agonists, opioids). Preemptive

analgesia has the benefit of decreasing drug requirements during the maintenance and recovery phases of anesthesia. Horses that are in pain before surgery will be in pain after surgery and should be treated for the anticipated severity of postoperative pain. Horses that are in pain and require nonemergency surgery should receive analgesics as soon as possible (preemptive) after diagnosis to improve their QOL and facilitate the induction, maintenance, and recovery of anesthesia. A multimodal therapeutic plan should be formulated that incorporates drugs directed toward the potential mechanisms responsible for pain.[12] Multimodal therapy generally reduces the dose of each drug used in the drug combination and therefore decreases the likelihood of side effects or toxicity. Many analgesic drug combinations (NSAIDs/opioids; α_2-adrenoceptor agonists/opioids) have additive or supra-additive (synergistic) effects when administered together. When drugs are synergistic, the combination of two or more drugs produces better analgesia and may allow the reduction of the dose, thereby decreasing the potential for side effects to occur. Coadministration of tranquilizers with analgesics can also potentiate analgesia, even if the tranquilizer (e.g., acepromazine) does not possess inherent analgesic efficacy. Preemptive and multimodal analgesia decreases intraoperative anesthetic drug requirements, thereby decreasing anesthetic risk. Postoperative analgesic requirements are likely to be reduced, and the potential for wind up and central sensitization is diminished.

Analgesic Therapies

Numerous approaches have been exploited for the treatment of pain in horses. Analgesic therapies range from pharmacological, nutritional-neutraceutical, and a host of so-called complimentary (e.g., acupuncture, chiropractic, physical, ultrasound, shock wave) therapies. Some of these therapies, most often pharmacological, have been assessed objectively in experimental pain models in conscious and anesthetized horses, but very few have been evaluated in naturally occurring disease.[20-24,33-51] The classes of analgesic drugs that have demonstrated efficacy in the treatment of perioperative pain in horses include NSAIDs, α_2-adrenoceptor agonists, opioids, and local anesthetics. These drugs are administered most frequently as intravenous boluses, intramuscularly, or by mouth but have also been administered by infusion, epidurally or spinally, and topically (Tables 20-3 to 20-5). Other classes of drugs may be useful when used alone or as adjuncts to those mentioned, although their efficacy is questionable and objective evidence to support efficacy remains to be demonstrated. These include dissociative anesthetics, anticonvulsants, and sedatives (see Table 20-3). Because of the severity and more acute nature of perioperative and surgical pain, emphasis here is placed on pharmacological approaches (other than corticosteroids) for pain management in horses.[52]

Nonsteroidal Antiinflammatory Drugs

NSAIDs are relatively weak analgesics; however, they are very effective inhibitors of inflammation, decreasing transduction of noxious stimuli, thereby helping to prevent peripheral sensitization. NSAIDs inhibit the cyclooxygenase (COX) enzyme, which metabolizes arachidonic acid to prostaglandins.[53] Prostaglandins are responsible for a variety of homeostatic (housekeeping) processes, particularly

---

Box 20–5 The Five Freedoms

- Freedom from thirst, hunger, and malnutrition
- Freedom from discomfort
- Freedom from pain, injury, and disease
- Freedom to express normal behavior
- Freedom from fear and distress

Table 20–3. Analgesic drugs administered to horses

Drug	Intravenous dose (mg/kg)	Dosing interval
Antiinflammatory drugs		
Corticosteroids		
Hydrocortisone sodium succinate	1-4	
Dexamethasone isonicotinate	0.015-0.050	
Methylprednisolone	0.1-0.5	
Prednisolone	0.25-1	
Nonsteroidal		
Phenylbutazone	2.2-4.4	sid-bid
Flunixin	1.1	sid-bid
Ketoprofen	2.2	sid-bid
Carprofen	0.5	sid-bid
Opioids		
Butorphanol	0.01-0.04	
Buprenorphine	0.01-0.04	
Morphine	0.05-0.1	
Methadone	0.05-0.1	
Meperidine	0.2-1	
Fentanyl	0.01-0.1	
α_2-Agonists		
Xylazine	0.5-1	
Detomidine	0.03-0.04	
Medetomidine	0.01-0.02	
Romifidine	0.04-0.08	
Neuroleptanalgesics*		
Acepromazine	0.05-1	
Butorphanol or	0.05-0.1	
Buprenorphine	0.005-0.01	
Acepromazine	0.02-0.05	
Xylazine	0.2-0.5	
Butorphanol	0.01-0.05	
Xylazine	0.5-1	
Morphine	0.1-0.5	
Other		
Gabapentin	2-5 mg/kg PO	bid
Tramadol	1-2	bid

*Larger doses of opioids must be administered with α_2-adrenoreceptor agonists (see Chapter 10).
bid, Twice a day; *sid,* once a day.
Note: Alternative α_2-adrenoceptor agonists can be administered.

those that involve the maintenance of normal gastrointestinal, reproductive, renal, and ophthalmological function. There are two important COX iso-enzymes that vary in importance from tissue to tissue (gut, kidney, skeletal muscle, brain). COX-1 is constitutive in most tissues, whereas COX-2 is constitutive in some (kidney, reproductive organs, eye). COX-2 is inducible, particularly when tissue damage and inflammation occur. Inhibition of both COX-1 and particularly COX-2 has been linked to analgesic effects.[54] Most NSAIDs inhibit both COX-1 and COX-2, although the COX-1:COX-2 inhibitory effects of individual NSAIDs vary considerably.[53] Some NSAIDs are believed or known to be more

Table 20–4. Loading doses and infusion rates of analgesic drugs administered to horses

Drug	Loading dose (mg/kg)	Infusion rate (mg/kg/hr)	Side effects
Lidocaine	1.3-2	1.5-3	Muscle fasciculations
Butorphanol	0.01-0.02	0.01-0.02	↓ Fecal piles
Fentanyl	0.002-0.005	0.005-0.01	↑ Locomotor activity
Detomidine	0.005-0.01	0.01-0.03	Ataxia; sedation
Medetomidine	0.005-0.01	0.01-0.03	Ataxia; sedation
Ketamine	100-200	5.0-1.0	Muscle fasciculations, ↑ locomotor activity, apprehension

Table 20–5. Epidural drugs and drug doses administered to horses

	Dosage (mg/kg)	Route	Duration of analgesia
Local anesthetics			
Mepivacaine HCl	0.20	S3-4, S4-5 (CE)	1-1.5 hr
	0.14-0.25	S2-3, S3-4, S4-5 (CE)	1.5-2 hr
Mepivacaine HCl	0.06	S2-3 (CSA)	20-80 min
	0.05-0.08	S2-3 (CSA)	1-1.5 hr
Lidocaine HCl	0.16-0.22	Co1-2 (CE)	30-60 min
	0.22-0.44		1-2.5 hr
	0.45		2-3 hr
Lidocaine HCl	0.28-0.37	S3-4, S4-5 (CE)	1.5-3 hr
α₂-Agonists			
Xylazine	0.03-0.35	Co1-2 (CE)	3-5 hr
Detomidine HCl	0.06	S4-5 (CE)	2-3 hr
Opioids			
Morphine	0.05-0.10	Co1-2 (CE)	8-16 hr
Methadone	0.1	Co1-2 (CE)	2-3 hr
Meperidine	0.8	Co1-2 (CE)	4-6 hr
Dissociative anesthetics			
Ketamine	0.1-2.0	Co1-2 (CE)	30 min-1.5 hr
Combinations			
Lidocaine	0.22	Co1-2 (CE)	5.5 hr
Xylazine	0.17		
Lidocaine	0.25	Co1-2 (CE)	2.5 hr
Butorphanol	0.04		
Morphine	0.20	S1-L6 (CE)	>6 hr
Detomidine	0.03		
Morphine	0.1	Co1-2 (CE)	1.5 hr
Romifidine	0.03-0.06		
Tramadol	1.0	Co1-2 (CE)	12-16 hr
Fentanyl	0.005		
Ketamine	1.0	Co1-2 (CE)	12-18 hr
Morphine	0.1		
Ketamine	1.0	Co1-2 (CE)	2-3 hr
Xylazine	0.5		

CE, Caudal epidural; *CSA,* caudal-sacral epidural.

COX-1 selective (aspirin, phenylbutazone, vedaprofen) in horses. Those that are more COX-2 selective (carprofen, meloxicam, deracoxib) or specific (firocoxib) are less likely to retard intestinal barrier function and produce gastrointestinal ulceration; however, all NSAIDs have the potential to be nephrotoxic.[55-57] Caution is recommended when considering the administration of NSAIDs to horses with coagulopathies or renal, hepatic, or gastrointestinal disease. In addition to their peripheral activity, NSAIDs have also been shown to be active in the CNS.[58] They are commonly used perioperatively in horses to decrease surgery-induced inflammation (phenylbutazone, ketoprofen, flunixin meglumine) or for their beneficial effects in cases of colic-related endotoxemia (flunixin meglumine).[54,55,59] Theoretically, NSAIDs that are more selective for inhibiting COX-2 should be particularly effective for the treatment of pain caused by acute inflammation, and some evidence suggests that the concurrent use of two NSAIDs ("stacking") is more effective than administering one NSAID alone.[60,61] The role of lipoxygenase and lipoxygenase inhibitors in the initiation of inflammation and treatment of pain in horses, respectively, has not been emphasized and requires investigation.

Opioids

Opioids are classified according to the opioid receptor subtype (mu, kappa, delta) they activate and the degree to which they do so. Mu opioid receptor agonists (morphine, fentanyl, meperidine, methadone) are generally considered to produce the most potent analgesic effects but may be more likely to induce unwanted side effects.[62,63] Kappa-agonist/mu-antagonist drugs (butorphanol) may not be as potent for providing analgesia for somatic pain but are considered to be excellent visceral analgesics.[64] Opioid receptors are concentrated in the brain and dorsal horn of the spinal cord but have also been identified in the synovial membranes of horses.[65] Therefore opioid agonist drugs have the potential to inhibit pain perception (brain) and central sensitization (dorsal horn) and produce local analgesic effects (periphery). Aside from providing analgesia and euphoria, opioids (particularly mu-agonists) can produce sympathetic stimulation, ileus, constipation, colic, urinary retention, and CNS stimulation if administered repeatedly in a short period of time.[22,63] Opioid-induced excitement, characterized by sweating, mydriasis, anxiety, and increased locomotor activity (stall pacing), has been observed after single albeit large doses of opioids (see Chapter 10). These side effects can be controlled or prevented by the concurrent administration of sedatives such as acepromazine or α_2-adrenoceptor agonists.[22,63] Unwanted side effects, the requirement for licensure, the potential for opioid abuse, and a relative absence of evidence regarding the production of analgesia in horses with naturally occurring disease have led to considerable controversy regarding the efficacy and clinical use of most opioids in horses, at least when administered as monotherapy.[63,66] For example, fentanyl is a short-acting mu opioid agonist that has been advocated for the treatment of pain in horses and is available as a transdermal drug delivery system, or patch (see Chapters 9, 10).[67-69] However, the drug plasma concentrations of fentanyl required to produce a consistent and clinically efficacious analgesic effect in horses remain speculative and have not been established in horses.[70] Furthermore, reports of opioid-induced hyperalgesia in other species have cast doubt on the clinical efficacy of opioids in horses, at least when administered as monotherapy for pain.[71] Regardless, the administration of butorphanol both intravenously as a bolus and by infusion has been advocated for the treatment of visceral pain (see Table 20-4).[72-74] The combination of sedatives and opioids (or *neuroleptanalgesia*) is known to produce profound clinical analgesic effects, permitting standing surgical procedures to be performed, thereby avoiding the risks inherent to general anesthesia in the horse (see Table 20-3).[74-76] Finally, the coadministration of opioids (morphine, methadone) and ketamine (0.5 to 1 mg/kg/hr) has been demonstrated to enhance analgesic effects and reduce the potential for side effects of opioids in humans.[71] The identification and verification of opioid efficacy in horses with acute or chronic pain requires continued investigation and may be partially achieved by using appropriate dosages, opioid rotation, adding adjunctive medications, or combining opioids with available NMDA-receptor antagonists.

α_2-Adrenoceptor Agonists

α_2-Adrenoceptor agonists (xylazine, detomidine, medetomidine, romifidine) produce sedation, muscle relaxation, and analgesia by activating α_2-adrenoceptors both centrally and in the periphery.[77] The stupor and analgesic effects of α_2-adrenoceptor agonists can be profound; it is for these reasons that they are commonly administered to horses with moderate-to-severe pain and during all phases (induction, maintenance, recovery) of the anesthetic experience (see Chapters 10, 13, and 21). α_2-Adrenoceptor agonists decrease inhalant anesthetic requirements, and their administration by constant-rate infusion has been used as an adjunct to general anesthesia (see Table 20-4; Chapter 13). α_2-Adrenoceptor agonists have a major impact on the cardiovascular system, commonly causing bradyarrhythmias, including second-degree atrioventricular block, initial hypertension, and ultimately hypotension as CNS depression decreases sympathetic output (see Chapter 10).[78] Respiratory depression may occur, which can be exacerbated if the horse's head also droops. Heavy sedation should be induced with care in horses with preexisting upper airway noise because relaxation of the upper airway and pharyngeal muscles, along with congestion of the nares and nasal passages, may lead to respiratory obstruction. Like opioids, α_2-adrenoceptor agonists cause decreased gut motility, which may lead to gas distention and colic during the postoperative period.[79,80] Excessive sedation may lead to severe ataxia. Other side effects include diuresis and in some individual horses unexpected aggression. Frequent administration of α_2-adrenoceptor agonists can mask the clinical signs of pain, suggesting the use of reduced dosages if pain is being used as a determinant for surgery. Yohimbine, tolazoline, and atipamezole are α_2-adrenoceptor antagonists that can be used to reverse the effects of α_2-adrenoceptors (see Chapter 10). α_2-adrenoceptor antagonists are particularly effective for the treatment of postoperative ileus.[80] Excitement is a potential side effect of α_2-adrenoceptor agonist reversal.

Local Anesthetics

Local anesthetics (lidocaine, bupivacaine, mepivacaine, ropivacaine) block sodium channels, thereby decreasing transduction and transmission of nervous impulses both in the periphery and in the spinal cord (see Chapter 11).[81,82] Traditionally, local anesthetics have been administered topically (cornea), locally (nerve block), regionally (paravertebral block, line block), or epidurally; although loss of motor control of the hindquarters in horses is undesirable because of the potential for anxiety or a panic response.[40,41,83] Intravenous infusions of lidocaine can be administered to decrease both visceral and somatic nociception, reduce inhalant anesthetic requirements, and improve postoperative gastrointestinal activity.[84-87] Large intravenous doses (i.e., >2 mg/kg of lidocaine) or rapid infusion of local anesthetics can cause hypotension and bradyarrhythmias in horses and should be avoided (see Chapter 11). Overdose produces CNS toxicity, with symptoms ranging from agitation and ataxia to grand mal seizures.[88]

Other Drugs

Experimental investigations and clinical antidotes continue to identify potential targets and suggestions, respectively, for the pharmacological alleviation of pain in animals. Nontraditional pharmacological therapies, including dissociative anesthetics (ketamine, tiletamine), clonidine, gabapentin, tramadol, and capsaicin, have been investigated in horses.[89-99] Evidence for their efficacy, although rational, is sparse and in some instances (tramadol: poor oral bioavailability) not supported by scientific investigation.[97] Some drugs are known to possess anesthetic or anesthetic-like effects and may be valuable when administered at markedly reduced doses or by infusion. For example, ketamine is known to possess NMDA-receptor antagonist properties that could help to decrease central sensitization, thereby providing analgesia to horses with severe or chronic pain.[90-92] Many of the aforementioned drugs are administered in combination (multimodal analgesia) in an attempt to produce greater analgesic efficacy by inhibiting a wider array of pain-initiating mechanisms (see Chapter 13).[63,69,74-76,99,100]

FUTURE ADVANCEMENTS

Theory often turns into practice long before ample evidence exists supporting the efficacy of a specific therapy. Although new analgesic drugs and complimentary therapies continue to emerge, the efficacy of most for producing analgesia in horses has yet to be verified. The administration of opioids as pain relief in horses provides no better example of this issue.[63] Other than the rampant use of NSAIDs in general equine practice, pain therapy in horses is in its infancy. There is a dearth of evidence-based, blinded, randomized controlled trials (RCTs) in horses with naturally occurring pain; and the ignorance of and general attitudes toward the topic of pain and pain therapy in horses need to be modernized. It is encouraging to witness the publication of research that addresses pain assessment tools and therapies in horses with naturally occurring pain. Hopefully current therapies and future developments in stem cell research and gene therapy will provide effective pain-relieving modalities.[101-103] In the meantime more evidence from clinically relevant RCT investigations is required if pain therapy in horses is going to advance.

References

1. Muir WW, Woolf CJ: Mechanisms of pain and their therapeutic implications, *J Am Vet Med Assoc* 219:1346-1356, 2001.
2. Muir WW: Anesthesia and pain management in horses, *Equine Vet Educ* 19(6):335-340, 1998.
3. Muir WW: Pain and stress. In Gaynor JS, Muir WW, editors: *Handbook of veterinary pain management*, ed 2, St Louis, 2008, Mosby.
4. Price J et al: Pilot epidemiological study of attitudes towards pain in horses, *Vet Rec* 151(19):570-575, 2002.
5. Watkins LR, Maier SF: Immune regulation of the central nervous system functions: form sickness responses to pathological pain, *J Intern Med* 257:139-155, 2005.
6. Craig AD: Interoception: the sense of the physiological condition of the body, *Curr Opin Neurobiol* 13:500-505, 2003.
7. Moberg GP: Problems in defining stress and distress in animals, *J Am Vet Med Assoc* 191(10):1207-1211, 1987.
8. Woolf CJ, Ma Q: Nociceptors—noxious stimulus detectors, *Neuron* 55(3):353-364, 2007.
9. Woolf CJ, Max MB: Mechanism-based pain diagnosis: issues for analgesic drug development, *Anesthesiology* 95(1):241-249, 2001.
10. Woolf CJ, Salter MW: Neuronal plasticity: increasing the gain in pain, *Science* 288:1765, 2000.
11. Woolf CJ: Central sensitization: uncovering the relation between pain and plasticity, *Anesthesiology* 106(4):864-867, 2007.
12. Kehlet H, Woolf CJ: Persistent postsurgical pain: risk factors and prevention, *Lancet* 367:1618-1625, 2006.
13. Anil SS, Anil L, Deen J: Challenges of pain assessment in domestic animals, *J Vet Med Assoc* 220:313-319, 2002.
14. Pritchett LC et al: Identification of potential physiological and behavioral indicators of postoperative pain in horses after exploratory celiotomy for colic, *Appl Anim Behav Sci* 80:31-43, 2003.
15. Price J, Welsh EM, Waran NK: Preliminary evaluation of a behavior-based system for assessment of post-operative pain in horses following arthroscopic surgery, *Vet Anesth Analg* 30:124-137, 2003.
16. Ashley FH, Waterman-Pearson AE, Whay HR: Behavioral assessment of pain in horses and donkeys: application to clinical practice and future studies, *Equine Vet J* 37:565-575, 2005.
17. Rietmann TR et al: The association between heart rate, heart rate variability, endocrine and behavioural pain measures in horses suffering from laminitis, *J Am Vet Med Assoc* 51:218-225, 2004.
18. Bussières G et al: Development of a composite orthopaedic pain scale in horses, *Res Vet Sci* 85:294-306, 2008.
19. Vinuela-Fernandez I et al: Pain mechanisms and their implication for the management of pain in farm and companion animals, *Vet J* 174:227-239, 2007.
20. Rédua MA et al: The preemptive effect of epidural ketamine on wound sensitivity in horses tested by using Von Frey filaments, *Vet Anaesth Analg* 32:30-39, 2005.
21. Owens JG et al: Effects of ketoprofen and phenylbutazone on chronic hoof pain and lameness in the horse, *Equine Vet J* 27:296-300, 1995.
22. Kamerling S: Narcotic analgesics, their detection and pain measurement in the horse: a review, *Equine Vet J* 21:4-12, 1989.
23. Haussler KK, Erb HN: Mechanical nociceptive thresholds in the axial skeleton on horses, *Equine Vet J* 38:70-75, 2006.
24. Haussler KK, Erb HN: Pressure algometry for the detection of induced back pain in horses: a preliminary study, *Equine Vet J* 38:76-81, 2006.
25. Mich PM, Hellyer PW: Objective, categorical methods for assessing pain and analgesia. In Gaynor JS, Muir WW, editors: *Handbook of veterinary pain management*, ed 2, St Louis, 2008, Mosby, pp 78-109.
26. Lerche P, Muir WW: Pain management in horses and cattle. In Gaynor JS, Muir WW, editors: *Handbook of veterinary pain management*, ed 2, St Louis, 2008, Mosby, pp 437-466.
27. Cepeda MS et al: What decline in pain intensity is meaningful to patients with acute pain? *Pain* 105:151-157; 2003.
28. Cooper JJ, Mason GJ: The identification of abnormal behaviour and behavioural problems in stabled horses and their relationship to horse welfare: a comparative review, *Equine Vet J* 27(suppl):5-9, 1998.
29. Wiseman-Orr ML et al: Quality of life issues. In Gaynor JS, Muir WW, editors: *Handbook of veterinary pain management*, ed 2, St Louis, 2008, Mosby, pp 578-587.
30. Rollin BE: Euthanasia and quality of life, *J Am Vet Med Assoc* 228:1014-1016, 2006.
31. Karanikolas M, Swarm RA. Current trends in perioperative pain management. *Anesthesiol Clin North America* 18(3):575-599, 2000.
32. Kissin: Preemptive analgesia at the crossroad, *Anesth Analg* 100:754-756, 2005.
33. Pippi NL, Lumb WV: Objective tests of analgesic drugs in ponies, *Am J Vet Res* 40:1082-1086, 1979.

34. Muir WW, Robertson JT: Visceral analgesia: effects of xylazine, butorphanol, meperidine, and pentazocine in horses, *Am J Vet Res* 42:1523, 1981.

35. Higgins AJ, Lees P: Tissue-cage model for the collection of inflammatory exudates in ponies, *Res Vet Sci* 36:284-289, 1984.

36. Lowe JE, Hilfiger J: Analgesic and sedative effects of detomidine compared to xylazine in a colic model using IV and IM routes of administration, *Acta Vet Scand* 82: 85-95, 1986.

37. Harkins JD et al: Determination of highest no effect dose (HNED) for local anaesthetic responses to procaine, cocaine, bupivacaine, and benzocaine, *Equine Vet J* 28:30-37, 1996.

38. Haussler KK: Chiropractic evaluation and management, *Vet Clin Equine* 15:195-209, 1999.

39. Alvarez CBG et al: Effect of chiropractic manipulations on the kinematics of back and limbs in horses with clinically diagnosed back problems, *Equine Vet J* 40:153-159, 2008.

40. Grosenbaugh DA, Skarda RT, Muir WW: Caudal regional anaesthesia in horses, *Equine Vet Educ* 11:98-105, 1999.

41. Robinson EP, Natalini CC: Epidural anesthesia and analgesia in horses, *Vet Clin North Am (Equine Pract)* 18(1):61-82, 2002.

42. Flemming R: Nontraditional approaches to pain management, *Vet Clin Equine* 18:83-105, 2002.

43. Wolf L: The role of complementary techniques in managing musculoskeletal pain in performance horses, *Vet Clin Equine* 18:107-115, 2002.

44. Spadavecchia C et al: Quantitative assessment of nociception in horses by use of the nociceptive withdrawal reflex evoked by transcutaneous electrical stimulation, *Am J Vet Res* 63:1551-1556, 2002.

45. Spadavecchia C et al: Comparison of nociceptive withdrawal reflexes and recruitment curves between the forelimbs and hind limbs in conscious horses, *Am J Vet Res* 64:700-707, 2003.

46. Skarda RT, Muir WW: Comparison of electroacupuncture and butorphanol on respiratory and cardiovascular effects and rectal pain threshold after controlled rectal distention in mares, *Am J Vet Res* 64:137-144, 2003.

47. Spadavecchia C et al: Investigation of the facilitation of the nociceptive withdrawal reflex evoked by repeated transcutaneous electrical stimulations as a measure of temporal summation in conscious horses, *Am J Vet Res* 64:901-908, 2004.

48. Oku K et al: The minimum infusion rate (MIR) of propofol for total intravenous anesthesia after premedication with xylazine in horses, *J Vet Med Sci* 67:569-575, 2005.

49. Xie H, Colahan P, Oh EA: Evaluation of electroacupuncture treatment of horses with signs of chronic thoracolumbar pain, *J Am Vet Met Assoc* 227:281-286, 2005.

50. Spadavecchia C et al: Effects of butorphanol on the withdrawal reflex using threshold, suprathreshold, and repeated subthreshold electrical stimuli in conscious horses, *Vet Anaesth Analg* 34:48-58, 2007.

51. Sullivan KA, Hill AE, Haussler KK: The effects of chiropractic massage and phenylbutazone on spinal mechanical nociceptive thresholds in horses without clinical signs, *Equine Vet J* 40:14-20, 2008.

52. Harkins JD, Corney JM, Tobin T: Clinical use and characteristics of the corticosteroids, *Vet Clin Equine* 9:543-562, 1993.

53. Lees P et al: Pharmacodynamics and pharmacokinetics of nonsteroidal antiinflammatory drugs in species of veterinary interest, *J Vet Pharmacol Ther* 27(6):479-490, 2004.

54. Raekallio M, Taylor PM, Bennett RC: Preliminary investigations of pain and analgesia assessment in horses administered phenylbutazone or placebo after arthroscopic surgery, *Vet Surg* 26:150-155, 1997.

55. Goodrich LR, Nixon AJ: Medical treatment of osteoarthritis in the horse: a review, *Vet J* 171:51-69, 2006.

56. Tomlinson JE et al: Effects of flunixin meglumine or etodolac treatment on mucosal recovery of equine jejunum after ischemia, *Am J Vet Res* 65:761-769, 2004.

57. MacAllister CG et al: Comparison of adverse effects of phenylbutazone, flunixin meglumine, and ketoprofen in horses, *J Am Vet Med Assoc* 202:71-77, 1993.

58. Samad TA, Sapirstein A, Woolf CJ: Prostanoids and pain: unraveling mechanisms and revealing therapeutic targets, *Trends Mol Med* 8(8):390-396, 2002.

59. Moore JN: Nonsteroidal antiinflammatory drug therapy for endotoxemia—we're doing the right thing, aren't we? *Compendium* 11:741, 1989.

60. Doucet MY et al: Comparison of efficacy and safety of paste formulations of firocoxib and phenylbutazone in horses with naturally occurring osteoarthritis, *J Am Vet Med Assoc* 1;232(1):91-97, 2008.

61. Keegan KG et al: Effectiveness of administration of phenylbutazone alone or concurrent administration of phenylbutazone and flunixin meglumine to alleviate lameness in horses, *Am J Vet Res* 69:167-173, 2008.

62. IUPHAR Receptor Database (Opioid Receptors) 34:10-15, 2007.

63. Bennett RC, Steffey EP: Use of opioids for pain and anesthetic management in horses, *Vet Clin Equine* 18:47-60, 2002.

64. Muir WW, Robertson JT: Visceral analgesia: effects of xylazine, butorphanol, meperidine, and pentazocine in horses, *Am J Vet Res* 42:1523, 1981.

65. Sheehy JG et al: Evaluation of opioid receptors in synovial membranes of horses, *Am J Vet Res* 62:1408-1412, 2001.

66. Bennett RC et al: Influence of morphine sulfate on the halothane sparing effect of xylazine hydrochloride in horses, *Am J Vet Res* 65(4):519-526, 2004.

67. Maxwell LK et al: Pharmacokinetics of fentanyl following intravenous and transdermal administration in horses, *Equine Vet J* 35:484-490; 2003.

68. Thomasy SM et al: Transdermal fentanyl combined with nonsteroidal antiinflammatory drugs for analgesia in horses, *J Vet Intern Med* 18:550-554, 2004.

69. Orsini JA et al: Pharmacokinetics of fentanyl delivered transdermally in healthy adult horses—variability among horses and its clinical implications, *J Vet Pharamcol Ther* 29: 539-546, 2006.

70. Sanchez LC et al: Effect of fentanyl on visceral and somatic nociception in conscious horses, *J Vet Intern Med* 21(5): 1067-1075, 2007.

71. Mao J: Opioid-induced hyperalgesia, *Pain: Clin Updates* 16(2):1-4, 2008.

72. Sellon DC et al: Pharmacokinetics and adverse effects of butorphanol administered by single intravenous injection or continuous intravenous infusion in horses, *Am J Vet Res* 62:183-189, 2001.

73. Sellon DC et al: Effects of continuous rate intravenous infusion of butorphanol on physiologic and outcome variables in horses after celiotomy, *J Vet Intern Med* 18:555-563, 2004.

74. Robertson JT, Muir WW: A new analgesic drug combination in the horse, *Am J Vet Res* 44:1667-1669, 1983.

75. Muir WW, Skarda RT, Sheehan WC: Hemodynamic and respiratory effects of xylazine-morphine sulfate in horses, *Am J Vet Res* 40(10):1417-1420, 1979.

76. Schatzman U et al: Analgesic effect of butorphanol and levomethadone in detomidine-sedated horses, *J Vet Med A Physiol Pathol Clin Med* 48:337-342, 2001.

77. England GCW, Clarke KW: Alpha2-adrenoceptor agonists in the horse: a review, *Br Vet J* 152:641-657, 1996.

78. Kamerling SG, Cravens WMT, Bagwell CA: Dose-related effects of detomidine on autonomic responses in the horse, *J Auton Pharmacol* 8:241, 1988.

79. Merritt AM, Burrows JA, Hartless CS: Effect of xylazine, detomidine, and a combination of xylazine and butorphanol on equine duodenal motility, *Am J Vet Res* 59:619-623, 1998.

80. Grubb TL et al: Use of yohimbine to reverse prolonged effects of xylazine hydrochloride in a horse being treated with chloramphenicol, *J Am Vet Med Assoc* 210:1771, 1997.

81. Whiteside JB, Wildsmith JAW: Developments in local anaesthetic drugs, *Br J Anaesth* 87:27-35, 2001.

82. Becker DE, Reed KL: Essentials of local anesthetic pharmacology, *Anesth Prog* 53:98-109, 2006.

83. Bidwell LA, Wilson DV, Caron JP: Lack of systemic absorption of lidocaine from 5% patches placed on horses, *Vet Anaesth Analg* 34(6):443-446, 2007.

84. Robertson SA et al: Effect of systemic lidocaine on visceral and somatic nociception in conscious horses, *Equine Vet J* 37:122-127, 2005.

85. Doherty TJ, Frazier DL: Effect of intravenous lidocaine on halothane minimum alveolar concentration in ponies, *Equine Vet J* 30:300, 1998.

86. Freary DJ et al: Influence of general anesthesia on pharmacokinetics of intravenous lidocaine infusion in horses, *Am J Vet Res* 66:574-580, 2005.

87. Brianceau P et al: Intravenous lidocaine and small-intestinal size, abdominal fluid, and outcome after colic surgery in horses, *J Vet Intern Med* 16:736-741, 2002.

88. Harkins JD et al: A review of the pharmacology, pharmacokinetics, and regulatory control in the US of local anesthetics in the horse, *J Vet Pharmacol Ther* 18:397, 1995.

89. Muir WW, Sams RA: Effects of ketamine infusion on halothane minimal alveolar concentration in horses, *Am J Vet Res* 53:1802-1806, 1992.

90. Pozzi A, Muir WW, Traverso F: Prevention of central sensitization and pain by N-methyl-D-aspartate receptor antagonists, *J Am Vet Med Assoc* 228(1):53-60, 2006.

91. Lankveld DPK et al: Pharmacodynamic effects and pharmacokinetic profile of a long-term continuous-rate infusion of racemic ketamine in healthy conscious horses, *J Vet Pharmacol Ther* 29:477-488, 2006.

92. Fielding CL et al: Pharmacokinetics and clinical effects of a subanesthetic continuous rate infusion of ketamine in awake horses, *Am J Vet Res* 67:1484-1490, 2006.

93. Lopez-Sanroman FJ et al: Evaluation of the local analgesic effect of ketamine in the palmer digital nerve block at the base of the proximal sesamoid (abaxial sesamoid block) in horses, *Am J Vet Res* 64:475-478, 2003.

94. Gomez De Segura IA et al: Epidural injection of ketamine for perineal analgesia in the horse, *Vet Surg* 27:384-391, 1998.

95. Kong VKF, Irwin MG: Gabapentin: a multimodal perioperative drug? *Br J Anaesth* 99:775-786; 2007.

96. Davis JL, Posner LP, Elce E: Gabapentin for the treatment of neuropathic pain in a pregnant horse, *J Am Vet Med Assoc* 231:755-758, 2007.

97. Shilo Y et al: Pharmacokinetics of tramadol in horses after intravenous, intramuscular, and oral administration, *J Vet Pharmacol Ther* 31:60-65, 2005.

98. Seino KK et al: Effects of topical perineural capsaicin in a reversible model of equine foot lameness, *J Vet Intern Med* 17:563-566, 2003.

99. Doria RGS et al: Comparative study of epidural xylazine or clonidine in horses, *Vet Anaesth Analg* 35:166-172, 2008.

100. Corletto F, Raisis AA, Brearley JC: Comparison of morphine and butorphanol as preanaesthetic agents in combination with romifidine for field castration in ponies, *Vet Anaesth Analg* 32:16-22, 2005.

101. Muir WW: Anaesthesia and pain management in horses, *Equine Vet Educ* 10:335-340, 1998.

102. Muir WW: Recognizing and treating pain in horses. In Reed SM, Bayly WM, editors: *Equine internal medicine*, ed 2, Philadelphia, 2004, Saunders, pp 1529-1541.

103. Backstrom KC et al: Response of induced bone defects in horses to collagen matrix containing the human parathyroid hormone gene, *Am J Vet Res* 65(9):1223-1232, 2004.

104. Frisbie DD, McIlwraith CW: Evaluation of gene therapy as a treatment for equine traumatic arthritis and osteoarthritis, *Clin Orthop Relat Res* 379(suppl):S273-S287, 2000.

21

Considerations for Induction, Maintenance, and Recovery

John A.E. Hubbell
William W. Muir

KEY POINTS

1. The quality of induction to anesthesia is influenced significantly by the horse's response to sedation. All horses should be sedated before producing anesthesia.
2. Horses that do not respond appropriately to sedation should be reevaluated and resedated if necessary.
3. Horses should be positioned, padded, bandaged, and monitored to minimize muscle and nerve damage associated with anesthesia.
4. Complications that occur during the induction and maintenance phases may not be recognized until the horse resumes consciousness.
5. Recovery is the least controllable phase of anesthesia.
6. Recovery should not be rushed. A muted environment allows the horse to gradually transition from unconsciousness to an awake state.
7. The goal during recovery is for the horse to be strong and coordinated enough to stand on its first attempt.
8. Head pads, leg wraps, special flooring, mattresses, air pillows, head and tail ropes, pools, and slings are used to facilitate recovery and prevent injury.
9. Some horses may require the administration of oxygen, a sedative, or the placement of a nasopharyngeal, nasotracheal, or orotracheal tube to facilitate recovery.

There are five steps to equine anesthesia (Box 21-1). Step one includes evaluation and preparation of the horse for anesthesia and surgery. This may or may not include the administration of anxiolytics (acepromazine) or sedatives (α_2-adrenoceptor agonists) to complete required tasks (see Chapter 6). Step two includes the administration and evaluation of preanesthetic medication, including sedatives and analgesics (see Chapters 10 and 20). Step three includes the administration of injectable anesthetic drugs to produce (transition from standing to recumbent) general anesthesia (induction phase; see Chapters 12 and 13). Step 4 includes the padding, positioning, and administration and monitoring of drugs used to maintain anesthesia (maintenance phase; see Chapters 7, 8, 14, and 15). Step 5 includes the discontinuation of anesthetic drugs, the implementation of procedures to ensure an uneventful recovery (transition from recumbent to standing), and individualized postanesthetic medical care (see Chapter 22). Recovery from anesthesia generally is considered complete once the horse is able to stand and walk with minimum assistance, although epidemiological studies consider anesthetic-related outcomes for up to 7 days after anesthesia.[1] Induction, maintenance, and recovery are critically dependent on a thorough evaluation and appropriate preparation of the horse before administering anesthetic drugs.[2] A predetermined, systematic, standardized anesthetic protocol should be developed for field or surgical facility anesthetic procedures and used to anesthetize all normal healthy horses. Modification of this plan should be based on the horse's behavior, physical condition, and medical history; the surgical procedure (complexity, duration); the facilities; and technical expertise. Familiarity and experience gained by the routine use of a standard anesthetic protocol in combination with reduced anesthetic time have been suggested to decrease the risk associated with general anesthesia in horses (see Chapter 6).[2] Familiarity with a standard (specific) anesthetic protocol also increases awareness of potentially troublesome events and generates methods for remedial therapy, thereby reducing the probability of an adverse outcome. Modifications to this protocol may be required in horses that are depressed, debilitated, sick, severely stressed, or exhibiting signs of severe pain (see Chapters 4, 6, 20, and 22). For example, after being examined, administered antibiotics and a nonsteroidal anti-inflammatory drug, and sedated with an α_2-adrenoceptor agonist, most normal healthy horses can be safely induced to general anesthesia by administering diazepam-ketamine drug combination (see Chapter 13).

Methods for producing (inducing), maintaining, and recovering horses from anesthesia should be designed to reduce risk.[1] Standardized monitoring and anesthetic procedures that are modifiable should be developed, applied routinely, and recorded (see Chapters 8 and 24). Accurate morbidity and mortality records should be kept and keyed to the horse's health status (see Chapter 6 and Table 6-4).

PRODUCING (INDUCING) ANESTHESIA

Inducing a horse to general anesthesia should be the most predictable and uneventful phase of anesthesia. Normal healthy horses usually respond appropriately to sedatives or can be administered additional drugs (e.g., diazepam, guaifenesin) when necessary to ensure adequate calming and immobilization before inducing anesthesia.[3] The horse's response (behavioral, physical, physiological) to the administration of sedatives is a major factor determining the quality of anesthetic induction (see Chapters 6 and 10). Horses that do not respond appropriately or respond adversely to sedative drugs should not be anesthetized until alternate strategies are developed. Horses that remain anxious or excitable after the administration of α_2-adrenoceptor agonists are likely to exhibit a poor or inadequate response

1. Evaluation, preparation
2. Preanesthetic medication
3. Induction to anesthesia
4. Maintenance of anesthesia
5. Recovery from anesthesia

to the administration of injectable anesthetics, necessitating the administration of additional anesthetic drug (e.g., valium-ketamine; thiopental) to prevent movement, thereby increasing the potential for drug-related side effects.[4]

There are circumstances when anesthesia cannot be delayed or avoided (e.g., colic, dystocia, severe trauma). Every effort should be made to normalize physiological values, minimize stress, provide pain relief, and reduce the duration between diagnosis and surgery in emergency and high-risk horses.[2] Anesthetic induction procedures that use drug titration (to effect) protocols that incorporate guaifenesin drug combinations are optimal in these circumstances (see Chapters 12, 13, and 24).

The four most popular methods used to assist recumbency in horses are free fall, pushing the horse against a wall, squeezing the horse between a wall and a large door or gate, and fixation to a surgical tilt-table (Figure 21-1). All four are acceptable methods to assist induction to anesthesia, although the first method (free fall) is not recommended if the horse is severely lame ("three-legged"), dangerous, or feral. Horses that are allowed to free-fall without assistance are more likely to make awkward movements, slam their head on the ground, or fall over backwards, increasing the potential for limb fractures and head trauma. The horse's head should always be controlled by an experienced attendant to minimize head trauma during induction to anesthesia and ensure lateral recumbency once attained (Figure 21-2). The door method (when available) is preferred for inducing anesthesia in horses. The door method minimizes the horse's movement, protects the horse and attendants, provides appropriate support while the horse is relaxing, and is controllable and highly predictable. Most horses demonstrate signs of muscle weakness (muscle fasciculations, ataxia) and sit down before relaxing to their sternum if their head is raised to a normal position as the anesthetic induction drugs begin to take effect. Once the horse is recumbent, an orotracheal tube should be placed,

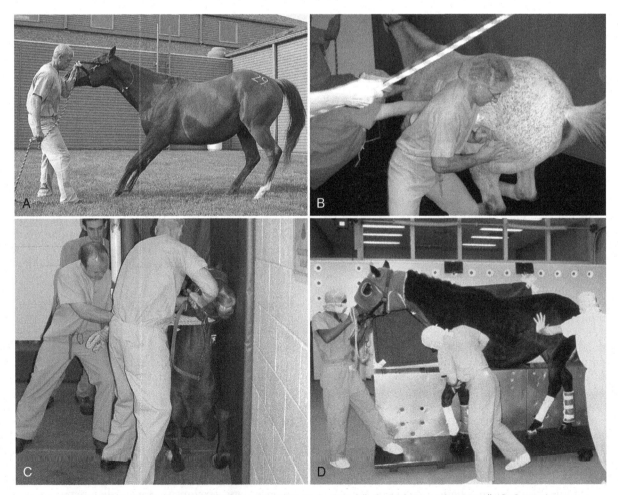

Figure 21–1. Methods used to facilitate recumbency. **A,** Free fall. **B,** Pushing against a wall. **C,** Squeezing behind a door. **D,** Tilt-table. All four methods require that the attendant maintain control of the horse's head at all times. (**B,** Courtesy of Dr. Paul Rothaug, Woodland Run Equine Facility. **D,** Courtesy of Dr. Robert Copelan Jr.)

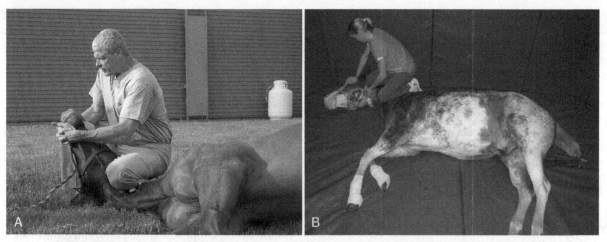

Figure 21–2. Controlling a recumbent horse. The horse's head should be controlled at all times. A horse that requires additional anesthetic (**A**) or is not ready to stand during recovery from anesthesia (**B**) can be controlled by kneeling across the its neck and lifting the muzzle vertically. (**B,** Courtesy of New England Equine MSC, Dover, NH.)

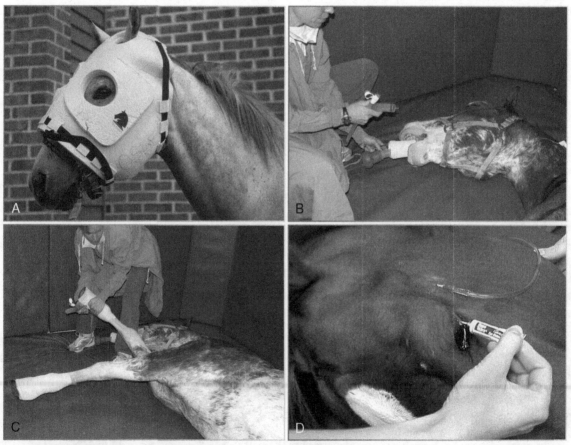

Figure 21–3. Equipment for procedures performed during induction should include protection of the head. **A,** Padded hoods. **B,** Placement of a cuffed endotracheal tube. **C,** Extending the down front limb forward. **D,** Placing lubricant (artificial tears) to protect the eyes. (**B** to **D,** Courtesy of New England Equine MSC, Dover, NH.)

protective eye lubricant administered, and the horse positioned to minimize muscle ischemia or nerve damage (see Chapter 14). The head should be protected, the down front leg (lateral recumbency) pulled forward to relieve pressure on the triceps muscle and radial nerve, and the limbs bandaged and secured (Figure 21-3).

MAINTAINING ANESTHESIA

Horses that are anesthetized for periods longer than 15 to 30 minutes should be placed on impervious, protective cushioned padding. The head should be protected (see preceding paragraph), and the nose slightly elevated if the horse is supine (dorsal recumbency). The head, limbs, and pressure points (shoulder, hip) should be positioned appropriately, padded, and protected (Figure 21-4). The halter should be removed during the maintenance phase to minimize the potential for facial nerve paralysis. The limbs should not be left in an extended position for prolonged periods. The bladder should be catheterized if a long (>2 to 3 hours) surgical procedure is anticipated to prevent urine accumulation on the padding and contamination of the surgical site or urination in the recovery phase, creating a slick surface during the horse's recovery. Appropriate monitoring, adjunctive medications, and ventilation should be used, depending on the anesthetic requirements (see Chapters 8, 13, and 22).

RECOVERY FROM ANESTHESIA

Prolonged recumbency is not a natural state for normal horses. Most horses lie down only 10% to 20% of the time and may not lie down when placed in an unfamiliar environment for the first 24 hours or longer.[5,6] The infrequency of recumbency in combination with the natural tendency for horses to flee when threatened results in many horses trying to rise before they have fully recovered from the effects of anesthetic drugs. Anesthetic drug–related effects can take hours to dissipate, particularly after prolonged periods of anesthesia.

Horses usually rise from sternal recumbency by placing their front legs forward and contracting the extensor muscles of their rear limbs to generate the force required to stand (Figure 21-5). This motion causes the horse to move forward as it rises. When positioning the horse for recovery, this forward motion, as well as the quality of the surface on which the horse will stand, should be considered carefully. The environment should be calm, quiet, and nonstressful.

Factors Affecting the Duration of Recovery

The quality and duration of recovery are determined by multiple factors, including but not limited to the horse's physical condition and temperament, the dose and route of anesthetic drug administration, the nature of the environment at the recovery site, the use of appropriate padding during recumbency, the duration of anesthesia, the occurrence of anesthetic events (hemorrhage, hypotension), the type of surgery (soft tissue, orthopedic), and administration of sedatives or drug antagonists during the recovery period (Box 21-2).[7-10]

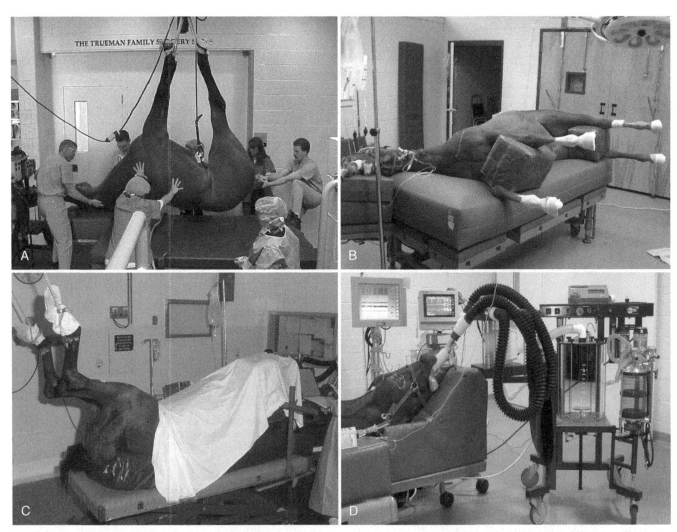

Figure 21–4. Padding and positioning. **A,** Thick foam rubber pads or air mattresses should be used to maximize the even distribution of the horse's weight. **B,** The down front leg should be extended forward, and pads positioned between the legs when horses are in lateral recumbency. **C,** The back and shoulders should be padded. **D,** The neck is slightly flexed in the supine horse. (**B,** Courtesy of New England Equine MSC, Dover, NH.)

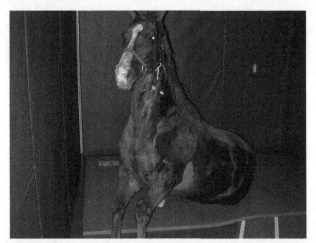

Figure 21–5. Horses usually begin to rise on their front legs first, which naturally moves them forward when attempting to stand.

Box 21–2	**Factors Affecting Recovery from Anesthesia**

- Age, breed, sex
- Temperament
- Size, weight
- Physical status
- Anesthetic drugs (dose, route)
- Positioning and padding during recumbency
- Surgical procedure (soft tissue, orthopedic)
- Duration of surgery
- Concurrent medications (antibiotics)
- Adverse events (hypotension, hypoxemia, electrolyte abnormalities)
- Recovery room (environment, dimensions, padding, flooring, procedures)
- Administration of sedatives or drug antagonists during the recovery period
- Personnel experience and training

Horses that have a poor induction to anesthesia and are stressed by exertion or disease frequently have a prolonged, poor recovery from anesthesia.[7] Horses that are in extreme pain (e.g., colic, fracture), physiologically impaired (e.g., hemorrhage, dehydration), or pregnant may be exhausted, weak, and hypocalcemic. This is particularly true in parturient mares that have been in prolonged labor and require anesthesia for repositioning of the foal or cesarean section. Horses that frequently lie down because of their disease (colic, laminitis, orthopedic injury) generally have prolonged recoveries from anesthesia and require frequent assessment and vigilant monitoring (see Chapters 8 and 22). Horses that develop hypotension (mean arterial pressure <50 mm Hg) during the maintenance phase of anesthesia or become hypotensive in recovery may develop myopathy or be too weak to stand and require supportive care.[11] Provision should be made for the continuation of oxygen, intravenous fluids, and cardiovascular stimulants (such as dobutamine) during recovery (see Chapter 22).

Horses that are anesthetized for prolonged periods (>3 hours) generally require a longer time to metabolize and eliminate drugs and recover from anesthesia (Figure 21-6; see Chapter 9).[7,9] However, horses anesthetized for 3 hours or less may recover in the same time as horses anesthetized for 1 hour. Historically, chloral hydrate anesthesia produced recoveries lasting for 90 minutes to 2 hours; but most studies investigating the duration of recovery from anesthesia report values of 60 minutes or less, independent of the method used to produce anesthesia (Table 21-1).[12-30] The desire to hasten recovery from anesthesia must be balanced with attempts to ensure that the horse has regained sufficient strength and coordination to stand and support itself. Conventional approaches to this problem

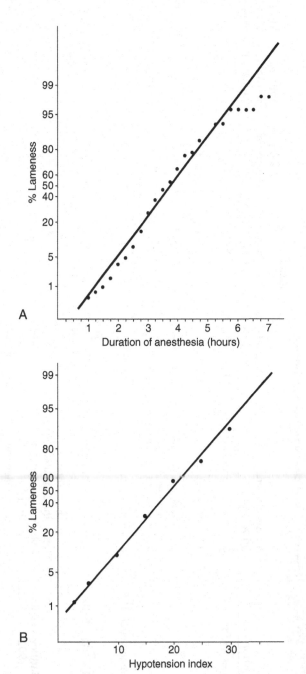

Figure 21–6. Longer durations of anesthesia **(A)** and hypotension **(B)** predispose to lameness.[9]

Table 21-1   Anesthetic recovery characteristics in horses

Author	Anesthetic drugs (induction)	Anesthetic drugs (maintenance)	Number of horses	Duration of anesthesia (min)	Time to sternal (min)	Time to standing (min)	Number of attempts	Quality of recovery
Auer 1978[12]	Acepromazine, guaifenesin, thiopental	Methoxyflurane	5	120	52	68	2	
	Acepromazine, guaifenesin, thiopental	Enflurane	5	120	25	33	1	
	Acepromazine, guaifenesin, thiopental	Isoflurane	5	120	18	37	1	
	Acepromazine, guaifenesin, thiopental	Halothane	5	120	30	42	1.75	
Greene et al, 1986[8]	Guaifenesin, xylazine, ketamine	Guaifenesin, xylazine, ketamine	8	120		15-30		Uneventful
McCarty, 1990[3]	Xylazine ± butorphanol, pentazocine, acepromazine, ketamine ± guaifenesin	Xylazine, ketamine, ± guaifenesin	60	34	30	31-55		Unsatisfactory in five horses
Matthews et al, 1992[13]	Xylazine, guaifenesin, thiamylal	Isoflurane	6	105	19	22	1	
	Xylazine, guaifenesin, thiamylal	Halothane	6	128	28	43	2	
Taylor and Watkins, 1992[14]	Detomidine, guaifenesin, ketamine	Guaifenesin, ketamine, detomidine	6	120	11	25		4-5 out of 5, 5 is best
Whitehair et al, 1993[10]	Halothane	Halothane	6	60		37	1.8	2.8 out of 3, 3 is best
	Halothane	Halothane	6	180		44	2	2.2 out of 3, 3 is best
	Isoflurane	Isoflurane	6	180		39	1.5	2.2 out of 3, 3 is best
Bettschart-Wolfensberger et al, 1996[15]	Acepromazine, xylazine, ketamine	Climazolam, ketamine, sarmazenil reversal	6	120		27	1-7	Good in 3, Fair in 1, Excited/ataxic in 2
Carroll et al, 1998[16]	Xylazine, ketamine	Sevoflurane	8	269	54	78	1-2	1-3 out of 6, 1 is best
Mama et al 1998[17]	Xylazine, guaifenesin, ketamine	Xylazine, ketamine	6	75	36	45		Good
	Xylazine, guaifenesin, propofol	Xylazine, propofol (low)	6	73	82	90		Excellent
	Xylazine, guaifenesin, propofol	Xylazine, propofol (high)	6	73	73	80		Excellent
Matthews, Hartsfield, and Mercer, 1998[18]	Xylazine, diazepam, ketamine	Isoflurane	9	90	12.6	17.4	4	2.9 out of 6, 1 is best
	Xylazine, diazepam, ketamine	Sevoflurane	9	90	10.3	13.9	2	1.7 out of 6, 1 is best

Study	Induction	Maintenance/protocol	n					Assessment
Grosenbaugh and Muir, 1998[19]	Xylazine, diazepam, ketamine	Sevoflurane with xylazine recovery	9	90	13.8	18	2	1.7 out of 6, 1 is best
	Xylazine, guaifenesin, ketamine	Sevoflurane	4	90	6	12	2	1 out of 4, 1 is best
	Xylazine, guaifenesin, ketamine	Sevoflurane with xylazine	4	90	15	27	2	1.5 out of 4, 1 is best
	Xylazine, guaifenesin, ketamine	Isoflurane	4	90	11	16	2	2 out of 4, 1 is best
	Xylazine, guaifenesin, ketamine	Isoflurane with xylazine	4	90	13	24	2	1.5 out of 4, 1 is best
	Xylazine, guaifenesin, ketamine	Halothane	4	90	18	28	2	1.5 out of 4, 1 is best
	Xylazine, guaifenesin, ketamine	Halothane with xylazine	4	90	19	30	1	1 out of 4, 1 is best
Donaldson et al, 2000[20]	Xylazine, guaifenesin, ketamine	Halothane	49	86	38	41	1 (1-4)	Better
	Xylazine, guaifenesin, ketamine	Isoflurane	50	87	25	28	1 (1-3)	Worse
Yamashita et al, 2000[21]	Medetomidine, diazepam, ketamine	Guaifenesin, ketamine, medetomidine, Sevoflurane	6	187	26	36	2.5	Excitement free
	Medetomidine, diazepam, ketamine	Sevoflurane	6	171	31	48	2.7	Excitement free
Taylor et al, 2001[22]	Acepromazine butorphanol, detomidine, ketamine	Detomidine, ketamine, guaifenesin	12	140		60		Good
Read et al, 2002[23]		Isoflurane	6 foals	134		12.5	1-2	1.7 out of 3, 1 is best
		Sevoflurane	6 foals	142		9.2		1.3 out of 3, 1 is best
Wagner et al, 2002[24]	Xylazine, thiopental		4	30	47	53	1-2	3 out of 5, 5 is best
	Xylazine, ketamine		4	13	22	25	1	4-5 out of 5, 5 is best
	Xylazine, thiopental, propofol		12	17-24	36-39	43-46	1-2	4-5 out of 5, 5 is best
	Xylazine, ketamine, propofol		12	26-32	26-32	29-39	1	4-5 out of 5, 5 is best
Spadavecchia et al, 2002[25]	Xylazine, methadone, guaifenesin. ketamine	Halothane	14	92	20	31		Acceptable
		Guaifenesin, ketamine, low halothane	14	92	23	32		Acceptable
Santos et al, 2003[31]	Xylazine, butorphanol, ketamine	Isoflurane	6	120	7.7	14.5	4.2	52, Lower is better

(Continued)

Table 21–1—Cont'd.

Author	Anesthetic drugs (induction)	Anesthetic drugs (maintenance)	Number of horses	Duration of anesthesia (min)	Time to sternal (min)	Time to standing (min)	Number of attempts	Quality of recovery
	Xylazine, butorphanol, ketamine	Isoflurane plus xylazine	6	120	19.7	30	2.2	27 Lower is better
	Xylazine, butorphanol, ketamine	Isoflurane plus detomidine	6	120	25.3	38.7	1.2	25 Lower is better
	Xylazine, butorphanol, ketamine	Isoflurane plus romifidine	6	120	23.2	37.3	1.2	22 Lower is better
Bettschart-Wolfensberger et al, 2005[26]	Medetomidine, diazepam, ketamine	Medetomidine, propofol	50	111 (46-225)	12	42	Most 1-2	All satisfactory
Mama 2005[27]	Xylazine, guaifenesin, ketamine	Xylazine, ketamine	5	66-73	23-58	33-69		4.3-5 out of 5 5 is best
Valverde et al, 2005[28]	Xylazine, midazolam, ketamine	Isoflurane, lidocaine	9	101	22	30		3.9 out of 6 1 is best
	Xylazine, midazolam, ketamine	Isoflurane, lidocaine (d/c last 30 min)	9	101	22	30		3.7 out of 6 1 is best
	Xylazine, midazolam, ketamine	Isoflurane	9	101	22	30		3.2 out of 6 1 is best
	Xylazine, midazolam, ketamine	Sevoflurane	9	101	22	30		3.2 out of 6 1 is best
	Xylazine, midazolam, ketamine	Sevoflurane, lidocaine (d/c last 30 min)	9	101	22	30		2.7 out of 6 1 is best
	Xylazine, midazolam, ketamine	Sevoflurane, lidocaine	9	101	22	30		4 out of 6 1 is best
Durongphcngtorn et al, 2006[29]	Romifidine, diazepam, ketamine	Halothane	8	57		63	1.3	1.3 out of 5 1 is best
	Romifidine, diazepam, ketamine	Isoflurane	8	83		56	1.9	1.8 out of 5 1 is best
Umar et al, 2006[30]	Medetomidine, midazolam, ketamine	Propofol	6	120	59	87	2.2	
	Medetomidine, midazolam, ketamine	Ketamine, medetomidine, propofol	6	120	36	62	1.7	

have centered on holding the horse in lateral recumbency or administering sedatives and tranquilizers to lengthen the period of recumbency, thus lengthening the time for exhalation of inhalant drugs or elimination of the injectable anesthetic drugs (see Figure 21-2).[31] The availability of α_2-adrenoceptor antagonists has increased the options for the management of horses that do not recover in an appropriate amount of time (Table 21-2).[32] Atipamazole or doxapram increases awareness in horses that are recovering too slowly ("sleeping" >60 to 90 minutes) and generally initiates attempts to rise and stand within 3 minutes of drug administration. The administration of morphine as preanesthetic medication (0.1 to 0.15 mg/kg) and infusion (0.1 mg/kg/hr) during anesthesia has been demonstrated to shorten the time from first movement to standing during recovery and to reduce the number of attempts to stand in halothane-anesthetized horses.[33] Whether or not this effect is similar following isoflurane or sevoflurane anesthesia has not been demonstrated. However, terminating isoflurane anesthesia while prolonging sedation and recumbency with a total intravenous anesthesia drug combination (xylazine-ketamine) does not positively influence recovery.[34]

The quality of recovery is difficult to predict, although older, calmer, properly padded, and trained horses generally have good recoveries because they are less excitable and easier to assist. The rate of return of consciousness and active reflexes (swallowing, palpebral) during recovery is predictable and can be predetermined by the experienced anesthetist.[10] Useful signs of recovery include eyelid and eyeball movement, ear movement, swallowing, head lift, and limb movement. If an endotracheal tube is present, most horses begin to swallow before they attempt to attain a sternal position. The observation of rapid nystagmus or rotary eyeball movement suggests delirium (Box 21-3). Horses that demonstrate these and other signs of poor recovery should be restrained in lateral recumbency until they regain a greater degree of consciousness (see Figure 21-2). Alternatively, a sedative can be administered to quiet the horse and prolong the recovery process. Many horses anesthetized with inhalant anesthetics with low blood gas solubilities (isoflurane, sevoflurane, desflurane) benefit from the administration of small doses of sedatives or analgesics immediately before or during recovery (see Table 21-2).[31-33] Sedation produces a longer period of lateral recumbency during which inhalant

| Box 21-3 | Signs Suggesting Poor Recovery |

- Uncoordinated limb movements
- Stretching
- Paddling
- Sweating
- Muscle fasciculations
- Trembling/shaking
- Rapid breathing
- Whinnying
- Rapid or rotary nystagmus
- Head slapping
- Muscle weakness
- Uncoordinated or immediate (premature) attempts to stand

anesthetics can be eliminated, resulting in more coordinated attempts to stand. The use of analgesics in the recovery period may make the horse more comfortable, resulting in a calmer transition to consciousness. Horses oxygenate better in sternal recumbency than in lateral or dorsal recumbency (see Chapter 2). Horses with low PaO_2, poor mucous membrane color, or labored respiration should be insufflated with high oxygen flow rates (>15 L/min), rolled into sternal recumbency, and supported in that position (see Chapter 22).[35] The horse should be allowed to remain in sternal recumbency as long as necessary before attempting to stand. Reduced lighting and quiet surroundings improve the transition to the awake state and reduce the horse's desire to stand. A clean towel can be placed over the eyes in horses that are recovering outside. Ventilation should be adequate to remove exhaled trace anesthetic gases for horses recovering from inhalant anesthesia.

Recovery Stall Design

Recovery box dimensions, padding, and flooring are key considerations when designing a recovery area. The floor should be a dry, nonslip, compressible surface and provide traction even if wet (Box 21-4). The use of deep straw or sawdust bedding does not overcome the deficiency of a slippery floor. When appropriate, horses can be recovered outdoors on a grass or an earthen surface. Turf provides

| Table 21-2. | Drugs that facilitate recovery |

Drugs that improve but slow recovery

Drug	Dose
Acepromazine	0.01-0.02 mg/kg IV during recovery
Xylazine	0.2-0.4 mg/kg IV during recovery
Detomidine	0.05-0.01 mg/kg IV during recovery

Drugs that improve and hasten recovery

Morphine	0.1-0.15 mg/kg IV premed; 0.1 mg/kg/hr

Drugs that speed recovery

Atipamazole	0.05-0.1 mg/kg
Doxapram	0.1-0.2 mg/kg

IV, Intravenously.

| Box 21-4 | Recovery Floor Surfaces |

- Lawn or sand
- Straw
- Wood chips
- Composites
  - Poured
  - Granular
- Wrestling of gymnastic mats
- Rubber mats

excellent footing for recovery and some padding should the horse fall. A floor drain should be incorporated to facilitate cleaning and disinfection. Recovery stall dimensions should be large enough to accommodate the average adult, 500-kg horse. Recovery boxes that are 4 × 4 m square are usually adequate. Oversized rooms do not provide any advantage since the horse may use the additional space to gather speed as it attempts to stand. The walls of the recovery stall should be at least 2.5 m high and padded. Metal rings (2 to 3 cm in diameter) capable of withstanding forces of greater than 1000 kg should be affixed to at least three walls of the box at the highest points permitted by the construction (Figure 21-7). Head and tail ropes can be passed through the rings to assist recovery and remove personnel from the immediate area. A ceiling hook capable of supporting a minimum of 1000 kg should be constructed over the center of the stall in case a sling is required.[36] An additional hook for the suspension of intravenous fluids should be available. An observation area, window, or large convex mirror from which personnel can watch and assist recovery should be incorporated into new construction (Figure 21-8). Alternatively, experienced personnel can remain in the recovery stall or use a mounted camera for remote monitoring.

The choice of floor surface is based on cost, anticipated frequency of use, and the type of procedures to be performed. Synthetic surfaces are more easily cleaned and disinfected should contamination from procedures such as an abdominal exploratory occur. The simple application of straw or wood shavings on top of a hard, slippery synthetic surface (rubber matt, concrete) is unsatisfactory. Alternatively, a composite surface can be applied to any surface beginning with a 3- to 5-cm layer of sand. An additional 3- to 5-cm layer of shredded bark and then straw is placed atop the sand to provide good traction and a "clean" environment. Straw should not be piled excessively high because it may cause the horse to stumble as it attempts to stand. The floor surface should provide some cushioning if the horse falls. The composite must be removed and replaced if infectious disease contamination is suspected and disinfection is required.

Most surfaces are rubber based or made of compressible synthetic materials. The surface of the material must either be roughened or compressible so that the horse's hoof can indent

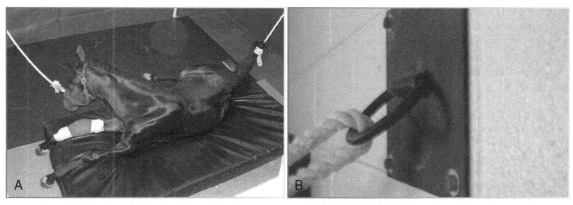

Figure 21–7. A, Horses should be recovered on padded or air-filled mattresses. **B,** Head and tail ropes that can be passed through rings markedly facilitate recovery.

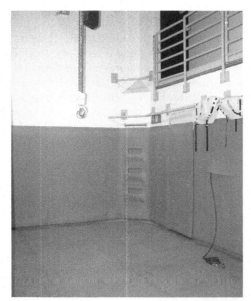

Figure 21–8. Specially designed recovery stalls that are fully padded and contain a nonslip compressible floor, a hoist, and an observation area are ideal. (Courtesy of Dr. Nora Matthews, College of Veterinary Medicine, Texas A&M University.)

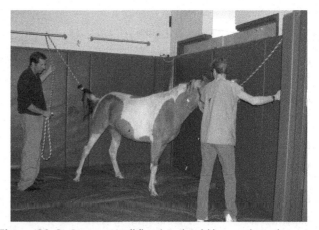

Figure 21–9. Recovery stall flooring should be roughened or compressible so that the horse's hoof can indent the surface to gain traction. Note the compressible floor. (Courtesy of New England Equine MSC, Dover, NH.)

the surface to gain traction (Figure 21-9). Wrestling or gymnastic mats, 3- to 5-cm thick, can be used for flooring. The mats are lightweight, compressible, and removed easily for cleaning.

Assisting Recovery

A number of techniques have been devised to improve recovery from anesthesia, but the risk of morbidity and mortality during the recovery phase of anesthesia remains comparatively high (Table 21-3 and Box 21-5). Recovery is improved if the horse is assisted. Horses can be recovered without assistance but should always be observed and assisted when necessary. A number of methods and protocols are available for the physical assistance of horses recovering from anesthesia (see Box 21-5).[37] If an orotracheal tube is placed, it may be removed when the horse swallows or when it stands; and the horse is left alone in a quiet environment. Experienced personnel should remain in the area until the horse stands, and a method of visualization (window, mirror, or camera) should be devised (see Figure 21-8). Unassisted recoveries carry greater risk to the horse but the least risk to personnel. Decisions regarding the best method for assisting recovery are influenced by the number of experienced personnel and facilities available. Safety can be enhanced by removing the horse's shoes before recovery and bandaging the horse's legs.

Box 21–5 Methods of Recovery from Anesthesia in Horses

- Field recovery
- Floor of padded stall
  - ± Head and tail ropes
- Mattress and padded stall
  - ± Head and tail ropes
- Inflating-deflating air pillow
  - ± Head and tail ropes
- Tilt-table recovery
- Anderson sling suspension system
- Pool-raft system
- Hydropool system

Equipment

Some simple basic equipment is useful for any recovery (Box 21-6). A dependable halter that is not too tight or too loose should be placed before the horse attempts to stand. Head and tail ropes provide a method for assisting the horse while allowing the assistant to be some distance from the horse.

Table 21–3. Indications and consequences of methods of recovery in horses

Method	Indication	Advantages	Disadvantages
Unassisted	Short-duration anesthesia Uncomplicated procedures Unbroken or obstreperous horses	Minimum risk to personnel	Greater potential for injury or airway obstruction Horse may take missteps "Capture" must be accomplished before assistance can be provided or tranquilization administered
Assisted (head and tail rope)[37]	Any procedure	Increased control Easy to provide assistance or tranquilization Ability to limit movement once standing	Risk to personnel Requires minimum of two people
Slings[40-44]	Procedures with increased risk of catastrophic injury	Places horse in a supported standing position Less force is required to attain a standing position Missteps minimized	Some horses resist sling restraint (improved with prior application) Equipment cost Requires minimum of three trained people
Tilt-table[39]	Procedures with increased risk of catastrophic injury	Places the horse in a supported, standing position	Equipment cost Space required (table should be fixed to the floor) Requires three to five people
Pool and raft[46]	Procedures with increased risk of catastrophic injury	Minimizes stress on weight-bearing tissues	Cost of equipment and maintenance Space required Horses are resedated or reanesthetized for removal from the pool Requires four to six people
Rectangular pool[45,47]	Procedures with increased risk of catastrophic injury	Minimizes stress on weight-bearing tissues Easier removal from pool (compared to pool and raft)	Cost of equipment and maintenance Space required Longer-duration recovery Pulmonary edema Requires three to five people

Box 21–6	**Recovery Equipment**

- Dependable halter
- Lead rope
- Tail rope (soft material 2.54 cm in diameter, 10 m in length)
- Eye lubricant
- Towel to cover the eyes
- Nasotracheal tube (12- to 14-mm internal diameter)
- Oxygen source (insufflation, demand valve)
- Emergency drugs (epinephrine, furosemide; see Chapter 22)

Optional
- Leg wraps
- Padded hood
- Ear plugs

A towel placed over the eyes and cotton to plug the ears reduce environmental stimulation. Padded hoods help to prevent head injury, but they occasionally rotate out of position and block the horse's vision (see Figure 21-3). A nasotracheal or orotracheal tube and oxygen source provide a method for ensuring an airway and supplementing the inspired oxygen tension during the recovery process (Figure 21-10).

Recovery from Anesthesia Outdoors

Recovery from anesthesia in the field after short anesthetic procedures is usually uncomplicated. A minimum of two trained and experienced attendants should stay with the horse until it stands. Horses should be recovered with the halter in place and lead rope attached (preferably one without a chain). Good-to-excellent footing is the primary requirement for choosing the site of recovery. Turf is ideal, but an indoor arena or stall can also be used. The area should be free of obstructions or machinery. Remember that most horses move forward as they stand (see Figure 21-5, Figure 21-11). Every attempt should be made to maintain a quiet, calm environment and minimize stimulation; the eyes should be covered, and the ears plugged. Most horses lie in lateral recumbency before rolling to sternal recumbency and attempting to stand. The attendant should keep the horse in lateral recumbency until the judgment is made that the horse is strong and coordinated enough to stand (see Figure 21-2). The attendant responsible for holding the lead rope should not attempt to pull the horse to its feet. The lead rope should be held closely but loosely so that the horse can use its head to stand. Once standing, the head should be held closely to limit movement until the horse is stable and coordinated. Grasping and pulling straight backward on the tail assists the horse during attempts to stand (see Figure 21-11). This action may lift a smaller horse, but the primary action is to slow forward momentum and prevent awkward movements as the horse rises. Cotton rope (2.5 cm diameter,

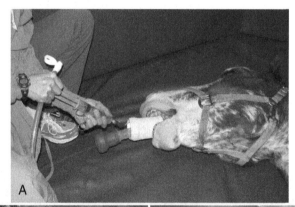

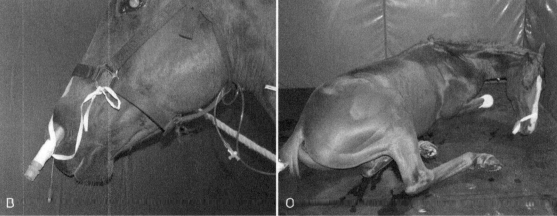

Figure 21–10. A, The orotracheal tube with cuff deflated should be removed when the horse begins to swallow. **B,** A nasotracheal tube or, **C,** uncuffed orotracheal tube provides a method to ensure an airway during recovery or in horses that demonstrate signs (snoring) of upper airway obstruction. (**A,** Courtesy of New England Equine MSC, Dover, NH.) (**C,** Courtesy of Dr. Claire Scicluna, Clinique du Plessis, Chamant, France.)

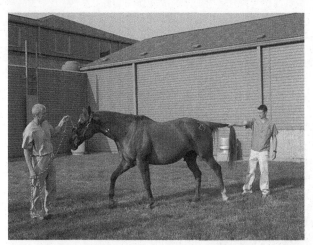

Figure 21–11. Controlling the head and grasping and pulling straight backward on the tail as the horse rises to a standing position can facilitate recovery.

7 m long) can be attached to the tail (see Chapter 5). The placement of a tail rope provides stability and increases safety to assisting personnel by moving them away from the hind legs of the horse. This method of aiding recovery is useful but is not totally without risk to personnel.

Recovery from Anesthesia in Specially Designed Facilities

Horses recovering in a recovery stall should be placed on a pad or air mattress. The attendant should keep the horse in lateral recumbency until the judgment is made that the horse is strong and coordinated enough to stand (see Figure 21-2). Thick pads or an inflatable mattress provide cushioning and may slow attempts to stand by requiring the horse to make a deliberate, coordinated effort to attain sternal recumbency.[37] Foam rubber pads (25 cm thick, 2 × 4 m in size) covered with impervious materials provide excellent padding (see Figure 21-7). The horse should be placed on the pad with its legs at the edge of the pad; it will usually roll off the pad during attempts to become sternal, at which point the pad can be removed.

Inflated Air Pillow Recoveries

Large inflatable pillows, 4.3 × 4.8 m in size and 45 cm deep, have been used to assist horses during recovery from anesthesia. The pillow covers the entire floor of the recovery stall (Figure 21-12).[38] The horse is placed on the deflated pillow with a nasotracheal tube in place, and the pillow is inflated using a fan system. The fan continues to run throughout the inflation period. No assistance is provided; and the horse must make strong, coordinated effects to attain sternal recumbency. The pillow is deflated rapidly once the horse has made three to four aggressive attempts to stand. Horses remain recumbent for a longer time when the pillow is used but usually require fewer attempts to stand than horses recovered without the pillow.[38] This study supports the opinion that restraining the horse in lateral recumbency until it has the strength to produce deliberate coordinated movements reduces attempts to stand and the potential for collapse once standing.

Tilt-Table Recoveries

Tilt-table recovery has been suggested for horses recovering from anesthesia after high-risk orthopedic procedures (Figure 21-13).[39] Horses are recovered on a 3 × 2 m padded table that is secured to the floor. They are placed on the table in the horizontal position. A custom-made halter and recovery hood are placed on the horse's head and secured to the table at three points. A tail rope is placed and secured to the table. Two heavy girths encircle the abdomen and the thorax, and protective bandages are placed on all four limbs. Each limb is secured independently to the table. Sedatives, tranquilizers, and analgesics are administered as necessary to control awakening. The leg straps are removed once the horse displays at least three forceful attempts to move its legs. The head and tail ropes remain secured, but the girths are loosened as the table is moved to the vertical position. Thirty-nine of 54 horses had good-to-excellent recoveries using this method.[39] One horse suffered a complete fixation failure, and six horses failed to adapt to the system.[39]

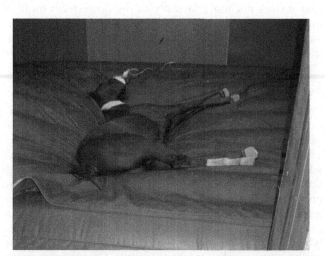

Figure 21–12. Large inflating-deflating air pillows can be used to assist horses during recovery from anesthesia. (Courtesy of Dr. David Hodgson, College of Veterinary Medicine, Kansas State University.)

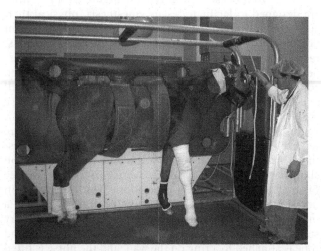

Figure 21–13. Tilt-table system for recovering horses at increased risk because of orthopedic-related procedures. (Courtesy Drs. Antonio Cruz and Carolyn Kerr, Ontario Veterinary College, University of Guelph, Canada.)

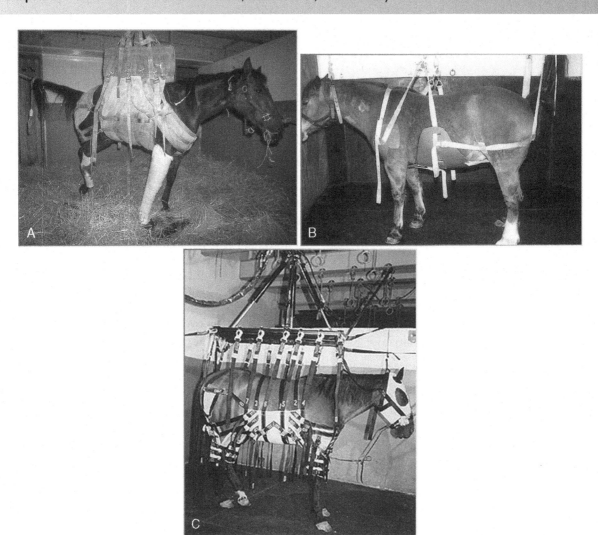

Figure 21–14. A, Slings can be used to assist recovery in horses. **B,** Shells and, **C,** girths (Anderson sling) attached to hoists decrease weight on the limbs once the horse stands.

Sling Recoveries

A variety of sling systems have been developed to assist recovery from anesthesia in horses (Figure 21-14). Slings are designed to facilitate rescue, anesthesia, physical therapy, immobilization, suspension, and reduction of weight bearing.[35,40,41] One system specifically designed to assist recovery from anesthesia uses a shell with girths and is suspended using a minimum of four hoists to allow improved adjustment of support (see Figure 21-14).[42-44] The shell and girths are positioned in the recovery stall. The horse is sedated and lifted to a standing position as soon as it begins to lift its head. Forty of 42 and 69 of 83 horses were reported to be recovered successfully from inhalant anesthesia using this approach.[42-44] Alternatively, an Anderson sling has been used for 32 recoveries in 24 horses (see Figure 21-14).[41] The sling is positioned with the horse in dorsal recumbency on the surgical table. It is attached to a metal frame, and the horse is transported to the recovery stall. The frame is fixed in the middle of the stall. A head rope is attached to a ring on the wall, and the horse is lifted until its feet just touch the ground. The horse is progressively lowered to the ground as it awakens. Successful sling recovery depends on the presence of trained experienced personnel, the use of appropriate equipment, a cooperative horse, and the judicious use of sedatives and tranquilizers. At a minimum, the hoist used should be fixed in place so that it does not move laterally as the horse recovers from anesthesia. Acceptance of the sling is improved if the horse can be accustomed to it before anesthesia. Slings are frequently used to assist horses that are weak or unable to stand without continuous assistance.

Swimming Pool and Raft Systems

Swimming pool and raft systems can be used to assist recovery from anesthesia in horses (Figure 21-15).[45-47] The horse is placed in a sling and lifted into a specially designed raft. The raft is comprised of sleeves for each of the four limbs, with additional support for the head. The horse, sling, and raft are placed into a pool using an overhead rail system. A head and tail rope are attached. Once the horse has recovered from anesthesia, it is sedated, hoisted from the pool, and transported to a recovery stall in the sling. The sling is removed when the horse is standing in the recovery stall with a head and tail rope attached to opposite walls. Complications associated with water recoveries include aspiration of water, pulmonary edema, abrasions, and incision infections.[45,46]

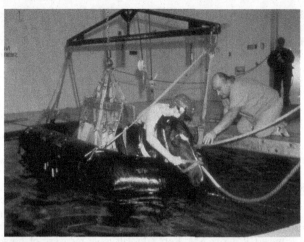

Figure 21–15. Pool and raft recovery systems for recovery. (Courtesy of Dr. Dean Richardson, College of Veterinary Medicine, University of Pennsylvania.)

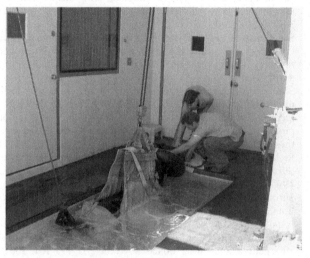

Figure 21–16. A hydropool system specifically designed to assist recovery in horses. The floor of the pool is raised to ground level as the horse awakens and gains strength. (Courtesy Dr. Douglas Herthel, Alamo Pintado Equine Clinic, Los Olivos, Calif.)

Rectangular (Hydropool System)

A rectangular hydropool (4 × 1.3 m) approximately 2.5 m deep has been specially designed to assist recovery from anesthesia in horses (Figure 21-16).[45] The floor of the pool is a stainless steel grate that can be raised rapidly by a hydraulic mechanism as the horse awakens.[45] The horse is placed in a sling and lowered into the pool with an air-inflated rubber tube around its head. The horse's body is completely submerged, with the head suspended by two ropes. Once the horse has recovered, the steel grate is raised until the horse can bear weight on its limbs. The steel grate is raised to ground level when the horse demonstrates the ability to support itself, and the sling and inner tube are removed. Of concern is the increased ventilatory effort required to overcome the extrathoracic hydrostatic effects of immersion. This effect may be responsible for the development of pulmonary edema associated with pool recovery.[45]

CONCLUSION

Most horses recover from anesthesia and stand within 60 minutes. Longer surgical procedures and anesthesia time coupled with hypotension are major factors determining recovery time and morbidity.[1,9,11,48,49] Horses that attempt to stand prematurely should be restrained or sedated (see Box 21-1). Horses should be visualized continuously, monitored (pulse quality and rate, color of mucous membranes, respiratory rate at 10-minute intervals), and assisted when necessary during the recovery period. Some horses may "dog sit" before standing (see Figure 21-5). Deviations from normal values should be evaluated and treated as soon as possible. Horses that attempt to stand too soon may require sedation, and those that do not stand within 60 minutes may require stimulation. Recovery is the time during which imperceptible complications directly or indirectly related to anesthesia and surgery make themselves apparent (see Chapter 22).

REFERENCES

1. Johnston GM et al: The confidential enquiry into perioperative equine fatalities (CEPEF): mortality results of phases 1 and 2, *Vet Anaesth Analg* 29:159-170, 2002.
2. Bidwell LA, Bramlage LR, Rood WA: Equine perioperative fatalities associated with general anaesthesia at a private practice—a retrospective case series, *Vet Anaesth Analg* 34(1): 23-30, 2007.
3. McCarty JE, Trim CM, Ferguson D: Prolongation of anesthesia with xylazine, ketamine, and guaifenesin in horses: 64 cases (1986-1989), *J Am Vet Med Assoc* 197(12):1646-1650,1990.
4. Trim CM, Adams JG, Hovda LR: Failure of ketamine to induce anesthesia in two horses, *J Am Vet Med Assoc* 190(2): 201-202, 1987.
5. McGreevy P, Hahn CN, McLean AN: *Equine behavior: a guide for veterinarians and equine scientists*, London, 2004. Saunders.
6. Houpt KA: The characteristics of equine sleep, *Equine Pract* 2:8-17, 1980.
7. Trim CM et al: A retrospective survey of anaesthesia in horses with colic, *Equine Vet J* 7:84-90, 1989.
8. Greene SA et al: Cardiopulmonary effects of continuous intravenous infusion of guaifenesin, ketamine, and xylazine in ponies, *Am J Vet Res* 47:2364-2367, 1986.
9. Richey MT et al: Equine post-anesthetic lameness: a retrospective study, *Vet Surg* 19:392-397, 1990.
10. Whitehair KJ et al: Recovery of horses from inhalation anesthesia, *Am J Vet Res* 54:1693-1702, 1993.
11. Grandy JL et al: Arterial hypotension and the development of postanesthetic myopathy in halothane-anesthetized horses, *Am J Vet Res* 48:192-197, 1987.
12. Auer JA et al: Recovery from anaesthesia in ponies: a comparative study of the effects of isoflurane, enflurane, methoxyflurane, and halothane, *Equine Vet J* 10:18-23, 1978.
13. Matthews NS et al: Comparison of recoveries from halothane versus isoflurane anesthesia in horses, *J Am Vet Med Assoc* 201: 559-563, 1992.
14. Taylor PM, Watkins SB: Stress responses during total intravenous anaesthesia in ponies with detomidine-guaiphenesin-ketamine, *J Vet Anaesth* 19:13-17, 1992.
15. Bettschart-Wolfensberger R et al: Physiologic effects of anesthesia induced and maintained by intravenous administration of a climazolam-ketamine combination in ponies premedicated with acepromazine and xylazine, *Am J Vet Res* 57:1472-1477, 1996.
16. Carroll GL et al: Maintenance of anaesthesia with sevoflurane and oxygen in mechanically ventilated horses subjected to exploratory laparotomy treated with intra- and post-operative anaesthetic adjuncts, *Equine Vet J* 30:402-407, 1998.

17. Mama KR et al: Comparison of two techniques for total intravenous anesthesia in horses, *Am J Vet Res* 59:1292-1298, 1998.
18. Matthews NS, Hartsfield SM, Mercer D: Recovery from sevoflurane anesthesia in horses: comparison to isoflurane and effect of postmedication with xylazine, *Vet Surg* 27:480-485, 1998.
19. Grosenbaugh DA, Muir WW: Cardiorespiratory effects of sevoflurane, isoflurane, and halothane anesthesia in horses, *Am J Vet Res* 59:101-106, 1998.
20. Donaldson LL et al: The recovery of horses from inhalant anesthesia: a comparison of halothane and isoflurane, *Vet Surg* 29:92-101, 2000.
21. Yamashita K et al: Combination of continuous intravenous infusion using a mixture of guaifenesin-ketamine-medetomidine and sevoflurane anesthesia in horses, *J Vet Med Sci* 62:229-235, 2000.
22. Taylor PM et al: Intravenous anaesthesia using detomidine, ketamine, and guaiphenesin for laparotomy in pregnant pony mares, *Vet Anaesth Analg* 28:119-125, 2001.
23. Read MR et al: Cardiopulmonary effects and induction and recovery characteristics of isoflurane and sevoflurane in foals, *J Am Vet Med Assoc* 221:393-398, 2002.
24. Wagner AE et al: Behavioral responses following eight anesthetic induction protocols in horses, *Vet Anaesth Analg* 29:207-211, 2002.
25. Spadavecchia C et al: Anaesthesia in horses using halothane and intravenous ketamine-guaiphenesin: a clinical study, *Vet Anaesth Analg* 29:20-28, 2002.
26. Bettschart-Wolfensberger R et al: Total intravenous anaesthesia in horses using medetomidine and propofol, *Vet Anaesth Analg* 32:348-354, 2005.
27. Mama KR et al: Evaluation of xylazine and ketamine for total intravenous anesthesia in horses, *Am J Vet Res* 66:1002-1007, 2005.
28. Valverde A et al: Effect of a constant rate infusion of lidocaine on the quality of recovery from sevoflurane or isoflurane general anaesthesia in horses, *Equine Vet J* 37:559-564, 2005.
29. Durongphongtorn S et al: Comparison of hemodynamic, clinicopathologic, and gastrointestinal motility effects and recovery characteristics of anesthesia with isoflurane and halothane in horses undergoing arthroscopic surgery, *Am J Vet Res* 67:32-42, 2006.
30. Umar MA et al: Evaluation of total intravenous anesthesia with propofol or ketamine-medetomidine-propofol combination in horses, *J Am Vet Med Assoc* 228:1221-1227, 2006.
31. Santos M et al: Effects of α_2-adrenoceptor agonists during recovery from isoflurane anaesthesia in horses, *Equine Vet J* 35:170-175, 2003.
32. Hubbell JA, Muir WW: Antagonism of detomidine sedation in the horse using intravenous tolazoline or atipamezole, *Equine Vet J* 38(3):238-241; 2006.
33. Clark L et al: The effects of morphine on the recovery of horses from halothane anesthesia, *Anaesth Analg* 35:22-29, 2008.
34. Wagner AE et al: A comparison of equine recovery characteristics after isoflurane or isoflurane followed by a xylazine-ketamine infusion, *Vet Anaesth Analg* 35:154-160, 2008.
35. Mason DE, Muir WW, Wade A: Arterial blood gas tensions in the horse during recovery from anesthesia, *J Am Vet Med Assoc* 190:989-994, 1987.
36. Ishihara A et al: Full body support sling in horses. Part 1: Equipment, case selection and application procedure, *Equine Vet Educ* 8:277-280, 2006.
37. Hubbell JAE: Recovery from anaesthesia in horses, *Equine Vet Educ* 11:160-167, 1999.
38. Ray-Miller WM et al: Comparison of recoveries from anesthesia of horses placed on a rapidly inflating-deflating air pillow or the floor of a padded stall, *J Am Vet Med Assoc* 229:711-716, 2006.
39. Elmas CR, Cruz AM, Kerr CL: Tilt-table recovery of horses after orthopedic surgery: fifty-four cases (1994-2005), *Vet Surg* 36:252-258, 2007.
40. Ishihara A et al: Full body support sling in horses. Part 2: Indications, *Equine Vet Educ* 8:351-360, 2006.
41. Taylor EL et al: Use of the Anderson sling suspension system for recovery of horses from general anesthesia, *Vet Surg* 34:559-564, 2005.
42. Schatzmann U et al: Historical aspects of equine suspension (slinging) and a description of a new system for controlled recovery from general anesthesia, *Proc Am Assoc Equine Pract* 41:62-64, 1995.
43. Schatzmann U: Suspension (slinging) of horses: history, technique and indications, *Equine Vet Educ* 10:219-223, 1998.
44. Liechti J et al: Investigation into the assisted standing up procedure in horses during recovery phase after inhalation anesthesia, *Pferdeheilkunde* 19(3):271-276, 2003.
45. Richter MC et al: Cardiopulmonary function in horses during anesthetic recovery in a hydropool, *Am J Vet Res* 62:1903-1910, 2001.
46. Sullivan EK et al: Use of a pool-raft system for recovery of horses from general anesthesia: 393 horses (1984-2000), *J Am Vet Med Assoc* 221:1014-1018, 2002.
47. Tidwell SA et al: Use of a hydropool system to recover horses after general anesthesia: 60 cases, *Vet Surg* 31:455-461, 2002.
48. Young SS, Taylor PM: Factors influencing the outcome of equine anaesthesia: a review of 1314 cases, *Equine Vet J* 25:147-151, 1993.
49. Duke T et al: Clinical observations surrounding an increased incidence of postanesthetic myopathy in halothane-anesthetized horses, *Vet Anaesth Analg* 33:122-127; 2006.

22

Anesthetic-Associated Complications

William W. Muir

John A.E. Hubbell

There are no safe anesthetic drugs, there are no safe anesthetic techniques, there are only safe anesthetists.

ROBERT SMITH

KEY POINTS

1. Horses have a higher incidence of morbidity and mortality in the perianesthetic period than other commonly anesthetized species.
2. The most common causes of mortality are cardiovascular arrest, fracture, and myopathy.
3. Most anesthetic-induced or related complications occur during the maintenance or recovery periods.
4. The incidence of complications increases in sick horses and is related to the duration of anesthesia and the complexity of the surgical procedure.
5. Anesthesia-associated morbidity and mortality rates are closely linked to the anesthetists' knowledge, skill, and experience.

Anesthetizing horses is risky business. Morbidity and mortality rates associated with equine anesthesia suggest that horses are at high risk for the development of a wide variety of anesthetic and anesthesia-associated complications.[1-7] Retrospective, prospective, and multicenter studies investigating anesthesia-associated adverse events and the various factors influencing the outcome of equine anesthesia suggest that horses are 10 times more likely to suffer an anesthesia-associated fatality than dogs and cats (>1 in 100 versus 1 in 1000) and 5000 to 8000 times more likely to die from anesthesia than humans (1 in 100 versus 1 in 500,000 to 800,000).[5,6,8,9] Fatality rates are even higher if the horse presents for anesthesia and surgery as an emergency (one in six) or for colic (one in three).[4,10-12] The largest prospective study to date, the Confidential Enquiry into Perioperative Equine Fatalities, evaluated over 40,000 equine anesthesias over a 6-year period and found an overall death rate of 1.9% within 7 days of anesthetic drug administration.[6] When horses with abdominal pain were excluded, the death rate fell to 0.9%. The leading causes of death were cardiac arrest or postoperative cardiovascular collapse, fractures, and myopathies.[2,6,8] Increased risk of death was associated with the type of surgery (fracture repair, colic), duration of anesthesia (higher risk for longer anesthesia time), timing of surgery (outside of regular hours), dorsal recumbency, not using a sedative for premedication, and age. Horses between the ages of 2 and 7 years old had a lower risk of death; foals younger than 1 month old had a greater risk.[6] The use of inhalant anesthetics increased the death rate in foals. Acepromazine and inject-able anesthetics were identified as potential risk-reducing agents.[6] However, the reduction of mortality when injectable anesthetic drugs were administered was confounded by shorter anesthesia times compared to those in which an inhalant anesthetic was administered. There was no difference in the death rate in adult horses administered halothane versus isoflurane.[7]

Although mortality rates are reported to be lower when equine anesthesia is performed in specialty surgery facilities or academic institutions, rates as high as 1 in 1000 to 1 in 10,000 are still reported.[5,8,9] Similarly, anesthesia-associated complications in otherwise normal horses range from 1 in 5 to 1 in 50, depending on the criteria used to judge anesthetic-associated events (Box 22-1).[3-5] Human error may be the most important cause for anesthetic-related complications, including death in horses; and one retrospective evaluation of equine mortality suggests that up to two thirds (>60%) of equine anesthesia–associated deaths are preventable.[3] Future studies should relate risk of morbidity and mortality to the horse's health status (see Table 6-4).

It is axiomatic that safe and effective equine anesthesia requires a thorough knowledge of the pharmacology of the drugs used to produce sedation, analgesia, and hypnosis and that the means to provide appropriate treatments are readily available. The horse's physical size, health status, and physiology notwithstanding, the most likely reasons for the aforementioned and unacceptably high anesthesia-associated morbidity and mortality rates are closely linked to the anesthetist's knowledge, skill, and experience; the duration and type of surgical procedure; the monitoring techniques used; and the availability of emergency therapies.

Anesthetic-related complications can occur at any time during induction, maintenance, or recovery from anesthesia. Eternal vigilance and incorporation of appropriate anesthetic monitoring techniques reduce the incidence of complications during all phases of anesthesia (see Chapter 8).

THE INDUCTION PHASE

Drug Administration

Trained and experienced personnel, appropriate facilities, and good equipment are key factors for providing safe anesthesia for horses. Inexperienced attendants assisting in the physical restraint of a horse may injure themselves, the veterinarian, and the horse. Mishaps from broken halters, ropes, or lead shanks can be avoided if high-quality equipment is used and kept in good repair. Complications associated with the administration of sedatives include broken needles, perivascular or intraarterial deposition of drugs, administration of inadequate doses, and unanticipated drug-related reactions.

| **Box 22–1** | **Anesthetic Complications** |

A. Induction phase
1. Injury to the horse or personnel
2. Incomplete or inadequate sedation
3. Excitement or startle responses
4. Perivascular or intraarterial injections
5. Intravenous air administration (air embolism)
6. Inability to place an orotracheal tube and laryngeal trauma
7. Hypoventilation/apnea/hypoxemia
8. Hypotension/poor perfusion
9. Cardiac arrhythmias
10. Incomplete or inadequate anesthesia
11. Drug reaction

B. Maintenance phase
1. Hypoventilation/apnea/hypoxemia
2. Hypotension/poor perfusion
3. Cardiac arrhythmias
4. Decreased tear production
5. Pain/tourniquet-induced hypertension
6. Inadequate anesthesia or alternating light and deep periods of anesthesia
7. Air embolism
8. Gastric reflux
9. Anesthetic equipment failure
10. Malignant hyperthermia-like reactions

C. Recovery phase
1. Hypoxemia/hypercapnia
2. Nasal edema or hemorrhage (labored breathing, "snoring")
3. Acute airway obstruction (laryngeal paralysis)
4. Hypotension/poor perfusion
5. Cardiac arrhythmias
6. Delirium or excitement
7. Pain
8. Hypocalcemia
9. Delayed recovery
10. Myopathy, myositis ("tying up")
11. Weakness, paralysis, paresis (facial, radial, femoral, nerves, myelopathies)
12. "Choke"
13. Colic
14. Acute hyperkalemic periodic paralysis
15. Pleuritis
16. Diarrhea
17. Temporary blindness
18. Cerebral necrosis

Perivascular and intraarterial injections are uncommon but generally produce disastrous results (see Chapter 7). The first indication of perivascular (extravascular) drug administration is a lack of drug effect (Figure 22-1). An intravenous catheter should always be preplaced and aspirated to ensure the appearance of venous blood before intravenous drug injection. If aspiration is unsuccessful, a large volume (500 to 1000 ml) of normal saline or a balanced electrolyte solution should be infused into the perivascular tissues to dilute any drug that was inadvertently administered and minimize tissue injury. The application of a hot pack may also help reduce swelling. The reaction to an intraarterial injection is immediate and described as the horse "falling off the needle." Intraarterial injection of sedatives or tranquilizers produces muscle rigidity followed by extensor rigidity, uncontrolled motor activity, recumbency, paddling, and convulsions. Therapy for intraarterial injections is symptomatic and supportive. The intravenous administration of diazepam (0.05 to 0.1 mg/kg) or the combination of guaifenesin (5%) and thiopental (0.4%) to effect may be required to control seizures and prevent self-induced trauma. If an inadvertent intraarterial injection occurs during induction to anesthesia, the procedure should be postponed.

Sedation

Producing adequate sedation may be the single most important factor determining safe and uneventful induction to anesthesia in horses. The appropriate use of sedatives, tranquilizers, and opioids alone or in combination decreases the potential for excitement and injury to the horse and personnel (see Chapter 10). The horse should be quiet and calm before attempting to produce anesthesia. Anesthetic drugs should never be administered to excited or stressed horses unless no other options are available (e.g., acute trauma, colic). Appropriate sedation markedly reduces the amount of anesthetic drug required to produce recumbency, thereby decreasing the potential for adverse events (see Chapters 11 and 13). Horses that are excited or stressed invariably require additional amounts of anesthetic drug, predisposing them to unnecessary cardiorespiratory depression. The choice of preanesthetic medication and route of administration is based on the horse's behavior, physical condition,

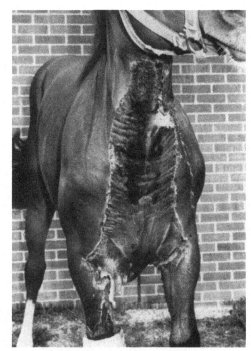

Figure 22–1. Sloughing of a horse's neck caused by the unintended perivascular administration of a 3-g bolus of thiopental.

and previous drug history. Hypotensive horses or horses that have hemorrhaged or lost an unknown quantity of blood should not be administered acepromazine unless adequately rehydrated. Acepromazine is more likely to cause hypotension and "fainting" in horses that are stressed and hypovolemic (see Chapter 10). Horses that are extremely lame or ataxic (fracture, "wobbler") should be moved or transported to the site of induction before the preanesthetic medication is administered to prevent falling and reduce the risk of self-inflicted trauma. Horses that remain excited can be administered incremental doses of xylazine (0.1 to 0.4 mg/kg intravenously [IV]) with or without infusions of guaifenesin (to effect; see Chapter 13). The anesthetic regimen and techniques chosen should produce a rapid transition from standing to recumbency.

The development of priapism has been and remains a major concern following the administration of phenothiazine tranquilizers to breeding stallions (see Chapter 10). This problem may have been more frequent when promazine and propriopromazine were more popular as sedatives in horses.[13-15] The dose of phenothiazine tranquilizer administered is likely to be related to the risk of priapism since it determines the magnitude and duration of drug effect, but no direct relationship has been established (see Figure 10-5).[14] Lower intravenous doses of acepromazine (5 mg or less) in adult horses are used to facilitate hand-walking and trailoring and allow cleaning of the penis and preputial cavity in breeding stallions. This dose is unlikely to produce either priapism or persistent flaccid penile prolapse since third eyelid prolapse, a more sensitive indicator of phenothiazine effect, is not observed. Nevertheless, the potential exists for acepromazine to cause priapism or flaccid paralysis of the penis in stallions and gelding. Horses that develop priapism should be treated symptomatically and promptly to prevent irreversible damage to the penis. Penile slings, bandaging, and massage are recommended as initial therapies. Flushing the corpus cavernosum penis with heparinized saline and the intravenous administration of benztropine mesylate (0.015 mg/kg; central acetylcholine antagonism) have been described as effective therapy for priapism.[16,17] Surgical treatment of priapism is a last resort.[18]

Producing Anesthesia

Failure to adequately respond to recommended doses of injectable anesthetics (thiopental, ketamine) can occur.[19] Inadequate sedation may be responsible for these occurrences. Other causes include extravascular administration of intravenous drugs, the administration of an insufficient dose, or loss of drug potency (see Figure 22-1 and Box 22-1). Extremely light levels of anesthesia are common during the first 10 to 20 minutes of inhalant anesthesia. Horses that hypoventilate or are apneic after administration of injectable anesthetics may not attain adequate alveolar concentrations of the inhalant anesthetic in a timely manner. The effects of the intravenous drugs may subside before inhalant anesthesia is established (see Chapters 9, 13, and 15). Surgical stimulation during this period may cause the horse to move, resulting in contamination of the surgical site or injury to the horse and attendants. The rapid administration of small doses of thiopental (0.5 to 1 mg/kg IV) or ketamine (0.2 to 0.4 mg/kg

IV) increases the depth of anesthesia within 30 to 90 seconds. Physical restraint (control of the head) may be required until intravenous drugs take effect (see Chapter 21). If the horse's muscle tone increases but the horse does not move, reduced doses of α_2-agonists (xylazine: 0.1 to 0.3 mg/kg IV) or valium-ketamine drug combination (0.025/ 0.5 mg/kg IV) may suffice, but their administration is unlikely to stop movement.

Breathing

Bolus injections of injectable anesthetic drugs can induce marked hypoventilation and apnea in horses (see Chapter 12). Drug-induced decreases in respiratory rate or volume (tidal or minute) produce hypoxemia (low PO_2) and hypercarbia (high PCO_2), leading to tissue acidosis (lactic acidosis, respiratory acidosis). Hypoventilation combined with decreases in pulmonary blood flow (low cardiac output) produces ventilation-perfusion mismatches in the lungs, compromising arterial PO_2 (PaO_2) and tissue oxygenation.[20] Ventilation-perfusion mismatching is exaggerated by both compression and absorption atelectasis once the horse becomes recumbent and especially when the horse is placed in a supine position.[21] Noxious stimuli (ear twist, slap on the neck, compression of the rib cage) can be used to initiate breathing in horses that become apneic, have normal pulses, and appear to be in a light plane of anesthesia. The use of a ventilatory assist device (demand valve, respirator) or the administration of doxapram (0.2 to 0.4 mg/kg IV) should be considered if cyanosis occurs or a normal breathing pattern (4 to 6 breaths/min) is not established within 3 to 5 minutes (see Chapter 17). A demand valve can be connected to an endotracheal tube (if available) or attached to a short length of tubing (10- to 15-mm diameter, 0.5 m in length) that is inserted into the ventral meatus of the nose (Figure 22-2). The demand valve is triggered manually while occluding both nostrils, causing the thoracic wall to rise. Release of the trigger and the nostrils after a suitable thoracic excursion allows the horse to expire. Alternatively, a nasogastric tube can be placed nasotracheally and attached to a compressed

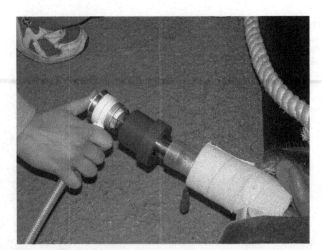

Figure 22–2. A demand valve can be attached to the endotracheal tube and used to ventilate adult horses and foals. Inspiratory time should be short (≤2 sec). The demand valve should be removed during exhalation so as not to impede expiration.

oxygen source. The nostrils are occluded as described previously. Excessive inspiratory pressures and times should be avoided, especially in foals.[22] Insufflation (>15 L/min) of oxygen (the instillation of oxygen flow into the airway) can be used to increase arterial oxygen tensions in ventilating horses but does not result in adequate oxygenation during apnea.[23]

Orotracheal intubation is easily performed blindly in most horses because the small diameter of the esophagus in comparison to that of the trachea provides dramatically greater resistance to advancement of the endotracheal tube. Proper placement of the endotracheal tube can be confirmed by feeling the passage of air at the end of the tube when the horse attempts to breathe, movement of the rebreathing bag if inhalant anesthetics are used, and capnometry (see Chapter 8). The distal end of the endotracheal tube should reach the midcervical trachea, anterior to the thoracic inlet. Overinflation of the endotracheal tube cuff can cause tracheal damage or the tube to collapse within the cuff (see Figure 14-9). Accidental endobronchial intubation is rare in adult horses but can occur in foals and miniature horses; it rarely produces abnormal blood gases.[24] The inability to place an orotracheal tube during a period of prolonged apnea is an emergency requiring tracheostomy (see Chapter 14). Finally, the head and neck should not be overextended (see Chapter 21). Overextension of the head and neck has been associated with laryngeal paralysis after surgery.[25] Kinking (e.g., overflexion of the head) or partial obstruction (e.g., mucus, blood) of the endotracheal tube

causes the horse to generate excessive pressures to breathe and can precipitate pulmonary edema.[26,27]

Blood Pressure and Tissue Perfusion

Hypotension and poor tissue perfusion can develop immediately after the bolus administration or inadvertent overdose of intravenous anesthetic drugs. Weak peripheral pulses; pale pink, pinkish-gray, or white mucous membranes; and an increased capillary refill time (>3 seconds) are signs of low arterial blood pressure and poor tissue perfusion (see Chapter 8). These clinical signs can be produced by poor cardiac contractile strength, vasodilation, or both and are exaggerated by preexisting disease. Occasionally cardiac arrhythmias, particularly bradycardia, are responsible for marked decreases in cardiac output and hypotension (see Chapters 3 and 8; Figure 22-3). α_2-Adrenoceptor agonists (xylazine, detomidine, romifidine) are noted for their ability to produce sinus bradycardia and second-degree atrioventricular block. Opioids may increase or decrease heart rate, depending on the dose and preexisting circumstances (pain, attitude). Acepromazine produces vasodilation, potentially decreasing arterial blood pressure and resulting in hypotension (see Chapter 10). Regardless of the cause, extended periods of hypotension and poor tissue perfusion must be avoided to prevent myopathy and shock. Mean arterial blood pressure should be maintained above 60 to 70 mm Hg. Treatment for an acute decrease in arterial blood pressure during induction to anesthesia includes fluids and vasopressors (ephedrine) if heart rate is normal or

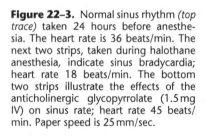

Figure 22–3. Normal sinus rhythm *(top trace)* taken 24 hours before anesthesia. The heart rate is 36 beats/min. The next two strips, taken during halothane anesthesia, indicate sinus bradycardia; heart rate 18 beats/min. The bottom two strips illustrate the effects of the anticholinergic glycopyrrolate (1.5 mg IV) on sinus rate; heart rate 45 beats/min. Paper speed is 25 mm/sec.

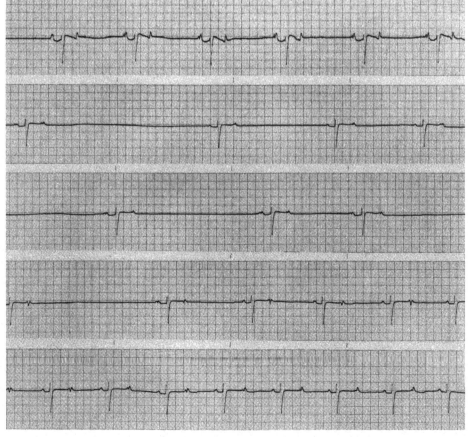

Table 22–1. **Pharmacological treatment of hypotension in horses**

Drug	Dose (IV)	Use	Effect
Fluids	20 ml/kg	Replace volume	Replace volume
Ephedrine	0.03-0.06 mg/kg	Treat hypotension	Increase force of cardiac contraction, vasoconstrictor
Dopamine	1-5 µg/kg/min	Treat hypotension Treat bradycardia	Increase force of cardiac contraction, vasoconstrictor, chronotope
Dobutamine	1-5 µg/kg/min	Treat hypotension	Increase force of cardiac contraction
Lidocaine	0.5-4 mg/kg	Treat cardiac arrhythmias	Antiarrhythmic
Glycopyrrolate	0.02-0.04 mg/kg	Treat bradycardia	Anticholinergic
Epinephrine	1-3 µg/kg/min	Treat severe hypotension and bradycardia	Inotrope, vasoconstrictor, chronotope

elevated and cardiovascular stimulants (epinephrine) when both arterial blood pressure and heart rate are decreased (Table 22-1).

THE MAINTENANCE PHASE

The maintenance phase of anesthesia is a balance between producing an adequate depth of anesthesia for surgery and preserving cardiorespiratory function. Allergic reactions to anesthetic drugs are rare. Some inhalant anesthetics are capable of producing toxic by-products (carbon monoxide [isoflurane], compound A [sevoflurane]) when they come in contact with outdated or exhausted CO_2 absorbents, depending on the temperature and moisture content of the absorbent and the inhalant anesthetic drug (see Chapter 15). However, concentrations of these metabolites are unlikely to reach clinical significance if the CO_2 absorbent is monitored and regularly replaced (Figure 22-4).[28,29] All injectable and inhalant anesthetics (halothane, isoflurane, sevoflurane, desflurane) are capable of producing decreases in heart rate (HR), bradyarrhythmias (sinus bradycardia, atrioventricular block), and vasodilation, resulting in hypotension (see Figure 22-3). Decreases in HR or cardiac contractile force decrease stroke volume (SV) and cardiac output (CO) (HR × SV = CO), further compromising arterial blood pressure (MAP = CO × vascular resistance). Injectable and inhalant anesthetics are also capable of producing a variety of supraventricular and ventricular arrhythmias, including the occasional development of atrial or ventricular premature depolarizations, atrial fibrillation, and ventricular tachycardia (Figures 22-5 and 22-6).[30,31] Systemic hypotension and hypotensive events (mean arterial blood pressure <50 to 60 mm Hg) are responsible for most drug-related complications during anesthesia in horses.[32,33] Marked reductions in mean arterial pressure and tissue blood flow (CO) are responsible for or contribute to the development of myopathy; myositis; rhabdomyolysis; "compartment syndrome"; spinal cord ischemia and degeneration; spinal cord malacia; cerebral necrosis; transient or permanent blindness; acute cardiac collapse; and, at the very least, prolonged and awkward recovery from anesthesia.[2,8,10,34-47] Optimum cardiorespiratory values should be maintained throughout maintenance and recovery from anesthesia (Box 22-2).

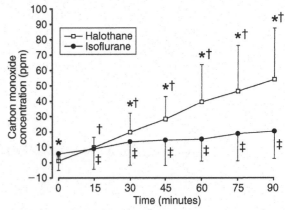

Figure 22–4. Carbon monoxide concentrations (ppm) in halothane- (□) isoflurane (•) anesthetized horses. Significant (P <0.05) difference between groups (∗). Significantly different (P<0.05) from time 0 (†,‡). (From Dodam JR et al: Inhaled carbon monoxide concentrations during halothane or isoflurane anesthesia in horses, *Vet Surg* 28:506-512, 1999.)

Breathing

Hypoventilation leading to arterial hypercapnia (high $PaCO_2$) is common during the maintenance phase of anesthesia followed by arterial hypotension. Most spontaneously breathing horses hypoventilate when anesthetized, especially when administered an inhalant anesthetic. Drug-induced decreases in respiratory rate or volume (tidal volume) produce hypercarbia, which, when severe, can result in hypoxemia, leading to acidosis (respiratory acidosis, lactic acidosis).[48,49] The $PaCO_2$ in most adequately anesthetized spontaneously breathing horses is routinely between 50 and 70 mm Hg. Interestingly, ponies trained to lie in lateral recumbency for 30 minutes do not develop significant increases in $PaCO_2$ and develop only minimal decreases in PaO_2, emphasizing the importance of consciousness on breathing and the depressant effects of anesthetic drugs.[50] The maximum value that the $PaCO_2$ should be allowed to increase before instituting controlled ventilation remains controversial, although values of 70 mm Hg are well tolerated (see Chapters 2 and 8). Increases in $PaCO_2$ have the potential to increase cardiac output, arterial blood pressure, and tissue perfusion secondary to sympathetic activation.[51,52]

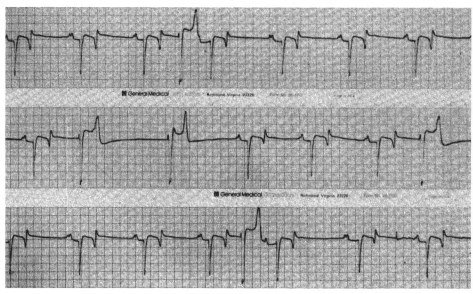

Figure 22–5. Interpolated premature ventricular depolarization *(top* and *bottom strips)* observed in a 510-kg Thoroughbred during halothane anesthesia during colic surgery. Three ventricular depolarizations are observed *(second, third,* and *last complexes)* in the middle strip. Ventricular premature depolarizations are very responsive to lidocaine (0.5 mg/kg IV) or quinidine (0.5 to1 mg/kg IV). Paper speed is 25 mm/sec.

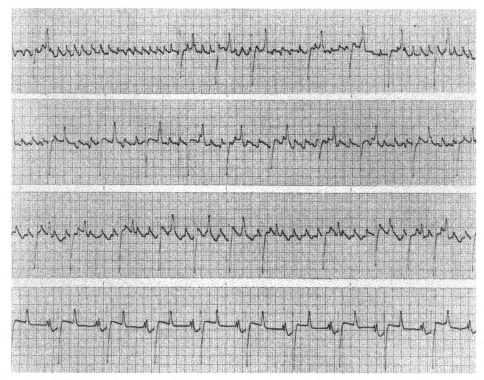

Figure 22–6. Electrocardiogram of atrial flutter-fibrillation that developed in a 518-kg Thoroughbred during halothane anesthesia and arthroscopic surgery. Note the flutter waves *(top three strips).* The ventricular rate varies between 35 and 60 beats/min. Normal sinus rhythm was produced *(bottom strip)* following the administration of three 200-mg bolus injections of intravenous quinidine gluconate. The heart rate is 55 beats/min. Paper speed is 25 mm/sec.

Arterial PCO_2 values greater than 70 mm Hg may activate the central nervous system, making it more difficult to maintain a stable plane of anesthesia, and result in signs that could be mistaken for insufficient anesthetic depth (muscle tensing, nystagmus, altered respiration).

Attempting to normalize $PaCO_2$ values in anesthetized adult horses by manually squeezing the rebreathing bag on an anesthetic machine is difficult because of operator fatigue. Assisted ventilation may increase tidal volume but does not always return $PaCO_2$ to normal values.[53] Initiating

Box 22–2 Goals During the Maintenance Phase of Anesthesia

- PaO_2 >200 mm Hg
- SpO_2 >90%
- $PaCO_2$ >35, <70 mm Hg
- Mean arterial blood pressure >70 mm Hg, <110 mm Hg
- pH >7.2, <7.45
- Temperature 37°-39° C
- Heart rate >30, <45
- Respiratory rate >4, <15
- Capillary refill time <2.5 seconds
- Pale pink mucous membranes
- Stable plane of anesthesia

Box 22–3 Methods Used to Improve PaO_2

- Increase the FiO_2 to 100%
- Control ventilation (f = 6-10 breaths/min; volume = 15 ml/kg)
- Increase cardiac output (reduce anesthetic, fluids, ephedrine, dobutamine)
- Change the horse's position
- Provide selective mechanical ventilation and PEEP
- Demand valve or Tygon tubing and >15 L/min O_2 (surgical facility or field anesthesia)

controlled ventilation early during the maintenance phase of anesthesia provides the best opportunity to rapidly transition to inhalant anesthesia, prevent hypercarbia, and maximize PaO_2 (see section on hypoxemia).[54] Controlled ventilation ensures the more consistent delivery of inhalant anesthetics, leading to a more stable plane of anesthesia. However, controlling ventilation does eliminate spontaneous breathing as an index of anesthetic depth and, if improperly performed, can decrease cardiac output and arterial blood pressure secondary to increases in intrathoracic pressure, which can decrease venous return.[53] Hypovolemia and arterial hypotension should be corrected before instituting positive-pressure ventilation (see Chapter 17).

Normal PaO_2 values in standing horses breathing air range from 95 to 110 mm Hg. The PaO_2 should approximate five times the inspired oxygen concentration. Thus an anesthetized horse breathing 95% oxygen should have a a PaO_2 value greater than 450 mm Hg (FiO_2 [95] × 5 = 475 mm Hg) and an SpO_2 value greater than 90%.[55] Potential causes for lower PaO_2 values in horses breathing 100% oxygen in the absence of hypoventilation include diffusion impairment, right-to-left vascular shunts, and ventilation-perfusion mismatching (see Chapter 2). Diffusion impairment and vascular shunts are unlikely to occur as the result of anesthesia. Cardiac output almost always decreases in anesthetized horses, contributing to ventilation-perfusion mismatch. Methods to increase cardiac output (intravenous fluids, inotropes) should be considered if hypoxemia is present but are not always effective therapy.[56,57]

Less than expected PaO_2 values occur in almost every anesthetized adult horse, whether or not O_2 is administered (Box 22-3). The insufflation of oxygen at a rate of 15 L/min marginally increases oxygen, with further improvements in PaO_2 produced by use of a demand valve. PaO_2 values are maximized by placing an endotracheal tube, sealing the airway, and attaching an oxygen source as described previously. A conventional anesthetic machine can be used to deliver oxygen. Currently the incorporation of a mechanical ventilator with oxygen concentrations in excess of 90% provides the highest alveolar oxygen tension possible. Selective endobronchial intubation and the application of selective positive end-expiratory pressure (PEEP), alveolar recruitment maneuvers, and bronchodilators offer alternative methods to increase PaO_2.[21] Conventional PEEP may increase PaO_2 and reduce atelectasis but can produce negative effects on cardiac output.[57-59] Alveolar recruitment

maneuvers produce marginal increases in PaO_2 in ponies; thus their use in horses deserves evaluation.[60] The use of bronchodilators such as salbutamol (2 µg/kg via the endotracheal tube) has been reported to increase PaO_2, but intravenous administration of clenbuterol has the opposite effect.[61,62] The only method that improves or restores PaO_2 to near-normal values in some horses is to change the horse's position from dorsal to lateral recumbency or from lateral to sternal recumbency.

Blood Pressure and Tissue Perfusion

Hypotension (mean arterial blood pressure <60 mm Hg) with or without hypoventilation is a common problem and can occur at any time in anesthetized horses. Hypotension is a direct result of the administration of anesthetic drugs, surgery (blood loss), and positioning and can be quantitatively assessed by indirect methods; but direct methods (cannulation of a peripheral artery) are more accurate and dependable (see Chapters 7 and 8; Table 22-2). Other factors contributing to hypotension include preexisting disease states (dehydration, hemorrhage, shock), acidosis and electrolyte abnormalities (hyperkalemia, hypocalcemia), and the development of cardiac arrhythmias. Adult horses anesthetized with halothane for 3.5 to 4 hours and with mean arterial blood pressures ranging from 50 to 65 mm Hg have marked increases in blood lactate and serum enzymes (creatine kinase, aspartate transaminase), indicative of muscle damage, and blood lactate.[33] These data suggest that the maintenance of mean arterial blood pressures below 60 mm Hg in conjunction with ineffective or poor padding is the likely cause of postanesthetic myopathies.

Hypotension during the maintenance phase of anesthesia should be treated immediately (see Tables 22-1 and 22-2; Table 22-3). The amount of anesthetic delivered should be evaluated and reduced when possible. The rate of fluid administration should be increased. Alternatively, colloidal solutions (5 to 10 ml/kg IV), hypertonic saline (7% saline, 4 ml/kg IV), or their combination may be administered (see Chapter 7).[63] Cardiovascular stimulants should be administered if fluid therapy is ineffective and anesthesia cannot be interrupted (see Table 22-3). Dobutamine is the preferred drug for increasing arterial blood pressure because of its rapid onset of action and controllability.[64-66] Dobutamine produces dose-dependent increases in cardiac output; arterial blood pressure; and renal, splanchnic, coronary, and skeletal muscle blood flow (Table 22-4 and Figure 22-7). Increases in heart rate usually do not occur in horses that have normal or near-normal circulating blood volume and may decrease when

Table 22–2.   Causes of and therapy for hypotension during anesthesia in horses

Cause	Therapy
Ineffective circulating volume	
1. Dehydration	1. Balanced electrolyte solutions
2. Hemorrhage	a. 10 ml/kg/hr increase as needed
3. Vasodilating drugs	b. 5-10 ml/kg 6% hetastarch for hypovolemia
	c. Maintain TP >3.5 g/dl
	d. Maintain PCV >20%
Anesthetic drugs	1. Reduce or terminate anesthetic drug administration
	2. Increase fluid administration (see preceding section)
	3. 1-5 µg/kg/min dopamine or dobutamine
	4. 10 mg IV boluses of ephedrine to effect
	5. 4 ml/kg IV 7% sodium chloride in 6% dextran 70
Acid-base and electrolyte abnormalities	
1. Metabolic acidosis	1. 1 mEq/kg NaHCO$_3$ to effect
2. Hyperkalemia	2. 0.9% NaCl to effect; 0.2 mg/kg calcium chloride
3. Hypocalcemia	3. 5-10 ml/100 kg calcium chloride 20 ml/100 kg calcium gluconate 0.1-0.2 g/kg IV calcium borogluconate
Cardiac arrhythmias	
1. Bradycardia (<25 beats/min)	1. 0.005 mg/kg IV glycopyrrolate (repeat twice)
2. Supraventricular arrhythmias	2. 1 mg/kg IV quinidine gluconate as needed to a total dose of 4 mg/kg
3. Ventricular arrhythmias	3. 0.5-4 mg/kg IV lidocaine HCl for ventricular arrhythmias only; 50 µg/kg/min

IV, Intravenously; *PCV,* packed cell volume; *TP,* total protein.

Table 22–3.   Hemodynamic effects of drugs used to increase blood pressure

Drug	Principal activity	Cardiac output	Arterial blood pressure	Heart rate	Vasoconstriction	Potential for arrhythmia	Diuresis
Epinephrine	β$_1$=β$_2$>α	↑↑	↑	↑↑	↑	↑↑↑	0
Dobutamine	β$_1$>β$_2$>α	↑↑	↑	0, ↑	High dose ↑	↑↑	0
Dopamine	D>β ↑ Dose α	↑↑	High dose↑	↑	↑	High dose↑	↑↑
Ephedrine*	α ≥ β$_2$	↑	↑	0, ↑	↑	↑	↑
Norepinephrine	β$_1$>α>β$_2$	0, ↑	↑↑	↑	↑↑	↑	↑
Phenylephrine	α	0	↑↑↑	0	↑↑↑	0	↓
Amrinone	Phosphodiesterase III	↑	↓, 0	0, ↑	0	↑	0
Milrinone	Inhibitors	↑	↓, 0	0, ↑	0	↑	0
Dopexamine	D>β$_2$>α	↑↑	↑	0, ↑	0	↑↑	↑

D, Dopamine receptors; ↑, increase; ↓, decrease; *0,* no change.
*Release norepinephrine from presynaptic storage sites.

lower infusion rates (<1 µg/kg/min) are used.[67] Larger doses (>3 µg/kg/min) usually produce marked increases in hemodynamic variables, including heart rate. Horses that are stressed, in pain, and hypovolemic (e.g., colic, trauma) may develop sinus tachycardia, suggesting the need for additional analgesic and fluid therapy, respectively. Finally, horses that require large doses (>5 µg/kg/min) of dobutamine or respond poorly to infusion rates greater than 5 µg/kg/min generally have a poor long-term prognosis. Dobutamine should be administered with a syringe infusion pump to minimize the potential for accidental overdose (Figure 22-8; see Table 22-4). It is capable of inducing ventricular arrhythmias, including ventricular tachycardia and ventricular fibrillation, although the probability of arrhythmias is less than when epinephrine is used. One study in which dobutamine was administered to 200 horses for the treatment of hypotension reported a 28% incidence of cardiac arrhythmias, which included sinus bradycardia, second-degree atrioventricular block, premature ventricular depolarizations, and isorhythmic dissociation.[67] Dobutamine should be used with caution in horses administered anticholinergics (atropine, glycopyrrolate) because of increased risk for the development of sinus tachycardia and ventricular arrhythmias.[68]

Table 22–4. Dobutamine in horses*

Dose (µg/kg/min)	Body weight (kg)								
	50	100	150	200	300	400	450	500	600
	Infusion rate (ml/hr)								
0.5	1.5	3	4.5	6	9	12	13.5	15	18
1.0	3	6	9	12	18	24	27	30	36
2.0	6	12	18	24	36	48	54	60	72
3.0	9	18	27	36	54	72	81	90	108
5.0	15	30	45	60	90	120	135	150	180

* These infusion rates (ml/hr) assume a dobutamine concentration of 1 mg/ml.
Infusion rate (ml/hr) = desired infusion rate µg/min ÷ concentration of the solution µg/ml (e.g., 1 µg/kg/min ÷ 1 mg [1000 µg/ml]
= 0.001 ml/kg/min × 60 = 0.06 ml/kg/hr; 0.06 ml/kg/hr × 450 = 27 ml/hr) (see chart).

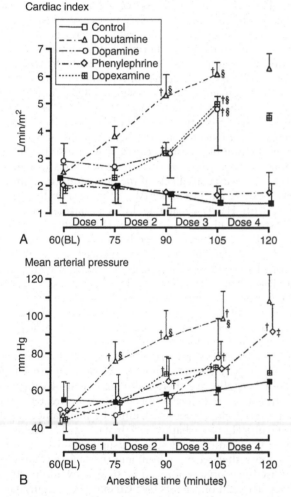

Figure 22–7. A, Change in cardiac index and **B,** mean arterial blood pressure in six halothane-anesthetized ponies. Dose 1 was 0.25, 2.5, 1, 0.5; Dose 2 was 0.5, 5, 2.5, 1; Dose 3 was 1, 10, 5, 5; Dose 4 was 2, 20, 10, 10 µg/kg/min for phenylephrine, dopamine, dobutamine, and dopexamine, respectively. Significantly (P=0.01) different from baseline *(BL)* (†). Significantly different (P<0.05) from saline (control) at the same time points (‡). Significantly different (P<0.01) from saline at the same time points (§). (From Lee Y-HL et al: Effects of dopamine, dobutamine, dopexamine, phenylephrine, and saline solution on intramuscular blood flow and other cardiopulmonary variables in halothane-anesthetized ponies, *Am J Vet Res* 59:1463-1472, 1998.)

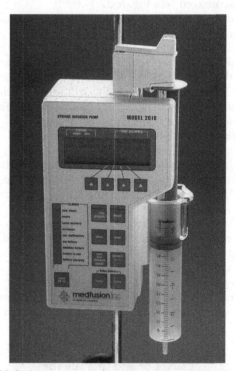

Figure 22–8. Battery-supported syringe infusion pumps simplify the administration of small quantities of drug once the machine is programmed with the animal's weight, the dose (µg/kg/min; µg/kg/hr; ml/hr), and the concentration of the solution (µg/ml; mg/ml).

Additional cardiovascular-stimulating drugs that have been advocated for the treatment of hypotension during anesthesia in horses include dopamine, calcium, ephedrine, epinephrine, dopexamine, milrinone, methoxamine, and phenylephrine (see Tables 22-1 and 22-3). Dopamine is more likely to induce tachycardia in horses and has been supplanted by dobutamine.[69-73] Ephedrine is effective therapy for the treatment of mild arterial hypotension but may take several minutes or repeated dosing to produce desired results.[74] Ephedrine increases heart rate, stroke volume, and arterial blood pressure.[75,76] The advantage of ephedrine is that it can be given as an intravenous bolus. Ephedrine crosses the blood-brain barrier and may decrease the depth of anesthesia secondary to increases in arterial blood pressure and central nervous system stimulating effects.

Calcium solutions (calcium chloride, calcium gluconate) improve cardiovascular function by increasing myocardial and vascular cytoplasmic calcium ion concentrations, but their effects are not pronounced and may not be immediate.[77] Dopexamine increases arterial blood pressure but offers no significant advantages over dobutamine and can produce profuse sweating and tachycardia.[78,79] Milrinone and similar drugs (inodilators) are phosphodiesterase III inhibitors, which inhibit the breakdown of cyclic adenosine monophosphate, thereby augmenting the force of cardiac contraction and producing arterial and venous vasodilation. To date the inodilators have not demonstrated advantages over dobutamine for the acute treatment of hypotension during anesthesia, although newer inotropes (levosimendan) require further investigation for this purpose. Methoxamine and phenylephrine increase arterial blood pressure but do not increase cardiac output or muscle blood flow; thus their use is discouraged (see Figure 22-7).[72,80,81]

Arterial hypertension is an infrequent but important complication that can occur during the maintenance phase of anesthesia. Inadequate anesthesia, increased $PaCO_2$, hypoxemia, pain, and hyperthermia individually or together can activate the sympathetic nervous system, resulting in hypertension. The use of a tourniquet to control hemorrhage can cause arterial hypertension.[82,83] Hypertension increases hemorrhage at the surgical site, triggers bradyarrhythmias, and makes it more difficult to keep horses anesthetized. Systolic arterial blood pressures in excess of 160 mm Hg should be avoided. Treatment of arterial hypertension should be directed toward the cause, although low doses of acepromazine (0.01 mg/kg IV) may facilitate a return to normal values without inducing hypotension (Table 22-5).

"Hot" horse and malignant hyperthermia-like reactions are reported to occur in anesthetized horses and can be triggered by stress, inhalant agents (especially halothane), and succinylcholine.[84-89] Horses that develop malignant hyperthermia-like reactions become tachycardic and tachypneic and sweat profusely. Their muscles become rigid, and myoglobin appears in the serum and the urine. They

develop severe metabolic and respiratory acidosis. Death follows with acute rigor mortis. The cause of the dramatic and rapid increase in body temperature has been linked to a gene mutation that produces an intracellular skeletal muscle membrane defect involving calcium and inappropriate binding and release of calcium by the sarcoplasmic reticulum.[88] The calcium release triggers a cascade of metabolic events leading to muscle contraction and heat production. Suggested treatments include discontinuation of anesthesia, isotonic fluids, external cooling, nonsteroidal antiinflammatory drugs, muscle relaxants, and dantrolene. Dantrolene decreases the amount of calcium released by the sarcoplasmic reticulum, but its use may result in excessive weakness and the inability to stand.[90,91]

Hyperkalemic periodic paralysis (HYPP) is a genetic disease of American Quarter Horses resulting in hyperkalemia caused by potassium efflux from skeletal muscle. Triggering events for HYPP include stress, sedation, and general anesthesia.[92] HYPP has been reported to occur during the maintenance and recovery phases of anesthesia.[93-95] Muscle fasciculations and sweating may occur. Heart rate may be decreased or normal but generally increases. Electrocardiographic signs associated with hyperkalemia (K^+ >6 to 7 mEq/L) include a reduced amplitude or absent P waves, a prolonged PR interval, widened QRS complex, and elevation of the ST segment. Differentials for HYPP include malignant hyperthermia and rhabdomyolysis. Treatment is directed toward decreasing the serum potassium concentration (sodium bicarbonate, dextrose with insulin) and the administration of calcium-containing solutions to counteract the cardiovascular effects of the potassium (calcium gluconate, 23%, 0.2 to 0.4 ml/kg IV).[94,95] Long-term therapy for horses with HYPP usually includes acetazolamide.[92] The HYPP status of all American Quarter Horses should be determined before anesthesia. Affected horses that are being administered acetazolamide can be anesthetized safely, although the risk of an HYPP episode remains. Calcium solutions should be available at all times when anesthetizing a horse with HYPP.

Less common complications associated with the maintenance phase of anesthesia include the development of cardiac arrhythmias, decreased tear production (dry cornea), and regurgitation.[31,94-98] The development of premature ventricular depolarizations and atrial fibrillation has been reported and may aggravate hypotension.[30,31] Lidocaine (1 to 2 mg/kg slowly IV) is effective therapy for treatment of ventricular arrhythmias. Atrial fibrillation need not be treated unless mean arterial blood pressure cannot be maintained greater than 60 mm Hg (see Chapter 3).[98] Instances of atrial fibrillation occurring during anesthesia usually resolve within 24 to 48 hours after recovery from anesthesia (see Chapter 3). Decreased tear production can be treated by administering tear replacement ointments (see Chapter 21). Regurgitation in the horse is rare and generally indicates gastric distention; it should be controlled by placing a nasogastric tube.

THE RECOVERY PHASE

The recovery phase of anesthesia is the least controllable component of the horse's overall anesthetic experience. The administration of intravenous fluids and oxygen and the use of assisted or controlled ventilation and quantitative monitoring devices (electrocardiogram, arterial blood pressure)

Table 22–5. Causes of and therapy for hypertension in horses

Cause	Therapy
Hypercarbia (↑$PaCO_2$)	Assist or control ventilation Check CO_2 absorbent
Hypoxemia (↓PaO_2)	Assist or control ventilation Increase FiO_2 and cardiac output
Pain (tourniquet)	0.1-0.3 mg/kg IV xylazine 0.01-0.03 mg/kg IV butorphanol 0.01-0.03 µg/kg IV fentanyl Administer a local anesthetic
Hyperthermia/stress	1-2 mg/kg IV dantrolene 0.02-0.05 mg/kg IV diazepam 1-2 mg/kg IV methocarbamol 0.1-0.3 mg/kg IV xylazine or 0.03-0.1 µg/kg IV detomidine 1-2 mEq/kg IV NaHCO₃ Fluid therapy

IV, Intravenously.

are usually stopped. Horses that recover unassisted require close observation (Figure 22-9). Previously established but inapparent problems, including but not limited to rhabdomyolysis, paresis, or upper airway obstruction, become manifest. Hypoventilation (hypercapnia), hypoxemia, hypotension, poor tissue perfusion, and cardiac arrhythmias are potential problems that argue strongly for close observation and frequent physical monitoring throughout the recovery phase (see Chapter 8; Table 22-6). Recovery should be observed at all times after discontinuation of anesthetic drugs and should occur with a minimum of external stimuli (noise, external manipulation) under subdued light (see Chapter 21). The recovery stall should be equipped with electrical, oxygen, and suction outlets and a means to provide continuous intravenous fluids. Emergency drugs and equipment should be organized and kept in close proximity to the recovery stall.

Breathing

Hypoventilation and hypoxemia can occur during the recovery phase, particularly if the horse was hypoxemic during the maintenance phase of anesthesia. It is difficult, inconvenient, and many times impractical to keep the horse attached to an anesthetic machine (if used) during recovery from anesthesia. Most horses begin to breath regularly once the $PaCO_2$ increases to values above 60 mm Hg.[48,99] Weaning the horse from a ventilator (if used) should occur before the horse is moved to the recovery stall. A demand oxygen delivery system can be used to ventilate horses that develop apnea or hypoventilate in the recovery stall (see Chapters 14 and 17). Oxygenation can be supplemented by a demand valve or with nasal or tracheal oxygen (15 l/min) insufflation.[23]

Nasal congestion leading to partial or complete airway obstruction becomes apparent once the orotracheal tube

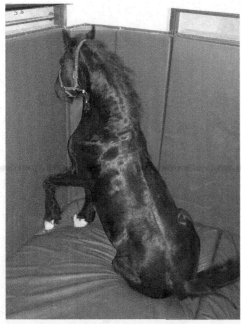

Figure 22–9. Some horses "dog sit" before standing. They may obstruct their nostrils (head in corner), which obstructs breathing and leads to hypoxia, excitement, and stress if they are not assisted or moved to a different position. (Courtesy of New England Equine MSC, Dover, NH.)

is removed (Table 22-7). Head edema is a sign that nasal congestion and edema may become problems during recovery. Nasal congestion occurs more frequently in horses that are positioned on their back (supine) and is exacerbated by the administration of α_2-adrenoceptor agonists during the recovery process.[100] The severity of congestion depends on the position of the head relative to the body (head down is worse) during the maintenance phase and the duration of anesthesia. The consequences of nasal congestion should not be underestimated.[27] Progressive or acute upper airway obstruction can occur any time during or after the recovery from anesthesia in horses with partial airway obstruction. The endotracheal tube should not be removed until the horse is swallowing actively or standing so that the horse will replace the epiglottis to its normal position above the soft palate. Although laryngeal paralysis or laryngospasm is relatively uncommon during recovery from anesthesia, both require an immediate response. Clinical signs of acute airway obstruction vary, depending on the depth of anesthesia at the time the horse is extubated; but labored breathing with inspiratory dyspnea (extreme abdominal lift), retraction of the nares and facial muscles, and tachycardia can progress to sweating and violent movements (thrashing, kicking). If adequate airflow is not restored, convulsions and pulmonary edema may occur before cardiovascular collapse and death. If attempts to place a nasotracheal or orotracheal tube are unsuccessful, a tracheostomy should be performed. Treatment includes placing an orotracheal tube or inserting a 12- to 14-mm internal diameter tube (20 to 30 cm in length) into one or both nares and administering oxygen (see Chapters 14, 17, and 21). The nasal tube should be advanced into the ventral meatus past the area of obstruction (15 to 20 cm) and secured to the halter. The tube can be removed after the horse stands. Spraying the nasal turbinates with phenylephrine has been suggested to reduce congestion and promote the passage of air, but the response is often inconsistent and inadequate.[101]

Pulmonary edema can occur in horses that experience respiratory obstruction during recovery.[26,27] The development of pulmonary edema is rapid and suggested by the development of tachypnea, tachycardia, hypoxemia, hypercapnia, and the discharge of pink fluid or foam from the nostrils or endotracheal tube. The pathogenesis is unclear but most likely related to the generation of significant negative intrathoracic pressures during the attempts to ventilate against an obstructed airway.[26,102] The obstruction should be relieved immediately by passing a nasotracheal tube or performing a tracheostomy. Oxygen and furosemide (1 mg/kg IV) should be administered to increase PaO_2 and redistribute fluid away from the lung, respectively. Sedation (acepromazine 0.02 to 0.04 mg/kg IV) may be required to reduce anxiety. Thoracic radiography and arterial blood gas analysis aid in determining the severity and consequences of edema and the response to therapy.

Postanesthetic neuromuscular damage is always a potential complication of anesthesia in horses and may become manifest as minor forelimb lameness, resulting in inconsequential ataxia during recovery to severe myopathy or bilateral hind limb paralysis.[35,36,43,103,104] Multiple factors are responsible for the development of neuromuscular abnormalities, including the duration of the anesthetic period, the horse's weight and nutritional status, the anesthetic

Table 22–6　Complications during recovery

Complication	Detection	Treatment	Results
Excitement premature attempts to stand	Flailing Disorganized attempts to stand Rapid nystagmus Rapid respirations Vocalization	Intravenous sedation (small doses, i.e., xylazine 0.2 mg/kg) Physical restraint until sedatives take effect	Recovery prolonged Subsequent attempts usually calmer and more controlled
Hypotension	Delayed awakening or deepening level of sedation Rapid heart rate/weak pulses Low blood pressure (if being measured)	Intravenous fluids (5 to 10 LRS) Vasoactive substances (dobutamine, ephedrine)	Recovery prolonged Support may need to be continued after standing
Hypoxia	Poor color Rapid respiratory rate	Oxygen supplementation Assisted ventilation Reversal of respiratory depressants	May be no long-term sequelae if brief Potential for blindness (temporary or permanent)
Respiratory obstruction	Increased respiratory noise Rapid respiratory rates Malposition of the head and neck (extreme flexion) Excitement	Relieve obstruction Place nasotracheal or endotracheal tube Tracheostomy (if not relieved by above) Correct malposition Supplement oxygen Assist ventilation	May be no long-term sequelae if brief
Pulmonary edema	Rapid respiratory rates Fluid from nostrils Increased bronchovesicular sounds	Anticipate pulmonary edema Supplement oxygen Administer diuretics (furosemide) Bronchodilators Suction to remove fluid as necessary	Mild cases resolve with diuretics and bronchodilators Extensive involvement may be fatal
Fracture/dislocation	Cracking noise Inability to use one or more legs Pain behavior Abnormal limb angulation	Reanesthetize if necessary for evaluation Immobilize injury if possible Treat pain	Dependent on the injury and prognosis
Weakness	Inability to stand despite appropriate placement of limbs	Increase cardiac output (fluids and inotropes) Consider antagonism of sedatives Check electrolytes (hypocalcemia, hyperkalemia) Check plasma glucose Hypothermia (sedate if necessary)	Prolonged recovery Depends on horse's demeanor (better prognosis with cooperative patient)

	Signs	Treatment	Prognosis
Rhabdomyolysis	Inability or unwillingness to stand on one or more legs Sweating Hardened muscle bellies Horse uses a limb for a brief period, then collapses (tachycardia) Pain behavior Coffee-colored urine	Large volumes of balanced electrolytes (produce diluted urine) Correction of acid-base abnormalities Diazepam (0.02-0.04 mg/kg, IV) for muscle relaxation Acepromazine (0.01-0.03 mg/kg) for calming Nonsteroidal antiinflammatory drugs Apply a sling/support bandages	Depends on demeanor Better if a single limb is affected Usually respond in 12 to 24 hours
Nerve paralysis	Inability or unwillingness to stand on one or more legs Inability to extend the legs or "fix" the stifle or the elbow Apparent anxiety	Nonsteroidal antiinflammatory drugs Support bandages Apply a sling Acepromazine (0.01-0.03 mg/kg) for calming Examination for location of dysfunction (apply dimethyl sulfoxide) Corticosteroids?	Depends on demeanor Better if a single limb is affected Usually respond in 12 to 24 hours
Hyperkalemic periodic paralysis	Quarter Horse Well muscled Trembling, fasciculations Weakness Recumbency Tachycardia or bradycardia Hyperthermia Altered electrolytes (increased potassium) Metabolic acidosis	Large volumes of normal saline (reduce serum potassium) Calcium supplementation Correction of acid-base abnormalities (sodium bicarbonate) Correct arrhythmias if present Epinephrine if bradycardic	Incurable Likely to recur with or without anesthesia Acetazolamide for maintenance
Spinal cord degeneration	Dorsal recumbency Flaccid paralysis Areflexia Absence of tail or anal tone Apparent analgesia of affected area Incontinence Loss of panniculus	Supportive care (fluids, correction of electrolyte abnormalities) Gauge response to therapy Rule out other diagnoses	No known effective therapy Diagnosis obtained at postmortem

IV, Intravenously; *LRS*, lactated Ringer's solution.

Table 22–7. **Causes of and therapy for acute partial or complete airway obstruction in horses**

Cause	Therapy
Pharyngeal, laryngeal, tracheal secretions	Suction
Displaced soft palate	Replace orotracheal tube
Nasal edema	Elevate head intraoperatively and during recovery
	Maintain tracheal intubation until standing
	Digitally hold the nostrils open
	1 mg/kg IV furosemide
	5-10 mg intranasal phenylephrine diluted in 10 ml of sterile water
Elongated soft palate	Maintain tracheal intubation until standing
Partial or complete laryngeal paralysis	Establish an airway
	Nasal or oral intubation
	Tracheostomy
	Symptomatic/supportive
	1 mg/kg IV furosemide
	1-3 mg/kg IV dexamethasone
	2-5 µg/kg IV epinephrine
	IV fluids to effect
	0.1-0.2 mg/kg IV xylazine

IV, Intravenously.

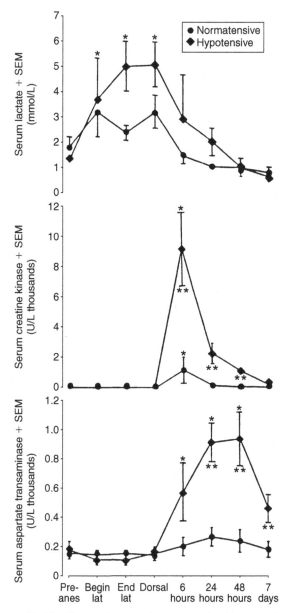

Figure 22–10. Changes in serum lactate, creatine kinase, and aspartate transaminase in horses subjected to normotensive (80 to 90 mm Hg) and hypotensive (50 to 55 mm Hg) halothane anesthesia. *Different from baseline; **different from normotensive. (Modified from Lindsay WA et al: Induction of equine post-anesthetic myositis after halothane induced hypotension, *Am J Vet Res* 50:404, 1989.)

drugs selected, position, padding, the use of restraining devices, dehydration, hemorrhage, electrolyte imbalances (hypocalcemia), hypoxemia, hypotension, and poor tissue perfusion. The development of hypotension during the maintenance phase of anesthesia is a major cause of neuromuscular problems during recovery (see Chapter 21 and Figure 21-6).[33,104] The incidence of postanesthetic rhabdomyolysis is unknown but is known to be linked to hypotension, although it can occur in the absence of hypotension (Figure 22-10). Furthermore, its occurrence may not be overly influenced by the underlying surface (Figure 22-11).[32] Rhabdomyolysis and nerve dysfunction may be difficult to differentiate, but both produce a horse that is weak and reluctant or incapable of supporting weight on one or more legs. Rhabdomyolysis produces hardened muscles, extreme pain, and the appearance of myoglobin in the plasma and urine (coffee-colored urine). Nerve paralysis can result in the development of rhabdomyolysis in the supporting limb. Therapy is directed toward the restoration of skeletal muscle perfusion. Dobutamine, intravenous fluids, muscle relaxants, mild vasodilation, and alkalinizing the urine help to improve skeletal muscle blood flow and promote diuresis, limiting the precipitation of myoglobin in the renal tubules (Figure 22-12). Other therapies include tranquilization, analgesics, and the use of slings (see Chapter 21; Table 22-8). Low doses of acepromazine (0.02 to 0.04 mg/kg IV) and fluid therapy are used to calm the horse and promote peripheral perfusion, respectively. Small doses of diazepam (0.04 to 0.05 mg/kg IV) help to relieve muscle cramping. Nonsteroidal antiinflammatory drugs (phenylbutazone, flunixin) relieve pain and inflammation but should be used with caution because of their potential to cause gastrointestinal ulceration and renal tubular damage. Dantrolene, a skeletal muscle relaxant that reduces calcium release from intracellular sites, may help to relax skeletal muscle and improve skeletal muscle blood flow but can cause muscle weakness, contributing to the horse's difficulty in standing.[90,91]

Facial, radial, or femoral nerve paralysis can occur in horses after anesthesia (Figure 22-13). Radial and femoral nerve paralysis may be difficult to differentiate from rhabdomyolysis and most likely results from inappropriate pressure on the affected nerve.[35-37] Horses that develop

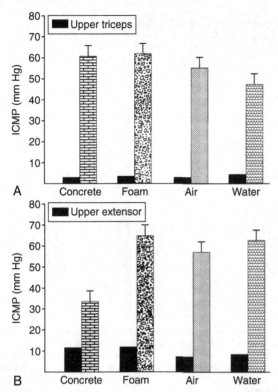

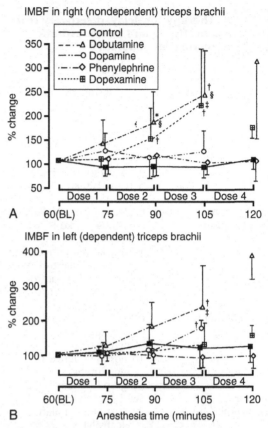

Figure 22–11. Intracompartmental muscle pressures *(ICMP)* within the upper (■) and lower long heads of **A,** the triceps brachii and **B,** the extensor carpi radialis muscles from eight horses. All pressures in the lower limbs exceeded the critical closing pressure (30 mm Hg), regardless of surface. Extension of the lower limb and elevation of the upper limb reduce ICMP and aid in venous return. (From Lindsay WA et al: Effect of protective padding on forelimb intro-compartmental muscle pressures in anesthetized horses, *Am J Vet Res* 46:688, 1985.)

Figure 22–12. Improvement in intramuscular blood flow *(IMBF)* in **A,** right (nondependent) and **B,** left (dependent) triceps brachii muscles of six halothane-anesthetized ponies. Note that only dobutamine produced significant increases in IMBF in the dependent limb at clinically relevant doses. Dose 1 was 0.25, 2.5, 1 0.5; Dose 2 was 0.5, 5, 2.5, 1; Dose 3 was 1, 10, 5, 5; Dose 4 was 2, 20, 10, 10 µg/kg/min for phenylephrine, dopamine, dobutamine, and dopexamine, respectively. Significantly different µ($P<0.05$) from baseline *(BL)* (∗). Significantly different ($P<0.05$) ($P=0.01$) from baseline (†). Significantly different from saline (control) at the same time points (‡). Significantly different ($P<0.01$) from saline at the same time points (§). (From Lee Y-HL et al: Effects of dopamine, dobutamine, dopexamine, phenylephrine, and saline solution on intramuscular blood flow and other cardiopulmonary variables in halothane-anesthetized ponies, *Am J Vet Res* 59:1463-1472, 1998.)

nerve paralysis and are not painful are less likely to have hot, hard, or swollen muscles. Facial (cranial nerve VII), forelimb (brachial plexus and radial nerve paralysis), and hind limb (femoral or peroneal nerve paralysis) extensor deficits can occur but have become less common with improved padding and position techniques (Figure 22-14).[35-37] Horses with unilateral neurological deficits usually begin to recover limb function within 24 to 48 hours but may remain noticeably lame for days. Treatment is supportive (fluids, slings, message, analgesics) and designed to keep the horse comfortable until function returns. The topical application of dimethylsulfoxide gel may help to reduce inflammation.

Spinal cord degeneration following general anesthesia in horses (particularly Draft breeds) has been reported.[38-42] The presumptive diagnosis is made on the basis of paraplegia, loss of hind limb deep pain, and a loss of anal tone. Definitive diagnosis is made during postmortem examination and includes ischemic neuronal changes in the spinal cord that resemble poliomyelomalacia. The lesion may occur because of compromised perfusion or oxygenation of the spinal cord during anesthesia, although a specific cause has not been identified. The disease is of low incidence; thus no preventive measures have been identified.

OTHER COMPLICATIONS

Equipment

Almost every piece of equipment that has been developed or used to produce anesthesia in horses has been responsible for the development of an anesthesia-associated complication. Hypodermic needles are responsible for inadvertent subcutaneous infections, intramuscular fibrosis, jugular vein thrombosis, venous and arterial hematomas, local and systemic infections and venous abscessation. Intravascular catheters have produced thrombophlebitis, jugular vein thrombosis, venous and arterial hematomas, local and systemic infections, arterial obstruction, and distal tissue infection and necrosis.[105,106] The orotracheal placement of an endotracheal tube has produced retroversion and trauma of the epiglottis; tracheal, pharyngeal, and laryngeal mucosal damage and ischemic damage to the tracheal wall; and laryngeal dysfunction and partial or complete bilateral arytenoid cartilage paralysis leading to acute or delayed upper airway obstruction.[107-109]

Problem	Therapy*
Prolonged recumbency	Physical therapy, massage Change position Sling Splint legs
Dehydration/acidosis/ hypocalcemia	10-20 ml/kg IV balanced electrolytes 1-2 mEq/kg IV NaHCO₃ 5-10 ml/100 kg IV calcium chloride (%)
Muscle damage/ rigidity/spasm	0.01-0.2 mg/kg IV diazepam 0.02-0.04 mg/kg IV acepromazine 1-2 mg/kg IV methocarbamol 1-2 mg/kg IV dantrolene 5-10 mg/kg PO dantrolene 1 mg/kg IV dimethylsulfoxide in 5% dextrose
Stress/excitement/ pain	0.1-0.2 mg/kg IV xylazine 0.05-0.1 μg/kg IV detomidine 10 mg/kg IV flunixin meglumine 5 mg/kg IV phenylbutazone
Hypotension/ hypoxemia/shock	See Tables 22-2 to 22-4 20-40 ml/kg IV balanced electrolytes 4 ml/kg IV 7% NaCl in 6% dextran or hetastarch 1-3 mg/kg IV dexamethasone Antibiotics

Table 22–8. Therapy for delayed recovery from anesthesia and postanesthetic myopathy in horses

IV, Intravenously; *PO*, orally.
*Therapy may be repeated as necessary.

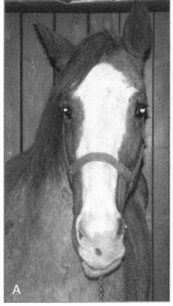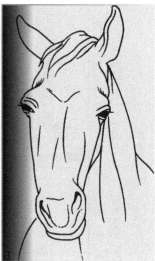

Figure 22–13. A and **B**, Paralysis of various branches (auricular, palpebral, buccal) of the right facial nerve. Pressure from improper padding or a halter could injure the buccal branches of the facial nerve, causing paralysis and distortion of the nose and lips. The ear and eyelid may droop because of pressure on the auricular and palpebral nerves, respectively.

Nasotracheal intubation or placement of a nasogastric tube can produce profuse bleeding, nasal and pharyngeal mucosal irritation, and laryngeal inflammation.[110,111]

Inhalant anesthetic machines may not function properly. Out-of-the-circle precision anesthetic vaporizers may deliver anesthetic concentrations that are too high or too low if used at temperatures and operated to flow rates that

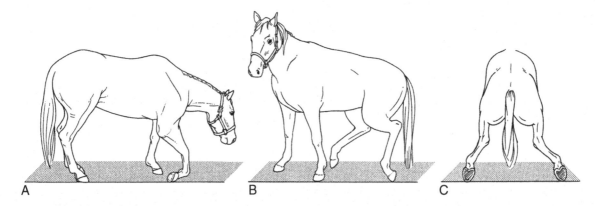

Figure 22–14. A, Horses with injury to the brachial plexus and radial nerve or with triceps myositis and partial radial nerve injury display a dropped elbow. The horse may not be able to bear weight and can advance the limb only by flipping the whole brachial region forward (brachial plexus or radial nerve injury). Partial weight bearing is observed during triceps myositis and preservation of partial radial nerve conduction. **B** and **C,** Horses with bilateral femoral nerve paralysis. The hock and fetlock are flexed, and the stifle cannot be fixed. Horses with either sciatic or peroneal nerve paralysis may demonstrate a similar posture. (Modified from Dyson S et al: Femoral nerve paralysis after general anesthesia, *Equine Vet J* 20:376, 1988.)

exceed their compensatory limits. Precision vaporizers that are left in cold environments frequently deliver less than the concentration on the vaporizer dial. Inhalation and, more important, one-way exhalation valves can become stuck in the open position, resulting in the rebreathing of exhaled gases, hypercarbia, abdominal breathing, and severe respiratory acidosis.[112] The horse's increased respiratory rate and efforts to breathe may be interpreted as a sign of "light" anesthesia, resulting in the inappropriate increase in the delivery of the inhalant anesthetic, potentially impairing cardiovascular function. The interaction of the inhalant anesthetic with exhausted CO_2 absorbent material (baralyme, sodalyme) is capable of producing carbon monoxide (isoflurane) or compound A (sevoflurane), both of which are potentially toxic (see Figure 22-4).[28,29] The use of a mechanical ventilator has the potential to decrease cardiac output and arterial blood pressure as a result of the production of positive pressure within the thoracic cavity during the inspiratory phase of ventilation, thereby limiting venous return.[53] Anesthetic machines that cannot hold a positive pressure when the pressure relief (pop-off) valve is closed or endotracheal tubes that do not seal the trachea and allow room air to enter the anesthetic circuit, thus diluting inhalant anesthetic concentrations, make it difficult to maintain steady-state anesthetic concentrations and a stable plane of anesthesia. Stuck pop-off valves and small holes in the ventilator bellows may allow anesthetic circuit pressures or driving gas pressures from the ventilator to produce overly high inspiratory pressures, increasing the potential for pulmonary barotrauma (see Chapter 17).

Hospitalization and Surgery

The invasiveness and duration of surgery, severity of pain, amount of blood lost, surgical technique (e.g., arthrotomy, arthroscopy, laparoscopy) and type of surgery (e.g., ocular, reproductive, gastrointestinal) independently or together can be responsible for anesthesia-associated adverse events (Table 22-9). Invasive and prolonged surgical procedures

Table 22–9.   Treatment of anesthesia-associated complications

Problem	Drug	Dose
Hypotension	Lactated Ringer's solution (LRS) and/or 6% hetastarch	10-20 ml/kg LRS IV; 5ml/kg 6% hetastarch (repeat if necessary)
Acepromazine	Phenylephrine	0.2-0.4 µg/kg/min IV Dilute; 20 µg/ml, 50-100 ml/min/500 kg IV
Anesthetic	Dobutamine	1-2 µg/kg/min IV to effect; 0.5mg/ml, 1-2ml/min
	Ephedrine	20-40 µg/kg IV bolus dilute; 5 mg/ml
	Calcium	0.1-0.2 mEq/kg IV or calculated extracellular deficit Undiluted; slowly over 5-30min
Sepsis	Norepinephrine	0.1-0.2 µg/kg/min dilute; 4 µg/ml, 25-50 ml/min
Cardiac collapse/arrest	Epinephrine	5-10 µg/kg IV bolus undiluted
Hemorrhage	Lactated Ringer's solution	10-20 ml/kg IV
	Hypertonic saline	4 ml/kg IV
	Hetastarch	5 ml/kg IV up to 20 ml/kg as needed
	Blood	
Cardiac arrhythmia	Atropine	0.01-0.02 mg/kg IV
Sinus bradycardia	Glycopyrrolate	0.005 mg/kg
Atrial fibrillation	Quinidine	4.0 mg/kg IV given 1 mg/kg every 10 min until a total of 4 mg/kg
Ventricular arrhythmias	Lidocaine	0.5 mg/kg IV, slowly; 50 µg/kg/min
Hypertension	Acepromazine	0.1 mg/kg IV
	Fentanyl	5-10 µg/kg/hr
Hypoxemia	O_2	15 L/min/450 kg
Hypoventilation	Ventilation	Tidal volume approx 10-15 ml/kg; respiration rate = 6 min
Ventilation-perfusion mismatch	Dobutamine	1-2 µg/kg/min dilute; 0.5 mg/ml, 1-2 ml/min
	Positive end-expiratory pressure (PEEP)	Temporary 10-15 cm H_2O PEEP
	Recruitment maneuver	Sustained lung expansion: 20-30 cm H_2O
Apnea/hypercarbia	Doxapram	0.2 mg/kg IV
	Ventilation	10-15 ml/kg
	Demand valve	
Laryngeal paralysis	Tracheotomy	
Nasal edema	Nasopharyngeal tube	
Pulmonary edema	Acepromazine	0.1 mg/kg IV
	Oxygen	15 L/min/450 kg
	Furosemide	0.2-0.5 mg/kg IV
Ileus	Lidocaine	2 mg/kg IV 50 µg/kg/min IV
	Metoclopramide	1 mg/kg IM

(Continued)

Table 22–9. Treatment of anesthesia-associated complications—Cont'd

Problem	Drug	Dose
Postoperative colic	α₂-Agonist	See below
	Mineral oil	
	Lidocaine	50 mg/kg/min IV
Postoperative tympany	Atipamazole	100 µg/kg IV
Myopathy	Lactated Ringer's solution	10-20 ml/kg/min IV
	Acepromazine	0.05 mg/kg IV
	Diazepam	0.05-0.1 mg/kg IV
	Furosemide	0.2-0.5 mg/kg IV
	Dantrolene	5-10 mg/kg PO
Pain	Xylazine	0.4-1 mg/kg
	Detomidine	0.01-0.02 mg/kg
	Medetomidine	5-20 µg/kg
	Romifidine	0.08-0.12 mg/kg
	Morphine	0.04-0.1 mg/kg
	Lidocaine	1-2 mg/kg slowly; 50 µg/kg/min
Hyperthermia	Lactated Ringer's solution	10-20 ml/kg/min IV
	Insulin/glucose	0.1 U/kg IV, 0.5-1 g/kg IV
	Dantrolene	1 mg/kg IV until body temperature and HR begin to decrease
		Given in increments of 2-3 mg/kg IV
Priapism	Benztropine	10-15 µg/kg IV
Allergic reaction	Tripelennamine	0.04 mg/kg/hr
	Ephedrine	20-40 µg/kg IV
	Epinephrine	0.05-1 µg/kg IV

HR, Heart rate; *IM,* intramuscularly; *IV,* intravenously; *PEEP,* positive end-expiratory pressure; *PO,* orally.

are more likely to result in nerve and muscle damage, require a longer time for drug metabolism and elimination, and are associated with a greater degree of stress-related and metabolic disorders (e.g., hypoglycemia, hypocalcemia, hyperlactatemia) than shorter, less invasive surgeries (Figure 22-15).[6,113] Hospitalization and/or surgery alone or together may predispose horses to ileus and colic.[114] The infusion of lidocaine (50 µg/kg/min) may help prevent postoperative ileus.[115] Surgical procedures involving the reproductive organs, bladder, or gastrointestinal tract predispose to increases in parasympathetic tone, resulting in sinus bradycardia, bradyarrhythmias, and hypotension. Visceral (e.g., gastric tympany, distended bladder) and orthopedic (e.g., fractured olecranon, arthrodesis) pain can produce premature and multiple attempts to stand during recovery. Pain activates the sympathetic nervous system, leading to tachypnea, tachycardia, anxiety, and stress.[116,117] Surgically induced blood loss (e.g., guttural pouch, nasal sinus) exceeding 20% of total blood volume (>15 mg/kg) predisposes to hypotension and reductions in tissue blood flow and tissue oxygenation, resulting in muscle weakness, myopathies, and a prolonged and challenging recovery from anesthesia. Excessive blood loss necessitates the administration of large volumes of fluid to maintain adequate tissue perfusion. The administration of large volumes of crystalloids (e.g., saline, lactated Ringer's) further dilutes red blood cells and total protein, resulting in anemia and hypoproteinemia, respectively. Large volumes of crystalloids can result in overhydration; cerebral, pulmonary and intestinal edema; and acid-base (nonrespiratory acidosis) and electrolyte disorders (e.g., hypokalemia). Finally, the surgical technique can predispose to multiple intraoperative and postoperative complications. Surgery for correction of cervical vertebral instability ("wobbler" surgery) can markedly reduce arterial PO₂ values, predisposing to reductions in tissue oxygenation, lactic acidosis, and myopathy. Laparoscopic procedures can compromise cardiovascular function by limiting venous return during abdominal insufflation with carbon dioxide or by restricting diaphragmatic movement and pulmonary function during head-down tilting.[118,119] Interestingly, ocular surgery was not associated with an increased incidence of the oculocardiac reflex, but horses were at greater risk for unsatisfactory recovery from anesthesia.[120] Surgical correction of colic has an exceptionally high complication and mortality rate because of the development of ileus, endotoxemia, laminitis, and pain.[121]

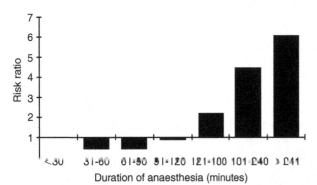

Figure 22–15. Risk ratio associated with increasing duration of anesthesia. (Data from Johnston GM et al: The confidential enquiry into perioperative equine fatalities [CEPEF]: mortality results of phases 1 and 2, *Vet Anaesth Analg* 29:159-170, 2002.)

Human Error

Human error is probably the most common cause for adverse events, including mortality associated with equine anesthesia. Human error is caused by a lack of knowledge, lack of experience, lack of adequate communication, lack of supervision, complacency, task saturation, and personal fatigue (see Chapter 1). Errors in drug selection and dose and route of administration (e.g., intracarotid injections) in conjunction with inadequate monitoring and a general lack of familiarity with resuscitation procedures all contribute significantly to human error–associated anesthetic complications and mortality. The issue is not whether human error occurs but how it can be minimized. Each of the aforementioned categories should be assessed individually, and action planes developed if anesthetic-associated complications are to be reduced.

References

1. Klein L: Anesthetic complications in the horse, *Vet Clin North Am (Equine Pract)* 6:665-692, 1990.
2. Young SS, Taylor PM: Factors influencing the outcome of equine anaesthesia: a review of 1314 cases, *Equine Vet J* 25:147-151, 1993.
3. Mee AM, Cripps PJ, Jones RS: A retrospective study of mortality associated with general anaesthesia in horses: elective procedures, *Vet Rec* 142:275-276, 1998.
4. Mee AM, Cripps PJ, Jones RS: A retrospective study of mortality associated with general anaesthesia in horses: emergency procedures, *Vet Rec* 142:307-309, 1998.
5. Jones RS. Comparative mortality in anaesthesia, *Br J Anaesth* 87:813-815, 2001.
6. Johnston GM et al: The confidential enquiry into perioperative equine fatalities (CEPEF): mortality results of phases 1 and 2, *Vet Anaesth Analg* 29:159-170, 2002.
7. Johnston GM et al: Is isoflurane safer than halothane in equine anesthesia? Results from a prospective multicentre randomized controlled trial, *Equine Vet J* 36:64-71, 2004.
8. Bidwell LA, Bramlage LR, Wood WA: Fatality rates associated with equine general anesthesia, *Proc Am Assoc Equine Pract* 50:492; 2004.
9. Bidwell LA, Bramlage LR, Rood WA: Equine perioperative fatalities associated with general anaesthesia at a private practice—a retrospective case series, *Vet Anaesth Analg* 34:23-30, 2007.
10. Pascoe PJ et al: Mortality rates and associated factors in equine colic operations—a retrospective study of 341 operations, *Can Vet J* 24:76-85, 1983.
11. Mair TS, Smith LJ: Survival and complication rates in 300 horses undergoing surgical treatment of colic. Part 1: Short-term survival following a single laparotomy, *Equine Vet J* 37:296-302, 2005.
12. Proudman CJ et al: Preoperative and anaesthesia-related risk factors for mortality in equine colic cases, *Vet J* 171:89-97, 2006.
13. Gerring EL: Priapism after ACP in the horse, *Vet Rec* 109:64, 1981.
14. Ballard S et al: The pharmacokinetics, pharmacological responses, and behavioral effects of acepromazine in the horse, *J Vet Pharmacol Ther* 5:21-31, 1982.
15. Nie GJ, Pope KC: Persistent penile prolapse associated with acute blood loss and acepromazine maleate administration in a horse, *Am J Vet Med Assoc* 211:587-589, 1997.
16. Sharrock AG: Reversal of drug-induced priapism in a gelding by medication, *Aust Vet J* 58:39-40, 1982.
17. Wilson DV, Nickels FA, Williams MA: Pharmacologic treatment of priapism in two horses, *J Am Vet Med Assoc* 199:1183-1184, 1991.
18. Schumacker J, Hardin DK: Surgical treatment of priapism in a stallion, *Vet Surg* 16:193-196, 1987.
19. Trim CM, Adams JG, Houda LR: Failure of ketamine to induce anesthesia in two horses, *J Am Vet Med Assoc* 190:201-202, 1987.
20. Day TK et al: Blood gas values during intermittent positive pressure ventilation and spontaneous ventilation in 160 anesthetized horses positioned in lateral or dorsal recumbency, *Vet Surg* 24:266-276, 1995.
21. Nyman G et al: Selective mechanical ventilation of dependent lung regions in the anaesthetized horse in dorsal recumbency, *Br J Anaesth* 59:1027-1034, 1987.
22. Dunkel B, Dolente B, Boston RC: Acute lung injury/acute respiratory distress syndrome in 15 foals, *Equine Vet J* 37:435-440, 2005.
23. Blaze CA, Robinson NE: Apneic oxygenation in anesthetized ponies and horses, *Vet Res Commun* 11:281-291, 1987.
24. Moens Y, Gootjes P, Lagerweij E: A tracheal tube-in-tube technique for functional separation of the lungs in the horse, *Equine Vet J* 24:103-106, 1992.
25. Abrahamsen EJ et al: Bilateral arytenoid cartilage paralysis after inhalation anesthesia in a horse, *J Am Vet Med Assoc* 10:1363-1365, 1990.
26. Tute AS et al: Negative pressure pulmonary edema as a post-anesthetic complication associated with upper airway obstruction in a horse, *Vet Surg* 25:519-523, 1996.
27. Kollias-Baker CA et al: Pulmonary edema associated with transient airway obstruction in three horses, *J Am Vet Med Assoc* 202:1116-1118, 1993.
28. Dodam JR et al: Inhaled carbon monoxide concentrations during halothane or isoflurane anesthesia in horses, *Vet Surg* 28:506-512, 1999.
29. Driessen B et al: Serum fluoride concentrations, biochemical and histopathological changes associated with prolonged sevoflurane anaesthesia in horses, *J Vet Med A Physiol Pathol Clin Med* 49:337-347, 2002.
30. Garber JL et al: Postsurgical ventricular tachycardia in a horse, *J Am Vet Med Assoc* 201:1038-1039, 1992.
31. Hubbell JAE, Muir WW, Bednarski RM: Atrial fibrillation associated with anesthesia a Standardbred Gelding, *Vet Surg* 15:450-452, 1986.
32. Young SS, Taylor PM: Factors influencing the outcome of equine anaesthesia: a review of 1314 cases, *Equine Vet J* 25:147-151, 1993.
33. Grandy JL et al: Arterial hypotension and the development of postanesthetic myopathy in halothane-anesthetized horses, *Am J Vet Res* 48:192-197, 1987.
34. McGoldrick TM, Bowen IM, Clarke KW: Sudden cardiac arrest in an anaesthetized horse associated with low venous oxygen tensions, *Vet Rec* 142:610-611, 1998.
35. Dodman NH et al: Postanesthetic hind limb adductor myopathy in five horses, *J Am Vet Med Assoc* 193:83-86, 1988.
36. Dyson S, Taylor P, Whitwell K: Femoral nerve paralysis after general anaesthesia, *Equine Vet J* 20:376-380, 1988.
37. Franci P, Leece EA, Brearly JC: Post anesthetic myopathy/neuropathy in horses undergoing magnetic resonance imaging compared to horses undergoing surgery, *Equine Vet J* 38:497-501, 2006.
38. Blakemore WF et al: Spinal cord malacia following general anesthesia in the horse, *Vet Rec* 114:569-570, 1984.
39. Yovich JV et al: Postanesthetic hemorrhagic myelopathy in a horse, *J Am Vet Med Assoc* 188:300-301, 1986.
40. Dunigan CE, Ragle CA, Schneider RK: Equine postanesthetic myelopathy, *Proc Am Assoc Equine Pract* 42:178, 1996.
41. Trim CM: Postanesthetic hemorrhagic myelopathy or myelomalacia, *Vet Clin North Am (Equine Pract)* 13:74-77, 1997.
42. Jouber KE, Duncan N, Murray SE: Post-anaesthetic myelomalacia in a horse, *J S Afr Vet Assoc* 76:36-39, 2005.

43. White NA, Suarex M: Change in triceps muscle intracompartmental pressure with positioning and padding of the lowermost thoracic limb of the horse, *Am J Vet Res* 47:2257-2260, 1986.

44. MacLeay JM et al: Heritable basis of recurrent exertional rhabdomyolysis in Thoroughbred Racehorses, *Am J Vet Res* 60: 250-256, 1999.

45. Edner A, Essen-Gustavsson B, Nyman G: Muscle metabolic changes associated with long-term inhalation anaesthesia in the horse analyzed by muscle biopsy and microdialysis techniques, *J Vet Med A Physiol Pathol Clin Med* 52:99-107 2005.

46. Duke T et al: Clinical observations surrounding an increased incidence of postanesthetic myopathy in halothane-anesthetized horses, *Vet Anesth Analg* 33:122-127, 2006.

47. Ripoll S et al: Postanaesthetic cerebral necrosis in five horses, *Vet Rec* 23:387-388, 2002.

48. Hubbell JAE, Muir WW: Rate of rise of arterial carbon dioxide tension in the halothane-anesthetized horse, *J Am Vet Med Assoc* 186:374-376, 1985.

49. Mason DE, Muir WW, Wade A: Arterial blood gas tensions in the horse during recovery from anesthesia, *J Am Vet Med Assoc* 190:989-994, 1987.

50. Hall LW: Cardiovascular and pulmonary effects of recumbency in two conscious ponies, *Equine Vet J* 16:89-92, 1984.

51. Wagner AE, Bednarski RM, Muir WW: Hemodynamic effects of carbon dioxide during intermittent positive-pressure ventilation in horses, *Am J Vet Res* 51:1922-1929, 1990.

52. Khanna AK et al: Cardiopulmonary effects of hypercapnia during controlled intermittent positive-pressure ventilation in the horse, *Can J Vet Res* 59:213-221, 1995.

53. Hodgson DS et al: Effects of spontaneous, assisted, and controlled ventilatory modes in halothane-anesthetized geldings, *Am J Vet Res* 47:992-996, 1986.

54. Day TK et al: Blood gas values during intermittent positive pressure ventilation and spontaneous ventilation in 160 anesthetized horses positioned in lateral or dorsal recumbency, *Vet Surg* 24:266-276, 1995.

55. Smale K, Butler PJ: Temperature and pH effects on the oxygen equilibrium curve of the Thoroughbred Horse, *Respir Physiol* 97:293-299, 1994.

56. Swanson CR, Muir WW: Dobutamine-induced augmentation of cardiac output does not enhance respiratory gas exchange in anesthetized recumbent healthy horses, *Am J Vet Res* 47: 1573-1576, 1986.

57. Swanson CR, Muir WW: Hemodynamic and respiratory responses in halothane-anesthetized horses exposed to positive end-expiratory pressure alone and with dobutamine, *Am J Vet Res* 49:539-542, 1988.

58. Wilson DV, McFeely AM: Positive end-expiratory pressure during colic surgery in horses: 74 cases (1986-1988), *J Am Vet Med Assoc* 199:917-921, 1991.

59. Moens Y et al: Influence of tidal volume and positive end-expiratory pressure on inspiratory gas distribution and gas exchange during mechanical ventilation in horses positioned in lateral recumbency, *Am J Vet Res* 59:307-312, 1998.

60. Wettstein D et al: Effects of an alveolar recruitment maneuver on cardiovascular and respiratory parameters during total intravenous anesthesia in ponies, *Am J Vet Res* 67:152-159, 2006.

61. Robertson SA, Bailey JE: Aerosolized salbutamol (albuterol) improves PaO2 in hypoxaemic anaesthetized horses—a prospective clinical trial in 81 horses, *Vet Anaesth Analg* 29: 212-221, 2002.

62. Dodam JR et al: Effects of clenbuterol hydrochloride on pulmonary gas exchange and hemodynamics in anesthetized horses, *Am J Vet Res* 54:776-782, 1993.

63. Hallowell GD, Corley KTT: Preoperative administration of hydroxyethyl starch or hypertonic saline to horses with colic, *J Vet Intern Med* 20:980-986, 2006.

64. Swanson CR et al: Hemodynamic responses in halothane-anesthetized horses given infusions of dopamine or dobutamine, *Am J Vet Res* 46:365-370, 1985.

65. Young LE et al: Temporal effects of an infusion of dobutamine hydrochloride in horses anesthetized with halothane, *Am J Vet Res* 59:1027-1032, 1998.

66. Gehlen H et al: Effects of two different dosages of dobutamine on pulmonary artery wedge pressure, systemic blood pressure, and heart rate in anaesthetized horses, *J Vet Med* 53:476-480, 2006.

67. Donaldson LL: Retrospective assessment of dobutamine therapy for hypotension in anesthetized horses, *Vet Surg* 17: 53-57, 1988.

68. Light GS, Hellyer PW, Swanson CR: Parasympathetic influence on the arrhythmogenicity of graded dobutamine infusions in halothane-anesthetized horses, *Am J Vet Res* 53:1154-1160, 1992.

69. Whitton DL, Trim CM. Use of dopamine hydrochloride during general anesthesia in the treatment of advanced atrioventricular heart block in four foals, *J Am Vet Med Assoc* 187: 1357-1361, 1985.

70. Robertson SA et al: Metabolic, hormonal, and hemodynamic changes during dopamine infusions in halothane-anesthetized horses, *Vet Surg* 25:88-97, 1996.

71. Gasthuys F, DeMoor A, Parmentier D: Influence of dopamine and dobutamine on the cardiovascular depression during a standard halothane anaesthesia in dorsally recumbent, ventilated ponies, *J Vet Med* 38:494-500, 1991.

72. Lee YL et al: Effects of dopamine, dobutamine, dopexamine, phenylephrine, and saline solution on intramuscular blood flow and other cardiopulmonary variables in halothane-anesthetized ponies, *Am J Vet Res* 59:1462-1472, 1998.

73. Young LE et al: Haemodynamic effects of a sixty-minute infusion of dopamine hydrochloride in horses anaesthetized with halothane, *Equine Vet J* 30:310-316, 1998.

74. Grandy JL et al: Cardiopulmonary effects of ephedrine in halothane-anesthetized horses, *J Vet Pharmacol Ther* 12:389-396, 1989.

75. Lee YL et al: The effects of ephedrine on intramuscular blood flow and cardiopulmonary parameters in halothane-anesthetized ponies, *Vet Anaesth Analg* 29:171-181, 2002.

76. Hellyer PW et al: The effects of dobutamine and ephedrine on packed cell volume, total protein, heart rate, and blood pressure in anaesthetized horses, *J Vet Pharmacol Ther* 21: 497-499, 1998.

77. Grubb TL et al: Hemodynamic effects of ionized calcium in horses anesthetized with halothane or isoflurane, *Am J Vet Res* 60:1430-1435, 1999.

78. Muir WW: Inotropic mechanisms of dopexamine hydrochloride in horses, *Am J Vet Res* 53:1343-1346, 1992.

79. Young LE, Blissitt KJ, Clutton RE: Temporal effects of an infusion of dopexamine hydrochloride in horses anesthetized with halothane, *Am J Vet Res* 58:516-523, 1997.

80. Dyson DH, Pascoe PJ: Influence of preinduction methoxamine, lactated Ringer solution, or hypertonic saline solution infusion or postinduction dobutamine infusion on anesthetic-induced hypotension in horses, *Am J Vet Res* 51:17-21, 1990.

81. Hardy J, Bednarski RM, Biller DS: Effect of phenylephrine on hemodynamics and splenic dimensions in horses, *Am J Vet Res* 55:1570-1578, 1994.

82. Abrahamsen EJ et al: Tourniquet-induced hypertension in a horse, *J Am Vet Med Assoc* 194:386-388, 1989.

83. Copland VS, Hildebrand SV, Hill T: Blood pressure response to tourniquet use in anesthetized horses, *J Am Vet Med Assoc* 195:1097-1103, 1989.

84. Klein L: Case report: a hot horse, *Vet Anesth* 2:41-42, 1975.

85. Waldron-Mease E, Klein LV, Rosenberg H: Malignant hyperthermia in a halothane-anesthetized horse, *J Am Vet Med Assoc* 179:896-898, 1981.

86. Hildebrand SV, Howitt GA: Succinylcholine infusion associated with hyperthermia in ponies anesthetized with halothane, *Am J Vet Res* 44:2280-2283, 1983.

87. Manley SV, Kelly AB, Hodgson D: Malignant hyperthermia-like reactions in three anesthetized horses, *J Am Vet Med Assoc* 183:85-89, 1983.

88. Aleman M et al: Equine malignant hyperthermia, *Proc Am Assoc Equine Pract* 50:51-54, 2004.

89. Aleman M et al: Malignant hyperthermia in a horse anesthetized with halothane, *J Vet Intern Med* 19:363-366, 2005.

90. Valverde A et al: Prophylactic use of dantrolene associated with prolonged postanesthetic recumbency in a horse, *J Am Vet Med Assoc* 197:1051-1053, 1990.

91. Edwards JG et al: The efficacy of dantrolene sodium in controlling exertional rhabdomyolysis in the Thoroughbred Racehorse, *Equine Vet J* 35:707-711, 2003.

92. Spier SJ et al: Hyperkalemic periodic paralysis in horses, *J Am Vet Med Assoc* 197:1009-1017, 1990.

93. Robertson SA et al: Postanesthetic recumbency associated with hyperkalemic periodic paralysis in a Quarter Horse, *J Am Vet Med Assoc* 201:1209-1212, 1992.

94. Cornick JL, Seahorn TL, Hartsfield SM: Hyperthermia during isoflurane anaesthesia in a horse with suspected hyperkalemic periodic paralysis, *Equine Vet J* 26:511-514, 1994.

95. Bailey JE, Pable L, Hubbell JAE: Hyperkalemic periodic paralysis episode during halothane anesthesia in a horse, *J Am Vet Med Assoc* 208:1-7, 1996.

96. Brightman AH et al: Decreased tear production associated with general anesthesia in the horse, *J Am Vet Med Assoc* 182:243-244, 1983.

97. Carpenter I, Hall LW: Regurgitation in an anaesthetized horse, *Vet Rec* 28:289, 1981.

98. Muir WW, Reed SM, McGuirk SM: Treatment of atrial fibrillation in horses by intravenous administration of quinidine, *J Am Vet Med Assoc* 197:1607-1610, 1990.

99. Wright BD, Hildebrand SV: An evaluation of apnea or spontaneous ventilation in early recovery following mechanical ventilation in the anesthetized horse, *Vet Anaesth Analg* 28:26, 2001.

100. Lavoie JP, Pascoe JR, Kurperschoek CJ: Effect of head and neck position on respiratory mechanics in horses sedated with xylazine, *Am J Vet Res* 53:1652-1657, 1992.

101. Lukasik V M et al: Intranasal phenylephrine reduces post anesthetic upper airway obstruction in horses, *Equine Vet J* 29:236-238, 1997.

102. Senoir M: Postanaesthetic pulmonary oedema in horses: a review, *Vet Anaesth Analg* 32:193-200, 2005

103. Ward TL et al: Calcium regulation by skeletal muscle membranes of horses with recurrent exertional rhabdomyolysis, *Am J Vet Res* 61:242, 2000.

104. Rasis AL: Skeletal muscle blood flow in anaesthetized horses. Part II: Effects of anaesthetics and vasoactive agents, *Vet Anaesth Analg* 32:331-337, 2005.

105. Dickson LR et al: Jugular thrombophlebitis resulting from an anaesthetic induction technique in the horse, *Equine Vet J* 22:177-179, 1990.

106. Dolente BA et al: Evaluation of risk factors for development of catheter-associated jugular thrombophlebitis in horses: 50 cases (1993-1998), *J Am Vet Med Assoc* 227:1134-1141, 2005.

107. Trim CM. Complications associated with the use of the cuffless endotracheal tube in the horse, *J Am Vet Med Assoc* 185:541-542, 1984.

108. Holland M et al: Laryngotracheal injury associated with nasotracheal intubation in the horse, *J Am Vet Med Assoc* 189:1447-1450, 1986.

109. Abrahamsen EJ et al: Bilateral arytenoid cartilage paralysis after inhalation anesthesia in a horse, *J Am Vet Med Assoc* 10:1363-1365, 1990.

110. Hardy J et al: Complications of nasogastric intubation in horses: nine cases (1987-1989), *J Am Vet Med Assoc* 201: 483-486, 1992.

111. Trim CM, Eaton SA, Parks AH: Severe nasal hemorrhage in an anesthetized horse, *J Am Vet Med Assoc* 210: 1324-1327, 1997.

112. Baxter GM, Adams JE, Johnson JJ: Severe hypercarbia resulting from inspiratory valve malfunction in two anesthetized horses, *J Am Vet Med Assoc* 198:123-125, 1991.

113. Richey MT et al: Equine post-anesthetic lameness: a retrospective study, *Vet Surg* 19:392-397, 1990.

114. Senior JM et al: Post anaesthetic colic in horses: a preventable complication? *Equine Vet J* 38:479-484, 2006.

115. Malone E et al: Intravenous continuous infusion of lidocaine for treatment of equine ileus, *Vet Surg* 35:60-66, 2006.

116. Taylor PM: Pain and analgesia in horses, *Vet Anaesth Analg* 30:121-123, 2003.

117. Muir WW. Pain therapy in horses, *Equine Vet J* 37:98-100, 2005.

118. Fischer AT, Vachon AM: Laparoscopic intraabdominal ligation and removal of cryptorchid testes in horses, *Equine Vet J* 30:105-108, 1998.

119. Fischer AT: Advances in diagnostic techniques for horses with colic, *Vet Clin North Am (Equine Pract)* 13:203-219, 1997.

120. Parviainen AKJ, Trin CM: Complications associated with anaesthesia for ocular surgery: a retrospective study 1989-1996, *Equine Vet J* 32:555-559, 2000.

121. Proudman CJ et al: Pre-operative and anaesthesia-related risk factors for mortality in equine colic cases, *Vet J* 171:89-97, 2006.

Cardiopulmonary Resuscitation

William W. Muir

John A.E. Hubbell

Most acute life-threatening complications associated with anesthesia involve failure of the lungs and cardiovascular system (see Chapters 2 and 3). Cardiopulmonary emergencies can occur as a result of interference or interruption of normal ventilation, tissue perfusion, or both. Abnormalities in tissue perfusion can be linked directly to hypovolemia, blood loss, depression of cardiac contractile force, cardiac arrhythmias, or disturbances in the regulation of vascular tone. The cardiovascular effects of anesthetic drugs combined with recumbency invariably lead to decreases in cardiac output and hypotension. Most anesthetized horses usually register cardiac outputs less than half ($\leq$40 ml/kg/min versus 70 to 80 ml/kg/min) that recorded in standing normal horses. The lower cardiac output is linked directly to the central nervous system and cardiovascular depressant effects of most anesthetic drugs (see Table 3-11). Reduced venous return caused by the weight of the abdominal viscera on the posterior vena cava is an additional complicating factor.

Cardiopulmonary resuscitation (CPR) is labor intense, expensive, and often unsuccessful. Inadequate or poor monitoring techniques, unfamiliarity with resuscitative procedures, overdependence on pharmacological therapies, and a general lack of clinically useful research are important reasons for limited success. Questions relating to the effectiveness of external cardiac massage, the optimum rate and method to perform chest compressions, and the optimum ventilatory strategy during chest compressions have not been answered as they relate to the horse.[1]

CAUSES OF CARDIOPULMONARY EMERGENCIES

A cardiopulmonary emergency is defined as any potentially life-threatening process that interferes with the delivery of oxygenated blood to peripheral tissues. The most common causes for cardiopulmonary emergencies in horses include severely debilitating diseases, colic, endotoxemia, pleuritis, pneumonia, heart failure (congenital or acquired), supraventricular and ventricular arrhythmias, severe dehydration, hemorrhage, and anesthesia (Box 23-1). Severe acid-base and electrolyte disorders may result in cardiovascular compromise but generally occur in conjunction with or as a result of other disease processes. Factors associated with anesthesia that predispose or are capable of producing a cardiopulmonary emergency include the administration of preanesthetic medications and anesthetic drugs, accidental intracarotid injections, body position, an obstructed airway, improper use of ventilatory assist devices, poor monitoring techniques, equipment failure, and human error (see Chapters 1 and 22). Any one or a combination of these factors can be responsible for impaired ventilation or cardiovascular failure, resulting in death. Tranquilizers, sedative analgesics, muscle relaxants, and intravenous or inhalation anesthetics are all potentially capable of producing cardiopulmonary emergency (see Table 3-11 and Chapters 4, 10-13, and 15; Figure 23-1).

DIAGNOSIS OF CARDIOPULMONARY EMERGENCIES

Cardiopulmonary emergencies can be minimized by a thorough familiarity with the drugs and anesthetic techniques used (a standardized anesthetic protocol; see Chapter 22), vigilant patient monitoring, and recognition of the signs associated with cardiopulmonary distress. Hypoventilation, apnea, and hypotension are indicated by infrequent or absent breathing efforts and weak or irregular peripheral pulses (Box 23-2).

Most horses that have just been anesthetized have pink or pale-pink mucous membranes. Thiobarbiturates and inhalation anesthetics (isoflurane, sevoflurane) produce pink mucous membranes with normal or rapid capillary refill time as a result of vasodilation. Dissociative anesthetics (ketamine, tiletamine) produce pale-pink mucous membranes because of mild peripheral vasoconstriction that may be intensified by the prior use or coadministration of an α_2-adrenoceptor agonist. Regardless of the anesthetic drug administered, most horses develop pale-pink or whitish-pink mucous membranes during prolonged anesthesia as a result of gradual increases in sympathetic tone, peripheral vasoconstriction, and redistribution of blood flow away from the skin. Cyanosis or bluish discoloration of the mucous membranes suggests hypoxemia. Hypoxemia is extremely important in an anemic horse but may be difficult to diagnose because of the reduced amount of hemoglobin. For example, horses with less than 5 g/dl

Box 23–1 Causes of Cardiopulmonary Emergencies in Horses

1. Drugs and idiosyncratic reactions
   a. Phenothiazines: hypotension
   b. α_2-Agonists: bradycardia
   c. Thiobarbiturates: Hypoventilation/apnea
   d. Inhalation anesthetics: Hypotension
   e. "Mycin" antibiotics: Neuromuscular paralysis, hypoventilation

2. Intracarotid injections
   a. Saline
   b. Drugs

3. Positional effects
   a. Dorsal recumbency

4. Airway related
   a. Airway obstruction (soft palate, laryngeal abnormality)
   b. Kinked or obstructed endotracheal tube
   c. Esophageal or endobronchial intubation
   d. Overinflated endotracheal tube cuff
   e. Nasal edema
   f. Partial or complete laryngeal paralysis

5. Pulmonary or thoracic
   a. Pneumonia
   b. Bronchitis/bronchiolitis
   c. Pleuritis
   d. Diaphragmatic hernia
   e. Improper use of restraining ropes

6. Volume depletion
   a. Dehydration
   b. Hemorrhage
   c. Third space losses

7. Cardiovascular abnormalities
   a. Hypotension
   b. Heart failure
   c. Cardiac arrhythmias
   d. Pulseless electrical activity
   e. Asystole
   f. Ventricular fibrillation

8. Acid-base abnormalities
   a. Hypokalemia
   b. Hyperkalemia
   c. Hypocalcemia
   d. Metabolic acidosis

9. Equipment failure
   a. Inaccurate vaporizer
   b. Stuck inhalation/exhalation valves
   c. Leaky bellows

10. Human error
   a. Drug overdose
   b. Administration of wrong drug or solution
   c. Poor monitoring
   d. Lack of recognition of warning signs

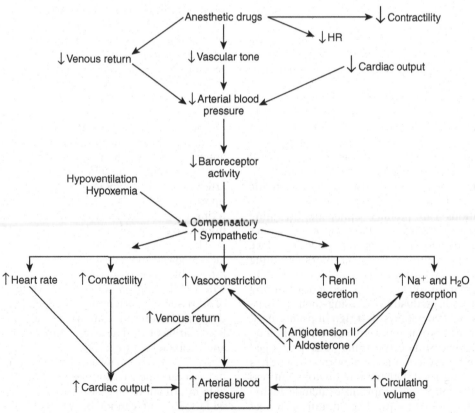

Figure 23–1. Hemodynamic responses induced by anesthetic drugs.

Box 23–2 **Signs and Symptoms of Cardiopulmonary Complications**

- Nervous system
  - Loss of consciousness
  - Loss of palpebral reflex
  - Loss of corneal reflex
  - Loss of anal pinch reflex
  - Loss of thoracic pressure reflex
  - Pupillary dilation
- Breathing
  - Hypoventilation (<4 beats/min)
  - Apnea
  - Tachypnea (>20 beats/min)
  - Dyspnea
  - Abnormal breathing patterns (apneustic, Biot's, Cheyne-Stokes)
  - Agonal gasps
- Heart and circulation
  - Cyanotic, injected (red), gray, or white mucous membranes
  - Prolonged capillary refill time (>2.5 seconds)
  - Weak or irregular peripheral pulse
  - Absence of bleeding
  - Rapid (>60 beats/min) or slow (<25 beats/min) heart rate
  - Muffled or absent heart sounds
  - Hypotension (MAP <70 mm Hg)
  - Abnormal electrocardiogram (ST-T segment depression, wide QRS, enlarging T waves)
  - Cardiac arrhythmias, asystole

MAP, Mean arterial blood pressure.

---

of circulating hemoglobin do not become cyanotic (see Chapter 8). Extremely red or injected mucous membranes in anesthetized horses may be a sign of endotoxemia or hypercapnia.

Short periods of apnea lasting 30 to 90 seconds are common immediately after induction to anesthesia but should not occur during the maintenance or recovery phases of anesthesia. Apneustic (inspiratory breath holding) and Biot's (intermittent) breathing patterns are not considered normal; they are signs of respiratory center depression and can be associated with the administration of anesthetic drugs. Ketamine or tiletamine and rapid infusion of 10% guaifenesin solutions can produce apneustic breathing and breath holding (Table 23-1). Deep stages and planes of intravenous or inhalation anesthesia frequently induce intermittent or Biot's breathing. However, Biot's breathing is observed occasionally during light planes of inhalation anesthesia, particularly in fit horses. Infrequent breathing efforts associated with gradually increasing then decreasing tidal volumes (Cheyne-Stokes) is a sign of pronounced respiratory center depression and decreased cerebral blood flow. Marked Cheyne-Stokes breathing and prolonged apnea (>90 seconds) are considered abnormal regardless of the anesthetic drug used. Other more obvious but less frequent signs of respiratory compromise include tachypnea, dyspnea, and agonal gasps. The administration of anesthetic drugs should be terminated, and ventilation should be controlled.

Cardiopulmonary emergencies caused by respiratory abnormalities alone are infrequent but can be insidious: the horse may appear to be in a stable state of anesthesia and breathing spontaneously but can develop significant hypercapnia and hypoxemia. The only accurate method for assessing gas exchange is the routine measurement of blood gas values. Arterial and venous blood gases (PCO_2, PO_2) are particularly helpful during circulatory failure, and the continuous evaluation of SpO_2 and $ETCO_2$ can be used as noninvasive methods to identify trends (see Chapter 8).[2,3] $ETCO_2$ and $PaCO_2$ values are indicative of pulmonary blood flow and cardiac output, respectively, thus serving as prognosticators of effective CPR (see Chapter 8).[4]

Changes in capillary refill time are frequently used to assess tissue perfusion. Prolonged capillary refill time can be caused by hypovolemia, poor cardiac function, and vasoconstriction, all of which decrease tissue perfusion. The assessment of the peripheral pulse digitally or by displaying and recording a peripheral pulse wave can provide important hemodynamic information. Changes in pulse rate and regularity are easily detectable in most horses by palpating the facial or dorsal metatarsal arteries. Increases in pulse rate suggest sympathetic activation caused by an increased level of consciousness during anesthesia, pain, hypoxemia, or severe hypotension. Decreases in heart rate suggest excessive depression by anesthetic drugs, increases in parasympathetic tone, or toxicity. Irregular pulses are indicative of cardiac arrhythmias and should be evaluated electrocardiographically. The loss of a palpable arterial pressure pulse or arterial pressure waveform can be caused by one of five abnormalities presented in descending frequency of occurrence: (1) hypotension, (2) profound bradycardia, (3) other cardiac arrhythmias, (4) cardiac asystole (arrest), and (5) pulseless electrical activity (normal electrocardiogram [ECG] but mean arterial blood pressure less than 40 mm Hg; see Box 23-1).

Muffled heart sounds during lateral and especially dorsal recumbency are a common finding in anesthetized horses and are caused by positional changes in the heart. A gradual decrease in the intensity of the heart sounds during anesthesia suggests a gradual decrease in cardiac contractile performance, low cardiac output, and the potential for the development of hypotension if not already present. The absence of heart sounds may indicate heart failure, cardiac arrest, or ventricular fibrillation. However, other signs of arrest (prolonged capillary refill time, absent pulse, dilated unresponsive pupils) should be evaluated before administering resuscitative therapy and emphasize the use of more informative (arterial blood pressure) monitoring techniques.

The absence of bleeding of bright red blood from cut surfaces suggests hypotension and poor tissue perfusion. Mean arterial blood pressures below 50 to 60 mm Hg may not provide the driving pressure necessary to maintain perfusion of all tissues. Transient or prolonged hypotension and poor tissue perfusion can result in cardiac arrhythmias, including bradycardia or cardiac arrest caused by myocardial ischemia and hypoxia (Figure 23-2).

An ECG is extremely useful for determining abnormalities in heart rate and rhythm (see Chapter 8). The ECG can provide information suggestive of poor cardiac function (e.g., wide QRS) but cannot be used to assess hemodynamics. Many horses have died with a normal ECG (pulseless electrical activity; electromechanical dissociation). The value of the

Table 23–1. Patterns of breathing

Respiratory pattern	Description	Potential causes
Eupnea tachypnea	Increased respiratory rate	Normal horse Excitement Fever Hypoxia Hypercapnia Hypotension Hyperthermia Airway obstruction Pneumonia Lesions of CNS respiratory centers
Bradypnea	Slow but regular respirations	Sleep Anesthesia α_2-Agonists Hypothermia CNS neoplasia Respiratory decompensation
Shallow breathing	Regular reduced rate of breathing or small tidal volume	Drug depression (barbiturates, inhalation anesthetics) Coma
Apnea	Absence of respiration; may be periodic	100% O_2 (transiently) Drug depression (barbiturates) Muscle paralysis Overventilation Increased cerebral blood pressure Shock
Hypercapnia or Kussmaul	Large (increased tidal volume) respirations; rate normal or increased	Pain Hypercapnia Surgical stimulation Pneumonia Metabolic acidosis Uremia Hypoxia Hyperthermia Increased cerebrospinal fluid pressure Sepsis Shock
Cheyne-Stokes	Respirations become faster with increased tidal volume, then slower with decreased tidal volume, followed by an apneic pause	Increased intracranial pressure Drug overdose Severe hypoxia Hypotension; heart failure Renal failure Meningitis
Biot's or Cluster	Respirations are faster and deeper than normal with abrupt pauses between them; each breath has approximately the same tidal volume	Anesthetic drugs in some normal horses and foals Hypotension Medullary (CNS) depression
Apneustic	Respirations characterized by an inspiratory hold and rapid expiration	Cyclohexamines (ketamine, tiletamine) Guaifenesin (large doses) Anoxia
Agonal respiration	Infrequent breathing characterized by rapid inspiration and expiration; exaggerated chest wall and abdominal effort	Terminal event; cerebral hypoxia

CNS, Central nervous system.

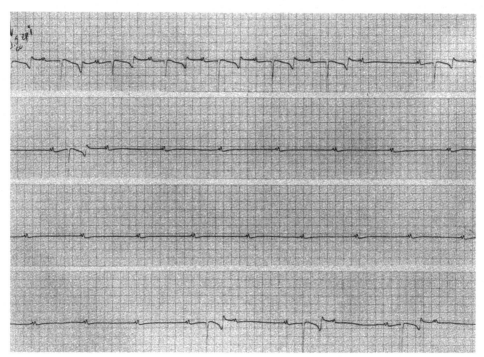

Figure 23–2. Complete atrioventricular block without ventricular escape in a 3-year-old Standardbred during halothane anesthesia. Note the regularity of P waves. Mean arterial blood pressure transiently decreased to 15 mm Hg. The horse responded favorably to epinephrine (1 µg/kg IV) followed by dopamine (3 µg/kg/min) (25 mm/sec paper speed).

ECG is its ability to provide heart rate, the electrical rhythm, and the timing and pattern of electrical activation of the atria and ventricles. For example, simple sinus bradycardia is treated considerably different than a wide QRS duration or a slow idioventricular rhythm, both of which could produce a palpable, albeit slow, peripheral pulse. Common ECG abnormalities in the anesthetized horse include wandering pacemaker, sinus bradycardia, sinus arrest, second-degree atrioventricular block, and interference dissociation (see Chapter 3). These rhythms usually are associated with

normal arterial blood pressure and are only treated when ventricular rate falls below 25 beats/min or mean arterial blood pressure falls below 50 to 60 mm Hg. Sinus tachycardia, atrial fibrillation, and atrial or ventricular premature depolarizations are considered abnormal but may not be treated, depending on the ventricular rate and hemodynamics. Ventricular rates >60 beats/min or hypotension suggests that therapy is indicated. Frequent ventricular depolarizations and ventricular tachycardia are considered abnormal and suggest cardiac electrical instability and should be

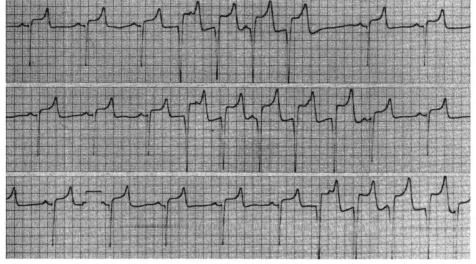

Figure 23–3. Ventricular premature depolarizations in a 5-year-old Thoroughbred Stallion during halothane anesthesia. Mean arterial blood ressure decreased from 94 mm Hg to 62 mm Hg during the episodes of ventricular tachycardia. The horse responded to quinidine (0.5 mg/kg IV) (25 mm/sec paper speed).

treated (Figure 23-3). Other ECG abnormalities suggestive of poor hemodynamics include marked ST-T segment deviation or QRS widening caused by myocardial ischemia; tented T waves and short QT intervals caused by hyperkalemia; and continuously irregular electrical tracing, indicating ventricular flutter. Finally, gradual trends in heart rate can be used to support decisions to modify anesthetic drug delivery or fluid therapy and to initiate hemodynamic support.

Measuring arterial blood pressure and assessing the arterial blood pressure waveform provide indirect information concerning cardiac contractile performance and vascular tone (see Chapter 8). The slope of the rate of rise of the arterial blood pressure curve is indicative of an increase or decrease in cardiac contractility. Similarly, gradual increases or decreases in arterial blood pressure caused by vasoconstriction or vasodilation, respectively, are usually associated with changes in the arterial waveform morphology (see Box 8-5). Mild decreases in vascular tone (peripheral vasodilation) can increase cardiac output and vice versa. This is why peripheral vasodilation may be preferred over peripheral vasoconstriction if arterial blood pressure can be maintained. However, mean arterial perfusion pressures less than 50 mm Hg can produce skeletal muscle or gut ischemia in some horses. Improper use of assisted or controlled ventilation can decrease venous return, cardiac output, and arterial blood pressure (see Chapter 17). Increases in pleural pressure (Ppl) decrease cardiac output by increasing the resistance to the forward flow of blood. Sustained collapse of low-pressure veins within the thoracic cavity decreases venous return.[5] The influence of Ppl and the corresponding decrease in cardiac output are generally greater when larger lung volumes, longer inspiratory times, and greater respiratory frequencies are used.

CHEST COMPRESSION IN HORSES

The traditionally accepted method for maintaining blood flow during cardiopulmonary arrest in horses is compression of the chest wall.[6-9] Studies conducted in dogs and humans suggest that chest compression produces blood flow by multiple mechanisms but that direct compression of the heart (heart pump) and increases in intrathoracic pressure (thoracic pump) are the most important.[10] External chest compression increases pressure in the thoracic cavity, creating a pressure gradient for blood flow into extrathoracic vessels to peripheral tissues. Retrograde blood flow is minimized by the heart valves, venous valves, and collapse of the great veins (Figure 23-4). When applied appropriately, this rationale argues for simultaneous ventilation and chest compression to maximize brief increases in intrathoracic pressure, although no controlled studies have been reported that demonstrate the benefit of simultaneous ventilation with chest compression in horses or foals. Studies conducted in euthanatized adult horses weighing from 410 to 530 kg suggest that increases in intrathoracic pressure induced by chest wall compression are effective in maintaining blood flow (Table 23-2).[9] Cardiac output may reach values in excess of 25 ml/kg/min, which may be adequate to sustain life until normal cardiac activity can be restored.[9] The optimum chest compression rate in horses is between 60 and 80 per minute, and the force applied during each chest compression is important. The addition of simultaneous

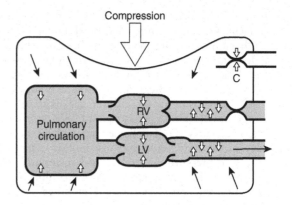

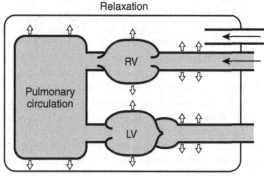

Figure 23–4. Thoracic pump mechanism for generating blood flow during cardiopulmonary resuscitation. Intrathoracic pressure increases during chest compression *(top)*, compressing low pressure veins and small airways *(C)* within the thorax. The intrathoracic veins and cardiac chambers fill during relaxation *(bottom)*. The one-way valves in the heart direct the flow of blood forward. Blood flow in foals is probably caused by both direct cardiac compression of the heart and the thoracic pump mechanism. *LV,* Left ventricle; *RV,* right ventricle. (Modified from Cooper JA, Cooper JD, Cooper JM: Cardiopulmonary resuscitation: history, current practice, and future direction, *Circulation* 114:2839-2849, 2006.)

Table 23–2.	Effects of chest compression rate, simultaneous ventilation-compression, and interposed abdominal compression on cardiac output in horses
Physical status	**Cardiac output**
Conscious standing horse	65-80 ml/kg/min
Anesthetized horse	30-50 ml/kg/min
Arrested horse	0 ml/kg/min
Arrested horse, during chest compression	
40 CPM	10-15 ml/kg/min
60 CPM	15-20 ml/kg/min
80 CPM	15-25 ml/kg/min
Arrested horse, during simultaneous ventilation-compression	
60 CPM	10-15 ml/kg/min
Arrested horse, during chest compression and interposed abdominal compression	
60 CPM	15-20 ml/kg/min

CPM, Compressions per minute.

ventilation and chest compression markedly reduces blood flow in horses and is not recommended.[9] Abdominal compression, whether timed during the release phase or arbitrarily applied, does not improve results, suggesting that horses do not respond like the dog or humans to newer and supposedly more beneficial modifications in CPR techniques (see Table 23-2). The reason for these differences is most likely linked to the lung inflation pressures and inspiratory times required to adequately ventilate horses versus their effects on pulmonary blood flow (quantity; distribution). Increases in intrathoracic pressure or a prolonged inspiratory time could increase pulmonary vascular resistance and impede blood flow from the periphery through the lungs.[5] The rate and degree of pooling of blood in the abdominal viscera of the horse after cardiac arrest are unknown and could limit the potential value of this and other suggested techniques for improving venous return.[10] Similar arguments can be used to explain the inability of abdominal compressions to increase blood flow. Compression of the abdominal viscera might increase intraabdominal aortic pressure, decreasing the driving pressure and flow of blood from the thoracic aorta. Increasing abdominal pressure could also compress abdominal veins, thereby trapping blood in abdominal organs. The benefits of chest compression and alternative techniques for improving cardiac output are greater in smaller horses, ponies, and foals because of a more compliant chest wall. Simultaneous ventilation, chest compression, and abdominal compressions, whether timed or arbitrary, provide questionable, if any, additional benefit to blood flow in large horses.

CARDIAC COMPRESSION

Direct cardiac compression is more effective than chest wall compression for increasing blood flow. Studies in dogs and humans suggest that direct cardiac compression generates blood flows that are at least twice those generated by chest wall compression.[10] The reasons for this are primarily related to more complete emptying of the ventricles. The influence of changes in intrathoracic pressure caused by lung inflation is not a factor once the chest is opened. Direct cardiac compression has been accomplished successfully in the adult horse. A 150-kg pony and 450-kg horse have been successfully resuscitated using direct cardiac compression at rates ranging from 30 to 40 times per minute.[11] The pony died, and the horse was euthanatized as a result of postresuscitative complications. Three additional horses weighing 123, 355, and 460 kg have been resuscitated successfully using direct cardiac compression.[12] The chest was opened within 5 minutes of cardiac arrest, and the heart was compressed approximately 30 times per minute. The 355-kg horse was euthanatized after resuscitation because of poor hemodynamic values and shock. The remaining two horses recovered but developed severe lameness on the operative side and pleuritis, which was treated successfully. The 460-kg horse was euthanatized after 7 days for humane reasons. These observations suggest that successful direct cardiac compression is possible; that early diagnosis of cardiac arrest is critical to success; and that sterility, patient size, and the amount of procedural trauma are key factors in determining long-term outcome. Direct cardiac compression is impractical for adult horses but is a consideration in foals because of their smaller size. The decision

to initiate CPR must not be delayed and should be based on the operative environment, the horse's physical condition at the time of arrest, and familiarity of the surgeon with CPR techniques. The practical aspects of cardiac compression remain formidable.

PERFORMING CARDIOPULMONARY RESUSCITATION IN THE HORSE

CPR is almost always a failure in adult horses once blood pressure becomes undetectable. Nonetheless, this does not mean that it should not be attempted and emphasizes the importance of developing a standardized anesthetic and emergency resuscitation protocol, using optimum monitoring techniques and keeping key emergency drugs and equipment readily available.[13,14] The approach to CPR in the horse is similar to that in other species and is based on the acronym ABCD, which stands for Airway, Breathing, Circulation, Drugs (Boxes 23-3 and 23-4; Figure 23-5).

Airway and Breathing

A constant-delivery animal resuscitator that includes specialized masks is available (Figure 23-6; www.mcculloch-medical.com) for ventilating neonatal and small foals. An

---

Box 23–3 Cardiopulmonary Resuscitation Techniques in Horses

A. Airway
1. Nasotracheal placement of Tygon tubing
2. Nasotracheal intubation
3. Orotracheal intubation
4. Tracheostomy

B. Breathing: 100% O_2
1. Alternating occlusion and release of nostrils and mouth during O_2 flow (see text) four to six times per minute
2. Demand valve or similar device (see Chapter 17)
3. Anesthetic machine
4. Pulmonary insufflation (< 200 kg; foals)
5. Administer 0.5-1 mg/kg IV doxapram

C. Circulation
1. Terminate anesthetic drugs if possible
2. Chest compression and 3-5 µg/kg IV epinephrine; 0.2-0.5 U/kg vasopressin (foals)
   a. 60-80 compressions per minute
3. Intrathoracic cardiac compression (foals) 1-5 µg/kg IV epinephrine (foals; small horses)*
4. Increase rate of fluid administration to maximum
   a. 20 ml/kg
5. Administer 1-5 µg/kg/min IV dobutamine for hypotension
6. Administer 0.005 mg/kg IV glycopyrrolate for bradyarrhythmias
7. 0.5-1.0 mg/kg IV lidocaine for ventricular arrhythmias
8. Administer 0.5-1 mEq/kg V NaHCO₃ for metabolic acidosis (pH < 7.2)
9. Administer 0.5-1 mg/kg IV furosemide for pulmonary edema
10. Administer 5-10 mg/kg dexamethasone for shock (?)

IV, Intravenously.
*When chest compression is ineffective.

airway is established very easily in larger horses by passing a nasal catheter into the trachea, placing an oral or nasal endotracheal tube, or performing a tracheotomy (see Chapter 14). A 2-cm inside diameter, 10-foot length of Tygon tubing can be adapted to a flow regulator of an E oxygen cylinder. The tubing is then passed by way of the nostril into the nasopharynx or trachea. The flow of oxygen is increased, and the nostrils and mouth of the horse are alternately held closed and released. Oxygen flow rate should be adjusted to cause moderate chest expansion in 2 to 3 seconds. Approximately 2 to 4 breaths/min maintain near normal PaO_2 values. Alternatively, an appropriately sized uncuffed (Cole catheter) or cuffed endotracheal tube (see Chapter 14) can be positioned in the trachea, and oxygen delivered as described previously or by attaching a field resuscitator or demand valve (see Chapter 22).[15] The horse should not be allowed to spontaneously trigger or exhale against a demand valve because of the high resistance offered to both inhalation and exhalation, respectively.[15] A tracheotomy can be performed when an endotracheal tube cannot be placed or when upper airway obstruction (laryngeal paralysis, fibrosis) is present (see Chapter 14).

After placement of an endotracheal tube, a large animal anesthetic machine (when available) can be used to ventilate horses or foals by manually or mechanically compressing the rebreathing bag 4 to 8 times per minute to pressures ranging from 20 to 30 cm H_2O. Decreased venous return

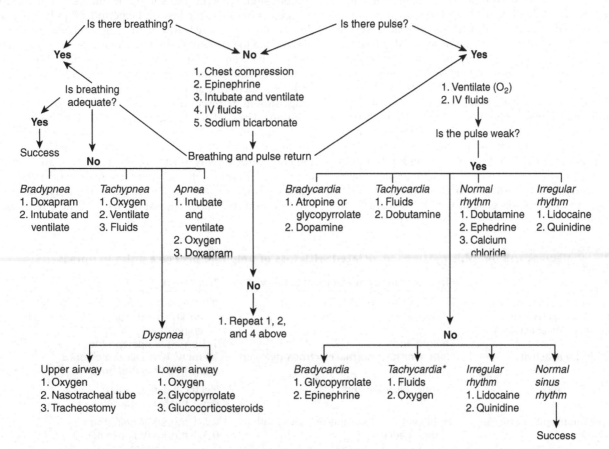

Figure 23–5. Patient evaluation during cardiopulmonary resuscitation in horses. (Modified from Muir WW, Bednarski RM: Equine cardiopulmonary resuscitation—Part II, *Compend Contin Educ* 5:S288, 1983.)

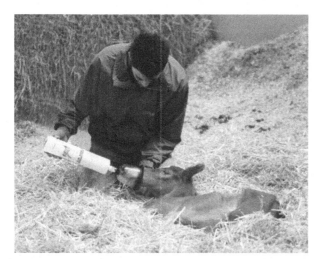

Figure 23–6. Foals can be resuscitated successfully using a constant-delivery resuscitator. (http://www.mccullochmmedical.com/.)

H_2O (open airway), which is considerably less than that produced by conventional ventilation (i.e., 20 to 30 cm H_2O) and would not be expected to compromise venous return and cardiac output.[18] The availability of equipment and practicality of this technique make its use in adult horses of limited value.

Respiratory stimulants are considered a last resort. Horses that do not respond to ventilatory techniques to improve arterial oxygenation usually do not respond to respiratory stimulants. Doxapram hydrochloride is the respiratory stimulant of choice in horses when hemodynamics have been normalized, when the $PaCO_2$ has been allowed to increase to values ranging from 60 to 70 mm Hg, or when apnea persists.[19,20] Doxapram can also be used to support breathing efforts in horses that have been anesthetized for extended periods of time with an inhalant anesthetic.[21] Arterial carbon dioxide tension decreases, and pH increases during doxapram infusion. Arterial blood pressure increases; pulse rate, ECG, and PaO_2 do not change. Anesthesia may lighten, necessitating an increase in the vaporizer setting to prevent arousal.[21] Doxapram administration during recovery is controversial and can cause a period of hyperventilation, lowering $PaCO_2$ and leading to hypoventilation. In rare instances repeated dosages of doxapram may cause tachycardia, muscle rigidity, and seizures.

Circulation

Restoration of blood flow and blood pressure is the principal goal of CPR. Techniques used to restore blood flow (chest compression, epinephrine) should be initiated immediately. Regardless of cause, the loss of the peripheral pulse; a mean arterial blood pressure below 50 mm Hg; or an electrocardiographic tracing that suggests severe bradycardia, ventricular tachycardia, ventricular asystole, or ventricular fibrillation requires an immediate response: (1) chest wall compression and (2) epinephrine administration (Table 23-3). Anesthetic drugs should be discontinued, and the rate of fluid administration increased to the maximum. Chest wall compression is accomplished with the horse in lateral recumbency (preferably right lateral recumbency) and performed by forcefully and rapidly thrusting the knee into the horse's chest just behind its elbow.[9] The force required depends on chest wall rigidity and the size of the patient. The palm of one hand can be placed against the back of the other hand,

and cardiac output leading to hypotension are potential disadvantages of these techniques and emphasize the importance of monitoring peak inspiratory pressure, inspiratory time, and appropriate fluid therapy. Pulmonary insufflation and high-frequency jet ventilation have been investigated in horses as alternative means of providing effective gas exchange and arterial oxygenation during anesthesia (see Chapter 17).[16-18] The potential advantage of both techniques is that the tube used to deliver gas need be no more than 1 cm in diameter. A tube this small can easily be passed into the trachea when orotracheal intubation is prevented (severe upper airway obstruction) or can be introduced through a small tracheostomy or laryngotomy incision. During pulmonary insufflation (apneic oxygenation), extremely high gas flows are necessary (>30 ml/kg) to promote diffusive gas exchange and may be effective for only short periods (less than 10 minutes).[16] Pulmonary insufflation does not maintain arterial $PaCO_2$ and PaO_2 values in large horses.[16] High-frequency jet ventilation is a technique whereby relatively small volumes of gas are delivered at very high respiratory frequencies (three times per second) through a small diameter tube. A suggested advantage of high-frequency ventilation is that airway pressures generally do not exceed 5 cm

Table 23–3. **Electrocardiographic patterns associated with loss of palpable pressure pulse in horses**

Rhythm	Electrocardiogram electrical activity	Treatment
Sinus, junctional, or ventricular bradycardia (can produce pulseless electrical activity)	Infrequent (less than 25) electrical complexes	0.005 mg/kg IV glycopyrrolate, 3-5 µg/kg/min dopamine, 1-5 µg/kg IV epinephrine
Asystole	Straight line	1-5 µg/kg IV epinephrine
Pulseless electrical activity	Normal or near normal electrocardiogram	10 ml IV 10% calcium chloride 1-5 µg/kg IV epinephrine
Ventricular fibrillation	Chaotic, disorganized	Electrical defibrillation 0.5-1 mg/kg IV lidocaine
Uniform or multiform ventricular tachycardia	Rapid ventricular complexes; saw-tooth in appearance	0.5-1 mg/kg IV quinidine 0.5-1 mg/kg IV lidocaine

IV, Intravenously.

and the same technique applied to small horses (less than 150 kg, ponies, or foals). Chest compression increases intrathoracic pressure, compressing compliant vascular structures within the thorax and resulting in blood flow (see Figure 23-4). Compression rates of 40 to 60/min in adult horses and 60 to 80/min in foals produce significant elevations in cardiac output (see previous discussion). Although chest compression is unlikely to support adequate tissue oxygenation for an extended period of time, it augments blood flow and facilitates the distribution of intravenous drugs (epinephrine) through the right ventricle and lungs to the coronary circulation. As pointed out, the benefits of simultaneous ventilation and abdominal compression to generate greater blood flow remain to be demonstrated in adult horses or foals and may decrease blood flow by decreasing venous return. Intrathoracic cardiac compression is difficult to perform, is an impractical option in adult horses, and is unlikely to produce a favorable outcome.[11,12] Direct cardiac compression may be an option in newborn foals but has not been advocated, most likely because of long-term consequences.[11] If direct cardiac compression is attempted, an incision is made perpendicular to the spine on the left thoracic wall at the level of the fifth rib. The fifth-to-sixth rib interspace is retracted, and manual compression of the left ventricle is initiated using the palm of either hand. The heart should be compressed at a rate of 40 to 60 compressions per minute until a normal beat is restored (see Table 23-2). Although potentially successful, intrathoracic cardiac compression is associated with a high incidence of postoperative complications, including pneumothorax, infection, and severe lameness. Intrathoracic cardiac compression is best performed on horses weighing less than 100 kg.

Drugs

All drugs should be administered into a central vein (jugular vein, anterior vena cava) (see Table 23-3; Table 23-4). Doxapram can be administered to treat apnea if no other means of supporting ventilation is available.[19,20] Epinephrine is the drug of choice for the treatment of most cardiovascular catastrophes. Epinephrine is a mixed α- and β-agonist that stimulates heart rate and the force of heart contraction (see Table 22-3). Ventricular tachycardia does not always produce a complete loss of ventricular function. The use of epinephrine in this situation frequently induces ventricular fibrillation because of increases in ventricular excitability during myocardial hypoperfusion. Similarly epinephrine is unlikely to produce a normal heart rhythm or restore arterial blood pressure during ventricular fibrillation. The treatment of choice during ventricular tachycardia and ventricular fibrillation is lidocaine in adult horses and defibrillation (2 to 4 J/kg), if available, in foals.[22-24] Electrical defibrillation has been applied successfully to a 350-kg horse, but this is not a clinically practical procedure in adult horses at this time.[25] If heart rhythm normalizes, dobutamine can be administered to sustain increases in cardiac contractility, cardiac output, and arterial blood pressure (see Chapter 22). Ventricular fibrillation in the horse rarely, if ever, converts to sinus rhythm after the administration of epinephrine or antiarrhythmic drugs. Epinephrine only makes the electrical activity coarser. Dobutamine is the drug of choice for maintaining cardiac output and arterial blood pressure once a normal rhythm has been restored (see Chapter 22).[26,27]

Alternatively, vasopressin, a nonadrenergic endogenous stress hormone, can be administered (0.4 to 0.6 U/kg) intravenously (IV) alone or in combination with epinephrine to enhance cardiac contractile function, increase arterial blood pressure, improve coronary artery perfusion pressure, and restore peripheral tissue perfusion.[24,28] Vasopressin is one of the most potent vasoconstrictors known. Acting at vasopressin (V_1, V_2) receptors, it stimulates catecholamine secretion from chromaffin cells in the adrenal medulla and may help to "sensitize" adrenergic receptors, improving the response to both endogenous and exogenous catecholamines. In addition, vasopressin may play a role in hemostasis. Studies in other species suggest that return to spontaneous circulation may be improved following vasopressin therapy.[28] Repeat doses are not necessary. The use and clinical benefits of vasopressin administration during CPR in adult horses have not been determined. Calcium may be beneficial in counteracting the effects of hypocalcemia, hyperkalemia, and inhalant anesthetics.[29,30]

Lidocaine, 1 to 2 mg/kg IV slowly and 20 to 50 µg/kg/min, has been used to treat ventricular arrhythmias, including ventricular tachycardia in adult horses and foals.[22-24] Lidocaine produces multiple potential beneficial actions, including mild sedation, analgesia, and promotility effects, but can suppress sympathetic tone, resulting in vasodilation and hypotension; therefore infusion requires close monitoring. Magnesium sulfate, 20 to 30 mg/kg diluted in 5% dextrose in water IV slowly, is occasionally used as therapy for the treatment of ventricular tachycardia in horses; but its clinical effectiveness has not been confirmed, and it can produce hypotension.[24]

Fluids and aggressive fluid therapy are an essential component of any cardiopulmonary resuscitation effort in the horse (see Chapter 7). The volume of fluid needed to sustain mean circulatory filling pressure in the adult horse ranges from 5 to 10 ml/kg/hr during anesthesia but should be increased to at least 20 ml/kg during resuscitation. Electrolyte solutions used to replace fluids lost during hemorrhage should be administered in volumes at least three times the volume of lost blood. The administration of large volumes of balanced electrolytes can lead to hemodilution, low packed cell volume, and low total protein, predisposing to edema (see Chapter 7). Packed cell volumes of less than 20% and total protein of less than 3.5 g/dl should be avoided when possible. The use of 7% hypertonic saline and 7% hypertonic saline in 6% dextran 70 or 6% hetastarch produces beneficial hemodynamic effects in hemorrhaged horses.[31,32] Combined with conventional fluid therapy, the administration of hypertonic saline improves tissue blood flow and reduces fluid sequestration in the gut without overdiluting the patient (see Table 23-4).[33]

The administration of sodium bicarbonate ($NaHCO_3$; 1 mEq/kg IV) during CPR is indicated to treat metabolic acidosis and combat hyperkalemia caused by tissue hypoxia and ischemia. Sodium bicarbonate therapy is not necessary if hemodynamics can be restored in a short time and may prove detrimental if given in large quantities. Sodium bicarbonate administration can cause hyperosmolality, hypernatremia, hypocalcemia, hypokalemia, and decreases in hemoglobin affinity for oxygen. Furosemide is administered to treat pulmonary edema; nonsteroidal antiinflammatory drugs and glucocorticosteroids may be useful for treating shock.

Table 23–4. Drugs used to treat complications in horses

Generic name (trade name)	Concentration	Recommended use	Dose, IV	Potential side effects
Cardiovascular stimulants				
Epinephrine	1 mg/ml	Initiate or increase heart rate Increase arterial pressure Increase cardiac contractility	1-5 µg/kg	Tachycardia, cardiac arrhythmias, hypertension, hypotension
Dopamine	40 mg/ml	Increase arterial pressure Increase cardiac contractility Increase heart rate	1-5 µg/kg/min*	Cardiac arrhythmias, hypertension
Dobutamine	12.5 mg/ml	Increase arterial pressure Increase cardiac contractility	1-5 µg/kg/min*	Cardiac arrhythmias, hypertension
Ephedrine	25 mg/ml	Increase arterial pressure	0.01-0.2 mg/kg in 10-mg boluses	Cardiac arrhythmias
Phenylephrine	10 mg/ml	Increase arterial pressure	0.01 mg/kg to effect	Bradycardia, cardiac arrhythmias
Calcium chloride	10% solution	Increase cardiac contractility	5-10 ml/100 kg (0.2 mg/kg)	Cardiac arrhythmias
Hypertonic saline	7%	Increase cardiac output and blood pressure	4 ml/kg	Hyperosmolality, hypokalemia
Antiarrhythmics				
Atropine	15 mg/ml	Increase heart rate	0.01-0.2 mg/kg	Tachycardia, arrhythmias
Glycopyrrolate	0.2 mg/ml	Increase heart rate	0.005 mg/kg	Tachycardia, arrhythmias
Quinidine	80 mg/ml	Supraventricular or ventricular arrhythmias	4-5 mg/kg total (given 1 mg/kg every 10 min)	Hypotension, tachycardia
Lidocaine	20 mg/ml	Ventricular arrhythmias	0.5 mg/kg; total 2 mg/kg	Convulsions
Respiratory stimulants				
Doxapram	20 mg/ml	Initiate or stimulate breathing (↑ frequency volume)	0.2 mg/kg	Respiratory alkalosis, hypokalemia, convulsions
Others				
Sodium bicarbonate		Treat metabolic acidosis (pH <7.20)	0.5 mEq/kg at 10-15 min intervals as required	Metabolic alkalosis, hypokalemia, hyperosmolality, paradoxical CSF acidosis
Furosemide	50 mg/ml	Promote diuresis, eliminate edema	1 mg/kg	Dehydration and decreased cardiac output, hypokalemic metabolic alkalosis
Prednisolone sodium succinate	10 mg/ml	Shock, ischemia	1-2 mg/kg	—
Dexamethasone	2 mg/ml	Shock, ischemia	2-4 mg/kg	—
Flunixin meglumine	50 mg/ml	Analgesic, antiinflammatory	0.5-1.1 mg/kg IM or IV	Gastric ulcers rarely Anorexia, decreased total protein

CSF, Cerebrospinal fluid; *IV,* intravenously; *IM,* intramuscularly.
*Doses up to 15 µg/kg intravenously are used in severe cardiovascular depression.
(Modified from Muir WW, Bednarski RM: Equine cardiopulmonary resuscitation—Part II, *Compend Contin Educ* 5:S292, 1983.)

Assessment of Cardiopulmonary Resuscitation and Prognosis

Successful CPR is indicated by a return of normal respiration and a strong palpable peripheral pulse. Active corneal and palpebral reflexes, response to auditory and physical stimuli, and other signs of increased consciousness should follow shortly thereafter. Mild sedation (xylazine, detomidine) may be required to prevent struggling and excitement. The rapidity with which these signs return is a reliable index of long-term prognosis. If normal ventilation and circulation can be restored (less than 3 to 5 minutes), most horses recover without significant complications. Resuscitation efforts longer than 5 minutes suggest a very poor prognosis because cerebral and peripheral tissue ischemia and hypoxia eventually result in cell death and lysis, regardless of the restoration of blood flow. The potential for neural deficits and seizures is increased after prolonged resuscitative efforts. Clinical studies in humans suggests that therapy to prevent cerebral edema (mannitol, diuretics, nonsteroidal antiinflammatory drugs, anticonvulsants) are not effective after resuscitation and that the administration of 7% hypertonic saline significantly lowers cerebral spinal pressure and reduces brain swelling after cardiac arrest (see Table 23-4).[34,35] Its potential benefit for these purposes in adult horses and foals has yet to be demonstrated.

In conclusion, the best way to treat cardiopulmonary emergencies in horses is to prevent them. A thorough history and physical examination must be obtained before administering anesthetic drugs (see Chapter 6). Vigilant and accurate patient monitoring and monitoring techniques must be utilized (see Chapter 8). The decision to quit CPR is guided by the duration of resuscitation, the horse's response, and practical considerations. Finally, all personnel should be familiar with emergency drugs and techniques and, most of all, be prepared should a cardiopulmonary emergency occur.

References

1. Schleien CL et al: Controversial issues in cardiopulmonary resuscitation, *Anesthesiology* 71:133-149, 1989.
2. Gazmuri RJ et al: Arterial $PaCO_2$ as an indicator of systemic perfusion during cardiopulmonary resuscitation, *Crit Care Med* 17:237-240, 1989.
3. Takasu A, Sakamoto T, Okada Y: Arterial base excess after CPR: the relationship to CPR duration and the characteristics related to outcome, *Resuscitation* 73: 394-399, 2007.
4. Hatlestad D: Capnography as a predictor of the return of spontaneous circulation, *Emerg Med Serv* 33(8):75-80, 2004.
5. Edner A, Nyman G, Essen-Gustavsson B: The effects of spontaneous and mechanical ventilation on central cardiovascular function and peripheral perfusion during isoflurane anaesthesia in horses, *Anaesth Analg* 32:136-146, 2005.
6. Frauenfelder HC et al: External cardiovascular resuscitation of the anesthetized pony, *J Am Vet Med Assoc* 179:673-676, 1981.
7. Goldstein MA et al: Cardiopulmonary resuscitation in the horse, *Cornell Vet* 71:225-268, 1981.
8. Kellagher REB, Watney GCG: Cardiac arrest during anaesthesia in two horses, *Vet Rec* 119:347-349, 1986.
9. Hubbell HAE, Muir WW, Gaynor JS: Cardiovascular effects of thoracic compression in horses subjected to euthanasia, *Equine Vet J* 25:282-284, 1993.
10. Cooper JA, Cooper JD, Cooper JM: Cardiopulmonary resuscitation: history, current practice, and future direction, *Circulation* 114:2839-2849, 2006.
11. Kellagher REB, Watney GCG: Cardiac arrest during anaesthesia in two horses, *Vet Rec* 119:347-349, 1986.
12. DeMoor A et al: Intrathoracic cardiac resuscitation in the horse, *Equine Vet J* 4:31-33, 1972.
13. Hodgson DS, Steffey EP: Intra-operative cardiac arrest routes to recovery, *Equine Vet J* 25(4):259-260, 1993.
14. Goldstein MA et al: Cardiopulmonary resuscitation in the horse, *Cornell Vet* 71:225-268, 1981.
15. Watney GCG, Watkins SB, Hall LW: Effects of a demand valve on pulmonary ventilation in spontaneously breathing, anaesthetised horses, *Vet Rec* 117:358-362, 1985.
16. Levy W, Gillespie JR: Emergency ventilator for resuscitating apneic horses, *J Am Vet Med Assoc* 161:57-60, 1972.
17. Blaze CA, Robinson NE: Apneic oxygenation in anesthetized ponies and horses, *Vet Res Commun* 11:281-291, 1987.
18. Young SS: Jet anaesthesia in horses, *Equine Vet J* 21:319-320, 1989.
19. Short CE, Cloyd GD, Ward JW: The use of doxapram hydrochloride with intravenous anesthetics in horses—Part I, *Vet Med Small Anim Clin* 65:157-160, 1970.
20. Wernette KM et al: Doxapram: cardiopulmonary effects in the horse, *Am J Vet Res* 47:1360-1362, 1986.
21. Taylor PM: Doxapram infusion during halothane anaesthesia in ponies, *Equine Vet J* 22:329-332, 1990.
22. McGuirk SM, Muir WW: Diagnosis and treatment of cardiac arrhythmias, *Vet Clin North Am (Equine Pract)* 1:353-370, 1985.
23. Muir WW, McGuirk SM: Pharmacology and pharmacokinetics of drugs used to treat cardiac disease in horses, *Vet Clin North Am (Equine Pract)* 1:335-352, 1985.
24. Palmer JE: Neonatal foal resuscitation, *Vet Clin North Am (Equine Pract)* 23(1):159-182, 2007.
25. Witzel DA et al: Electrical defibrillation of the equine heart, *Am J Vet Res* 29(6):1279-1285, 1968.
26. Swanson CR, Muir WW: Dobutamine-induced augmentation of cardiac output does not enhance respiratory gas exchange in anesthetized recumbent healthy horses, *Am J Vet Res* 47:1573-1576, 1986.
27. Young LE et al: Temporal effects of an infusion of dobutamine hydrochloride in horses anesthetized with halothane, *Am J Vet Res* 59:1027-1032, 1998.
28. Aung K, Htay T: Vasopressin for cardiac arrest, *Arch Intern Med* 165:17-24, 2005.
29. Grubb TL et al: Hemodynamic effects of calcium gluconate administered to conscious horses, *J Vet Intern Med* 10(6):401-404, 1996.
30. Grubb TL et al: Hemodynamic effects of ionized calcium in horses anesthetized with halothane or isoflurane, *Am J Vet Res* 60(11):1430-1435, 1999.
31. Moon PF et al: Effects of a highly concentrated hypertonic saline-dextran volume expander on cardiopulmonary function in anesthetized normovolemic horses, *Am J Vet Res* 52(10):1611-1618, 1991.
32. Hallowell GD, Corley KTT: Preoperative administration of hydroxyethyl starch or hypertonic saline to horses with colic, *J Vet Intern Med* 20:980-986, 2006.
33. Radhakrishnan RS et al: Hypertonic saline resuscitation prevents hydrostatically induced intestinal edema and ileus, *Crit Care Med* 34(6):1713-1718, 2006.
34. Ziai WC, Toung TJ, Bhardwaj A: Hypertonic saline: first-line therapy for cerebral edema, *J Neurol Sci* 261(1-2):157-166, 2007.
35. Tyagi R et al: Hypertonic saline: a clinical review, *Neurosurg Rev* 30(4):277-289, 2007.

Anesthetic Protocols and Techniques for Specific Procedures

John A.E. Hubbell

William W. Muir

KEY POINTS

1. Standard drug protocols should be developed and used routinely to produce anesthesia in horses.
2. Protocols must be modifiable on the basis of the medical history, age, and physical status of the horse; the procedure to be performed; and the severity of pain.
3. Injectable anesthetic drugs should always be available for horses that wake up unexpectedly or for those requiring an extension of general anesthesia.
4. Physical monitoring techniques should be used and recorded regularly in every horse.
5. Technological monitoring techniques should be used in longer, more involved surgical procedures.
6. Normal values for an anesthetized adult horse are: heart rate >25 beats/min; mean arterial blood pressure >70 mm Hg; respiratory rate >4 breaths/min; SpO_2 >90%; $ETCO_2$ <60 mm Hg.

New anesthetic drugs and anesthetic techniques continue to evolve. This evolution, combined with clinical research, provides the basis for improved anesthesia in horses. The anesthetic protocols described are used frequently and provide a basis for discussion of commonly encountered surgical procedures requiring anesthesia. Every anesthetic protocol should be capable of being modified or adjusted to meet each horse's individual requirements. Each case discussion addresses common occurrences or predicaments that can occur during equine anesthesia and provides potential solutions.

CASTRATION (Box 24-1)

A 400-kg 2-year-old Standardbred colt is presented for elective castration. The colt has not been fed today but has had free access to water. Preanesthetic physical examination and blood work (hemogram, fibrinogen) are normal. Both testicles are palpable in the scrotum. A grassy paddock is available for the surgical procedure, which is anticipated to require 20 minutes. A 14-g catheter is percutaneously placed in the left jugular vein and sutured to the skin after local infiltration with 2 ml of 2% lidocaine. The catheter will be used for administration of anesthetic drugs and will not be removed until the horse has recovered from anesthesia.

The colt was walked to the grassy paddock before being administered xylazine (400 mg [1 mg/kg] intravenously [IV]). Approximately 3 minutes later the colt became indifferent to its surroundings, reluctant to move, and ataxic; the head was lowered to a position where its nose was below its knees. It knuckled on its front legs and

swayed from side to side. The colt's mouth was rinsed with water to remove any foreign material; ketamine (900 mg [≈2.2 mg/kg]) and then diazepam (40 mg [0.1 mg/kg]) were drawn into a syringe (17 ml total) and administered rapidly IV (see Chapters 12 and 13). The halter was held securely, and the head elevated in an attempt to make the colt "sit down" before becoming recumbent. The colt sat down, fell in sternal recumbency 50 seconds after ketamine/diazepam administration, and was rolled into right lateral recumbency. A rope was placed around the left hind leg ankle, and an attendant lifted the leg to expose the scrotum. The horse's eye signs (depth of anesthesia), heart rate, respiratory rate, mucous membrane color, and capillary refill time were monitored for the duration of the procedure. The scrotum was surgically scrubbed, and 20 ml of 2% lidocaine was injected into the base of each testicle and spermatic cord to reduce the reaction to clamping and transfixation of the spermatic cord during "closed" castration. The castration was completed within 10 minutes (≈15 minutes from induction). The gelding rolled to a sternal position 30 minutes after induction of anesthesia and stood 7 minutes later. Phenylbutazone paste (1 g po, bid) was administered for 5 days.

Predicament 1

The colt does not respond satisfactorily to preanesthetic medication.

Solution 1

Administer additional xylazine (0.3 to 0.5 mg/kg IV) and wait for an appropriate response.

Solution 2

Administer a 5% or 10% solution of guaifenesin to effect (depression, ataxia, unable to support weight) and then induce anesthesia.

Box 24-1   Anesthesia for Castration

Sedation

Xylazine (1 mg/kg IV) (wait for full effect)

Anesthesia

Diazepam (0.1 mg/kg IV) combined with ketamine (2.2 mg/kg IV)

Lidocaine (2%; 20 ml into the spermatic cord)

Postoperative Analgesia

Phenylbutazone (2 mg/kg bid per os)

Predicament 2

The surgical procedure takes longer than expected.

Solution 1

Administer an additional 3 ml of a 2:1 (vol:vol) ketamine (100 mg/ml)-xylazine (100 mg/ml) drug combination IV.

Solution 2

Prepare a 5% solution of guaifenesin in a 500-ml bag of 5% dextrose to which 500 mg of ketamine and 250 mg of xylazine have been added and administer IV to effect.

ARTHROSCOPY (Box 24-2)

A 450-kg three year old female Thoroughbred Racehorse is presented for surgical removal of bilateral distal radial chip fractures. Preanesthetic physical examination and blood work (hemogram, fibrinogen) are within normal limits. The anticipated duration of surgery is 75 minutes. Food but not water is withheld for 8 hours before surgery, and the mouth is rinsed with water to remove any foreign material. Detomidine (10 mg [≈20 μg/kg]) is administered intramuscularly (IM) 30 minutes before induction to facilitate clipping and shaving of the surgical sites. A 14-g catheter is percutaneously introduced into the left jugular vein after local infiltration with 2 ml of 2% lidocaine to facilitate administration of anesthetic drugs and isotonic fluids. The intravenous catheter is sutured to the skin to prevent inadvertent removal during subsequent procedures. Phenylbutazone (2 g IV) is administered 20 minutes before producing anesthesia.

The filly was brought to the induction stall and positioned with its hindquarters in a corner and its body along a wall. Additional detomidine (3 mg IV) was administered, followed 4 minutes later by ketamine (1g [≈2.2 mg/kg]) and diazepam (45 mg [0.1 mg/kg]) drawn into a syringe (17 ml total) and administered rapidly IV. The head was elevated to a normal position as the filly relaxed first to a sitting and then a sternal position 40 seconds after drug administration. The filly was rolled to lateral recumbency. A bite block was placed (5 cm polyvinylchloride [PVC] pipe; see Chapter 14), and a 26-mm diameter cuffed endotracheal tube was passed

| Box 24–2 | **Anesthesia for Arthroscopy** |

Sedation
Detomidine (22 μg/kg IM) (T–30 min)
Detomidine (6.6 μg/kg IV) (T–3 min)

Anesthesia
Diazepam (0.1 mg/kg IV) combined with ketamine (2.2 mg/kg IV)
Isoflurane in O_2 (3% then 2% in oxygen); controlled ventilation

Recovery
Detomidine (4.4 μg/kg IV)

Preoperative and Postoperative Analgesia
Preop: Phenylbutazone (2 mg/kg IV)
Postop: Phenylbutazone (2 mg/kg bid per os)

into the trachea. The endotracheal tube cuff was inflated and connected to a large animal circle anesthetic machine. The initial oxygen flow rate was 10 L/min, and the isoflurane vaporizer setting was 3%. The filly was positioned in dorsal recumbency on a 25-cm thick foam rubber pad. The filly's eye signs (depth of anesthesia), heart rate, respiratory rate, mucous membrane color, and capillary refill time were monitored and recorded for the duration of the procedure. A 21-g catheter was placed in the facial artery for continuous determination of arterial blood pressure and periodic collection of anaerobic arterial blood samples for pH and blood gas analysis. Lactated Ringer's solution (LRS), 10 ml/kg/hr, was administered IV. The oxygen flow rate was reduced to 3 L/min, and isoflurane concentration to 2% 15 minutes after induction when the palpebral reflex became depressed, voluntary blinking stopped, and nystagmus was absent. The arterial blood pressure was 112/58/76 (systolic/diastolic/mean) mm Hg 20 minutes after induction, and the mean arterial blood pressure did not change more than 7 mm Hg throughout the procedure. An arterial blood gas sample obtained 30 minutes after induction to anesthesia produced the following values: pH 7.28, $PaCO_2$ 65 mm Hg, and PaO_2 175 mm Hg. Primary respiratory acidosis was diagnosed ($0.25 \times 0.05 = 0.125$; $7.40 - 0.125 = 7.28$; see Chapter 8); and controlled ventilation was initiated at a tidal volume of 7 L (inspiratory time of 1.3 seconds), respiratory rate of 6 breaths/min, producing an inspiratory pressure of 24 cm H_2O for the remainder of anesthesia. An arterial blood gas sample obtained just before stopping controlled ventilation was pH 7.38, $PaCO_2$ 45 mm Hg, and PaO_2 225 mm Hg. Bandages were applied at the completion of surgery, and detomidine (2 mg IV) was administered as the filly was moved to the recovery stall. Head and tail ropes were attached to assist recovery (see Chapter 21). The filly rolled to sternal recumbency 30 minutes after being placed in the recovery stall, remained in sternal recumbency for 10 minutes, and then stood on the first attempt. Phenylbutazone paste (1 g) was administered twice a day for 5 days.

Predicament 1

The horse becomes "light" while transitioning to inhalant anesthesia.

Solution 1

Administer an additional 4 ml of a 1:1 (vol:vol) ketamine (100 mg/ml)-diazepam (5 mg/ml) drug combination.

Solution 2

Administer thiopental (0.5 to 1 mg/kg IV) to improve hypnosis and relaxation and stop movement. Thiopental is an excellent hypnotic and muscle relaxant and markedly facilitates orotracheal intubation in horses administered ketamine-diazepam.

Solution 3

The inhalation anesthetic circuit can be primed with a 2% (maintenance) concentration of isoflurane by closing the pop-off valve, putting a stopper in the end of the Y piece, and turning the isoflurane vaporizer to 2% and the oxygen flow to 6 to 10 L/min. The oxygen flow rate is turned off once the rebreathing bag is filled. Once the horse is anesthetized, the stopper is removed from the Y piece, and the endotracheal tube is attached. This procedure causes the horse to breathe maintenance concentrations of isoflurane from the beginning of inhalant anesthesia and avoids the potentially prolonged times of 10 to 20 minutes generally required to equilibrate the anesthetic circuit with oxygen and inhalant anesthetic.

Predicament 2

The horse does not begin to breathe spontaneously when controlled ventilation is stopped.

Solution 1

Wean the horse from the ventilator by reducing the respiratory rate to 2 breaths/min. Most horses begin to breathe spontaneously as anesthesia is lightened and the $PaCO_2$ becomes >50 to 55 mm Hg or the $ETCO_2$ becomes >55 to 60 mm Hg.

Solution 2

Administer doxapram (0.05 to 0.1 mg/kg IV). Doxapram initiates spontaneous breathing in lightly anesthetized horses recovering from anesthesia.

ARTHRODESIS (Box 24-3)

A 425-kg 6-year-old American Quarter Horse that is used for barrel racing is presented for pastern arthrodesis of the right front limb. Preanesthetic physical examination and blood work (hemogram, fibrinogen, and chemistry profile) are within normal limits. The horse has been administered phenylbutazone (1 g bid) for the past 7 months. Food but not water is withheld for 6 hours, and the mouth is rinsed with water to remove residual debris. A 14-g catheter is introduced transcutaneously into the left jugular vein to facilitate administration of anesthetic drugs and isotonic fluids. The anticipated duration of anesthesia is 180 minutes.

Thirty minutes before induction, detomidine (10 mg IM [≈20 µg/kg]) was administered to facilitate clipping and preparation of the surgical site. The horse was moved to the

---

Box 24–3	**Anesthesia for Arthrodesis**

Sedation
Detomidine (22 µg/kg IM) (T –30 min)
Detomidine 96.6 µg/kg IV) (T –3 min)

Anesthesia
Diazepam (0.1 mg/kg IV) combined with ketamine
  (2.2 mg/kg IV)
Isoflurane in O_2 (3% then 2% then 1.25%); controlled
  ventilation

Intraoperative Analgesia with 1.25 % Isoflurane
Lidocaine (2 mg/kg IV bolus over 15 minutes), infusion
  (3 mg/kg/hr)
Morphine (0.1 mg/kg IV)

Recovery
Detomidine (4.5 µg/kg IV)

Postoperative Analgesia
Phenylbutazone (2 mg/kg bid IV; then PO for 5 days)
Morphine (0.1 mg/kg IM bid for 3 days)

---

induction stall and administered detomidine (2 mg IV) to augment sedation. Anesthesia was produced by administering ketamine (1g [≈2.2 mg/kg]) and diazepam (50 mg [≈0.1 mg/kg]) drawn into a syringe (20 ml total) and administered rapidly IV. A speculum (PVC pipe) was placed between the incisors, and a 26-mm diameter cuffed endotracheal tube was positioned in the trachea. The endotracheal tube was connected to a large animal circle anesthetic machine. The horse's eye signs (depth of anesthesia), heart rate, respiratory rate, mucous membrane color, and capillary refill time were monitored and recorded for the duration of the procedure. The horse was positioned in right lateral recumbency on a 25-cm thick foam rubber pad. The right (down) front limb was pulled forward, and pads were placed between the front and rear legs. The initial oxygen rate was set at 10 L/min with an initial isoflurane vaporizer setting of 3%. A 21-g catheter was placed in the facial artery for continuous determination of arterial blood pressure and periodic collection of anaerobic arterial samples for pH and blood gas analysis. The initial mean arterial blood pressure was 85 mm Hg. Intravenous LRS, 10 ml/kg/hr, was administered. Controlled ventilation was instituted: tidal volume 7 L (inspiratory time 1.2 sec); respiratory rate of 6 breaths/min produced an inspiratory pressure of 26 cm H_2O. Fifteen minutes after induction the oxygen flow rate was reduced to 3 L/min. The isoflurane vaporizer setting was reduced to 2% when the palpebral reflex slowed, voluntary blinking stopped, and nystagmus was absent. Lidocaine was administered as a bolus (850 mg [2 mg/kg]) IV over 10 minutes and infused (3 mg/kg/hr) throughout anesthesia (see Chapter 13). Morphine (45 mg [0.1 mg/kg]) was administered IM immediately before the beginning of the surgical procedure and was infused (0.1/kg/hr) throughout anesthesia (see Chapter 13). The isoflurane vaporizer setting was reduced to deliver 1.25% 15 minutes beginning the infusion of morphine. The arterial blood pressure stabilized at 107/58/77 (systolic/diastolic/mean) mm Hg 15 minutes after reducing the isoflurane vaporizer to 1.25% and did not change more than 9 mm Hg throughout the procedure. Arterial blood gases analyses were pH 7.38, $PaCO_2$ 45 mm Hg, and PaO_2 325 mm Hg 30 minutes after initiating controlled ventilation.

Surgery was completed uneventfully, and the horse was moved to the recovery stall and administered detomidine (2 mg IV) to facilitate inhalant anesthetic elimination and calm the recovery process. A demand valve was used to assist ventilation and augment oxygenation, and head and tail ropes were used to assist attempts to stand. The horse stood on its second attempt 55 minutes after being placed in the recovery stall and was administered phenylbutazone (2 mg/kg IV) and morphine (0.1 mg/kg IV) for postoperative analgesia.

Predicament 1

Maintaining a stable plan of anesthesia without producing hypotension. Many horses become hypotensive (mean arterial blood pressure <60 mm Hg) at inhalant anesthetic concentrations required to perform major (orthopedic, abdominal) surgical procedures. Reducing inhalant anesthetic concentrations improves arterial blood pressure but often results in too light a plane of anesthesia and the possibility that the horse could move.

Solution

The administration of an analgesic or anesthetic analgesic adjunct improves analgesia without producing significant additional cardiovascular depression. Inhalant anesthetic concentration can be reduced by 25% to 50% in most horses, resulting in marked improvement in arterial blood pressure and blood flow. Unimodal (lidocaine, medetomidine, detomidine, butorphanol, morphine) or multimodal (morphine-lidocaine-ketamine drug combination) therapies can be administered to augment inhalant anesthesia (see Chapter 13). The use of morphine-lidocaine-ketamine is very effective in reducing inhalant anesthetic requirements and improving hemodynamics in horses (see following paragraph). The infusion is stopped after 3 hours.

Add 60 ml of lidocaine + 3 ml of morphine + 7 ml of ketamine to 5 L of LRS and administer 10 ml/kg/hr. This infusion rate delivers morphine: 0.1 mg/kg/hr; lidocaine: 3 mg/kg/hr; ketamine: 1.5 mg/kg/hr.

NASAL SEPTUM REMOVAL (Box 24-4)

A 650-kg 10-year-old warm-blooded gelding is presented for removal of the nasal septum because of neoplasia. Preanesthetic physical examination and blood work (hemogram, fibrinogen, and chemistry profile) are within normal limits with the exception of the packed cell volume, which is 24% (reference range 35% to 45%). A blood donor has been identified, and major and minor cross-match performed. Eight liters of whole blood have been collected. Food but not water is withheld for 8 hours, and the mouth is rinsed with water to remove residual debris. A 14-g catheter is introduced percutaneously into each jugular vein after local infiltration with 2 ml of 2% lidocaine to facilitate administration of anesthetic drugs, isotonic fluids, colloids, and blood if needed. The ventral surface of the neck is clipped in anticipation of a tracheostomy. Total anesthesia time is anticipated to be 90 minutes.

The horse was moved to the induction stall, and xylazine (325 mg [0.5 mg/kg] IV) was administered. The horse became moderately sedate, but additional xylazine (150 mg

---

Box 24-4 Anesthesia for Nasal Septum Removal

Sedation
Xylazine (0.5 mg/kg IV)
Xylazine (0.2 mg/kg IV)

Anesthesia
Diazepam (0.07 mg/kg IV) combined with ketamine (1.8 mg/kg IV)
Tracheostomy
Sevoflurane in O_2 (3% then 2%-3% as needed)

Fluid Therapy for Blood Loss
Hetastarch in lactated Ringer's solution (Hextend)
Hypertonic saline (7%) in 6% hetastarch: 3 ml/kg IV
    Add 1 ml of 23.4% Na+Cl− to 2 ml of 6% hetastarch
    Dose this combination at 3 ml/kg
Whole blood (8 L IV)

Postoperative Analgesia
Phenylbutazone (2 mg/kg bid IV)

IV) was administered to optimize sedation. Anesthesia was produced by administering ketamine (1.3 g [≈2 mg/kg]) and diazepam (50 mg [≈0.1 mg/kg]) drawn into a syringe (23 ml total) and administered rapidly IV. A speculum (PVC pipe) was placed between the incisors, and a 26-mm diameter cuffed endotracheal tube was positioned into the trachea. The endotracheal tube cuff was inflated, and the endotracheal tube was connected to a large animal circle anesthetic machine. The inhalation anesthetic circuit had been primed with a 3% (maintenance) concentration of sevoflurane by closing the pop-off valve, putting a stopper in the end of the Y piece, and turning the isoflurane vaporizer to 3% and the oxygen flow to 6 L/min. The oxygen flow rate was turned off once the rebreathing bag was filled. Initial fresh gas flow rates were set at 3 L/min with an initial sevoflurane vaporizer setting of 3%. The horse's eye signs (depth of anesthesia), heart rate, respiratory rate, mucous membrane color, and capillary refill time were monitored and recorded for the duration of the procedure. The horse was positioned in dorsal recumbency, and a midcervical tracheostomy was performed. The orotracheal endotracheal tube was removed, and a 24-mm diameter endotracheal tube was placed into the trachea. Anesthesia was maintained for the duration of the procedure via this airway. The horse was positioned in right lateral recumbency on a 25-cm thick foam rubber pad. The right (down) front limb was pulled forward, and pads were placed between the front and rear legs. LRS (10 ml/kg/hr) was administered IV. A 21-g catheter was placed in the dorsal metatarsal artery of the left hind limb for continuous determination of arterial blood pressure and periodic collection of anaerobic arterial samples for pH and blood gas analysis. The initial mean arterial blood pressure was 75 mm Hg. The sevoflurane vaporizer setting was adjusted periodically between 2% and 3%, and the oxygen flow rate was adjusted to 3 L based on the palpebral and corneal reflexes and the presence of nystagmus. Spontaneous ventilation was 8 breaths/min. Estimated blood loss associated with surgical removal of the horse's nasal septum was 15 L. The mean arterial blood pressure decreased to a value of 55 mm Hg during hemorrhage. The sevoflurane concentration was deceased to 2.25%, the rate of IV fluid administration was increased to 30 ml/kg/hr, and 2 L of 7% hypertonic saline in 6% hetastarch was administered IV in 15 minutes. Eight liters of blood was administered IV after the initial fluid resuscitation. The mean arterial blood pressure increased to 79 ± 5 mm Hg and remained stable for the remainder of surgery and anesthesia. The nose was packed with gauze, and the incisions were closed. The horse was moved to the recovery stall with the endotracheal tube in place. Head and tail ropes were attached to assist recovery. The horse rolled to its sternum and immediately stood on its first attempt 35 minutes after being placed in the recovery stall. The endotracheal tube was replaced with a standard J type tracheostomy tube when the horse was returned to its stall.

Predicament 1

Blood loss is common during many surgical procedures. Blood volume is approximately 70 ml/kg in adult horses (650 × 70 = 45.5 L total blood volume). The horse's packed cell volume (PCV) and total protein (TP) may not change appreciably during acute blood loss but are decreased by anesthesia, crystalloid (LRS) administration, and hypotension (see Chapter 3: Starling forces). Blood loss greater than 15% to 20% of the estimated total blood volume usually triggers compensatory responses (tachycardia, vasoconstriction) that can be blunted by anesthetic drugs. This horse suffered moderate blood loss totaling 33% (15/45.5; 23 ml/kg) of its total blood volume. Moderate hemorrhage can result in intestinal and skeletal muscle ischemia, predisposing this horse to myopathy, diarrhea, and endotoxemia.

Solution

The PCV and TP should be monitored and recorded in all horses anticipated or experiencing significant blood loss before and during anesthesia. Horses that have initial PCV and TP values within normal limits at the start of surgery that acutely fall to PCV <20% and TP <3.5 g/dl should be administered blood, albumin, or an alternate colloidal solution if blood is not available. Crystalloids (LRS; 0.9% Na$^+$Cl$^-$) are relatively ineffective for treating hypotension induced by blood loss or inhalant anesthetics because of their short retention time in the vascular fluid compartment. Crystalloids have no oncotic value and rapidly redistribute into the interstitial fluid compartment (see Chapter 7). Arterial blood pressure may increase when crystalloids are administered rapidly (>20 ml/kg/hr) but decrease to original values or below once fluid rate is slowed or discontinued. In addition, crystalloids dilute PCV, TP, electrolytes (e.g., K$^+$), and H$^+$ buffers (dilutional acidosis). Hypertonic saline (7%; 3 to 4 ml/kg IV) is hypertonic compared to plasma, produces beneficial hemodynamic effects, and is administered in small volumes (3 ml/kg IV). Hetastarch (6%; in 0.9% Na$^+$Cl$^-$ or LRS [Hextend]; 5 ml/kg [20 ml/kg total dosage]) has a colloid osmotic pressure approximately twice that of plasma. Both fluids produce an immediate and sustained increase in plasma volume, resulting in an increase in arterial blood pressure and blood flow.

Predicament 2

This horse recovered with an endotracheal tube placed through a tracheostomy into the trachea. Horses that are intubated orotracheally and develop low PCV and TP values during anesthesia because of hemodilution (LRS administration), blood loss, or hypotension have an increased incidence of nasal edema and upper airway obstruction. once the orotracheal tube is removed, signs of nasal edema include increased respiratory effort (abdominal lift), reduced air passage through the nose, snoring, and stress (apprehension, fear).

Solution

A nasopharyngeal or nasotracheal tube should be placed and secured to the horse's halter. The tube can be removed once there is evidence for airflow through the opposite nares (see Chapter 22).

ABDOMINAL EXPLORATORY FOR COLIC PAIN (Box 24-5)

An 18-year-old 475-kg Arabian gelding is presented for abdominal pain of at least 4 hours' duration. The horse had been found recumbent in a stall at 8:00 AM and was

---

Box 24–5   Anesthesia for Abdominal Exploratory

Sedation
Xylazine (0.5 mg/kg IV)
Xylazine (0.4 mg/kg IV)

Anesthesia
Guaifenesin (40 mg/kg IV) followed by ketamine (1.5 mg/kg IV)
Sevoflurane (4% then 2%); controlled ventilation

Intraoperative Analgesia
Lidocaine (2 mg/kg bolus over 15 minutes), infusion 3 mg/kg/hr

Fluid Therapy for Hypotension
Hetastarch in LRS (Hextend): 5 L (10 ml/kg IV)
Dobutamine (1-2 µg/kg/min IV)

Recovery
Xylazine (2 µg/kg IV)

Postoperative Analgesia
Flunixin (1 mg/kg sid)

---

transported for surgery because it was unresponsive to therapy and had unrelenting pain. A nasogastric tube had been placed at the farm, and a large quantity of green fluid was removed from the stomach. The nasogastric tube was removed before the horse was transported for surgery. On presentation, the horse is standing but depressed. The pulse rate is 70 beats/min, and respiratory rate is 30 breaths/min. The abdomen is distended, and multiple loops of small intestine were palpated during rectal examination. A nasogastric tube was passed, and an additional quantity (approximately 5 L) of green fluid retrieved. The nasogastric tube was left in place. A hemogram indicated hemoconcentration (packed cell volume 65) and leukocytosis. A 14-g catheter was percutaneously introduced into each jugular vein after local infiltration with 2 ml of 2 % lidocaine, and 10 L of LRS was rapidly administered. The horse was administered xylazine (250 mg [≈ 0.5 mg/kg] IV) and scheduled for an immediate exploratory laparotomy. The anticipated duration of surgery and anesthesia is 180 minutes.

The horse was moved to an induction stall, and additional xylazine (200 mg IV) was administered. The horse became adequately sedated within 2 minutes. Guaifenesin (5% in 5% dextrose) was administered (to effect, 20 g) until the horse's head dropped below its knees and it demonstrated signs of weakness (the knee buckled) and ataxia. Ketamine (725 mg [≈1.5 mg/kg]) was administered IV. The horse became recumbent 45 seconds later and was rolled to lateral recumbency. A 26-mm cuffed endotracheal tube was passed through a PVC mouth speculum and into the trachea. The horse was positioned in dorsal recumbency and connected to a circle anesthesia machine with an attached ventilator. The horse's eye signs (depth of anesthesia), heart rate, respiratory rate, mucous membrane color, and capillary refill time were monitored and recorded for the duration of the procedure. The initial oxygen flow rate was 10 L/min, and a sevoflurane vaporizer was adjusted to deliver an anesthetic concentration of 4%. The ventilator was set to deliver

2 breaths/min to an inspiratory pressure of 30 cm H_2O until the abdomen was opened surgically or the arterial blood pressures were known. A 21-g catheter was placed in the facial artery for continuous determination of arterial blood pressure and periodic collection of anaerobic arterial samples for pH and blood gas analysis. The initial heart rate was 62 beats/min, and arterial blood pressure values were 75/30/45 mm Hg (systolic/diastolic/mean). Every time the ventilator cycled on (inspiration), the systolic arterial blood pressure increased by 8 mm Hg above and then fell 5 mm Hg below the average systolic value of 75 mm Hg (determined when the ventilator was not cycling). Ten liters (20 ml/kg) of LRS and 5 L (10 ml/kg) of 6% hetastarch were administered during the next 30 minutes, and a dobutamine infusion (1 µg/kg/min) was started. The mean arterial blood pressure increased to a value of 73 mm Hg over the next 5 minutes. The ventilator rate was increased to 6 breaths/min, and tidal volume increased to 6 L once the abdomen was opened. Lidocaine (1 g [2 mg/kg] intravenous bolus over 5 minutes, 3 mg/kg/hr) was administered, the sevoflurane concentration was decreased to 2%, and the oxygen flow rate was reduced to 3 L/min. The mean arterial blood pressure decreased to 62 mm Hg 5 minutes after beginning the lidocaine infusion. An arterial blood gas sample (pH, 7.26; $PaCO_2$, 59 mm Hg; PaO_2, 75 mm Hg; BE, –7 mEq/l) was interpreted as mixed acidosis with low oxygen tension. The tidal volume was increased to 7 L in an attempt to lower $PaCO_2$; and the dobutamine infusion was increased to 2 µg/kg/min to improve arterial blood pressure, improve pulmonary blood flow, and potentially reduce ventilation-perfusion mismatch and thus increase oxygen delivery. The mean arterial blood pressure increased to 76 mm Hg; and an arterial blood gas sample revealed pH of 7.31, $PaCO_2$ of 42 mm Hg, and PaO_2 of 80 mm Hg. Dobutamine (1 µg/kg/min) maintained mean arterial blood pressure between 71 and 76 mm Hg for the remainder of surgery and anesthesia. Approximately 15 feet of small intestine was removed as a result of a strangulating obstruction. Polymyxin B (3 million units in 1 L of LRS per 450 kg) was administered to combat endotoxemia. The horse was moved to the recovery stall, became anxious, and attempted to stand within 5 minutes but was physically restrained. Xylazine (100 mg IV) was administered to slow recovery, and flunixin meglumine (1 mg/kg IV) was administered for pain.

Predicament 1

Cyclical variation in the systolic arterial blood pressure associated with the inspiratory phase of ventilation. Systolic pressure variation (SPV) associated with mechanical ventilation is a sign of poor cardiac performance or, more commonly, volume depletion (see Figure 17-11).

Solution 1

Fluid therapy is indicated when SPV is greater than 10 mm Hg. The choice of fluids is critical since crystalloids produce minimum and only temporary increases in arterial blood pressure because of their rapid redistribution into the extravascular (interstitial) space. Both colloids (5 to 10 ml/kg, 6% hetastarch) and hypertonic saline (3 ml/kg, 7%) produce an immediate and sustained increase in vascular volume and translocation of fluid from the interstitial space to the vascular compartment (autotransfusion) as a result of their colloid osmotic pressure and tonicity, respectively.

Solution 2

Dobutamine is the drug of choice for increasing arterial blood pressure in anesthetized horses (see Table 22-4). Dobutamine produces dose-dependent increases in arterial blood pressure, cardiac output, and intestinal and skeletal muscle blood flow without increasing heart rate in otherwise normal or moderately ill horses that become hypotensive during anesthesia. Dobutamine may produce sinus tachycardia or ventricular arrhythmias if administered too rapidly (>3 to 5 µg/kg/min) or to severely stressed and markedly hypotensive (shock) horses, suggesting the need for fluids to restore vascular volume and myocardial and tissue perfusion. Horses that respond poorly to dobutamine doses in excess of 3 to 5 µg/kg/min or do not respond at all have a poor prognosis.

Solution 3

Ephedrine can be administered as an intravenous bolus (0.03 to 0.06 mg/kg) to increase arterial blood pressure and cardiac output. The increase in arterial blood pressure is gradual and usually delayed. Ephedrine is best administered to prevent hypotension in horses with low normal (60 to 70 mm Hg) mean values or in anticipation of decreases in arterial blood pressure associated with increases in anesthetic depth for surgical purposes (e.g., enucleation, arthrodesis).

Predicament 2

Premature attempts to stand. It is normal and common for horses to attempt to attain a sternal position and stand before they have recovered fully from anesthesia and are capable of supporting their weight. Most horses require 30 to 40 minutes to eliminate the effects of inhalant anesthetics after a surgical/anesthetic procedure lasting more than 3 hours. Horses that are in pain during recovery are more likely to attempt to stand prematurely. however, premature attempts to rise can result in multiple failed attempts to stand, producing delirium and fear and predisposing the horse to stress, abrasions, and potentially fractures.

Solution 1

α_2-Adrenoceptor agonists (e.g., xylazine, 0.1 to 0.2 mg/kg IV) slow all phases of the recovery process, providing additional time for the elimination of inhalant and injectable drugs.

Solution 2

Morphine sulfate, 0.1 mg/kg IM, provides analgesia and may shorten recovery time.

OPHTHALMOLOGICAL SURGERY (Box 24-6)

A 350-kg yearling Appaloosa colt is presented for removal (phacoemulsification) of a cataract in the right eye. Preanesthetic physical examination and blood work (hemogram, fibrinogen, and chemistry profile) are within normal limits. The total anesthesia time is estimated to require 45 to 60 minutes, and complete relaxation of the muscles of the eye is required for optimum surgical exposure. The colt is difficult to restrain and resists handling. Detomidine (7 mg IM [≈20 µg/kg]) is administered 20 minutes before induction of anesthesia to facilitate intravenous catheter placement and washing of the mouth.

Box 24–6   Anesthesia for Ophthalmologic Surgery

Sedation
Detomidine (20 μg/kg IM) (T–20 min)

Anesthesia
Guaifenesin to effect (42 mg/kg IV) then thiopental
    (3 mg/kg IV)
Isoflurane (2%-3%); controlled ventilation

Peripheral Skeletal Muscle Relaxation (Paralysis)
Atracurium (0.05 mg/kg, IV)
Reversal of atracurium (if needed): glycopyrrolate
    (5 μg/kg IV); neostigmine (0.05 mg/kg IV) or edrophonium
    (0.5 mg/kg IV)

Recovery
Xylazine (1.5 μg/kg IV)

Postoperative Analgesia
Phenylbutazone (2 mg/kg IV) was administered before surgery

The colt was moved to the induction stall and administered 5% guaifenesin (15 g total dose) to effect (muscle weakness, ataxia) IV. A bolus of thiopental (1 g IV [≈3 mg/kg]) was administered at the point of maximum skeletal muscle relaxation. The colt collapsed within 20 seconds of thiopental administration and was rolled to lateral recumbency. A PVC speculum was placed between the incisors, and a 22-mm ID cuffed endotracheal tube was passed through the mouth and into the trachea. The endotracheal tube was connected to a standard large animal anesthetic machine with attached ventilator. The colt was then positioned in left lateral recumbency on a padded surgical table, the head was positioned and padded, the left front limb was pulled forward, and pads were placed between the front and hind limbs. The vaporizer was adjusted to deliver an initial concentration of 3% isoflurane, and the oxygen flow rate was set at 10 L/min. The horse's eye signs (depth of anesthesia), heart rate, respiratory rate, mucous membrane color, and capillary refill time were monitored and recorded for the duration of the procedure. Controlled ventilation was initiated at a frequency of 6 breaths/min and a tidal volume of 5 L. A 21-g catheter was placed in the dorsal metatarsal artery of the right hind limb for measurement of arterial blood pressures and anaerobic collection of arterial blood samples for pH and blood gas analysis. The initial mean arterial blood pressure was 63 mm Hg and was gradually increased during the first 15 minutes of anesthesia to 78 mm Hg. The vaporizer was adjusted to deliver 2% isoflurane, and the oxygen flow was readjusted to deliver 3 L/min.

Atracurium (35 mg IV [≈0.1 mg/kg]) was administered to produce relaxation of the muscles of the eye, thereby facilitating positioning of the globe. Cataract removal (phacoemulsification) was completed in 25 minutes, and anal tone and corneal reflex responses returned 5 minutes after completion of the surgery. An arterial blood gas revealed a pH of 7.38, $PaCO_2$ of 42 mm Hg, and a PaO_2 of 463 mm Hg. The respiratory rate was decreased to 2 breaths/min, and spontaneous ventilation with adequate thoracic and abdominal excursions resumed within 6 minutes. The colt was moved to the recovery stall and administered xylazine (50 mg IV) to produce sedation and prolong the recovery process. The colt stood unassisted on its first attempt 45 minutes after being disconnected from the anesthetic machine.

Predicament 1

Failure to resume spontaneous breathing when the ventilator rate is decreased to 2 breaths/min. Neuromuscular blocking drugs (NMBDs) produce skeletal muscle paralysis (see Chapter 19). Their effects can be potentiated and prolonged by injectable and inhalant anesthetic drugs, aminoglycoside antibiotics, hypotension, hypothermia, and acidemia. Atracurium is the preferred nondepolarizing NMBD because it produces a dose-dependent and predictable duration of effect and is reversible (see Table 19-1).

Solution 1

Controlled ventilation can be maintained until the colt begins to breathe spontaneously. It is important to monitor the colt's respiratory rate, tidal volume, and ideally arterial blood gas values ($PaCO_2$, PaO_2) to ensure adequate ventilation and prevent hypoxemia.

Solution 2

All nondepolarizing NMBDs can be antagonized (reversed) by administering an acetyl cholinesterase inhibitor (see Table 19-1). This colt could be administered neostigmine (0.02-0.04 mg/kg IV) or edrophonium (0.3-0.5 mg/kg IV) to reverse the effects of atracurium and hasten the return of spontaneous breathing. An anticholinergic (glycopyrrolate [0.005 mg/kg IV]) should be administered before the acetyl cholinesterase inhibitor to prevent the cholinergic (vagal) effects of acetyl cholinesterase inhibition.

ANESTHESIA OF A DRAFT HORSE (Box 24-7)

A 5-year-old 900-kg Clydesdale gelding is presented for surgical treatment of left laryngeal hemiplegia. Respiration is normal at rest, but the horse makes an audible noise during exercise. The physical examination and blood work (hemogram, fibrinogen) are within normal limits. Food but not water is withheld for 6 hours, and the mouth is rinsed with water to remove any residual debris. Thirty minutes before induction, xylazine (900 mg IM [1 mg/kg]) is administered to facilitate clipping of the surgical site and intravenous catheter placement. This dose of xylazine causes the horse

---

Box 24–7   Anesthesia of a Draft Horse

Sedation
Xylazine (1 mg/kg IM) (T–30 min)
Xylazine (0.3 mg/kg IV) at induction

Anesthesia
Diazepam (0.05 mg/kg IV) combined with ketamine
    (1.7 mg/kg IV), sevoflurane in O_2 (5% then 3%)

Therapy for Hypotension
Dobutamine (1-2 μg/kg/min IV)

Recovery
Xylazine (0.1 mg/kg IV) on way to recovery

Postoperative Analgesia
Phenylbutazone (2 mg/kg IV)

to lower its head and become minimally ataxic. A 14-g catheter is introduced percutaneously into the right jugular vein after local infiltration with 2 ml of 2% lidocaine to facilitate administration of anesthetic drugs and isotonic fluids. The anticipated duration of anesthesia is 90 minutes.

The horse was moved to the induction stall, and an additional dose of xylazine (300 mg IV [≈0.3 mg/kg]) was administered, resulting in profound sedation (lowered head, reluctance to move, ataxia, stumbling). Anesthesia was produced by administering a diazepam (50 mg IV[≈0.05 mg/kg])-ketamine (1500 mg IV [≈1.5 mg/kg]) drug combination (25 ml total volume). The horse sat down and relaxed to sternal recumbency within 50 seconds of drug administration and was positioned in right lateral recumbency and orotracheally intubated with a 30-mm cuffed endotracheal tube. Anesthesia was initially maintained with 5% sevoflurane delivered in 10 L/min of oxygen; and (LRS), 10 ml/kg/hr, was administered IV. The horse's eye signs (depth of anesthesia), heart rate, respiratory rate, mucous membrane color, and capillary refill time were monitored and recorded for the duration of the procedure. A 21-g catheter was placed in the dorsal metatarsal artery of the left hind limb for measurement of arterial blood pressures and anaerobic collection of arterial blood samples for pH and blood gas analysis. The sevoflurane concentration was reduced to 3% in 5 L/min of oxygen. The mean arterial blood pressure was 67 mm Hg and was maintained at or above 75 mm Hg by administering dobutamine (1 μg/kg/min IV). The surgical procedure included a laryngeal prosthesis for the treatment of left laryngeal hemiplegia. The horse was rolled into dorsal recumbency after prosthesis placement, the endotracheal tube cuff was deflated, and the endotracheal tube was withdrawn into the pharynx. A ventriculectomy was performed via the cricothyroid membrane. The endotracheal tube was replaced with the cuff deflated, and the horse was moved to a recovery stall and administered xylazine (100 mg IV [≈0.1 mg/kg]). A head rope was attached to the horse's halter and used to assist recovery, but there was not sufficient tail for a tail rope. The horse rolled to a sternal position 15 minutes after being disconnected from the anesthetic machine and stood on its second attempt 4 minutes later.

Predicament 1

Providing adequate time to complete additional surgical procedures after stopping the delivery of inhalant anesthesia. Newer inhalant anesthetics (isoflurane, sevoflurane, desflurane) are pharmacologically safer and have lower blood gas solubility coefficients than halothane (see Chapter 15). A lower blood gas solubility coefficient provides greater control of anesthetic depth by producing faster induction and recovery from anesthesia. Sevoflurane has a lower blood gas solubility coefficient than halothane and isoflurane and can provide more control over anesthetic depth and a more rapid recovery, particularly in Draft Horses. Horses administered sevoflurane for general anesthesia may require alternative methods to maintain anesthesia if additional surgical procedures (e.g., ventriculectomy, cast application) are required.

Solution 1

Total intravenous anesthesia can be used to supplement and extend inhalant anesthesia. The addition of 2.2 g of ketamine and 500 mg xylazine to a 1-L bag or bottle of 10%

guaifenesin can be administered IV to effect until surgical procedures are completed.

Solution 2

A ketamine (0.4 mg/kg IV)-xylazine (0.2 mg/kg IV) drug combination can be administered to extend the duration of anesthesia 5 to15 minutes.

Solution 3

Thiopental (0.4 mg/kg) can be administered as incremental intravenous boluses as needed to extend the duration of anesthesia 5 to 10 minutes.

ANESTHESIA OF A FOAL (Box 24-8)

A 3-week-old 75-kg Andalusian filly is presented for bilateral periosteal elevation of the distal metatarsi for treatment of valgus abnormalities of the hind limbs. Preanesthetic physical examination and blood work (hemogram, fibrinogen, chemistry profile) are within normal limits, with the exception of increased bronchovesicular sounds bilaterally and an elevated plasma fibrinogen. The anticipated duration of the surgical procedure and anesthesia is 45 minutes. The foal is allowed to nurse until its mouth is rinsed with water to remove debris. An 18-g catheter is placed in the left jugular vein to facilitate administration of antibiotics, anesthetic drugs, and isotonic fluids. A standard small animal anesthesia machine is used to deliver isoflurane and oxygen.

The foal was accompanied by a 500-kg mare to the induction area. The mare was administered a xylazine (250 mg [≈0.5 mg/kg])-acepromazine (10 mg [≈0.02 mg/kg]) drug combination IV to reduce the stress of being separated from the foal. The foal was administered xylazine (35 mg IV [≈0.5 mg/kg]) for sedation and induced to anesthesia with ketamine (150 mg IV [≈2 mg/kg]). A 14-mm cuffed endotracheal tube was passed through a 4-cm ID PVC speculum and positioned in the trachea. The endotracheal tube was attached to the small animal anesthesia machine. The foal's eye signs (depth of anesthesia), heart rate, respiratory rate, mucous membrane color, and capillary refill time were monitored and recorded for the duration of the procedure. The isoflurane vaporizer was adjusted to deliver 3%, and the oxygen flow rate was set at 3 L/min; the foal was

---

Box 24–8   Anesthesia of a Mare/Foal

Sedation
Mare: Xylazine (0.5 mg/kg IV) then acepromazine (0.02 mg/kg IV)
Foal: Xylazine (0.5 mg/kg IV)

Anesthesia
Ketamine (2 mg/kg IV)
Isoflurane (small animal anesthesia machine) in O_2 (3% then 2%)

Recovery
Manually assisted

Postoperative Analgesia
Butorphanol (0.05 mg/kg IM tid)

positioned in dorsal recumbency for surgery. The isoflurane concentration was reduced to 2%, and the oxygen flow rate to 1.5 L/min 10 minutes later. The foal's heart rate was 52 beats/min, and the pulse was regular and easily palpated. LRS was administered IV at a rate of 10 ml/kg/hr. The foal was "hand" recovered by placing one arm around its neck and grasping tail as it attempted to stand. The foal stood unassisted 15 minutes after being placed in the recovery stall.

Predicament 1

Determination of arterial blood pressure. Technically, arterial catheterization is more difficult in foals because of smaller vessel diameter and may be deemed unnecessary because of the short duration of the surgical procedure and anesthesia. Regardless, hypotension may occur and can result in hypothermia and prolonged recovery.

Solution

Noninvasive indirect blood pressure can be determined by placing an appropriately sized inflatable cuff (0.4 to 0.5 times circumference) around the base of the tail. Oscillometric determination of systolic arterial blood pressure is reliable and accurate in foals. Systolic blood pressure should be maintained greater than 90 mm Hg (see Chapter 8).

ANESTHESIA OF A FOAL WITH A RUPTURED BLADDER (Box 24-9)

A 3-day-old 45-kg Missouri Fox Trotter colt is presented with a distended abdomen. The colt was normal at birth and nursed enthusiastically. Two days later the foal becomes inappetent and depressed, and the abdomen became progressively distended. Diagnostic ultrasound identifies free fluid in the abdomen and establishes a presumptive diagnosis of a ruptured bladder. The abdomen is distended, and the foal is tachypneic and tachycardic. A hemogram reveals an increased packed cell volume and a mild leukocytosis. Serum chemistry reveals hypochloremia (80 mEq/l), hyponatremia (115 mEq/l), and hyperkalemia (6.3 mEq/l). The serum creatinine is 4.1 mg/dl, and blood urea nitrogen concentration is 66 mg/dl. An abdominocentesis is performed, and a large quantity of yellow fluid is removed. The catheter is left in place. An electrocardiogram is unremarkable except for tachycardia (HR 70 beats/min). An 18-g intravenous catheter is placed in the left jugular vein, and 2 L of 0.9% saline in 5% dextrose is administered. An abdominal exploratory is scheduled for surgical correction of a ruptured bladder. The foal is allowed to nurse until taken to the anesthetic induction area where its mouth is rinsed with water to remove debris. The anticipated duration of surgery and anesthesia is 90 minutes.

Repeated serum chemistry revealed a plasma sodium concentration of 125 mEq/l and serum potassium concentration of 5.5 mEq/l. The foal was less depressed but continued to strain to urinate. Xylazine (20 mg IV [≈0.05 mg/kg]) was administered, and the foal was nasotracheally intubated with an 8-mm internal diameter cuffed endotracheal tube. The nasotracheal tube was connected to a small animal anesthetic machine. The initial oxygen flow was adjusted to 3 L/min, and the sevoflurane vaporizer to 4%. Ventilation was assisted manually. The foal was placed in dorsal recumbency, and the nasotracheal tube was replaced with a 12-mm

---

Box 24–9   Anesthesia of a Foal with a Ruptured Bladder

Sedation
Xylazine (0.4 mg/kg IV)

Anesthesia
Nasal intubation
Sevoflurane (small animal anesthesia machine) in O_2 (4% then 2.5%)

Therapy for Hyperkalemia
Calcium chloride or calcium gluconate (20 mg/kg IV)
Sodium bicarbonate (1 mEq/kg IV)
Glucose (4-5 mg/kg/min); monitor blood glucose

Recovery
Manually assisted

Postoperative Analgesia
Butorphanol (0.05 mg/kg IM) as needed

ID orotracheal tube. The foal's eye signs (depth of anesthesia), heart rate, respiratory rate, mucous membrane color, and capillary refill time were monitored and recorded for the duration of the procedure. A 21-g Teflon catheter was placed in the transverse facial artery just caudal to and below the eye. The initial systolic and mean arterial pressures were 78 and 50 mm Hg, respectively. The sevoflurane concentration was reduced to 2.5%, and calcium (0.2 ml/kg IV, 10% CaCl) was added to the balanced electrolyte solution. The electrocardiogram was monitored for signs of hyperkalemia: sinus bradycardia, flattened or absent P waves, widened QRS complexes, and large peaked T waves with a shortened QT interval. A ruptured bladder was discovered during surgery and repaired. The foal recovered uneventfully.

Predicament 1

Metabolic acidosis and hyperkalemia are common problems associated with ruptured bladder in foals. Arterial pH values below 7.20 and serum K^+ values greater than 6 mEq/L can exaggerate anesthetic drug effects, resulting in decreases in cardiac contractility, vasodilation, vascular hyporesponsiveness, and ultimately in shock and cardiovascular collapse.

Solution 1

Metabolic (nonrespiratory) acidosis should always be treated by directing therapy toward the cause. Surgical correction of the ruptured bladder and restoration of blood pressure, blood flow, and tissue perfusion rapidly normalize acid-base and electrolyte abnormalities.

Solution 2

Metabolic acidosis (pH < 7.20) should be treated by administering Na^+ bicarbonate (1 mEq/kg, IV).

Solution 3

Calcium chloride or calcium gluconate improves cardiovascular function (0.2 ml/kg IV, 10% CaCl). Epinephrine is administered in emergency situations (see Chapter 23).

Solution 4

Glucose infusion, 4 to 5 mg/kg/min, while monitoring blood glucose.

Anesthetic Risk and Euthanasia

Lori A. Bidwell

John A.E. Hubbell

William W. Muir

KEY POINTS

1. Morbidity and mortality rates are higher in horses than in other commonly anesthetized species.
2. There is no substitute for a vigilant, educated, trained, and experienced person to perform and monitor anesthesia.
3. Development of standardized (yet modifiable) protocols and procedures, accurate and detailed records, and open communication helps to prevent adverse events.
4. The term euthanasia connotes a "good" or painless death.
5. Euthanasia ideally incorporates stress reduction, analgesia, and unconsciousness followed by death.
6. An intravenous overdose of pentobarbital is preferred for producing euthanasia in horses in North America. Captive bolt and gunshot can be used, when appropriate, but only by trained and experienced personnel.
7. Two-stage euthanasia (induction of anesthesia followed by production of death) is preferred for aesthetic reasons.
8. Prompt and proper disposal of pentobarbital-euthanized horses is critical because of the risk of consumption by wildlife.
9. All regulatory issues; legal authorizations; documentation; and public, personnel, or welfare concerns should be considered carefully before performing euthanasia.

ANESTHETIC RISK

Unintended or untoward reactions to anesthetic drugs are common occurrences in veterinary practice and are responsible for an estimated incidence of 30% of all adverse events associated with general drug use.[1] The reported morbidity and mortality rates for horses subjected to general anesthesia are higher than for other domestic species, regardless of inclusion and exclusion criteria (Boxes 25-1 and 25-2).[2,3] Numerous studies have concluded that between 2% and 4% of all horses have an unexpected or adverse event associated with anesthesia and that approximately 0.5% to 2% of otherwise normal healthy horses die under general anesthesia.[2-14] Studies investigating anesthetic mortality in horses have included cases from private equine practices, veterinary teaching hospitals, and a variety of anesthetic protocols, where both formally and informally trained anesthetists have provided anesthesia. A major prospective multicenter study concluded that the use of acepromazine administered before surgery followed by total intravenous anesthesia (TIVA) reduced the risk of anesthetic fatalities.[14] The most commonly reported postoperative morbidity is colic (13.7%), which, when associated with hypoxia in pregnant

mares, resulted in abortion or delivery of severely compromised foals that did not survive.[15,16] Mortality associated with anesthesia and surgery for colic and other emergency situations approaches 30% to 35%.[17-19] The most common causes for death include cardiac arrest, myopathy and/or neuropathy, fractures in the recovery, and emergency cases in which the disease process is exacerbated by anesthesia (see Box 25-2).[3,13-15] Factors that increase the risk of death include emergency cases, particularly those performed after regular hours, and the lack of administration of preanesthetic medication (i.e., use of only inhalant anesthetic).[11,15,18,19] Stress was indicated as a potential risk factor for death associated with anesthesia (see Chapter 4).[20]

A recent study conducted at a single private equine referral practice analyzed anesthetic fatalities in elective and emergency situations and reported a fatality rate of 0.12% of equine cases under general anesthesia, a rate significantly lower than previously reported in other studies.[20] The lower mortality rate was attributed to the abilities of the local farm managers in recognizing emergency situations earlier, the relatively young and healthy population of horses anesthetized, the consistency and relative safety of a familiar anesthetic protocol, and regularity of monitoring by trained veterinarians and anesthetic technicians. The administration of a 1-L mixture of guaifenesin (50 g), xylazine (500 mg), and ketamine (1 g) to a 450-kg horse for TIVA of 1 hour or less was associated with no anesthetic fatalities. This finding was likely because the drug combination was administered to healthy horses for elective surgical procedures and because most procedures were completed in less than 1 hour. Procedures longer than 2 hours involving arthrodesis or osteotomy carried the highest crude mortality rate (66.7 deaths per 1000).[20] Although horses have a large muscle mass that increases the risk of neuropathy or myopathy and a rigid rib cage that complicates cardiopulmonary resuscitation, proper anesthetic management can minimize the risk of general anesthesia in horses. The disease process and physical status of the horse may be the most important determinants of outcome, all other factors being equal.[2,15,19,20]

EUTHANASIA

Euthanizing a horse is never easy; the decision is often made on the basis of the horse's perceived quality of life and is greatly influenced by perceived outcomes and economics.[21] The decision-making process involves the owner making an informed decision after consulting a veterinarian and may require confirmation from an insurance company.

Box 25–1 Morbidity and Anesthesia in Horses

Morbidity

6.4%	1990[2]
1.4-1.8%	1990[3]
13.7%	2007[15]

Morbid Events

Prolonged and uncoordinated recovery

Wounds in recovery

Lameness, myopathy, neuropathy

Thrombophlebitis

Pyrexia, depression, leukopenia

Colic

Postoperative ileus

Colitis, diarrhea

Respiratory distress

Fractures

Factors Influencing Morbidity

Human error

American Society of Anesthesiologists: Category

Age

Duration of anesthesia/surgery: Myopathy

Position

   Supine: Nasal edema

   Lateral body position: Myopathy

Severity of pain

Hypotension

Increased packed cell volume

Hypoxia in pregnant mares

New environment: Colic

Small intestinal lesion: Postoperative ileus

Box 25–2 Mortality and Anesthesia in Horses

Mortality

0.3%	1961 (chloral hydrate)[5]
5.0%	1969[6]
5.1%	1973[7]
1.18%	1982[8]
2.2%	1983[9] 1.5% when sick animals excluded
0.68%	1993[3]
0.63%	1998[10] 0.08% anesthesia only
31.4%	1998[11] overall emergencies (nonabdominal 15.3%); surg/anesth death rate: 4.3% abdominal; 2% nonabdominal
0.08%	1999[12] (nonemergency; nonabdominal)
0.9%	2002[13] 1.6% overall
0.12-0.24%	2007[15]
0.12%	2007[20]

Colic

35.3%	1983[17]
35.5%	1998[11]
7.9%	2002[13]
16.9-29.7%	2005[18] (end of anesthesia to discharge)
12%	2006[19]

Causes of Death/Euthanasia

Cardiac arrest	32.8%
Fractures	25.6%
Abdominal (colic; colitis)	13.1%
Postoperative myopathies	7.1%
Central nervous system	5.5%
Respiratory complications	3.7%

Factors Influencing Mortality

Human error

American Society of Anesthesiologists: Category

Age

Duration of anesthesia/surgery

More invasive/extensive surgical procedures

Colic

Heart rate (↑ or ↓)

PCV ((↑ or ↓)

Horses that become nonpainful

Older horses

The American Association of Equine Practitioners has developed criteria for veterinarians to consider when deciding whether to recommend euthanasia (Box 25-3).[22] In addition to these criteria, veterinarians should ask and discuss the following questions with the owner before finalizing a decision to euthanize: (1) Can the owner financially handle the cost of treatment or surgical intervention and postoperative care without the situation becoming a burden? (2) Is the horse insured and does the insurance company need to be contacted before care?[23] Euthanasia requires an organized, thorough, professional approach by a compassionate and caring veterinarian that has considered all of the mitigating factors (Box 25-4).

The veterinarian and owner must consult with the insurance company, if applicable, before making a decision to euthanize unless the horse is in uncontrollable pain. In the latter situation the carcass should be saved for necropsy until

the insurance company has been informed. The insurance company may elect to consult a second veterinarian to verify the medical findings before euthanasia can be performed, unless humanitarian reasons are more important. Details for euthanasia vary among insurance companies and are the responsibility of the owner. Cooperation with the insurance company's representative or agent helps ensure a satisfactory settlement.[23] Laws regarding movement, slaughter, and disposal of horses in the United States are currently under scrutiny.[24,25] The limitation on horse slaughter in the United States has resulted in the shipment of horses outside of the

<table>
</table>

Box 25–3 American Association of Equine Practitioners' Guidelines for Recommending Euthanasia Criteria 2007

1. Is the condition chronic or incurable, and does it produce excessive or inhumane pain and suffering?
2. Does the immediate condition present a hopeless prognosis for life?
3. Is the horse a hazard to itself or its handlers?
4. Will the horse require continuous medication for the relief of pain for the remainder of its life?

The justification of euthanasia of a horse for humane reasons should be based on medical, not economic considerations; the same criteria should be applied to all horses, regardless of age, sex, or potential value.

Box 25–4 Considerations Before Performing Euthanasia

- Professionalism: Reflective listening; owner communication and attachment
- Permission: Verbal and written consent
- Welfare: Quality of life, welfare organizations
- Legal issues: State and local ordinances regarding methods, burial or disposal, insurance, justification, second opinion, permission
- Special circumstances: Emergency, hospital, farm
- Euthanasia technique: Chemical, physical
- Written records: Signed, dated, archived
- Confirmation of death: Methods
- Postmortem examination
- Disposal: Burial, incineration, rendering, others

Box 25–5 Steps, Drugs, and Methods for Euthanasia in Horses

Step 1
Tranquilization/Sedation
1. Acepromazine: 0.08 mg/kg IV
2. Xylazine: 1.1 mg/kg IV
3. Detomidine: 5-10 µg/kg IV

Step 2
Production of Unconsciousness (Anesthesia) and/or Death
1. Barbiturate (high doses can result in euthanasia)
   a. Pentobarbital: >50 mg/kg IV for euthanasia
   b. Thiopental: >20-30 mg/kg IV for euthanasia

Production of Unconsciousness (After Step 1)
1. Guaifenesin: 5% or 10% plus a barbiturate (3 mg/ml IV to effect) (recumbency)
2. Ketamine: 2-3 mg/kg IV
3. Telazol: 1-2 mg/kg IV
4. Chloral hydrate-magnesium sulfate-pentobarbital preparation to effect IV (recumbency)

Step 3: Only After Unconsciousness Is Achieved by Step 2
Induction of Respiratory and/or Cardiac Arrest and Death
1. Succinylcholine: 100-200 mg IV
2. Potassium chloride: 50 ml saturated solution
3. Penetrating captive-bolt
4. Free-bullet
5. Electrocution
6. Exsanguination

IV, Intravenously.

United States, where slaughter practices may not be regulated. Alternatively, thousands of unwanted horses are subjected to improper care or abandonment. Fortunately rescue organizations help to care for these unwanted horses, although the end result is often humane euthanasia for horses that are not adopted (www.unwantedhorsecoalition.org).

The major objective of humane euthanasia is to produce unconsciousness as rapidly and painlessly as possible.[23] Once an unconscious state has been achieved, intravenous or physical methods that produce death may be administered. The aesthetic effects of euthanasia are also important, especially when performed in the presence of the owner or lay people. The veterinarian should strive to project a professional image by evidencing a caring attitude and performing the procedure expediently. These attributes promote client confidence and establish respect for the veterinarian.[21]

A two- or three-step approach should be used to euthanize horses (Box 25-5). The first step is designed to produce sedation or tranquilization, thus relieving stress and render-

ing the horse manageable. The second step should produce rapid and painless unconsciousness. The third step (death) can be produced by increased doses of the drugs used to produce unconsciousness or can be produced by physical methods.

AMERICAN VETERINARY MEDICAL ASSOCIATION GUIDELINES FOR EUTHANASIA

The American Veterinary Medical Association (AVMA) committee on euthanasia (June 2007) has developed guidelines for appropriate management of euthanasia in horses.[26] The guidelines define euthanasia (pain and stress-free death), provide a description of appropriate staff and training required, describe the neural and emotional components of euthanasia, and suggest appropriate methods for euthanasia and the mechanisms of how each method works (Box 25-6).

It is the responsibility of the veterinarian to know and understand the benefits and risks of the methods recommended by the AVMA. State and local regulations should

Box 25–6 Considerations for Methods of Euthanasia*

1. Ability to induce loss of consciousness and death without causing pain, distress, anxiety, or apprehension
2. Compatibility with species, age, and health status
3. Compatibility with requirement and purpose
4. Drug availability and human abuse potential
5. Time required to induce loss of consciousness and death
6. Reliability
7. Safety of personnel
8. Irreversibility
9. Emotional effect on observers or operators
10. Compatibility with subsequent evaluation, examination, or use of tissue
11. Ability to maintain equipment in proper working order
12. Safety for predators/scavengers should the carcass be consumed
13. Environmental and human safety

*Modified from *AVMA guidelines* on *euthanasia*, 2007.

also be consulted to ensure compliance with local ordinances. Regardless of the technique chosen, the major requirement is rapid, painless, and stress-free induction of unconsciousness before death.

MODES OF ACTION OF DRUGS USED FOR EUTHANASIA

Euthanasia can be produced by: (1) hypoxemia, direct or indirect; (2) direct depression of neurons vital for life; and (3) physical damage to brain tissue (Table 25-1).[26] The arrest of oxygenated blood flow to vital tissues is ultimately responsible for the cause of death, regardless of the category into which a particular method is placed. Unconsciousness should always precede cessation of blood flow to the brain but may not always precede cessation of muscular activity. Excitatory responses (i.e., involuntary muscle activity) frequently occur during the early stages of anesthesia (i.e., between stage 2 and stage 3) and are generally mistaken as purposeful movement by lay or uninformed persons. Furthermore, an agonal response characterized by exaggerated inspiratory efforts can occur and may be misinterpreted as a painful response.

Uncontrolled movement in an unconscious horse during euthanasia may be misinterpreted as pain. In contrast, lack of movement does not necessarily denote unconsciousness, particularly if muscle relaxants are incorporated into the euthanasia protocol. For example, a horse administered a massive dose of a peripheral muscle relaxant (e.g., succinylcholine; see Chapter 19) may rapidly develop skeletal muscle paralysis and appear peaceful, although the horse is conscious but unable to move or breathe. Although

muscle relaxation is a desirable feature of euthanasia solutions, peripheral muscle relaxants (e.g., succinylcholine, curare, gallamine, pancuronium, atracurium) and drugs that produce muscle relaxation (e.g., magnesium sulfate, guaifenesin, diazepam) or immobilization (e.g., strychnine, potassium chloride, nicotine sulfate) do not produce anesthesia and are "absolutely condemned" as sole euthanizing drugs.[26] This strong statement is supported by the fact that most muscle relaxants (immobilizing drugs) do not produce unconsciousness and are not analgesics. Their administration as single therapies to produce euthanasia is considered cruel since asphyxia occurs in a conscious horse that can feel pain but cannot move.

Instantaneous destruction of brain tissue or electrocution may be used to humanely euthanize a horse. Destruction of brain tissue is most often by gunshot or penetrating captive bolt. Application of these techniques should only be performed on properly restrained horses by skilled veterinarians.

CHEMICAL METHODS OF EUTHANASIA

Approved chemical methods for euthanizing horses include barbiturates and chloral hydrate (conditionally acceptable). Conditionally acceptable methods are those that might not consistently produce humane death or are not adequately documented in the scientific literature (e.g., gunshot, electrocution). Choral hydrate produces death by hypoxemia resulting from progressive depression of the respiratory center and should be preceded by heavy sedation and/or anesthesia. Although penetrating captive bolt, gunshot, and electrocution, if humanely performed, can be used to produce euthanasia, they are not generally recommended because of the negative perception of lay personnel and the skill required to perform these techniques.

INHALANTS

Inhalant anesthesia can be combined with injectable anesthetic drugs to produce euthanasia. Inhalant anesthetics are expensive, require specialized equipment, and are not rapidly effective when administered alone.[26]

INJECTABLE DRUGS

A wide variety of injectable drugs have been administered to euthanize horses.[27,28] Many drugs are no longer acceptable or available, such as T-61, a nonbarbiturate, nonnarcotic mixture of three drugs; and some drugs are illegal when used as the sole euthanizing drug (e.g., nicotine alkaloids and succinylcholine).[29] Discussion of euthanizing drugs is limited to barbituric acid derivatives, chloral hydrate, potassium chloride (KCl), and chloral hydrate-magnesium sulfate-pentobarbital. The dissociative anesthetics (ketamine, tiletamine) can be administered to immobilize the horse and induce anesthesia but rarely are used to produce death. Xylazine or other α_2-adrenoceptor agonists should be included as adjuncts for the purpose of sedation (see Chapter 10). Succinylcholine or KCl is not satisfactory when used alone but may be administered to induce respiratory and cardiac arrest, respectively, after producing general anesthesia.[26]

Table 25–1. Methods of euthanizing horses

	Site of action	Classification	Comments
Hypoxic agents			
Curariform drugs:* Curare Succinylcholine Atracurium	Paralysis of respiratory muscles; oxygen not available to blood	Hypoxic, hypoxemia, and hypercarbia	Unconsciousness develops slowly, preceded by anxiety and fear; no motor activity **(NOTE: should be used only after the horse is anesthetized)**
Direct neuron depressing agents			
Barbituric acid derivatives	Direct depression of cerebral cortex, subcortical structures, and vital centers; direct depression of heart muscle	Ultimate cause of death is hypoxemia caused by depression of vital centers	Unconsciousness reached rapidly; no anxiety; no excitement period; no motor activity; best to administer by intravenous or intracardiac administration
Chloral hydrate and chloral hydrate combinations	Direct depression of cerebral cortex, subcortical structures, and vital centers; direct depression of heart muscle	Ultimate cause of death is hypoxemia caused by depression of vital centers	Transient anxiety; unconsciousness occurs rapidly; no motor activity **(NOTE: should be used only after the horse is anesthetized)**
T-61* (no longer available in United States)	Direct depression of cerebral cortex, subcortical structures, and vital centers; direct depression of heart muscle	Hypoxemia caused by depression of vital centers	Transient anxiety and struggling may occur before unconsciousness when given too rapidly; tissue damage may occur; must be given intravenously at recommended dosage and rates
Physical agents (NOTE: should be used only after the horse is anesthetized)			
Penetrating captive bolt or gunshot into brain	Direct concussion of brain tissue	Hypoxemia caused by depression of vital centers	Instant unconsciousness; motor activity may occur after unconsciousness
Exsanguination*	Direct depression of brain	Hypoxemia	If this method is preceded by unconsciousness, there should be no struggling or muscle contraction
Electrocution through brain	Direct depression of brain	Hypoxemia	Violent muscle contractions occur at same time as unconsciousness

* Not acceptable as the sole means of producing euthanasia in the horse.
Modified from *The AVMA guidelines on euthanasia,* June 2007.

Barbituric Acid Derivatives

Barbiturates are controlled substances, and complete records are required. Barbiturate anesthetics, even in small doses, depress the central nervous system (CNS), with the higher centers being affected first. A descending depression of the CNS occurs as the dose increases, producing unconsciousness and general anesthesia. Death occurs from respiratory arrest and myocardial hypoxia. The rapidity of death after respiratory arrest depends, to a large extent, on the state of oxygenation of the horse at the time of respiratory arrest. For example, cardiac arrest occurs more slowly in horses breathing oxygen than in horses breathing room air. Although most barbiturates can be used for euthanasia, pentobarbital is the most popular and effective. A tranquilizer or sedative (acepromazine, xylazine, detomidine, romifidine) is administered to the horse and given time to act before injecting the barbiturate. This approach calms a fractious, excited, or apprehensive horse and facilitates a smooth transition from standing to recumbency. The dose required to euthanize a 450-kg adult horse is approximately 100 ml of a 20% solution.[30] The recommendation in the United States is to administer 100 ml of 39% solution (390 mg/ml) to a 450-kg horse (86.7 mg/kg). If thiopental is substituted for pentobarbital, it should be put into solution just before injection to ensure maximum potency. The dose of a thiobarbiturate required to euthanize a horse depends on the health of the horse; but doses ranging from 30 to 50 mg/kg are usually sufficient, particularly if followed by succinylcholine (100 to 200 mg intravenously [IV]).[27] The dose of thiobarbiturate should be increased in young, healthy horses. A technique using a concentrated solution of thiopental (2.5 to 5 g in 10 to 20 ml of water) injected into the carotid artery of horses has been described as effective and humane.[31] Immobilization occurs within 5 seconds; thus the injection must be made rapidly, with the veterinarian prepared to move quickly out of danger. Sudden or unexpected movement of the horse can be avoided by prior administration of a tranquilizer or a sedative.

Barbiturates have the distinct advantages of a rapid onset of action and a relatively uneventful induction to anesthesia, and they produce minimal unacceptable side effects. The effectiveness of barbiturates or any other injectable anesthetic drug administered for euthanasia can be increased with supplemental drugs. For example, succinylcholine (100 to 200 mg IV) induces respiratory arrest and helps to eliminate movement, including agonal breaths. Potassium chloride (50 to 100 ml, saturated solution) produces cardiac arrest. Injecting a combination of drugs that includes succinylcholine or potassium chloride simultaneously is not recommended because of the potential for discordant effects and unexpected results.

There are some disadvantages to the use of barbiturates. For example, intravenous injection is required for satisfactory results. Barbiturates must not be used to euthanize horses intended for human or animal consumption. Consumption of the carcass by predators or scavengers can be fatal and can result in severe fines.[32,33] Transition from a standing position to recumbency may be preceded by the horse rearing or collapsing to the ground unexpectedly unless it is properly sedated or restrained. Terminal gasps resulting from loss of blood flow to the respiratory centers frequently occur after unconsciousness in pentobarbital euthanized horses.

Chloral Hydrate

Chloral hydrate is a controlled substance, and complete records regarding its use are required. It can be administered as a sedative/narcotic and has been used as an anesthetic. It is not presently recommended as a sole euthanizing drug, but prior administration of a sedative makes it conditionally acceptable. Slow intravenous injection of chloral hydrate induces narcosis. Continued administration results in unconsciousness and recumbency, but at a slower rate than that produced by barbiturates. The slow onset of action is partially the result of the necessity for metabolic conversion of chloral hydrate to its corresponding alcohol (trichloroethanol) before becoming effective (see Chapter 12).[26] Severe ataxia, incoordination, and delirium may occur before the horse is recumbent and immobilized. These problems are minimized by administering a sedative dose of α_2-adrenoceptor agonist or acepromazine and producing anesthesia before administering chloral hydrate. Three to five times the dose (300 to 500 mg/kg) required for narcosis must be administered for euthanasia.[27] Agonal breaths (i.e., terminal gasps) may occur and are objectionable to observers. Choral hydrate is most effective when combined with a barbiturate.

Magnesium Sulfate

Magnesium sulfate ($MgSO_4$) should not be administered alone to produce euthanasia. It is not an anesthetic but can produce neuromuscular blockade, resulting in respiratory muscle paralysis and cardiac arrest. Cortical activity continues and is only minimally depressed before respiratory arrest occurs. Death results from hypoxia. A saturated solution of $MgSO_4$ can be combined with injectable anesthetic drugs (e.g., chloral hydrate and a barbiturate) to facilitate respiratory arrest.

Potassium Chloride

Potassium chloride (KCl) should not be used as the sole method for euthanasia because it does not produce anesthesia or analgesia. Intravenous administration of 50 to 100 ml of a saturated solution of KCl rapidly produces cardiac arrest. Cessation of blood flow occurs immediately, and death ensues as a result of tissue hypoxia. KCl is effective, economical, and humane when administered to euthanize unconscious or anesthetized horses. Succinylcholine or some other peripheral muscle relaxant can be administered before administering KCl to prevent agonal respirations.

Chloral Hydrate, Magnesium Sulfate, and Sodium Pentobarbital

Combinations of chloral hydrate, magnesium sulfate, and sodium pentobarbital were used for many years to produce general anesthesia in horses. Although seldom used today, they are still available as individual drugs. Their combination (chloral hydrate, 30 g; magnesium sulfate, 15 g; and sodium pentobarbital, 6.6 g dissolved in 1 L of water) induces an anesthetic state that is accompanied by profound CNS depression and muscle relaxation as the dose is increased. Continued administration results in death from respiratory and cardiac arrest. Fifty to 100 ml of saturated KCl solution may be injected rapidly IV, once the horse is unconscious, to ensure rapid death from cardiac arrest.

Peripheral Muscle Relaxants

Peripheral muscle relaxants are "absolutely condemned as euthanizing drugs when administered alone" because they do not produce anesthesia or analgesia.[26,30] Drugs in this group include tubocurarine, succinylcholine, gallamine, pancuronium, vecuronium, and atracurium (see Chapter 19). They are approved for humane euthanasia in horses only when combined with general anesthesia.[26] When a fractious horse cannot be handled safely for euthanasia, a dose of a muscle relaxant such as succinylcholine can be administered for immobilization if immediately followed by an intravenous anesthetic drug that renders the horse unconscious.[26,30]

Strychnine

The AVMA Panel on Euthanasia has underscored the statement that *"strychnine is absolutely condemned for euthanasia."*[26]

Strychnine competitively blocks the inhibitory effects of the CNS neurotransmitter glycine on motor neurons, producing activation of striated muscle groups. The extensor muscle groups all tend to contract at once, causing diffuse, painful, and uncontrollable muscle cramps.[26] Death results from respiratory arrest and suffocation. The physical signs of strychnine toxicity are revolting, making it one of the most inhumane methods for euthanizing any animal.

Nicotine Sulfate

The AVMA Panel on Euthanasia recommends that *nicotine sulfate be condemned for euthanasia.*[26] Furthermore the report of the Euthanasia Study Committee for the American Association of Equine Practitioners has stated that "in light of the FDA's recent ruling, the use of nicotine alkaloids and/or succinylcholine for the purpose of *euthanasia* is not only pharmacologically inadvisable but illegal."[34] Concentrated nicotine sulfate in any form is considered extremely dangerous. Intravenous administration stimulates the CNS, producing a short period of excitement followed by autonomic blockade and skeletal muscle relaxation as the dose is increased. Respiratory muscle paralysis occurs, and death results from hypoxia. Salivation, vomiting, defecation, and convulsions occur at frequent occurrences in some species before death.

PHYSICAL METHODS OF EUTHANASIA

The following physical methods are acceptable for special circumstances as alternatives to chemical euthanasia. The only approved physical method of euthanasia is a penetrating captive bolt, and conditionally approved methods include gunshot and electrocution.

Captive Bolt

The captive bolt is a stunning device that has been used to euthanize large and small animals.[26] Its use for euthanasia of horses is controversial. The sight for entrance of a penetrating captive bolt is approximately where lines drawn from the base of an ear to the medial canthus of the opposite eye cross on the horse's forehead.[35-37] Stunning with a captive bolt is accompanied by a "15-second period of tetanic spasm followed by slow hind limb movements of increased frequency."[36] Although the captive bolt damages the cerebral hemispheres and causes immediate destruction of brain tissue and collapse, evaluation of unconsciousness is difficult.[26] Results of a study using auditory evoked potential (AEP) measurements and an electroencephalogram (EEG) to determine the time of onset of unconsciousness in rabbits and dogs support use of the captive bolt as a humane device for euthanasia. This study demonstrated that organized AEP activity could not be detected above the medulla within 15 seconds of the pistol firing and that EEG activity became isoelectric.[36] Bolt penetration of the cranium may elicit a sudden upward movement of the head in the standing horse before it falls to the ground. The penetrating bolt can become lodged tightly in the horse's cranium and difficult to remove. The operator must be prepared to release his or her grip from the pistol quickly to avoid personal injury.[36] Many features of captive bolt stunning are aesthetically unacceptable to the uninformed. Use of a captive bolt can be combined with pithing or exsanguination. Pithing is performed by inserting a surgical scalpel through the foramen magnum into the level of the spinal cord and moving it back and forth until the cord is completely severed. Exsanguination, as described later, may be more appropriate.

Gunshot

Under some circumstances gunshot with a free bullet (pistol, rifle, or slug from a shot gun) may be the only practical method for euthanizing a horse.[38-42] Shooting requires skill and should be performed by a trained person because the bullet must strike and damage the brain.[39,41] Other animals and bystanders must be cleared from the immediate area to avoid injury should the bullet ricochet. The bullet from a rifle used for deer hunting or a pistol of 32 calibers or larger easily kills a horse if properly placed in the brain. The sight for entrance of a bullet or a penetrating captive bolt is approximately where lines drawn from the base of an ear to the opposite eye cross on the horse's forehead.[38] When possible, gunshot should be followed by a supplemental method of euthanasia such as pithing, exsanguination, or electrocution.[26]

Exsanguination

Exsanguination should be performed only after unconsciousness has been produced by some other method and is most commonly performed by severing one or both of the carotid arteries. Another method in larger horses is to cut the posterior aorta. The aorta is located by rectal palpation. A handheld scalpel is advanced into the rectum. The aortic pulse is palpated dorsally along the spine, at which point it is severed. Blood spill occurs within the abdominal cavity, which is more aesthetic than severing the carotid arteries. Exsanguination in the conscious horse is accompanied by agonal gasps and limb paddling once hypotension and hypoxia become pronounced. The occurrence of these reactions before death is unsightly and stressful to the horse. As a single method, exsanguination is inhumane and cannot be recommended for use in the conscious horse.

Electrocution

The application of electrical current to induce ventricular fibrillation is an effective, humane, and economical method of ensuring death when a horse is rendered unconscious by an anesthetic.[23] It is inhumane to euthanize any animal by placing electrodes so that current passes between forelimbs and hind limbs or from the neck to a forelimb because cardiac arrest (ventricular fibrillation) precedes unconsciousness. The equipment consists of a heavy extension cord. The electrodes, attached to the horse, may be clamps similar to those used on automobile battery jumper cables. The electrodes must be placed (on the skull) so that current passes directly through the brain and instantaneously induces unconsciousness. Signs of effective electrocution include extension of the limbs, opisthotonos, downward rotation of the eyeball, and tonic spasms changing into a clonic spasm, with eventual muscle flaccidity. It is recommended that electrocution be followed by exsanguination or some other appropriate method to ensure cardiac arrest and death.[26]

The disadvantages of electrocution are:

1. Electrocution can be hazardous to personnel.
2. The current must be applied for several minutes; thus the danger is compounded in vicious or unruly horses.
3. Profound body contortions characterized by violent extension and stiffening of the limbs, head, and neck are aesthetically objectionable.
4. When used in the standing horse, one or both of the electrodes can easily be dislodged when the horse falls to the ground.

Appropriate equipment must be used to ensure safety to personnel. Electrode attachments must provide good skin contact and must not be easily dislodged. Although electrocution is an accepted method of euthanasia, the disadvantages may outweigh the advantages under most circumstances.[26]

METHODS OF CONFIRMING AND ENSURING DEATH

Death should be confirmed by multiple methods, including the loss of the corneal reflex, the absence of respiration over a 5- to 10-minute period, and the inability to palpate a peripheral pulse or hear cardiac contractions. The findings should be confirmed initially and then be reaffirmed 5 to10 minutes later. An electrocardiogram, if applied, may reveal electrical activity in the absence of cardiac contractions for 10 to15 minutes after death.

USE OF EUTHANIZED HORSES FOR FOOD

Meat from euthanized horses must be residue free if intended for consumption by humans or animals. The carcass of horses euthanized with barbiturates or other injectable drugs (e.g., chloral hydrate) must be disposed of properly. Wild or domestic carnivores could easily die if permitted to consume large amounts of drug-contaminated meat.[32,33] Stunning, gunshot, and electrocution followed by exsanguination or carbon dioxide insufflation are the only humane methods of killing animals to provide residue-free meat.

REFERENCES

1. Ndiritu CG, Enos LR: Adverse reactions to drugs in a veterinary hospital, *J Am Vet Med Assoc* 171: 335-339, 1977.
2. Richey MT et al: Equine post-anesthetic lameness: a retrospective study, *Vet Surg* 19(5):392-397, 1990.
3. Young SS, Taylor PM: Factors influencing the outcome of equine anaesthesia: a review of 1314 cases, *Equine Vet J* 25:147-151, 1993.
4. Jones RS: Comparative mortality in anaesthesia, *Br J Anaesth* 87:813-815, 2001.
5. Wright JG, Hall LW: *Veterinary anaesthesia and analgesia*, ed 5, London, 1961, Baillière Tindall & Cox, p 161.
6. Mitchell B: Equine anaesthesia: an assessment of techniques used in clinical practice, *Equine Vet J* 1: 261-274, 1969.
7. Lumb WV, Jones EW: *Veterinary anaesthesia*, ed 2, Philadelphia, 1973, Lea & Febiger, pp 611-629.
8. Perkens D, Heath RB, Lumb WV: Unpublished data Fort Collins, Co, 1982, Colorado State University.
9. Tevik A: The role of anaesthesia in surgical mortality in horses, *Nord Vet Med* 35:175-179, 1983.
10. Mee AM, Cripps PJ, Jones RS: A retrospective study of mortality associated with general anaesthesia in horses: elective procedures, *Vet Rec* 142:275-276, 1998.
11. Mee AM, Cripps PJ, Jones RS: A retrospective study of mortality associated with general anaesthesia in horses: emergency procedures, *Vet Rec* 142:307-309, 1998.
12. Muir WW et al: Unpublished data, Columbus, Oh, 1999, The Ohio State University.
13. Johnston GM et al: The confidential enquiry into perioperative equine fatalities (CEPEF): mortality results of phases 1 and 2, *Vet Anaesth Analg* 29:159-170, 2002.
14. Johnston GM et al: Is isoflurane safer than halothane in equine anesthesia? Results from a prospective mulitcentre randomized controlled trial, *Equine Vet J* 36:64-71, 2004.
15. Senoir JM et al: Reported morbidities following 861 anaesthetics given at four equine hospitals, *Vet Rec* 160:407-408, 2007.
16. Santschi EM et al: Types of colic and frequency of postcolic abortion in pregnant mares: 105 cases: (1984-1988), *J Am Vet Med Assoc* 199:374-377, 1991.
17. Pascoe PJ et al: Mortality rates and associated factors in equine colic operations—a retrospective study of 341 operations, *Can Vet J* 24:76-85, 1983.
18. Mair TS, Smith LJ: Survival and complication rates in 300 horses undergoing surgical treatment of colic. Part 1: short-term survival following a single laparotomy, *Equine Vet J* 37:296-302, 2005.
19. Proudman CJ et al: Pre-operative and anaesthesia-related risk factors for mortality in equine colic cases, *Vet J* 171:89-97, 2006.
20. Bidwell LA, Bramlage LR, Rood WA: Equine perioperative fatalities associated with general anaesthesia at a private practice—a retrospective case series, *Vet Anaesth Analg* 34:23-30, 2007.
21. Buelke DL: There's no good way to euthanize a horse, *J Am Vet Med Assoc* 196:1942-1944, 1990.
22. American Association of Equine Practitioners euthanasia guidelines, Accessed 1/15/2008 from www.aaep.org/images/files/2007_%20Euthanasia%20Guidelines.pdf.
23. Barkley JE: Euthanasia—two sides of the story, *Equine Pract Mod Vet Pract*, 63(8):662-664, 1982.
24. Otten DR: Advisory on proper disposal of euthanatized animals (Letter), *J Am Vet Med Assoc* 219:1677-1678, 2001.
25. Lenz TR: An overview of acceptable euthanasia procedures, carcass disposal options, and equine slaughter legislation, *Proc Am Assoc Equine Pract* 50:191-195, 2004.
26. AVMA guidelines on euthanasia. June 2007, Accessed from http://www.avma.org/issues/animal_welfare/euthanasia.pdf.
27. Austin FH: Chemical agents for use in the humane destruction of horses, *Irish Vet J* 27:45-48, 1973.
28. Brewer NR: The history of euthanasia, *Lab Anim* 11:17-19, 1982.
29. Barocio LD: Review of literature on use of T-61 as an euthanasic agent, *Inst Anim Prob* 4:336-342, 1983.
30. Oliver DF: Euthanasia of horses, *Vet Rec* 105:224-225, 1979.
31. Littlejohn A, Marnewich JJ: Euthanasia of horses, *Vet Rec* 6:420, 1980 (correspondence).
32. Euthanatized animals can poison wildlife: veterinarians receive fines, *J Am Vet Med Assoc* 220:146-147, 2002.
33. Secondary pentobarbital poisoning of wildlife. United States Fish and Wildlife Service Fact Sheet., Accessed 1/15/2007 from www.fws.gov/mountain-prairie/poison.pdf.
34. Hoffman PE: Report: euthanasia study committee, *AAEP Newsl* 1:48-49, 1979.
35. Nuallian TO: Euthanasia of horses, *Irish Vet J* 30:51, 1985.
36. Dennis MB et al: Use of captive bolt as a method of euthanasia in large laboratory animal species, *Lab Anim Sci* 38:459-462, 1988.
37. Blackmore DK: Energy requirements for the penetration of heads of domestic stock and the development of a multiple projectile, *Vet Rec* 116(2):36-40, 1985.
38. Dodd K: Humane euthanasia. 1. Shooting a horse, *Irish Vet J* 39:150-151, 1985.
39. Longair J et al: Guidelines for euthanasia of domestic animals by firearms, *Can Vet J* 32:724-726, 1991.
40. California Department of Food and Agriculture, Sacramento, and University of California Veterinary Medical Extension, Davis, Ca: *The emergency euthanasia of horses*, 1999.
41. Millar GI, Mills DS: Observations on the trajectory of the bullet in 15 horses euthanised by free bullet, *Vet Rec* 146:754-757, 2000.
42. House CJ: Euthanasia of horses, *Vet Rec* 147:83, 2000.

Respiratory Abbreviations

Abbreviation	Definition
a	arterial
A	Alveolar
C	Content of gas in blood, or when appropriate, Compliance (V/P)
D	Difusing capacity
F	Fractional concentration of gas
P	Pressure, tension or partial pressure of gas. NOTE: 1kPa = 7.5 mm Hg = 10.2 cm H_2O; 1 mm Hg = 1.36 cm H_2O
Q	Volume of blood
R	Respiratory exchange ratio (RQ)
S	Saturation of hemoglobin (Hb) with oxygen
V	Volume of gas
v	Venous
·	a time derivative; used as an overdot above V or Q indicating flow
$(Ca-Cv)O_2$	Arterial to mixed venous difference in blood oxygen concentration
Cdyn	Dynamic compliance
Cstat	Static compliance
ΔPplmax	Maximal change and pleural pressure during tidal breathing
$ETCO_2$	End-tidal carbon dioxide partial pressure
f	Respiratory frequency
$FACO_2$	Alveolar fraction of carbon dioxide
FiO_2	Fraction of oxygen in inspired air
FRC	Functional residual capacity
$PA-aO_2$	Alveolar-arterial oxygen difference
$PaCO_2$	Arterial partial pressure of carbon dioxide
$PACO_2$	Alveolar partial pressure of carbon dioxide
PaO_2	Arterial partial pressure of oxygen
PAO_2	Alveolar partial pressure of oxygen
PO_2	Partial pressure of oxygen (pressure is measured in mm Hg or kPa where 7.5 mm Hg = 1 kPa)
PCO_2	Partial pressure of carbon dioxide
PvO_2	Venous partial pressure of oxygen
PB	Barometric pressure
Ppl	Pleural pressure
$\dot{Q}$	Cardiac output
R	Pulmonary (airway) resistance
RV	Residual volume
SaO_2	Percent saturation of arterial blood with oxygen
SpO_2	Percent saturation of blood with oxygen obtained by pulse (p) oximetry
TLC	Total lung capacity
VA	Alveolar ventilation
VC	Vital capacity
$\dot{V}CO_2$	Elimination of CO_2 per minute
VD	Deadspace ventilation
VD/VT	Dead space/tidal volume ratio
Vmin	Minute ventilation (MV)
$\dot{V}/\dot{Q}$	Ventilation/perfusion ratio
VT	Tidal volume

Drug Schedules

Scheduled drugs	Controlled substances (or classes)	Description	Examples
Schedule I	C-I	No accepted medical use High potential for abuse	Heroin, dihydromorphine
Schedule II	C-II	Accepted medical uses in United States (may include severe restrictions) High potential for abuse, which may lead to severe psychological or physical dependence	Morphine, meperidine, oxymorphone, etorphine, pentobarbital
Schedule III	C-III	Accepted medical uses in United States Lesser degree of abuse potential than C-II Abuse may lead to moderate or low physical dependence or high psychological dependence	Thiopental, tiletamine/zolazepam, buprenorphine
Schedule IV	C-IV	Accepted medical uses in United States Low potential for abuse relative to C-III Abuse may lead to limited physical or psychological dependence (relative to C-III)	Chloral hydrate, diazepam, pentazocine
Schedule V	C-V	Accepted medical uses in United States Low potential for abuse relative to C-IV Abuse may lead to limited physical or psychological dependence (relative to C-IV) Some over-the-counter items included in this class (as determined by the Federal Food, Drug, and Cosmetic Act) may be dispensed without prescription subject to overriding state regulations and provisions on the buyer	

All references and laws from Ohio Drug Laws handbook. In Code of Federal Regulations and Selected Provisions and Controlled Substance Act, 1987.

Controlled substances are obtained by prescription. They must be used for legitimate medical purposes, and there must be a valid veterinarian-client/patient relationship. Prescriptions may not be written to receive and dispense from one's own office. A controlled substance may be prescribed only if the prescriber has authorization from appropriate legal authorities (usually the Attorney General). Always check state and other local regulations.

CLASS I AND CLASS II

Class I (C-I) and Class II (C-II) drugs must be ordered from a wholesaler by filling out an official order form, which is obtained by contacting the Drug Enforcement Agency (DEA). Power of attorney may also be given to one or more people to obtain and use the forms; any theft or loss of these forms must be reported.

If prescriber registration expires, all unused forms must be returned. All or part of an order may be canceled if both buyer and supplier are informed.

For all controlled substances, the prescription must be dated and signed (as any legal document) on the date of issue. The full name and address of the patient and prescriber name, address, and DEA number must be on the written prescription.

CLASS II

These drugs may be dispensed or administered by a practitioner (subject to the preceding rules).

Oral orders for C-II drugs are permitted in *emergencies* but only for the amount needed for the emergency period; oral orders must be followed up with a written, signed prescription issued to the providing pharmacy within 7 days for the emergency quantity dispensed. The date of the oral order and *Authorization for emergency dispensing* must be written on the follow-up prescription. Failure to do this will cause action to void all "dispensing without a written prescription" rights.

Oral orders are not permitted in nonemergency situations. Indelible pencil, ink, or typewriter may be used; the prescription should be signed manually. Prescriptions may be prepared by a secretary or agent, but the prescriber is responsible for all directions and information on the prescription.

Class II drugs may not be refilled. A new prescription is required for each filling.

CLASS III, CLASS IV, AND CLASS V

Class III (C-III), Class IV (C-IV), and Class V (C-V) drugs may be prescribed by written or oral prescription or may be dispensed or administered by the practitioner.

An institutional practitioner may directly administer or dispense (but not prescribe) C-III, C-IV, or C-V drugs only if the prescribing physician has:

1. Written and signed the prescription,
2. Given an oral order and had the pharmacist make it into a written order, or
3. Ordered for immediate administration to the ultimate user.

Refills

C-III and C-IV drugs may not be filled or refilled more than 6 months after the original date of issue of the prescription. They may not be refilled more than five times.

Refills may be entered on the back of the original prescription or other appropriate document (medication record or computer).

When retrieving the prescription number, the following information should be available: patient's name, dosage form, date filled or refilled, quantity dispensed, initials of the registered pharmacist for each refill, and total number of refills for that prescription to date.

Written and Oral Refills (C-III, C-IV, and C-V)

The total number of refills (quantity) allowed, including the amount of the original, may not exceed five refills or 6 months from the original date.

The quantity of each refill must be less than or equal to the original quantity authorized.

A new and separate prescription must be issued for anything more than five refills or after 6 months. Prescriptions cannot be predated.

All of the above information may be kept on the computer. The physician's name, telephone number, DEA number, and patient's name and address must also be kept on the computer.

Partials (C-III, C-IV, and C-V)

These must be recorded in the same manner as refills.

The total quantity of partials may not exceed the total quantity prescribed.

C-III, C-IV, and C-V drugs may not be dispensed more than 6 months past the original date of the prescription.

Labeling

All controlled substances must be labeled with the pharmacy name and address, serial number and date of initial filling, the patient's and physician's names, directions for use, and any cautionary statements. All prescription bottles containing controlled substances that are dispensed to a client must contain the following statement:

Caution: Federal law PROHIBITS the transfer of this drug to any person other than the patient for whom it was prescribed.

Disposal

Contact your local DEA office for proper disposal requirements for outdated or unusable medications. They may send you the appropriate form used for disposal along with instructions on how to handle the disposal. Some states allow returns to a reverse distributor. Check with the state where you are practicing.

Equine Anesthesia Record and Recovery Sheet

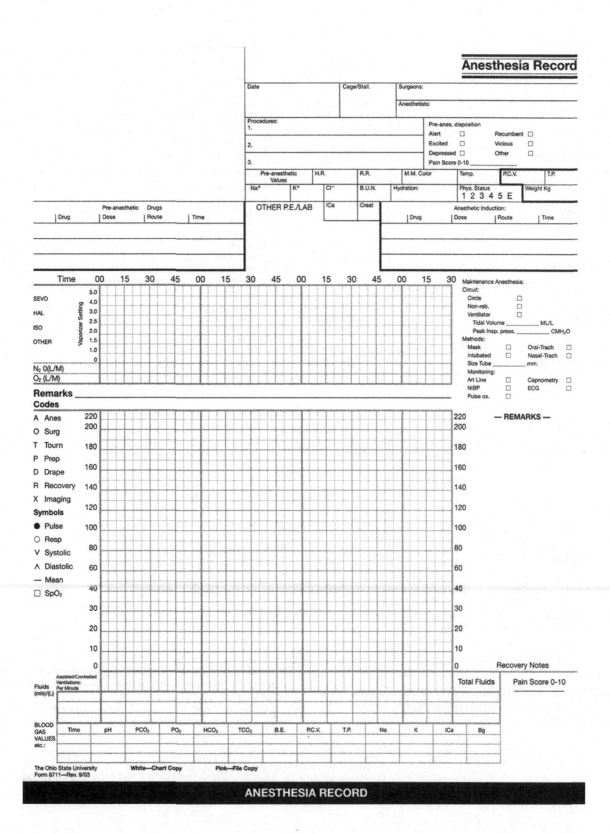

EQUINE RECOVERY SHEET
(Attach Anesthesia Record)

Date _____ Horse # _____   Premed _____ Route _____ Dose _____ Clock Time _____

Wt. _____ Age _____ Breed _____   Premed _____ Route _____ Dose _____ Clock Time _____

Quantitative Variables[1]			Qualitative Variables[2,3]		
Observation	Clock Time	Time (min)	Observation	Scale	Score
End of anesthesia			Overall attitude (1-10)	1 - calm 5 - anxious/disoriented 10 - frantic/aggressive	
First move Ex: Head, neck, limbs*			Activity in recumbency (1-10)	1 - quiet, occasional stretch, head lift 3 - tense, hyperactive/hypersensitive 5 - flailing	
Move ear*			Move to sternal (1-10)	1 - smooth, methodical 5 - uncoordinated but controlled 10 - considerable effort, flopping over/ uncontrolled	
Move limbs*			Sternal phase (1-10)	1 - an organized pause 3 - prolonged (>10 min) 6 - multiple attempts 10 - continues to struggle (can't attain)	
Swallow*			Move to stand (1-10)	1 - methodical (unassisted) 3 - an organized scramble (some assistance) 6 - uses walls for support (required support) 10 - repeated attempts due to weakness (requires support)	
Extubation*			Strength (1-10)	1 - strong 3 - minimally weak and ataxic 6 - dog sitting before standing 10 - repeated attempts due to weakness	
Head lift*			Balance and coordination (1-10)	1 - solid 3 - moderate dancing 5 - stumbling 8 - careening 10 - falls back down	
First sternal posture attempt*			Knuckling (1-4)	1 - none 2 - hindlimbs or forelimbs mild 3 - hindlimbs or forelimbs marked 4 - all four moderate	
No. of attempts to sternal	# _____		**OVERALL QUALITATIVE SCORE (70 points max.)**		
No. of attempts to stand	# _____		Person evaluating _____		
First stand*			Recovery stall and type _____ Head and tail ropes Yes _____ No _____		
Remains standing*			Disposition before anesthesia _____ Antipamazole (100 μg/kg) _____ ml Clock time _____ Comments:		

[1]Modified from Whitehair et al. based upon variables most likely to discriminate between drug effects upon recovery.
[2]Modified from Donaldson et al. based upon discriminative capabilities.
[3]Modified from Santos et al. based upon discriminatory capabilities.
*Minutes from end of inhalant anesthesia

REFERENCES

1. Donaldson LL et al: The recovery of horses from inhalant anesthesia: a comparison of halothane and isoflurane, *Vet Anesth* 29:92-101, 2000.

2. Santos M et al: α-Adrenoceptor agonists during recovery from isoflurane anaesthesia in horses, *Equine Vet J* 35:170-175, 2003.

3. Whitehair KJ et al: Recovery of horses from inhalation anesthesia, *Am J Vet Res* 54:1693-1702, 1993.

Pain Management Plan

PAIN MANAGEMENT PLAN

"Pain assessment is considered part of every patient evaluation, regardless of presenting complaint."

PATIENT ID CARD

Date: _____ Department: _____

Pulse rate:		Temperature:	°C/°F	
Respiratory rate:		Weight:	lbs/kg	Attitude:

Is pain present upon admission? ☐ Y ☐ N   Pain on palpation only? Y ☐ N ☐   Cause of pain:

Signs of pain (Check all that apply):

									Descriptors (Circle):	
Behavior:	Normal ☐	Depressed ☐	Excited ☐	Agitated ☐	Guarding ☐	Aggressive ☐			Restless	Fearful
Vocalization:	None ☐	Occasional ☐	Continuous ☐	Other ☐					Agitated	Obtund
Posture:	Normal ☐	Frozen ☐	Rigid ☐	Hunched ☐	Recumbent ☐	Reluctant to move ☐			Trembling	Inappetant
Gait:	Sound ☐	Lame weight bearing ☐		Lame non-weight bearing ☐		Non-ambulatory ☐			Nervous	Biting or licking area

Other signs of pain: _____   Previous analgesic history: _____

Classification of pain (Check):

Acute ☐
Acute recurrent ☐
Chronic (>weeks) ☐
Chronic progressive ☐

Superficial ☐
Deep ☐
Visceral ☐

Inflammatory ☐
Neuropathic ☐
Both (Infl/neuro) ☐
Cancer ☐

Primary hyperalgesia ☐
Secondary hyperalgesia ☐
Central analgesia ☐

Anatomical location of pain (Circle):

Ventral   Dorsal

Left

Right

Comments:

Diagnosis:

SEVERITY OF PAIN: VISUAL ANALOG SCALE

Indicate event(s) on VAS: Initial/date

No Pain   Worst Possible Pain

Event:	Time (HH:MM):	Date:	Comments:
1			
2			
3			
4			

PAIN THERAPY (Pharmacologic and complementary)

	Date:	Dose/Route:	Efficacy/Duration:	Comments:	ADDITIONAL THERAPY
Current					Surgery ☐
					Chemotherapy ☐
Prescribed					Radiation ☐
					Physical therapy ☐

RESPONSE TO THERAPY: VISUAL ANALOG SCALE

Indicate event(s) on VAS

No Analgesia   Complete Analgesia

Event:	Time (HH:MM):	Date:	Comments:
1			
2			
3			
4			

Clinician: _____   Release date: _____

Anesthesia Equipment Companies

Equine Anesthetic Machines

Burtons Manufacture
www.burtons.uk.com
01622 832919
Units 1-6, Guardian Industrial Estate
Pattenden Lane
Marden, Kent TN12 9QD England

Hallowell EMC
www.hallowell.com
413-496-9254
63 Eaglet Street
Pittsfield, MA 01201

JD Medical Distributing Co., Inc.
www.jdmedical.com
602-997-1758
1923 West Peoria Avenue
Phoenix, AZ 85029

Mallard Medical, Inc.
www.mallardmedical.net
530-226-0727
20268 Skypark Drive
Redding, CA 96002

Smiths Medical
www.smiths-medical.com/veterinary/
www.surgivet.com
1-800-258-5361
5200 Upper Metro Place
Dublin, OH 43017

Vetland Medical Sales & Services LLC
www.vetland1.com
877-329-7775
2601 Holloway Road
Louisville, KY 40299

Oxygen Concentrator

Airsep Corporation
www.airsep.com
716-691-0202
401 Creekside Drive
Buffalo, NY 14228

Jorgensen Laboratories, Inc.
www.jorvet.com
970-669-2500
1450 Van Buren Avenue
Loveland, CO 80538

Vaporizers

Burtons Medical Equipment Limited
www.burtons.uk.com
01622832919
Units 1-6, Guardian Industrial Estate
Pattenden Lane
Marden, Kent TN12 9QD England

Draeger Medical, Inc.
www.draeger.com
215-721-5400
3135 Quarry Road
Telford, PA 18969

Intermed Penlon Limited
www.penlon.com
+44 (0) 1235 547000
Abingdon Science Park
Barton Lane
Abingdon OX14PH, United Kingdom

Jorgensen Laboratories, Inc.
www.jorvet.com
970-669-2500
1450 Van Buren Avenue
Loveland, CO 80538

Smiths Medical
www.smiths-medical.com/veterinary
1-800-258-5361
5200 Upper Metro Place
Dublin, OH 43017

Vetland Medical Sales and Services LLC
www.vetland1.com
877-329-7775
2601 Holloway Road
Louisville, KY 40299

Slings

Anderson Sling
www.equisling.com
707-743-1300
Care for Disabled Animals
P.O. Box 53
Potter Valley, CA 95469

Liftex Corporation
www.liftex.com/
215-967-0810
443 Ivyland Road
Warminster, PA 18974

Protective Padding

A&A Pad Co.
www.aapadco.com
865-970-7400
803 West Faye Drive
Maryville, TN 37803

Dandy Products Inc.
www.dandyproductsinc.com
3314 State Road 131
Goshen, OH 45122
513-625-3000

Snell Packaging and Safety Ltd.
www.snell.co.nz
09-622-4144
6-8 Goodman Place
Penrose 1061
Auckland, New Zealand

Air-dunnage bag

The Goodyear Tire & Rubber Company
www.goodyear.com
330-796-2121
1144 East Market Street
Akron, OH 44316

C.V. Harold Rubber Co.
504-821-5944
4431 Euphrosine Street
New Orleans, LA 70125

Surgical Tables

Kimzey, Inc.
www.kimzeymetalproducts.com
164 Kentucky Avenue
Woodland, CA 95695

Shanks Veterinary Equipment, Inc.
www.shanksvet.com
815-225-7700
505 East Old Mill Street
Milledgeville, IL 61051

Endotracheal Tubes

Silicone Adult and Foal Nasotracheal Tubes

Jorgensen Laboratories, Inc.
www.jorvet.com
970-669-2500
1450 Van Buren Avenue
Loveland, CO 80538

Bivona distributed by Smiths Medical
www.smiths-medical.com/veterinary
1-800-258-5361
5200 Upper Metro Place
Dublin, OH 43017

Tracheostomy Tubes

Silicone

Jorgensen Laboratories, Inc.
www.jorvet.com/
970-669-2500
1450 Van Buren Avenue
Loveland, CO 80538

Smiths Medical
www.smiths-medical.com/veterinary
1-800-258-5361
5200 Upper Metro Place
Dublin, OH 43017

Foal Resuscitator

McCulloch Medical
www.mccullochmedical.com
64-9-444 2115
90 Hillside Road
PO Box 100-990
North Shore Mail Centre
Auckland, New Zealand

Monitoring Devices

Abbott Laboratories
847-937-6100
100 Abbott Part Road
Abbott Park, IL 60064-3500

Columbus Instruments
www.colinst.com
614-276-0861
950 N. Hague Avenue
Columbus, OH 43204

Criticare Systems, Inc.
www.csiusa.com
262-798-8282
20925 Crossroads Circle
Waukesha, WI 53186

Datascope Corp.
www.datascope.com
201-995-8000
800 MacArthur Boulevard
Mahwah, NJ 07430

Digicare Biomedical Technology Inc.
(Animal Health Division)
Digicarebiomedical.com
561-689-0408
107 Commerce Road
Boynton Beach, FL 33426

DRE, Inc.
www.dremed.com
1-502-244-4444
1800 Williamson Court
Louisville, KY 40223

Intermed Penlon Limited
www.penlon.com
+44 (0) 1235 547000
Abingdon Science Park
Barton Lane
Abingdon OX14PH, United Kingdom

ITC
www.itcmed.com
732-548-5700
8 Olsen Avenue
Edison, NJ 08820

Parks Medical Electronics, Inc.
www.parksmed.com
503-649-7007
19460 SW Shaw
Aloha, OR 97007

Philips Respironics
www.respironics.com
1010 Murry Ridge Lane
Murrysville, PA 15668

Sharn Veterinary Inc.
866-447-4276/813-962-6664
12950 N. Dale Mabry Highway
Tampa, FL 33618

Smiths Medical
www.smiths-medical.com/veterinary
1-800-258-5361
5200 Upper Metro Place
Dublin, OH 43017

Vetland Medical Sales and Services LLC
www.vetland1.com
877-329-7775
2601 Holloway Road
Louisville, KY 40299

Infusion Catheter and Pumps

ReCathco LLC
Recathco.com
412-487-1482
2853 Oxford Boulevard, Suite 106
Allison Park, PA 15101-2443

Smiths Medical
Smiths-medical.com
Waukesha, WI

Index

Note: Page numbers followed by "f" indicate figures, "t" indicate tables, and "b" indicate boxes.

A

Abaxial sesamoidean nerve block, 224, 224f
Abdominal distention, preoperative, 127
Abdominal exploration
  anesthesia for, 434–435, 434b
  ventilatory support and, 348–350
Abdominal muscles in ventilation, 12
Absolute refractory period, 42f, 43
Accumulation of drug, 180
Acepromazine, 186–187, 255–256, 256t
  applied pharmacology of, 187–188, 200f
  biodisposition of, 188–189
  for chemical restraint, 189t
  chloral hydrate and thiopental combined
    with, 255t
  clinical use and antagonism of, 189, 189t
  complications, side effects, and toxicity
    of, 189–190, 398–399
  etorphine combined with, 256t
  in euthanasia, 441b
  mechanism of action, 187
  for pain management, 375t
  pharmacokinetic parameters for, 178t
  for recovery facilitation, 389t
  recovery from, 386t
  for total intravenous anesthesia, 262t
  xylazine combined with, 197f
Acetylcholine, 358–359, 359–360, 359f
Acid-base balance
  in anesthetic monitoring, 166–169, 167t,
    168t
  hypotension and, 404t
  neuromuscular blocking drugs and, 364
Acidosis
  metabolic, 167t, 168
    bicarbonate supplementation for,
      145–146
    due to colic, 126–127
    hypotension due to, 404t
  respiratory, 167t, 168
Actin, cardiac, 39–40
Action potential, 41, 41f, 41t, 43, 210, 211f
Activated charcoal canister, 328–329, 329f
Active zones in motor nerve terminal,
  358–359, 359f
Acute-phase response, 102b
Adenosine triphosphate (ATP), 29
Administration sets, 138f
Adrenergic response to stress, 102
α_2-Adrenoceptors, 192, 218, 377
  applied pharmacology of, 192–193,
    193–195, 195–196
  biodisposition of, 196
  for chemical restraint, 189t
  clinical use and antagonism of, 196–198
  for colic, preoperative, 126
  complications, side effects, and clinical
    toxicity of, 198–199
  hemodynamic effects of, 93t
  history of use of, 6–7
  ketamine combined with, 250–251

α_2-Adrenoceptors (*Continued*)
  location and function of, 192t
  mechanism of action of, 192
  respiratory effects of, 33t, 34
A fibers, 210–211, 211t, 212–213
Afterdepolarization, 77–78
Afterload, 51
Age, pharmacokinetics and, 181
Agonal respirations, 421t
Air embolism, 139t
Air pillow recovery, 393, 393f
Airway
  cardiopulmonary resuscitation and,
    424–426
  conducting, 11, 12f
    ventilatory support and, 332–333
  dynamic compression of, 15
  hyperresponsive, 15
  obstruction of during recovery, 408t, 410t
  receptors in, 31
  resistance, 15
  smooth muscle of, 15
    effects of anesthesia on, 15
Alcohol, ethyl, 218
Alfentanil, 262t
Alkaline phosphatase, 125t
Alkalosis
  metabolic, 167t, 168
  respiratory, 167t, 168
Allergy
  lidocaine, 216
  postanesthesia, 413t
  procaine, 215
Allodynia, 369, 370b
Alpha 400, 343
Alphazalone/alphadolone, 256–257
Altitude, oxygen partial pressure and, 23t
Alveolar-arterial oxygen difference
  (PA-aO_2), 26–27
Alveolar concentration, minimum, of inhalation
  anesthetic, 290–291, 290b, 291t, 291b
Alveolar gas, composition of, 23–24, 291b
Alveolar hyperventilation, 24
Alveolar hypoxia, 20
Alveolar partial pressure of carbon dioxide.
  See Partial pressure of carbon dioxide
  (PCO_2)
Alveolar partial pressure of inhaled
  anesthetic, 293–295, 293b
Alveolar partial pressure of oxygen. *See* Partial
  pressure of oxygen (PO_2)
Alveolar ventilation (VA), 11
American College of Veterinary
  Anesthesiologists monitoring
  guidelines, 149–150, 150b
American Society of Anesthesiologists
  (ASA) physical status classification, 126t
American Veterinary Medical Association
  (AVMA) guidelines for euthanasia,
  441–442, 442b
Amides, local anesthetic, 211–212, 213t

4-Aminopyridine, 364
Amrinone, 404t
Analgesics, 185, 374, 375t
  for colic, preoperative, 126
  for donkeys and mules, 353–357
  epidural, 218, 219t, 376t
  loading doses and infusion rates of, 376t
  multimodal, 374
  nonopioid sedative, 186t, 192–199, 192b
    applied pharmacology of, 192–196
    biodisposition of, 196
    clinical use and antagonism of,
      196–198, 197b
    complications, side effects, and clinical
      toxicity of, 198–199
    in drug combinations, 203–204
    mechanism of action, 192t
  opioid (*See* Opioid analgesics)
  preemptive, 370b, 374
Anal reflex in anesthesia depth
  evaluation, 150
Anatomic dead space. *See* Conducting airways
Anemia, arterial oxygen content during, 158b
Anesthesia
  cardiovascular effects of, 93, 93t
  defined, 1
  depth of, 150–153, 152t, 291–292,
    292t, 292b
  for donkeys and mules, 353–357
  as emerging science, 1–4
  equipment for (*See* Equipment)
  evolution of, 4–6, 4f
    recent developments in, 6–9, 7f
    resistance to change in, 5b
  future of, 9
  history of, 1–10
  inhalation (*See* Inhalation anesthetics)
  intravenous (*See* Intravenous anesthetics)
  key components of, 3f
  local (*See* Local anesthetics)
  monitoring during, 149–170
  morbidity and mortality associated with,
    8t, 9b
  phases of, 381–396
  planes of, 152t
  preparation of horse for, 128–130,
    128f, 128b
  risks associated with, 439, 440b
    physical status assessment and, 126
  stress response to (*See* Stress response)
  total intravenous (*See* Total intravenous
    anesthesia [TIVA])
  types of procedures in, 3f
Anesthesia record, 150, 151f, 152b
Anesthetic machine
  cleaning and disinfection of, 329
  commercially available, 325–326,
    325t, 326f
  companies associated with, 452
  complications related to, 328, 328t
  components of, 318–325

459

Printed in the United States
By Bookmasters